# Occupational & Environmental Medicine

*a LANGE medical book*

# Occupational & Environmental Medicine

second edition

**Edited by**

**Joseph LaDou, MS, MD**
Clinical Professor and Director
International Center for Occupational Medicine
University of California, San Francisco

Appleton & Lange
Stamford, Connecticut

97 98 99 00 01 / 10 9 8 7 6 5 4 3 2 1

Prentice Hall International (UK) Limited, *London*
Prentice Hall of Australia Pty. Limited, *Sydney*
Prentice Hall Canada, Inc., *Toronto*
Prentice Hall Hispanoamericana, S.A., *Mexico*
Prentice Hall of India Private Limited, *New Delhi*
Prentice Hall of Japan, Inc., *Tokyo*
Simon & Schuster Asia Pte. Ltd., *Singapore*
Editora Prentice Hall do Brasil Ltda., *Rio de Janeiro*
Prentice Hall, *Upper Saddle River, New Jersey*

ISSN: 1047-4498

Acquisitions Editor: Shelley Reinhardt
Development Editor: Cara Lyn Coffey
Production Editor: Christine Langan
Associate Art Manager: Maggie Belis Darrow

ISBN 0-8385-7216-2

9 780838 572160   90000

PRINTED IN THE UNITED STATES OF AMERICA

# Contents

# The Authors

**Robert M. Adams, MD**
Clinical Professor of Dermatology (Emeritus), Stanford University, School of Medicine, Stanford, California.
*Occupational Skin Disorders*

**Daniel C. Adelman, MD**
Associate Adjunct Professor of Medicine, University of California, San Francisco; Clinical Scientist, Genentech, Inc., South San Francisco, California.
*Clinical Immunology*

**John R. Balmes, MD**
Associate Professor of Medicine, University of California, San Francisco; Chief, Division of Occupational and Environmental Medicine, San Francisco General Hospital, San Francisco, California.
*Occupational Lung Diseases; Outdoor Air Pollution*

**Neal L. Benowitz, MD**
Professor of Medicine, Department of Medicine, University of California, San Francisco, San Francisco, California.
*Cardiovascular Toxicology; Smoking & Occupational Health*

**Paul D. Blanc, MD, MSPH**
Associate Professor of Medicine and Chief, Division of Occupational and Environmental Medicine, University of California, San Francisco, San Francisco, California.
*Gases & Other Inhalants*

**Nancy N. Byl, MPT, PT, PhD**
Professor and Director, Graduate Program in Physical Therapy, University of California, San Francisco, California.
*Musculoskeletal Injuries*

**Richard Cohen, MD, MPH**
Associate Clinical Professor, Division of Occupational and Environmental Medicine, University of California, San Francisco, San Francisco, California.
*Injuries Due to Physical Hazards; Occupational Infections*

**James E. Cone, MD, MPH**
Assistant Clinical Professor, Department of Medicine, University of California, San Francisco, San Francisco, California.
*Solvents*

**Lloyd E. Damon, MD**
Associate Clinical Professor of Medicine, University of California, San Francisco, San Francisco, California.
*Occupational Hematology*

**Rupali Das, MD, MPH**
Assistant Clinical Professor of Medicine, University of California, San Francisco; Public Health Medical Officer, Office of Environmental Health Hazard Assessment, California Environmental Protection Agency, Berkeley, California.
*Routine Industrial Emissions, Accidental Releases, & Hazardous Waste*

**Michael L. Fischman, MD, MPH**
Assistant Clinical Professor and Assistant Chief, Division of Occupational and Environmental Medicine, Department of Medicine, University of California, San Francisco, San Francisco, California.
*Occupational Cancer; Building-Associated Illnesses*

**Douglas P. Fowler, PhD, CIH**
Visiting Lecturer in Industrial Hygiene, Department of Medicine, University of California, San Francisco; Fowler Associates, Redwood City, California.
*Industrial Hygiene*

**Ernest K. Goodner, MD**
Clinical Professor of Ophthalmology, University of California, San Francisco, San Francisco, California.
*Eye Injuries*

**Robert J. Harrison, MD, MPH**
Associate Clinical Professor of Medicine, University of California, San Francisco, San Francisco, California.
*Liver Toxicology; Chemicals; Biological Monitoring; Multiple Chemical Sensitivity*

**Franklin T. Hoaglund, MD**
Professor of Orthopaedic Surgery, University of California, San Francisco, San Francisco, California.
*Musculoskeletal Injuries*

**John J. Howard, MD, JD**
Chief, Division of Occupational Safety and Health, California Department of Industrial Relations, San Francisco, California.
*Environmental Exposures & Controls*

**Robert K. Jackler, MD**
Professor of Otolaryngology and Head and Neck Surgery, University of California, San Francisco, San Francisco, California.
*Hearing Loss*

**Richard J. Jackson, MD, MPH**
Assistant Clinical Professor of Epidemiology and International Health, University of California, San Francisco, San Francisco, California; Director, National Center for Environmental Health, Centers for Disease Control & Prevention, Atlanta, Georgia.
*Environmental Exposures & Controls*

**Ira L. Janowitz, PT, CPE**
Ergonomist, University of California, San Francisco; Berkeley Ergonomics Program, Berkeley, California.
*Ergonomics & the Prevention of Occupational Injuries*

**Elizabeth A. Katz, MPH, CIH**
Associate Industrial Hygienist, Occupational Health Branch, California Department of Health Services, Berkeley, California.
*Solvents*

**Ware G. Kuschner, MD**
Fellow, Division of Pulmonary and Critical Care Medicine; Division of Occupational and Environmental Medicine; Cardiovascular Research Institute, University of California, San Francisco, San Francisco, California.
*Gases & Other Inhalants*

**Joseph LaDou, MS, MD**
Clinical Professor and Director, International Center for Occupational Medicine, University of California, San Francisco, San Francisco, California.
*The Practice of Occupational Medicine; Approach to the Diagnosis of Occupational Illnesses; Workers' Compensation; Disability Evaluation; Environmental Exposures and Controls*

**Kelvin C. Lee, MD**
Chief of Otolaryngology, Head and Neck Surgery, San Francisco General Hospital, San Francisco, California.
*Facial Injuries*

**Richard Lewis, MD, MPH**
Assistant Clinical Professor, Department of Medicine, University of California, San Francisco, San Francisco, California; Consultant to industry, Cleveland, Ohio.
*Metals; Plastics; The Rubber Industry*

**Melanie A. Marty, PhD**
Chief, Air Risk Assessment Unit, Office of Environmental Health Hazard Assessment, California Environmental Protection Agency, Berkeley, California.
*Routine Industrial Emissions, Accidental Releases, & Hazardous Waste*

**Andrew H. Murr, MD**
Assistant Professor of Otolaryngology, Head and Neck Surgery, University of California, San Francisco, San Francisco, California.
*Facial Injuries*

**Michael A. O'Malley, MD, MPH**
Assistant Clinical Professor, Division of Occupational Medicine, University of California, Davis, Davis, California.
*Pesticides*

**Kevin W. Olden, MD**
Assistant Clinical Professor of Medicine and Psychiatry, University of California, San Francisco, San Francisco, California.
*Substance Abuse & Employee Assistance Programs*

**Ana Maria Osorio, MD, MPH**
Assistant Clinical Professor, Division of Occupational and Environmental Medicine, University of California, San Francisco; Chief, Division of Environmental and Occupational Disease Control, California Department of Health Services, Emeryville, California.
*Female Reproductive Toxicology; Male Reproductive Toxicology*

**Dennis J. Paustenbach, PhD, DABT, CIH**
Adjunct Professor, Environmental Health/Science Program, University of Massachusetts, Amherst; Visiting Professor (1996), Center for Risk Analysis, Harvard University School of Public Health, Boston, Massachusetts; President and Chief Executive Officer, McLaren/Hart ChemRisk, Alameda, California.
*Health Risk Assessment*

**Franklyn G. Prieskop, MS, CSP**
Lecturer in Occupational Safety, University of California, San Francisco, San Francisco, California.
*Occupational Safety*

**David M. Rempel, MD, MPH**
Associate Professor of Medicine, Division of Occupational Medicine, University of California, San Francisco, San Francisco, California.
*Ergonomics & the Prevention of Occupational Injuries*

**Peggy Reynolds, PhD, MPH**
Chief, Environmental Epidemiology and Geographic Information Section, California Department of Health Services, Emeryville, California.
*Use of Population-Based Disease Registries in Occupational & Environmental Medicine*

**Scott T. Robinson, MPH, CIH, CSP**
Assistant Clinical Professor, Department of Medicine, University of California, San Francisco, San Francisco, California.
*Hearing Loss*

**Rudolph A. Rodriguez, MD**
Assistant Clinical Professor, Department of Medicine, University of California, San Francisco, San Francisco, California.
*Renal Toxicology*

**Jon Rosenberg, MD**
Assistant Clinical Professor of Medicine, University of California, San Francisco, San Francisco, California.
*Clinical Toxicology; Solvents; Pesticides; Biological Monitoring*

**Hope S. Rugo, MD**
Associate Clinical Professor of Medicine, Adult Leukemia and Bone Marrow Transplant Program, University of California, San Francisco, San Francisco, California.
*Occupational Hematology; Occupational Cancer*

**Cornelius H. Scannell, MB, Bch, BAO, MPH**
Assistant Professor of Medicine, Divisions of Occupational and Environmental Medicine and Pulmonary Medicine, University of California, San Francisco, San Francisco, California.
*Occupational Lung Diseases; Outdoor Air Pollution*

**Marc B. Schenker, MD, MPH**
Professor and Chair, Department of Epidemiology and Preventive Medicine, University of California, Davis, Davis, California.
*Appendix A: Biostatistics & Epidemiology*

**David N. Schindler, MD**
Clinical Professor of Otolaryngology and Head and Neck Surgery, University of California, San Francisco, San Francisco, California.
*Hearing Loss*

**James P. Seward, MD, MPP**
Associate Clinical Professor of Medicine, University of California, San Francisco, San Francisco, California.
*Occupational Stress*

**Richard S. Shames, MD**
Assistant Professor of Pediatrics and Co-Director, Pediatric Allergy/Immunology, Stanford University Medical Center, Stanford, California.
*Clinical Immunology*

**Dennis Shusterman, MD, MPH**
Associate Clinical Professor, Division of Occupational and Environmental Medicine, University of California, San Francisco, San Francisco, California.
*Occupational & Environmental Disorders of the Upper Respiratory Tract*

**Yuen T. So, MD, PhD**
Associate Professor of Neurology, Oregon Health Sciences University, Portland, Oregon.
*Peripheral Nerve Injuries; Neurotoxicology*

**Daniel Thau Teitelbaum, MD**
Associate Clinical Professor of Preventive Medicine, University of Colorado School of Medicine; Adjunct Professor of Environmental Sciences, Colorado School of Mines, Denver, Colorado.
*Water Pollution*

**Dan J. Tennenhouse, MD, JD**
Lecturer in Legal Medicine, University of California, San Francisco, San Francisco, California.
*Liability Issues in Occupational Medicine*

**Marilyn C. Underwood, PhD**
Staff Toxicologist, California Department of Health Services, Environmental Health Investigations Branch, Emeryville, California.
*Routine Industrial Emissions, Accidental Releases, & Hazardous Waste*

**Gayle C. Windham, MSPH, PhD**
Epidemiologist, Reproductive Epidemiology Section, California Department of Health Services, Emeryville, California.
*Female Reproductive Toxicology*

**Herman Woessner, BS, MSS, MA**
Lecturer in Occupational Safety, University of California, San Francisco, San Francisco, California; President, SafeRisk Corporation, New Orleans, Louisiana.
*Occupational Safety*

# *Preface*

This second edition of *Occupational & Environmental Medicine,* bearing an expanded title, continues to serve as a concise yet comprehensive resource for health care professionals in all specialties who are called on to diagnose and treat occupational injuries and occupational and environmental illnesses. The text's broad coverage and emphasis on fundamental concepts make it an ideal text for students and residents.

## COVERAGE & APPROACH TO THE SUBJECT

The book provides a complete guide to common occupational injuries and occupational and environmental illnesses, their diagnosis and treatment, and preventive and remedial measures in the workplace and community. Our aim is to help physicians understand and deal with the complexities of occupational and environmental medicine and at the same time provide useful clinical information on common illnesses and injuries. The book contains eight new chapters, expanding the coverage of environmental medicine well beyond that of the first edition.

## SPECIAL AREAS OF EMPHASIS

- Detailed coverage of diagnosis and treatment of a broad spectrum of occupational injuries and occupational and environmental illnesses.
- Chapters on basic toxicology and immunology, providing the foundation necessary for a solid understanding of occupational and environmental disease.
- Practical information on toxic properties and clinical manifestations of common industrial materials.
- Techniques to prevent workplace-related accidents and illness.

## SPECIAL SUBJECTS IN SUPPORT

- Although epidemiologic data are not presented in the text, much of the clinical information is drawn from epidemiologic studies, and the reader will learn epidemiologic and biostatistical principles

by studying the text. (Previous knowledge of these principles is not necessary for an understanding of the information in this text.) **Appendix A** presents a basic introduction to biostatistics and epidemiology.
- The role of non-physician health and safety professionals and their interaction with physicians is examined; the importance of a team effort in developing health and safety programs in the workplace is emphasized.
- Chapters on the legal aspects of occupational and environmental medicine round out the book's comprehensive approach.

## ORGANIZATION & HIGHLIGHTS OF EACH SECTION

**Section I** (Chapters 1 through 5) focuses on the health professional's role in the occupational health and safety team. It offers guidance for identifying workplace and community exposures to toxic materials—putting this information to immediate clinical use and applying it toward better health and safety practices in the workplace. This section also orients physicians to the special nature of disability examinations required for workers' compensation insurance settlements and considers some of the legal issues important in the practice of occupational and environmental medicine.

**Section II** (Chapters 6 through 12) concisely discusses common occupational injuries and their treatments. Noise-induced hearing loss and the impact of other physical hazards, such as heat, cold, and radiation, are examined. It also emphasizes the importance of ergonomics and discusses how ergonomic principles can be instituted in the workplace to prevent further work loss associated with injury and illness.

**Section III** (Chapters 13 through 26) is a comprehensive discussion of clinical toxicology arranged by organ system, with special emphasis on the environmental as well as workplace origins of toxic exposure. It thoroughly reviews commonly recognized environmental and occupational illnesses and highlights many clinical problems not often thought to be work-related. Chapter 16, "Occupational Infections," includes an up-to-date discussion of AIDS and its implications in the workplace.

**Section IV** (Chapters 27 through 33) presents the most common toxic materials encountered in the workplace and community and the diagnostic and treatment recommendations appropriate to illnesses related to these materials. This section is designed to serve as an immediate reference source and clinical guide for the practicing health care professional. The discussion on pesticides, in particular, emphasizes the environmental as well as occupational exposures that may lead to illness. The chapter on biologic monitoring provides the information necessary for institution of medical surveillance programs and for interpretation of data obtained in such programs.

**Section V** (Chapters 34 through 38) presents the roles and responsibilities of other, nonphysician occupational health and safety professionals, including the industrial hygienist and the safety professional. The chapter on industrial hygiene includes a discussion of recommended exposure limits for common industrial materials. Chapters on occupational stress and drug and alcohol abuse in the work setting consider programs for controlling and treating these problems.

**Section VI** (Chapters 39 through 47)—new to this second edition—provides a comprehensive discussion of environmental medicine and some of the complex societal issues that accompany industrialization and technologic advances throughout the world. Emphasis is placed on recognizing that some common "occupational" exposures are found also in homes and public locations and require the same high index of suspicion that is assumed when encountered in the workplace. Chapter 40, which includes discussion on accidental releases and hazardous waste, will be of particular interest to health care professionals.

**Appendix A** concisely introduces biostatistics and epidemiology. These principles are important not only in research but also in clinical practice. Ultimately, all occupational and environmental physicians serve as clinical epidemiologists.

**Appendix B**—new to the second edition—contains a selected portion of *Acute Low Back Problems in Adults: Assessment and Treatment: Clinical Practice Guideline* to introduce the important contribution the Agency for Health Care Policy and Research (AHCPR) is making in assisting health care professionals with patient-related decisions.

## ACKNOWLEDGMENTS

I wish to thank the many *Occupational & Environmental Medicine,* second edition, contributors. This book brings together their combined experience of more than 20 years of teaching at UCSF the course entitled "Occupational and Environmental Medicine." It is the result of working with the many attendees of our courses that we could compile a text that emphasizes information vital to clinicians.

## TO OUR READERS

The guidance of our readers is essential to our continuing efforts to maintain this book as a major resource for education and reference in this important field of medicine. Address suggestions and comments to Joseph LaDou, MS, MD, Division of Occupational and Environmental Medicine, UCSF, Box 0924, San Francisco, CA 94143.

Joseph LaDou, MS, MD

San Francisco, California
June 1997

# Section I.
# Occupational Health

# The Practice
# of Occupational Medicine

# 1

*Joseph LaDou, MS, MD*

The rapid proliferation of new industrial materials, new production methods, and new commercial products in the 20th century—particularly since World War II—has gone forward with too little attention paid to assessment of their effects on the environment and on human health. Only about 12,000 of the estimated 70,000 chemicals commonly used in industry have been tested for toxicity in animals.

While toxicity testing lags far behind the rate of new developments, the incidence of work- and environment-related illnesses in humans increases. Similarly, the number of trained professionals in occupational safety and health is much lower than what is needed to prevent and treat these illnesses.

The result is that private physicians must assume the burden of diagnosing, treating, and if possible preventing work-related illnesses and injuries. In the United States, there are more than 6 million business establishments with 117 million employees. Nearly 90% of the businesses employ fewer than 100 workers, and it is in these smaller workplaces that many of the more serious occupational safety and health problems exist. The National Institute for Occupational Safety and Health (NIOSH) estimates that only 2% of employees in these businesses have access to industrial hygiene services and workplace monitoring programs, and only rarely is an occupational health nurse available to the small employer.

## TRAINING IN OCCUPATIONAL MEDICINE

With additional postgraduate training in occupational medicine, physicians in many specialties could provide the occupational health care required by most employers. The Institute of Medicine (IOM) estimates that the United States alone has a need for 3100–5500 occupational physicians. To accomplish the objective of expanding general medical practice to cover the shortage of occupational health professionals, three conditions must be met: (1) Primary care physicians must be trained in the disciplines of occupational and environmental medicine; (2) they must be dedicated to learning and practicing new skills in prevention, diagnosis, and treatment of occupational injuries and illnesses; and (3) they must be familiar with the skills provided by other members of the occupational health and safety team and make a commitment to working with those professionals in a team context.

Medical schools generally offer only a few hours of formal instruction in occupational medicine. Only 40 medical schools in the United States offer residency training in occupational medicine, and fewer than that offer postgraduate courses for practicing physicians. This means that most training in occupational and environmental medicine will have to be gained through individual study and practical experience.

Reasons for incorporating occupational health care into the training and practice of general medicine include the following:

(1) Large numbers of people are exposed to toxic materials, and the extent of exposure is important information physicians must have in evaluating their patients' complaints. Millions of workers have exposures sufficient to result in demonstrable health problems. Fortunately, the adverse effects are reversible in a significant number of cases when the toxic material is identified and exposure is held thereafter to an acceptable level.

(2) Early recognition by physicians of unusual patterns of illnesses in their patients can alert the plant authority and local public health officials to the need for further industrial and environmental control measures.

(3) New chemicals introduced into the industrial setting require toxicologic testing as well as the development of a medical literature data base. Physicians can contribute to this data base by reporting their observations in the occupational and environmental health literature. Case reports often prompt industry-wide epidemiologic studies.

(4) A multidisciplinary occupational health and

safety team must include physicians with training and experience in recognizing, treating, and preventing occupational illness. When broadly trained and experienced, the physician can serve as the health and safety team leader.

(5) Physicians in general practice will continue to encounter problems in managing patients with work-related health problems. In such cases, the physician must ask questions about all aspects of the patient's life, including the past and present occupational history. The physician must have the training needed to consult perceptively with specialists in occupational and environmental medicine and with other occupational health professionals, including safety professionals and industrial hygienists.

## Board Certification
## in Occupational Medicine

In 1955, occupational medicine became a recognized specialty under the American Board of Preventive Medicine (ABPM). The ABPM has certified 2200 occupational physicians, but only about half that number are currently practicing the specialty. Residencies in occupational medicine require from 1–3 years of full-time training depending on the level of academic achievement of the trainee. Residency training can be done in parallel programs with family medicine, internal medicine, physical medicine, pulmonology, dermatology, or toxicology. The ABPM prefers that candidates for certification complete an accredited residency program. However, the ABPM provides an equivalency pathway for physicians who graduated from medical school before 1984, who demonstrate competency in occupational medicine through practice and experience, and who complete educational courses at the postgraduate level in four required core subjects (epidemiology, biostatistics, environmental health, and health services administration). For details on board certification, contact

The American Board of Preventive Medicine
9950 W. Lawrence Avenue, Suite 106
Schiller Park, IL 60176
(708) 671-1750
FAX (708) 671-1751

## EVOLUTION OF THE FIELD
## OF OCCUPATIONAL MEDICINE

Recognition of work-related disease has been slow in evolving. In the early part of this century, efforts to focus attention on occupational health hazards were largely ignored.

A tunnel was being constructed through a nearby mountain to divert water from two rivers to a planned hydroelectric plant farther south.

Plans at first called for the tunnel to be 32 ft wide, but when the rock was found to have a high content of quartz, the width was expanded to 46 ft. Dust in the tunnel was so thick that workers often could not see beyond 10 ft, and the silica content of the dust ranged between 90% and 95%. The workers had trouble breathing, and as conditions worsened, they began to drop dead in the tunnel. Within a few months, 50% had died or were suffering from silicosis.

This disaster at Gauley Bridge, West Virginia, in the 1930s—which eventually claimed the lives of 476 men and disabled an additional 1500—focused government and public attention on the neglected problem of occupational disease as a public health concern.

Through much of the 20th century, Dr Alice Hamilton was a pioneer in the field of occupational medicine and environmental toxicology. Her descriptions of lead poisoning in factories, silica exposure in quarries, and mercury poisoning in quicksilver mines—as well as her demands for preventive health care in US industry—served as initial steps toward recognizing occupational diseases and dealing with them.

The pervasiveness of potentially toxic contaminants both in the workplace and in the home and community environment is a source of ongoing concern. Public concern has resulted in the development of a number of governmental activities to protect the health of workers and of the community. Passage of the Occupational Safety and Health Act in 1970 created the Occupational Safety and Health Administration (OSHA) and NIOSH. These and other government agencies, including the Environmental Protection Agency (EPA), and private organizations concerned with occupational and environmental health are reviewed in Chapter 2.

## PREVENTION OF OCCUPATIONAL
## & ENVIRONMENTAL ILLNESSES

Preventing work-related and environmental illnesses is made difficult by the following features of life in an industrialized society:

(1) The uninterrupted flow of new and untested chemicals into the workplace and subsequently into the environment.

(2) The paucity of data about the toxicologic and environmental effects of most of these substances, including their interactions, their metabolites, and their cumulative effects.

(3) Diagnostic difficulties related to the sometimes protracted intervals between the exposure and the onset of disease or occurrence of overt symptoms.

(4) The problems of safe disposal of hazardous

wastes and the often prohibitive costs of detoxification of the most hazardous materials.

## Health Surveillance Techniques

Health surveillance techniques frequently include preplacement and periodic physical examinations of workers. Preventive health examinations—including batteries of screening laboratory tests—are parts of many occupational health and safety programs. Major advances in molecular biology make it possible to identify genes and enzymes that play an important role in many diseases. Identification of chemical adducts to deoxyribonucleic acid (DNA) in various worker groups may be taken both as a marker of exposure and as a sign of early effect. Other tests, such as specific enzyme patterns, activated oncogenes, or inactivated suppressor genes, may identify susceptible individuals. Debate over the legal and ethical issues inherent in genetic testing is resulting in a gradual acceptance of these practices.

## Worker Population Surveillance Systems

Studies of illnesses and causes of death of workers in various industries in the United States have often been flawed by failure to sort information by industry or specific occupation or to include information about exposure of workers to toxic substances. Because the death certificates in only about a dozen of the 50 states include information about the deceased worker's occupation and employment history, it is impossible to evaluate occupational mortality patterns at the national level. Work history is not usually part of the hospital record either. This further restricts the efforts of worker health surveillance groups to determine the extent of occupational illnesses and to identify workplace hazards that need to be controlled or eliminated.

## Epidemiologic Studies

Epidemiologic methods can be used to (1) identify subgroups of the population at high risk for given diseases and injuries, (2) detect hazardous exposures and their adverse effects, (3) determine the effectiveness of control measures instituted in the workplace, and (4) evaluate the efficiency of screening tests for occupational diseases or substance abuse in the workplace. A brief introduction to basic epidemiologic methods is presented in the Appendix.

## OCCUPATIONAL ILLNESSES

### Scope of the Problem

Each year in the United States, over 2 million people suffer permanent or temporary disability from various causes. Although the number of people with disabilities resulting from occupational illness is not known, it has been estimated that there are at least 400,000 new cases of disabling occupational illness and as many as 100,000 deaths from occupational diseases each year. Yet one study suggested that because of the difficulty of diagnosis and the likelihood that occupational illness claims will be disputed by employers, only 3% of workers with occupational illnesses were receiving compensation under the workers' compensation insurance system.

Workers in manufacturing have the largest number of occupational illnesses. Although they constitute only 20% of total employees, they account for 35% of occupational illnesses, with ergonomic disorders and skin rashes representing most cases. A major cause of occupational illnesses among production workers is exposure to toxic chemicals, such as solvents, acids, and those chemicals found in soaps, petroleum fractions, paints, plastics, and resins. Additional problems occur from exposure to dusts, gases, and metals.

Occupational stress is becoming more widely recognized among workers and, consequently, is beginning to add to the total number of occupational disease cases receiving workers' compensation benefits. Heart disease has become a major source of workers' compensation stress claims in many states, and cerebrovascular accidents and other vascular diseases are common occupational illnesses and suitable claims for compensation in some states. Furthermore, occupational illnesses resulting from repeated exposure to stressors such as noise, heat, repetitive movements, and years of heavy lifting now result in "cumulative injury" claims. About three-fifths of workplace illnesses are disorders associated with repeated trauma such as carpal tunnel syndrome. Although such cases account for only a small percentage of total claims, their treatment and settlement costs are high.

### Major Occupational Illnesses

NIOSH has developed a priority list of the 10 leading work-related illnesses and injuries. Three criteria were used to develop the list: (1) the frequency of occurrence of the illness or injury, (2) its severity in individual cases, and (3) its potential for prevention.

Occupational lung disease is first on the list. NIOSH estimates that 1.2 million workers are exposed to silica dust and that about 60,000 exposed workers will suffer some degree of silicosis. Among some 20 million living men and women exposed to asbestos, between 75,000 and 300,000 are expected to develop exposure-related cancer in the next 50 years. Longitudinal studies of exposed shipyard workers show that 10–18% die of asbestosis. Byssinosis has already disabled an estimated 35,000 current and retired textile workers. About 4000 deaths each year are attributed to legislatively defined "black lung disease." The prevalence of occupational asthma varies from 10% to nearly all of workers in certain high-risk occupations.

NIOSH considers occupational cancer to be the second leading work-related disease, followed by cardiovascular diseases, disorders of reproduction, neurotoxic disorders, noise-induced hearing loss, dermatologic conditions, and psychologic disorders.

## Occupational Illnesses Resulting From Exposure to Toxic Materials

Many occupational illnesses result from exposure to toxic substances about which little is known. As high-technology industries replace traditional forms of manufacture, the use of new and often toxic materials increases. Microelectronics manufacturers, for example, use hundreds of chemicals developed specifically for their product lines. Industrial hygiene services are in many cases unavailable to workers in these companies, and information on the toxic effects of the materials used is often inadequate or nonexistent.

Although industry spends an estimated 2% of corporate revenues on health and safety programs, very little of this outlay is for toxicologic studies or for worker health problems. As a result, there is little information about the possible toxicity of most of the commonly used industrial chemicals, and the long-term effects of these chemicals on the environment and on community health are generally unknown.

The National Research Council of the National Academy of Sciences concluded from a recent study that toxicologists have fairly complete information on health hazards for only 10% of pesticides and only 18% of drugs in use today. Moreover, at least one-third of pesticides and drugs have never been tested for toxicity. The problem with common commercial chemicals is even more serious, since nearly 80% of them have never been tested, and little is known about many that have been studied.

Occupational health professionals and government officials thus anticipate that there will be more deleterious effects on worker and community health in the future. A further area now being studied by toxicologists is the interaction of toxic materials, in which one substance may potentiate the toxicity of other chemicals or in which new chemicals may be created by interaction with others.

## OCCUPATIONAL INJURIES

Every year, American workers suffer an estimated 1 million eye injuries, 400,000 fractures, 21,000 amputations, and more than 2 million lacerations severe enough to require medical treatment. Hospital emergency rooms alone treat at least 3 million occupational injuries each year. Work-related injuries occur at a rate more than twice that of injuries in the home or public places and account for more than 200 million lost workdays annually at a cost in excess of $25 billion.

The most common occupational injuries involve the musculoskeletal system, with over 1 million workers sustaining back injuries each year.

Many studies of injury reporting systems in industry indicate that occupational injuries are grossly underreported. When employers assign injured workers to "light duty," they sometimes feel relieved of the obligation to report the injuries. Similarly, occupational injuries and illnesses are often not reported if no loss of work time occurs. Comparisons of national reporting with that of individual states, such as California, have led some investigators to conclude that occupational illnesses are at least 50% underreported nationally.

There may be as many as 10 million injuries, 30 million separate bouts of illness, between 20,000 and 75,000 deaths, and, cumulatively, 2 million disabled each year in the United States.

Nonetheless, injury rates have been declining as a result of a fundamental change in US industry and employment patterns: The service sector is growing fairly rapidly, while many traditional manufacturing industries are in decline. Because service employment (eg, food and clothing sales, banking, insurance) is generally safer than labor or trade work with heavy equipment and mechanized processes, the injury rate for all industries decreased from 11 injuries per 100 workers in 1975 to 8 injuries per 100 workers in 1995. Injury rates may continue to decline because of continuing expansion of the service sector relative to manufacturing.

The major causes of occupational deaths are work-related motor vehicle accidents, assaults, falls, trauma, and electric shock. The industries with the highest rates of fatal injury are mining and quarrying, construction, and agriculture.

# REFERENCES

Auer CM, Nabholz JV, Baetcke DP: Mode of action and the assessment of chemical hazards in the presence of limited data: Use of structure-activity relationships (SAR) under TSCA, Section 5. Environ Health Perspect 1990;87:183.

Axelson O: Some recent developments in occupational epidemiology. Scand J Work Environ Health 1994;20(special issue):9.

Castorina J, Rosenstock L: Physician shortage in occupational and environmental medicine. Ann Intern Med 1990;113:983.

Cullen MR, Cherniack MG, Rosenstock L: Medical progress: Occupational medicine, part I. N Engl J Med 1990;322:594.

Cullen MR, Cherniack MG, Rosenstock L: Medical progress: Occupational medicine, part II. N Engl J Med 1990;322:675.

Ducatman AM: Occupational physicians and environmental medicine. J Occup Med 1993;35:135.

Landrigan PJ, Baker DB: The recognition and control of occupational disease. JAMA 1991;266:676.

Söderkvist P, Axelson O: On the use of molecular biology data in occupational and environmental epidemiology. J Occup Environ Med 1995;37:84.

US Department of Labor, Bureau of Statistics: Workplace Injuries and Illnesses in 1995. US Government Printing Office, 1996.

Van Damme K et al: Individual susceptibility and prevention of occupational diseases: Scientific and ethical issues. J Occup Environ Med 1995;37:91.

Van Damme K, Casteleyn L, Heseltine E (editors): Seminar: Current medical surveillance and pre-employment practices. Int. J Occup Environ Health 1996;2(3):supplement.

# 2

# Approach to the Diagnosis of Occupational Illnesses

*Joseph LaDou, MS, MD*

Diagnosing occupational illnesses is often difficult because the illnesses are often the result of acute as well as chronic exposures to multiple agents and may be confounded by other nonoccupational factors.

For example, a patient has frequent respiratory infections that appear to be caused by long-term exposure to fumes and vapors at work. The problem does not subside during his annual vacations away from the plant. He is also a heavy smoker.

How can the physician determine which contaminant is making the patient ill? When common illnesses are ruled out after thorough assessment, the physician must question whether the patient's problem stems from exposure to toxic materials in the workplace, conditions in the home, or environmental exposure. A useful tool in this regard is the medical history and, more importantly, the occupational and environmental medical history. A visit to the workplace may be in order, as well as a review of the health records of the worker.

## THE OCCUPATIONAL MEDICAL HISTORY

The most important diagnostic skill in the practice of occupational medicine is the taking of a comprehensive occupational medical history. The importance of this skill cannot be overemphasized in the training of medical students and in the everyday practice of physicians. The questions and topics outlined in Figure 2–1 are intended to uncover associations between work and the patient's chief symptoms. If answers to these questions result in positive associations, more detailed follow-up questioning is necessary.

One method of speeding up the process of screening for associations between work and symptoms is to add specific occupational history questions to primary health questionnaires. Table 2–1 lists the important additions to such a questionnaire survey. Figure 2–2 provides a more complete history form to be used in the evaluation of occupational and environmental exposures. The detailed occupational and environmental history can be enhanced by a number of information sources.

## EMPLOYEE DOCUMENTS

Medical records should be obtained from the treating physician. These may contain clues as to previous occupational or environmental history, predisposing factors for the illness, previous similar episodes of illness, and information regarding the course and causes of the illness.

If the physician suspects that the workplace is the source of the health problem, the employer should be asked to produce the patient's records pertaining to sick leave, accidents, and job performance. The physician should also ask to see the workers' compensation insurance carrier's files describing all medical care rendered to the patient for previous occupational illnesses and injuries. The company should cooperate in answering questions about similar illnesses occurring in coworkers.

The physician must indicate on the insurance form whether the illness is related to work. Neglecting to state this opinion early in the course of treatment may cause delays in benefits to the worker and may also create problems with statute of limitations provisions that would later deny payments to the worker.

## THE OCCUPATIONAL HAZARD

When a patient's medical history indicates that occupational or environmental factors may be a cause of illness, the physician should identify all potentially toxic materials to which the worker is exposed, both in the workplace and at home or elsewhere. Technical data pertaining to the chemical properties, uses, and toxicity of many industrial materials are available to treating physicians.

Three excellent books cited below should be in the

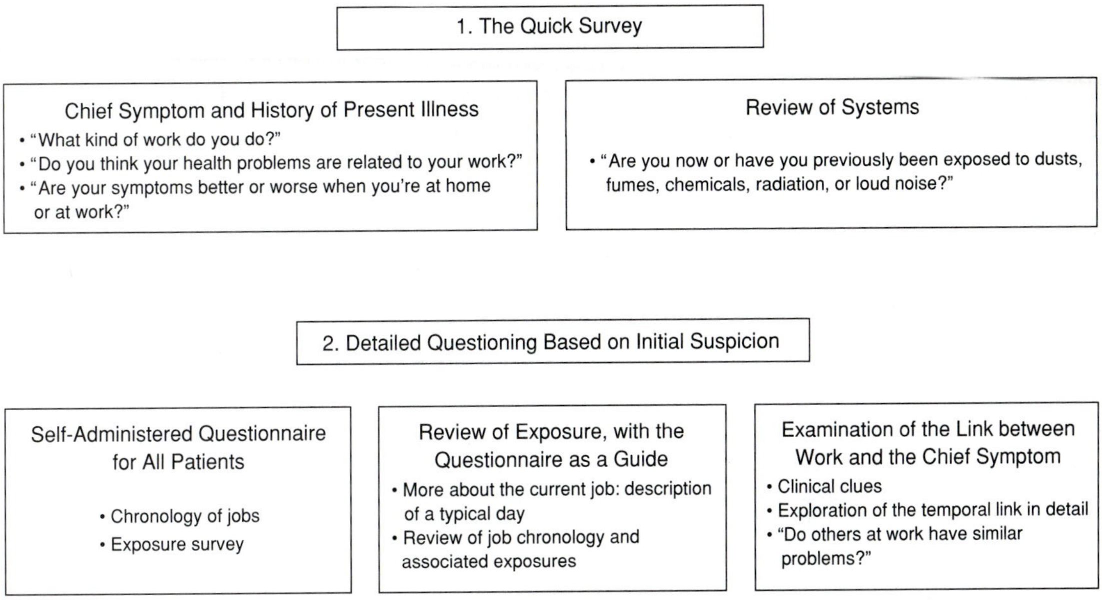

```
┌─────────────────────────────────────────┐
│           1. The Quick Survey            │
└─────────────────────────────────────────┘
```

**Chief Symptom and History of Present Illness**
- "What kind of work do you do?"
- "Do you think your health problems are related to your work?"
- "Are your symptoms better or worse when you're at home or at work?"

**Review of Systems**
- "Are you now or have you previously been exposed to dusts, fumes, chemicals, radiation, or loud noise?"

```
┌─────────────────────────────────────────────────┐
│  2. Detailed Questioning Based on Initial Suspicion  │
└─────────────────────────────────────────────────┘
```

**Self-Administered Questionnaire for All Patients**
- Chronology of jobs
- Exposure survey

**Review of Exposure, with the Questionnaire as a Guide**
- More about the current job: description of a typical day
- Review of job chronology and associated exposures

**Examination of the Link between Work and the Chief Symptom**
- Clinical clues
- Exploration of the temporal link in detail
- "Do others at work have similar problems?"

**Figure 2–1.** The initial clinical approach to the recognition of illness caused by occupational exposure. (Modified and reproduced, with permission, from Newman LS: Occupational illness. N Engl J Med 1995;333:1129.)

**Table 2–1.** Essential elements of the occupational history and questionnaire.[1]

**Current or most recent work and exposure history**
Job title; type of industry; name of employer
Year work started and year work finished (if not currently employed)
Description of job (what is a typical workday), especially the parts of the job the patient believes may be potentially hazardous
Current work hours and any shift changes
Current exposure to dust, fumes, radiation, chemicals, biologic hazards, or physical hazards
Protective equipment used (clothes, safety glasses, hearing protection, respirator, or gloves)
Other employees at the workplace who have similar health problems
**Earlier employment history**
Job chronology, working backward from the current or most recent job
The same information as above for each job previously held
**Major types of exposure associated with clinical illness**

| | |
|---|---|
| Gases | Solvents |
| Corrosive substances (acids, alkalis) | Petrochemicals (coal, tar, asphalt, petroleum distillates) |
| Dyes and stains | |
| Dusts and powders | Physical factors (noise, lifting, thermal stress, vibration, repetitive motion) |
| Asbestos, other fibers | |
| Infectious agents | |
| Insecticides and pesticides | Emotional factors (stress) |
| Metals and metal fumes | Radiation (electromagnetic fields, x-ray radiation, ultraviolet radiation) |
| Organic dusts (cotton, wood, biologic matter) | |
| Plastics | |

[1]Modified and reproduced, with permission, from Newman LS: Occupational illness. N Engl J Med 1995; 333(17):1129.

library of every practicing occupational physician. They are sources of information on potential health hazards in a wide variety of industries and serve as guides to identification or recognition of hazards of hundreds of industrial processes. The books cover major industries, in which large numbers of workers are employed, and various hazard potentials are presented.

Burgess WA: *Recognition of Health Hazards in Industry: A Review of Materials and Processes*, 2nd ed. John Wiley, 1995.
Grayson M (editor): *Kirk-Othner Concise Encyclopedia of Chemical Technology*, 4th ed. John Wiley, 1995 (also available on CD-ROM).
Harris RL, Cralley LJ, Cralley LV (editors): Patty's Industrial Hygiene and Toxicology, John Wiley, 1994.

## THE MATERIAL SAFETY DATA SHEET (MSDS)

An important step in obtaining information is often to request an MSDS—a written evaluation of a hazardous chemical, generally prepared by the substance manufacturer and given to the employer with the purchase of the substance—on each of the suspected materials. The Occupational Safety and Health Administration (OSHA) requires suppliers to include these data sheets with each shipment of in-

# Exposure History Form

## Part 1. Exposure Survey

*Please circle the appropriate answer.*

Name: _____ Date: _____

Birthdate: _____ Sex:  M     F

1. Are you currently exposed to any of the following?

   metals
     no     yes

   dust or fibers
     no     yes

   chemicals
     no     yes

   fumes
     no     yes

   radiation
     no     yes

   loud noise, vibration, extreme heat or cold
     no     yes

   biologic agents
     no     yes

2. Have you been exposed to any of the above *in the past?*
     no     yes

3. Do any household members have contact with metals, dust, fibers, chemicals, fumes, radiation, or biologic agents?
     no     yes

If you answered *yes* to any of the items above, describe your exposure in detail—how you were exposed; to what you where exposed. If you need more space, please use a separate sheet of paper.

4. Do you know the names of the metals, dusts, fibers, chemicals, fumes or radiation that you are/were exposed to?
     no     yes ——————————————————————→ If *yes,* list them below.

5. Do you get the material on your skin or clothing?
     no     yes

6. Are your work clothes laundered at home?
     no     yes

7. Do you shower at work?
     no     yes

8. Can you smell the chemical or material you are working with?
     no     yes

9. Do you use protective equipment such as gloves, masks, respirator, hearing protectors?
     no     yes ——————————————————————→ If *yes,* list the protective equipment used.

10. Have you been advised to use protective equipment?
     no     yes

11. Have you been instructed in the use of protective equipment?
     no     yes

12. Do you wash your hands with solvents?
     no     yes

13. Do you smoke at the workplace?     At home?
     no     yes          no     yes

14. Do you eat at the workplace?
     no     yes

Developed by ATSDR in cooperation with NIOSH, 1992.     Page 1

**Figure 2–2.** The exposure history form. (Modified and reproduced with permission, from ATSDR: *Case Studies in Environmental Medicine*: Taking an Exposure History. Appendix in Environmental Medicine: Integrating a Missing Element into Medical Education. Pope AM, Rall DP [editors]. National Academy Press, 1995.)

15. Do you know of any coworkers experiencing similar or unusual symptoms?

     *no*    *yes*

16. Are family members experiencing similar or unusual symptoms?

     *no*    *yes*

17. Has there been a change in the health or behavior of family pets?

     *no*    *yes*

18. Do your symptoms seem to be aggravated by a specific activity?

     *no*    *yes*

19. Do your symptoms get either worse or better at work?

     *no*    *yes*

at home?

     *no*    *yes*

on weekends?

     *no*    *yes*

on vacation?

     *no*    *yes*

20. Has anything about your job changed in recent months (such as duties, procedures, overtime)?

     *no*    *yes*

If you answered *yes* to any of the questions, please explain.

**Figure 2–2.** Continued

## Part 2. Work History

**Name:** ______________________ **Date:** __________

### A. Occupational Profile

**Birthdate:** ____________________ **Sex: M F**

The following questions refer to your current or most recent job:

Job title: ______________________

Type of industry: ______________________

Name of employer: ______________________

Date job began: ______________________

Are you still working in this job?
Yes No

If no, when did this job end? ______________________

Describe this job:
______________________

Fill in the table below listing all jobs you have worked including short-term, seasonal, part-time employment, and military service. Begin with your most recent job. Use additional paper if necessary.

| Dates of Employment | Job Title and Description of Work | Exposures* | Protective Equipment |
|---|---|---|---|
| | | | |
| | | | |
| | | | |
| | | | |

* List the chemicals, dusts, fibers, fumes, radiation, biologic agents (i.e., molds, viruses) and physical agents (i.e., extreme heat, cold, vibration, noise) that you were exposed to at this job.

Have you ever worked at a job or hobby in which you came in contact with any of the following by breathing, touching, or ingesting (swallowing)? If yes, please check the box beside the name.

- ❑ Acids
- ❑ Alcohols (industrial)
- ❑ Alkalies
- ❑ Ammonia
- ❑ Arsenic
- ❑ Asbestos
- ❑ Benzene
- ❑ Beryllium
- ❑ Cadmium
- ❑ Carbon tetrachloride
- ❑ Chlorinated naphthalenes
- ❑ Chloroform
- ❑ Chloroprene
- ❑ Chromates
- ❑ Coal dust
- ❑ Dichlorobenzene
- ❑ Ethylene dibromide
- ❑ Ethylene dichloride
- ❑ Fiberglass
- ❑ Halothane
- ❑ Isocyanates
- ❑ Ketones
- ❑ Lead
- ❑ Manganese
- ❑ Mercury
- ❑ Methylene chloride
- ❑ Nickel
- ❑ PBBs
- ❑ PCBs
- ❑ Perchloroethylene
- ❑ Pesticides
- ❑ Phenol
- ❑ Phosgene
- ❑ Radiation
- ❑ Rock dust
- ❑ Silica powder
- ❑ Solvents
- ❑ Styrene
- ❑ Talc
- ❑ Toluene
- ❑ TDI or MDI
- ❑ Trichloroethylene
- ❑ Trinitrotoluene
- ❑ Vinyl chloride
- ❑ Welding fumes
- ❑ X rays
- ❑ Other (specify)

Developed by ATSDR in cooperation with NIOSH, 1992. Page 3

**Figure 2–2.** Continued

## B. Occupationnal Exposure Inventory    *Please circle the appropriate answer.*

1. Have you ever been off work for more than one day because of an illness related to work?     *no*    *yes*

2. Have you ever been advised to change jobs or work assignments because of any health problems or injuries?     *no*    *yes*

3. Has your work routine changed recently?     *no*    *yes*

4. Is there poor ventilation in your workplace?     *no*    *yes*

# Part 3. Environmental History    *Please circle the appropriate answer.*

1. Do you live next to or near an industrial plant, commercial business, dump site, or nonresidential property?     *no*    *yes*

2. Which of the following do you have in your home?
   *Please circle those that apply.*

   | | | |
   |---|---|---|
   | Air conditioner | Air purifier | Central heating (gas or oil?) |
   | Gas stove | Electric stove | Fireplace |
   | Wood stove | Humidifier | |

3. Have you recently acquired new furniture or carpet, refinished furniture, or remodeled your home?     *no*    *yes*

4. Have you weatherized your home recently?     *no*    *yes*

5. Are pesticides or herbicides (bug or weed killers; flea and tick sprays, collars, powders, or shampoos) used in your home or garden, or on pets?     *no*    *yes*

6. Do you (or any household member) have a hobby or craft?     *no*    *yes*

7. Do you work on your car?     *no*    *yes*

8. Have you ever changed your residence because of a health problem?     *no*    *yes*

9. Does your drinking water come from a private well, city water supply, or grocery store?
   _____

10. Approximately what year was your home built? _____

---

If you answered *yes* to any of the questions, please explain.

Page 4

**Figure 2–2.** Continued

dustrial materials and requires employers to maintain them and make them available to physicians and workers. An MSDS can be obtained by telephone or by written request to either the employer or the supplier. If the product or process is a trade secret, the physician or worker may be required to sign a confidentiality agreement before receiving sensitive information. The Chemical Manufacturers' Association CHEMTREC, at (800) 262-8200, (202) 463-1596, will also assist you in obtaining MSDSs.

The MSDS primarily assists company personnel in the event of emergencies. Although it seldom provides adequate clinical information for the treating physician, the MSDS often serves as a starting point in the assessment of the worker's possible exposure to toxic substances. Each MSDS is required to have an emergency company phone number for information regarding toxicologic information often missing from the MSDS. MSDSs are also available from the Canadian Centre for Occupational Health and Safety, either on-line or on CD-ROM (800) 668-4284, (905) 570-8094, FAX (905) 572-2206, e-mail at cust-serv@ccohs.ca.

The Internet now has several on-line databases of MSDSs that are freely available. They may be found by using any one of the searching services on the Internet (eg, http://www.yahoo.com/) and searching for the term MSDS.

## ADDITIONAL SOURCES OF TECHNICAL INFORMATION

Because of the shortcomings of the MSDS, additional information on toxic materials is often needed. Sources include the following:

(1) The employer may have information beyond what is written on the MSDS. As discussed below, it is helpful to establish a line of communication with the person in charge of health and safety at the company.

(2) Poison control centers, county and state health departments, regional offices of the National Institute for Occupational Safety and Health (NIOSH), and other government agencies and local academic institutions with departments of occupational medicine, toxicology, industrial hygiene, or safety engineering may be helpful.

(3) Workers' compensation insurance carriers often employ specialists in safety, industrial hygiene, and occupational medicine and occupational health nursing. They may already be familiar with the workplace where the exposure occurred.

(4) Occupational physicians and industrial hygienists practicing in the area can often assist in evaluating the incident and may have information about other incidents of a similar nature.

(5) Medical libraries in academic centers and local hospitals can provide computer searches regarding toxic materials.

## DATABASES

The databases described in the following section can be reached through National Library of Medicine (NLM), MEDLARS Management Section, 8600 Rockville Pike, Bethesda, MD 20894; (301) 496-6095 or 496-6193; (800) 638-8480; e-mail: mms@nlm.nih.gov.

**MEDLARS (MEDical Literature Analysis and Retrieval System)** is the computerized system of databases based at the National Library of Medicine. The databases may be accessed by more than 120,000 universities, medical schools, hospitals, government agencies, commercial and nonprofit organizations, and private individuals. MEDLARS contains some 20,000,000 references to journal articles and books in the health sciences published after 1965. An individual user may search the store of references to produce a list pertinent to a specific question.

A number of on-line databases are available on the MEDLARS system. Each is described in a section below, beginning with MEDLINE (MEDlars onLINE), the largest and most frequently used, with approximately 7,000,000 references to biomedical journal articles. Essentially *Index Medicus* on-line, MEDLINE enables individuals and organizations with computer terminals to query NLM computers for journal article references on specific topics.

**TEHIP (Toxicology and Environmental Health Information Program)** provides the following on-line databases:

**ChemID** (Chemical Identification File) serves as an authority file for the identification of over 260,000 chemical substances cited in NLM databases. For a given substance, ChemID provides Chemical Abstract Service (CAS) Registry Numbers and chemical names, both of which can be used as search terms to enhance retrieval in the subsequent search of other NLM databases. ChemID also contains SUPERLIST, a collection of lists of chemical organizations.

**CHEMLINE** (Chemical Dictionary Online) is a chemical dictionary with nearly 1.5 million records on chemical substances found in various NLM files, as well as in the Environmental Protection Agency (EPA) Toxic Substances Control Act Inventory. It contains chemical names, synonyms, CAS registry numbers, molecular formulas, NLM file locators and, when appropriate, ring structure information.

**TOXLINE (Toxicology Information Online) and TOXLIT (Toxicology Literature from Special Sources)** are bibliographic databases covering the pharmacologic, biochemical, physiologic, and toxicologic effects of drugs and other chemicals. TOXLINE and TOXLIT, and their respective backfiles, TOXLINE65 and TOXLIT65, together contain more than 4 million citations, almost all with abstracts, index terms, or both, and CAS Registry Numbers.

**DIRLINE (Directory of Information Resources Online)** is an on-line directory file with nearly 18,000 records on resource centers, primarily health-science related. The service is willing to respond to public inquiries in their specialty areas. DBIR (Directory of Biotechnology Resources) is included as a component of DIRLINE.

**HSDB (Hazardous Substances Data Bank)** is a comprehensive, scientifically reviewed, factual database containing records for more than 4500 toxic or potentially toxic chemicals. It contains extensive information in such areas as toxicity, environmental fate, human exposure, chemical safety, waste disposal, emergency handling, and regulatory requirements. The data are taken from a core set of monographs augmented with government documents, special reports, and primary journal literature.

**RTECS (Registry of Toxic Effects of Chemical Substances)** contains toxic effects data on some 130,000 chemicals. It is built and maintained by the NIOSH and covers such areas as skin/eye irritation, carcinogenicity, mutagenicity, reproductive consequences, and multiple dose studies.

**CCRIS (Chemical Carcinogenesis Research Information System)** is sponsored by the National Cancer Institute. It contains scientifically evaluated data derived from carcinogenicity, mutagenicity, tumor production, and tumor inhibition tests on almost 7000 chemicals.

**DART (Developmental and Reproductive Toxicology)** is a bibliographic database covering teratology and developmental toxicology. It contains 26,000 citations to literature published since 1989. It is a continuation of ETICBACK.

**ETICBACK (Environmental Teratology Information Center Backfile)** is a bibliographic database covering teratology literature published from 1950–1989. It is continued by DART.

**EMIC and EMICBACK (Environmental Mutagen Information Center and its Backfile)** are bibliographic databases covering agents tested for genotoxic activity in the literature from 1950 to the present, over 75,000 citations.

**GENE-TOX** is a data bank created by the EPA with genetic toxicology test results on more than 3000 chemicals. In the field of genetic toxicology, selected mutagenicity assay systems and the source literature are reviewed by work panels of scientific experts for each of the test systems under evaluation, and the GENE-TOX data bank is the product of these data review activities. Each test system in GENE-TOX has been peer reviewed and is referenced.

**IRIS (Integrated Risk Information System)** is an on-line database built by the EPA. It contains EPA carcinogenic and noncarcinogenic health risk assessment and regulatory information on over 600 chemicals. The risk assessment data have been scientifically reviewed by groups of EPA scientists and represent EPA consensus. IRIS also contains EPA Drinking Water Health Advisories and references.

**TRI (Toxic Chemical Release Inventory)** contains information on the annual estimated releases of toxic chemicals to the environment. This series of files is mandated by the Emergency Planning and Community Right-to-Know Act and is based on data submitted to the EPA from industrial facilities around the country. These data include names and addresses of the facilities, and the amount of certain toxic chemicals they release to the air, water, or land or transfer to waste sites. In 1991 facilities were also required to report on source reduction and recycling activities as well.

**TRIFACTS (Toxic Chemical Release Inventory Facts)** supplements the environmental release data on chemicals in the TRI series of files, with information related to the health and ecologic effects, and safety and handling of these chemicals. There is a TRIFACTS record for most TRI chemicals. The data may be especially useful to workers, employers, community residents, and health professionals. TRI 1987–1994 is available on CD-ROM and on the web: http://rtk.net For assistance with TRI, contact TRI-US, 401 M Street, SW (7407), Washington, DC 20460, (202) 260-1531, FAX (202) 401-2347, E-mail: tri.us@epamail.epa.gov

## TEHIP Contact

Inquiries about the Toxicology and Environmental Health Information Program or any of its products or services should be addressed to:

National Library of Medicine
Specialized Information Services
8600 Rockville Pike
Bethesda, MD 20894
(301) 496-1131
e-mail: tehip@teh.nlm.nih.gov

## Other Resources

**NLM** has a program for assisted searching via the Internet through the World Wide Web (WWW). Called Internet Grateful Med (IGM), the program helps a user create, submit, and refine a search of MEDLINE, NLM's database of citations—most with abstracts in English—from some 3700 of the world's leading medical journals. The NLM home page uniform resource locator (URL) is http://www.nlm.nih.gov/ and off-line information is available at (800) 638-8480.

The equipment needed to access the National Library of Medicine MEDLARS system is rapidly becoming standard in almost every hospital, medical library, clinic, and doctor's office. All you need is a computer terminal or a personal computer, a modem, a printer, and the appropriate software.

The National Library of Medicine will send you

an on-line services application along with a helpful brochure describing Grateful Med for people who want easy access to the Library's vast collection of medical and health science information. Telephone (credit card) orders for Grateful Med may be made directly to the National Technical Information Service at (800) 423-9255.

**The Canadian Centre for Occupational Health and Safety (CCOHS)** offers a number of databases on CD-ROM (CCINFOdisc). An enhanced version of the RTECS database is available in English and French for an annual subscription, which includes quarterly updates. TOXLINE on CCINFOdisc is also available from the same source, as is NIOSHTIC, CHEM Source, and MSDSs. Contact: (800) 668-4284, (905) 570-8094, FAX (905) 572-2206, e-mail: custserv@ccohs.ca

Another useful resource is Richard J. Lewis, Sr: *Sax's Dangerous Properties of Industrial Materials*, 9th ed. Van Nostrand Reinhold, 1995, available in a three-volume set and CD ROM annual subscription service (with three quarterly updates); (800) 842-3636 (set), or (800) 575-5886 (CD-ROM), FAX (212) 780-6205, e-mail: http://www.vnr.com/vnr.html

## FEDERAL AGENCIES ON THE WORLD WIDE WEB

The entire **Code of Federal Regulations** can be accessed and searched on the web: http://www.pls.com:8001/his/efr.html

**NIOSH**—http://www.cdc.gov/niosh/whatsnew.html provides numerous documents on the Internet, including a list of approved respirators under 42 CFR Part 84.

**OSHA**—http://www.osha.gov/wutsnew.html provides industrial hygiene publications, recognizing and controlling hazards, examples of job hazards, booklets on "Employee Rights" and "Employer Rights and Responsibilities," etc.

**CDC**—http://www.cdc.gov/ provides a journal on the web. Emerging Infectious Diseases (EID) was begun to promote the recognition of new and re-emerging infectious diseases.

**ATSDR**—http://atsdr1.atsdr.cdc.gov:8080/atsdr home.html provides CLUSTER version 3.1 software for the epidemiologist working with cancer, birth defects, or environmental and occupational exposures, and many case studies such as lead and radon.

**EPA**—http://www.epa.gov/ provides a wealth of information on the Internet.

A useful resource to help discover Internet access to government documents, medical references, practice guidelines is Ronald S. Leopold: 1997 OEM Internet Companion. OEM Press, 1997.

## COMMERCIAL SOFTWARE

The American College of Occupational and Environmental Medicine (ACOEM) publishes a Directory of Occupational Health and Safety Software. The 500-page directory provides descriptions, uses, hardware requirements, training, user support, cost, and other information for software programs. Categories include integrated health data management, chemical and environmental, clinic management, decision support/loss control, health screening and surveillance, ergonomics and health promotion, and disability management and other software. Features include "The Use of Computers in Occupational Medicine," an updated guide to "Selecting and Purchasing PC-Based Hardware and Generic PC Software," articles on "Drug Test Data Management Software" and "Accessing Databases and Information Networks Through CD-ROM and Telecommunications," and software comparison tables. ACOEM, 55 W. Seegers Road, Arlington Heights, IL 60005; (847) 228-6850; FAX (847) 228-1856.

## ASSESSMENT OF THE WORKPLACE

The physician should become familiar with the patient's work and the environment in which the work is done. This often necessitates a visit to the workplace. A review of the working conditions requires the cooperation of company managers. Physicians who deal with these problems should learn whom to contact and should have some understanding of their roles in the company's health and safety program.

### Working With Safety Professionals

By law, all companies must have a designated safety officer at every office or plant. In small companies, this person may have little or no formal training in safety matters and may have a variety of other responsibilities. In larger companies, the safety professional is more likely to be trained in safety science and to deal solely with health and safety matters. Some companies are large enough to maintain a medical office staffed by one or more physicians and the services of occupational health nurses and other professionals.

The safety professional is the first person the physician should seek out during the visit to the work site. The working relationship between the safety professional and the occupational physician must be founded on mutual respect. If the physician shows little respect for the level of professionalism of the health and safety team members, their full cooperation cannot be assured.

The safety professional should be able to provide a description of the company's activities, products, and processes to give the physician information about past injuries and illnesses in the work force and take the physician on a tour of the general work areas and the specific areas where the patient has been working. See Chapter 36 for further information on the role of the safety professional.

## Working With Industrial Hygienists

Industrial hygienists are skilled health and safety professionals who are trained to measure and control the levels of exposure of workers to toxic materials, physical hazards, and infectious agents. Only the largest companies with well-developed health and safety programs have an industrial hygienist on the staff. Nonetheless, industrial hygiene data can be made available to smaller companies by consultants or by industrial hygienists from a workers' compensation insurance carrier. If the company employs an industrial hygienist or a consultant, the physician should work with that individual to the maximum extent possible. Industrial hygiene data are invaluable in proving or ruling out many occupational disease possibilities. These data are also important in the development of control measures and in the eventual monitoring of the effectiveness of such measures. Industrial hygiene is discussed further in Chapter 37.

## Case Example of the Team Approach to Occupational Safety & Health

A physician observed a number of severe chemical burns in patients who worked for a semiconductor manufacturer in his area. He telephoned the company's safety professional and asked whether a tour of the work area could be arranged. The company was small and did not have an industrial hygienist, but as a result of the rapport developed during the telephone conversation, the safety professional arranged for an industrial hygienist from a larger semiconductor company nearby to join the tour.

When the physician toured the workplace, he was introduced to the occupational health nurse. He learned that there had been a significant number of burns from hydrofluoric acid, used in an etching process. The nurse explained that the workers were required to immerse racks of silicon wafers into acid tanks and that the resulting burns developed slowly because the acid was diluted with water. Most burns were being seen half a day later by private physicians, who were not always told by the workers that the burns were associated with chemical exposure at work.

The hygienist had previously measured the airborne levels of hydrofluoric acid in the work area, and he gave the physician a copy of these data. Although he had recommended changes in the hoods and vents of the area, he had not found evidence that illness would result from inhalation of vapors at the levels measured. The physician was surprised to learn that the industrial hygienist was familiar with systemic effects of exposure to hydrofluoric acid. The patients seen by the physician showed no evidence of such effects.

The company safety professional gave the physician a copy of the MSDS for hydrofluoric acid and reported that the company had already instituted corrective measures to vent the acid tanks and to provide splash guards over the tanks. Protective clothing and a different type of glove were being distributed to workers.

As a result of his trip to the workplace, the physician learned that he was dealing with an occupational injury and with the possibility of an occupational illness in more severe cases of exposure to hydrofluoric acid. He also learned that the health and safety professionals at the company would begin an education program with the workers and were taking other measures to prevent further injuries.

Most importantly, the physician was included as a member of the health and safety team and was asked to consult on any future cases suspected to be the result of exposure to toxic materials by the company's workers.

## ASSESSMENT OF FACTORS OUTSIDE THE WORKPLACE

When a review of the workplace has offered no clues to the source of the patient's health problem, the physician must consider the possibility that the illness is due to exposure to toxic materials or emissions in the home or in various hobby activities. These include disinfectants, cleaning agents, paint removers, wax strippers, solvents, and pesticides; emissions from heating or cooling devices; sunlamps; and a wide variety of materials used in painting, ceramics, printmaking, sculpture and casting, welding, stained glass, woodworking, photography, and many forms of commercial art.

The timing of the onset of symptoms is important in determining whether an illness is work-related. Symptoms that occur during the workweek and subside over weekends certainly suggest an occupational cause. Conversely, those that appear only when away from the workplace could well be associated with home exposure or hobby activities.

## GOVERNMENT AGENCIES & PRIVATE ORGANIZATIONS CONCERNED WITH OCCUPATIONAL HEALTH

The occupational physician needs to become familiar with government organizations that provide information about occupational health and safety—in particular with OSHA regulations and with technical reports from OSHA and NIOSH dealing with specific questions. Many aspects of occupational medicine are directly determined by OSHA standards (eg, biological monitoring and medical surveillance examinations). Still other aspects of occupational medicine are indirectly determined by OSHA policies and procedures. Thus, the occupational medicine practitioner should take time to understand the regulatory milieu of occupational medicine.

## Occupational Safety & Health Administration (OSHA)

OSHA (US Department of Labor, Room N3647, 200 Constitution Avenue NW, Washington, DC 20210; [202] 219-8021) is the primary regulatory agency for occupational safety and health. However, the federal Occupational Safety and Health Act (OSH Act) of 1970 allows states to operate their own safety and health program if the state program meets its standards and is approved. Twenty-one states,[1] Puerto Rico, and the Virgin Islands operate their own occupational health and safety programs. In states without approved plans, jurisdiction remains at the federal level. Even in states covered by federal OSHA, however, jurisdiction for public sector employees (state, county, and city employees) always rests with the state or territory.

In order for a state to maintain approval by OSHA for its own occupational safety and health program, it must adopt (and enforce) occupational safety and health standards that are "as effective as" those adopted by federal OSHA. After federal OSHA has adopted or changed a regulation, state programs have 6 months to adopt a regulation that is at least as effective as the federal one. Most states simply adopt identical standards. But some states like California, Michigan, Oregon, Hawaii, Minnesota and Washington have adopted standards that are more stringent than their federal counterparts. On occasion, these states have even developed and adopted occupational safety and health standards that federal OSHA does not yet have.

Workplace safety and health standards are enforced by federal and state compliance officers—usually these are safety professionals and industrial hygienists. These standards have the force of law and employers must comply with the requirements contained in them. Compliance officers have the right to inspect any workplace at any time to determine if employers are complying with specific OSHA standards and regulations. OSHA inspections may be triggered by an employee complaint or an accident involving a fatality or serious injury or can be conducted as part of a high hazard industry program—a so-called programmed inspection. During an inspection, an employer found to be in violation of an OSHA standard may receive a citation carrying a

monetary penalty. Fatal accidents resulting in willful violations may also result in criminal charges being brought by federal or state criminal prosecutors.

All states offer employers consultative assistance in developing a worksite safety and health program and in complying with safety and health standards. Consultation services are provided free of charge and are a good source of information for all safety and health professionals, including occupational medicine physicians.

Finally, the OSH Act also requires that each federal agency develop and maintain a safety program consistent with OSHA standards. OSHA has entered into various Memoranda of Understanding with other federal agencies to assist them in providing occupational safety and health enforcement equal to that provided by federal OSHA.

If you need information about occupational safety and health standards, and your state has its own occupational safety and health program, call your nearest state occupational safety and health office. If you are in a state under federal OSHA jurisdiction, contact the nearest OSHA Regional Office (see below). For specific information about federal OSHA publications, including informational materials on standards and regulations, contact OSHA's Publications Office, 200 Constitution Avenue, NW, Room N3101, Washington, DC 20210, (202) 219-4667; FAX (202) 219-9266.

The Department of Labor publishes a document entitled *All About OSHA*, 1995 (Revised), OSHA 2056. The pamphlet is available at any OSHA Regional Office. The pamphlet explains the provisions of the 1970 Act and the policies of the agency.

To keep up on new standards and regulations, you can consult the federal government's regulatory newspaper, the *Federal Register*. The *Federal Register* publishes all federal OSHA standards as well as all amendments, corrections, insertions, or deletions when adopted. The *Federal Register* is available in all law libraries and also in many public libraries, which are repositories of federal documents. Annual subscriptions are available from the Superintendent of Documents, US Government Printing Office, Washington, DC 20402. For information about how to obtain copies of state occupational safety and health standards, contact your state occupational safety and health office, usually a part of the state's labor department.

The Federal OSHA Subscription Service provides all federal standards, interpretations, regulations, and procedures in loose-leaf form. The service also is available from the Superintendent of Documents. (Contact the nearest federal OSHA Regional Office for information.) Individual volumes of the OSHA Subscription Service are available as follows:

Volume I: General Industry Standards and Interpretations

---

[1]Alaska, Arizona, California, Hawaii, Indiana, Iowa, Kentucky, Maryland, Michigan, Minnesota, Nevada, New Mexico, North Carolina, South Carolina, Oregon, Tennessee, Utah, Vermont, Virginia, Washington, Wyoming.

Volume II: Maritime Standards and Interpretations
Volume III: Construction Standards and Interpretations
Volume IV: Other Regulations and Procedures
Volume V: Field Operations Manual
Volume VI: Industrial Hygiene Field Operations Manual

## OSHA Regional Offices

**Region I** (CT, ME, MA, NH, RI, VT)
JFK Federal Building, Room E340
Boston, MA 02203
(617) 565-9860

**Region II** (NY, NJ, PR, VI)
201 Varick Street, Room 670
New York, NY 10014
(212) 337-2378

**Region III** (DC, DE, MD, PA, VA, WV)
Gateway Building, Suite 2100
3535 Market Street
Philadelphia, PA 19104
(215) 596-1201

**Region IV** (AL, FL, GA, KY, MS, NC, SC, TN)
1375 Peachtree Street, NE, Suite 587
Atlanta, GA 30367
(404) 347-3573

**Region V** (IL, IN, MN, MI, OH, WI)
230 South Dearborn Street
32nd Floor, Room 3244
Chicago, IL 60604
(312) 353-2220

**Region VI** (AR, LA, NM, OK, TX)
525 Griffin Street, Room 602
Dallas, TX 75202
(214) 767-4731

**Region VII** (IA, KS, MO, NE)
City Center Square
1100 Main Street, Suite 800
Kansas City, MO 64105
(816) 426-5861

**Region VIII** (CO, MT, ND, SD, UT, WY)
1999 Broadway, Suite 1690
Denver, CO 80202-5716
(303) 844-1600

**Region IX** (CA, AZ, NV, HI, Guam, Samoa, Pacific Trust Territories)
71 Stevenson Street, Room 420
San Francisco, CA 94105
(415) 975-4310

**Region X** (AK, ID, OR, WA)
1111 Third Avenue, Suite 715
Seattle, WA 98101-3212
(206) 553-5930

## Other OSHA Offices

**OSHA Training Institute**
OSHA Office of Training and Education
1555 Times Drive
Des Plaines, IL 60018
(708) 297-4810

**Cincinnati Laboratory**
435 Elm Street, Suite 500
Cincinnati, OH 45202
(513) 684-3721

**Salt Lake City Laboratory**
OSHA Analytical Laboratory
PO Box 15200
Salt Lake City, UT 84115
(801) 487-0680

**Health Response Unit**
OSHA Analytical Laboratory
PO Box 15200
Salt Lake City, UT 84115
(801) 487-0521

## NATIONAL INSTITUTE FOR OCCUPATIONAL SAFETY & HEALTH (NIOSH)

NIOSH is the workplace safety and health research agency within the US Department of Health and Human Services and the Centers for Disease Control and Prevention that conducts studies to develop and recommend safety and health standards to OSHA. It does not have legal authority to adopt or enforce regulations. Rather, OSHA determines which of the standards proposed by NIOSH will be adopted and enforced.

Like OSHA, however, NIOSH has the authority to conduct investigations into workplace safety and health problems, to question employers and employees, and even to include the use of warrants to gain information on workplace conditions and to examine workers. Generally, though, NIOSH conducts health hazard surveys with the cooperation of employers and employees. NIOSH also provides services to employers and employees, including telephone consultations and on-site evaluations in many areas of the country.

### NIOSH Offices

**Director's Office**
Room 715H, Humphrey Building
200 Independence Avenue, SW
Washington, DC 20201
(202) 401-6997

### Office of the Deputy Director
Centers for Disease Control and Prevention
1600 Clifton Road, NE
Building 1, Room 3007
Atlanta, GA 30333
(404) 639-3771

### Education and Information Division (EID)
Robert A. Taft Laboratories
Technical Information Branch
4676 Columbia Parkway, MS C14
Cincinnati, OH 45226
(513) 533-8302
FAX (513) 533-8588

### Division of Surveillance, Hazard Evaluations & Field Studies (DSHEFS)
Alice Hamilton Laboratories
4676 Columbia Parkway, MS R12
Cincinnati, OH 45213
(513) 841-4428
FAX (513) 841-4483

### Division of Safety Research (DSR)
1095 Willlowdale Road, MS 1172
Morgantown, WV 26505-2888
(304) 285-5894

## Field Offices
### NIOSH New England Field Office
P.O. Box 87040
South Dartmouth, MA 02748
(508) 997-6126
FAX (617) 565-9860

### CDC/NIOSH Field Office
1600 Clifton Road
Atlanta, GA 30333
(404) 639-4171
FAX (404) 730-9641

### NIOSH Denver Field Office
P.O. Box 25226
Denver, CO 80225-0226
(303) 236-6032
FAX (303) 236-6072

## NIOSH Information Services
NIOSH offers a toll-free technical information service that provides convenient public access to NIOSH and its information resources. The toll-free number is (800) 356-4674. This service combines an automated voice-mail system with direct access to NIOSH technical information staff and the NIOSH Publications Office. The automated system operates 24 hours a day and provides recorded messages on a variety of topics, including NIOSH publications and computerized databases, NIOSH Educational Re-

source Center training programs and grants, Health Hazard Evaluation (HHE) program, and such selected topics as carpal tunnel syndrome, indoor air quality, and homicide in the workplace.

Requesters may speak with a technical information specialist or a publications representative from 9 AM until 4 PM (Eastern Time).

NIOSH information is also available in electronic form through the Internet on the World Wide Web. The NIOSH Home Page, http://www.cdc.gov/niosh/homepage.html, includes recent full-text publications, notices of meetings, conferences, and symposia, as well as technical notices such as respirator information, employment opportunities, database information, NIOSH directory, research fellowship information, and other specialized safety and health topics. Users may also access the e-mail reply system to request NIOSH publications and to post questions and other messages about the National Institute for Occupational Safety and Health.

For a comprehensive list of NIOSH publications (with instructions on purchasing them from the Government Printing Office or the National Technical Information Service), request a copy of the NIOSH Bookshelf. Write or FAX your publication requests to: NIOSH Publications, 4676 Columbia Parkway, MS C13, Cincinnati, OH 45226-1998; FAX (513) 533-8573; e-mail: Pubstaff@cdc.gov

The following is a partial list of free publications currently available from NIOSH:

**Criteria Documents (CD)** are developed to provide the basis for comprehensive occupational safety and health standards. These documents generally contain a critical review of the scientific and technical information available on the prevalence of hazards, the existence of safety and health risks, and the adequacy of control methods. Recommendations for minimizing safety and health risks include medical monitoring, exposure assessment, worker training, control technology, personal protective equipment, and record keeping, as well as recommended exposure levels when appropriate.

**Current Intelligence Bulletins (CIB)** review and evaluate new and emerging information about occupational hazards. They may draw attention to a previously unrecognized hazard, report new data on a known hazard, or disseminate information about hazard control.

**NIOSH Alerts (NA)** briefly present new information about occupational illnesses, injuries, and deaths. Alerts provide urgent assistance in preventing, solving, and controlling newly identified occupational hazards. Workers, employers, and safety and health professionals are asked to take immediate action to reduce risks and implement controls.

**Updates** are brief, nontechnical publications that

are intended to provide information about NIOSH findings and recommend preventive measures. The information is presented in a format that can be easily used by the media and other organizations.

**Miscellaneous Publications (MP)** and **Bibliographies (Bib)** are documents not assigned a publication number. When ordering a miscellaneous publication or a bibliography, be sure to include the full title for positive identification. Some publications are also available in Spanish.

## FOOD & DRUG ADMINISTRATION (FDA)

The FDA is concerned with the safety and health of workers in those industries producing and distributing foods, drugs, cosmetics, medical devices, animal feed, and biological and some electronic products. Inquiries can be made to Food and Drug Administration, National Center for Toxicological Research, 5600 Fishers Lane, Rockville, MD 20857; (301) 443-3170.

## ENVIRONMENTAL PROTECTION AGENCY (EPA)

The EPA was established in 1970 in the executive branch as an independent agency. The EPA endeavors to abate and control pollution systematically, by proper integration of a variety of research, monitoring, standard-setting, and enforcement activities. It coordinates and supports research and antipollution activities by state and local governments, private and public groups, individuals, and educational institutions. The EPA enforces the Toxic Substances Control Act (TSCA), the Federal Insecticide, Fungicide, and Rodenticide Act (FIFRA), and the Noise Control Act (NCA). It is responsible for regulating the quality of air and water and almost all other environmental problems. Through FIFRA, EPA has primary responsibility for regulating the use of pesticides, including the health of agricultural workers, and establishing safe pesticide levels in agricultural products. OSHA has jurisdiction over the manufacturing and formulation of pesticides (see Chapter 32). Through the TSCA, the agency plays a major role in regulating the output of the nation's chemical industry. Thus, it affects the health and safety of workers as well as public health. It also works with other agencies in collecting and disseminating information on hazardous materials. Finally, it has considerable regulatory authority, even to the point of prohibiting the manufacture of materials it considers dangerous to workers or to the public health. Toxicologic reviews are published as health assessment documents and water criteria documents. Inquiries can be made to the Environmental Protection Agency, 401 M Street SW, Washington, DC 20460; (202) 260-2090. For specific contaminants, the following Assistant Administrators may be contacted directly: Water (202) 260-5700, Solid Waste and Emergency Response (202)260-4610, Air and Radiation (202) 260-7400, Prevention, Pesticides, and Toxic Substances (202) 260-2902, Enforcement and Compliance Assurance (202) 260-4134.

Regional Administrators are responsible for the execution of EPA programs, developing and implementing regional programs for integrated environmental protection activities, conducting regional enforcement and compliance programs, and providing technical program direction and evaluation at the regional level.

Information on EPA regulatory programs can be obtained from Toxic Substances Control Act Assistance Office (TAO), EPA (TS-799), Washington, DC 20460. TSCA line: (202) 554-1404. RCRA line: (800) 424-9346.

The EPA's Integrated Risk Information System (IRIS) is available on CD-ROM. The IRIS database is helpful with risk assessment and management decisions. Contact Government Institutes, 4 Research Place, Rockville, MD 20850, (301) 921-2355, FAX (301) 921-0373, E-mail: giinfa@aol.com

EPA Region I is in Boston, Region II in New York, Region III in Philadelphia, Region IV in Atlanta, Region V in Chicago, Region VI in Dallas, Region VII in Kansas City, Region VIII in Denver, Region IX in San Francisco, and Region X in Seattle.

## OTHER RELEVANT GOVERNMENT AGENCIES

**The Department of Transportation (DOT)** enforces the Hazardous Materials Transportation Act (HMTA). DOT also licenses and regulates drivers engaged in interstate commerce. Other agencies with authority in the area of occupational safety and health include the Mine Safety and Health Administration and a variety of state departments of public health as well as other state agencies.

Agencies of interest to those concerned with occupational safety and health are the following:

**Agency for Toxic Substances and Disease Registry (ATSDR)**, Public Health Service, US Department of Health and Human Services, was created under CERCLA (Superfund). Its mission is to prevent exposure and adverse human health effects from exposure to hazardous substances from waste sites, accidental releases, and other sources of pollution.

**Divison of Toxicology** has developed a National Priorities List (NPL) of more than 1300 sites with more than 275 hazardous substances, with fact sheets and toxicologic profiles. It also provides clinically useful environmental health case studies. (404) 639-6300, FAX (404) 639-6315.

**Division of Health Education** provides public health statement notebooks on 80 hazardous substances commonly found at waste sites. It publishes *Hazardous Substances and Public Health* on a quarterly basis and is available for free. (404) 639-6205, FAX (404) 639-6207 or 6208.

> **Agency for Toxic Substances and Disease Registry (ATSDR)**
> 1600 Clifton Road, MS E28, room 3726
> Atlanta, GA 30333
> (404) 639-0700
> FAX (404) 639-0744
> **Bureau of Labor Statistics**
> Department of Labor, Room 3180
> 2 Massachusetts Avenue, NE
> Washington, DC 20212
> (202) 606-6179
> FAX (202) 606-6196
> **Department of Transportation**
> 400 7th Street SW
> Washington, DC 20590
> (202) 366-4000
> **Department of Energy**
> 1000 Independence Avenue SW
> Washington, DC 20585
> (202) 586-5000
> **Mine Safety and Health Administration**
> Department of Labor, Room 601
> 4015 Wilson Boulevard
> Arlington, VA 22203
> (703) 235-1452
> **National Cancer Institute/Cancer Information Service**
> 9000 Rockville Pike
> Bethesda, MD 20892
> (301) 496-5583; (800) 422-6237
> **National Institute of Environmental Health Sciences**
> 111 Alexander Drive
> Research Triangle Park, NC 27709
> (919) 541-3345
> **National Technical Information Services (NTIS)**
> (A central source for sale of federal publications.)
> US Department of Commerce
> 5285 Port Royal Road
> Springfield, VA 22161
> (703) 487-4650 or 4780
> (800) 423-9255

# PRIVATE AGENCIES & ORGANIZATIONS

## American College of Occupational and Environmental Medicine (ACOEM)

ACOEM is the largest organization of member occupational physicians. It sponsors an annual meeting in the spring, the American Occupational Health Conference. Numerous committees research topics of interest to members. For helpful publications, contact the American College of Occupational and Environmental Medicine, 55 West Seegers Road, Arlington Heights, IL 60005; (847) 228-6850. (Membership in the organization provides subscription to the *Journal of Occupational and Environmental Medicine*.)

## American Public Health Association (APHA)

APHA sponsors an Occupational Health and Safety Section that meets annually and receives publications relevant to occupational health. The address is 1015 15th St NW, Suite 300, Washington, DC 20005. (202) 789-5600. (Membership provides subscription to the **American Journal of Public Health.**)

## Association of Occupational & Environmental Clinics (AOEC)

AOEC is a network of academically based occupational/environmental medicine clinics throughout the United States that provide training, community education about toxic substances, exposure and risk assessment, clinical evaluation, and consultation. For patient referral information, contact AOEC at 1010 Vermont Street, Suite 513, Washington, DC, 20005; (202) 347-4976. AOEC sponsors the Occ-Env-MedL Listserver on the Internet (via Duke University). To subscribe, send a single line message that reads: SUBSCRIBE Occ-Env-Med-L "your First then Last Name" to mailserv@duke.edu

## Society for Occupational & Environmental Health (SOEH)

SOEH has a large, multidisciplinary, international membership, including occupational physicians and others interested in occupational and environmental health. The organization sponsors an annual conference in the fall in Washington, DC. For information on meetings and publications, contact the society at 6728 Old McLean Village Drive, McLean, VA 22101; (703) 556-9222, FAX (703) 556-8729. (A full subscription to the *Archives of Environmental Health* is included with membership dues. Membership provides reduced rate subscription to the *American Journal of Industrial Medicine* and *Annual Reviews of Public Health*.)

## International Commission on Occupational Health (ICOH)

ICOH is an international scientific and professional society that aims to foster the scientific progress, knowledge, and development of occupational health and safety. It sponsors triennial World Congresses on Occupational and Environmental Health. ICOH directs the work of 30 scientific committees that share scientific advances internationally. For information on meetings and publications, contact: ICOH Secretariat, Division of Occupational Medicine, National University of Singapore, Lower Kent Ridge Road, Singapore 0511; 65 772-4290; FAX 65 779-1489; e-mail: cofsec@leonis.nus.sg

## International Labor Office (ILO)

ILO is a major source of publications in international occupational and environmental health. They are available from the ILO Publications Center, 49 Sheridan Avenue, Albany, NY 12210; (518) 436-9686; FAX: (518) 436-7433. ILO also provides a variety of information services through CIS, International Occupational Safety and Health Information Centre, ILO-CIS, CH-1211, Geneva 22 Switzerland; Tel. 41 22 799 67 40, Telefax 41 22 798 62 53; e-mail: 100043.2440@compuserve.com

## Other National Organizations & Sources of Information

**American Association of Occupational Health Nurses (AAOHN)** provides training and certification to occupational health nurses. 50 Lenox Pointe, Atlanta, GA 30325; (404) 262-1162.

**American Conference of Governmental Industrial Hygienists (ACGIH)** lists various publications in a Publications Catalog available from ACGIH at 1330 Kemper Meadow Drive, Cincinnati, OH 45240; (513) 742-2020.

**American Industrial Hygiene Association (AIHA)** provides information and communication services pertaining to industrial hygiene. The address is 2700 Prosperity Avenue, Suite 250, Fairfax, VA 22031; (703) 849-8888.

**American Society of Safety Engineers** is the major association of safety professionals in the United States. It publishes a monthly magazine, *Professional Safety,* and sponsors many meetings and training sessions. The address is 1800 E. Oakton Street, Des Plaines, IL 60018-2187; (847) 699-2929.

**National Safety Council** also publishes numerous books and pamphlets and sponsors training programs and an annual conference. The address is 1121 Spring Lake Drive, Itasca, IL 60143; (630) 285-1121.

**Chemical Manufacturer's Association** provides information on the most widely used chemicals. The address is 1300 Wilson Boulevard, Arlington, VA 22209; (703) 741-5000. For nonemergency services, call (800) 262-8200; (202) 463-1596.

**Chemical Transportation Emergency Center (CHEMTREC)** provides information for emergencies involving hazardous materials. (800) 424-9300. Based on information provided by the caller, CHEMTREC relays immediate emergency response information to the incident scene using any of several databases, including over 1 million MSDSs, numerous reference texts, and a network of chemical industry contacts. International callers will need to use (202) 483-7616.

**National Council for Radiation Protection and Measurements (NCRP)** provides information on the common sources of radiation exposure. The address is 7910 Woodmont Avenue, Suite 800, Bethesda, MD 20814; (301) 657-2652.

**National Pesticide Telecommunications Network (NPTN)** provides pesticide product information, information on recognition and management of pesticide poisonings, safety information, health and environmental effects, and cleanup and disposal procedures. The network is located at Oregon State University; (800) 858-7378. A priority number for physicians is (800) 858-7377.

**Teratogen Exposure Registry and Surveillance (TERAS)** maintains information networks for consultation and evaluations concerning the effects of toxic agents on the fetus. Department of Pathology, Brigham and Women's Hospital, 75 Francis Street, Boston, MA 02115, (617) 732-6507.

**Toxicology Information Response Center**, Oak Ridge National Laboratory, provides information about toxic compounds and industrial processes, conducts literature searches, and compiles bibliographies. The Center is located at 1060 Commerce Park, MS 6480, Oak Ridge, TN 37830; (423) 576-1746.

## SOURCES OF INFORMATION ON OCCUPATIONAL HEALTH

Recommended reading is included with each chapter of this book. A recommended library of textbooks and reference materials for physicians practicing in the field of occupational medicine is as follows:

### BOOKS

ACGIH: *Threshold Limit Values for Chemical Substances and Physical Agents in the Work Environment.* American Conference of Governmental Industrial Hygienists, 1997.

Adams RM: *Occupational Skin Disease,* 3rd ed. Saunders, 1998.

Amdur MO, Doull J, Klaasen CD: *Casarett and Doull's Toxicology,* 4th ed. Macmillan, 1991.

Brooks SM, Gochfeld M, Herzstein J, Jackson R, Schenker M: *Environmental Medicine.* Mosby, 1995.

Ellenhorn MJ: Ellenhorn's Medical Toxicology 2nd ed. Williams & Wilkins, 1997.

Harber P, Schenker M, Balmes J: *Occupational and Environmental Respiratory Disease.* Mosby, 1995.

Herington TN, Morse L: Occupational Injuries: *Evaluation, Management, and Prevention.* Mosby, 1995.

Levy BS, Wegman DH: *Occupational Health: Recognizing and Preventing Work-Related Diseases,* 3rd ed. Little, Brown, 1995.

McCunney R: *A Practical Approach to Occupational and Environmental Medicine,* 2nd ed. Little, Brown, 1994.

*NIOSH Registry of Toxic Effects of Chemical Substances.* US Government Printing Office, 1992. (order from Superintendent of Documents, US Government Printing Office, Washington D.C. 20402)

Raffle PA, Adams H, Baxter PJ, Lee WR: *Hunter's Diseases of Occupations,* 8th ed. Little, Brown, 1994.

Rom WN: *Environmental and Occupational Medicine,* 3rd ed. Lippincott-Raven, 1997.

Rosenstock L, Cullen MR: *Textbook of Clinical Occupational and Environmental Medicine.* Saunders, 1994.

Sullivan JB, Krieger GR: *Hazardous Materials Toxicology: Principles of Environmental Health.* Williams & Wilkins,1992.

Zenz C, Dickerson OБ, Horvath EP: *Occupational Medicine,* 3rd ed. Mosby, 1994.

## JOURNALS

*American Industrial Hygiene Association Journal.* AIHA, 2700 Prosperity Avenue, Suite 250, Fairfax, VA 22031. Monthly.

*American Journal of Epidemiology.* The Johns Hopkins University School of Hygiene and Public Health, 111 Market Place, Suite 840, Baltimore, MD 21202-6709. Monthly.

*American Journal of Industrial Medicine.* Wiley-Liss, Inc., 605 Third Avenue, New York, NY 10158-0012. Monthly.

*American Journal of Public Health.* APHA, 1015 Fifteenth Street, NW, Washington, DC 20005. Monthly.

*Archives of Environmental Health.* SOEH, Heldref Publications, 1319 Eighteenth Street, NW, Washington, DC 20036-l802. Bimonthly.

*Environmental Health Perspectives.* NIEHS, Superintendent of Documents, P.O. Box 271954, Pittsburgh, PA 15250-7954. Monthly.

*International Archives of Occupational and Environmental Health.* Springer-Verlag, Heidelberger Platz 3, D-14197 Berlin, Germany. Monthly.

*International Journal of Occupational and Environmental Health.* Hanley & Belfus, Inc., 210 S. 13th Street, Philadelphia, PA 19107. Quarterly.

*Journal of Occupational and Environmental Medicine.* ACOEM, Williams & Wilkins, 351 West Camden Street, Baltimore, MD 21201-2436. Monthly.

*Occupational and Environmental Medicine.* BMJ Publishing Group, BMA House, Tavistock Square, London WC1H 9JR, UK. Monthly.

*Occupational and Environmental Medicine Report.* OEM Health Information Inc., 181 Elliott Street, Suite 814, Beverly, MA 01915. Monthly.

*Occupational Medicine.* Elsevier Science, Ltd., The Boulevard, Langford Lane, Kidlington, Oxford OX5 1GB, UK. Monthly.

*Occupational Medicine: State of the Art Reviews.* Hanley & Belfus, Inc., 210 S. 13th Street, Philadelphia, PA 19107. Quarterly.

*Scandinavian Journal of Work, Environment & Health.* Topeliuksenkatu 41aA, FIN-00250 Helsinki, Finland. Monthly.

*Yearbook of Occupational and Environmental Medicine.* Mosby-Year Book, Inc. 200 N. LaSalle Street, Suite 2500, Chicago, IL 60601. Annual.

## REFERENCES

Mullan RJ, Murthy LI: Occupational sentinel health events: An updated list for physician recognition and public health surveillance. Am J Ind Med 1991;19:775.

Murphy LI, Halperin WE: Medical screening and biological monitoring: A guide to the literature for physicians. J Occup Environ Med 1995;37:170.

Newman LS: Occupational illness. N Engl J Med 1995; 333:1128.

Pope AM, Rall DP (editors): *Environmental Medicine: Integrating a Missing Element into Medical Education.* National Academy Press, 1995.

Schwartz DA et al. The occupational history in the primary care setting. Am J Med 1992;90:315.

# Workers' Compensation

# 3

*Joseph LaDou, MS, MD*

Virtually every country provides some form of entitlements to workers or their survivors to assist them in the event of an occupational injury or illness. Workers' compensation is the form of social insurance broadly accepted in industrially developed countries. Most commonly, workers' compensation is embedded in a country's social security system. In the United States, however, the workers' compensation insurance system has almost no linkages with the social security system. The workers' compensation system in the United States is an increasingly costly burden on individual employers. US employers incur more than $60 billion in direct workers' compensation costs each year, triple the amount spent a decade earlier. Counting other costs—production delays, damage to equipment, and recruiting and training replacement workers—the total cost is about $350 billion.

Workers' compensation laws share many characteristics on an international basis. There are, however, many important differences between the several federal and state systems in the United States. Workers' compensation systems are designed to ensure the injured worker prompt but limited benefits and to assign to the employer sure and predictable liability. Physicians and other health care providers who render care for work-related injuries and illnesses must (1) **understand the requirements** of their state's workers' compensation system and (2) **provide the necessary services** both to treat the condition appropriately and efficiently and to ensure the flow of benefits to the worker.

## WORKERS' COMPENSATION LAW

The financial responsibility of the employer for the injury or death of an employee in the workplace was first established under Bismarck in Germany in 1884. Great Britain followed in 1897 with legislation requiring employers to compensate employees or their survivors for an injury or death regardless of who was at fault. Thus, workers' compensation laws

are the result of a historic compromise in which the employee gave up the right to sue the employer for negligence in exchange for the employer's agreement to pay the cost of medical care and to compensate the worker for time lost from work. By the turn of the century, all European countries had workers' compensation laws. The workers' compensation movement did not begin in the United States until 1908 when a forerunner of the Federal Employees Compensation Act was passed. In 1911, the first states enacted their laws. These initial workers' compensation systems were far from the array of programs that deal with disability income loss, medical care, accident prevention, and vocational rehabilitation that characterize contemporary workers' compensation programs.

One of the major deficiencies in workers' compensation law is that its roots are in the past century at a time when occupational disease was not recognized. The system operates with relative success in the recognition and compensation of work-related injuries. But far less than half of all occupational disease is compensated under workers' compensation systems, and the reporting of occupational diseases by government agencies is also woefully inadequate. Consequently, preventive measures aimed at occupational diseases receive less attention than those directed at the causes of occupational injury.

## Worker Benefits

The objectives of workers' compensation systems are to provide injured employees with an income following an injury and during recovery, to ensure injured workers a competitive position in the employment market, and to avoid lengthy and costly legal action. In the event of death, survivors are compensated for the loss of their income provider. An injured employee is automatically entitled to medical treatment and compensation, whether the incident is the fault of the employee or the employer. The cost of workers' compensation benefits is considered to be a cost of doing business and is passed on to purchasers of the product or service. In the case of governmental workers' compensation systems, the costs are included in the taxes collected by federal, state, and local governments.

To be compensable, an injury usually must "arise out of and in the course of employment (AOE/COE)." A work injury that activates or aggravates a pre-existing condition also is compensable. Recurrence of an earlier compensable injury is compensable as well. Depending on the jurisdiction, judicial action may be necessary to resolve questions of liability for self-inflicted injuries and suicidal acts. Similar determinations may be necessary for injuries occurring under the influence of alcohol or drugs, during entirely personal activity (not AOE/COE), and for fights at work.

Occupational diseases are the direct result of work or exposure to toxic substances in the workplace. Occupational disease claims have proliferated in recent decades. In some states, this resulted from judicial interpretations. In other jurisdictions, the increase is the result of "presumptions" that lead to the automatic acceptance of workers' compensation liability for certain diseases in designated worker groups. An example is the presumption in California law that heart disease in police and fire personnel, and some other uniformed services, is work-related and is covered by workers' compensation. In all areas of the United States, occupational disease claims are increasing as physicians become more familiar with the discipline of occupational medicine and more confident of their diagnoses of occupational diseases and understand the causes of multifactorial diseases.

Many states recognize cumulative injury claims as occupational illnesses when the worker has sustained repeated small physical or psychic injuries that eventually result in a disability. These broadened interpretations of illness and disability open workers' compensation systems to numerous claims of occupational stress. They also bring many new cases of repetitive motion disorders, cardiovascular diseases, hearing loss, and emotional disturbance into the system. Occupational physicians play key roles in many states where their medical opinions are necessary to resolve issues surrounding compensability of such contentious cases as myocardial infarction and cerebrovascular accident, occupational and environmental exposure to toxic materials, and the occurrence of birth defects and other reproductive and developmental problems. Many physicians devote their practices to such forensic activities.

Benefits to workers or their families are of several types: (1) permanent total disability, (2) temporary total disability, (3) permanent partial disability, (4) temporary partial disability, (5) survivors' benefits, and (6) vocational rehabilitation benefits.

**A. Permanent Total Disability:** Permanent total disability covers those workers who are so disabled that they will never be able to work again in an open labor market and for whom further treatment offers no hope of recovery. Most states compensate such individuals with two-thirds of their average wages subject to minimum and maximum limits. Since benefits are not taxed, this can amount to about 85–90% of take-home wages. States may also provide additional funds for dependents. Although some states limit the duration of payments, others provide compensation for the remainder of the injured worker's life.

**B. Temporary Total Disability:** The majority of injured workers fall under the temporary total disability classification—that is, the worker is expected to recover with treatment but is unable to work for a time. Benefits are paid during the recovery period on the basis of the worker's average earnings. Minimum and a maximum limits apply and benefits of as much as two-thirds of gross or 80% of take-home wages are paid until the individual is able to return to work or reaches maximum recovery. There is a waiting period for this type of compensation, but it is paid retroactively if the worker cannot work for a certain number of days or if hospitalization is necessary. The waiting period serves as an incentive to return to work after less serious injuries. Thus, it is like a deductible provision in other forms of health insurance.

**C. Permanent Partial Disability:** Permanent partial disability occurs when an injured worker is disabled to the point that he or she has lost some ability to compete in the labor market. In some jurisdictions, benefits compensate the injured worker for losses in future earnings and are divided into two categories: (1) scheduled injuries (eg, loss of a limb, an eye, or hearing) and (2) nonscheduled injuries (eg, back injury, tenosynovitis). The first is paid according to a schedule fixed by statute. Under this category, benefits are paid whether or not the individual is working. Payment is usually provided for a specified number of weeks, the length of which depends on which part of the body is damaged. Benefits are based on a percentage of earnings at the time of injury and again are subject to a minimum and a maximum amount. Nonscheduled injuries receive weekly benefit payments based on a wage-loss replacement percentage. The percentage is derived from the difference between wages earned before and after injury. In some states, however, nonscheduled permanent partial disabilities are compensated as a percentage of the total disability benefits.

**D. Temporary Partial Disability:** Temporary partial disability occurs when a worker is injured to the degree that he or she cannot perform his or her usual work but is still capable of working at some job during convalescence. Modified duty is viewed by many insurers and employers as a critical element of the treatment plan and rehabilitation of these injured workers. Under this category, the injured worker is compensated for the difference between wages earned before the injury and wages earned during the period of temporary partial disability, usually at two-thirds of the difference. Modified duty may save the worker from wage differentials by stopping the temporary partial disability payment.

**E. Survivors' Benefits:** Dependent survivors of employees killed on the job are paid death benefits under workers' compensation. The method and size of payments vary widely among the various states, but all systems provide for a death benefit and some reimbursement for burial expenses.

**F. Vocational Rehabilitation Benefits:** Some level of rehabilitation is provided in all states even if unspecified by statute. Vocational and psychological counseling or retraining and job placement assistance are typical benefits. The goal is returning the injured worker to suitable, gainful employment.

## Benefits From Other Sources

A number of benefits are available to workers from other sources.

**A. Social Security Disability Insurance (SSDI):** Social Security supplements workers' compensation with monthly benefits for disability. Such benefits are available only after a 5-month waiting period and are calculated as if the disabled individual had reached Social Security retirement age. To be considered disabled, the injured person must be unable to work in substantial gainful employment. Furthermore, the disability must be expected to last more than 1 year or to result in premature death. Social Security Disability combined with workers' compensation cannot exceed 80% of the worker's average earnings or the total family benefit under Social Security before the injury. If this is the case, Social Security benefits are reduced accordingly, although some states will reduce workers' compensation benefits by all or part of the Social Security payments.

**B. Second Injury Funds:** Second injury funds compensate workers for injuries that are exacerbated by a subsequent injury. Some states' second injury funds compensate workers for flare-ups that do not necessarily lead to total disability. These funds are established and maintained by most states in the hope that the outcome will encourage employers to hire the handicapped or previously injured workers. Payments are made for the second injury by the employer's compensation carrier, and the fund reimburses the carrier for the additional costs.

## Employers' Responsibilities

Employers are responsible for providing medical treatment and compensation benefits for employees injured at work or made ill from exposure to the workplace environment. The system is based on a premise of liability without fault—that is, regardless of whether the worker, the employer, or neither is at fault, the employer is still responsible for providing medical treatment and compensation benefits to the injured employee.

Workers' compensation insurance coverage is compulsory for most private employment except in New Jersey, South Carolina, and Texas. In those states, employers may decline coverage, but, in turn, they lose the customary common-law defenses against suits filed by employees (the "exclusive remedy" is the quid pro quo under which the employer enjoys immunity from being sued in exchange for accepting absolute liability for all work-connected injuries). Employees most likely to be exempt from coverage include domestic workers, agricultural workers, and casual laborers. Coverage may also be limited for workers in small companies with only a few employees (this number varies by state), nonprofit institutions, and state and local governments. About 87% of all wage and salary workers are covered by workers' compensation laws.

**A. Demonstration of Ability to Pay Benefits:** Unless exempted by the law, employers must demonstrate their ability to pay workers' compensation benefits. There are three ways of accomplishing this: (1) insurance with a state fund, (2) insurance through a private carrier, or (3) self-insurance.

**1. State insurance funds**–The states have adopted two methods of meeting the problem of workers' compensation coverage. Some states require that employers insure through a state fund that operates as the exclusive provider of insurance. Other states operate their funds in competition with private carriers. A few states do not permit an employer to be self-insured.

**2. Private insurance carriers**–Private workers' compensation insurance contracts have two purposes: (1) to satisfy the employer's obligation to pay compensation and (2) to ensure that the injured employee receives all the benefits provided by law. Once the contract is signed, the insurer is responsible for compensating the injured worker. The carrier's liability is not relieved by either the insolvency or death of the employer or any disagreement the carrier may have with the employer. Most state funds are similarly restricted.

**3. Self-insurance**–Large employers may decide to serve as their own insurers. This approach includes the responsibility for adjusting claims and paying benefits, although it is possible to contract these tasks out to companies that provide such services. To qualify as a self-insurer, a company must demonstrate that it has the financial ability to pay all claims that may reasonably be expected. The state agency may require that a bond or other security be posted. Since this form of insurance is both time-consuming and requires financial reserves, smaller companies can seldom self-insure.

Companies choose to self fund to reduce costs and to maximize cash flows. Since costs of benefits, claim reserves, litigation, and attendant administrative costs have spiraled in recent years, many companies have concluded that they could do as well as independent carriers while saving the cost of commissions and premium taxes, and take advantage of greater cash flow and increased investment income rates. Self-insured employers are more likely to contest injury and illness claims than are privately insured employers and state insurance funds. This tendency to litigate may erase some of the cost savings that are realized by self-insurance.

**B. Penalties for Not Having Insurance:** Employers often failed to provide workers' compensation insurance coverage for their employees. The cost of even one serious injury can deplete a company's entire annual income or even bankrupt it. Consequently, all but three states have made workers' compensation insurance mandatory. Otherwise, a company could be out of business even before a seriously injured employee is fully recovered.

There are heavy penalties for uninsured employers. They can be subject to fines, loss of common-law defenses, increases in the amount of benefits awarded, and payment of attorneys' fees. The biggest financial deterrent is suit at common law. A number of states will force closure of an uninsured business. All states have established uninsured employer's funds to which the injured employee can apply for benefits. Applying to such a fund does not preclude the individual from also bringing action against the employer for penalties and legal fees. The uninsured employer may also be required to reimburse the fund for benefits paid the injured worker.

## Insurance Costs
## & Claims Expenses

The cost of workers' compensation insurance is rate adjusted for all but the smallest employers—a process known as experience rating. When fewer injuries and illnesses occur, the employer profits from lowered workers' compensation insurance costs. Experience modification provides an automatic financial incentive for employers to provide their employees a work environment free from the hazards that may result in compensation claims. The results of economic studies on the value of experience rating are conflicting, and there are numerous problems in the interpretation of available data. Nonetheless, it is a hallowed provision of workers' compensation systems. Most large employers are experience rated, whereas small employers are typically insured in groups of similar companies. As the definitions of compensable injury are broadened, the intent and the benefits of experience rating are diluted.

About three-fourths of all compensable claims for workers' compensation benefits and one-fourth of all cash payment benefits involve temporary total disability. Permanent total disability occurs in less than 1% of all compensable workers' compensation claims. Benefits paid in cash compensation are nearly equaled by medical and hospitalization benefits.

State and federal funds and self-insured employers

each pay about one-fifth of all regular benefits, while private insurance companies pay the remaining three-fifths. The total costs to employers include the expenses of policy writing, claims investigation and adjustment, allocation to reserves to match increases in accrued liabilities, payroll auditing, commissions, premium taxes, and other administrative expenses and profit.

Employers are required to provide medical treatment as well as compensation benefits. The injured or ill employee is required to report the injury or illness as soon as possible. There is typically a statute of limitation that limits the employer's liability when an injury or illness is not promptly reported. It is considered that the requirement has been met if the employer is informed by someone other than the injured individual. The employer must then provide all medical care reasonably required to alleviate the problem. In fact, the law allows for treatment even when recovery is not possible—that is, palliative care that does not cure but only relieves.

In most states, there are no statutory limitations on the length of time or the cost of treatment although a number of cost containment strategies are being implemented by states and private insurers. These include (1) utilization review of inpatient and outpatient care, (2) hospital bill auditing of inpatient services, (3) medical bill auditing of practitioner and other services, and (4) preferred provider networks for inpatient care (where fees are discounted) and outpatient care (where the emphasis is on optimization of outcome measures). Some jurisdictions are considering the disallowance of services provided by physicians who own facilities where patients are referred for testing or treatment.

## THE ROLE OF THE OCCUPATIONAL
## HEALTH PROFESSIONAL

Health professionals are involved in many of the required activities of workers' compensation systems since medical treatment involves the services of physicians and nurses and, frequently, that of physical therapists. Hospitalization, medicines, prosthetic appliances, and surgical supplies are all paid for by workers' compensation. Many states also allow treatment by licensed psychologists, dentists, optometrists, podiatrists, osteopaths, and chiropractors. Some states even permit treatment by acupuncturists, naturopaths, and Christian Science practitioners.

Workers in many states are permitted by state workers' compensation regulations to choose their own physicians. The choice may be any licensed physician or may be made from a list maintained by the employer or the state workers' compensation agency. Regardless of how the physician is chosen, the worker must submit to periodic examinations by a physician of the employer's choice. If either the employer or the worker is dissatisfied with the progress under the chosen physician's treatment, he or she can request and often be allowed to change physicians. Typically, an employee is permitted one such change for subjective reasons alone. In contrast, the employer can be required to prove to the state agency that a change is needed. Reasons for discharging a physician include incompetence, lack of reasonable progress toward recovery, inadequate or insufficient reporting by the physician, and inconvenience of the physician's practice location. If the employer selects the physician, an employee who is not satisfied with the treatment and progress may be permitted consultation with another physician at the employer's expense.

Although the employer must provide medical treatment for the injured employee, if the employee refuses reasonable treatment or surgery without justifiable cause, the employer is relieved of responsibility for any benefits related to injuries caused by the delay in or refusal of any treatment. When the suggested treatment or surgery entails a significant risk, the worker's refusal is usually considered justified.

When a compensation case results in litigation, occupational health professionals become important witnesses in settling disputes.

## Claims Disputes

Differences of opinion often arise over workers' compensation claims. Such disputes often result from issues of insurance coverage, work-relatedness of the injury or illness, provision of medical treatment, the worker's earnings capacity, and the extent of the disability. The last is the most common cause of disputes, which require the physician to provide expert medical opinion. Although the system was designed to be "no fault," a large number of claims are subject to disputes among the employer, the insurance carrier, and the worker. Because adjudication is cumbersome, costly, and time-consuming, tribunals have been established to hear claims disputes in the minimum time possible and at the least cost.

In most states, the initiation of a claim is by the worker, and the initial review is by the insurer. When there is a disagreement on the result, either party can apply for a hearing before the workers' compensation agency or court. If there is still dissatisfaction with the hearing officer's decision, an appeal can be made.

The states vary widely in their methods of hearing disputes, but the most commonly used methods are (1) a court-administered system, (2) a wholly administrative system, and (3) a combination of the two. The last is rapidly becoming almost as unwieldy as the common-law approach that it was designed to replace.

**A. The Court-Administered System:** The court-administered system is closest to common-law procedure and is based on the hypothesis that the parties of a dispute are more likely to receive justice from a court than from a referee or commission.

In this type of system, the employer may be covered either by a carrier or by self-insurance. All injuries or illnesses resulting in more than 6 days of disability must be reported within 14 days, usually accompanied by a physician's report. (Time periods, exact procedures, fee percentages, and so on are drawn from one state for the purposes of example.) The state Department of Labor, through its workers' compensation division, decides whether or not the worker should receive compensation other than medical treatment. A form letter is then sent to the worker informing him or her of rights in case additional benefits are decided upon. Unless there is a complaint, the compensation agency takes no further action to ensure prompt payment, but the carrier must file notice when the claim is first paid. The system also requires that a settlement agreement be filed even if the worker refuses to sign it. A trial court reviews that agreement to determine whether the worker is receiving his or her just benefits. If so, the agreement is approved and payments are made accordingly.

The employer has 10 days thereafter to file with the division certified copies of all relevant documents from the worker's file. If the division decides that the agreement does not provide sufficient benefits to the worker, the insurance carrier is required to adjust the agreement and have the court order modified. If the carrier refuses, the division advises the worker to take court action. Once a settlement has been approved by the court, it is binding on all parties if not contested within 30 days. However, the worker may go to trial court to contest the settlement at any time within 1 year of the injury. Compensation cases receive priority and are usually completed within 10 weeks. The case is heard by a trial judge and may be appealed to a circuit court and even to the state supreme court if the judge's finding is unacceptable to the worker. The attorney may receive 20% of the award for his or her services.

**B. The Wholly Administrative System:** Under a wholly administrative system, the workers' compensation board reviews claims made against covered employers. Injuries must be reported as soon as possible, and benefits or the denial of benefits is determined by a claims adjudicator of a board located closest to the worker's home (again, using one state's system as an example). If the claim is denied, the worker is informed of the reason for denial and how to appeal. Either the government, without charge, or the worker's union assists in the appeal. Judgments can be appealed, in turn, to a board of review in all cases except those related to a rehabilitation decision.

The review boards are part of the Department of Labor but are totally disassociated from the workers' compensation division. They consist of a chairman and two members, one chosen by an employers' group and the other by an organization of workers in this state's example.

The claimant must make an appeal within 90 days after the claims adjudicator's report has been received. The appeal may be in the form of a letter stating the claimant's objections, or it may be submitted on a two-page form used for that purpose. The review board studies the workers' compensation board file and any new information the board obtains in the course of its decision-making. There is no hearing on the matter unless the claimant requests it, and such a request will be denied if the board decides that an appeal is not justified. If the board agrees to a hearing, it is held at a location most convenient for the worker. The worker may have an attorney, but the appeals process does not include payment of the attorney's fees, that being the responsibility of the worker.

Although the decision of the review board is usually binding, it can be appealed further to the commissioners of the workers' compensation board within 60 days by a labor union on behalf of the injured worker or by an organization of employers on behalf of the injured worker or employer. If the chairman of the review board believes that an important principle underlies the appeal, he or she may allow the worker to make an appeal within 30 days. Furthermore, if the decision of the review board is not unanimous, the worker is permitted to appeal to the commissioners on his or her own behalf within 60 days. The decision of the commissioners is binding and may not be appealed to the courts.

A medical review panel exists for *medical issues only*. This panel consist of a chairman appointed by the government and two physicians, one selected by the worker and one by the employer. Decisions by this panel are final. Many states sponsor less formal panels of physicians who interview and examine the claimant, then render opinion on disability, work restrictions, treatment, and prognosis.

**C. The Combination System:** The workers' compensation agency under the combination system consists of a seven-member appeals board that is responsible only for reviewing appeals and an administrative director who is responsible for the administrative functions of the agency. In California, for example, eight individuals are appointed by the governor and confirmed by the state senate.

First reports of worker injury or illness must be filed with the state Division of Labor Statistics and Research by both the employer and the attending physician. They are usually submitted through the employer's compensation carrier or adjusting agent and constitute the initiation of a claim. Furthermore, within 5 days of the injury, the employer must inform the injured worker in simple terms not only about the benefits he or she is entitled to but also about the services available from the state Division of Workers' Compensation. The employer is further required to inform the compensation system administrator, as well as the worker, concerning commencement and termination dates of benefits, nonpayment of benefits, or rejection of claims. The worker must also be informed that he or she can obtain an attorney, if desired. The worker must further be advised that any action must be taken promptly to avoid loss of compensation.

Thus, the worker is informed of his or her rights, and since there are penalties for the unwarranted rejection of compensation, most claims are paid automatically. The Division of Workers' Compensation becomes involved only if either the employer or the employee seeks adjudication from the workers' compensation appeals board. Such adjudication is initiated by the filing of a simple one-page form. The application must be filed within 1 year of the injury or by the date of the termination of benefits, whichever is longer. If the adjudication claim is related to further trauma resulting from the original injury, the application requirement is 5 years from the date of the original injury.

Although the system anticipates that a hearing will be held within 30 days after the application, that is seldom possible because of backlog. The hearings are conducted at several locations throughout the state and are assigned to a workers' compensation judge who makes the decision. Usually, each judge reviews about 90 cases per month.

The hearings are designed to be informal, but often they cannot be distinguished from a nonjury court trial. The judges are knowledgeable in the workers' compensation process and are required to develop additional information if the evidence provided by the parties is inadequate. Medical information is usually presented in written reports. Once all the evidence is presented, the judge must present a written decision within 30 days.

If the employer or the employee is unhappy with the decision, he or she may file an appeal. This appeal is called a petition for reconsideration and must be filed within 20 days of the posting of the original decision. It is heard by a panel of three members of the appeals board. The panel is authorized to approve or deny reconsideration, issue a different decision on the original evidence, or seek additional information, including consultation with an independent medical specialist.

The decision of this panel is final unless the dissatisfied party seeks a review by an appellate court within 45 days by submitting a petition for a writ of review to the appeals court. The court is empowered to deny the review without explanation. If a review is permitted, the appeals court studies the evidence, hears oral arguments, and presents a written decision. If the party bringing the appeal is still dissatisfied, he or she may petition the state supreme court for a further hearing. However, the supreme court will rarely accept more than a few workers' compensation cases each year.

In the most contested cases, both parties are represented either by attorneys or by expert lay representatives. On average, those representing the worker receive 9–15% of the award.

## Reopening of Claims

Workers' compensation proceedings differ from civil law suits in one important aspect—the body that originally decided the award may alter its decision if the worker's condition changes or there is other reasonable cause. This process may be limited under certain conditions by state compensation laws, and most states establish a time limit beyond which a modification cannot be made. If the requirements of the law cannot be met, final decisions in compensating cases are as binding as those in any judicial proceeding.

There is a wide divergence among states as to benefit amounts, conditions that are compensable, processing of claims, settlement of disputes, and general economics of each system. Consequently, physicians who expect to be treating patients with occupational injuries and illnesses are well advised to learn how the workers' compensation system operates in the state in which they are practicing.

## LEGISLATIVE REFORM

Many health policy experts consider the separate workers' compensation insurance system to be one of the more serious dysfunctional elements of the US health care system. In the current climate of health care reform, the goal of almost all legislative proposals is to extend health care coverage to all citizens. In addition, there are "single-payer" legislative approaches that include medical coverage for occupational injuries and illnesses in their national health insurance schemes. The "24-hour medical coverage" proposal defines an insurance system that combines the health care benefits under workers' compensation and group health insurance through coordinated claims management or through the development of a comprehensive insurance package.

By integrating public and private health insurance plans to cover medical expenses for occupational injuries and illnesses, worker access to care will be enhanced and administrative costs will be decreased. This approach may circumvent the cost shifting that complicates "twenty-four-hour medical coverage" as patients find the benefits more attractive with workers' compensation coverage than those provided by group health insurance. Cost shifting occurs when health care providers (1) bill a nonworkers' compensation payer for the care of an occupational injury or illness because they wish to receive a payment rate higher than workers' compensation payers provide, or (2) bill workers' compensation when the patient does not have group health insurance or participates in a managed care health plan that pays the physician less than workers' compensation rates.

Regardless of which reform proposal is enacted, the workers' compensation insurance system will still need to be maintained to provide nonmedical benefits. Medical costs reflected in rate modification will no longer provide the employer with an incentive to provide health and safety in the workplace. This loss would require some new form of cost incentive for employers. Expanded payments of scheduled injury benefits that reflect the employer's injury and illness experience has been advanced as an alternative. Employer disability insurance is another concept being discussed.

Because there is an increasing number of uninsured workers in the United States, these legislative proposals are likely to increase the costs of health insurance. Cost increases may be mitigated to some extent by savings resulting from increased efficiency and lowered administrative costs. But the same powerful forces that seek to continue the current US health care system will be at work to maintain the workers' compensation insurance system with as few fundamental changes as is politically possible.

## REFERENCES

Barth PS: Compensating workers for occupational disease: an international perspective. Int J Occup Environ Health 1995;1:147.

Greenwood J, Taricco A (editors): *Workers' Compensation Health Care Cost Containment.* LRP Publications, 1992.

Larson A: *The Law of Workmen's Compensation.* Matthew Bender, 1982.

National Council on Compensation Insurance. *Issues Report, 1996.* NCCI, 1996.

Nelson WJ: Workers' compensation: coverage, benefits, and costs, 1989, Social Security Bulletin 55(1):51-56, Spring 1992.

*Occupational Injuries and Illnesses in the United States by Industry,* 1995. Bureau of Labor Statistics, US Department of Labor, 1996.

Social Security Administration: Social Security Programs throughout the World–1993. SSA Publication 13-11805, Research Report #63, Washington, DC: Government Printing Office, 1994.

US Chamber of Commerce: *Analysis of Workers' Compensation Laws–1996 Edition,* US Chamber of Commerce, 1996.

US Department of Labor: *State Workers' Compensation Laws.* US Department of Labor, Employment Standards Administration, Office of Workers' Compensation Programs, Branch of Workers' Compensation Studies, January 1996.

# 4

# Disability Evaluation

*Joseph LaDou, MD*

## IMPAIRMENT & DISABILITY

Medical judgment is necessary to the proper settlement of workers' compensation cases. The physician evaluates the degree of "impairment" (measured by anatomic or functional loss) and supplies an opinion to disability raters, workers' compensation judges, commissioners, or hearing officers. These nonmedical people make the decision as to "disability." Disability, unlike impairment, depends on the job and one's ability to compete in the open job market. Impairment does not necessarily imply disability. For example, the loss of the distal phalanx of the second digit on the left hand results in the same impairment rating in a concert violinist and a roofer, but the disability would be much greater for the musician. It is important to discuss impairment and disability separately. An individual with carpal tunnel syndrome may be disabled when considered for a job with repetitive hand movements, but not for a job that does not require extensive use of the hands.

Insurers frequently ask the physician to determine work restrictions (eg, no overhead lifting for someone with shoulder problems, no working around moving machinery or at unprotected heights for someone with a balance problem, etc) in order to match the impairment to specific jobs. In some instances, the exact physical restrictions are best determined by a functional capacity evaluation. There are growing numbers of specialized centers that can assist physicians with both detailed job analyses and functional capacity evaluations. These evaluations range from very sophisticated computerized measurements to very unsophisticated tests not requiring any special training to conduct. The insurer may authorize referral to such centers before your evaluation of the employee.

When an impairment evaluation is requested, the examining physician should utilize the most current *AMA Guides to the Evaluation of Permanent Impairment* or the guides utilized in the physician's jurisdiction. Standards for disability evaluation can be found in the *AMA Guides* and in schedules provided by the Social Security Administration, the Veterans Administration, and some states. Physicians who perform impairment evaluations should make sure that they know which schedule is applicable in each case. Many states will send medical examiners their recommended guidelines for general medical and psychiatric assessments.

Handicap, under the Americans with Disabilities Act (ADA) definition, is "a physical or mental impairment that substantially limits one or more of the major life activities of such individual," but also includes the individual who "has a record of such an impairment or is regarded as having such an impairment." Therefore, an individual who has an abnormality on a preplacement lumbosacral spine film and has been excluded from heavy lifting jobs because of the radiographic finding could be considered handicapped even though he or she has no symptoms or prior back problems and would have neither an impairment rating nor a disability.

Addressing the issue of employability is complex but not usually part of a medical disability evaluation. Does the medical condition preclude traveling to and from work, being at work, or performing required essential functions of the job? Motivation is a factor in determining return to work status, but not for the purpose of determining employability.

## WRITTEN REPORT

Physicians who are experienced with submission of current status and progress reports to employers and insurance companies can expand their experience to include disability evaluations. All physicians who treat injured workers should develop the experience and confidence to undertake impairment and disability evaluations. The physician who has been asked to do a disability evaluation should understand exactly what the requesting party wants to know and obtain and completely review copies of all relevant medical records, reports, and test results. In a workers' compensation case, the patient will probably see reports written by the physician. All details should be presented in unambiguous terms and in appropriate detail. Use of abbreviations and other time-savers are not appropriate in this form of medical record. Be sure to explain technical terms for the benefit of non-medical readers.

## History

The history of the injury or exposure to toxic materials at work should be detailed, and there should be a complete and careful description of the activities of the job. All historical information should be obtained by the physician and not by office personnel. The history should also include information about all previous employment and all nonwork activities, with particular attention to factors that might have some relation to the present complaints. An example occurs in claims of toxic exposure in which the claimant has a cognitive deficit corroborated by neuropsychologic testing. In these cases, individuals may have had preexisting problems secondary to head injuries, hypoxia at birth, etc, and it may be necessary to review school records as well as previous medical history.

**History of Present Illness or Injury:** The history of the illness or injury should include a review of all preexisting conditions. The injured employee's complaints and symptoms should be listed. Many examiners quote these verbatim, without comment, to capture the flavor of the words and avoid misinterpretation. Be precise about temporal relationships between work and the injury or between exposures and the illness.

**Occupational History:** In obtaining the occupational history, physicians may need to have information in addition to that contained in the medical file. This may be requested from the workers' compensation judge or the appropriate governmental agency, eg, the Division of Industrial Accidents in the state. Additional medical reports and other evidence can often be obtained. The physician may need to talk with the claimant's family and with coworkers and friends. Be aware of the legal implications of telephone calls to or from supervisors or company management. Allegations of collusion between management and occupational physicians are not infrequent in workers' compensation actions.

The history should be as complete as necessary, yet as brief as possible. In the "Occupational History," summarize all jobs and note any work-related illnesses and injuries chronologically. Discuss required activities in the last job, including hours worked, shift work or other assignments that might have caused excessive fatigue or a circadian desynchronosis, changes in work routine that might interfere with safety and hygiene practices, and chemical and other toxic exposures in great detail. If industrial hygiene measurements are available to determine dose of exposure, these are vital to the evaluation of the health risk to the employee.

It is important to mention any preexisting condition that limited the ability to work or to compete in the job market, including work limitations or preclusions imposed by a physician. In the case of an injured employee reporting a back injury, for example, determine exactly what the person has done throughout his career that might affect his back. The job title is less useful information than a detailed description of the work activity and its duration. In a hearing loss case, a description of the work environment from an auditory standpoint might be needed to support an opinion that the disability was probably the result of the claimed injury. Some toxic agents have long latent periods, and it may be necessary to go back 25 or 30 years in taking the history. Formal job descriptions are often available and can be very useful in documenting the occupational history.

**Past Medical History:** Describe other coworkers involved in both injuries and illnesses. The "Past Medical History" should include relevant previous as well as concurrent conditions or complaints if there are no physical findings. List medications taken for these conditions. The "Social and Family History" should always include information on use of alcohol, recreational drugs, cigarettes, and family history of similar or related problems when relevant. Obtain data on workers' compensation claims and settlements. In some instances, historical data on major medical insurance utilization may be relevant as well. In the "Review of Systems," list pertinent positives and negatives without resorting to long lists.

Differences between the histories obtained by various physicians should be noted and explained. List and summarize the reports you reviewed to document having read them. The total time spent with the patient should be stated.

## Physical Examination

When examining patients with musculoskeletal problems, the physical examination requires precise, objective measurements of joint motion and any other objective signs of impairment. The ultimate rating of disability will reflect the findings more exactly if nonmedical raters are presented with terms that are readily understandable. If the uninjured limb to which the injured limb is being compared is itself not normal, use an estimated "range of normal" value. These can be found in the diagrams in the *AMA Guides*.

In some cases, the injured worker may not be making a maximal effort with, for example, a grip strength measurement. You should note that the "worker appears not to be putting in a maximal effort." Explain the reasons for the apparent lack of maximal effort if you can. Report the loss of grip strength, eg pain, limited joint motion, nerve injury, lack of maximal effort. Then, record an estimate of the disability percentage for each different factor. The *AMA Guides* contain specific tables for this purpose.

## Conclusions

Draw no medical conclusions that are not reasonably supported by your medical record. Your conclusions should include the following:

**A. Diagnoses:** Differential diagnosis should not be included in the report. References, unless they are critical to your conclusions, should not be cited. When stating the diagnosis, the opinions should be logically and adequately conveyed.

**B. Causation:** Is there a causal relationship between the condition(s) found and the claimed injury or occupational exposure? In this and in other answers give reasons for the opinion, and be as definite as possible. "Possibly" or "maybe" are not helpful terms. "Probably" or "more likely than not" is appropriate phrasing if it applies. In determining causation in workers' compensation, if the condition found would not now exist *but for* the occupational injury or exposure—even though there may have been other contributing nonoccupational causes—the occupational injury or exposure will be considered to be the cause of the condition. Nonetheless, do not attempt to make legal determinations. Do not say, "Impairment is due to an industrial injury." Say, "Impairment is more likely than not the result of the injury described that occurred on January 10, 1993."

**C. Disability:** During what periods of time was the injured employee unable to work as a result of the medical conditions you have found? Temporary disability requires careful attention to questions of when and how long.

Is the condition(s) "permanent and stationary" and on what date did it become so? A practical working definition of permanent and stationary is that "the condition is not going to get significantly better or worse with further medical treatment." In some states, a person has reached "permanent and stationary" or "maximum medical improvement" if symptoms have been stable for 6 months and additional therapy will not significantly change the impairment rating. If the worker is not permanent and stationary, when will the condition become so? What medical treatment(s) and anticipated benefits are recommended?

Has the injury resulted in permanent disability? "Disability" in this context means anything that causes decreased potential earning capacity, decreased function of a limb, eye, etc, or may result in a competitive handicap in the open labor market. "Impairment" may include subjective factors such as pain that limits the ability to work, or objective factors such as limitation of joint motion, or both. "Disability" may include work preclusion as well. Psychiatric factors must also be considered.

Summarize the factors of impairment, listing subjective symptoms and objective losses and limitations. In California, disabling symptoms such as pain should be referred to as "minimal," "slight," "moderate," or "severe," which are defined as follows:

- **Minimal pain** constitutes an annoyance, but causes no handicap in the performance of the particular employment activity.
- **Slight pain** can be tolerated but would cause some handicap in the performance of the employment activity bringing about the pain.
- **Moderate pain** can be tolerated but would cause marked handicap in the performance of the employment activity precipitating the pain.
- **Severe pain** would preclude the employment activity precipitating the pain.

Some other words often have special meaning. In California, "occasional" means 25% of the time, "intermittent" means 50% of the time, "frequent" means 75% of the time, and "constant" means 100% of the time.

In giving an opinion, do not use the words "guess" or "speculate." Instead, say "Based on my experience, my opinion is . . ." The physician is the medical expert.

Work restrictions should be stated in exact terms. If the injured employee *should not* do certain things at work, this should be reported in the same way as if he or she *cannot*.

**D. Apportionment:** Some jurisdictions request the physician to determine apportionment. Apportionment is a legal device for distributing financial responsibility. It is intended to assure that employers are only responsible for those injuries or illnesses caused in their workplace. Apportionment applies only to permanent disability. The examining physician does not apportion causation, disease, or pathology. The person being examined may have disability other than that resulting from the work injury. There may be disability resulting from congenital defects, from previous work- or nonwork-related injuries, from aging, from subsequent injuries, or from the natural progression of preexisting disease.

There is a relatively simple way for physicians to address apportionment that avoids legal complications. The physician should write two paragraphs, the first describing the existing disability factors (objective and subjective) and work restrictions and the second describing the disability factors and work restrictions that would exist in the absence of the occupational injury. The hearing officer can then decide the extent of the disability represented by each of the two paragraphs and, by subtraction, can decide the disability each employer is responsible for. Do not attempt to figure out the percentage of impairment that is represented by either of the paragraphs. The hearing officer and trained raters will do this.

**E. Medical Treatment:** Further medical treatment is an important consideration. Many workers' compensation cases are settled with "continuing medical treatment" provided either within limits or as a lifelong benefit. The opinion as to the value of continued medical treatment and for what purpose it is to be rendered should be stated, along with recommendations for current treatment should it be different from treatment already given the employee by other physicians.

**F.   Vocational Rehabilitation:** Vocational rehabilitation may be recommended for employees who cannot return to their former job. Unless experienced in vocational rehabilitation, physician comments on this subject should be limited to identifying the possible need for rehabilitation services for the worker. It should be left to vocational rehabilitation specialists to determine whether the worker will benefit from such services. If conclusions about the extent of disability have been stated clearly, experts on the physical requirements of various occupations will be able to make an appropriate decision regarding rehabilitation.

## REFERENCES

American Medical Association: *AMA Guides to the Evaluation of Permanent Impairment*, 4th ed. revised. American Medical Association, 1993.

Anderson GBJ: Impairment evaluation issues and the disability system. In: Mayer TG, Mooney V, Gatchel RJ (editors): *Contemporary Conservative Care for Painful Spinal Disorders*. Lea & Febiger, 1991.

Aylward M, Locascio JJ: Problems in the assessment of psychosomatic conditions in Social Security benefits and related commercial schemes. J Psychosom Res 1995;39(6):755.

Babitsky S, Sewall HD: Understanding the AMA guides. In: *Workers' Compensation*. Wiley Law Publications, 1992.

Balsam A: Evaluation of disability under workers' compensation. In: Balsam A and AP Zabin: *Disability Handbook*. Shepard's/McGraw-Hill, 1990.

Frymoyer JW, Haldeman S, Andersson GBJ: Impairment rating—the United States perspective. Chapter 16 in: Pope MH et al: *Occupational Low Back Pain: Assessment, Treatment and Prevention*. Mosby, 1991.

Smith GL: *How to Write a Winning Workers' Compensation Report*. OEM Press, 1995.

Turk DC, Melzack R: *Handbook of Pain Assessment*. Guilford Press, 1992.

Vasudevan SV: Impairment, disability, and functional capacity assessment. In: Turk DC, Melzack R: *Handbook of Pain Assessment*. Guilford Press, 1992.

Waddell G, et al: Objective clinical evaluation of physical impairment in chronic low back pain. Spine 1992;17:617.

# 5

# Liability Issues in Occupational Medicine

*Dan J. Tennenhouse, MD, JD*

Laws are different in different states, and this chapter must necessarily be limited to legal principles that are applicable everywhere. Every occupational provider (licensed health care professional) must make an effort to become familiar with their local and state laws that regulate the practice of medicine in general and occupational medicine in particular. For example, every state has its own occupational safety and health regulations and knowledge of these regulations can help the provider to better protect both employers and employees. Every state also has specific reporting statutes that may create very strict legal duties for the provider (eg, reporting of disorders characterized by lapses in consciousness or periods of confusion, reporting of pesticide poisoning, reporting of work-related injuries).

## NEGLIGENCE

A professional negligence action against a health care provider cannot succeed unless the following four elements are proved in a court of law:

1. The existence of legal duty on the part of the provider to protect the victim (plaintiff) from harm.
2. A breach of that duty meeting the legal definition of "negligence."
3. Legal "damages" (harm) to the victim (plaintiff).
4. A causal relationship between the negligence and the harm (ie, that the negligent act substantially contributed to the harm suffered by the victim [plaintiff]).

A legal duty to the plaintiff exists when the provider makes a contract with the plaintiff to provide medical care and the plaintiff relies on that contract, or when the plaintiff is a foreseeable victim of the provider's negligence toward a patient. In some circumstances, there may be no legal duty to the patient (employee) when the provider is required by a contract with the employer to perform a job-related evaluation of the employee without providing any treatment. In contrast, there may be a legal duty to persons *other* than the employee if the provider failed to protect them from injury caused by the employee. For example, prescribing a psychoactive medication for the employee without warning the employee not to drive or operate heavy equipment could expose the provider to liability from a coworker or from any member of the public who is injured by the medication-impaired employee.

Professional negligence, or "malpractice," occurs when the provider fails to have and use the necessary care and skill ordinarily possessed and used in similar circumstances by other reputable providers with similar training and experience. The degree of care and skill ordinarily used in similar circumstances is a theoretical concept sometimes called the "standard of care." In a lawsuit, the standard of care is determined by the "trier of fact" (jury, panel of arbitrators, or judge in a nonjury trial) usually based on the testimony of expert witnesses. Any failure to meet this "standard of care" is professional negligence.

"Damages" are based on legally compensable harm to the plaintiff that may include monetary compensation for medical care, occupational rehabilitation, loss of full enjoyment of life, pain, emotional suffering, psychiatric injury, loss of occupational income, loss of future earning capacity, etc. The purpose of a malpractice (civil) lawsuit is not to "do justice" or to "right a wrong" as happens in a criminal case, but instead is to compensate the plaintiff for injuries suffered. Inadequate as it may be, the law makes provision only for monetary compensation.

A causal relationship between the negligence and the harm exists when the negligence was a *substantial* (even if small) contributing factor to the plaintiff's injury. If the injury would have occurred to the same degree without the negligence, then there is no causal relationship and the lawsuit must fail. For example, assume a physician negligently fails to investigate an employee's chronic cough, exposing the employee to a risk of delayed diagnosis of lung cancer. Lung cancer is nevertheless discovered within one month but is in an advanced stage, and the employee soon succumbs to the cancer. There is little likelihood that the negligent delay in diagnosis would be found by a jury to be a legal cause of the employee's death. A 1-month's delay in a diagnosis of terminal lung cancer would probably not affect the outcome in this case; however, there might be a very different legal outcome if the delay in diagnosis was 6 months.

If the plaintiff *contributed* to the injury by negligent noncompliance, the plaintiff's own negligence would diminish the provider's negligence. Most states follow a scheme of proportionate fault, or "comparative negligence," whereby fault is allocated on a percentage basis between provider and plaintiff. The verdict, based on the extent of the plaintiff's injury, is reduced by the percentage the plaintiff was at fault.

## DISTINCTIONS BETWEEN EMPLOYEE & INDEPENDENT CONTRACTOR

The nature of the provider-employer relationship is paramount in determining the provider's own liability for negligence. The essential question is whether the provider is an employee or an independent contractor. If the provider is clearly an employee, negligence toward a fellow employee is usually encompassed by workers' compensation.

The workers' compensation system is the "exclusive remedy" available to employees who suffer job-related injuries, and they cannot ordinarily sue their employers or co-workers for injuries sustained on the job. Because workers' compensation is the "exclusive remedy," the employee also cannot sue for medical malpractice, but must accept the workers' compensation award as the *only* compensation. Compared with a workers' compensation award, the money damages awarded in a medical malpractice lawsuit could be many times greater.

If the provider is an independent contractor, however, the provider can be sued directly by the employee for medical malpractice. The courts have not been eager to incorporate medical malpractice into the traditional areas encompassed by the workers' compensation exclusive remedy scheme. Only if the provider is clearly and unequivocally a fellow employee are the courts likely to apply the exclusive remedy provision of the workers' compensation system. For example, if the provider is giving medical services to the employee *outside* of the scope of the employment arrangement, then an independent contractor status may be found by the court thereby opening up the potential for a malpractice lawsuit.

Two tests are sometimes used by the courts in order to resolve the question of whether an occupational provider is an employee or an independent contractor. The **"control" test** determines how much independent decision making and control of actions is exercised by the provider. For example, the

provider who is conducting a routine predetermined physical examination or providing care predetermined and formulated with management is deemed to be acting under the control of the employer and is therefore an employee. The provider who is making independent judgments as any provider in private practice does and who is not following preapproved functions or procedures is deemed an independent contractor. The **"indicia" test** determines whether the provider is treated as and functions as any other employee and so is actually under company control. Indicia of employee status are present if providers are required to keep regular working hours, are receiving the same benefits received by other employees, are required to report regularly to superiors, and must request and obtain authorization before acting outside existing protocols.

Due to the complexity of these rules and differences among the states (eg, the "dual capacity" doctrine that applies in some states), the provider is well advised to consult with local legal counsel familiar with this area of law before making decisions that may affect his or her status as an employee.

## HARASSMENT/WRONGFUL TERMINATION ACTIONS

Lawsuits against companies for harassment of or discrimination against employees or prospective employees is becoming epidemic with many very large monetary awards. Lawsuits against companies for wrongful termination of employees is also reaching epidemic proportions. These legal actions usually involve poor judgment on supervisorial or executive levels within a company depriving an employee of job benefits by demotion, undesirable job assignment, termination, or constructive termination (creating impossible conditions under which to work). Sometimes they involve retaliation against an employee for taking time off work or filing a workers' compensation claim.

A convenient reason for depriving an employee of job benefits is medical findings. If a provider states that an employee is unable to carry out essential job functions for medical reasons, the company has an excuse for taking action against the employee. This is not a legal problem for the provider unless evidence of some conspiracy can be shown. Unfortunately, evidence supporting a conspiracy is common.

A conspiracy may be established if there is evidence of both of the following:

1. A company official or supervisor suggested to a provider what medical findings would be desirable or should be reported (eg, finding a reason to demote or get rid of the employee, finding nothing wrong and returning the employee prematurely to work). This suggestion could take

the form of a telephone call, memo, fax, or other communication with the provider and often is recorded as a memo in the official's own files.

2. The provider then gave an opinion or made a recommendation against the employee's interests without clear and well documented medical reasons supporting that opinion or recommendation.

Providers implicated in such conspiracies may be liable not only for economic harm to the employee, but also for "punitive damages" (extra damages awarded as punishment) for intentional misconduct. Examples of situations in which conspiracies might be shown include the following:

1. A company official asks the provider to write up an overstated report describing the employee as not medically fit to continue the job or to assume responsibilities of a new job.
2. A company official asks the provider to return the employee prematurely to work.
3. A company official insists employees who take time off work for illness get an unnecessary psychiatric or other type of consultation (as harassment for the purpose of discouraging claimed illness).

Providers should be cautious of situations in which such recommendations or suggestions are made by company officials. They should refuse to discuss the possibility of providing opinions or recommendations for the convenience of the company. They should *always* have a reasonable medical basis and also clear documentation in support of all of their opinions and recommendations.

## MISREPRESENTATIONS

**A. Misrepresentations to Insurers:** A fraudulent letter is a letter that misrepresents a patient's condition or misrepresents the benefits of proposed care and that tends to support or deny medical insurance coverage or a workers' compensation claim that might otherwise be denied. This practice violates fraud laws and may constitute a basis for both civil *and criminal* action against the provider.

For example, a provider wrote a letter to an insurer stating that the patient needed surgery on a scar, that the surgery was "reconstructive" rather than "cosmetic," and would improve the patient's function. The patient's medical record and the patient's understanding of the purpose for the scar revision did not correlate with the provider's letter in regard to any improved function. In another example, a psychiatrist represented to an insurer that a patient with a chronic alcohol abuse disorder required hospitalization for acute psychotic manifestations related to alcohol

abuse. The hospitalization was in fact for alcohol dependence in an alcoholism recovery facility. In both of the above situations, the provider was aware that the proposed care was not covered by the patient's insurance and that the misrepresentation could result in payment by the insurer.

Criminal fraud actions must have a statutory basis. For example, California Penal Code Section 550 makes it a felony to present any written or oral statement in support of or in opposition to a claim for payment or any other insurance policy benefit knowing that the statement contains false or misleading information. Similar statutes exist in other states.

Letters to insurers that are inconsistent with the medical records, with reports from other providers, or with the patient's understanding of the medical needs may create suspicion of fraud. Also, multiple inconsistent letters from the same provider may trigger suspicion of fraud.

**B. Misrepresentations to Parties in Litigation:** There is also a legal risk when a provider gives supporting evidence for parties who plan to call that provider as a witness or expert witness. For example, a physician was influenced by attorneys representing various parties in a lawsuit between the patient and her insurer over coverage. The physician reversed himself in his testimony. The patient lost her case, blamed the physician for making false statements that caused her to lose her case against her insurer, and sued the physician for the benefits she had sought from her insurer. The court said a physician has a duty to the patient of honest testimony on the patient's behalf. Providers can avoid this type of liability by *always* giving honest opinions in the first place, and rejecting any prejudicial influences from self-serving attorneys, insurers, employers, or patients.

The litigation privilege protecting expert witnesses from lawsuit for statements made during testimony does not protect the witness from a lawsuit brought by the party that called the witness, only from a lawsuit by an adverse party (*Mattco Forge v. Arthur Young*, 6 Cal Rptr 2d 781, 1992). A party could sue its own witness for professional malpractice, fraud, breach of contract, etc, if dissatisfied with the expert witness' performance in support of the litigation. This usually means the witness' testimony changed without good reason in the course of the litigation, surprising the attorney who called the witness.

Providers who write letters for insurance, workers' compensation, or litigation purposes should be certain that their statements are supported by and consistent with their medical record documentation. Once a provider takes a position, it is unwise to change that position without new documented information that clearly supports such a change. Patients should be informed of the content of a provider's letter so they are not confused about the basis for any approval or denial of insurance benefits, or about the medical issues in their workers compensation claim or other litigation. If multiple providers are involved in a patient's care, review of another provider's report, or even a telephone call to another provider prior to writing a letter, can prevent dangerous inconsistencies.

Examples of situations creating an increased risk of fraud actions against providers include the following:

1. The provider is asked to write up an overstated report describing the employee as not medically fit to continue the job or to assume responsibilities of a new job.
2. The provider is asked to write up an understated report describing the employee's on-the-job injury as inconsequential so as to devalue a workers' compensation claim.
3. The treating provider always directs referrals to selected defense-oriented specialists in order to reduce workers' compensation risk.
4. The treating provider is told by someone who is not medically trained or who has not seen the patient to deny diagnostic or treatment services to an injured worker in order to reduce cost. The treating provider believes the services are medically indicated.
5. The provider is asked to mislead an employee about a job-related injury or illness so as to prevent a workers' compensation claim.

## EMPLOYEE RECORDS

Employee health information obtained through the efforts of the occupational health provider at the request of the company is the property of the company. Employers who pay for health care often believe they are entitled to all information obtained and demand it from the provider. However, the occupational provider has certain responsibilities in regard to confidentiality. Employee medical information is not to be disclosed to third parties without the consent of the employee. Releasing information from a employee's medical records without the employee's permission or other legal justification can result in an action by the employee for invasion of privacy and possibly an action by the provider's licensing board for unauthorized disclosure of a professional confidence.

Sometimes the distinction between employer and health care provider is blurred because the employer maintains a medical department with confidential files on its employees. If these medical files are not accessible to nonmedical personnel for nonmedical purposes, such a medical department may be considered part of the health care team and, by implication, entitled to medical information without express written authorization of the employee. The provider who shares medical information with an employer's med-

ical department *knowing* that in fact the information is being misused may, however, be violating the employee's right of confidentiality.

Employers often provide employees with medical examinations for the employer's own purposes. In such cases, information divulged to the employer should be limited to workplace-related findings. This includes the employee's ability to perform job functions, but does not usually include medical diagnoses or other specific medical findings.

An employee who acquiesces to examination by company health providers may or may not be agreeing to disclosure of confidential medical information. To be certain that confidentiality requirements are met, it is prudent to have a written authorization from the employee before any release of information to the employer. If such an authorization is always obtained prior to any evaluation, disputes over an employer's right to confidential information without the employee's authorization can be avoided.

An employer who permits false or confidential employee information to be disseminated to company personnel can be liable to the employee for defamation or invasion of the employee's right to privacy. The provider may share liability with the employer if confidential medical information was disclosed without authorization.

In many states the employee's own right of access to health records is provided for by statute. Providers should be familiar with the laws in their state allowing patients to examine or receive copies of their records. Occupational Safety and Health Administration (OSHA) regulations require employers dealing with toxic materials to make their records available to employees within 15 days after an employee's request to examine them. Documents that must be accessible include not only the employee's medical records but also environmental data about the workplace. An employee may even have access to the toxic exposure record of a fellow employee if such information is relevant to his or her own likelihood of toxic exposure.

## LEGAL IMPLICATIONS OF THE AMERICANS WITH DISABILITIES ACT

The Americans With Disabilities Act (ADA) is intended to prevent discrimination against employees or applicants on the basis of a disability. The primary risks of a claim are to the employer rather than the occupational provider; however, the provider can do much to help protect the employer. The ADA requires that employers not discriminate against a qualified individual with a disability because of the disability in regard to job application procedures, hiring, advancement, discharge, compensation, job training, and other privileges of employment. The ADA also requires the employer to make reasonable accommodations for a known impairment unless it would cause undue hardship (involve significant difficulty or expense).

The following definitions apply to the above ADA requirements:

"Discriminate" includes limiting an applicant or employee so as to adversely affect job status or opportunities.

"Qualified individual with a disability" is an individual with a disability who, with or without reasonable accommodation, can perform the essential functions of the employment. To determine what are "essential work functions," the employer's judgment is considered along with any job description prepared before interviewing job applicants.

"Disability" is a physical or mental impairment that substantially limits one or more of the major life activities of an individual. It does not include individuals currently engaged in illegal use of drugs, but does include those erroneously regarded as engaging in such use. "Disability" as used in the ADA includes emotional or psychiatric instability, a history of having filed workers compensation claims, and even having disabled family members who require assistance necessitating rearrangement of work schedules. The definition of disability given in the ADA is so general and so vague that *any* chronic medical or psychiatric disorder should be considered a disability. New injuries and acute illnesses are probably not disabilities, but any residual impairment would be.

"Reasonable accommodation" includes making existing facilities accessible to and usable by disabled employees, job restructuring, modifying work schedules, reassignment, acquiring or modifying equipment, etc.

The ADA also requires that employers not inquire of or medically examine a job applicant about the nature or severity of a disability. Employers may, however, require a medical examination after an offer of employment to determine the applicant's ability to perform job-related functions. The employer may condition the job offer on the results if all persons offered the same job are required to be examined, and medical information is kept separate and confidential (except for notification of supervisors as to job restrictions, accommodations, and emergency care). Employers shall not, as a requirement, inquire of or medically examine an employee about the nature or severity of a disability unless the examination is shown to be job related and consistent with business necessity.

If jobs or benefits are denied to individuals with disabilities, the employer must show the "qualification standards" are job-related, consistent with business necessity, and not correctable by reasonable accommodation. "Qualification standards" may require that the individual pose no direct threat to others in the workplace. "Direct threat" means a significant risk to the health or safety of others that cannot be eliminated by reasonable accommodation.

An employer may prohibit use of illegal drugs and use of alcohol in the workplace, as well as being under their influence. Testing for illegal drugs is not a medical examination under the ADA. "Use of illegal drugs" is use, possession, or distribution of controlled substances except under supervision by a licensed health care professional.

The occupational provider can help protect the employer by disclosing only the employee's ability to perform essential functions of employment and not disclosing any diagnosis of a chronic medical or psychiatric disorder. If the employer does not possess knowledge of the disability, it cannot discriminate against the employee because of the disability. The occupational provider can also help the employer by assisting in determining if a reasonable accommodation can be offered. Employers may have little idea about what measures might be effective in enabling a disabled employee to perform the essential functions of employment.

## CONTRACTUAL ISSUES BETWEEN PROVIDER & EMPLOYER

Careful consideration of provisions in the contract between an occupational provider and an employer can offer an excellent opportunity to prevent legal problems. The use of legal counsel familiar with occupational medicine issues, will assist in the preparation of these contracts. Consider addressing the following issues in the contract:

### 1. LEGAL RESPONSIBILITY

**A. There is no "exclusive remedy" protection** under workers compensation law for independent contractors. The provider's relationship to the employer should be made clear in the contract.

**B. Who is bearing liability cost?** Employers who bear no cost may believe they have nothing to lose and have strong economic incentives to increase the providers' liability risk by pressuring them to write misleading letters, return employees to work prematurely, select medically inappropriate care to reduce time off work, etc. The contract should address such issues.

### 2. ILLEGAL EMPLOYER ACTIVITY

The provider's unwillingness to participate in actions that may constitute harassment, discrimination, wrongful termination, or fraud, can prevent involvement in major litigation against the employer. Some supervisors may attempt to misuse providers to harass or discriminate against employees, to assist them in wrongfully terminating employees, or to fraudulently deceive employees. The contract should prohibit such conduct.

## 3. CONFIDENTIAL PATIENT INFORMATION

A frequent problem that is seldom addressed in contracts is the employer's right of access to confidential medical information about its employees. By specifying the employer's degree of access to information and how it may utilize such information, the contract negotiation becomes an opportunity to clarify the provider's right to protect patient confidentiality.

## 4. COMPLIANCE WITH THE AMERICANS WITH DISABILITIES ACT (ADA)

Because of the risks of ADA claims against the employer, the contract should address such issues as the following:

**A. If or how a diagnosis that could constitute a disability should be disclosed to the employer.** Employers should be reminded that the ADA prohibits them from inquiring about an employee's or applicant's disabilities, therefore they should not request a diagnosis of a chronic medical disorder.

**B. How information about the employee's job functions will be made available to the provider.**

**C. How the provider should participate in decisions about reasonable accommodations to disabled employees.**

## OCCUPATIONAL HEALTH NURSING

Nurses practicing in occupational settings are usually company employees. They commonly have more autonomy, however, than hospital-based nurses and frequently act without direct physician supervision. Because of this autonomy, the above discussions of the legal obligations and liabilities of occupational providers generally apply to occupational health nurses. To ensure that occupational health nurses are not operating outside the scope of licensed nursing practice or outside the umbrella of workers' compensation, the following guidelines should be followed:

1. The course and scope of the occupational health nurse's professional duties and activities should be defined by protocols outlining standardized nursing procedures. Each protocol should be in writing and should be jointly approved, dated, and signed both by a physician and by a company executive.
2. Each protocol for a function or duty of the occupational health nurse should clearly describe the specific procedure and the circumstances under which the procedure may be performed.
3. Protocols for occupational health nurses should not include functions that are restricted by law to other health care professionals, such as prescribing or dispensing medications where limited by state law, or performing surgical procedures.
4. Any special training or experience required of the occupational health nurse in order to perform a particular function or procedure should be described.
5. Procedures that require direct physician orders or supervision should be identified.
6. Circumstances requiring immediate notification of or referral to a physician or emergency department should be specified.
7. Circumstances requiring physician review of the nurse's actions, and when such review must take place, should be specified.
8. Protocols should be reviewed on a scheduled periodic basis.

# Section II.
# Occupational Injuries

# Ergonomics & the Prevention of Occupational Injuries

**6**

*David M. Rempel, MD, MPH, & Ira L. Janowitz, PT, CPE*

Ergonomics—also called human factors engineering—is the study of the physical and cognitive demands of work to ensure a safe and productive workplace. The function of specialists in ergonomics is to design or improve the workplace, workstations, tools, equipment, and procedures of workers so as to limit fatigue, discomfort, and injuries while also efficiently achieving personal and organizational goals.

## Approach to Job Design

Ergonomists, occupational physicians, and other health and safety professionals frequently work together to improve the design of jobs and work stations that have unsafe qualities or have caused injury. Controlling errors, wasted movements, and tool and materials damage and improving quality are also important goals. The principles of job design and redesign discussed in this chapter are relevant to both the office and the factory floor, and examples are drawn from both areas. This chapter presents ergonomics approaches that can be applied in the workplace to prevent musculoskeletal disorders. Although the methods may be useful for employees with musculoskeletal problems, a review of approaches to the medical management of these disorders has been published elsewhere.

## Approach to Prevention of Occupational Injuries

Health professionals should seek frequent opportunities to tour work areas and evaluate job procedures, equipment, and working conditions. The concepts and suggestions presented in this and related chapters should be kept in mind during these tours, and problem areas and activities should be noted for later study and possible job redesign. Such tours should focus on work areas and tasks where injuries, high turnover, excessive absenteeism, or other signs of a mismatch between workers and their jobs occur.

In addition to redesigning unsafe and unhealthy jobs, consideration might be given to restructuring a job at a new skill level or new mechanization level. This may involve employing the techniques of job simplification (reduction of physical complexity of the job) or job enlargement (broader use of skills or greater variety of tasks), and the aid of an ergonomist or an industrial engineer will often be necessary. These professionals are concerned with employee health and safety as well as productivity, since the two are closely interrelated.

## Structure of an Ergonomics Program

Almost all ergonomics programs contain the elements, in one form or another, laid out in Figure 6–1. Health surveillance, the review of existing health data (eg, workers' compensation data, OSHA logs, nursing logs) or walk-throughs to identify jobs with excessive risk factors are used to identify and prioritize jobs or tasks associated with the highest risk of injury. Meetings with employees and checklists may be used in risk factor surveillance. The next step is to perform a detailed analysis of the high-risk job or task to identify and prioritize the risk factors. Then, specific engineering or administrative solutions that will modify the most important risk factors are identified and implemented on a pilot basis. The pilot intervention, which should last for two weeks to two months, will ensure that the intervention is effective and does not cause additional health problems or interfere with productivity. In addition to the components in Figure 6–1, involved employees, supervisors, engineers, and health and safety staff need appropriate initial training in the components of an effective program and basic ergonomic methodologies.

The health professional should also work with a committee within the organization to plan health and safety reviews and follow-up activities and to act as a resource for management. Ergonomists, industrial or process engineers, health and safety personnel, maintenance personnel, the affected employees and their

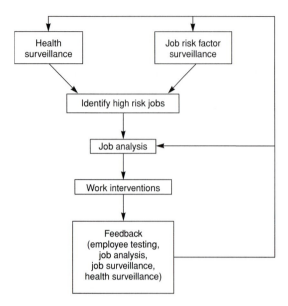

**Figure 6–1.** Components of an ergonomic program.

supervisors, and risk management personnel should all be encouraged to participate in these committees. Management support and appropriate assignment of tasks with follow-up are critical for success.

### Cost-Effectiveness of Preventive Activities

Indirect costs of musculoskeletal disorders, such as replacement employee wages and training costs, productivity reduction, and quality reduction are often three to four times as high as the direct costs of medical, disability, and rehabilitation expenses. Improvements in workstation design and procedures may have a pay back period of less than one year when the costs of the intervention are compared with the total costs of musculoskeletal disorders. Although job redesign usually focuses on reducing risk factors for classic musculoskeletal disorders (eg, tendinitis and carpal tunnel syndrome), secondary benefits are a reduction in acute injuries (fractures, bruises, and strains).

### PHYSICAL STRESS DUE TO POOR WORKPLACE OR EQUIPMENT DESIGN

### Use of Anthropometric Data

One of the primary reasons for physical stress on the job is the mismatch in size between the worker and the workplace, equipment, or tools. This mismatch may result in excessive forward bending and reaching for tools or materials, having to work bent over, having to work with one or both arms and shoulders held high for long periods, having to hold a power tool at some distance for long periods, or having to sit on a stool or bench that is too low or too high.

Figures 6–2 and 6–3 show the body dimensions of adult men and women in the United States. Workplaces and machines should be designed so that larger workers (up to the 95th percentile) and smaller workers (down to the 5th percentile) can function appropriately. That is, an ideal work space not only accommodates the larger worker's body size, height of viewing, location of hands and feet, etc, but it also keeps control levers within comfortable reach and activation of the smaller workers and accommodates their height of viewing.

Anthropometry data are used to place **visual targets** and **points of operation** (eg, materials or tools used by the hands) in appropriate locations. There may be more than one visual target (eg, computer screen, hard copy, workpiece) and the targets should be prioritized and placed on the basis of frequency of use. Frequently viewed targets should be directly in front of the operator and between eye level and 45 degrees below eye level. Similarly, continuously used tools, workpieces, or controls should be near elbow height and require little reach. The heavier the tool or workpiece, the closer it should be to elbow height.

### Improvement of Work & Workplace Design

**A. Elimination of "Waist Motion":** The most important physical design rule for a sedentary job is that the operator be able to reach all parts and supplies, keyboards, tools, controls, etc, without leaning, bending, or twisting at the waist. Frequent reaching should be restricted to movements of the arm, if possible. Figure 6–4 illustrates the forearm-only (preferable) and full-arm (satisfactory) reach limits for men and women in the United States. Task designs that require movements outside the full-arm reach limits increase the risk for shoulder, neck, and low back problems. These reach limits, called reach envelopes, are based on the dimensions outlined in Figures 6–2 and 6–3 and thus must be modified for special applications or different populations.

The reach envelope rules are particularly important if significant forces or weights are involved, though repetitive movement of the upper body without load may also become fatiguing. For example, employees at risk include assembly workers who must reach to a high shelf or reach behind them to retrieve parts and bus drivers who must lean forward across a steering wheel and then pull it laterally in the direction they wish to turn.

Although some movements of the waist and shoulders may be unavoidable even in well-designed jobs, the design rule still applies: the less required bending and twisting of the waist and torso, the better the job design.

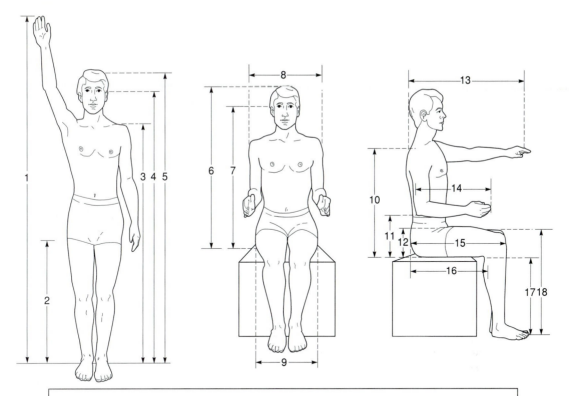

## Male Body Dimensions (cm)

| Dimension Number | Dimension Name | 5th Percentile | 50th Percentile | 95th Percentile | Standard Deviation |
|---|---|---|---|---|---|
| 1 | Vertical reach | 195.6 | 209.6 | 223.5 | 8.46 |
| 2 | Crotch height | 75.4 | 83.1 | 90.7 | 4.67 |
| 3 | Shoulder height | 133.6 | 143.6 | 154.1 | 6.22 |
| 4 | Eye height | 152.4 | 163.3 | 175.0 | 15.29 |
| 5 | Stature | 163.8 | 174.4 | 185.6 | 6.61 |
| 6 | Height, sitting | 84.5 | 90.8 | 96.7 | 3.66 |
| 7 | Eye height, sitting | 72.8 | 78.8 | 84.6 | 3.57 |
| 8 | Shoulder breadth | 41.5 | 45.2 | 49.8 | 2.54 |
| 9 | Hip breadth, sitting | 30.7 | 33.9 | 38.4 | 2.38 |
| 10 | Shoulder height, sitting | 57.1 | 62.4 | 67.6 | 3.18 |
| 11 | Elbow height, sitting | 18.8 | 23.7 | 28.0 | 2.78 |
| 12 | Thigh clearance | 13.0 | 14.9 | 17.5 | 1.36 |
| 13 | Thumb tip reach | 74.9 | 82.4 | 90.9 | 4.85 |
| 14 | Elbow-fingertip length | 44.3 | 47.9 | 51.9 | 2.31 |
| 15 | Buttock-knee length | 54.9 | 59.4 | 64.3 | 2.85 |
| 16 | Buttock-popliteal length | 45.8 | 49.8 | 54.0 | 2.50 |
| 17 | Popliteal height | 40.6 | 44.5 | 48.8 | 2.50 |
| 18 | Knee height, sitting | 49.7 | 54.0 | 58.7 | 2.73 |

**Figure 6–2.** Body dimensions for men. Corresponding weights are as follows: 5th percentile, 57.4 kg (126.3 lb); 50th percentile, 71 kg (156.2 lb); and 95th percentile, 91.6 kg (201.5 lb). Appropriate weights must be added for clothing and shoes. (Source of data: *Anthropometry of US Military Personnel.* DOD Handbook–743, 3 October 1980; and also as appears in modified form in *The Measure of Man and Woman.* Alvin R. Tilley & Henry Dreyfuss Associates, Whitney Library of Design, New York, 1993.)

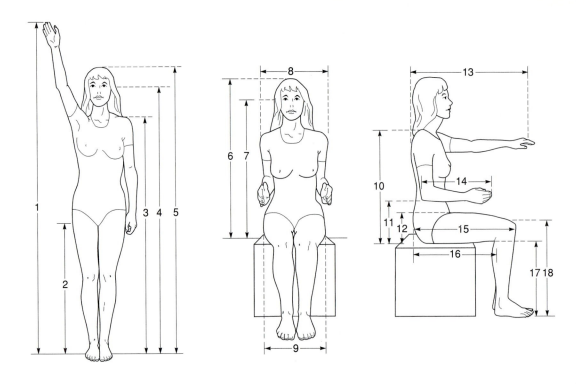

## Female Body Dimensions (cm)

| Dimension Number | Dimension Name | 5th Percentile | 50th Percentile | 95th Percentile | Standard Deviation |
|---|---|---|---|---|---|
| 1 | Vertical reach | 185.2 | 199.1 | 213.4 | 8.64 |
| 2 | Crotch height | 68.1 | 74.4 | 81.3 | 4.06 |
| 3 | Shoulder height | 123.9 | 133.3 | 143.7 | 6.00 |
| 4 | Eye height | 142.2 | 149.9 | 158.8 | 6.35 |
| 5 | Stature | 152.6 | 162.8 | 174.1 | 6.52 |
| 6 | Height, sitting | 79.0 | 85.2 | 90.8 | 3.59 |
| 7 | Eye height, sitting | 67.7 | 73.8 | 79.1 | 3.46 |
| 8 | Shoulder breadth | 38.4 | 42.0 | 45.7 | 2.24 |
| 9 | Hip breadth, sitting | 33.0 | 38.2 | 43.9 | 3.27 |
| 10 | Shoulder height, sitting | 53.7 | 57.9 | 62.5 | 2.66 |
| 11 | Elbow height, sitting | 16.1 | 20.8 | 25.0 | 2.74 |
| 12 | Thigh clearance | 13.2 | 15.4 | 17.5 | 1.31 |
| 13 | Thumb tip reach | 67.7 | 74.2 | 80.5 | 3.88 |
| 14 | Elbow-fingertip length | 40.0 | 43.4 | 47.5 | 2.28 |
| 15 | Buttock-knee length | 53.1 | 57.7 | 63.2 | 3.06 |
| 16 | Buttock-popliteal length | 43.5 | 47.5 | 52.6 | 2.76 |
| 17 | Popliteal height | 38.0 | 41.6 | 45.7 | 2.35 |
| 18 | Knee height, sitting | 46.9 | 50.9 | 55.5 | 2.60 |

**Figure 6–3.** Body dimensions for women. Corresponding weights are as follows: 5th percentile, 46.6 kg (103.5 lb); 50th percentile 59.6 kg (131.1 lb); and 95th percentile, 74.5 kg (163.9 lb). Appropriate weights must be added for clothing and shoes. (Source of data: *Anthropometry of US Military Personnel.* DOD Handbook–743, 3 October 1980; and also as appears in modified form in *The Measure of Man and Woman.* Alvin R. Tilley & Henry Dreyfuss Associates, Whitney Library of Design, New York, 1993.)

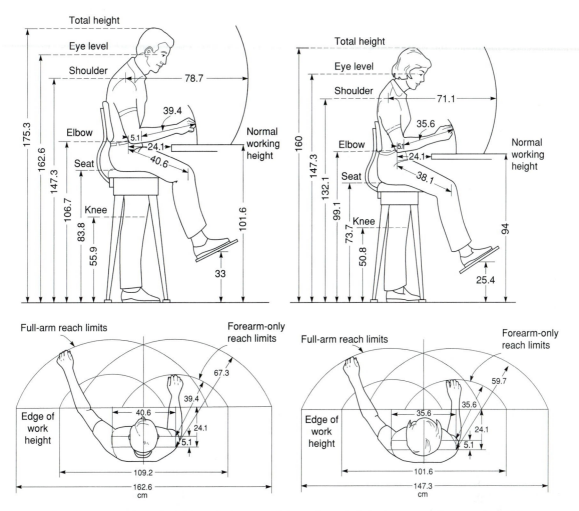

**Figure 6–4.** Forearm-only (preferable) and full-arm (satisfactory) reach limits for men and women in working areas shown in the horizontal and vertical planes. All dimensions are in centimeters. (Adapted from Farley, 1955. Modified and reproduced, with permission, from Dad B, Grady RM: Industrial workplace layout and engineering anthropometry. In: *Ergonomics of Workstation Design.* Kvalseth TO [editor]: Butterworth, 1983; and also as appears in modified form in *The Measure of Man and Woman.* Alvin R. Tilley & Henry Dreyfuss Associates, Whitney Library of Design, New York, 1993.)

Example: Women of average dimensions (50th percentile) can reach horizontally only about 74 cm (29 in), and short women (5th percentile) can reach horizontally only about 68 cm (27 in), as measured from the back of the chair when they are seated in an upright position. If a shelf of supplies or a panel of controls is 91 cm (36 in) in front of them (also measured from the back of the chair), they will have difficulty obtaining the supplies or manipulating the controls even with bending and twisting at the waist. If these activities are frequent, a potential health and safety problem exists resulting from the repetitive loading of the back, neck, and shoulder areas. Productivity will also be affected. The work area should be redesigned to reduce the re-quired reaching distances to within comfortable ranges.

**B. Avoidance of Static Positions:**

**1. Static holding positions**–A production task might involve holding an object rigidly in one hand and working on it with the other, or a maintenance job might involve holding a hand tool or power tool tightly in one hand for extended periods. In either case, sustained muscle tension reduces vascular flow to the muscles and hastens the onset of local fatigue. Reduction of fatigue may be accomplished by using a holding clamp or bench vise or, in the case of hand or power tools, by alternating hands or using self-locking tools. When sustained holding is still necessary, redesigning the tools or tool handles to achieve maximum comfort is helpful. For example, power tools can be suspended from cables or articulated with antitorque bars to decrease grip force and the transfer of vibration to the worker's hands.

> Example: In a quality control task, each part being checked was picked up and supported by the worker's left hand and forearm while testing clamps were attached and adjustments made. The job was redesigned so that each part was placed on a waist-high rolling rack that was pulled along by the worker, who then made attachments and adjustments with both hands. Muscle cramping in the left wrist, forearm, and hand was eliminated.

**2. Static body positions**–Workers who operate computers, calculators, laboratory equipment, telephone control panels, etc, tend to hold their bodies in a fixed position for protracted periods in order to maintain a consistent physical relationship with the equipment. For example, typists must maintain a fixed spatial relationship between their shoulders and the keyboard in order to strike the proper key each time without looking. In addition to maintaining a fixed shoulder position, they often maintain a rigid neck position required by looking for long periods at the copyholder or the computer monitor.

In jobs of this sort, measures must be taken to prevent chronic pain and cumulative trauma disorders in the shoulders, neck, and upper back. Workers should be encouraged to stretch or move the particular muscle groups that remain most static (eg, by an occasional shrug and relaxation of the shoulders). To promote posture changes, it may be preferable for workers to leave their chairs every 20–60 minutes to collect the next batch of work rather than have it delivered.

> Example: Keyboard operators in a large office used a break reminder software to remind them to perform a walking task every 20 minutes. Operators were encouraged to take their regular rest breaks and to do a few quick stretching exercises whenever a shoulder, wrist, or other part of the body started to bother them.

### Improvement of Equipment Design

Machine operation is most productive and least stressful when the machine does the work and the operator does the thinking.

**A. Proper Design of Controls:** Controls (eg, levers, switches, joysticks, and pedals) enable the operator to give a machine "orders" or feed it information. They also provide feedback to the operator. Primary controls—those of greatest importance or used most often—should be located within the forearm-only (preferable) reach limits, and other controls should be located within the full-arm (satisfactory) reach limits of the workstation, as shown in Figure 6–4.

**B. Proper Placement of Displays:** Primary displays (screens and/or hard copy) should be located in front of the operator and slightly (not more than 30 degrees) below eye level. If hard copy is used, a document holder should be placed either to one side of the screen or between the monitor and the keyboard. This allows the operator to monitor the displays from a position most comfortable for the head (ie, with the head balanced on top of the spine). Positioning the display higher or lower can lead to fatigue of the muscles of the neck and increased pressure on joints and other structures in the neck and shoulder area. Locating the display or other primary visual target to one side or the other of the operator causes stress on the rotation muscles of the neck.

Bifocal lens users are an exception to this monitor placement recommendation; they usually need the primary display lower. Bifocal lens users may benefit from special monofocal lenses for computer use; these lenses permit a greater range of head postures.

**C. Appropriate Control-Display Relationships:** The design rules for controls and displays generally allow them to be placed in the most convenient position for the operator, but they also must be integrated with each other on a logical basis.

> Example: If a steam turbine is to be monitored and operated, the displays will be in front of and below the eye level of the operator, and the turbine controls generally will be in front of and near the operator's hands. However, the control for rotational speed should be adjacent to and linked logically with its speed indicator display (eg, the control and display should both be contained in a box on the panel or linked by means of a color-coded line). Movement of the speed control upward or to the right should move the speed indicator display also upward or to the right. This will increase the stimulus-response compatibility of the two devices and improve the control capability of the operator.

Logical linkages of this sort suggest simple responses to the information displayed to the operator, and more sophisticated logical linkages can indicate more complex responses. In this manner, the control-display relationships can reduce the information-processing load on the operator and thus reduce stress and the rate of errors.

## VISUAL PROBLEMS DUE TO POOR ILLUMINATION OR TO GLARE

One or more of the following symptoms and signs may accompany a general feeling of tiredness of the eyes: oculomotor changes (esophoria, exophoria), ocular pain, itching, tearing, reduced ability of the eyes to accommodate and converge properly, headache, and complementary color reversals. "Eye fatigue" can result from visual stress due to rapid accommodation, extended viewing at short focal lengths, poor contrast between target and background, direct or reflected glare, or improperly fitted corrective lenses. It is commonly associated with extended use of video display terminals (see below) whose screens have reduced contrast, poor text resolution, or reflection on the screen. Glare is a common problem and can be reduced by limiting light from the source (eg, by using window coverings or parabolic lenses on fluorescent lights) or by moving the monitor relative to the light source.

As far as we know, ocular symptoms from overwork do not cause permanent eye damage. However, these symptoms can affect productivity and an employee's sense of well-being.

## Adequate Illumination of the Workstation

The amount of light required to perform a specific task without feeling visual fatigue is a function of the visual difficulty of the task at the desired work speed and quality, and the visual acuity of the worker. Degree of visual difficulty is typically determined by (1) the contrast between the target and its back-

grounds, (2) the spatial resolution, and (3) the size of the target. Visual acuity, even with corrected vision, varies with age. The recommended ranges of illumination for various types of tasks are shown in Table 6–1.

## Reduction of Workstation Glare

Glare may emanate directly from a bright light source or may be reflected off the shiny surfaces of machines, work tables, windows, displays, tools, etc. It can be reduced or eliminated by limiting light from the source or covering shiny surfaces with dull or nonreflective coatings.

> Example: In a garment plant, sewing machine operators complained of headaches and tired and itching eyes after lamps were installed on the other side of their machines. The purpose of the lamps was to improve visibility, but they had the opposite effect because their light reflected off the polished wood and metal sewing tables and the sewn material. Moving the lamps eliminated the glare and relieved the visual symptoms and headaches.

## Proper Design of Chairs

Common complaints that stem from improper seating include fatigue or cramping in the lower legs

Table 6–1. Recommended ranges of illumination for various types of tasks.[1]

| Type of Activity or Area | Range of Illumination[2] | |
| --- | --- | --- |
| | Lux | Footcandles |
| Public areas with dark surroundings | 20–50 | 2–5 |
| Simple orientation for short temporary visits | >50–100 | >5–9 |
| Working spaces where visual tasks are only occasionally performed | >100–200 | >9–19 |
| Performance of visual tasks of high contrast or large size: reading printed material, typed originals, handwriting in ink, good xerography; rough bench and machine work; ordinary inspection; rough assembly | >200–500 | >19–46 |
| Performance of visual tasks of medium contrast or small size: reading pencil handwriting, poorly printed or reproduced material; medium bench and machine work; difficult inspection, medium assembly | >500–1000 | >46–93 |
| Performance of visual tasks of low contrast or very small size: reading handwriting in hard pencil on poor-quality paper, very poorly reproduced material; very difficult inspection | >1000–2000 | >93–186 |
| Performance of visual tasks of low contrast and very small size over a prolonged period: fine assembly, highly difficult inspection, fine bench and machine work | >2000–5000 | >186–464 |
| Performance of very prolonged and exacting visual tasks: the most difficult inspection, extra fine bench and machine work, extra fine assembly | >5000–10,000 | >464–929 |
| Performance of very special visual tasks of extremely low contrast and small size: some surgical procedures | >10,000–20,000 | >929–1858 |

[1]Adapted from Flynn, 1979. Reproduced, with permission, from Eastman Kodak Company: *Ergonomic Design for People at Work.* Vol 1. Van Nostrand Reinhold, 1983.
[2]The choice of a value within a range depends on task variables, the reflectance of the environment, and the individual's visual capabilities.

or thighs and pain in the gluteal area, lower back, or upper back (Table 6–2).

The primary purpose of a chair is to provide comfortable but solid support for the weight of the body without localized pressure points. The chair must support the employee in the posture best suited for the task (eg, slightly reclined for computer work or slightly forward-leaning for writing). Shifting about, leaning to one side, etc, are natural ways to reduce loads on the lumbar spine and maintain circulation in the buttocks and thighs, and chair design needs to accommodate these postural variations.

If the seat pan is too long (>41 cm [16 in]), it cuts off circulation at the popliteus muscle, particularly in short women. For shorter people, a shallow seat or a smoothly curved "waterfall design" front edge helps eliminate pressure points. The seat should be soft enough to be comfortable but not so soft that changing posture or standing up is difficult. The seat pan should be not so concave that it restricts occasional changes of position. Many current chair designs have size adjustment features (eg, sliding seat pans and different size seat pans) for better fit.

Seat design must also provide sufficient lumbar support to maintain a comfortable degree of lordosis of the spine and assist in supporting the weight of the back. A chair should be easily adjustable while the operator is seated to offer a full range of back curvatures, seat heights, and recline of seat pan and backrest. Without good support, general fatigue is much more likely, muscular stress in the upper back tends to occur, and lower back pain may result.

The base of chairs should have five legs to reduce the likelihood of tipping over if the occupant leans backward. For comfort, the texture of material on the back and seat should be rough or nubby to allow some air circulation between the material and the body. If the chair has arms, they should fit the employee or be adjustable in height and distance apart to provide good arm support and should not strike the work table or bench during normal chair movements.

If it is necessary to adjust the chair to such a sitting height that short people's feet do not touch the ground, a sturdy large footrest must be provided to prevent the legs from dangling. A chair seat that is too high restricts circulation in the lower legs and makes it difficult to lean forward.

### Types of Chairs

**A. Chairs vs Stools:** People generally prefer chairs with a seat height of 38–46 cm (15–18 in). Occasional sitting for a highly mobile worker is best done on a stool with a seat height of 74–81 cm (29–32 in) with a large surface available for footrests. For people who move about frequently, it saves a lot of effort to perch on a stool whose height is about the length of the legs, so that the upper body is not repeatedly raised and lowered whenever they sit and stand. The advantages of this type of sit-stand stool are reduced fatigue and reduced compression on the spine. Sometimes even stationary workers prefer to alternate between sitting and standing to changed fixed postures, improve leg circulation and restore lumbar lordosis.

**B. Chairs With Forward-Sloping Seats:** Chairs that have forward-sloping seats and backrests but do not use knee rests to support the legs hold promise for various classes of jobs and preferences of users. Forward-sloping seats are especially advan-

**Table 6–2.** Common complaints that stem from improper seating.

| Complaint | Possible Causes |
|---|---|
| Pain in the gluteal area | 1. Extended sitting without break, especially constrained sitting.<br>2. Chair padding too hard, especially under ischial tuberosities and trochanters.<br>3. Seat not contoured (too flat).<br>4. Chair design restricting movement and periodic adjustment of position. |
| Pain in the lower back | 1. Inadequate lumbar support.<br>2. Improper adjustment of chair for lumbar support.<br>3. Excessive bending or twisting of worker while seated (poor location of chair in workspace or poor location of some job items).<br>4. Lifting while seated. |
| Pain in the upper back | 1. Chair too low for work area.<br>2. Frequent reaching from chair location, particularly at or above the shoulder.<br>3. Sitting in a static, rigid position for extended periods of time.<br>4. Arms held too high.<br>5. Chair back too small, poorly contoured, or improperly adjusted. |
| Poor circulation in the lower legs | 1. Anterior edge of seat pan cutting off circulation because edge too sharp (not curved or "waterfall" design), seat adjusted too high, or lack of footrest to prevent short legs from dangling.<br>2. High-heeled shoes causing plantar flexion of feet.<br>3. Inadequate foot and leg room causing excessive flexion at knees. |
| Poor circulation in the thighs | 1. Anterior edge of seat pan cutting off circulation (see above).<br>2. Seat padding too soft.<br>3. Excessive seat pan contouring in frontal plane (rolls thighs inward). |

tageous for users who must be extremely close to or hovering over their work, as is the case with some office workers, repairmen, air traffic controllers, dentists, surgeons, etc. In addition to having adjustable heights and back positions, these chairs should have an easily adjustable degree of slope and should provide for additional support to prevent slipping out of the chair (eg, high-friction seat material, seat pan contouring, or "saddle" shaping).

**C. Chairs That Recline:** Chairs with a back support that reclines can preserve lumbar lordosis. Reclining backwards up to 20 degrees from vertical can also unload the lower spine by transferring the weight of the upper body to the back support. Greater angles of reclining can lead to neck tension unless the visual target and controls of input devices are well-positioned and a headrest is provided.

### Proper Selection of Chairs

There are many well-designed types and models of chairs. The employer should obtain samples of two or three appropriate chairs for the task (adjustable forearm rests, locking or rocking seat and backrest, etc) that meet the requirements of the workers (appropriate seat pan depth, backrest shape, wheels, etc) and ask the workers to try them out for at least a week. A briefer period for chair testing is usually not sufficient, since initial impressions often differ from long-term impressions. The opinion of the workers should be considered when a supply of new chairs is ordered. If opinions are divided, it is best to order some of each type of chair.

### SETTING UP & USING COMPUTER WORKSTATIONS

Computer operators often complain of fatigue in the neck, upper back, shoulders, arms, or wrists, especially when they use the computer for long hours. They also can experience visual problems from long-term viewing of the computer monitor. Appropriate set-up and use of the computer workstation can help reduce these aches and pains.

### Adjust Chair First

The first step in adjusting a computer workstation is to adjust the seating. The seat height should be adjusted low enough that the operator's feet are firmly supported on the floor but not so low that the operator's weight is not evenly distributed over the seat pan. A large and solid footrest should be used only when attempts to adjust the chair and workstation fail. The arm supports should comfortably support the forearms and remove loading from the neck and shoulders. Some computer operators prefer to switch from sitting to standing during the day to promote posture changes; these operators will require workstations that adjust to a wide range of heights. Employees with low back problems will often benefit from the ability to alternate between sitting and standing.

### Position Monitor & Documents

The monitor will usually be placed directly in front of the operator, with the display screen below eye level approximately an arm length away. This works well for data acquisition, editing, and programming tasks in which the monitor is the primary source of information. The monitor should be positioned so that glare is minimized.

For word processing and data entry, in which the monitor may not be the primary source of information, the workplace layout will vary. Operators of word processors may require primary visual access to hard copy, and data entry clerks may look almost exclusively at the original data records (invoices, checks, etc) they are recording. In this situation, it is the copy stand or the pile of data records that should be in front of the operator, and the monitor should then be positioned to one side or the other. Continual looking to one side to view copy may result in muscle stress and pain in the neck and upper back.

For word processors, the copy stand should be directly adjacent to the monitor, at about the same height (up to 30 degrees below horizontal) and at the same viewing distance. This will reduce head rotation (side to side and up and down) and eliminate the need for frequent accommodation.

For data entry clerks, manual handling is often required to turn pages, lay aside checks or invoices, etc. In this case, it is necessary to compromise between optimal handling location and optimal viewing area.

> Example: In a data processing office, checks were turned over one by one with the left hand while their amounts were entered on a computer keyboard with the right hand. The pile of checks was placed in front of the operator and near the screen. However, to turn the checks, the operators had to reach over the keyboard and suspend their arms in space, which caused shoulder pain. Moving the checks closer to the operator would have meant more twisting to the left. The checks were left in the same position and padded armrests were provided to support the left forearm and take the load off the shoulder. Use of a numeric only (smaller) keypad allows for still better placement of the checks.

### Control of Screen Glare

Monitors provide their own illumination from the intensity of the cathode ray impinging on the phosphor used in the display screen. Because of technical limitations of this illumination, the brightness of the screen is often lower than that of a printed page, and the contrast may be much lower (about 3:1 for the screen compared with 10:1 for the printed page). In addition, the screen's characters consist of a matrix of tiny dots rather than continuous lines, and thus the characters may appear fuzzy to some computer operators. Screens should refresh themselves at least 72 times every second, so that operators with sensitive vision are not bothered by flicker.

Light from sources as bright as or brighter than the screen can cause glare. Not only is this irritating to the eyes, but it also represents "visual noise" that interferes with perception of the information on the screen. The operator must either try to "read through" this glare by focusing behind it or try to ignore it.

There are several ways to reduce the glare:

(1) Change the location of the monitor so that the light source is to the side of or above the operator, not directly behind or in front of the operator.

(2) Reduce the general illumination in the room to about 500 lux. This can be achieved by reducing the amount of overhead lighting (eg, removing every other bulb or fluorescent tube); by installing parabolic louvers for the fluorescent lights to direct the illumination straight downward; or by controlling window illumination with shades, louvered blinds, and/or tinted window film.

(3) Provide more illumination where needed with desk lamps ("task lighting") directed at the appropriate visual target. The goal is to have lighting as uniform as possible with a maximum ratio of 1:3 between the brightness of the computer screen and its immediate surroundings.

(4) If steps 1 through 3 fail, use glare-reducing filters on computer screens. These filters are available in several designs, although the principal two are coated filters (eg, polarized filters) and fine black nylon mesh filters. Polarized filters trap light reflections internally but should have treated surfaces to prevent their own reflections. Mesh screens reduce character resolution and tend to gather dust.

Another source of visual irritation is bright lights or unshaded windows. In addition to taking measures to reduce glare, employers should encourage computer operators to look up from the screen from time to time to allow the ciliary muscles to relax and thus prevent visual fatigue and pain. Computer operators who lean forward to see the screen may need their vision checked or the monitor moved closer.

## Position Input Devices

The keyboard and pointing device (eg, mouse, trackball) should be positioned directly in front of and close to the computer operator to prevent sustained reach to the front or side. The input devices should be as low as possible without touching the legs, so that the shoulders are not elevated during use. The slope of the keyboard may have to be adjusted so that the wrists are not held in extension during keying; it may be necessary to tilt the keyboard away from the user by a few degrees to achieve a straight wrist posture. The use of wrist rests is somewhat controversial. They can lead to pressure points at the wrist and promote wrist deviations to strike keys. One suggestion is to have operators use the wrist rests only between typing periods, not during typing. The computer operator should avoid resting the wrist or forearm on a sharp edge. Chair armrests that are height and width adjustable are a better form of arm support than are wrist rests.

People who use the computer for long hours and do not know how to touch type should take typing lessons. A good typist does not have to flex the neck forward constantly to see the keys and has learned to relax the fingers and arms during typing. To reduce hand motions during typing, keystroke shortcuts can be used for frequently repeated character sequences.

## Alternative Keyboards & Pointing Devices

Most computers have detachable keyboards, which allow more freedom in workplace arrangement, but most have linear keyboard layouts (keys in straight rows) that can cause ulnar deviation of the wrist, which may contribute to the development of tendinitis or carpal tunnel syndrome in long-term keyboard users. Modeled after the typewriter, these keyboards utilize the Scholes (QWERTY) layout. A recent proposal to prevent wrist deviation and such problems as carpal tunnel syndrome and tendinitis is to arrange the keyboard in a V shape so that the keys operated by each hand are in rows perpendicular to the long axis of each forearm.

To prevent radial deviation of the right wrist, for clerks who work mostly with numbers, the keyboard should include a 10-key numeric keypad arranged in adding-machine format on the right side of the alphabetic keys. The keypad may be part of the primary keyboard or may be on a separate keyboard off to the side but directly in front of the numeric shoulder. The keypad saves the clerk from having to reach a single row of numbers on the top row of a standard keyboard.

New keyboard designs that split the keyboard in half can reduce wrist ulnar deviation and full forearm pronation. Whether these designs prevent musculoskeletal problems in the arms and hands is currently unknown. In addition, keyboards vary in the "feel" of their keys, and the "feel" may influence the comfort and productivity of computer operators. As with chairs, it is suggested that employees evaluate the different keyboards while performing their usual tasks for at least one week. A systematic evaluation by a group of employees can be used to identify an appropriate set of keyboards for use at the company.

Similar evaluations may be valuable for pointing devices. In some workplaces, such as engineering

CAD work and graphics work, pointing devices are used more than the keyboard. There are a number of different types and styles of pointing devices: mice, trackballs, touch pads, short sticks, joysticks, etc. Devices that are comfortable and efficient to use can be identified by a systematic evaluation by employees. Many computer users will benefit from using the pointing device with the left hand, or alternating between the right and left hands.

If frequent telephone calls must be placed while using the keyboard, a 10-key telephone keypad should also be included. However, since the adding machine layout differs from the telephone layout, the keypad chosen will probably depend on the relative frequency of data entry and telephone calls, operator preference, and other factors.

### Task Variations & the Role of Exercises

Designing alternative tasks that can be performed every 20–60 minutes of computer use can help break up static postures. These can be short tasks (eg, retrieving printouts, getting new hard copy, returning reports, or performing other work) that involve a few minutes of walking or standing. It may be necessary to use a timer or reminder software to remind the operator to get up out of the chair.

Exercises designed specifically to relieve physical stress and strain and to be conducted at the workstation may be helpful in reducing musculoskeletal discomfort. Specific exercises chosen for a given work area should be based on removing the static postures and using muscles opposing those required to do the tasks. General guidelines based on a report by Sauter include the following:

(1) Exercises should be designed to relieve stress associated with awkward postures, highly repetitive tasks, and sedentary work or static effort.

(2) Exercises should target musculoskeletal stress in the upper and lower extremities, the shoulder girdle, the neck, and the lumbar and thoracic regions of the back.

(3) Exercises should be designed to be performed at the workstation. They should not be so conspicuous that they call attention to the worker or cause embarrassment, nor should they significantly disrupt task performance.

(4) Exercises should be performed during the times the musculoskeletal stress builds up, so that stress relief is timely and continuing. It is better to have many short exercise breaks than to have a few longer breaks; a scattering of micropauses as short as 90–120 seconds is considered healthy. If exercises are performed only at the beginning of the day or at lunchtime, there can be considerable stress buildup before relief.

(5) Exercises should not present any obvious biomechanical or safety hazards. In the absence of musculoskeletal disease, there should be no contraindications.

## CONTROLLING RISK FACTORS FOR UPPER EXTREMITY DISORDERS

Epidemiologic studies have identified risk factors associated with upper extremity musculoskeletal disorders, such as tendinitis, carpal tunnel syndrome, and neck tension syndrome. These risk factors apply to all workplaces that involve sustained hand/arm postures or repeated hand/arm motions, from assembly and packaging work to working with hand tools. The risk factors are:

- Sustained or repeated hand force
- Sustained awkward postures
- Rapid, repeated motions
- Contact stress
- Vibration

### Reduce Hand Force

The repeated application of high grip force to hold material or to grip power tools has been associated with tendon disorders of the forearm, muscle fatigue, and carpal tunnel syndrome. A classic example of a high-risk task is the sustained grip maintained by meat packers to a wet and slippery knife. Sustained or repeated pinch grip puts tendons at even greater risk than a power grip because the tendon generated in the tendons is 2–5 times higher than the force applied at the fingertips. Tasks and tools can be redesigned to reduce the force required to perform the tasks and to reduce the duration that force is applied during the task cycle.

The use of tools or parts that weigh more than 9 lb/4 kg can be modified to reduce sustained loading by suspending tools on mechanical arms or counterbalances. Parts can be held by jigs, so that the nondominant hand is not applying a constant grip force. Assembling parts with screws is usually performed with in-line drivers—the high force required to hold the driver when the screw seizes can be reduced by using a driver adjusted to the proper torque, antitorque clutches or bars, or screws appropriate for the task.

### Reduce Sustained Awkward Postures

Tasks, tools, and workstations should be designed to prevent sustained awkward postures. There is nothing wrong with moving joints through their full range of motion at work. Here, we are concerned primarily with awkward postures that are sustained over several hours or throughout the workday. Working with the hands above shoulder height for long periods can lead to shoulder, upper back, and neck musculoskeletal disorders. Some examples of work involving sustained awkward shoulder postures are electrical or plumbing work, automobile assembly and repair, and mail sorting. Other upper extremity structures can be similarly affected by long periods of work in non-neutral postures. Specifically, work should be designed to prevent sustained:

- Neck flexion or rotation
- Shoulder abduction or flexion
- Shoulder elevation
- Elbow flexion
- Wrist extension or flexion
- Wrist ulnar or radial deviation
- Finger extension
- Wide finger reach.

Awkward postures occur as a result of the worker's anthropometry with the hand locations of the task or the visual target. Nearby machinery or material may get in the way of legs or arms, increasing reach distances. In general, the operation point (the primary hand location for work) should be between waist and shoulder height. The operating point should be in the lower area of this envelope if the materials or tools handled are heavy or if the hands have to be held in one area for a long period.

## Reduce Rapid, Repeated Motions

Tasks which require rapid hand and shoulder movements or movements that are repeated every few seconds throughout the day have been associated with tendon disorders. Exposures to these tasks can be controlled by limiting the number of hours per day that an employee performs these movements or by rotating employees between different tasks so that the same muscle-tendon-bone unit is not loaded all day.

Consideration should also be given to redesigning the task so that the distance moved is minimized, thereby reducing the speed necessary to complete the task. Experienced workers know how to perform these tasks with smooth motions that reduce wasted energy and sudden impacts. Therefore, the experienced workers should be involved in teaching new hires the best work techniques.

## Reduce Contact Stress

Sharp or hard surfaces and edges may make convenient sites to rest the arm, but they can put pressure on tendons, nerves, bones, or bursa and lead to sore spots. If support surfaces are necessary (eg, supporting arms during prolonged microscope use), they should be rounded and padded to minimize the risk of contact stress and located so that they do not apply pressure over sensitive tissues.

## Avoid Use of the Hand as a Tool

The palm of the hand should never be used as a hammer. Even frequent light tapping with the heel of the hand can cause injury to the nerves, arteries, hand, and wrist (eg, hypothenar hammer syndrome). In addition, the shock waves may travel up the arm to the elbow and shoulder, causing additional physical problems. In assembly work, for example, the palm of the hand has been used for hitting electrical parts to tighten them after inserting and for hitting cabinet doors to align them after assembly. A mallet should be used instead.

## Effect of Vibrating Hand Tools

Vibration of the hand and arm for extended periods, as occurs in the operation of hand power tools such as hand saws, riveting hammers, sanders, pneumatic drills, and grinders, may be a continuing source of pain and physical trauma. While not all workers exposed to vibratory hand tools experience trauma, some develop vibration-induced whitefinger disease. In this disease, constriction of the blood vessels leads to a reduction in blood flow to the fingers and hand and causes them to blanch, tingle, and feel numb. Such vascular attacks seem to be exacerbated by cold working conditions. Workers afflicted with whitefinger disease have reduced blood flow to the skin and reduced skin temperature even when no longer working with vibratory tools, and they may also have a decrease in touch sensitivity, fine finger dexterity, and grip strength. Although the disease usually is not debilitating, advanced cases have led to gangrene of the fingertips. Diagnosis, prevention, and treatment of vibration-induced whitefinger disease are discussed in Chapter 12.

Other conditions linked to the use of vibratory hand tools include neuritis and decalcification and cysts of the radial and ulnar bones.

## Proper Design of Tool Handles

To avoid tissue compression stress in the hands, tool handles should be designed so that the force-bearing area is as large as practicable and there are no sharp corners or edges. This means that handles should be either round or oval. A compressible gripping surface is best, but handles should at least have a high coefficient of friction in order to reduce hand-gripping forces needed for tool control. Pinch points should be eliminated or guarded.

Rigid, form-fitting handles with grooves for each finger usually do not improve the grip function unless they are sized to the individual's hand. Form-fitting handles, which presumably are designed for the hand of a worker in the 50th percentile, will spread the fingers of a small (5th percentile) hand too far apart for efficient gripping and will cause uncomfortable ridges under the fingers of a large (95th percentile) hand. If finger grooves are on both handles of a tool held in one hand (eg, grass trimmers), the handle that fits into the palm of the hand causes added discomfort because of the ridges between the grooves.

Many power tools (eg, drills, sanders, and chain saws) are operated and controlled with two hands, and there is generally a primary handle with a trigger to provide for gripping by the dominant hand. If there is a secondary, stabilizing handle, it should be adjustable to either side of the tool to permit use by either left-handed or right-handed people. It will also have the added advantage of permitting the user to change the trigger hand from time to time to reduce fatigue.

Excessive use of a single finger for operating triggers on hand tools causes local fatigue and may result in a condition called "trigger finger." Triggers can be designed to be operated by several fingers or by a switch triggered by the foot. Locking buttons can reduce sustained loading.

## BIOMECHANICS OF LIFTING, PUSHING, & PULLING

Although a detailed biomechanical analysis of lifting, pushing, and pulling is beyond the scope of this chapter, some principles of these movements are included here to illustrate basic muscular activity of the body and suggest ways to prevent injuries.

### Principles of Lifting

Figure 6–5 illustrates the forces on the base of the spine (L5/S1) that result from two different methods of lifting a load of 150 N (approximately 15 kg or 34 lbs; 1 lb force = 4.44 N). When the lifting is done with the legs relatively straight (lifting in a stooped position), there is an L5/S1 shear force of 500 N and a spinal compression force of 1800 N. When the lifting is done with the knees bent (lifting in a squatting position, or "lifting with the legs"), the L5/S1 shear force is only 340 N, but the spinal compression force is 2700 N. This assumes that the load is too bulky to fit between the knees, as is often the case in practice. A commonly repeated safety rule is to "lift with the legs" and keep the load close to the body, but a deep squat often makes it difficult, if not impossible, to do both. In the example illustrated in Figure 6–5, the horizontal distance (H) from the spine to the center

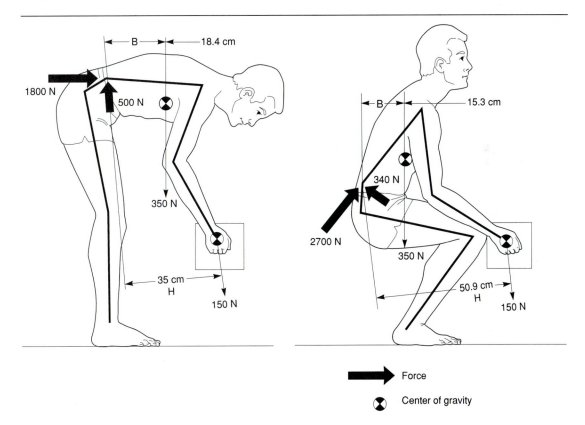

**Figure 6–5.** Forces on the base of the spine (L5/S1 forces) that result from two different methods of lifting a load weighing 150 N. When the lifting is done with the legs relatively straight, there is an L5/S1 shear force of 500 N and a spinal compression force of 1800 N. When the lifting is done with the knees bent, the L5/S1 shear force is only 340 N, but the spinal compression force is 2700 N. B = horizontal distance from the L5/S1 joint to the body's center of gravity; H = horizontal distance from the L5/S1 joint to the load's center of gravity. (Adapted from Park and Chaffin, 1974. Modified and reproduced, with permission, from Chaffin BD, Andersson GB: *Occupational Biomechanics*. Wiley, 1991.)

of gravity of the load is longer in the squatting position than it is with a stooped lift. This causes the load to exert more torque on the spine, increasing the compressive force on the lower lumbar disks. Also, workers avoid deep squats when lifting because squatting takes more time, requires more energy, and often results in poor balance. Optimal lifting styles (Figure 6–6) are those that:

- Allow the load to be kept as close as possible to the spine
- Offer a broad base of support for good balance
- Allow the worker to see ahead and avoid obstacles
- Allow the worker to retain a comfortable position ("neutral posture") of the spine, avoiding extremes of bending or twisting.

If possible, twisting should be avoided by turning the shoulders and hips together, as a unit.

## Principles of Pushing & Pulling

The forces involved in pushing and pulling loads are illustrated in Figure 6–7. As is shown, pulling a load causes more strain on the lower back than pushing a load. Pulling with a force of 80 lbs/350 N (the weight of the cart times its coefficient of rolling friction) at a height of 66 cm (26.4 in) above the floor causes a compression force on the lower spine of about 8000 N, which is substantially above the highest value (6400 N) that most workers can tolerate without injury.

The following are general guidelines to prevent injuries when pushing or pulling heavy loads: (1) Make certain that the area ahead of the load is level and clear of obstacles. If it is not level, some system of braking should be available. (2) Push the load, rather than pull it. This will reduce spinal stress, and in most cases will improve the visibility ahead. (3) Wear shoes that provide good foot traction. The coefficient of friction between the floor and the sole of

---

- Test the load; get help if needed.
- Plan the lift and the path you will take.
- Keep the load as close to the body as possible.

- Pivot and move your feet with a broad base of support to avoid twisting.
- Try to keep your movements smooth and coordinated.
- Keep the back in a straight line from "head to tail."

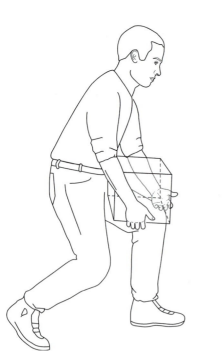
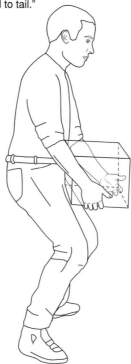
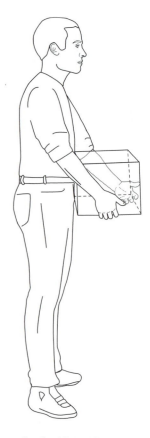

**Figure 6–6.** With good lifting technique, the spine is kept stable even when it must be tilted forward.

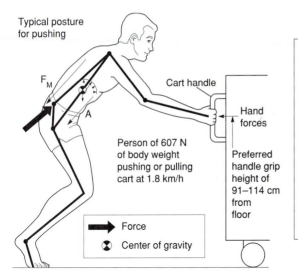

Typical posture for pushing

$F_M$

A

Person of 607 N of body weight pushing or pulling cart at 1.8 km/h

Cart handle

Hand forces

Preferred handle grip height of 91–114 cm from floor

➡ Force

⊗ Center of gravity

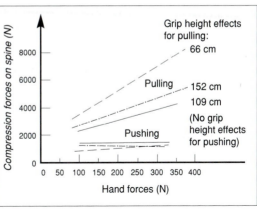

Grip height effects for pulling:

66 cm

Pulling

152 cm

109 cm

(No grip height effects for pushing)

Pushing

Compression forces on spine (N)

Hand forces (N)

**Figure 6–7.** Forces involved in pushing and pulling loads. Pulling a force of 350 N (the weight of the cart times its coefficient of rolling friction) at a height of 66 cm above the floor causes a compression force on the lower spine of about 8000 N, which is substantially above the highest value (6400 N) that most workers can tolerate without injury. (Adapted from Lee, 1982. Modified and reproduced, with permission, from Chaffin BD, Andersson GB: *Occupational Biomechanics.* Wiley, 1991.)

the shoes should be at least 0.8 wherever heavy loads are moved. (4) When starting to push a load, brace the rear foot and shift the body weight forward. If the load does not start to move when a reasonable amount of force is applied, get help from a coworker or use a powered vehicle. (5) Pushing or pulling is easier when the handles of the loaded cart are at about hip height (91–114 cm, or about 36–47 in, for men) than when they are at shoulder height or above. Handles lower than the hips are awkward and unsafe to use. Two vertical handles, or two sets of handles at different heights, allow workers of different stature to grasp the load at optimal points.

## EVALUATING LIFTING TASKS

Jobs in which lifting (as opposed to pushing, pulling, or carrying) is the predominant activity can be analyzed by using the Revised NIOSH Lifting Equation, published in 1993 by the National Institute for Occupational Safety and Health. It considers that a person's ability to lift may be limited by either biomechanical or metabolic factors. That is, the limiting factor may be the resultant forces on the body (biomechanical) or the energy expenditure (endurance) demanded by repeated lifting.

The NIOSH guidelines aim to provide recommended weight limits (RWL) that are protective of at least 75% of working women and 99% of working men (Figure 6–8). Even lifts falling within the RWL may exceed the capabilities of some workers, espe-

cially older women. The 1991 lifting guidelines are restricted to lifting that is:

- A two-handed lift of a stable (nonshifting) load
- Performed in a smooth manner
- Of objects no wider than 30 inches
- In an unrestricted posture
- With good traction underfoot
- With no extreme temperatures

In situations in which the NIOSH guidelines are applicable, it provides a ratio called the lifting index. The lifting index (LI), calculated by taking the actual weight lifted (AWL) divided by the RWL, provides a simple ratio to determine if a specific lift is within the NIOSH guidelines. An LI of 0–1.0 is considered within the guidelines.

**LI = AWL/RWL**

**RWL = Load Constant × HM × VM × DM × AM × FM × CM**

The NIOSH formula considers that the following factors reduce a worker's ability to lift. Each of these "modifiers" is a number between 0 and 1 that, when entered into a mathematical formula, reduces the lifting weight which is acceptable under the guidelines. An example of dimensions used in the formula is presented in Figure 6–9.

Horizontal Modifier: This factor, HM, considers the leverage exerted by the load being lifted from the fulcrum, the L5–S1 disk, to the center of gravity of

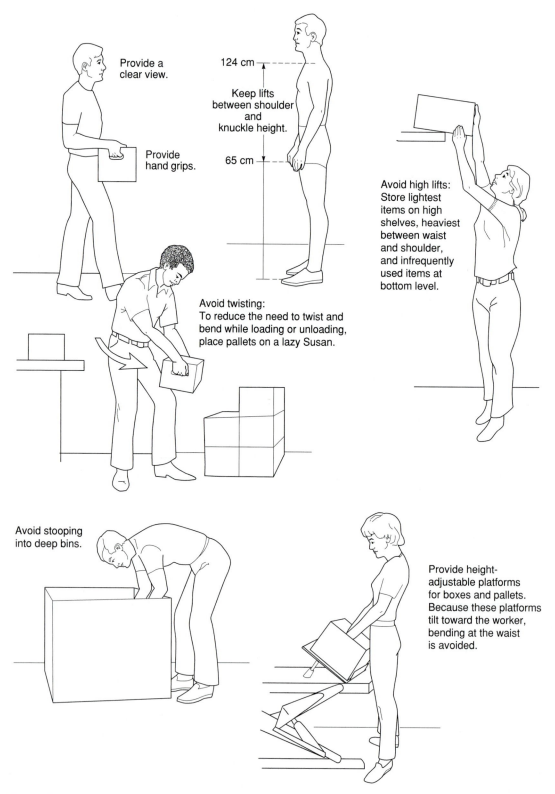

**Figure 6–8.** Suggestions for safe lifting. (Modified and reproduced, with permission, from Webb RD: *Industrial Ergonomics.* Industrial Accident Prevention Association, 1982.)

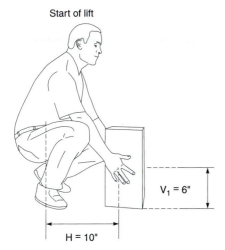

Start of lift

$V_1 = 6"$

H = 10"

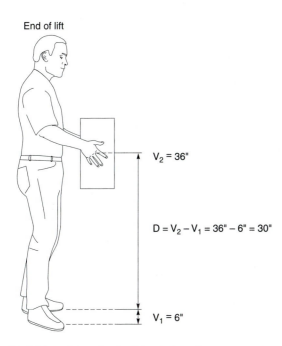

End of lift

$V_2 = 36"$

$D = V_2 - V_1 = 36" - 6" = 30"$

$V_1 = 6"$

**Figure 6–9.** Example of a lifting task and measurements used in the lifting model. The origin of H is taken from the point halfway between the ankles. H = horizontal modifier; V = vertical modifier; D = distance modifier (in this case, D = 30 in).

the load. For ease of measurement, HM is approximated by the midpoint of a line between the ankles and the location of the hand hold. It should be determined at both the origin and destination of the lift. Higher horizontal distances, of course, reduce the weight that would be safe to lift.

Vertical Modifier: This factor, VM, takes into account the amount of forward or backward bending

necessary to originate the lift. Lifts that originate below or above knuckle height (30 in [76 cm] from the floor for the average person) are more difficult, so the recommended weight would be reduced accordingly.

Distance Modifier: DM represents the vertical travel distance from the origin to the destination of a lift. Higher travel distances increase both the biomechanical and metabolic loads of the lift.

Asymmetry Modifier: This factor, AM, takes into account the twisting of the body needed to grasp the object, up to a maximum of 135 degrees of rotation. The greater the amount of twisting, the higher the probability of an injury. This modifier should be calculated at both the beginning and the end of the lift.

Frequency Modifier: This factor, FM, is calculated from the average frequency of the lift, in lifts per minute, and is used to take fatigue into account. See Table 6–5.

Coupling Modifier: This factor, CM, characterizes the grip as good, fair, or poor (Table 6–3). A poor coupling, for example, would result in a modifier of

**Table 6–3.** Coupling modifier table.

| | Coupling Modifier For: | |
|---|---|---|
| Couplings | V<75 cm (30 in) | V≥75 cm (30 in) |
| Good[1] | 1.00 | 1.00 |
| Fair[2] | 0.95 | 1.00 |
| Poor[3] | 0.90 | 0.90 |

[1]For containers of optimal design, such as some boxes and crates, a "good" hand-to-object coupling would be defined as handles or hand-hold cutouts of optimal design. An optimal handle design has 0.75–1.5 in (1.9–3.8 cm) diameter, ≥4.5 in (11.5 cm) length, 2 in (5 cm) clearance, cylindrical shape, and a smooth, nonslip surface. An optimal hand-hold cutout has 3 in (2.5 cm) height, 4.5 in (11.5 cm) length, semioval shape, ≥2 in (5 cm) clearance, smooth nonslip surface, and ≥0.43 in (1.1 cm) container thickness. An optimal container design has ≤16 in (40 cm) frontal length, ≤12 in (30 cm) height, and a smooth nonslip surface. For loose parts or irregular objects, which are not usually containerized, such as castings, stock, supply materials, etc, a "good" hand-to-object coupling would be defined as a comfortable grip in which the hand can be easily wrapped around the object.
[2]For containers of optimal design, a "fair," hand-to-object coupling would be defined as handles or hand-hold cutouts of less than optimal design. For containers of optimal design with no handles or hand-hold cutouts or for loose parts or irregular objects, a "fair" hand-to-object coupling is defined as a grip in which the hand can be flexed about 90°. A worker should be capable of clamping the fingers at nearly 90° under the container, such as required when lifting a cardboard box from the floor.
[3]Containers of less than optimal design with no handles or hand-hold cutouts or loose parts or irregular objects that are bulky or hard to handle. A less than optimal container has a frontal length ≥16 in (40 cm), height ≥12 in (30 cm), rough or slippery surface, sharp edges, asymmetric center of mass, and/or unstable contents; gloves are required when handling these.

**Table 6–4.** Values of factors used to compute recommended weight limits.[1]

| Modifier | U.S. Customary | Metric |
|---|---|---|
| **Load constant** | 51 lb | 23 kg |
| HM | (10/H) | (25/H) |
| VM | $(1 - [0.0075 V - 30])$ | $(1 - [0.003 V - 75])$ |
| DM | $(0.82 + [1.8/d])$ | $(0.82 + [4.5/d])$ |
| FM | From Table 6–6 | From Table 6–6 |
| AM | $(1 - 0.0032A)$ | $(1 - 0.0032A)$ |
| CM | From Table 6–3 | From Table 6–3 |

[1]Modified and reproduced from LaDou J (editor): *Occupational Health and Safety*, 2nd ed. National Safety Council, 1994.

0.90, which would reduce the acceptable weight of a lift by 10%.

The load constant represents the weight that would be acceptable under optimal conditions, and it is multiplied by each modifier to reduce it by an appropriate amount.

In United States customary and metric units, these factors are shown in Table 6–4.

The Frequency Multiplier Table (Table 6–5) divides the work duration into three categories: up to 1 hour per shift, up to 2 hours per shift, and up to 8 hours per shift. These are based on the body's ability to recover from fatigue better after short-duration tasks (less than 1 hour, and between 1 and 2 hours) than after lifting that takes place over a greater proportion of an 8-hour shift. Lifting periods of more than eight hours are beyond the scope of applicability of the equation.

Other approaches to guidelines for lifting, some of which include consideration of awkward and unusual postures, have been developed. Data published by Snook, Ayoub, and others present recommended limits for a variety of lifting, pushing, and pulling tasks, based on psychophysical testing. This involves having uninjured workers replicate a task for a few hours or days and report to the researchers what they could comfortably perform over an 8-hour shift, for a 5-day week (Table 6–6).

The University of Michigan has published two- and three-dimensional biomechanical models that are designed to make lifting, pushing, and pulling analyses easy to calculate on a personal computer. The estimated compression on the lower lumbar spine is estimated, as is the proportion of the industrial population capable of exerting a given force in a given direction. This model (and most in current use) is static and does not consider the additional force required to accelerate the object or the fatigue generated by repeating the activity over time. It is based on static strength testing of a large sample of working men and women (Table 6–7).

## Preplacement Tests

For jobs requiring strength for materials handling or other tasks, preemployment screening tests may be established to determine which applicants are likely to possess sufficient physical strength and work capacity to perform the necessary tasks without injury to themselves or others. However, any such screening tests must evaluate size, strength, and work capacity traits relevant to the tasks actually to be performed by the applicants. Otherwise, the test may be discriminatory against women or other physically

**Table 6–5.** Frequency multiplier table.

| Frequency (Lifts/min) | Frequency Modifier for Work Duration (Continuous): | | | | | |
|---|---|---|---|---|---|---|
| | ≤8 hours | | ≤2 hours | | ≤1 hour | |
| | V<75 cm (<30 in) | V≥75 cm (≥30 in) | V<75 cm (<30 in) | V≥ 75 (≥30 in) | V<75 cm (<30 in) | V≥75 cm (≥30 in) |
| 0.2 | 0.85 | 0.85 | 0.95 | 0.95 | 1.00 | 1.00 |
| 0.5 | 0.81 | 0.81 | 0.92 | 0.92 | 0.97 | 0.97 |
| 1 | 0.75 | 0.75 | 0.88 | 0.88 | 0.94 | 0.94 |
| 2 | 0.65 | 0.65 | 0.84 | 0.84 | 0.91 | 0.91 |
| 3 | 0.55 | 0.55 | 0.79 | 0.79 | 0.88 | 0.88 |
| 4 | 0.45 | 0.45 | 0.72 | 0.72 | 0.84 | 0.84 |
| 5 | 0.35 | 0.35 | 0.60 | 0.60 | 0.80 | 0.80 |
| 6 | 0.27 | 0.27 | 0.50 | 0.50 | 0.75 | 0.75 |
| 7 | 0.22 | 0.22 | 0.42 | 0.42 | 0.70 | 0.70 |
| 8 | 0.18 | 0.18 | 0.35 | 0.35 | 0.60 | 0.60 |
| 9 | 0.00 | 0.15 | 0.30 | 0.30 | 0.52 | 0.52 |
| 10 | 0.00 | 0.13 | 0.26 | 0.26 | 0.45 | 0.45 |
| 11 | 0.00 | 0.00 | 0.00 | 0.23 | 0.41 | 0.41 |
| 12 | 0.00 | 0.00 | 0.00 | 0 21 | 0 37 | 0.37 |
| 13 | 0.00 | 0.00 | 0.00 | 0.00 | 0.00 | 0.34 |
| 14 | 0.00 | 0.00 | 0.00 | 0.00 | 0.00 | 0.31 |
| 15 | 0.00 | 0.00 | 0.00 | 0.00 | 0.00 | 0.28 |
| >15 | 0.00 | 0.00 | 0.00 | 0.00 | 0.00 | 0.00 |

**Table 6–6.** Psychophysical limits for load lifting.[1]

| Height of Lift (cm) | Sagittal Plane Box Dimensions (cm) | Mean Lifting Limits[2] (N) | |
|---|---|---|---|
| | | Men | Women |
| Floor to knuckle height when erect | 30.5 | 296 | 194 |
| | 45.7 | 261 | 171 |
| | 61.0 | 236 | 152 |
| Knuckle to shoulder height when erect | 30.5 | 263 | 141 |
| | 45.7 | 233 | 129 |
| | 61.0 | 205 | 127 |
| Shoulder to reach height when erect | 30.5 | 221 | 120 |
| | 45.7 | 204 | 110 |
| | 61.0 | 195 | 112 |

[1]Reproduced, with permission, from Ayoub MM et al: Development of strength and capacity norms for manual materials handling. *Hum Factors* 1980;22:271.
[2]The values represent acceptable lifitng limits (N) based on lifting frequency of once per minute sustained for 8 hours.

small applicants. Validation studies may be conducted to establish job relevance for tests or other hiring criteria.

## Estimating Work Capacity

For workers who must expend high levels of energy (eg, materials handlers, sanitation crews, and furnace tenders), maximum work capacity is usually defined in terms of their aerobic capacity. Maximum aerobic capacity can be determined by measuring heart rate or oxygen uptake. Table 6–8 lists the maximum heart rate and oxygen uptake for men and women in average physical condition. Heart rate monitoring of employees or various models can be used to estimate the energy requirements of a job to assess the likelihood of causing excessive fatigue.

If there is ever a question about whether an observed employee is exceeding his or her maximum work capacity on a given job, attention should also be paid to modifying the task, improving the work environment, or both.

**Table 6–7.** Static strengths demonstrated by workers when lifting, pushing, and pulling with both hands on a handle placed at different locations relative to the midpoint between the ankles on the floor.[1]

| Test Description | Handle Location[2] (cm) | | Mean Strength (N)[3] | |
|---|---|---|---|---|
| | Vertical | Horizontal | Men | Women |
| Lift—legs in partial squat | 38 | 0 | 903 | 427 |
| Lift—torso stooped over | 38 | 38 | 480 | 271 |
| Lift—arms flexed | 114 | 38 | 383 | 214 |
| Lift—shoulder high and arms out | 152 | 51 | 227 | 129 |
| Lift—shoulder high and arms flexed | 152 | 38 | 529 | 240 |
| Lift—shoulder high and arms close | 152 | 25 | 538 | 285 |
| Lift—floor level, close (squat) | 15 | 25 | 890 | 547 |
| Lift—floor level, out (stoop) | 15 | 38 | 320 | 200 |
| Push down—waist level | 118 | 38 | 432 | 325 |
| Pull down—above shoulders | 178 | 33 | 605 | 449 |
| Pull in—shoulder level, arms out | 157 | 33 | 311 | 244 |
| Pull in—shoulder level, arms in | 140 | 0 | 253 | 209 |
| Push out—waist level, stand erect | 101 | 35 | 311 | 226 |
| Push out—chest level, stand erect | 124 | 25 | 303 | 214 |
| Push out—shoulder level, lean forward | 140 | 64 | 418 | 276 |

[1]Modified and reproduced, with permission, from Chaffin DB, Andersson GB: *Occupational Biomechanics,* Wiley, 1984.
[2]Handle locations are measured in midsagittal plane, vertical from the floor and horizontal from the midpoint between the ankles.
[3]1 lb. = 4.45 N.

**Table 6–8.** Maximum heart rate and oxygen uptake for men and women in average physical condition.

| Age (yr) | Heart Rate (beats/min) | | Oxygen Uptake (mL/kg/min) | |
|---|---|---|---|---|
| | Men | Women | Men | Women |
| 20–29 | 190 | 190 | 34–42 | 31–37 |
| 30–39 | 182 | 182 | 31–33 | 25–33 |
| 40–49 | 179 | 179 | 27–35 | 24–30 |
| 50–59 | 171 | 171 | 25–33 | 21–27 |
| 60–69 | 164 | 164 | 23–30 | 18–23 |

## THE ROLE OF ENVIRONMENTAL FACTORS IN OCCUPATIONAL INJURIES

The environment affects worker performance, health, and safety in a variety of ways. This discussion will focus primarily on physical aspects of the environment, although the social characteristics of the workplace (eg, isolation versus overcrowding, being undervalued versus being appreciated, organizational flexibility versus rigidity) often play a significant role in stress-related injuries. For additional information on injuries due to noise, temperature, and vibration, see Chapters 11 and 12.

### Physical Hazards

Hazards come in many forms, including unguarded moving machinery or equipment, missing or poorly designed railings to protect workers from dangerous areas, and slippery or obstructed floors. The safety and health standards prepared by the Occupational Safety and Health Administration (OSHA) outline the requirements for hazard elimination, as do most company safety regulations. Rigid and consistent enforcement of these safety standards is essential.

### Noise

Workers frequently complain that there is too much noise and that this distracts them from their jobs. Loudness is directly related to the mechanical pressure transmitted to the eardrum, although the sound frequency and other characteristics of sound determine the degrading effect it has on performance. At a given intensity, lower frequencies are more likely to produce hearing impairments while high frequencies are more apt to interfere with concentration and thought processes. The less predictable and controllable the sound, the more annoying it is.

In quiet areas, some sound (eg, soft music) may be preferable as a means of masking nearby conver-

sations that might otherwise be distracting. "White noise" (sound spread uniformly over the full hearing spectrum) is sometimes used successfully in lieu of music but is occasionally found to be objectionable.

Sound levels above 50 dB may become increasingly intrusive, objectionable, and fatiguing, depending on their frequency and predictability. Sound levels that exceed 85 dBA (as recorded on a sound level meter's A-weighted scale of frequency bands) and continue for as long as 8 hours may cause hearing loss. If noise levels routinely exceed 85 dBA, it is necessary to control the sound source or provide other means of hearing protection. Figure 6–10 shows the recommended maximum duration of human exposure to various noise levels. Workers should not be exposed to sounds above 115 dBA. Table 6–9 lists examples of the sound levels satisfying various communications needs.

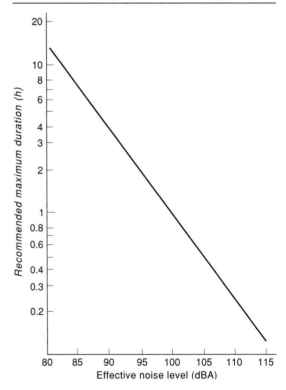

**Figure 6–10.** Recommended maximum duration of human exposure to various noise levels. Workers should not be exposed to sounds above 115 dBA. (ACGIH: Threshold Limit Values for Chemical Substances and Physical Agents in the Work Environment. American Conference of Governmental Industrial Hygienists, 1996.)

**Table 6–9.** Preferred noise criterion (PNC) curves and sound pressure levels recommended for several categories of activity.[1]

| | PNC Curve[2] | Approximate Sound Pressure Level (dBA)[3] |
|---|---|---|
| Listening to faint musical sounds or using distant microphone pickup | 10–20 | 21–30 |
| Excellent listening conditions | ≤20 | ≤30 |
| Close microphone pickup only | ≤25 | ≤34 |
| Good listening conditions | ≤35 | ≤42 |
| Sleeping, resting, relaxing | 25–40 | 34–47 |
| Conversing or listening to radio or TV | 30–40 | 38–47 |
| Moderately good listening conditions | 35–45 | 42–52 |
| Fair listening conditions | 40–50 | 47–56 |
| Moderately fair listening conditions | 45–55 | 52–61 |
| Just acceptable speech and telephone communication | 50–60 | 56–66 |
| Speech not required but no risk of hearing damage | 60–75 | 66–80 |

[1]Adapted from Beranck, Blazier, and Figwer, 1971. Modified and reproduced, with permission, from Eastman Kodak Company: *Ergonomic Design for People at Work,* vol 1. Van Nostrand Reinhold, 1983.
[2]PNC curves are used in many installations for establishing noise spectra.
[3]Voice sound frequencies are used to determine the approximate sound pressure levels. These levels are to be used only for estimates, since the overall sound pressure level does not give an indication of the spectrum.

## Lighting

See Visual Problems Due to Poor Illumination or to Glare (above) and Table 6–1.

## Temperature & Humidity

An elevated ambient temperature or humidity level increases the cardiovascular load of a materials handler, and a low temperature can substantially reduce finger flexibility and accuracy. The thermal comfort zone (Figure 6–11) is characterized by the ideal temperature and humidity conditions for work. The comfort zone is affected by a number of factors in addition to temperature and humidity. Among these are air velocity (producing a windchill effect), work load, radiant heat sources, and amount and type of clothing. In general, the body's core temperature should not vary by more than 1°C in either direction, and the above factors should be adjusted to accommodate this range.

## Vibration

With the increasing interaction between workers and mechanical tools, vibration at critical frequencies and accelerations has become an important source of injury and is associated with loss of equilibrium, nausea, Raynaud's phenomenon, and carpal tunnel syndrome. In addition, truck drivers and heavy equipment operators have a high incidence of lumbar spinal disorders, hemorrhoids, hernias, and digestive and urinary tract problems, which may be due to a combination of vibration, extended sitting, and truck loading and unloading.

The types of vibration that are of most concern to occupational health and safety analysts are those associated with operation of vehicles (eg, buses, forklifts, and heavy construction equipment) and with operation of machinery (eg, large punch presses, conveyors, and furnaces). The effect of vibration depends on its frequency, acceleration, duration, and direction (vertical or lateral) (Figure 6–12).

The lower intensities (measured by surface-mounted accelerometers) can be tolerated for longer periods without pain or injury than the high intensities can, and low-intensity vibrations of less than 1 Hz may in fact have a soothing effect.

Whole-body vertical vibration is a continuing problem for vehicle operators. The critical range of the torso's natural resonant frequency is 3–5 Hz, but discomfort can occur in the range of 2–11 Hz. Well-designed seats for bus and truck drivers will diminish the vibration in this critical frequency range by as much as 70%, but many older seats tend to have an amplification effect of as much as 20%. Moreover, the lateral acceleration intensity may be twice the vertical intensity in some buses or trucks. Visual performance is generally impaired in the range of 10–25 Hz. Truck and bus seats usually do not transmit vertical vibrations in this frequency range, but other equipment (eg, overhead cranes, lumber mill saws, and conveying machinery) may do so.

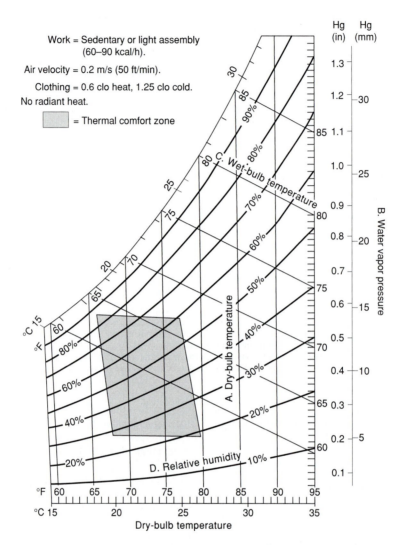

Work = Sedentary or light assembly (60–90 kcal/h).

Air velocity = 0.2 m/s (50 ft/min).

Clothing = 0.6 clo heat, 1.25 clo cold.
No radiant heat.

= Thermal comfort zone

**Figure 6–11.** Thermal comfort zone. The dry-bulb temperature and humidity combinations that are comfortable for most people doing sedentary of light work are shown as the shaded area on the psychometric chart. The dry-bulb temperature range is 19–26 °C (66–79 °F), and the relative humidity range (shown as parallel curves) is 20–85%, with 35–65% being the most common values in the comfort zone. On this chart, ambient dry-bulb temperature *(A)* is plotted on the horizontal axis and indicated as parallel vertical lines; water vapor pressure *(B)* is on the vertical axis. Wet-bulb temperatures *(C)* are shown as parallel lines with a negative slope; they intersect the dry-bulb temperature lines and relative humidity curves *(D)* on the chart. In the definition of the thermal comfort zone, assumptions were made about the work load, air velocity, radiant heat, and clothing insulation levels. These assumptions are given in the top left corner of the chart. (ACGIH: Threshold Limit Values for Chemical Substances and Physical Agents in the Work Environment. American Conference of Governmental Industrial Hygienists, 1996.)

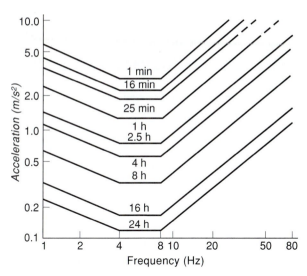

**Figure 6–12.** Maximum acceptable whole-body vertical vibration exposure times to various frequencies and accelerations. The shorter the vibration exposure, the higher the acceleration levels that can be tolerated. The least acceptable range of frequencies at all accelerations and durations of exposure is from 4 to 8 Hz. (ACGIH: Threshold Limit Values for Chemical Substances and Physical Agents in the Work Environment. American Conference of Governmental Industrial Hygienists, 1995–1996.)

## REFERENCES

Chaffin DB, Andersson GB: *Occupational Biomechanics.* John Wiley, 1991.

Corlett EN, Clark TS: *The Ergonomics of Workspaces and Machines,* 2nd ed. Taylor & Francis, 1995.

Eastman Kodak Company: *Ergonomic Design for People at Work.* Vol 1, 1983; Vol 2, 1986, Van Nostrand Reinhold.

Erdil M, Dickerson OB (editors): *Cumulative Trauma Disorders: Prevention, Evaluation and Treatment.* Van Nostrand Reinhold, 1997.

Gassett RS, Hearne B, Keelan B: Ergonomics and body mechanics in the work place. Orthop Clin North Am 1996;27(4):861.

Gordon SL, Blair SJ, Fine SJ (editors): *Repetitive Motion Disorders of the Upper Extremity.* American Academy of Orthopedic Surgeons, 1994.

*Handbook of Fundamentals. American Society of Heating, Refrigerating, and Air-Conditioning Engineers (ASHRAE),* 1989.

Janowitz IL, White AH: Preventing back injury. In: LaDou (editor): *Occupational Health and Safety,* 2nd ed. National Safety Council, 1994.

Lueder K, Noro K (editors): *Hard Facts about Soft Machines: The Ergonomics of Seating.* Taylor & Francis, 1994.

Maizlish N, Rudolph L, Dervin K, Sankaranarayan M: Surveillance and prevention of work-related carpal tunnel syndrome: An application of the sentinel events notification system for occupational risks. Am J Ind Med 1995;27(5):715.

Oxenburgh M: *Increasing Productivity and Profit Through Health and Safety.* Commerce Clearing House, 1991.

Rempel D, Harrison RJ, Barnhart S: Work-related cumulative trauma disorders of the upper extremity. JAMA 1992;267:838.

Stobbe TJ: Occupational ergonomics and injury prevention. Occup Med 1996;11(3):531.

Waters TR et al: Revised NIOSH equation for the design and evaluation of manual lifting tasks. Ergonomics 1994;36(7):749.

# 7

# Musculoskeletal Injuries

*Franklin T. Hoaglund, MD, & Nancy N. Byl, MPT, PT, PhD*

## Definitions of Common Orthopedic Conditions

The following definitions are suggested for the common occupational injuries.

**A. Strain:** A strained muscle, ligament, or tendon insertion has been pushed or pulled to its extreme by forcing the joint beyond its normal range of motion. It commonly results from lifting a heavy weight or bearing an external force—usually traction force. By definition, the symptoms of strain should resolve within a few days to a week.

**B. Sprain:** A sprain is an injury in which a ligament has been stretched so far that a few fibers within the substance of the ligament or its attachment may be torn. Reactive inflammation with associated edema and local venous and lymphatic congestion develops over hours to days. A complete tear of the ligament is sometimes called a third-degree sprain.

**C. Tendinitis:** Tendinitis is inflammation of a tendon. It may be the result of a primary inflammatory lesion, such as rheumatoid arthritis, or it may be secondary to a mechanical injury.

**D. Tenosynovitis:** Tenosynovitis is inflammation of a tendon sheath.

**E. Bursitis:** Inflammation of a bursa is know as bursitis. A common site is the subacromial bursa (the bursa between the rotator cuff and the coaracoacromial ligament).

**F. Myositis:** Myositis is inflammation of muscle. The inflammation may be primary, as in polymyositis, or secondary to mechanical injury, as when a muscle has been overstretched.

**G. Arthritis:** Arthritis is a condition in which a joint is inflamed or abnormal. Examples include post traumatic arthritis, osetoarthritis, and rheumatoid arthritis.

**H. Repetitive Strain Injures:** Repetitive strain injuries are related to cumulative trauma (primarily end range, repetitive movements which involve a forceful or a vibratory component). These cumulative traumas may lead to pain and acute or chronic inflammation of the tendon, the muscle, the capsule or the nerve. Eventual scarring and stenosis can entrap tendons, nerves and vascular tissues. Cumulative trauma may involve the extremity (commonly the hand, wrist, elbow, or shoulder) or the trunk (low back strain).

## Physical Agents & Electrotherapeutic Modalities in Physical Therapy

A variety of physical agents and electrotherapeutic modalities may be used to supplement physical therapy education, exercise, and retraining programs for patients with occupational-related musculoskeletal conditons (Table 7–1). These modalities can be paired with therapeutic exercise programs to relieve pain, increase tissue extensibility, facilitate healing or aid functional retraining. Cold is particularly beneficial to facilitate vasoconstriction after an acute injury, but it also can be used to decrease inflammation and pain after exercise. Ultrasound, high volt galvanic stimulation, diathermy, pulsed galvanic microcurrent, and electromagnetic fields can increase blood flow, facilitate the delivery of oxygen, and accelerate healing. Contrast baths and whirlpool can impact circulation and facilitate active range of motion. Iontophoresis and phonophoresis can facilitate the delivery of a topical drug such as a steroidal or a nonsteroidal anti-inflammatory agent. Transcutaneous electrical nerve stimulation may help manage pain and reduce the need for medications. Functional electrical stimulation and biofeedback can reduce the need for medications. Functional electrical stimulation and biofeedback can be used to decrease muscle tension, encourage strengthening, and restore motor control.

### INJURIES OF THE NECK

Neck problems are common among workers. For most young workers with single episodes of neck pain and stiffness, rapid recovery is expected based on the natural history of soft tissue injuries. Careful evaluation with specific treatment is appropriate. Radiographic studies are seldom helpful but should be done to rule out significant pathology and reassure the patient.

**Table 7–1.** Agents and modalities in physical therapy.

| Agent/Modality | Discussion |
|---|---|
| Diathermy and electro-magnetic fields | The use of high frequency waves from the electromagnetic spectrum to reduce pain, increase tissue flexibility, and increase blood flow to promote healing. |
| Iontophoresis | The use of electrical current to enhance the local delivery of topically applied drugs; effective when the polarity of the electrode is opposite to the polarity of the drug molecule. |
| Microcurrent neuromuscular electrical stimulation (MNES) | The use of pulsed, low intensity (less than 1 mA) galvanic current to promote healing. |
| Neuromuscular electrical muscle stimulation (NEMS) | The use of a faradic, electrical stimulation aided with voluntary contraction to facilitate the contraction of normal muscle fibers through its nerve to stimulate the muscle strengthening post surgery or post injury. Galvanic current can be used to stimulate muscle contraction directly, but is no longer recommended for treating deenervated muscles. |
| Phonophoresis | The use of ultrasound as an enhancer of topically applied drugs. |
| Traction | The use of manual or mechanical forces (including gravity) to retract the tissues, usually in a joint or in the spine to relieve pressure on a nerve and facilitate relaxation of the muscle. |
| Transcutaneous electrical nerve stimulation (TENS) | The use of milliamperage faradic current to stimulate large cutaneous receptors to counter the pain from nociceptors. This modality may decrease pain, but does not alter the underlying source of the pain. |
| Ultrasound | The use of high frequency sound waves (850 kc–3 mhz) to increase blood flow, increase oxygen availability, and increase collagen deposition. |

## Cervical Degenerative Disk Disease

Cervical degenerative disk disease is common in both men and women after age 40. The cause is unknown. The most common site of degenerative change is at C5-6, but more than one disk may be involved. In patients yougner than 40 years, pain usually occurs before radiographic changes are evident. Soft disk protrusion not seen by plain film x-ray can account for true radioculopathy, with resulting pain in the arms. Long-standing and more severe changes can eventually produce encroachment on the spinal canal and cervical myelopathy. Most people over 40 have significant degenerative changes in their cervical spine and have no symptoms.

## Clinical Findings

**A. Signs and Symptoms:** Neck pain may be first noted after a whiplash injury or after an incident in which the neck has been put in an extreme position or held flexed or extended for long periods. Onset of pain can be acute or gradual. The work history may include awkward and prolonged positions such as driving or working at a computer terminal. History of prior injury with specific statement of dates and job relationship is very important. Psychological factors such as job dissatisfaction and monotony may affect recovery from recurrent or chronic neck problems.

A common symptom is posterior neck pain or high interscapular pain after prolonged sitting with the head fixed in one position. Symptoms may be severe at night during recumbency. There is often little in the way of physical findings. Upper extremity reflexes, circulation, and sensation are usually normal. Patients demonstrate some restrictions of motion and pain with the head in extreme extension, in full flexion, in chin rotation, or in lateral flexion. Local tenderness in the posterior cervical spine is very nonspecific. It probably reflects extensor muscle overload. Upper extremity symptoms and reflex changes are infrequent but may be present.

Certain key physical findings may raise suspicion of a possible serious underlying condition of the spine. With age greater than 50 years, there is a greater potential for cancer. Unexplained weight loss, neck pain not improved with rest, fever, immunosuppression, intravenous drug use, or history of urinary infection may suggest disc space infection. Constant pain may indicate cancer, infection, symptom magnification, or drug abuse. Spinal fracture should be suspected with a history of significant trauma such as a fall from height or motor vehicle accident, prolonged use of corticosteroids or alcohol, or other substance abuse. Inflammatory arthritis of the spine can cause neck symptoms. Erythrocyte sedimentation rate is a useful laboratory test to help rule out nonmechanical sources of neck pain. A bone scan is also a useful survey test.

The remaining patients can be separated into two diagnostic categories based on location and characteristics of their symptoms.

1. The symptoms are regional or nonspecific neck problems are located in the neck, shoulder, and upper arm. Often there can be a nonspecific

headache. The neurological examination is typically normal.

2. Radicular cervical spine problems are those with significant radiation of pain or numbness into several fingers, but not the whole hand. The pattern should be along known neurologic patterns. Pain drawings and analog pain scales may be useful for baseline comparisons.

**B. Imaging:** AP/lateral x-ray of the cervical spine is indicated when serious underlying condition is suspected. It may reveal narrowing of the disk space and production of osteophytes. The most frequently affected levels are C5 and C6, but any level may be affected. Flexion-extension x-rays may be used to identify abnormal segmental motion. Patients in their 30s occasionally have symptoms before radiographic signs are present; this is especially true for patients who have sustained rear-end auto collisions. Specialized imaging studies, such as computed tomography (CT), magnetic resonance imaging (MRI), and myelography are not indicated in the early months of treatment unless there is a suspicion of serious spinal pathology which may lead to surgery or biopsy.

### Differential Diagnosis

In patients with pain limited to the interscapular area, the possibility of dorsal spine disease, tumor, or infection should be considered. The more common cause is referral from cervical strain. Bone tenderness over the dorsal spine processes should alert the examiner to the need for a dorsal spine x-ray, although this may also be referral from the cervical spine. Tumors or infection of the cervical spine can produce constant pain symptoms but are much less common. Pancoast's tumor or brachial neuritis may produce upper extremity radiculopathy, mimicking cervical pathology.

Electrophysiologic tests are utilized to identify dysfunction of a spinal nerve root or to identify a primary muscle abnormality. These tests may also differentiate entrapment problems of the brachial plexus and median and ulnar nerve, as well as the presence of neuropathy on the basis of metabolic abnormalities such as diabetes.

### Treatment

Treatment methods are the same for radicular and regional neck problems for the first month. Patients should be instructed to avoid prolonged sitting with the neck in a fixed position, extreme positions of the head or neck, and activities that bring on symptoms, such as driving, which sometimes requires sudden and extreme head movement. They should be taught to perform gentle range-of-motion exercises while at work, and as symptoms abate, to do resistance exercises.

A soft cervical collar provides rest for neck mus-

cles by supporting the head, especially late in the day, and will also limit extremes of motion. Soft collars may be of benefit in the first week of treatment, but are of no benefit longer term.

In more severe cases, cervical traction in slight flexion is helpful. A nonsteroidal anti-inflammatory drug in conjunction with heat and massage is generally useful. There is no evidence that oral corticosteroids are effective in treating acute spinal pain. Muscle relaxants and sedatives are not warranted. Occasionally, the patient needs acetaminophen with 30 mg of codeine at bedtime. There is usually no justification for the use of oral opioids beyond the first two weeks of treatment. Sleeping in an easy chair, sitting up or with the torso at a 45-degree angle, minimizes discomfort associated with turning over from the recumbent position. Pain usually subsides with time and proper rest, and gradual increase of motion of the neck.

Physical therapy in the form of heat, ultrasound, massage, etc. may reduce pain and muscle spasm, and help to restore normal range of motion. Job modifications including administrative and engineering controls (eg, job rotation, workstation adjustment) to limit work activities that might aggravate or lead to neck problems should be instituted in the workplace to promote a return to work. Traction (either manual or home pulley systems) may be of benefit in the first week of treatment for acute neck problems, but are of limited benefit longer term.

Patients with persistent radicular neck problems and continued and/or progressive neurologic deficits may require more aggressive therapeutic efforts. Further neurologic deterioration requires more definitive imaging tests with possible surgical intervention. When patients have upper extremity radiculopathy and do not respond to conservative treatment, disk excision and anterior interbody fusion should be considered. Cervical spine fusions for cervical degenerative disk disease have unpredictable results, if the specific pain generator has not been identified. Surgical care after failure of a purely passive physical therapy program has a poor prognosis.

### INJURIES OF THE SHOULDER

Pain complaints in the neck or upper thoracic spine are frequently referred to the shoulder. The comprehensive evaluation of shoulder pain includes the careful examination of the cervical and thoracic spine (Figure 7–1).

### 1. IMPINGEMENT SYNDROME OF THE SHOULDER

The term impingement syndrome has replaced more diffuse diagnostic terms such as bursitis and

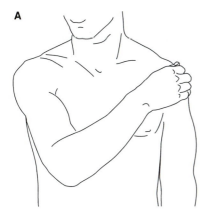

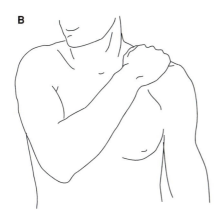

**Figure 7–1.** *A:* Patient putting opposite hand on side of pain to indicate shoulder pain. *B:* Patient identifying pain location in upper trapezius and upper interscapular area: although patients sometimes refer to this area as their shoulder, the pain is usually arising from the cervical spine.

tendinitis in the definition of shoulder pain following either repeated overuse or sudden overload. This pathology accounts for the vast majority of shoulder pain coming on spontaneously or associated with occupational stresses.

In the normal shoulder, the coracoacromial ligament crosses the supraspinatous tendon of the rotator cuff. In some individuals, when a hand is brought from the side to an overhead position in forward flexion or abduction, there may be contact pressure or impingement of the acromion and coracoacromial ligament on the rotator cuff or the intervening bursa. The pathology starts with a subacromial bursitis and may progress to an irritation of the tendon or tendonitis. Further progression leads to the beginning of ulceration of the tendon which can lead to a full thickness discontinuity or rupture of the rotator cuff. The long head of the biceps projecting across the

joint beneath the cuff to its origin on the supraglenoid tubercle may rupture. With more advanced disease, the anterior inferior aspect of the acromion develops osteophytic lipping with further encroachment on the subacromial space.

## Clinical Findings

**A. Signs and Symptoms:** The onset of anterior shoulder pain may be gradual or acute. Occasionally the onset coincides with the start of new repetitive motion work activities, especially overhead use of the shoulder. The patients are unaware of the inciting activity. The pain may be expressed generally over some aspect of the anterior shoulder. In some cases, pain is limited to the lateral arm about the deltoid insertion on the humerus. Occasionally pain is referred to the distal arm, elbow, and rarely to the hand.

All levels of pain occur including severe pain at rest due to a tense subacromial bursa. Night pain is a frequent complaint which brings the patient to medical treatment.

On physical examination patients begin to experience anterior shoulder pain when the arm is abducted at 30–40 degrees of elevation or brought above 90 degrees in a position of forward flexion. With the elbow flexed at 90 degrees, active external rotation does not usually cause discomfort. However, internal rotation (when the patient attempts to place his thumb on the opposite inferior angle of the scapula) is painful. With significant disruption of the rotator cuff, a patient may have no active elevation past 90 degrees of flexion. However, patient's can have full thickness tears of the rotator cuff without lost motion. Point tenderness anterior to the acromion over the subacromial bursa is common. Acute abduction can be improved by infiltration of local anesthetic in the subacromial area.

Post traumatic impingement syndrome may occur after a minor injury to the arm or shoulder. The self imposed immobilization of the shoulder predisposes the patient to the impingement syndrome due to imbalanced rotator cuff muscle function secondary to painful inhibition of normal balanced function.

**B. Differential Diagnosis:** Acute shoulder sepsis may mimic acute bursitis because of the comparable severity of pain. Sepsis is usually associated with systemic signs, such as an elevated sedimentation rate and white blood cell count, but is in fact quite rare. Osteoarthritis of the shoulder is also rare and may be indistinguishable from some aspect of the impingement syndrome until plain x-rays are obtained. Pain from symptomatic degenerative arthritis of a damaged acromial clavicular joint may be diagnosed or resolved by steroid injection into the joint.

**C. Imaging:** Plain x-rays include anteroposterior (AP) of the shoulder taken in internal and external rotation, an axillary and an outlet view. These may show some sclerotic change at the greater tuberosity or evidence of acromioclavicular (AC) joint degenerative arthritis. With massive disruptions of the cuff, the humeral head may be elevated in relationship to the glenoid cavity.

Rupture of the cuff will be clearly demonstrated by arthrography. Dye injected into the glenohumeral joint easily escapes into the subacromial space and is seen lateral to the greater tuberosity which indicates a cuff disruption or tear. Using MRI to determine the state of the cuff is less sensitive. However, it is not necessary to make a specific diagnosis of cuff tear if the patient gets over the pain. With progressive age there is an increasing incidence of asymptomatic, partial or full thickness cuff tear so that after age 70 most people have cuff tears.

## Treatment

The goals of treatment are to resolve the patient's pain and restore normal muscle balance around the shoulder. This can usually be accomplished with nonoperative treatment. Patients with less severe symptoms can be started on anti-inflammatory medications, pendulum exercises, and shoulder rotator cuff exercises. Pendulum exercises are performed with the individual flexing at the waist, relaxing all shoulder girdle musculature, and dangling the involved arm in a pendulum like fashion. This reduces the pressure on the impinged area and may increase the vascular supply to the tendon. Selective contraction of the internal and external rotator cuff muscles depresses the humeral head and reduces the pressure in the subacromial space. Patients are taught to do this using resistance exercises such as an elastic band (theraband), with the arm at the side, elbow flexed 90 degrees, applying force in internal and external rotation.

The fastest way to resolve impingement symptoms is to inject the subacromial space with corticosteroid and local anesthetic (eg, 40 mg of triamcinalone and 4 cc of 1% lidocaine) (Figure 7–2). This mixture is injected with a 25 degree needle directed at the point of the shoulder toward the greater tuberosity, 2.5 cm inferior to the anterior lateral quarter of the acromion. The diagnosis is made when the patient's symptoms are immediately relieved. The patients are then started on progressive resistance exercises. Ultrasound can enhance local tissue metabolism of the tendon and muscles.

Patients who respond only temporarily to the injection or who develop recurrence after two or three injections and who have participated in proper exercises may be candidates for surgery to decompress the subacromial space. The goal of the surgery is to resect the coracoacromial ligament and remove bone from the under surface of the acromion. The distal 2 cm of the clavicle is resected with acromioclavicular joint arthritis. At the time of surgery, cuff disruption can be identified and usually repaired.

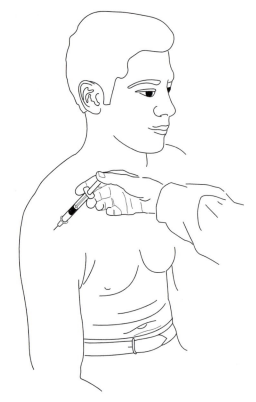

**Figure 7–2.** Lateral approach for subacromial injections. Needle should be positioned at an angle 45 degrees down and directed 45 degrees medially.

## 2. SHOULDER DISLOCATIONS

The anatomy of the shoulder contributes to the ease with which shoulder dislocations can occur. Stability of the large humeral head in the shallow 5 cm by 2.5 cm glenoid depends on shoulder capsule and specific ligament attachments to the margins of the glenoid. Excessive force applied in any direction may cause a dislocation. With forces applied to the arm held in a position of abduction, external rotation, the humeral head is driven forward tearing the anterior and middle glenohumeral ligaments and capsule from the margin of the glenoid. The humeral head is driven out anteriorly and rests in a position anterior and inferior to the glenoid. The humeral head can dislocate posteriorly rarely with automobile accidents, grand mal seizures, or electroshock therapy without proper muscle relaxation. In young people with lax ligaments and psychiatric disabilities, it may be dislocated intentionally.

## Clinical Findings

**A. Signs and Symptoms:** Acute anterior shoulder dislocation results from a specific injury and is associated with severe anterior shoulder pain.

The patients may be aware of a configurational change in the shoulder. Patients guard against shoulder motion by holding the elbow flexed with the ipsilateral forearm in the opposite hand. Any attempts at motion are associated with severe pain. Posterior dislocations are less obvious.

**B. Imaging:** AP and axillary x-rays are obtained in all suspected dislocations. Anterior dislocations will show the humeral head displaced inferiorly to the glenoid, confirming the diagnosis. In posterior dislocations the humeral head is at the same level as the glenoid. The diagnosis can be confirmed with an axillary view, which shows the humerus posterior to the glenoid. Posterior dislocations are frequently missed in initial screening x-rays.

### Treatment

Anterior and posterior dislocations are reduced by closed techniques immediately. Anterior dislocations can be reduced by various methods which include the Hippocratic maneuver. This technique involves gradual axial distraction to the arm in a position of forward flexion. Counter traction is applied to the axilla with the patient under intravenous and intraarticular analgesia medication (such as 40–l00 mg Demerol). Gentle rotation of the arm into internal rotation frequently assists reduction. Confirmatory x-rays are obtained after reduction.

Following reduction, patients are treated with a sling until symptoms subside (1–2 weeks), and then are allowed to return to their usual activities at 6–8 weeks. Three to six weeks of immobilization in internal rotation to allow the anterior capsular detachment to heal has not been successful in reducing the incidence of recurrent dislocation. Strengthening exercises for adduction and internal rotation may help stabilize the shoulder. Ten percent of patients will become recurrent dislocators necessitating shoulder surgery. Operations where there is a direct repair of the torn capsular attachment from the labrum of the glenoid anteriorly, has a high rate of success. Acute posterior dislocations usually require temporary immobilization in a position of slight abduction, shoulder extension, and external rotation to keep the humeral head reduced.

### 3. ANTERIOR SHOULDER SUBLUXATION

With a similar mechanism of force application to the abducted external rotated shoulder, a partial capsular tear, or a partial tear of the capsule glenoid attachment occurs in which the humeral head subluxes anteriorly and spontaneously reduces. The injury is usually associated with sporting activities. Some patients continue to have anterior shoulder pain with light activities or use of the arm overhead. If the patient is not responding to strengthening exercises of the shoulder internal rotators (pectoralis major and

subscapularis muscles), shoulder reconstruction, such as repair of the capsule-glenoid attachment as in the Bankhart procedure, may be required.

### 4. MULTI-DIRECTIONAL INSTABILITY

People with ligamentous laxity may have shoulder joints which easily sublux in anterior, posterior, or inferior directions. In the absence of injury, patients are asymptomatic. Following a minor injury, in which the shoulder joint is forcibly subluxed, the patients may continue to have shoulder pain with daily activities and symptoms of instability with different positions of the shoulder and arm.

Physical examination may demonstrate evidence of ligamentous laxity in the wrists, elbows, and knees. Shoulder examination will reveal laxity, and excessive translation of the humeral head anterior and posterior. Patients may demonstrate the instability voluntarily.

Treatment is directed at educating the patient to adjust to the problem, altering their lifestyle, strengthening the shoulder and delaying symptomatic activities. In some patients surgical repair is directed at correcting the dominant directional instabilities.

### 5. THORACIC OUTLET SYNDROME

Thoracic outlet syndrome is a group of symptoms and signs caused by compression of the neurovascular structures passing out of the chest, neck, and beneath the clavicle to the axilla. Cervical ribs or congenital fibrous bands, and rarely a nonunion or malunion of the clavicle, can lead to thoracic outlet compression. The condition is uncommon and the diagnosis is frequently missed. Women are more frequently affected, usually before the age of 30.

### Clinical Findings

**A. Signs and Symptoms:** Patients have pain and paresthesia radiating from the neck or shoulder, down to the forearm and fingers. They usually have difficulty with overhead activities. The hand may feel swollen or heavy. The lower trunk of the brachial plexus is more commonly involved producing signs of numbness, tingling, and weakness in the ulnar innervated intrinsic muscles. Sometimes patients also may have venous compression or arterial insufficiency from the outlet.

**B. Imaging:** Plain x-rays of the cervical spine should be studied for congenital differences such as cervical ribs and long transverse processes or even hypoplastic first ribs. Apical lordotic chest views are indicated to rule out Pancoast type tumors.

**C. Differential Diagnosis:** The diagnosis can be confused with cervical disc disease at the C7-T1 level (which is rare) that may produce a C8 radiculopathy. Compression of the ulnar nerve in the cubital tunnel or Guyon's canal can usually be distinguished by appropriate electromyographs (EMG). Provocative maneuvers such as overhead exercise or standing in the military brace position will obliterate the ipsilateral radial pulse. More importantly, one should look for the reproduction of symptoms of neural tension with specific controlled movements, eg, controlling the stretch on the brachial plexus through scapular depression, shoulder abduction (to 90 degrees), and external rotation, wrist/finger extension, followed by elbow extension with supination.

### Treatment

The initial treatment is conservative and depends on appropriate postural strength training to reduce the mechanism of thoracic outlet compression. In addition, the reduction of obesity and general physical fitness are encouraged. Overhead activities or carrying heavy loads should be minimized.

Patients should be taught that posture is a primary cause of impingement. Patients need to stand tall, using the obliques to pull the rib cage high (but without shoulder elevation), relax the scalenes and the pectoralis minor, and breathe using the diaphragm (breathing in while extending the spine and breathing out while flexing the spine). These patients should do gentle shoulder exercises, moving the trunk over the humerus to maintain full range of motion, and a gentle range of motion of the neck in the supine position. Patients must be taught to avoid stressful use of the arms, preferably using the arms while they are comfortably at the side.

Rarely patients may require surgery that may include surgical release of the anterior scalene muscles and resection of the first rib or fibrous band.

### 6. CLAVICLE FRACTURES

Clavicle fractures usually occur from a direct blow onto the shoulder and rarely from a falling on an outstretched hand. Middle third fractures are most common. Distal third fractures are infrequent.

### Clinical Findings

**A. Signs and Symptoms:** The proximal fragment of the clavicle is elevated by the action of the sternocleidomastoid; the weight of the shoulder displaces the distal fragment downward. Local swelling occurs from bleeding from the fracture site. The patient supports the involved extremity with the opposite hand. Rarely a proximal fragment can perforate the skin producing an open fracture. Plain x-rays of the clavicle are sufficient for diagnosis.

### Treatment

Immobilization of the fracture is provided by the application of a figure of eight bandage or sling and swath. It is doubtful that a figure of eight sling or even a plaster bolero will influence the fracture position. Nonunions are rare but some mild cosmetic deformity is usually present. Open reduction with internal fixation is seldom indicated and carries an increased risk of nonunion.

### 7. FRACTURES OF THE PROXIMAL HUMERUS

Isolated fractures of the proximal humerus can occur after a direct fall onto the arm or elbow.

### Clinical Findings

**A. Signs and Symptoms:** Clinical symptoms include pain experienced over the proximal shoulder region or radiating the length of the arm. Local swelling is noted on examination from bleeding at the fracture site. Dissection of the hematoma may be noted onto the anterior chest after a few days. Evaluation is with plain x-rays of the scapula and shoulder. These include an A/P radiograph of the scapula, proximal humerus, lateral scapular view. An axillary view is necessary to rule out a dislocation of the head fragment. If present, this requires reduction, usually by operative methods. Most proximal humeral fractures are minimally displaced.

### Treatment

The four part classification of proximal humeral fractures of Neer is helpful in deciding treatment. Undisplaced or minimally displaced fractures of the surgical or anatomical neck greater or lesser tuberosities can be treated by temporary immobilization. Displaced fractures of one or both tuberosities is indicative of a rotator cuff tear. Displaced fractures may require surgical treatment by open reduction and internal fixation. Four part fractures result in lost blood supply to the humeral head and may require prosthetic replacement. Instruction in early shoulder motion is required both for unfixed or operated fractures. The goal of physical therapy is to restore normal range of motion and strength around the shoulder. Patients should be progressed from active range of motion to resistive exercises beginning with isometrics and progressing to isotonic exercises.

### 8. FROZEN SHOULDER SYNDROME (Adhesive Capsulitis)

In patients with frozen shoulder syndrome, there is marked restriction of glenohumeral joint motion, presumably in response to diffuse capsular inflammation. Etiology is unknown.

### Clinical Findings

**A. Signs and Symptoms:** These patients may

be comfortable at rest, and symptoms are produced when they attempt to move the glenohumeral joint beyond that allowed by the inflammation and adhesions. All ranges of motion are limited. Loss of axial humeral rotation (internal and external rotation) with the elbow at the side is diagnostic.

## Treatment

Treatment for frozen shoulder syndrome is a short period of immobilization to accomplish complete pain relief, followed by range-of-motion exercises. Shoulder motion will recover gradually over 6–18 months. Intra-articular cortisone may be necessary for initial pain relief. Occasionally manipulation under anesthesia is used to break up the adhesions.

## 9. ACROMIOCLAVICULAR JOINT SEPARATION

Acromioclavicular joint injuries may result from falls or from direct trauma to the arm or shoulder. They are common in contact sports such as ice hockey and football.

Stability across the acromioclavicular joint is provided primarily by the conoid and trapezoid ligaments. These ligaments, which are connected to the undersurface of the clavicle, suspend the scapula in the upright position by their attachment at the base of the coracoid process. The less robust acromioclavicular ligaments and the attachments of the deltoid musculature between the clavicle and the arm provide additional stability. In minor injuries, the ligaments of the acromioclavicular joint are stretched, and with increased force the coracoacromial ligaments are injured as well. In severe injuries, the deltoid can be partially avulsed from its origin at the clavicle or acromion.

## Clinical Findings

**A. Signs and Symptoms:** These include pain and tenderness over the acromioclavicular joint and deformity of the joint.

X-rays of the injured shoulder will rule out fracture of the clavicle or proximal humerus. Displacement of the acromioclavicular joint can usually be demonstrated on an anteroposterior view of the joint. Shoulder x-rays taken with the patient holding a weight or with traction applied to the humerus are rarely necessary.

## Treatment

Treatment for most injuries consists of relieving symptoms by using a sling to immobilize the shoulder and support the weight of the arm. Patients may resume activity as comfort returns. Once the shoulder is stable in terms of decreased pain (4–6 weeks), physical therapy may be helpful for increasing strength.

If there is severe disruption of the acromioclavicular joint with detachment of the deltoid, surgery may be indicated. One repair option is the Weaver-Dunn procedure, in which the coracoacromial ligament is detached from the acromion and inserted into the distal end of the clavicle, which has been shortened by 1–2 cm. There is no urgency in deciding upon surgical reconstruction, since repair need not be done immediately. In general, the conservative and surgical approaches to treatment yield equivalent results, at least for the less severe disruptions.

## INJURIES OF THE ELBOW, WRIST, & HAND

## 1. LATERAL HUMERAL EPICONDYLITIS (Tendinitis of Common Extensor Origin, or Tennis Elbow)

Lateral humeral epicondylitis received the designation "tennis elbow" because it was a common complaint among tennis players. The lesion can occur with any type of repetitive wrist dorsiflexion activity, as may be suffered by any worker whose work calls for repeated forceful wrist extension such as in a power grasp. The pathologic process is thought to represent collagen necrosis at the attachment of the extensor carpi radialis brevis to the lateral humeral epicondyle and the extensor carpi radialis longus origin along the supracondylar line.

## Clinical Findings

Patients may have ill-defined elbow symptoms or pain radiating into the dorsal aspect of the forearm. Symptoms may occur at night and at rest, but they usually are related to activity, especially grasping or wrist dorsiflexion. There is local tenderness over the lateral humeral epicondyle or distal to it in the common extensor origin. Sometimes there is pain at the distal one-third of the humerus at the origin of the extensor carpi radialis brevis.

On clinical examination, symptoms can be reproduced by asking the patient to dorsiflex the wrist against resistance (as in grasping the back of a chair and lifting) or to apply resistance against wrist dorsiflexion (Figure 7–3). X-ray findings are normal. Tenderness at the lateral epicondyle is expected.

## Differential Diagnosis

The symptoms of radial head osteoarthritis, which is rare, can resemble those of tennis elbow. Plain films will usually distinguish the two disorders.

A fractured radial head or neck caused by falling on an outstretched hand may cause similar symptoms. The history of the injury and plain film anteroposterior and lateral x-ray views will establish the diagnosis of fracture.

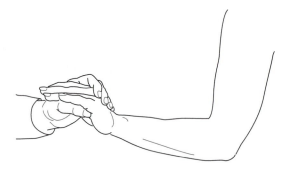

**Figure 7–3.** Physician testing dorsiflexion of the patient's wrist against resistance. Resulting lateral humeral epicondylar pain suggests tennis elbow.

## Prevention

General strengthening of elbow and forearm musculature and proper instruction in the use of hand tools and/or modification of the hand tool may prevent lateral humeral epicondylitis in workers at risk (see Chapter 6).

## Treatment

**A. General Measures:** The lesion usually heals if the harmful activity is eliminated. Patients should be instructed to avoid dorsiflexion activities and carrying heavy objects with the elbow extended (some women carry their purses in that manner). Nonsteroidal anti-inflammatory drugs are helpful, especially for patients with night pain.

**B. Specific Measures:** A 40-mg injection of triamcinolone acetonide into the most tender area of the epicondyle or common extensor origin is usually effective in relieving symptoms. Occasionally, a second injection is necessary. Complications of this treatment include fat necrosis and local skin atrophy. Loss of pigmentation (usually temporary) in darker-skinned patients may result from the injection.

Rarely is release of the common extensor origin or extensor carpi radialis brevis necessary. As patients recover from an acute episode, forearm muscle strengthening is helpful. A Velcro sleeve around the proximal forearm to minimize contraction of the extensor tendon of the extensor muscle mass, as used by some tennis players, also appears to be beneficial.

## 2. OLECRANON BURSITIS

Olecranon bursitis is irritation and swelling in pre-existing (normally occurring) bursa over the olecranon prominence. It is much more common in men, and trauma is usually a factor. Occasionally, the cause of the swelling is a low-grade infection, which must be considered prior to treatment. Swelling that develops over the olecranon process after hospitalization for any surgery may be gouty in origin.

Patients usually present with a history of gradual swelling and pain, though these symptoms may be acute after a direct blow to the olecranon process. Signs of increased warmth suggest a septic process. Sepsis can be present when symptoms are quite mild. Localized fluctuant swelling will be present with or without sepsis.

The use of a protective pad to avoid reinjury is sufficient treatment in most cases, and simple immobilization is adequate in mild cases. Aspiration and culture are indicated when sepsis is suspected. Aspiration is best performed by introducing the needle at least 2.5 cm away from the bursa and then tunneling beneath the skin before actual penetration. This technique may prevent secondary infection of a sterile bursa, which is a risk when direct penetration through overlying skin is used.

## 3. DE QUERVAIN'S TENOSYNOVITIS (First Dorsal Wrist Extensor Compartment Tenosynovitis)

De Quervain's tenosynovitis involves the first dorsal compartment of the wrist. Onset is usually associated with overuse of the thumb, as in repetitive grasping. Rarely, an aberrant or extra tendon may be present in the sheath, which normally contains the abductor pollicis longus and the extensor pollicis brevis. The tenosynovial lining will show low-grade inflammation.

### Clinical Findings

Patients in new job activities or those who engage in repetitive grasping complain of pain in an ill-defined area along the radial side of the thumb, occasionally extending as far as the interphalangeal joint. Local swelling is usually present over the lateral aspect of the distal radius and may be present in the absence of pain. When the patient grasps the fully flexed thumb into the palm and then ulnar deviates the hand at the wrist, exquisite pain develops and reproduces the patient's complaint (a positive Finkelstein test; Figure 7–4). Crepitus is frequently present over the involved tendon sheath. There are no specific laboratory or x-ray findings.

### Differential Diagnosis

Old nonunion of the navicular bone occasionally produces similar symptoms. Pain associated with osteoarthritis of the first carpometacarpal joint, which occurs in about 15% of white women over the age of 55 years, may mimic De Quervain's tenosynovitis, which occurs in younger patients. Plain film anteroposterior x-rays of the wrist will rule out carpometacarpal osteoarthritis (see below) and nonunion of the navicular bone.

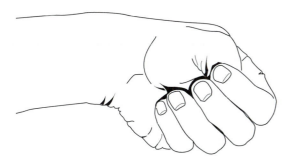

**Figure 7–4.** Finkelstein's test. With the thumb clasped in the palm as shown, the wrist is deviated toward the ulnar, producing pain over the first dorsal extensor compartment.

## Treatment

Most patients learn to limit their grasping activities, and the symptoms then resolve. Patients are instructed to decrease gripping activities and avoid unnecessary extension and abduction of the thumb. Patients who do heavy cutting as part of their job (gardeners, seamstresses, painters) are instructed to use the hand in alternate ways (eg, cutting using two hands, painting by using dorsi/palmar flexion or the wrist rather than radial deviation, and cutting by having the finger flexors and extensors open and close the scissors while leaving the thumb in a stable position. Padding to remove tension of the instrument against the tendons of the thumb may be helpful.

The standard treatment is 1 mL of lidocaine delivered locally with a 25-gauge needle to the common first dorsal extensor sheath; this is followed by 20 mg of triamcinolone acetonide. With the needle in the proper position, no resistance to injection is encountered. Immobilization of the thumb in a splint can be helpful, as are nonsteroidal anti-inflammatory drugs.

In the rare patient who does not respond to local injection, surgical decompression of the common extensor sheath by incision may be necessary. This procedure may inadvertently injure the sensory branch of the radial nerve, even when it is performed with the aid of magnification. Pain associated with a sensory branch radial nerve neuroma is at least as bad as and usually worse than the original tenosynovitis. Symptoms in the majority of patients with tenosynovitis resolve after one cortisone injection.

## 4. MEDIAL EPICONDYLITIS OR FLEXOR PRONATOR SYNDROME

Medial epicondylitis or flexor pronator syndrome is due to overuse of the finger flexors and the wrist flexors/pronators, and occurs in sportsmen such as golfers and baseball pitchers, as well as manual workers doing repetitive work with the elbow flexed.

Patients have exercise pain on the medial aspect of the elbow radiating to the forearm.

Physical findings include local tenderness over the medial epicondyle or common proximal flexor origin. The symptoms can be reproduced by resisted active wrist flexion. If symptoms are severe, the ulnar nerve can be irritated as it passes through the flexor carpi ulnaris.

Treatment is based on rest of the involved tissues and modified activity. The proximal forearm band to limit muscle contraction may be helpful. Steroid injection is useful. The need for surgical relief is rare.

## 5. CUBITAL TUNNEL SYNDROME

The ulnar nerve may be trapped, irritated, or subluxed in its anatomical course through the cubital tunnel and its entrance to the forearm through the arch of origin of the flexor carpi ulnaris. Compression of the nerve in the canal may be related to old elbow injuries with enlarging osteophytes, cubitus valgus, or a nerve that subluxes out of the groove.

### Clinical Findings

**A. Signs and Symptoms:** Patients present with aching pain in the medial aspect of the elbow and pain and recurrent paraesthesias in the distribution of the ulnar nerve into the ulnar fingers. Symptoms are frequently aggravated by position of elbow flexion or resting the elbow on a work table.

Physical examination may reveal minimal findings. There may be a Tinel's sign over the ulnar nerve in the cubital tunnel, weakness of the interossei and thumb adductor. Atrophy of these muscles is uncommon.

The differential diagnosis must exclude compression of the nerve in Guyon's canal. This diagnosis is excluded by the absence of numbness or history of numbness on the dorsum of the small finger and ulnar half of the ring finger.

### Treatment

Treatment is initially conservative and patients are taught to avoid pressure on the flexed elbow, flexion at night, or while working. Patients need to be taught the effect of elbow flexion on the ulnar nerve. When the elbow is flexed more than 90 degrees, the ulnar nerve is stretched and can sublux from the ulnar groove. While this is normal for much of the population, it does put the ulnar nerve at risk for injury. Thus, if a patient works with the elbow significantly flexed (eg, a violinist, a guitarist, or an interpreter of the deaf) it is necessary to reduce excessive flexion in non work-related activities. In particular, most people sleep in the fetal position and keep the elbow fully flexed while sleeping. It is helpful to reduce this period of flexion by making a tunnel splint (roll up a pillow and stitch it with elastic thread) and then slip the arm into the splint prior to going to bed. In addition, every effort should be made to facilitate job performance with less elbow flexion.

For patients with muscle atrophy of the inerossei and those not responding to conservative management, surgical decompression of the nerve in the canal or transposing the nerve submuscularly anteriorly, is indicated.

## 6. ANTERIOR INTEROSSEI SYNDROME

The anterior interosseus branch of the median nerve innervates the radial half of the flexor digitorum profundus, the flexor pollicis longus, and the pronator quadratus. The sydrome occurs when there is injury or compression of this nerve.

### Clinical Findings

The physical findings demonstrate the inability to pinch between the thumb and index finger. When there is involvement of the pronator teres, patients will have weakness of pronation against resistance. The diagnosis can be confirmed by EMG. Patients may present with an ill-defined pain in the anterior forearm, frequently with a history of a single strong contraction of the anterior forearm muscles resulting in subsequent motor loss.

### Treatment

Tension must be released in the involved muscles to help decrease the impingement. Forearm pronation and thumb adduction movements should be minimized. If conservative treatment is not successful, surgical decompression may be needed.

## 7. TRIGGER FINGER OR THUMB

Stenosing tenosynovitis of the flexor tendon to a finger or of the flexor pollicis longus to the thumb may produce pain when the digit or thumb is forcibly flexed or extended (Figure 7–5). Motion of the proximal interphalangeal (PIP) joint of the finger or the interphalangeal (IP) joint of the thumb produces the symptoms, which is a painful snap. This causes the joint to suddenly collapse much like a trigger.

The cause of the tenosynovitis may be repetitive finger flexion or direct trauma over the site of the stenosis on the metacarpal head. It is also associated with De Quervain's disease, carpal tunnel syndrome, and rheumatoid arthritis. The patient's work history may reveal the source of the irritation.

### Treatment

Kenalog (20 mg) with 1 cc of 1% lidocaine is directly injected into the synovial sheath at the point of greatest tenderness and is usually curative. Patients

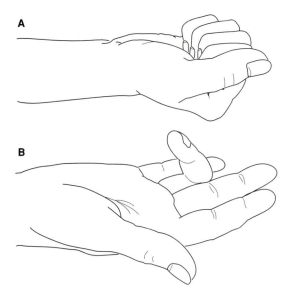

**Figure 7–5.** Trigger finger. **A:** The profundus tendons are completely flexed. **B:** An attempt at extension after flexion produces triggering or locking in flexion.

not responding or developing recurrent symptoms may require surgical release of the tendon sheath.

## 8. SCAPHOID FRACTURES

Scaphoid fractures occur in younger people from a fall on the outstretched hand. The scaphoid fractures against the unyielding anterior radiocarpal ligament. In elderly patients with osteoporosis the same mechanism of injury will produce a Colles fracture.

**A. Signs and Symptoms:** The patient complains of wrist pain which may not be localized. On physical examination there is tenderness to direct pressure over the tuberosity of the scaphoid.

**B. X-ray Diagnosis:** For any suspected carpal bone fracture or wrist sprain, three x-ray views are obtained and include a postero-anterior, lateral, and oblique x-ray (Figure 7–6). With any wrist injury subluxation of the scaphoid should be looked for in addition to scaphoid fracture or other fractures. If a scaphoid fracture is suspected and the x-rays are negative, the wrist is immobilized for 7–l0 days and repeat x-rays obtained.

### Treatment

When the scaphoid fracture is in proper alignment, treatment includes a thumb spica cast with a sugar tong extension around the elbow to limit pronation and supination. Immobilization is continued until the fracture union is definite based on x-ray examination. Most scaphoid fractures require 4 months of proper

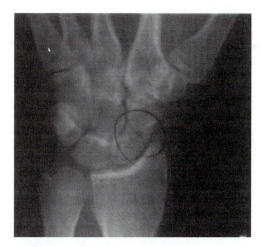

**Figure 7–6.** Fractured scaphoid in a 34-year-old man.

plaster immobilization. Open reduction and internal fixation may be necessary for some displaced scaphoid fractures. When out of the cast, the patient needs to restore sensory awareness, motor reaction time, normal range of motion, and strength of both the intrinsic and extrinsic muscles of the hand and wrist.

## 9.  NONUNION OF A SCAPHOID

Symptoms from a scaphoid nonunion may occur long after the original injury. Late onset symptoms may occur after a minimal wrist strain or reinjury. X-rays are necessary in patients with complaints of repeated wrist injury because of this possibility. If the diagnosis is made within 4 months of the original trauma, treatment by immobilization may suffice. However, surgical treatment with bone grafting is usually necessary.

## 10.  OCCUPATIONAL HAND CRAMPS

This is a repetitive injury problem that involves the loss of motor control in specific target tasks (eg, writing, keyboard work). It usually arises after a period of high rate of repetitive hand use under conditions of high cognitive drive. Pain, fatigue, or weakness from tendinitis, postural tension, or entrapment may precede the development of writer's cramp, but usually the pain has gone before the involuntary movement develops.

### Clinical Findings
**A.  Signs and Symptoms:** Patients usually will complain of an involuntary contraction of the flexors

or the extensors when they grasp a pen or place their hand on the target instrument. The hand may slowly be pulled into full flexion (of fingers and wrist) or the fingers may fly off the surface into extension. The traditional sensory and neurological examination is normal, but cortical sensory processing skills may be abnormal.

### Treatment
The most important principle of treatment is to stop doing the activity that causes the dystonia. Continued performance reinforces learning the abnormal strategy. If the patient can find a position in which the target activity can be done without the dystonia, then this position should be identified and normal performance should be encouraged. It is critical to work on reducing general tension in the affected limb, improving postural alignment with gravity.

## 11.  CARPAL TUNNEL SYNDROME

Carpal tunnel syndrome is a traumatic or pressure neuropathy of the median nerve as it passes through the carpal tunnel volar to the nine flexor tendons. The canal boundaries are the rigid transverse carpal ligament on the volar side and the carpal bones on the dorsal side.

Carpal tunnel syndrome affects patients of any age or either sex. Symptoms may appear after an injury, such as a direct blow to the dorsiflexed wrist or an injury associated with Colles' fracture. Rheumatoid arthritis, which causes inflammation in the sheath surrounding the flexor tendons, is one example of a space-occupying lesion that produces the encroachment. Rare hypothyroid patients with myxomatous tissue in this area are at risk for bilateral symptoms. While the cause of the syndrome is unknown in most cases, repetitive wrist and finger movements involved in work and hobby activities are frequently implicated. Computer operators and other workers with complaints of repeated trauma such as carpal tunnel syndrome account for most cases of occupational illness.

### Clinical Findings
In the absence of injury, patients can gradually and spontaneously develop paresthesias in the median nerve distribution (the distribution in the volar surface of the thumb and the index and long fingers). With progression of the syndrome, patients may be awakened at night with pain or paresthesia. Characteristically, they tend to stand up and massage the area or shake the wrist and fingers. Untreated carpal tunnel syndrome with progressively worsening symptoms may result in permanent damage to the median nerve with consequent persistent skin sensory deficit and thenar motor weakness.

When patients are seen early, there is no evidence of thenar atrophy, and sensation remains intact. If a blood pressure cuff on the arm is inflated midway between arterial and venous pressure, venous engorgement occurs and elicits the symptoms. Patients who hold their wrists maximally flexed will also develop symptoms (Phalen's sign). The diagnosis is confirmed by nerve conduction studies performed in an electrodiagnosis laboratory.

### Differential Diagnosis

Pain in the median nerve distribution with compression of the carpal tunnel should be distinguished from full median nerve compression. Occasionally, C6 radiculopathy from cervical disk disease may resemble this condition, but a properly performed neurologic examination should distinguish between the two.

### Treatment

Use of anti-inflammatory drugs and sometimes the use of dynamic wrist splints may minimize local inflammation. Injections of cortisone into the carpal tunnel (with care to avoid injection into the median nerve) are also helpful. Patients who fail to respond to the preceding measures may require surgical carpal tunnel release, which is a well-documented and standardized procedure.

Patients with carpal tunnel syndrome should be taught about the biomechanical causes of pressure on the median nerve. They should look at the way they use their hands in work activities (eg, excessive articulation of the fingers, excessive ulnar deviation, excessive wrist extension). Physical therapy needs to retrain the patient to use the hand with less stress.

### 12. OSTEOARTHRITIS OF THE FIRST CARPOMETACARPAL JOINT

Osteoarthritis of the first carpometacarpal (CMC) joint occurs in about 15% of women over the age of 55 years. The cause is unknown. Although the condition is frequently asymptomatic, some patients are aware of pain at the base of the thumb when grasping, as when unscrewing large glass jars, and there may be a clinical deformity of "squaring" of the base of the thumb at the carpometacarpal joint. Plain film x-rays will demonstrate the osteoarthritic changes in the joint.

The differential diagnosis includes De Quervain's tenosynovitis (see above), in which tenderness and swelling are more proximal, and old nonunions or fractures of the navicular bone. These conditions occur in younger patients and can be ruled out by plain films.

Wearing an orthosis to immobilize the thumb can minimize symptoms. Educating patients about keep-

ing the CMC joint in neutral position (eg, avoiding hyperextension at the CMC joint). Teaching the patient to stabilize the wrist by contracting the flexor/extensor carpi ulnaris when using the thumb may be helpful.

Anti-inflammatory drugs are helpful for patients who experience pain at night. For those rare patients who do not respond to conservative treatment, a surgical procedure such as an arthroplasty may be considered.

## INJURIES OF THE SPINE

Low back problems affect virtually everyone at some time during their life. Surveys indicate a yearly prevalence of symptoms in 50% of working age adults; 15–20% seek medical care. Low back problems rank high among the reasons for physician office visits and are costly in terms of medical treatment, lost productivity, and nonmonetary costs such as diminished ability to perform or enjoy usual activities. In fact, for persons under age 45, low back problems are the most common cause of disability.

Acute and subacute low back problems are defined as activity intolerance due to lower back or back-related leg symptoms of less than 3 months' duration. About 90% of patients with acute and subacute low back problems spontaneously recover activity tolerance within 1 month. The approach to a new episode in a patient with a recurrent low back problem is similar to that of an acute episode.

### Initial Assessment

Seek potentially dangerous underlying conditions. In the absence of signs of dangerous conditions, there is no need for special studies since 90% of patients will recover spontaneously within 4 weeks. If the initial onset is associated with a lot of muscle spasm, it is helpful to relax the muscles (eg, using cold or gentle stretching) and then consider heating modalities after the first 48 hours. These patients will generally recover with minimal intervention. However, they should be instructed in proper lifting techniques and back care.

Potentially serious spinal conditions, eg, tumor, infection, spinal fracture, or a major neurologic compromise such as cauda equina syndrome, are suggested by a red flag. Diagnosis and treatment guidelines for a variety of musculoskeletal injuries have been developed. A good example of a treatment guideline is: Bigos SJ et al. *Quick Reference Guide for Clinicians Number 14: Acute Low Back Problems in Adults.* US Department of Health and Human Services, Public Health Service, Agency for Health Care Policy and Research, AHCPR Publication No. 95-0643, December 1994, which is reproduced in part in Appendix B.

## 1. LOW BACK PAIN DUE TO DISK DISEASE OR INJURY
### (Spinal Degenerative Disk Disease)

Injuries to the lower lumbar intervertebral disks, preexisting degenerative disk disease, or both are responsible for many low back problems, occupational or otherwise. In the United States, a specific identifiable injury is associated with the onset of symptoms in only 15% of workers. Symptoms may begin at any age, with a peak incidence in the third or fourth decade. Over half of the population under the age of 65 have had experience with backache, with half of those having lost time from work. By 60 years of age, two-thirds of all adults have some radiographic evidence of degenerative disk disease.

Disks become increasingly less resilient with age, and degeneration may cause the posterior annulus to bulge into the spinal canal. The nucleus pulposus within the annulus may also protrude or herniate through a weakened portion of the annulus or be frankly sequestered in the spinal canal. Pressure of a disk or disk fragment on a nerve root may produce pain or sensorimotor weakness in the distribution of the nerve root. The cause of pain in the absence of direct nerve root pressure is not well understood; it may be due to inflammation in response to injury to the degenerated disk. There are free nerve endings in the posterior third of the annulus.

### Clinical Findings
**A. Signs and Symptoms:** The onset of symptoms may be gradual or sudden. Patients sometimes wake with back pain after a day of strenuous activity, or symptoms may be directly related to a specific fall or lifting incident. Pain is usually, but not always, associated with motion and may be located in the lower lumbar region, the lumbosacral angle, midline, the sacroiliac joint region, or the medial buttock. With associated radiculopathy, patients may experience leg pain independently of back pain. Pain from an S1 radiculopathy may be felt in the posterior calf and lateral border of the foot. L4 radiculopathy produces pain below the knee or in the medial part of the leg, and L5 radiculopathy produces pain in the lateral calf and dorsum of the foot or in the great toe.

Restriction of back motion, common to all patients, is demonstrated on forward bending. Sciatic scoliosis, which is a list to the opposite side of a disk protrusion, may occur. Patients with severe disk problems avoid sitting and prefer standing or recumbency because intradiskal pressure is lower in the latter two positions.

With a disk that produces radiculopathy, straight leg raising carried out passively by the examiner with the patient recumbent will cause back or leg pain, and the patient will guard against further elevation of the leg; this is considered a positive test (Figure 7–7).

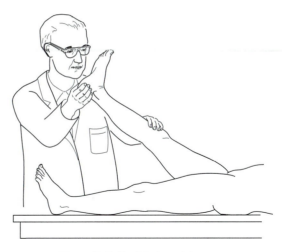

**Figure 7–7.** Straight leg raising test.

The degree of positivity is the angle of the elevated leg from the table, eg, 45 degrees. S1 radiculopathy causes decreased or absent ankle jerk or decreased sensation along either the lateral border of the foot or the lateral three toes. L4 radiculopathy, which is less common, causes decreased or absent knee jerk and/or decreased sensation in the medial surface of the leg or pretibial region. L5 radiculopathy produces weakness of dorsiflexion of the great toe, hypoesthesia on the dorsum of the foot or great toe, or both (Figure 7–8).

**Imaging:** Plain film lateral and anteroposterior x-ray views of the entire lumbar spine are obtained with the patient standing. In addition, spot anteroposterior and lateral views of the two lowest disks are obtained with the patient recumbent and are used to rule out infection, tuberculosis, tumor, or fracture. Computerized axial tomography (CAT) scan or MRI should be performed to confirm the level of the lesion prior to surgery.

### Differential Diagnosis
Almost any pathologic process involving the spine, meninges, abdomen, pelvis, or retroperitoneal area can cause low back pain. Physical examination should include evaluation for costovertebral angle tenderness, urinalysis to rule out renal disorders, abdominal examination for aneurysm, and evaluation of peripheral pulses to determine if there are vascular causes of back pain. If pyogenic infection of the disk space is suspected, gallium and technetium bone scans and an erythrocyte sedimentation rate are helpful in making this diagnosis; plain film x-rays usually show no pathologic changes during the first 2 weeks of back pain due to pyogenic sepsis. In tuberculosis of the spine, which has an insidious onset, plain films will show disk space collapse and endplate loss at the initial examination.

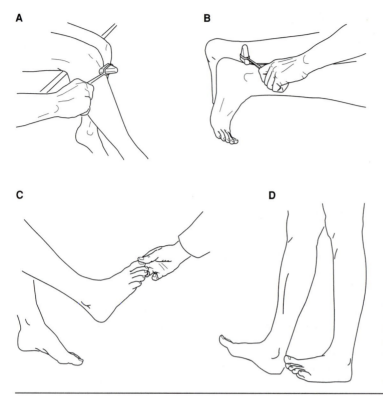

**Figure 7–8.** Reflex motor power physical examination checks L4, L5, and S1 radiculopathy. Knee jerk *(A),* ankle jerk *(B),* and big toe dorsiflexion *(C)* are shown. *D.* Patient walking on heels to demonstrate tibialis anterior motor power.

Ankylosing spondylitis (see below), which is more common in males, may start in the latter part of the second decade. Chest expansion measured at the nipple line will be less than 2 cm. Plain x-rays will show sacroiliitis or early "squaring" of the lumbar vertebral bodies.

Deposits of tumor or multiple myeloma in the pedicles of vertebral bodies usually present with an early compression fracture. Technetium bone scans will reveal the former, and immunoelectrophoresis can be used to diagnose the latter.

A large or massive disk protrusion may produce cauda equina syndrome. Symptoms include urinary retention, sphincter paralysis, and perineal numbness. Patients with suspected cauda equina syndrome should be hospitalized, studied, and treated immediately.

### Prevention

Proper instruction about prevention of symptoms of degenerative disk disease should be mandatory for all new employees, regardless of their activity level. Education about body mechanics, lifting, bending, the hazards of prolonged sitting, and the deleterious effects of lack of exercise should be emphasized (see Chapter 6). Industrial workers with any degree of low back pain should be given an opportunity for early medical evaluation to minimize progressive changes. Job activity should be designed to minimize prolonged sitting or standing and to avoid sitting while leaning forward and rotating. Employee selection using strength performance criteria may be useful (see Chapter 6). There is no evidence that preemployment x-rays are helpful to either the employer or the employee in identifying individuals who may be at risk for developing low back injuries. However, appropriate evaluation and counseling of individuals with previous back injury or surgery are valuable.

### Treatment

**A. Conservative Measures:** Symptoms in 80–90% of patients with acute low back pain or radiculopathy will resolve with conservative measures such as temporary bed rest, time, and avoidance of reinjury. Patients with severe pain should be instructed to remain in bed in the semi-Fowler position for a few days. Patients should be encouraged to be as active as possible. There is no evidence that bed rest speeds the healing process or that early gentle activity is destructive. If necessary, acetaminophen with 30 mg of codeine or a standard anti-inflammatory drug such as ibuprofen may be taken. For any patient with significant initial radiculopathy, return to full-time work should be based on resolution of symptoms. Progressive sitting as tolerated is appropriate as long as radiculopathy does not increase. For those who perform heavy labor, this prescription may be as long as 3–4 months. Strength testing should be done before return to heavy work is allowed.

Patients whose occupations involve light labor or who are self-employed and can adjust their work schedules may be allowed to work part-time and then be encouraged to be recumbent during leisure time. Initial use of a lumbosacral corset is especially helpful for those whose occupations call for prolonged sitting or driving. As symptoms resolve, corset use is gradually tapered, and patients are taught progressive exercises.

At the appropriate time, a swimming program in which the individual uses either the backstroke or the sidestroke is encouraged.

**B. Exercise:** Exercise with early mobilization in the painfree directions should be implemented as soon as possible. A stepwise program using exercise goals which are gradually increased over time is appropriate in uncomplicated cases of low back problems. All individuals should have an aerobic conditioning program integrated into their usual activities. Aerobic exercises (eg, paced walking, treadmill walking, biking [stationary or regular], and swimming) complemented with stretching exercise can begin early and can be used to increase endurance and mobility. Progressive strengthening exercises for abdominal and back muscles may promote recovery and prevent prolonged disability due to deconditioning. The focus of back exercises should be first to restore normal mobility and then restore normal strength and specific endurance in the abdominals, back extensors, spinal rotators, knee extensors, and knee flexors.

**C. Surgical Measures:** Patients with radiculopathy who fail to respond to conservative treatment (as evidenced by persistent pain and persistently positive results in the straight leg raising test or by sciatic scoliosis with evidence of disk protrusion) are candidates for surgery. Surgery may consist of percutaneous nuclectomy, or diskectomy to relieve nerve root pressure. In rare cases, spinal fusion is added to the procedure if post laminectomy instability is expected.

## 2. SPINAL STENOSIS

Spinal stenosis may be the result of congenitally short pedicles but is more frequently due to progressive degenerative disk and facet joint encroachment into the spinal canal and or neuroforamia. It may be the most common cause of leg pain in the elderly.

Disk degeneration at multiple levels with secondary hypertrophy of the ligamenta flava and facet joints causes narrowing of the thecal sac and nerve root impingement. Although involvement at more than one level is evident radiographically, patients usually present with single-root involvement. Standing and walking with the lumbar spine in extension further decrease the already compromised space in the spinal canal. With the spine flexed, as it is when seated, there is more space for the neural contents and relief of symptoms.

### Clinical Findings

**A. Signs and Symptoms:** Neurogenic claudication may be accompanied by an ill-defined pain in the lower extremity or by pain that is distributed along a specific nerve root and felt while walking. Patients may experience difficulty in standing, as when shopping or waiting in line. The symptoms are typically relieved with sitting, recumbency, or even standing with one hip and knee flexed and one foot raised on a stair or footstool.

There may be no physical findings, or there may be unilateral reflex changes affecting the involved root, such as decreased ankle jerk (S1), decreased knee jerk (L3 or L4), or decreased power in the great toe extensor (L5). In some cases, there are symmetric signs with generalized areflexia. Patients should be asked to walk to reproduce symptoms and then be reexamined for reflex changes (the Gill walk test). They may not have limitation of spine motion and usually have negative results in the straight leg raising test.

**B. Imaging:** Plain film x-rays may show scoliosis or degenerative disk changes with associated osteophytic hypertrophy of the facet joints at one or more levels. In younger patients with congenital spinal stenosis, shortening of the pedicles may be seen on lateral x-ray views of the spine; however, this shortening may best be seen on CT scans.

CT scan or MRI of the spine will show encroachment on the theca or nerve roots caused by a combination of disk degeneration, osteophytic overgrowth of the facet joints, and ligamentous hypertrophy at one or more levels. Myelography will show stenosis at one or more levels or even spinal block.

### Differential Diagnosis

Patients with degenerative disease of the spine may also have degenerative arthritis of the hips or knees. The source of groin pain upon hip motion is more likely to be the hip joint rather than lower lumbar spinal stenosis. Knee pain associated with degenerative arthritis is more localized. Vascular claudication can mimic neurogenic claudication but is associated with altered pulses and will require assessment by Doppler ultrasonography and treatment by vascular surgery. Tumors or infections of the spine may produce leg pain from radiculopathy.

Patients who have bladder or bowel dysfunction and are suspected of having cauda equina syndrome will require immediate investigation. If the diagnosis is confirmed, surgical decompression is indicated on an emergent basis.

### Treatment

Epidural corticosteroids are frequently effective

for varying periods of time. Braces that keep the spine in flexion during walking or standing may be tried but tend to further weaken the paraspinal musculature. Those who do not respond to epidural steroids after further time may require surgical decompression. Interlaminar decompression, laminectomy, foraminotomy, or facetectomy may be necessary at one or more levels. Preoperative spinal instability with spondylolisthesis or postdecompression instability must be assessed. If instability is significant, single or multiple-level spinal fusion may be necessary by the lateral transverse process fusion technique. Currently internal fixation with pedicle screws offers the best fusion rate for pre or post decompression instability.

## 3. COCCYGODYNIA

The coccyx consists of three small segments of bone with articulations between them. The segments are connected to the sacrum by the sacrococcygeal joint. A direct fall onto the coccyx or a direct blow to the area can injure any of the articulations and cause coccygodynia. Pain at the lower tip of the spine may persist if the joint is aggravated by sitting. Symptoms can be reproduced by manual palpation of or direct pressure over the coccyx. Plain films will rule out fracture.

Patients should be instructed to sit with a small pillow under the mid thighs so that the buttocks are raised from the chair. Anti-inflammatory drugs are helpful in relieving pain at night. A few patients require local anesthesia and cortisone delivered into the articulation.

## 4. SPONDYLOLYSIS AND SPONDYLOLISTHESIS

Spondylolysis, a defect in the pars interarticularis, may develop during childhood as a congenital anomaly or from an unhealed stress fracture. The defect may be familial, but most cases are associated with trauma (as when a football lineman performs a blocking maneuver and puts the spine into forceful extension). The defect may allow spondylolisthesis, or forward displacement of one vertebra on the next. In the older age group, spondylolisthesis may also result from degenerative disk disease or facet arthritis. Displacement of L5 on S1 is the most common level seen in isthmic spondylolisthesis; displacement of L4 on L5 is most common in degenerative spondylolisthesis. Individuals with backache have no greater incidence of isthmic spondylolysis and spondylolisthesis than do individuals without backache. The presence of the lesion may not necessarily be the cause of the patient's back pain.

## Clinical Findings

**A. Signs and Symptoms:** Spondylolysis and spondylolisthesis may cause symptoms similar to those of degenerative disk disease. Patients with spondylolisthesis occasionally have bilateral posterior thigh pain and may experience radiculopathy caused by irritation of the nerve root as it passes the fibrocartilaginous buildup at the pars interarticularis (most commonly, the fifth root in L5-S1 spondylolisthesis). In degenerative spondylolisthesis there is no defect in the pars interarticularis, and the leg complaints emerge from secondary spinal stenosis and neuroforaminal narrowing.

Patients may have tight hamstring muscles in both legs, as demonstrated on straight leg raising. This occurs in pars defect spondylolisthesis. Local point tenderness over the spinous process of the involved vertebrae may produce exquisite tenderness or even radiation of pain in the distribution of the fifth nerve root (doorbell sign).

**B. Imaging:** An angled anteroposterior x-ray (upshot view) of the two lowest vertebrae should demonstrate the defect in the pars interarticularis. Oblique views can also demonstrate the pars defect, but they expose the patient to a large amount of radiation. Spondylolisthesis is obvious on lateral view x-rays.

CT scans will show the pars defect (double facet sign) in spondylolysis and the elongated spinal canal in spondylolisthesis.

## Treatment

Patients with spondylolisthesis or spondylolysis may or may not have other lumbar problems. The goal is to teach these patients about good postural alignment with gravity including a posterior tilt of the spine. These patients also need to do a general spinal stabilization program and general posture exercises. The abdominal wall must be strong and the knee flexors and extensors should be strong to enable pain free and stress free lifting.

Patients with spondylolysis or spondylolisthesis should be treated with conservative measures similar to those recommended for patients with disk disease (see above). For those who do not respond to conservative treatment, surgery may be indicated. This may consist of decompression of the root, and transverse process fusion or anterior interbody fusion. For adolescent spondylolisthesis of minimal degree, lateral fusion alone is sufficient. For degenerative spondylolisthesis, the addition of internal fixation enhances the success rate.

## 5. ANKYLOSING SPONDYLITIS

Ankylosing spondylitis affects about 1% of the white population and may be more prevalent in other groups such as the southern Chinese. It is much more prevalent among males than females. About 90% of affected patients have a genetic predisposition to the disease, as evidenced by the presence of HLA-B27, and symptoms develop in one out of seven white patients who test positive for HLA-B27.

## Clinical Findings

**A. Signs and Symptoms:** Patients experience spontaneous and gradual onset of low back pain with associated restriction of spine motion. Symptoms frequently begin during the second decade and, apparently, are more frequently missed during this period. Occasionally, patients will develop a markedly stiffened spine and not remember experiencing any pain. Rarely, the disease presents like sciatica, with back and leg pain.

Restricted back motion can usually be demonstrated on forward flexion, but muscle spasm from disk disease may also do this and is more common. Even in the early stages of disease, maximal chest expansion measured at the nipple line will be less than 5 cm. Stiffening of the spine becomes more obvious as the disease progresses, and normal dorsal kyphosis increases with flattening of the lumbar region and reduction of the normal lumbar lordosis. There may be involvement of the glenohumeral joints or hip joints, and, rarely, a patient will have more peripheral joint involvement.

**B. Imaging:** On plain film x-rays of the back, the sacroiliac joints show erosions, sclerosis, and, in more advanced cases, frank bony fusion. Lateral views of the lumbar spine in the early stages show "squaring" of the vertebrae (in which the normal slight anterior concavity has been filled with new bone as a result of inflammation beneath the anterior longitudinal ligament). In later stages, the classic bony bridging, or "bamboo spine," is evident.

## Treatment

It is not possible to predict the extent of the spondylosis that will occur, but the goal of treatment must be to maintain a good spinal position with gravity and to avoid progression of thoracic kyphosis. The greatest risk of deformity is kyphosis and the exercise programs must emphasize deep breathing and spinal excursion as well as spinal extension strengthening. The patients should be taught to lay prone, as well as over a longitudinal roll to facilitate spinal extension. Treatment is aimed at relieving pain and preventing deformity. Patients should be given anti-inflammatory medication (eg, aspirin, naproxen, or Voltaren or Relafen).

A patient with a stiff, ankylosed spine who complains of pain after a fall should be considered to have a fracture until it is proved otherwise. The fracture could increase the patient's spinal deformity, usually in flexion. Common fracture locations are the dorsolumbar junction and the cervicothoracic junction. It is necessary to obtain bone scans or repeat x-rays or to take special views and immobilize the patient to protect against flexion deformity. Immobilization may involve use of a halo jacket device at the cervicothoracic junction or a brace at the dorsolumbar junction.

## INJURIES OF THE HIP

### 1. TROCHANTERIC BURSITIS

Trochanteric bursitis is an uncommon disorder which may be due to local contusion that causes bleeding into the trochanteric bursa. More commonly, however, the onset of symptoms is spontaneous. Symptoms consist of local tenderness and persistent pain with activity.

Trochanteric bursitis is often confused with hip arthritis because of referred joint pain from the latter, and sometimes low back pain. The diagnosis can be confirmed by administering an anesthetic into the trochanteric bursa.

## Treatment

Local cortisone injection is usually successful in resolving the symptoms.

### 2. OSTEONECROSIS OF THE FEMORAL HEAD

Classic osteonecrosis was described in caisson workers subjected to severe atmospheric pressure changes creating vascular blockage in the femoral head. However, standards for the rate of barometric pressure change (from data on navy divers) have been effective in eliminating pressure change as a cause. Today, osteonecrosis occurs in several groups: in patients with subcapital fractures that interrupt the blood supply; in a small number of patients taking high doses of cortisone (eg, in 1% or 2% of those who undergo renal transplantation with concurrent cortisone therapy) and, less frequently, in patients taking low doses of cortisone; in patients with asthma; in patients with lupus erythematosus; and in drug abusers. It also occurs idiopathically. An association with high alcohol consumption has been demonstrated.

One theory of pathogenesis is that a clotting abnormality or increased level of lipoprotein obstruct the small vessels of the femoral head producing an infarct. Increase in marrow pressure of the proximal femur have been documented in early osteonecrosis. As revascularization of the ischemic bone occurs, weakening of subchondral bone at the interface of viable and dead bone produces a fracture and accounts for the mechanical symptoms secondary to deformity of joint contours.

## Clinical Findings

**A. Signs and Symptoms:** The onset of pain associated with activity is usually insidious. Occasionally, a specific event (eg, putting the lower extremity in an extreme position) will precipitate pain. Infrequently, pain occurs at night. Patients limp with an antalgic gait on the affected side, and hip motion may be slightly restricted compared with a lesser involved or uninvolved opposite side. Symptoms can be elicited by movements at the extremes of hip motion—especially rotation.

Some patients with osteonecrosis have involvement of the opposite hip, the knees, or the shoulders. Involvement of both knees and shoulders may occur in the absence of hip disease.

**B. Imaging:** An anteroposterior x-ray of the pelvis in the early stages of osteonecrosis will show mottling changes in the femoral head. Findings on plain film x-rays are rarely normal. With progression of the disease, there is flattening of the femoral head (Figure 7–9). This flattening is due to settling of a quadrant of the head—because of the fracture—between the vascular and avascular bone. The cartilage, which receives its nutrients via the surface from the synovial fluid, remains normal until late and secondary osteoarthritic changes occur.

MRI may show abnormalities before they are evident on CT scans or plain films.

## Differential Diagnosis

Symptoms of osteonecrosis may be confused with those of early degenerative arthritis of the hip. The two disorders can be distinguished with plain films.

## Treatment

Partial relief of symptoms may result from use of measures such as body weight reduction, walking with

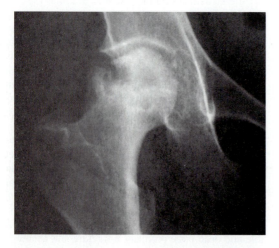

**Figure 7–9.** Advanced osteonecrosis of the femoral head.

a cane in the hand on the unaffected side, or walking with crutches. It is important to maintain normal range of motion and strength about the hip joint.

Attempts to decompress the proximal femur by early drilling and bone grafting of the femoral head and neck, which revascularizes the head and enables it to support the necrotic and compressed area, have been tried and found ineffective in all but the very early stages.

Surgical treatment is indicated in symptomatic patients in whom the weight-bearing dome of the femoral head has collapsed. At the time of surgery, it is difficult to be certain of the damage to the acetabular cartilage, which, if present, would necessitate total hip replacement. Hemiarthroplasty, cemented or uncemented, can also be used. In younger patients, realignment femoral osteotomies may be used.

The complications of hip replacement and hemiarthroplasty include loosening of the femoral or acetabular prosthesis, which is the most frequent adverse consequence, and infection on rare occasions. Sciatic or femoral nerve injury can occur rarely. Loose prostheses can be revised. An infected arthroplasty requires debridement of the prosthesis, appropriate antibiotics, and, depending on whether or not the infection has been eradicated, reinsertion of a prosthesis.

## 3. OSTEOARTHRITIS OF THE HIP

The cause of primary osteoarthritis of the hip is unknown. Secondary osteoarthritis results from mechanical stress related to deficient acetabular coverage, as in congenital hip disease, the femoral head deformity in Legg-Perthes disease, or slipping capital femoral epiphyses. The disease is unrelated to occupation, but it may be first noticed in the workplace. There is no evidence that repeated subliminal trauma to or overuse of the hip is a causative factor.

Osteoarthritis of the hip occurs in 3–8% of whites, in whom most cases are primary. It is rare among Asians and blacks. Osteoarthritis secondary to congenital hip disease is quite common among native Japanese and is more likely to be symptomatic in the fourth, fifth, and sixth decades (younger patients than in primary osteoarthritis.

The earliest pathologic changes occur in the articular cartilage, with fibrillation, fissuring, and surface cartilage loss. This is followed by the body's attempt at repair through proliferation and replication of existing chondrocytes. Low-grade inflammatory changes occur in the synovium secondarily and in response to the cartilage surface degeneration. As the disease progresses, osteophytic projections occur at the margins of the articular cartilage and the periosteum, and there is cartilage loss down to eburnated subchondral bone. This results in an incongruous relationship between the femoral head and acetabulum. Synovial and capsular thickening, occurring along with the incongruous bony relationship, contributes to restricted joint motion.

### Clinical Findings

**A. Signs and Symptoms:** Patients gradually become aware of pain with activity. The pain may be felt in the groin, proximal thigh, trochanteric region, or lateral buttock. Rarely, patients complain of pain only in the distal thigh or knee. Early in the course of the disease, patients may not be aware of a subtle hip limp (antalgic gait, or abductor lurch over the affected side). As the disease progresses, they may be awakened at night with hip pain, which is usually what causes them to seek medical evaluation.

Restricted hip motion is seen on clinical examination. The earliest loss is internal rotation, followed by loss of abduction and flexion. With long-standing symptoms, patients may have obvious thigh atrophy.

**B. Imaging:** Plain film x-rays demonstrate the characteristic changes of osteoarthritis, (ie, joint space narrowing, subchondral sclerosis, and marginal osteophytes).

### Treatment

In the early stages of the disease, an anti-inflammatory drug such as Voltaren (diclofenac sodium) (50 mg twice daily) or ibuprofen (800 mg three times daily) may provide symptomatic relief. Using a cane in the hand on the unaffected side or protecting the hip by using two crutches is beneficial. Patients who experience unrelieved pain at night or increasing symptoms will require total hip replacement.

## INJURIES OF THE KNEE, ANKLE, & FOOT

### 1. KNEE LIGAMENT INJURIES

Knee ligament injuries can result from indirect force such as a fall or misstep or from a direct blow. They are seen most commonly in young athletes who engage in contact sports, but they also occur in the workplace. The injuries range from simple strain to frank disruption in which the ligament is torn in its substance or avulsed from its bony attachment.

First-degree injury is a tear involving a few fibers of the ligament. The knee is tender on palpation but shows no instability and demonstrates no excessive motion when force is applied. Second-degree injury, which is a partial tear of the ligament, also causes no instability. Third-degree injury is a complete tear or disruption of the ligament and does result in joint instability. The different ligaments of the knee can be injured individually or in combination.

### Diagnosis

Accurate diagnosis of knee ligament injuries re-

quires considerable experience and depends on a careful history, a detailed physical examination of the joint, and special imaging techniques. Severe pain may interfere with proper physical examination, in which case MRI imaging is indicated.

The most common knee ligament injuries are to the medial collateral and anterior cruciate ligaments or some combination of the two. Lateral collateral ligament and posterior cruciate ligament injuries are less common. Plain film x-rays are obtained and are usually negative for bone injury. MRI can specify the nature and location of ligament disruption as well as provide evidence of injury to the meniscus, articular cartilage, and bone.

In addition to the usual evaluation of knee motion, and the detection of presence of ecchymosis and local swelling, the various ligaments in the knee are tested by stressing the joint in different directions. Such stress can manifest instability and indicate which ligaments are involved. Valgus and varus stresses with the knee flexed at 15 degrees test the medial and lateral collateral ligaments, respectively. Anterior cruciate stability is tested by the anterior drawer, Lachman, and pivot shift tests. The posterior drawer test is specific for the posterior cruciate ligament. Stress tests that can demonstrate opening of the joint may also be necessary. The reader is referred to Chapman's *Operative Orthopaedics* (1994) for the technique of test administration and the interpretation of test results.

### Common Types of Knee Ligament Injury

**A. Injuries of the Medial Collateral Ligament:** The most frequent mechanism of injury is indirect force that applies valgus stress to the knee. On examination, there may be evidence of local hemorrhage or effusion into the joint (Figure 7–10). Tenderness can usually be demonstrated at the site of ligamentous injury, at the site of attachment of the

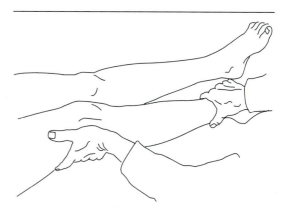

**Figure 7–10.** Collateral ligament testing for valgus stress to the knee.

ligament in the region of the medial epicondyle, or along the ligament one handbreadth below the joint line at its distal attachment on the tibia. The degree of instability can be determined by applying valgus stress to the joint in full extension and at 20 degrees of flexion. Any instability detected by opening of the medial joint space is indicative of medial collateral ligament injury. Instability noted in full extension indicates medial collateral ligament injury plus additional injury involving the anterior cruciate ligament, the posterior capsule, or both.

**B. Injuries of the Anterior Cruciate Ligament (ACL):** The mechanism of injury of the ACL is that of a force applied to a decelerating and twisting knee or sudden hyperextension. At the time of injury, patients experience a precipitable pop, followed by an effusion (bloody that arises slowly and is maximal at 24 hours). The anterior cruciate ligament is stretched over the posterior cruciate ligament or torn against the outlet of the bony intercondylar notch. The ligament is usually torn in its substance (interstitial) and rarely avulsed from either bony insertion. Anterior cruciate ligament injuries commonly accompany medial collateral ligament injuries when significant force is applied to the knee in abduction, flexion, and internal rotation. Medial menisci may be injured along with the medial collateral and anterior cruciate ligaments.

**1. Signs and Symptoms:** Physical examination reveals evidence of an intra-articular (bloody) effusion and pain with limited knee motion. Lachman's test will be positive. This involves flexing the knee 20 degrees and manually translating the leg forward (Figure 7–11). The amount of displacement will depend on whether there is a partial or complete tear and whether there is disruption of other joint capsule restraints.

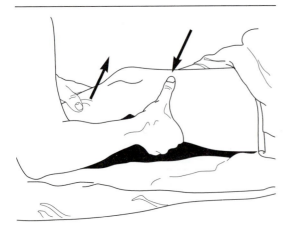

**Figure 7–11.** Lachman's test for anterior cruciate ligament insufficiency. The thigh is stabilized with a posteriorly directed force, and the tibia is subluxed anteriorly.

**2. Imaging:** An MRI can confirm specific ACL or other joint pathology.

### Treatment

First- and second-degree medial collateral injuries can be treated symptomatically with crutches and a knee immobilizer. Third-degree injuries have been effectively treated with cast immobilization or cast bracing and are rarely treated by open surgical repair. The goal of treatment for medial collateral ligament tear is to restore normal range of motion and increase the strength of the muscles around the knee, particularly the vastus medialis.

With a tear of the anterior cruciate ligament, emphasis must be placed on strengthening the hamstrings. It is desirable to restore complete range of motion as soon as possible with active exercises. The treatment protocol will vary by the type of repair and patient status prior to injury. The rehabilitative treatment including resisted knee extension is not started until the surgical repair is stable. As soon as the surgical repair is stable, eccentric and concentric training for the quadriceps and hamstrings are recommended with increasing emphasis on proprioception and dynamic balance training.

In patients who remain symptomatic with episodes of giving-way pain, swelling, or catching, arthroscopic, arthroscopic intra-articular, or open extra articular ACL repair can be done. Physical therapy is important after ACL repair.

### 2. PREPATELLAR & INFRAPATELLAR BURSITIS

Local trauma, such as that resulting from a direct blow or from kneeling repeatedly (eg, scrubbing floors), can produce prepatellar bursitis, characterized by pain, tenderness, and irritation of or bleeding into the pancake-shaped bursa overlying the patella. In no form of prepatellar bursitis is there evidence of knee joint effusion indicating intra-articular involvement.

Priests, carpenters who lay flooring, and other workers who kneel over the region of the tibial tubercle may experience similar trauma resulting in infrapatellar bursitis. Superficial infrapatellar bursitis causes diffuse swelling over the tibial tubercle and lower portion of the patellar ligament. Deep infrapatellar bursitis is dumbbell-shaped because the patellar ligament compresses its center.

The treatment of prepatellar or infrapatellar bursitis is usually symptomatic. Knee flexion and kneeling are avoided, and the knee may be splinted in extension when symptoms are severe. Occasionally, prepatellar bursitis may be septic and require diagnostic aspiration, antibiotic treatment, and surgical drainage.

## 3. CHONDROMALACIA PATELLAE

Chondromalacia patellae is characterized by fibrillation or roughening of the undersurface of the patellar articular cartilage, usually on the medial facet. It occurs much more frequently in growing females than in growing males, but it may also occur during the young adult years. The articular cartilage changes are generally nonprogressive.

Symptoms of anterior knee pain may begin spontaneously or with a direct blow to the patella. They tend to be intermittent and are not usually associated with knee joint effusion. The pain occurs with activity, is usually more severe when descending than when ascending stairs, and is relieved by rest. It can be reproduced during clinical examination by depressing the patella at the patellofemoral groove against active quadriceps contraction. Other causes of knee disorders need to be ruled out by physical examination of the knee and plain film x-rays.

For treatment of most cases of chondromalacia, patients should be instructed to do active isometric quadriceps exercises with the knee in extension and to protect the knee by avoiding kneeling, squatting, and activities that cause discomfort. An elastic patella support may be helpful. Tracking of the patella should be noted. Controlled contractions of the quadriceps with emphasis on the vastus medialis can be helpful. Symptoms are generally self-limited, lasting for just a few weeks. However, if the patella is frankly subluxing and causing articular damage at the patellofemoral joint, patellar realignment surgery may be necessary.

## 4. TEARS & INTERNAL DERANGEMENTS OF THE MENISCUS

Traumatic injury to the meniscus may occur at any age, though it occurs most commonly in young male athletes. Some meniscal injuries result from an apparent minor twisting of the lower extremity or even from sudden twisting of the knee while squatting. Injuries are much more common in the medial than in the lateral, more mobile meniscus and can range in severity from those which cause little damage and manifest relatively minor pain to those that displace the large bucket handle of the meniscus and cause frank catching and locking of the joint. The meniscus becomes stiffer with age, and symptoms may result from degenerative tears that occur in the fourth or fifth decade.

About 20% of patients with excised menisci develop radiographic changes of joint space narrowing and some progress to degenerative arthritis in the vacant compartment. Postmortem studies demonstrate that torn menisci left in place are unrelated to degenerative arthritis of the knee joint—and, conversely, that degenerative arthritis of the knee joint can occur in the absence of meniscal injury. Therefore, there is no late risk of osteoarthritis from leaving a torn but asymptomatic meniscus in place.

### Clinical Findings

Symptoms and signs of a torn meniscus include pain at the extremes of motion and local tenderness at the joint line over the involved meniscus. McMurray's sign (rotation of the tibia on the femur when moving the knee from flexion to extension) is rarely positive. Diagnosis can be confirmed by MRI and, more definitively, by arthroscopic examination.

### Treatment

After the initial pain decreases from the acute injury, active range of motion exercises should be progressed to resistance exercises. Patients who continue to manifest symptoms after a prolonged period of conservative therapy require surgery. When the tear is located peripherally, where there is vascularity and healing is possible; repair is accomplished through arthroscopy, followed by immobilization with a cast or brace. Arthroscopic debridement is performed for marginal lesions.

Because long-term osteoarthritis has been associated with total meniscal excision, this procedure should be avoided.

## 5. POPLITEAL CYST (Baker's Cyst)

A cystic swelling medial to the head of the gastrocnemius muscle in the popliteal fossa is almost always related to intra articular pathology. Osteoarthritis and meniscal disease are common causes. The cysts are the result of the overflow of synovial fluid from the knee joint.

### Signs & Symptoms

Symptoms include pain and a feeling of fullness in the popliteal fossa. Patients may not be aware of any anterior joint symptoms, ie, the torn meniscus, osteoarthritis, rheumatoid arthritis, etc. Swelling from the cyst may wax and wane along with the amount of joint fluid in the anterior knee joint.

### Treatment

Treatment is directed at the primary intra-articular problem.

## 6. PES ANSERINUS BURSITIS & TIBIAL COLLATERAL LIGAMENT BURSITIS

Bursitis can occur beneath the tibial collateral ligament or beneath pes anserinus insertion. The usual cause is kneeling or direct trauma.

Signs and symptoms include local pain and tenderness. Swelling may be minimal. The symptoms are frequently attributed to meniscal pathology since a torn meniscus produces similar symptoms. Plain radiographs are taken to rule out other bone lesions. The diagnosis can be confirmed by a local injection of 3 cc of lidocaine with 40 mg of Kenalog (triamcinolone acetonide), which may also be curative.

## 7. ANKLE SPRAINS
### (Sprains of the Lateral Collateral Ligament Complex)

The lateral collateral ligament complex of the ankle consists of seven ligaments that attach the fibula to the tibia, talus, and calcaneus. An inversion injury with or without the foot in plantar flexion may strain or sprain the anterior talofibular ligament, which is the ligament most commonly injured. When this happens, tenderness will be present, as will local swelling at either the anterior lateral neck of the talus or the tip of the fibula. A stronger external force may disrupt the posterior talofibular ligament, the calcaneofibular ligament, or the tibiofibular ligaments that account for the ligamentous stability of the ankle mortise.

### Clinical Findings
Depending on the seriousness of the injury, pain can range in severity from minimal upon weight bearing to severe enough to make walking impossible. Local swelling and tenderness will be present at the site of ligament damage. Fibular fractures or tibiofibular ligament disruptions can be ruled out with plain film x-rays. Stress films of the ankle to determine the degree of tilt of the talus can be obtained but are not usually indicated.

### Treatment
Treatment of ankle sprains usually consists of relieving the symptoms by supporting the ankle with an elastic bandage or adhesive strapping. Decreased weight bearing with crutches while maintaining a normal pattern of gait is usually successful. In more severe cases, the patient is immobilized for 4–6 weeks in a short leg walking cast. Surgery does not achieve results superior to those attained by conservative treatment.

Ligamentous injury causing disruption of the ankle mortise usually requires surgical treatment.

In rare cases, a patient will have a persistent instability that is impossible to predict at the initial evaluation. When this instability occurs, secondary end-to-end repair of the the anterior talo-fibular ligament (Brostrom procedure) may be indicated.

## 8. AVULSION FRACTURES OF THE FIFTH METATARSAL

Avulsion fractures of the tip of the fifth metatarsal are produced by inversion injuries to the foot and the ankle, usually when the ankle is flexed. They occur commonly in athletes and dancers but may also occur in anyone who, for example, steps into a hole or trips.

In contrast with ankle sprain, avulsion fracture does not cause tenderness about the fibular malleolus. Instead, it causes local tenderness and swelling over the base of the fifth metatarsal. Location of the fracture site can be confirmed by x-ray.

Treatment consists of relieving symptoms. Wearing a stiff-soled shoe, including a doughnut pad to relieve the pressure on the fracture site, is sufficient for patients whose symptoms are minimal. More severe injuries and symptoms may call for immobilization in a short leg walking cast for 4–6 weeks. Nonunion of this fracture is rare, though a true Jones fracture—a transverse fracture across the full base of the metatarsal—can result in delayed union and even nonunion.

## 9. PLANTAR FASCIITIS
### (Medial Calcaneal Tubercle Bursitis)

Pain affecting the plantar aspect of the medial heel may develop spontaneously or may occur after direct trauma to the area or after impact on the heel. Patients are comfortable at rest, but pain returns with weight bearing and is especially severe when the patient gets out of bed in the morning.

Clinical examination reveals exquisite local tenderness over the medial calcaneal tubercle, which is the site of plantar fascial attachment. Lateral x-rays usually show a spur that projects from the calcaneus and has been present for many years. This suggests that the more recent local symptoms are due to bursitis in the area or to traction on the plantar fascia.

Wearing heel cushions can minimize impact on the heel and relieve symptoms. Use of a soft heel cup or local cortisone injection is helpful, as is the use of a shoe insert, with a medial wedge that maintains the heel in a slightly varus angle and reduces traction on the plantar fascia. Ultrasound plus exercises to increase hind and mid foot inversion may be helpful. Running with the foot slightly towed-in also may be helpful.

## 10. MORTON'S NEUROMA

Morton's neuroma is usually found on the common plantar digital nerve branches to the third and fourth toes. It occurs more frequently in women. Pain is produced by direct pressure on the neuroma, which is located between the third and fourth metatarsal heads, and is aggravated by dorsiflexing the toe such as during the push-off phase of gait or when wearing high-heeled shoes. Patients frequently describe the pain as radiating into the toes.

On clinical examination, a small "click" can usually be felt as pressure is applied to the third and fourth metatarsal heads while the examiner passively dorsiflexes the toes. The click may temporarily disappear after the initial manipulation. Diagnosis can sometimes be confirmed by local nerve block.

Treatment with metatarsal bars or low-heeled, well-fitting shoes is rarely rewarding but should be tried. Surgical excision of the neuroma is frequently necessary.

## 11. OSTEOCHONDRITIS DISICCANS OF THE TALUS

Osteochondrotic lesions of the medial or lateral aspect of the dome of the talus are the result of previ-ous trauma. Symptoms include pain, swelling, and catching about the ankle. Typical findings may include signs and symptoms similar to a lateral or medial ankle sprain.

### Imaging

Standard plain x-rays of the ankle will usually identify the osteochondral defect. An MRI may be necessary for the diagnosis.

### Treatment

When osteochondral acute fractures are recognized initially these are treated by immobilization. Chronic lesions are treated expectantly with temporary mobilization and observation. Those patients not responding may require surgical treatment such as fragment excision, replacement, drilling, or bone grafting.

## REFERENCES

### INJURIES OF THE NECK

Fechter JD, Kuschner SH: The thoracic outlet syndrome. Orthopedics 1993;16(11):1243.

Koes BW et al: The effectiveness of manual therapy, physiotherapy and treatment by the general practitioner for nonspecific back and neck complaints. A randomized clinical trial. Spine 1992;17:28.

Pennie BH, Agambar LJ: Whiplash injuries. J Bone Jt Surg 1990;72B:277.

### INJURIES OF THE SHOULDER

Hawkins RJ, Bokor DJ: Clinical evaluation of shoulder problems. In: Rockwood CA, Matsen FA (editors): *The Shoulder*. Saunders, 1990.

Luck JV, Andersson GB: Occupational shoulder disorders. In: Rockwood CA, Matsen FA (editors): *The Shoulder*. Saunders, 1990.

Milgram C, Schaffler M, Gilbert S, Van Holsbeck M: Rotator cuff changes in asymptomatic adults. J Bone & Jt Surg 1995;77B:296.

Rockwood CA, Matsen FA: Muscle ruptures affecting the shoulder girdle. In Post M (editor) *The Shoulder*. Mosby-Year Book, 1990.

Rockwood CA, Lyons FR:L Shoulder impingement syndrome: diagnosis, radiographic evaluation, and treatment with a modified Neer acromioplasty. J Bone Jt Surg 1993;75A:409.

### INJURIES OF THE ELBOW, WRIST, & HAND

American Academy of Orthopedic Surgeons: Clinical policies—lateral epicondylitis of the elbow. AAOS 1–3, 1992.

Dawson DM: Entrapment neuropathies of the upper extremities. New Engl J Med 1993;329:2013.

Gupta A, Kleinert HE: Evaluating the injured hand. Hand Clinics 1993;9:195.

Hagberg M, Morgenstern H, Kelsh M: Impact of occupations and job tasks on the prevalence of carpal tunnel syndrome: A review. Scand J Work Environ & Health 1992;18:337.

Harter BT et al: Carpal tunnel syndrome: surgical and nonsurgical treatment. J Hand Surg. American Volume, 1993;18:734.

Newport ML, Lane LB, Stuchin SA: Treatment of trigger finger by steroid injection. J Hand Surg 15A:748.

Rempel DM, Harrison R, Barnhart S: Work-related cumulative trauma disorders of the upper extremity. JAMA 1992;267:838.

Thorson E, Szabo Rm: Common tendonitis problems in the hand and forearm. Orthopedic Clinics of North America 23:65.

### INJURIES OF THE SPINE

Battie MC, Bigos SJ: Industrial back pain complaints. A broader perspective. Orthopedic Clinics of North America. 1991;22:273.

Bigos S et al: Acute Low Back Problems in Adults. Clinical Practice Guideline. U.S. Department of Health and Human Services, Public Health Service, Agency for Health Care Policy and Research, AHCPR Pub. No. 95-0643. December 1994.

Deyo RA, Loeser JD, Bigos SJ: Herniated lumbar intervertebral disk. Ann Int Med 1990;112:596.

Deyo RA, Rainville J, Kent DL: What can the history and physical examination tell us about low back pain? JAMA 1992;268:760.

Indahl A, Velund L, Reikeraas O. Good prognosis for low back pain when left untampered: A randomized clinical trial, Spine 1995;20:473–477.

Lancourt J, Kettelhut M: Predicting return to work for lower back pain patients receiving workers' compensation. Spine 1992;17:629.

Lindstrom I et.al: Mobility, strength, and fitness after a graded activity program for patients with subacute low back pain. Spine 1992;17(6):641.

Malmivaara A et al: The treatment of acute low back pain-bed rest, exercises, or ordinary activity? New Engl J Med. 1995;332:351.

Mayer TG, Polatin P, Smith B, Smith C, Gatchel R, Herring SA, Hall H, Donelson RG, Dickey J, English W. Contemporary concepts in spine care: Spine rehabilitation: Secondary and tertiary nonoperative care. Spine 1995;20:2060–2066.

Mitchell RI, Carmen GM. The functional restoration approach to the treatment of chronic pain in patients with soft tissue and back injuries. Spine 1994;19: 633–642.

Nachemson AL: Newest knowledge of low back pain. A critical look. Clinical Orthopedics and Related Research. 1992 Jun 279:8.

Pope MH, Andersson GBJ, Chaffin DB: The workplace. In: Post MH et al (editors): *Occupational Low Back Pain.* Mosby-Year Book, 1991.

## INJURIES OF THE HIP

Guerra JJ: Destructive transient osteoporosis from avascular necrosis of the hip. J Bone and J Surg 1995; 77H:616.

Mont MA, Hungerford DS: Nontrochanter avascular necrosis of the femoral head. J Bone & J Surg 1995;77A:459.

## INJURIES OF THE KNEE, ANKLE, & FOOT

Crenshaw AH (editor): *Campbell's Operative Orthopedics*, 8th ed. Mosby, 1993.

Karr SD: Sub calcaneal heel pain. Ortho Clinic North America 1994;25 1:161.

Pfeffer GB, Frey C: Current Practice in foot and ankle surgery. Mc Graw-Hill, Inc. New York, 1994.

Scheck M: Miscellaneous joint disorders. In: *Operative Orthopaedics,* 2nd ed. Lippincott, 1994.

## RECOMMENDED READING

Chapman MW (editor): *Operative Orthopaedics*, 2nd ed. Lippincott, 1994.

Herington TM, Morse LH (editors): *Occupational Injuries: Evaluation, Management, and Prevention.* Mosby, 1995.

Kilbom A et al: Musculoskeletal disorders: Work-related risk factors and prevention. Int J Occup & Environ Health 1996;2(3):239.

Kuorinka I, Forcier L (editors): *Work-related Musculoskeletal Disorders: A Reference Book for Prevention.* Taylor & Francis, 1995.

# Peripheral Nerve Injuries

# 8

*Yuen So, MD, PhD*

Dysfunction of sensory, motor, or autonomic nerve fibers leads to a **peripheral neuropathy**. The term encompasses a wide spectrum of clinical disorders associated with a large number of possible causes. Clinically important diseases include nerve trauma, nerve entrapment, genetic disorders, nerve ischemia and infarction, inflammatory neuropathies, and neuropathies associated with systemic diseases such as diabetes, alcoholism, uremia, and hypothyroidism.

Occupational exposures affect peripheral nerves in two possible ways. First, excessive exposure to many industrial or environmental chemicals causes a generalized nerve disorder. This is characterized typically by simultaneous involvement of numerous peripheral nerves manifestating as a diffuse and symmetric clinical syndrome. Second, many occupations predispose workers to physical injuries to peripheral nerves. Single nerves or spinal roots are affected in these instances, leading to a more focal or localized pattern of neurological symptoms and signs. The term **polyneuropathy** is often used to refer to the former, in contrast to **mononeuropathy** or **focal neuropathy**, which is more often a result of physical injuries. Neurotoxins, diabetes, and alcoholism are common causes of polyneuropathy. Neuropathies related to toxins are discussed in Chapter 24, Neurotoxicology. The present chapter is devoted instead to focal neuropathies.

## GENERAL PRINCIPLES

The symptoms of focal neuropathies may be separated into two categories—motor and sensory disturbances. When severe enough, focal nerve injury leads to weakness and atrophy of muscles innervated by the affected nerve. The pattern of weakness is frequently the most useful clue for anatomical localization of nerve injuries. Sensory symptoms include hypesthesias (diminished sensation), paresthesias (altered sensation), and pain. The distribution of sensory dysfunction often follows the cutaneous innervation of the involved nerve. This also provides a

useful clue for anatomical localization. A notable exception is pain, which is the most nonspecific of the sensory symptoms. Pain may be caused by tendinitis, arthritis, or other rheumatological or orthopedic diseases. Even when pain is caused by a nerve injury, its location may be distant from the site of nerve involvement ("referred" pain).

Very minor derangement of peripheral nerve causes paresthesias. It has been shown experimentally that abnormal firing of single sensory nerve fibers leads to perceptible paresthesias. Paresthesias are therefore a sensitive indicator and are present in nearly all focal neuropathies (unless the affected nerve contains only motor nerve fibers). Isolated complaint of pain without paresthesias is seldom due to a neuropathy. Except in very severe nerve injuries, severe or total loss of sensation is encountered rarely in the occupational medicine setting. Patients often use the term "numbness" to refer to paresthesias. Genuine loss of sensation (ie, an elevated threshold of stimulus detection) is not easy to demonstrate by bedside examination without elaborate tools. Like sensory symptoms, the perception of weakness is very observer-dependent. Pain and sensory disturbances often mislead a patient to report weakness even when true weakness is absent. Complaints of weakness should always be followed by attempts at verification through careful clinical examination.

The temporal pattern of sensory symptoms provides useful diagnostic clues. The sensory symptoms of entrapment neuropathies such as carpal tunnel syndrome and ulnar neuropathy at the elbow fluctuate characteristically through the course of a day. Experimental evidence indicates that the pressure within an anatomically confined space (carpal tunnel for median nerve and cubital tunnel for ulnar nerve) increases with flexion or extension of the joints. Increased pressure contributes to mechanical irritation and ischemia of the nerve. Careful inquiry frequently reveals a strong correlation between symptoms and physical activities or postures of the involved limb (Table 8–1). Such a history of exacerbation is useful in distinguishing entrapment neuropathies from the

**Table 8–1.** Occupational entrapment neuropathies.

| Syndrome | Entrapment Site | Occupational Predisposition |
|---|---|---|
| Carpal tunnel syndrome | Carpal tunnel (just distal to wrist crease) | Repetitive/forceful finger flexion or wrist movements<br>Sustained abnormal wrist posture<br>Vibration |
| Ulnar neuropathy at elbow | Cubital tunnel or condylar groove | Elbow flexion<br>Repetitive elbow movements<br>Leaning on elbow |
| Ulnar neuropathy at wrist | At or near Guyon canal | Leaning on wrist<br>Repetitive pounding with hands |
| Thoracic outlet syndrome | Anomalous cervical rib or fibrous band compressing lower trunk of brachial plexus | Carrying heavy objects (eg, suitcases, bags)<br>Sustained arm raising above shoulder |

polyneuropathy of systemic diseases (eg, diabetic neuropathy). The latter tends to present with paresthesias that are relatively constant.

Some patients may be inherently more susceptible to physical injuries of peripheral nerves. Women, for example, on the average have smaller carpal tunnel size than men; the difference explains in part the increased incidence of carpal tunnel syndrome in women. Some polyneuropathies predispose peripheral nerves to mechanical injuries. The most dramatic example is a hereditary disorder of peripheral nerve myelin called by the descriptive name of "hereditary neuropathy with increased liability to pressure palsy" or HNPP. A far more common example is encountered in patients with diabetes mellitus. Not only do many diabetic patients develop a polyneuropathy, these patients are more susceptible to entrapment neuropathies than the general population.

## Approach to Patients

History taking should focus on the nature of sensory and motor symptoms. Paresthesias should be distinguished from pain and hypesthesias. "Numbness," "tingling," "prickly," and "pins and needles" are often used interchangeably by patients for paresthesias. Pain, if present, should be documented by its character and location. The term "weakness" may mean different symptoms to different observers and should never be taken at face value. Most importantly, the history taking must include a detailed probe of all possible exacerbating factors. For upper extremity symptoms, these may include neck turning, coughing, driving, sleeping, carrying a heavy shoulder bag, or any prolonged or forceful use of the hands or arms. For lower extremity symptoms, these may include bending, twisting, valsalva maneuver, or prolonged walking or standing.

Physical examination should include assessment of sensation, strength, and tendon reflexes in the af-

fected limbs. Cutaneous sensation is tested by stimuli of light touch, pin prick, or cold temperature. Altered sensation in the distribution of an affected nerve can be very helpful. However, the sensory examination is largely subjective and is entirely dependent on a patient's ability to observe and report. The clinician should resist the temptation to depend excessively on published maps of cutaneous innervation. They provide rough guidance at best. Muscle strength testing is probably more important in the hands of skilled clinicians, as it provides more objective information. Lack of effort due to pain or malingering can usually be identified by its giveaway quality in the manual muscle testing, and can be readily distinguished from true weakness. Each muscle should be tested individually. Focal weakness, if present, provides perhaps the best clinical sign for localization of nerve lesion. Readers should refer to many excellent texts on peripheral neuroanatomy.

## Diagnostic Tools

**Nerve conduction study** and **electromyography (EMG)** are important laboratory tools in the evaluation of focal neuropathies. Nerve conduction studies are performed by electrical stimulation of a nerve at different sites along its course. Parameters such as nerve conduction velocity and response amplitude provide quantitative measures of peripheral nerve function. In many focal neuropathies, the site of lesion is identified by focal slowing in nerve conduction velocity or by reduction in amplitude of the nerve response. Electromyography is performed by inserting a needle electrode into skeletal muscles to record their electrical activities. Fibrillation potentials and positive sharp waves are seen in denervated muscle fibers. Denervation may also be indicated by a reduction in the number of recorded motor unit action potentials. There are also electromyographic signs of reinnervation to help identify chronic denervation; in such cases, the amplitude and duration of the motor unit action potentials are abnormally increased. Nerve conduction studies and EMG are often performed together. The term EMG has often been used loosely to refer to both tests, even though strictly speaking, EMG means only the needle electromyographic examination of muscles.

There are several drawbacks to nerve conduction and EMG studies. These tests are uncomfortable at best, and occasionally patients tolerate them poorly. Another drawback of nerve conduction and EMG studies is the need to use specialized and expensive equipment. Although simplified electronic devices have been advocated, especially in the setting of occupational health screening (eg, screening for carpal tunnel syndrome), they invariably result in some compromise in measurement precision and diagnostic accuracy. Proper interpretation and performance of these tests requires specialized training. Unfortunately, the clinical and technical expertise of providers varies greatly. When carried out properly, these procedures provide valuable and reliable information. All too frequently, misleading conclusions result from improper performance and interpretation of these tests.

**Quantitative sensory testing** employs specially designed equipment for delivery of calibrated vibratory, light touch, thermal, or electrical stimuli. The subject is asked to report perception of the stimuli according to a specific test paradigm. Like the bedside sensory examination, it is dependent on a patient's cooperation. Therefore, it does not provide truly objective information. There are two major advantages to quantitative sensory testing. First, it reduces the interobserver variability and may be administered successfully by paramedical personnel. Second, it provides quantitative data that are suitable for comparison with normal population and for longitudinal assessment of patients. Thermal sensation testing has an additional benefit of assessing small-diameter sensory nerve fibers that are not tested at all by conventional EMG and nerve conduction studies.

**Magnetic resonance imaging (MRI)** and **computed tomography (CT)** are important adjunctive tools to evaluate focal neuropathies. They are most frequently employed to assess cervical and lumbar radiculopathies, conditions that mimic entrapment neuropathies. The advancement of technology has permitted unprecedented visualization of the spinal cord, nerve roots, and bony structures. The main limitation is their relative lack of specificity in diagnosing symptomatic disease. Asymptomatic but radiologically significant spondylitic disease is frequently seen in the normal population. Varying degree of MRI or CT abnormalities are encountered in over 50% of asymptomatic subjects over the age of 50, and in about 20% of those under 50. Thus, imaging studies should never replace a careful clinical evaluation.

# OCCUPATIONAL FOCAL NEUROPATHIES

## CARPAL TUNNEL SYNDROME

Carpal tunnel syndrome is by far the most common entrapment neuropathy in occupational medicine. The median nerve along with the flexor digitorum tendons pass through the carpal tunnel. The transverse carpal ligament, a fibrous structure, forms the roof of the tunnel. Symptomatic median nerve entrapment is associated with reduced carpal tunnel size, increased nerve susceptibility, extrinsic masses compressing the median nerve, and a number of systemic diseases (Table 8–2). The dominant hand is disproportionately affected in most patients. It is clear that repetitive and forceful use of the hands and fingers exacerbate symptoms of carpal tunnel syndrome. As one might imagine, a variety of occupations predispose workers to increased symptoms. It is also clear that a substantial proportion of cases occur in patients who do not have "at risk" occupations or any other identifiable risk factors. The pathogenesis of carpal tunnel syndrome is therefore multifactorial. Carpal tunnel size, hormonal factors, trauma, physical activity, as well as factors yet to be defined, all play important roles.

If patient reporting is reliable, a confident diagnosis can often be made on the basis of the history. The most diagnostically useful feature is intermittent paresthesias of the hand and fingers. Paresthesias may be worse at night, awakening the patient from sleep, or may be exacerbated after prolonged use of the hands. Paresthesias are often most prominent in the median-

**Table 8–2.** Causes of carpal tunnel syndrome.

**Reduced carpal tunnel size**
Fractures
Gout
Rheumatoid arthritis
Tenosynovitis
**Increased nerve susceptibility**
Diabetes mellitus
Hereditary neuropathy with liability to pressure palsy
Uremia
Possibly other polyneuropathies
**Extrinsic masses at or near carpal tunnel**
Ganglia
Hematoma
Osteophytes
**Other conditions**
Acromegaly
Amyloidosis
Hypothyroidism
Pregnancy

innervated fingers (the first three digits and the lateral half of the ring finger), although about half of all patients report symptoms in all five fingers. Even the latter group of patients often name the index or middle fingers as the most symptomatic, if asked specifically. Sensory changes in the distribution of the median nerve with sparing of the thenar eminence are often demonstrable on physical examination.

Pain is usually localized to the hand and wrist, but may also be referred to the forearm and even the shoulder. The presence of prominent pain may suggest another superimposed condition like tenosynovitis or arthritis.

Although it is not uncommon for patients to complain of hand weakness or an increased tendency to drop objects held in the hand, objective weakness is either absent or mild in the majority of cases. The long flexor muscles responsible for hand grip are supplied by branches of the median nerve in the forearm and are invariably normal on formal strength testing. Weakness is detectable in the median-innervated thenar muscles (abductor pollicis brevis and opponens pollicis) in severe cases. Likewise, thenar atrophy is seen only in advanced disease.

Increased paresthesias to percussion of the median nerve at the carpal tunnel (Tinel sign) or to 1-minute flexion of the wrist (Phalen sign) are present in about two-thirds of patients with carpal tunnel syndrome. These should not, however, be considered pathognomonic signs of carpal tunnel syndrome as false positives are common in the normal population. Tendon reflexes, as well as the remainder of the neurological examination, are normal unless a superimposed cervical radiculopathy or polyneuropathy is present.

### Diagnostic Investigations

Nerve conduction and EMG studies play several roles in the clinical management of carpal tunnel syndrome. They can document the disorder when the history is uncertain, assess the severity of the nerve pathology, and provide confirmation as well as a baseline prior to surgery. Focal slowing of sensory nerve conduction velocity at the carpal tunnel is the earliest and most specific sign. Other median nerve conduction abnormalities are present in more severe cases. Ulnar nerve conduction studies should be performed as a control. The ulnar nerve should be normal unless a polyneuropathy or a concurrent ulnar neuropathy is present. Sometimes, cervical radiculopathy may be present as a confounding factor. Needle EMG evaluation of the cervical myotomes should be carried out in such cases. Electrodiagnostic studies are abnormal in about 70–90% of patients with unequivocal carpal tunnel syndrome. The yield is probably lower in patients with only mild symptoms, although the true sensitivity of the test is difficult to ascertain because of the absence of a suitable gold standard for comparison. Electrodi-

agnostic parameters permit quantitative assessment of nerve pathology, and are particularly useful in assessing failed response to therapy. Quantitative sensory testing (vibrometry, Neurometer, etc) and thermography have been used as alternatives to routine electrodiagnostic studies. Present data are inconclusive and do not support their routine use in patient management.

### Treatment

The choice of treatment depends on the certainty of the diagnosis and the severity of symptoms and neurological deficits. Most symptomatic patients benefit from prophylactic work restrictions in combination with the use of wrist splints. Additional benefits may be provided by injection of corticosteroids near the carpal tunnel. This should be performed by experienced personnel, as injection injury to the median nerve is a rare but well-recognized complication. Relapse after injection is common, and multiple injections (greater than three) are to be avoided, as corticosteroids weaken the flexor tendons and predispose them to later rupture. Oral nonsteroidal antiinflammatory agents provide only minor benefits. Likewise, oral corticosteroids are of little benefit and their long-term use should be discouraged because of side effects.

Persistent and disabling symptoms, neurological deficits on physical examination, or moderate to severe nerve conduction abnormalities all suggest moderate or advanced disease. These patients may benefit from conservative therapy, but most eventually require surgical treatment. All that is required in surgery is the division of the transverse carpal ligament. Surgical dressings are typically removed in a few days, and most patients fully recover from the procedure within six weeks. Recent advances in endoscopic surgical technique may speed post-operative recovery, but endoscopic carpal tunnel release should be performed only by experienced surgeons.

Many surgical series reported satisfactory results in more than 90% of patients. Incomplete relief of symptoms after surgery may be due to incorrect preoperative diagnosis, incomplete section of the transverse ligament, or multicausal etiologies that are untreated. Some patients develop recurrent symptoms after a period of initial success. Possible causes include post-surgical fibrosis and progressive tenosynovitis. Reflex sympathetic dystrophy, degenerative arthritis, iatrogenic injury to the median nerve, and other complications are also possible after surgery. Patients on workers' compensation may have less favorable treatment outcome.

## ULNAR NEUROPATHY

Ulnar nerve dysfunction usually manifests as weakness and atrophy of the intrinsic hand muscles and paresthesias in the little and ring fingers. The presenting history is quite variable. Some patients present solely with paresthesias, whereas others present only with weakness and atrophy. Frequently, patients come to medical condition only after someone else, frequently a medical provider, notices atrophy of the intrinsic hand muscles. Paresthesias are the most common symptoms. Sensory disturbances are often intermittent and vary from day to day. They may worsen with prolonged elbow flexion or with repetitive elbow flexion and extension. Most ulnar neuropathies are associated with little or no pain. Pain, if present, is usually referred to the elbow. Some patients may awaken at night with elbow pain and hand numbness. These nocturnal symptoms may be confused with those of carpal tunnel syndrome. Weakness of hand grasp and thumb pinch may occasionally be part of the presenting syndrome. Most patients, however, are only aware of a generalized loss of dexterity or strength and are unable to identify the specific weak muscles.

Advanced cases are readily diagnosed on physical examination. Muscle atrophy involves all the intrinsic hand muscles with the exception of those in the thenar eminence (innervated by the median nerve). Weakness is easily demonstrable with pinching using the thumb (adductor pollicis and first dorsal interosseous), abduction of the index finger (first dorsal interosseous), and abduction of the little finger (abductor digiti minimi). Most ulnar neuropathies are due to a lesion at the elbow. In such cases, flexion of the ring and little fingers may be also be weak (ulnar portion of flexor digitorum profundus). Diagnosis is much more difficult in milder cases. Sensory alteration may not be demonstrable on examination, or the sensory complaints may extend beyond the ulnar distribution. In most instances, it is difficult to distinguish with certainty an ulnar neuropathy from a C8 radiculopathy. The distributions of sensory complaints are nearly identical in the two conditions. The motor deficits of C8 radiculopathy theoretically also involve the thenar muscles innervated by the median nerve. Other conditions such as polyneuropathy and amyotrophic lateral sclerosis may also be confused with ulnar neuropathy.

## Diagnostic Investigations

Although most ulnar neuropathies are due to an elbow lesion, the nerve can also be compressed at the palm or wrist (Table 8–3). Electrodiagnostic studies provide the only reliable means for further anatomical localization. Nerve conduction study may reveal focal slowing of nerve conduction velocity at the site of the lesion. The pattern of denervation on EMG studies complements the clinical examination and anatomic localization. These studies are also invaluable in differentiating ulnar neuropathy from other conditions that cause hand weakness and numbness.

**Table 8–3.** Causes of ulnar neuropathy.

**Ulnar neuropathy at the elbow**
  Entrapment at cubital tunnel syndrome
  External compression (during anesthesias, repeated leaning on elbow)
  Ulnar nerve prolapse
  Bony deformity near the elbow (old fractures, supracondylar spur, rheumatoid arthritis, osteoarthritis)
  Acute trauma (dislocation, fracture)
  Soft tissue constriction (scar tissue, tumors, masses)
  Leprosy

**Ulnar neuropathy at or near the wrist**
  Entrapment at Guyon canal
  External compression (repeated pressure on the palm— eg, bicycling, certain occupations)
  Bony deformity near the wrist (old fractures, rheumatoid arthritis, osteoarthritis)
  Acute trauma (dislocation or fracture)
  Soft tissue constriction (ganglia, scar tissue, tumors, masses)

## Treatment

For mild intermittent symptoms, a change of activity and avoidance of leaning on the elbow or the palm may be the only necessary treatment. Elbow pad or splint may help those with a lesion at the elbow. Conservative therapy should be accompanied by careful follow-up. More severe cases and those that fail conservative therapy are candidates for surgery. Surgery should be preceded by electrodiagnostic confirmation and localization. For those with a lesion at the elbow, the most commonly used procedures are medial epicondylectomy, simple decompression at the cubital tunnel, or anterior transposition of the ulnar nerve. Regardless of the chosen procedure, the most important determinant of outcome is the severity of ulnar neuropathy at the time of surgery. Success rates vary widely, and is highest in those with minimal neurological deficits.

## THORACIC OUTLET SYNDROME

This is likely to be a heterogenous syndrome. The classic neurological syndrome is often called the **true neurogenic thoracic outlet syndrome**. This is a rare disorder with paresthesias in the ulnar aspect of the hand and forearm, selective wasting of the thenar eminence and, to a lesser extent, wasting of other intrinsic muscles of the hand. Prior to the advent of electrodiagnostic testing, most patients said to have this syndrome probably had either carpal tunnel syndrome or ulnar neuropathy. Another rare syndrome is caused by angulation and compression of the subclavian artery over an anomalous cervical rib. This is often called **vascular thoracic outlet syndrome**. Typical manifestations are intermittent arm claudication, coldness of the limb, and occasional embolic phenomena in the distal upper extremity.

The most common entity, however, does not fit

the true neurogenic or vascular syndromes. These patients present with intermittent pain and paresthesias poorly localized in the arm. Symptoms may worsen with carrying heavy objects in the arm or holding the arm overhead for a prolonged period. There is little evidence to support that vascular compression plays a significant role in this syndrome. Popular clinical tests such as supraclavicular bruit, Adson maneuver, hyperabduction maneuver, and costoclavicular maneuver are all tests for vascular compression and are of dubious value. Moreover, positive tests occur in many normal individuals. The remaining clinical examination is usually normal. The diagnostic utility of electrodiagnostic studies is controversial. Most clinicians agree that electrodiagnostic tests are abnormal only in the true neurogenic thoracic outlet syndrome. Testing is primarily used to exclude or confirm other entrapment neuropathies or cervical radiculopathy.

Surgical decompression of the thoracic outlet should be reserved for those with true neurogenic or vascular syndromes. For most patients, treatment begins with avoidance of activities that worsen symptoms. Exercises designed to promote proper shoulder and neck posture may help. These consist of strengthening exercises of shoulder girdle muscles and full range of movements of the shoulder and neck.

## REFERENCES

American Academy of Neurology, American Association of Electrodiagnostic Medicine, American Academy of Physical Medicine and Rehabilitation: Practice parameter for electrodiagnostic studies in carpal tunnel syndrome. Neurology 1993;43:2404.

Baker EL, Ehrenberg RL: Preventing the work-related carpal tunnel syndrome: Physician reporting and diagnostic criteria. Ann Intern Med 1990;112:317.

Dellon AL, Hament W, Gittelshon A: Nonoperative management of cubital tunnel syndrome: An 8-year prospective study. Neurology 1993;43:1673.

Jablecki CK et al: Literature review of the usefulness of nerve conduction studies and electromyography for the evaluation of patients with carpal tunnel syndrome. Muscle Nerve 1993;16:1392.

Jensen MC et al: Magnetic resonance imaging of the lumbar spine in people without back pain. N Engl J Med 1994;331:69.

Katz JN et al: The carpal tunnel syndrome: Diagnostic utility of the history and physical examination findings. Ann Intern Med 1990;112:321.

LeRoux PD, Ensign TD, Burchiel KJ: Surgical decompression without transposition for ulnar neuropathy: Factors determining outcome. Neurosurgery 1990;27:709.

Panegyres PK et al: Thoracic outlet syndromes and magnetic resonance imaging. Brain 1993;116:823.

Quantitative sensory testing: A consensus report from the Peripheral Neuropathy Association. Neurology 1993;43:1050.

Wilbourn AJ: Thoracic outlet syndromes: A plea for conservatism. Neurosurg Clin North Am 1991;2:235.

### SUGGESTED READINGS

Aminoff MJ: *Electrodiagnosis in Clinical Neurology,* 3rd ed. Churchill Livingstone, 1992.

Dawson DM, Hallett M, Millender LH: *Entrapment Neuropathies.* Little, Brown, 1990.

Stewart JD: *Focal Peripheral Neuropathies,* 2nd ed. Raven Press, 1993.

# Eye Injuries

# 9

*Ernest K. Goodner, MD*

The personal tragedy and economic loss associated with impaired vision or even blindness due to occupational eye injuries can be prevented by identifying workers at risk and instituting appropriate safety programs. Proper maintenance of tools and equipment by the employer and effective use of protective devices such as safety glasses or face shields by the employee will reduce the number of injuries such as ocular contusions, trauma due to penetrating and nonpenetrating foreign bodies, conjunctival and corneal abrasions, lid lacerations, and optic nerve damage.

Recognition of the toxic effects of chemical agents and protection from those that may be splashed into the eyes are vital for prevention of visual damage. The ready availability of facilities for cleansing and irrigation of the face and eyes in the workplace is of the utmost importance, since initial steps for treatment of chemical burns—especially those due to strong alkalis and acids—must be carried out immediately by the employee, fellow workers, or anyone else near at hand. There is no time to wait for specialized medical care, so employee education programs for emergency care of chemical burns are essential.

The risks of ocular damage for x-ray technicians, glassblowers, welders, and other workers exposed to ionizing, infrared, and ultraviolet radiation have long been known, but damage due to exposure to excessive amounts of visible light has only recently been recognized. Wearing protective lenses that filter the most offending wavelengths of visible light may become commonplace in the future.

## Anatomy & Physiology
## (Figure 9–1)

A brief review of ocular anatomy and function will be helpful in understanding the mechanisms of several kinds of eye injuries and how they affect the visual system.

The orbit, eyelid, and conjunctiva are protective mechanisms for the eye. The **orbit** and its bony rim offer excellent mechanical protection from injuries with the exception of those coming from the direct anterior or temporal directions. The **eyelid** and **conjunctiva** are essential for normal maintenance of the smooth, moist, clear anterior surface of the **cornea**, which in turn is essential for clear vision. The normal blinking mechanism depends on the third cranial nerve to open the lids and the seventh to close them. Moistening of the conjunctiva by lacrimal fluid depends in part on activation of the reflex arc between the sensory fifth innervation of the anterior eye and the parasympathetic secretomotor fibers that accompany the seventh cranial nerve along the petrous temporal bone into the middle fossa and thence through the orbit to the lacrimal gland. Moistening of the **corneal epithelium** is aided by mucus from the goblet cells of the conjunctiva, particularly those on the tarsus of the upper lid. Reflex tear production by the **lacrimal gland** helps dilute and wash away irritating substances that find their way into the conjunctival sac. The rich blood supply of the conjunctiva and lid also helps in resisting and limiting infections of the anterior eye.

Internal structures of the eye can be conveniently divided into anterior and posterior segments. The **anterior segment** includes the cornea, anterior chamber, iris, lens, and ciliary body. These structures comprise the essential optical elements of the eye. The regular pattern of the collagen fibers and posterior endothelial layer of the **cornea** maintain its optical clarity. Since the cornea and **lens** are avascular, they require a specialized source of nutrition, which is provided by aqueous humor. The **ciliary body** produces aqueous humor at a nearly constant rate, bathing the lens and posterior surface of the cornea and then draining near the base of the cornea through the structures associated with Schlemm's canal. A normal rate of production and drainage of aqueous humor maintains the intraocular pressure between 10 and 21 mm Hg. Injuries causing sustained elevation of pressure can lead to significant glaucomatous visual field loss. The **iris** and its **pupil** adjust the amount of light entering the eye. Contraction of the ciliary muscle changes the shape of the lens, thereby allowing for accommodation (adjustment of focusing for seeing at different distances).

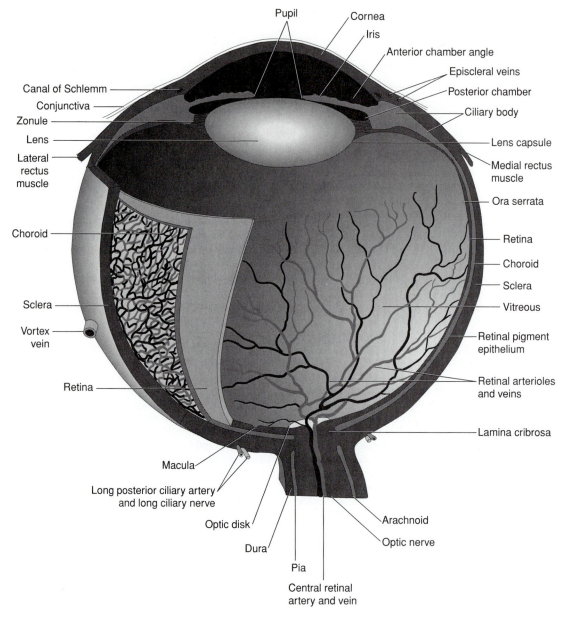

**Figure 9–1.** View of the inferior half of the right eye.

The **posterior segment** of the eye is the light-sensing portion of the visual system and contains the **retina** and its supporting vascular layer, the **choroid**. The retina has over 1 million nerve fibers that arise from the ganglion cells and collect in the optic disk to form the **optic nerve**, which transmits visual information to the posterior visual system. These nerve fibers are second-order neurons similar to the myelinated sensory tracts of the spinal cord and are not capable of healing with restoration of visual function following injuries such as penetrating wounds of the

orbit or posterior orbit fractures involving the optic canal. Depending on the severity of the injury, the fibers may disappear partially or completely resulting in either partial or complete atrophy of the optic disk (optic nerve). The optic chiasm, optic tracts, and visual radiations to the cortex usually are not involved directly in eye injuries except those involving the bones of the head and the intracranial structures.

Visual acuity depends on the optical clarity of the cornea, lens, and vitreous, and proper functioning of the **fovea**, which is the avascular center of the retinal

**macula** and is composed entirely of specialized cones that are color-sensitive and capable of resolving the finest images. If this small area (< 0.5 mm in diameter) is damaged, no adjacent portion of the retina is capable of assuming the fine function that provides maximum visual acuity.

Eye injuries causing retinal detachment or vitreous hemorrhage can lead to loss of peripheral vision, and injuries of the extraocular muscles or their nerves can produce diplopia ("double vision").

### History & Eye Examination

*Caution:* For chemical burns (see page 100), emergency treatment should be started immediately, and the history and examination of the patient can proceed in due course. In cases of suspected ruptured or lacerated globe (see below), care must be taken to prevent further damage to the eye during transport to the hospital and initial evaluation.

**A. History:** As outlined in Table 9–1 and discussed in Chapter 2, the occupational medical history should include a variety of questions not always considered pertinent to general histories. In addition, the worker should be asked about vision before and after the injury and whether any visual loss was sudden or gradual. Sudden loss of vision without obvious injury may be caused by central retinal artery occlusion or ischemic damage to the optic nerve occasionally due to giant cell arteritis. These problems require emergency treatment. Progressive loss of vision following facial bone fractures or head injuries is sometimes due to optic nerve damage, which may respond to surgery if recognized in time.

In cases of mechanical injury, the worker should be asked about previous tetanus inoculations and about the nature of the forces involved during the injury. Was the eye struck with a small, rapidly moving object that may have penetrated the globe, as sometimes occurs when a steel hammer strikes a steel

**Table 9–1.** Classification of chemical burns of the eye.[1]

| Classification | Clinical Findings |
| --- | --- |
| Mild | Erosion of the corneal epithelium. Faint haziness of the cornea. No ischemic necrosis of the conjunctiva or sclera. |
| Moderate | Corneal opacity blurring details of the iris. Minimal ischemic necrosis of the conjunctiva and sclera. |
| Severe | Corneal opacity blurring the pupillary outline. Severe ischemic necrosis and blanching of the conjunctiva and sclera. |

[1]Modified and reproduced, with permission, from Thoft RA, Dohlman CH: Chemical and thermal burns of the eye. In: *Ocular Trauma.* Freeman HM (editor). Appleton-Century-Crofts, 1979.

tool? Or was the eye hit by a large, slowly moving object that may have caused a contusion injury or rupture of the globe? If the presence of a foreign body is suspected, the worker should be asked about the type of material that might be involved (a magnetic metal such as iron or steel, a nonmagnetic metal such as aluminum or copper, or an organic material such as wood), since this information is helpful for determining the method of treatment and for prognosis. Soluble metallic salts from iron- or copper-containing foreign bodies can cause irreversible toxic damage to the retina, best prevented by their prompt removal. Less soluble materials such as aluminum, plastic, or glass are associated with a better prognosis. Organic foreign bodies such as pieces of wood or splinters of plant material may introduce an intraocular infection that is frequently difficult to treat and has a very poor prognosis.

If a chemical burn is present or suspected, the type of chemical (alkali or acid) will influence how quickly and deeply it penetrates the eye. If eye injuries are thought to be due to long-term exposure to chemicals, the various substances to which the worker is exposed should be identified and a material safety data sheet (MSDS) obtained for each, as described in Chapter 2. The worker should also be asked about exposure to aerosols, surfactants, detergents, dust, and smoke, which can damage the corneal epithelium.

**B. Examination:** Even if an injury is thought to have affected only one eye, both eyes should be carefully examined. If swelling prevents easy opening of the eyes for inspection, a sterile topical anesthetic can be instilled through nearly closed eyelids by applying the drops along the lid fissure. After a few minutes, smooth sterile retractors may be carefully used to lift the lids for eye examination.

**1. External eye examination–**

**a. Eyelids–**Note symmetry of the lids of both eyes. Look for lacerations that cross the lid margins and for perforating wounds through the skin of the lid above or below the lid margin. Except in the case of a suspected ruptured or lacerated globe, the lid can be everted to search for foreign bodies on the upper tarsus. To evert the lid, the patient is asked to look down while the physician pulls gently on the lashes and applies mild pressure on the upper surface of the lid.

**b. Orbits–**Palpate the orbital rims, and note discontinuities and crepitus due to subcutaneous air from fractures of the paranasal sinuses. In orbital fractures, injury to the inferior or superior orbital nerves as they pass through the floor or roof of the orbit can cause decreased sensibility of the lids and face.

**c. Conjunctiva–**To examine the conjunctiva, evert the lids by applying gentle pressure over the superior orbital rim of the upper lid or over the malar eminence of the lower lid, thereby avoiding direct pressure on the globe. Look for foreign bodies, hemorrhage, laceration, and inflammation.

Inflammation caused by trauma usually produces a watery discharge (tears), in contrast to the purulent mucoid discharge of bacterial conjunctivitis. Viral or chlamydial conjunctivitis is characterized by lymph follicles in the inferior fornix of the conjunctival sac along with a watery discharge. Preauricular lymph nodes are also frequently present.

**d. Corneas–**With a bright light, look at the light reflection on the normally smooth corneal surface. Irregularities indicate disruptions of the corneal epithelium. Because the cornea is normally clear and lustrous, the surface texture of the iris is easily and clearly seen. A corneal wound with incarceration of the iris may also be indicated by asymmetry of the pupil. A fluorescein paper strip moistened with sterile saline or a topical anesthetic can be used to stain the tears on the surface of the cornea. The stain diffuses into any area of disrupted epithelium and stains it bright green. The color is enhanced with a blue light. Details of the cornea and the anterior eye are much more easily examined with magnification such as a 2- to 4-power loupe or (and preferably) with a slit lamp and microscope if one is available.

**e. Anterior chambers–**The anterior chambers should appear deep and clear. Hyphema (hemorrhage into the anterior chamber) is almost always a sign of significant injury. Hypopyon (purulent material in the anterior chamber) is characterized by a white or gray layer of inflammatory cells at the chamber bottom. Hypopyon is usually caused by an infection following a penetrating injury or a bacterial or fungal corneal ulcer.

**f. Pupils–**The pupils should appear round, black, and equal in size. Pupillary reactions to light should be carefully noted. Normally, both pupils constrict and dilate equally and simultaneously when one pupil is stimulated by light. While the illuminated pupil is demonstrating the direct light response, the unilluminated pupil is showing the consensual light response. The direct light responses of the two eyes can be compared by moving a flashlight back and forth between the eyes and pausing a few seconds at each eye to observe the pupil. Normally, each pupil constricts when illuminated; failure of one of the pupils to constrict but to dilate instead indicates the presence of an afferent pupillary defect (Marcus Gunn pupil), which may be due to an optic nerve injury or extensive retinal damage on that side.

**2. Test of ocular motility–**If there are no severe eye injuries, the ocular movements may be safely tested by comparing the excursions in all directions to make sure that they are the same in both eyes. Limitation of upward or downward gaze occurs frequently in orbital floor fractures and may be the result of accompanying edema or mechanical restriction of the ocular muscles. It can also result from direct trauma to a muscle when a penetrating injury of the orbit occurs.

**3. Ophthalmoscopic examination–**

**a. Red reflex–**The presence of a good bright red reflex demonstrates normal optical clarity of the eye. A direct ophthalmoscope with a good bright light is used to observe the red reflex (the red glow reflected from the fundus). Examination should take place in a darkened room with the instrument set at 0 or + 1, and the eyes should be observed arm's length, about 60 cm (2 ft) so that the reflex in both of them can be seen at the same time and compared. An opacity in the cornea, anterior chamber, lens, or vitreous or a gross change in the color of the retina will appear as a dark form against a red background or as a dull or absent red reflex.

**b. Optic disks–**The examiner should be as close to the patient as possible to maximize the relative size of the pupil. The optic disks should be examined for the presence of papilledema (choked disk). Optic disks are usually well-vascularized and have a good pink color. When nerve fibers in the optic nerve die as the result of various injuries, the blood supply to the disks decreases in proportion to the loss of fibers. The disk will show a faint pallor if only a few fibers are missing, or it may appear completely white as a result of optic atrophy following total destruction of the nerve.

**c. Optic cups–**The width of each optic cup is usually one-third or less of the diameter of the whole optic disk. If it is as large as half the diameter, there is an increased risk for glaucoma. Therefore, estimating the cup size is useful for screening patients for glaucoma.

**d. Retinal vessels–**The vessels should be examined along the upper and lower arcades proceeding from the optic disk, and the presence of hemorrhages, exudates, and other alterations in the appearance of the retina should be noted.

**e. Maculas and foveas–**Each macula should be checked for alterations in its usual relatively featureless appearance. Its center, the fovea, can always be located 2.5 disk diameters temporal to the optic disk. Its concave center usually shows a small, bright foveal light reflex.

**4. Measurement of intraocular pressure–**If a lacerated or ruptured globe is suspected, intraocular pressure should not be measured. In other injuries, pressure can be measured with a Schiotz tonometer or with an applanation tonometer if one is available on a slit lamp. If a tonometer is not available, a general impression of extremely high or low intraocular pressure can be obtained by gently palpating each globe in turn with one finger of each hand through the closed upper eyelid. Comparison of the firmness of the two eyes is occasionally useful when the intraocular pressure is extremely high, as in angle closure glaucoma.

Angle closure glaucoma accounts for only about

5% of all glaucoma, it usually presents with acute aching pain in the involved eye with moderate redness of the globe and blurred vision, sometimes described as colored halos around bright lights. It occurs when the iris root touches the back of the cornea blocking the aqueous outflow and causing intraocular pressure to rise very rapidly, thus leading to the symptoms. Angle closure glaucoma can occur only in eyes with anatomically shallow anterior chambers and narrow chamber angles. An attack of angle closure glaucoma requires prompt treatment. The first approach is to lower the pressure medically with topical miotics such as pilocarpine 1–4% every 15 minutes for 1–2 hours. The production of aqueous humor is reduced with a topical ophthalmic beta-adrenergic blocker such as Timolol. Intraocular pressure can be lowered quickly by increasing the osmolarity of the blood that moves fluid out of the eye, thus reducing the ocular volume and the pressure. Intravenous urea or mannitol infusions are effective, but oral ingestion of glycerine is as effective, safer, and more easily available. Subsequent attacks are prevented by making an opening in the peripheral iris (iridectomy), which passes aqueous humor directly from the posterior chamber, to the anterior chamber keeping the filtration angle open. The iridectomy usually is made with a laser.

Open-angle glaucoma accounts for most cases of glaucomatous visual loss (90%). Its onset is insidious, there is no pain, and visual symptoms are noticed only after severe irreversible loss of visual field has occurred. Therefore, it becomes the physician's responsibility to see changes in the optic cup. Cups as large as one-half the disk diameter are suspicious. Such changes are an indication to measure intraocular pressure. Early lowering of elevated intraocular pressure is the only way to prevent loss of visual field. All adults should be encouraged to have their intraocular pressures measured every few years.

The remaining 5% of cases of glaucoma have a variety of causes. Contusion injuries to the eye can tear the iris root and the ciliary body's attachment to the sclera, damaging the filtration angle, reducing aqueous outflow, and raising pressure. This is called angle recession glaucoma. Blood in the anterior chamber (hyphema) and inflammatory cells in cases of chronic inflammation, such as uveitis, can block aqueous outflow channels, causing secondary glaucoma.

The only effective treatment of open-angle and secondary glaucoma is lowering of the elevated intraocular pressure. This is usually done by medically reducing the production of aqueous humor with a topical beta-adrenergic blocker and sometimes with a systemic carbonic anhydrase inhibitor such as acetazolamide (Diamox). Miotic drops such as pilocarpine increase the outflow of aqueous humor. If these measures fail to adequately lower the pressure, an external surgical fistula can be made to increase the drainage of aqueous humor, usually into the potential space under the conjunctiva.

**5. Test of visual acuity–**Visual acuity should always be tested and the results recorded before treatment is instituted. This is important both from the point of view of good care and for medicolegal reasons, since patients do not always remember the amount of visual loss that occurred at the time of a severe injury. Visual acuity should be measured with a Snellen chart if possible or with a near-acuity card and recorded appropriately. Each eye should be tested separately, first without correction (glasses or contact lenses) and then with correction; each acuity measurement should be recorded for the right eye followed by the left. If a near-acuity card is used, it is important to record the distance at which the measurements were made and whether they were made with or without the patient's glasses. If visual acuity is poor and a refractive error is suspected, the chart or card can be read through a pinhole as a substitute for corrective lenses; an improvement in acuity will confirm the presence of a refractive error. If acuity is less than 20/200, the greatest distance at which fingers can be counted should be noted for each eye. If the patient cannot see the fingers well enough to count them, the greatest distance at which hand movements can be seen should be recorded. If vision is poorer than this, light perception can be tested with a bright flashlight held as close to the eye as possible, and the ability to perceive light in each of the four quadrants is recorded. If there is no light perception, it should be recorded as such. Visual acuity measured with a Snellen chart is based on a visual angle of 1 minute of arc; this is considered the best resolving power of the eye and is the standard used to design of all types of test charts. The 20/20 letters are formed of black lines separated by white spaces, each 1 minute of arc wide; the whole letter is 5 minutes of arc high, measuring 8.7 mm (Figure 9–2). When letters of this size are accurately read at a distance of 20 ft (6 m), 20/20 vision is determined. Other letters on a chart increase in multiples of this standard dimension. The 20/200 letter is 10 times larger or 87 mm high and would appear the same size as a 20/20 letter when seen at a distance of 200 ft. Metric visual acuity charts use 6 m as the standard test distance; therefore, 6/6 = 20/20. The peak of the light sensitivity curve of the eye is at a wavelength of about 555 nm. This means that our best vision is in yellow-green light.

There are two techniques for objectively estimating visual acuity—optokinetic nystagmus and visual evoked response—that may be useful in certain situations, particularly when the patient is unable or unwilling to respond to the usual subjective measures of visual acuity.

**Optokinetic nystagmus** is a visually stimulated response to relatively large targets. These eye movements are observed in the intact visual system by

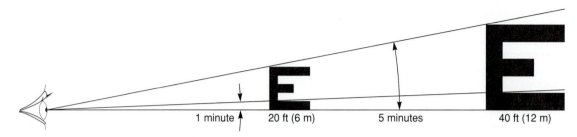

1 minute | 20 ft (6 m) | 5 minutes | 40 ft (12 m)

**Figure 9–2.** Measurement of visual acuity. Visual acuity measurements are based on a visual angle of 1 minute of arc subtending each part of a test letter. Each letter is made up of five equally sized black or white parts, therefore, the whole letter subtends a visual angle of 5 minutes of arc. The 20/20 letters are 8.7 mm high, the 20/40 letters are twice as large, or 17.4 mm high. This drawing is not to scale.

passing an alternating series of dark and light stripes of equal width before the patient's eyes. Involuntary nystagmus is produced—slow following movement in the direction of movement of the stripes alternating with a quick recovery movement. The stimulus is usually presented as a series of vertical stripes 1–2 cm in width on a handheld drum 10–15 cm in diameter. The drum is held 20–30 cm from the patient and turned slowly while observing the patient's eyes to see the induced nystagmus. The stripes can also be presented on a 50-cm long cloth strip with the stripes running across the 10–12 cm width. Normally, the nystagmus can be induced in any direction, and its rate will vary with the speed of the stimulus.

The **visually evoked response** is an electroencephalographic recording over the visual cortex (occipital lobe) in response to visual stimuli. The stimulus can be a simple light flash giving an on-off response, or an estimate of visual acuity can be made by presenting an alternating pattern of dark and light squares in a checkerboard pattern on a television screen. The squares can be made progressively smaller until the response is no longer recorded and the size of the smallest squares eliciting a cortical recording can be related to standard visual acuity measurements. The responses are involuntary and cannot be controlled by the subject; acuity measurements in the range of 20/400 to 20/20 have been recorded even in infants younger than 1 year of age. This technique is usually available through neuroophthalmologic or neurologic consultation. It can be particularly valuable when evaluating patients with compensation or forensic problems.

**6. Test of visual fields**–Visual fields should be tested, especially in patients with suspected head injury or a significant decrease in visual acuity. Each eye is tested separately by confrontation. The patient is asked to look at the examiner's eye while the examiner's hand moves toward the center of the visual field. The point at which the patient can accurately count fingers in each of the four quadrants is determined, and the results in the two eyes are carefully compared.

**7. Tests for malingering**–When a patient claims poor vision or blindness in one or both eyes, the presence of normal pupillary light responses (in the absence of an afferent pupillary defect) objectively demonstrates a functioning retina and optic nerve in each eye. The following tests will frequently help reveal the presence of normal fusion.

**a.** Utilizing the refractor, place a strong convex lens in front of the good eye and a weak convex lens in front of the "blind" eye. If the patient reads small letters on the test chart, the eye under consideration is not blind. This test can be more subtly done with the refractor than with the trial frame, since the strong convex lens is not visible to the patient when the refractor is used.

**b.** Place a 1-diopter base-out prism in front of the "blind" eye. If there is sight in the eye, diplopia will result and the eye will be seen to move inward to correct the diplopia.

**c.** Place a pair of red-green glasses on the patient, with the red lens in front of the right eye and the green lens in front of the left eye. Ask the patient to read from a chart of red and green letters. If the left eye is the suspected eye and the patient can read green letters with this eye, the eye is not blind; the green letters will not be transmitted through the red lens in front of the right eye.

## CHEMICAL BURNS OF THE EYE

### Etiology & Pathogenesis

Strong alkalis and acids cause the most severe and damaging chemical injuries that can be sustained by the eye. Alkali burns are commonly due to sodium and potassium hydroxide used as cleaning agents, to calcium hydroxide used in mason's mortar and plaster, and to anhydrous ammonia used in fertilizer. Battery acids and the strong acids used to clean metal in the electroplating industry are also common causes of severe eye injury.

Alkalis affect the lipid in cell membranes and thereby reduce the normal barriers to diffusion. This allows the chemical to rapidly penetrate the interior of the eye. Because alkalis are not quickly neutralized by tissue, their destructive action can continue for hours if they are not diluted and removed immediately by irrigation of the eye. In contrast, acids tend to be fixed by protein in tissues, and this neutralizes them in a relatively shorter period and keeps them from penetrating as deeply.

The corneal endothelium, which is essential to the normal function and survival of the cornea, is particularly vulnerable to chemical insult. There is often severe damage within the anterior chamber, including the aqueous outflow pathways, and this can lead to glaucoma. Obliteration of the blood vessels of the conjunctiva and sclera can cause severe ischemia of the anterior eye, including the periphery of the cornea and the underlying ciliary body and iris. Ischemia is one of the major causes of the poor prognosis in patients with severe chemical burns.

## Clinical Findings

The skin on the face and eyelids shows edema and erythema, sometimes with sloughing of the surface. Eye examination may require use of a topical anesthetic, depending on whether pain is noted or nerve damage is severe enough to cause anesthesia. The conjunctiva may be mildly hyperemic, show small hemorrhages, or be blanched and have the appearance of white marble (Figure 9–3). Testing the pH of the conjunctival surface with indicator paper will help confirm the cause of the injury. The severity of injury (Table 9–1) is usually judged by the degree of corneal opacity, using the normal clarity of the pupil as a guide. The cornea may appear gray or cloudy because of epithelial and stromal edema. If the cornea is not cloudy, the anterior chamber can be clearly seen. In some cases, the iris and pupil appear hazy and indistinct. Visual acuity is decreased in proportion to the severity of corneal damage.

Injuries of the nasopharynx and upper respiratory passages are frequently found in association with aspiration of the chemical irritant.

## Prevention

Chemical burns can be prevented by safety measures such as keeping chemicals in unbreakable containers and providing splash protection shields and eyeglasses for employees who must handle them. Workers at risk should be taught emergency treatment measures for themselves and their fellow workers.

## Treatment

Emergency treatment (Table 9–2) should be started in the workplace by the patient or anyone immediately available. Any source of water (drinking fountain, hose, etc) is adequate and should be used immediately to wash the eyes with copious amounts of water until the patient can be taken to an emergency facility. At least 1 L of saline or other isotonic solution should then be used to irrigate each eye carefully, with the lids held open to thoroughly cleanse the conjunctival sac. Use of a sterile topical anesthetic may be necessary.

Moist cotton-tipped applicators should be used to sweep the conjunctival surface free of particulate matter, such as the granules found in drainpipe cleaners and plaster. The pH of the conjunctival surface should be tested with pH test paper strips or urine pH test strips and irrigation repeated until the pH approaches the normal level of 7.0. As a general rule, there is no practical limit to the amount of irrigation that may be helpful. If there is any doubt about its efficacy, irrigation may be repeated for several hours while waiting for ophthalmologic consultation.

During irrigation, the gray color or cloudiness of the cornea may appear to clear, giving a false impression of improved clinical status. The change is usually due to sloughing of the damaged corneal epithe-

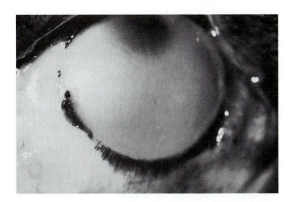

**Figure 9–3.** Severe alkali burn. The cornea is opaque, with the exception of a small dark area of corneal epithelium protected by the upper lid. The conjunctiva and sclera are blanched and ischemic.

**Table 9–2.** Emergency treatment of chemical burns of the eye.

(1) **In the workplace:** Wash the eyes with copious amounts of water until the patient can be taken to an emergency facility.

(2) **In the emergency facility:**
  (a) Irrigate each eye with at least 1 L of saline or other isotonic solution, with the lids open to flush the conjunctival sac.
  (b) Use sterile topical anesthetic as necessary.
  (c) Remove particulate matter with cotton-tipped applicators.
  (d) Test the pH of the conjunctival surface, and continue irrigation until the pH approaches neutral.
  (e) Remove loose or damaged epithelium from the cornea and conjunctiva.
  (f) Dilate the pupil with cyclopentolate or scopolamine.
  (g) Give topical antibiotic drops, patch the eyes, and refer the patient to an ophthalmologist.

lium, which reveals the clearer corneal stroma underneath.

After irrigation is completed, cycloplegic drops (eg, cyclopentolate or scopolamine) may be instilled to dilate the pupil and thus prevent posterior synechiae (adhesions between iris and lens). Antibiotic drops should be instilled before the eye is patched. The patch prevents blinking and should provide some comfort. The patient should be referred to an ophthalmologist.

Specific ophthalmologic treatment may include the use of topical corticosteroids and antibiotics to reduce the severe inflammatory response that occurs shortly after injury. These medications—particularly the corticosteroids—must be used with caution since they enhance the possibility of secondary infection and discourage the formation of new vessels in ischemic areas. The topical and systemic use of ascorbic acid (vitamin C) may be useful in lowering the intraocular pH and helping to promote healing of the conjunctival and corneal epithelium. Irrigation of the anterior chamber with saline solution may help restore the pH to more normal levels. After the initial reaction subsides and the conjunctiva and cornea have epithelialized, the severity of the injury can be judged. A scarred cornea can be replaced by a corneal transplant, and a damaged lens (cataract) can be surgically removed. Glaucoma due to scarring of aqueous outflow pathways may be medically controlled—and, if not, a surgical fistulization procedure may be done.

## Prognosis

Emergency treatment of chemical burns is usually followed by a period of weeks or months of effort to rehabilitate the damaged ocular tissues. The degree of blanching or ischemia of the conjunctiva is an important factor influencing the final outcome. Ischemic damage even in the presence of apparent healing makes ultimate restoration of vision difficult. The survival of a corneal transplant depends on normal function of structures in the anterior eye. The survival of the cornea and the anterior segment of the eye are directly related to the degree of damage to the corneal endothelium, aqueous drainage pathways, and ciliary body. If the ciliary body fails to produce enough aqueous humor, the entire eye becomes soft and ultimately atrophies. In patients with severe burns, deep penetration and extensive destruction of ocular tissues can lead to perforation of the globe, infection, and loss of the eye. Milder burns in which chemical penetration is more shallow may heal with little scarring.

## THERMAL BURNS OF THE EYE & EYELID

Thermal burns of the eyelids and upper face may involve the eyes. However, in cases of flash burn caused by a sudden gas explosion, most individuals forcibly close their eyes, and this reflex lid closure usually protects the ocular surface. Direct contact with molten metal or glass can cause severe injury to the lids and even to the open eye. Thermal injury occurs rapidly at the time of contact. Tissue destruction is not progressive, as is the case with some chemical burns.

Eye examination may require topical anesthesia and careful use of lid retractors. Irrigation may be necessary to remove particulate matter, especially in injuries caused by explosions.

Depending on their severity, thermal burns of the eye structures are treated in the same manner as burns occurring elsewhere on the body (see Chapter 12). Extensive loss of lid skin can lead to exposure and drying of the cornea. This can be prevented by covering the eye with a transparent plastic sheet and sealing it to the surrounding skin with a sterile antibiotic ointment, thus producing a humidity chamber over the eye. Healing of lid skin is frequently followed by scarring, contraction, and distortion of the lids, which results in some degree of exposure of the globe. Plastic surgery with skin grafting may be necessary to restore lid function.

## MECHANICAL INJURIES OF THE EYE & EYELID

Mechanical injuries range from superficial abrasions to complete disruption of the globe, depending on the nature of the force striking the eye. Small, sharp, fast-moving objects can penetrate or lacerate the globe, whereas larger objects may exert enough compressive force to cause contusion injury or to rupture the eyeball.

### Laceration of the Eyelid

Lid lacerations result from two common mechanisms: (1) contact with sharp, fast-moving objects such as glass or metal parts, which cut the skin and subcutaneous tissues (partial-thickness lacerations) or involve the posterior layers, the tarsus, and the conjunctiva (full-thickness lacerations); and (2) avulsion injuries, which are due to blunt trauma (eg, a blow to the malar eminence) and cause abrupt traction of the lid and tear it from its attachment to the medial canthal ligament. The type and extent of injury determine the method of treatment.

Partial-thickness lacerations can be closed by direct suturing with generally good results. Full-thickness lacerations require meticulous repair in two layers by an ophthalmic surgeon to accurately restore the continuity of the lid margin. If notching of the margin occurs with healing, the cornea may not be adequately moistened by tears and protected from abrasions and other trauma. Deep stabwounds above the upper lid may sever the levator muscle of the lid.

The cut end of the levator is easier to retrieve and repair if surgery is performed immediately after injury. Inadequate repair can result in chronic ptosis. Severe damage to the upper lid and blinking mechanism can also place the patient at risk for superficial corneal injuries.

In avulsion injuries, lid structures that have pulled away from the globe should be carefully examined and placed as close to their anatomic positions as possible to protect the eye while the patient is awaiting treatment by an ophthalmic surgeon. Retention of avulsed lid structures is important. They can frequently be repaired and usually heal well because of their rich blood supply. It is difficult to substitute skin grafts or skin flaps for the normal lid structures, particularly the tarsal and conjunctival structures that are essential for normal functioning of the lid. Avulsion of the medial canthal ligament sometimes disrupts the lacrimal drainage system, and failure to repair it will result in epiphora (the overflow of tears).

### Injuries of the Iris

Injuries to the iris can be caused indirectly by contusion and directly by perforating or penetrating injuries of the eye.

Contusion of the globe transmits force to the iris by the rapid displacement of aqueous humor. Since water is incompressible and the eye is essentially inelastic, these forces can be very large and destructive.

**Iridoplegia** is caused by damage to the pupillary sphincter. The pupil may react to light either directly or consensually and only slightly or not at all. The iris root, where it attaches to the ciliary body, may be torn, producing an iridodialysis. Sometimes the ciliary body with the iris root intact is torn away from its scleral attachment, producing an angle recession that can damage the aqueous outflow, causing a form of glaucoma.

Penetrating injuries, foreign bodies, stab wounds, corneal lacerations, and ruptured globes all may perforate, tear, or disrupt the iris. Iris tissue frequently herniates through corneal or scleral wounds.

Iris injuries do not usually require treatment other than that incidental to repair of the associated major injuries. Except for an increase in the amount of light entering an eye, it may have quite useful vision without an iris or with an iris with multiple holes. An eye with more than one pupil still sees only one image.

### Injuries of the Retina

Retinal injuries are caused by both blunt trauma (contusion) and penetrating wounds.

When the eye is struck in a contusion injury, the force is transmitted by the fluid contents throughout the interior of the globe. Posteriorly, the retina may become edematous in a discrete area, frequently including the macula—a condition called commotio retinae, or Berlin's edema. Vision is reduced but may improve to nearly normal when the edema clears. This process may require several weeks to a month to complete. Contusion injuries also cause forceful displacement of the vitreous, resulting in traction at its anterior attachment on the surface of the retina at the posterior edge of the ciliary body. This may disinsert the retina from the ciliary body or tear a hole in the peripheral retina. Hemorrhage may result, clouding the vitreous for a time.

Retinal tears or holes frequently cause retinal detachments, which require prompt surgical repair.

Visual prognosis depends on macular involvement. If the macula is intact, vision is usually good; if the macula is detached for even a few days, the prognosis is apt to be poor.

Penetrating injuries cause direct perforations and tears in the retina, causing hemorrhage and detachments.

Treatment of retinal detachments requires localization and closure of the tears or holes. This is done by creating an adhesion and scar between the retina and the choroid surrounding the hole. A freezing probe placed on the scleral surface over the hole will cause an inflammatory reaction in the choroid that will adhere to the retina. Sometimes it is necessary to bring the scleral, choroidal, and retinal surfaces together. This is usually done by placing an encircling band of silicone rubber around the entire globe; it may also be done by pushing them together from the inside by injecting a gas bubble into the vitreous space.

### Ruptured or Lacerated Globe

If a ruptured or lacerated globe is present or suspected, placing a metal shield or other protective covering (eg, the bottom half of a paper cup) over the injured eye will prevent external pressure from causing further damage during transport to the hospital. Patching the other eye will reduce ocular movements and thus help prevent further trauma to the injured eye.

Visual acuity should be measured and recorded. Severe injuries are almost always associated with some degree of visual loss, lid swelling, orbital swelling, exophthalmos, and hemorrhage. If lid swelling is extreme, it may be necessary to use a sterile topical anesthetic and lid retractors to lift the lids away from the globe during initial examination.

If the cornea is clear and the pupil is round and reacts to light, the globe is probably intact (Figure 9–4). Global rupture (Figure 9–5) is usually characterized by the presence of brownish or grayish tissue beneath the conjunctiva (subconjunctival hemorrhage), which is due to exposure or herniation of uveal tissue; an irregular or disrupted corneal surface; or the presence of blood or gross alteration in the appearance of the iris and pupil. Pupillary light reflexes may be abnormal. The pupil pulled or peaked toward one side of the cornea usually indi-

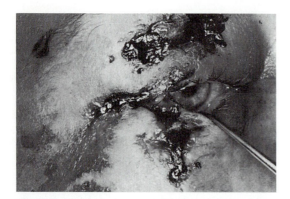

**Figure 9–4.** Injury in a patient with multiple facial lacerations. Eye examination with the use of a topical anesthetic and lid retractor reveals that the cornea is clear and the pupil is round and reacts to light. The globe is probably intact. (Reproduced, with permission, from Singleton BJ: *Eye Trauma and Emergencies: A Slide-Script Program.* American Academy of Ophthalmology, 1995.)

cates that the iris has herniated through a laceration in that direction.

Ophthalmoscopic examination may be difficult because of corneal irregularities and hemorrhage in the anterior chamber and vitreous. If the fundus can be examined and the disk and vessels appear relatively normal, gross disruption of the globe is unlikely. A bright red reflex usually indicates that the interior of the globe is intact.

Intraocular pressure should not be measured if a reptured or lacerated globe is suspected.

An x-ray for detection of any radiopaque material in the region of the globe is an essential part of the initial examination.

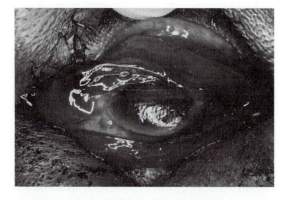

**Figure 9–5.** Ruptured globe, characterized by a large subconjunctival hemorrhage, grossly distorted cornea, and irregular corneal light reflection. (Reproduced, with permission, from Singleton BJ: *Eye Trauma and Emergencies: A Slide-Script Program.* American Academy of Ophthalmology, 1995.)

Definitive examination and treatment should be performed by an ophthalmic surgeon. Until a surgeon is available, both eyes should be covered again, with a sterile eye pad used on the injured eye to minimize contamination. The patient should be supported with parenteral fluids and be considered a candidate for general anesthesia. The repair of a ruptured globe or corneal laceration is usually done under general anesthesia. A local anesthetic is not considered safe, because the distortion from its injection might cause additional damage.

The eye is safely examined under anesthesia, usually with an operating microscope, and the repair is carried out by suturing the torn sclera or lacerated cornea. Exposed intraocular structures such as the iris or ciliary body may be replaced in the eye or excised depending on their condition. When the repair is complete, the eye is filled with saline or an electrolyte solution that simulates aqueous humor. Antibiotics are injected subconjunctivally after the globe is closed and continued intravenously for 4 or 5 days to prevent infection that may have been introduced by the injury.

A ruptured globe has a grave prognosis for restoration of vision. Corneal lacerations have a better prognosis, since their surgical repair is usually easily accomplished. If scarring occurs, corneal transplant can be performed.

### Contusion Injuries

Blunt trauma to the eye causes various contusion injuries ranging in severity from ecchymosis of the eyelids (black eye) to major intraocular damage.

**Compression injuries of the anterior eye** are characterized by corneal edema, anterior chamber hemorrhage, and increased intraocular pressure. These symptoms usually resolve without treatment. In some cases, however, return of normal intraocular pressure is followed several weeks or months later by another increase, which indicates the presence of angle recession glaucoma. This is caused by a tear of the attachment of the iris and ciliary body from the internal surface of the sclera at the anterior chamber angle, damaging the aqueous outflow pathway. Patients with compression injuries should always receive follow-up care at the hands of an ophthalmologist so that angle recession glaucoma can be detected and treated to prevent progressive damage to the optic nerve. Treatment usually begins with twice-daily drops of an ophthalmic beta-blocker.

**Hyphema** (hemorrhage into the anterior chamber) frequently clears spontaneously, but secondary hemorrhage occurs after several hours or days in up to one-third of cases as a result of lysis of the thrombus in the injured vessels of the iris or ciliary body. Secondary hemorrhage frequently continues until the anterior chamber is completely filled with blood, during which time the intraocular pressure may rise to 50–60 mm Hg (normal = 12–20 mm Hg). Lysis and reabsorption of this blood clot may take many days and cause damage to the aqueous filtration pathways and subsequent glaucoma. Breakdown products of blood can also diffuse into the cornea, stain it, and cause long-term reduction of vision. If reabsorption of the blood clot is prolonged, it can sometimes be successfully aspirated. If not, the anterior chamber is opened, and the clot is directly removed. Secondary hemorrhages may require surgical treatment. The prognosis for good vision in patients with secondary hemorrhage is poor.

The prevention of secondary hemorrhages is difficult. Bed rest with binocular patching has been a standard treatment for many years. More recent experience comparing patients treated with bed rest and others allowed normal activity showed no significant difference in the incidence of secondary hemorrhages.

Aminocaproic acid has been used to retard fibrinolysis in the injured vessels to prevent secondary hemorrhages to the benefit of many patients. This treatment slows the lysis of the primary hyphema but when given for 5–7 days does reduce the occurrence of secondary hemorrhages. There are significant side effects, so that use of aminocaproic acid must be carefully considered and monitored.

**Retinal edema,** particularly in the macula, causes acute reduction of vision. Vision usually improves with clearance of edema in a few days to several weeks. Clearance is not always complete, and there may be permanent damage to the macula.

In **ruptures of the choroid,** blood spreads beneath the retina at the time of injury, and reabsorption of blood will reveal a crescent-shaped scar concentric with the optic disk. There is no treatment.

Other contusion injuries include **dislocation of the lens** (partial or complete); **traumatic cataracts**; and tears in the region of the anterior attachment of the retina to the ciliary body, which lead to vitreous hemorrhages and **detachment of the retina**.

A damaged lens—either dislocated or cataractous—may reduce vision or may be displaced anteriorly, causing increased intraocular pressure by closing the aqueous filtration angle. In either case, the lens is removed using one of the cataract surgery techniques.

Vitreous hemorrhages are removed with a suction-cutting vitrectomy instrument. Following this procedure, the retinal detachment is repaired by creating an adhesive scar between the choroid and retina, usually by freezing through the scleral surface (cryotherapy) over the area of the retinal tear or hole. The sclera may then be buckled inward to push the adhesion against the retina. This is usually done by compressing the globe with an encircling band of silicone rubber. Sometimes, an intraocular gas bubble is used to push the retina, choroid, and sclera into contact.

## Intraocular Foreign Bodies

An intraocular foreign body should be suspected on the basis of the occupational history, particularly if the worker complains of an irritating sensation in the eye and no superficial foreign body is found. For example, when steel tools are used to hammer other steel objects, the hammered steel work-hardens to a glassy surface from which small, sharp chips can fly and penetrate the globe with a minimum of discomfort at the moment of impact. Vision may be nearly normal if the entry wound is small. In cases such as this, in which a radiopaque foreign body is suspected, an x-ray should be taken. Ultrasound will usually demonstrate nonradiopaque objects (eg, glass and plastic). If a foreign body is found, referral to an ophthalmologist for further evaluation and early treatment is essential.

Failure to remove iron or copper foreign bodies can cause severe impairment or loss of vision, owing to their toxic effects on ocular tissue. A retained iron or copper foreign body may dissolve away in several months to a year, but the damage done to the retina by the soluble metallic salts is irreversible, and marked visual loss—even blindness—results. The prognosis for these foreign bodies is good if they are removed before they have time to dissolve. Inert materials such as glass or plastic may cause mechanical damage to the eye, but in the absence of a local toxic reaction, the long-term prognosis is better. It is not necessary to remove every foreign body made of inert material; some of them may be left in place depending upon their position in the globe and their effect on visual function. Iron-containing magnetic foreign bodies are usually removed with an ophthalmic magnet—sometimes through the entry wound or through a surgical incision made as close as possible to the foreign body. Nonmagnetic foreign bodies are removed with grasping instruments specially designed for ophthalmic microsurgery. Penetrating wounds caused by potentially contaminated objects such as agricultural implements or by wood fragments thrown from woodworking machinery can introduce severe intraocular infections that lead to complete disruption and loss of the globe; therefore, microbiologic studies and treatment with appropriate systemic and local antibiotics are required.

## Injuries to the Orbit & Optic Nerve

Orbital floor ("blowout") fractures (see Chapter 10) are frequently associated with herniation of intraorbital contents into the fracture line. There usually is severe edema within the orbit, which restricts eye movements for 7–10 days. If restriction continues, surgical repair of the fracture may be indicated to free the entrapped extraocular muscles.

Facial bone and orbital fractures that extend to the posterior orbit may involve the optic canal, with damage to the optic nerve indicated by the presence of an afferent pupillary defect. Initial and later evaluations of the patient should include documentation of visual acuity. If there is progressive loss of vision, surgical decompression of the optic nerve in the canal may preserve or, occasionally, even improve the remaining vision.

Orbital injuries may cause severe hemorrhage, marked exophthalmos of the globe, and a dramatic and abrupt increase in intraocular pressure due to compression. Although this increased pressure is usually relieved by the normal dissipation of interstitial fluid in a short period of time, it occasionally results in occlusion of the central retinal artery or vein. Pressure can sometimes be reduced by applying gentle external massage to the globe through the closed lids. Surgical lysis of the lateral canthus of the lids may be required.

Penetrating wounds can directly damage the optic nerve by advancing through the funnel-shaped orbit to reach its apex, where the nerve and its blood supply are trapped by the optic canal. Contusion of the nerve causes severe visual impairment and is sometimes treated with large doses of systemic corticosteroids in a manner similar to treatment of spinal cord injuries.

## Injuries of the Corneal Epithelium (Abrasions & Superficial Foreign Bodies)

Abrasions of the corneal epithelium can be caused by superficial mechanical trauma (eg, prolonged wearing of contact lenses), by the presence of a foreign body, or by exposure to ultraviolet radiation, chemicals, aerosols, dust, smoke, and other irritants. The occupational medical history should be taken, as described in an earlier section.

**Photokeratoconjunctivitis ("welder's flash")** is a specific ocular injury caused by unprotected exposure to ultraviolet radiation with wavelengths shorter than 300 nm (actinic rays). This radiation is generated by the welder's arc and damages the exposed corneal and conjunctival epithelium. Injuries are caused not only by direct observation of the arc but occur also in persons nearby who are often not wearing protective filters.

In the first few hours after exposure, there may be only mild discomfort and slight conjunctival redness. After a latent period of several hours—even as long as 6–8 hours—the injured epithelial cells slough, causing an acute onset of severe pain sometimes said to be "as though someone had thrown hot sand in my eyes." Marked tearing, photophobia, and blepharospasm (tightly closed lids) are usual.

Examination requires a sterile topical anesthetic, which may be introduced through nearly closed eyelids by placing several drops along the lid margins. When the eyes open, more anesthetic may be instilled, along with fluorescein from a sterile paper strip. The fluorescein will diffuse over the cornea where the epithelium has sloughed, staining it bright green—best observed with a blue light. Epithelial loss is confined to the area exposed in the lid opening.

Treatment consists of instillation of an antibiotic ointment and patching the eye or eyes to prevent lid movement or blinking. The epithelium will not heal rapidly and in some cases not at all if it is frequently wiped and disturbed by blinking. It will require 12–24 hours for healing to occur, and in some cases several days may be necessary. The eyes should be examined daily. Anesthetic drops and fluorescein help in following progress of reepithelialization. Continue to patch with antibiotic ointment until healing has occurred. Corneal epithelium heals without scarring. Antibiotic solutions or ointments containing corticosteroids are sometimes recommended for the treatment of welder's flash burns. The steroids may speed clearing of the associated hyperemia and edema, but they increase the incidence of secondary bacterial, viral, and fungal infections. If steroids are used, frequent examination (every 12–24 hours) is essential to detect early signs of infection until healing occurs. In addition, prolonged use of topical steroids (10–14 days or more), even in low doses, can raise intraocular pressure and in time can cause significant glaucomatous field loss. This unpredictable response occurs in about 10% of the population. It is therefore probably best to avoid the routine or frequent use of topical corticosteroids in the treatment of corneal and conjunctival injuries and infections.

The patient should not be given anesthetic drops or ointment to use at home. Anesthetics slow and may even prevent epithelial healing, and when used in these circumstances they have led to severe scarring of the cornea and even the loss of an eye.

These injuries are easily prevented by wearing adequate protective filters in the face masks for the welder and goggles or ultraviolet filter glasses by visitors and workers in nearby areas where the welding flash can be seen.

Symptoms and signs of **corneal abrasions** include severe ocular pain, tearing, and blurring of vision. Inspection of the anterior eye with a flashlight usually shows irregular light reflections on the corneal surface in the area of the abraded epithelium. Use of sterile topical anesthetic and fluorescein paper strips is helpful for further examination. The fluorescein dye diffuses into the area of disrupted epithelium, stains it bright green, and can be easily observed with a blue light. If further evaluation reveals normal pupillary reactions, a bright red reflex, and no disruption of the anterior segment, the injury is usually confined to the anterior external layer of the cornea.

Small **foreign bodies** on the surface of the cornea or conjunctiva may be seen directly or detected by evidence of damaged epithelium from the fluorescein stain.

Foreign bodies can usually be removed with a cotton-tipped applicator, but a sharp instrument is occasionally helpful. The side bevel of a disposable hypodermic needle can be used to gently detach foreign bodies that are firmly attached to the corneal surface. Rust deposited in the anterior layers of the cornea frequently can be removed by the same gentle scraping maneuver. If all the foreign body or rust is not removed easily, it can usually be left to slough or absorb by itself without causing damage. After foreign bodies are removed, treatment is as for abrasions.

**Abrasions** are treated by applying a sterile ophthalmic antibiotic ointment effective against both gram-positive and gram-negative organisms (eg, gentamicin, tobramycin, or a mixture containing bacitracin, polymyxin, and neomycin) and covering the affected eye with a patch dressing to keep the lids closed. Corneal epithelium usually heals promptly if the surface of the cornea is allowed to rest without blinking the lid. The initial process of healing is one in which the normal epithelial cells slide from the edge of the wound over the smooth surface of the cornea to fill the gap. The eyes should be inspected in 12–24 hours to determine if healing has occurred and to rule out corneal infection, which appears as a white or gray haze in the area of the wound. If the abrasion is not completely healed, a second application of the ointment and patch dressing for an additional 12–24 hours may be required. This process should be continued until the epithelial defect is healed. Scarring usually does not occur, and vision is restored to normal.

*Caution:* After the initial examination with topical anesthetic, sharp pain may return until the epithelium begins to heal. Under no circumstances should the patient be supplied with anesthetic drops or ointment to use during the healing process, since topical anesthetics will delay healing and place the patient at risk for severe corneal infection and scarring. Antibiotic mixtures containing corticosteroids should not be used for treatment, because they provide inadequate protection against bacterial infection and enhance the growth of viral and fungal pathogens.

Abrasions caused by fat-soluble petroleum products splashed into the eyes are treated initially by copious irrigation with water or saline solution to remove any remaining material. Staining with fluorescein will demonstrate the amount of epithelial loss, which may vary from a few punctate areas to complete denudation of the cornea. In either case, treatment is the same as outlined above. If the abraded area is large, the corneal stroma may appear slightly gray, owing to some degree of edema. This clears rapidly with healing of the epithelium.

Exposure to aerosols (eg, paint sprays), detergents, surfactants, dust, smoke, and vapors can produce both acute and chronic symptoms of abrasion. Acute symptoms almost invariably include marked tearing and blepharospasm, which act to protect the eyes and wash away the offending material. Treatment for acute symptoms is as for other abrasions (see above).

Chronic exposure to low-level irritants causes fatigue of the lacrimal reflex and subsequent sensations of dryness and burning of the eyes. Some degree of redness is common. Irrigation with saline solution prevents most of these chronic symptoms. Adequate ventilation and avoidance of irritants in the workplace are obviously the best preventive measures.

Exposure to some chemical substances causes a delayed loss of corneal epithelium. For example, formaldehyde fumes cause diffuse damage to epithelial cells, leading to their accelerated sloughing with normal blinking. Fortunately, the abrasion will heal without scarring when the fumes are subsequently avoided. The long list of other substances that produce this effect includes butylamine, diethylamine, hydrogen sulfide, methyl silicate, mustard gas, osmium tetroxide, podophyllum resin, and sulfur.

## INDIRECT INJURIES TO THE EYE

In massive crush injuries, compression of the abdominal and chest vessels can cause sudden vascular engorgement of the retina. This leads to marked edema and diffuse hemorrhages in the fundus and can result in permanent ocular damage. **Purtscher's retinopathy** is one form of this condition. There is no treatment. The prognosis for vision depends on the amount of damage done to the macula or optic nerve. Slow improvement in vision occurs as hemorrhages absorb for periods up to several months.

In fractures of the long bones, fat emboli can migrate to the retina and produce small embolic changes that have the appearance of cotton-wool spots and are sometimes associated with flame-shaped hemorrhages in the fundus. Fat emboli, thrombi from heart valve disease and endocarditis, and emboli from a variety of sources occasionally obstruct branches of the retinal artery and cause infarction of a segment of the retina. Cholesterol crystals shed from atheromatous plaques in the carotid arteries may also migrate to the retina and appear as glistening intra-arterial bodies. In intravenous drug abuse, the injected drugs frequently contain inert substances such as talc, which may be seen in the retina as small white deposits. The prognosis for each of these conditions depends entirely on their location and whether or not the macula is involved. There is no ocular treatment. Clearing of the effects of these emboli—hemorrhages and edema—requires several weeks to a month. Cholesterol crystal emboli are an indication to investigate the patency of the carotid arteries.

Rarely, a septic embolus from a distant systemic infection causes endophthalmitis. Endophthalmitis has a generally poor prognosis. Specific diagnosis requires aspiration of vitreous fluid and sometimes aqueous humor for the isolation of organisms. Periocular injection of antibiotics adjacent to the scleral surface, occasionally intravitreal injection of appropriate doses of antibiotics, and intravenous antibiotics are the usual methods of treatment. The poor prognosis is due to delay in diagnosis while the infection advances and to the unpredictable and sometimes poor ocular penetration of antibiotics.

## SYMPATHETIC OPHTHALMIA

If the uveal tract (ie, the iris, ciliary body, or choroid) of one eye is injured, the uninjured (sympathizing) eye may show inflammation. This rare disorder is thought to be an autoimmune inflammatory response and can be prevented by prompt, adequate treatment of the initial injury to minimize continuing trauma to the damaged uveal tissue. Sympathetic ophthalmia can cause complete loss of vision in both eyes if unrecognized and untreated early in its course. As soon as inflammation is seen in the sympathizing eye, treatment of both eyes with local corticosteroids (topical and periocular injections) and mydriatics should be started. Large doses of systemic corticosteroids are also frequently used.

## OCCLUSION OF THE CENTRAL RETINAL ARTERY

Occlusion of the central retinal artery is characterized by sudden painless loss of vision and is considered an **ocular emergency**. Permanent loss of vision will result if the retina is deprived of blood for 30–60 minutes; therefore, arterial circulation must be restored as soon as possible.

Diagnosis is based on the history and eye examination. Occlusion is usually seen in older patients with arteriosclerosis or following embolism from the great vessels. It can also be caused by pressure from an unusually tight dressing over the eye, particularly when there is orbital edema or hemorrhage. If the visual loss is incomplete, the patient may be able to detect some light. Ophthalmic examination reveals a bloodless retina with thin and thready arteries. Early findings include a faint retinal edema that appears as a grayish or white discoloration and is particularly noticeable around the macula, allowing the normal red color of the choroid in the fovea to show through as a cherry-red spot. Later, red cells in the blood column of the arteries may separate into segments and appear as "boxcars." The veins also appear thinner than normal. The optic disk retains its normal pink color for several weeks, but the retinal edema becomes more apparent.

Although central retinal artery occlusions are not usually associated with increased intraocular pressures, the most effective treatment is immediate reduction of the normal intraocular pressure in an attempt to dislodge the embolus or thrombus thought

to be obstructing the artery at a restricted area of the vessel as it passes through the scleral shell just posterior to the optic disk. The pressure can be reduced by using two fingers to alternately massage and press the globe through the closed lids. This maneuver should be repeated four or five times over 10–15 minutes to accelerate the expression of aqueous humor and applies intermittent pressure on the artery. The patient's use of a rebreathing bag will increase the amount of carbon dioxide in the cerebral and ocular blood vessels, sometimes effecting vascular dilation.

If these maneuvers fail, paracentesis of the anterior chamber may be indicated. After a topical anesthetic is given, the conjunctiva is grasped with fine-tooth forceps. An incision is made through the clear cornea at the periphery of the anterior chamber, with the sharp scalpel blade held in the plane of the iris so as not to touch either the iris or the lens. The blade is then turned slightly to allow some of the aqueous humor to escape abruptly. This lowers the intraocular pressure and sometimes restores circulation to the retina.

## Anterior Ischemic Optic Neuropathy

This condition is characterized by an acute, painless loss of vision in individuals 50–70 years old. The ischemia of the optic nerve is in or just behind the disk. The disk appears swollen or edematous at first, clearing with time and leaving various amounts of optic atrophy and usually a severe loss of vision. The same process in the 70- to 80-year age group may be due to giant cell arteritis, frequently associated with temporal arteritis. Systemic steroids are sometimes helpful in the latter group to prevent involvement of the second eye.

## OCCLUSION OF THE CENTRAL RETINAL VEIN

Occlusion of the central retinal vein produces painless visual loss and is most commonly seen in older patients with diabetes, hypertension, or other vascular occlusive diseases. Findings include a swollen optic disk, distended and tortuous retinal veins, and an edematous retina with flame-shaped hemorrhages.

There is no effective emergency treatment, although anticoagulants have occasionally been tried. Patients should be followed for specific care by an ophthalmologist.

The prognosis for improvement of vision is slightly better in patients with an occluded retinal vein than in those with an occluded retinal artery.

# EYE INJURIES DUE TO RADIATION EXPOSURE

See Chapter 12 for a description of the electromagnetic spectrum and a discussion of methods to prevent occupational exposure to radiation.

## Injuries Due to Ionizing Radiation

X-rays, beta rays, and other radiation sources in adequate doses can cause ocular injury. The eyelid is particularly vulnerable to x-ray damage because of the thinness of its skin. Loss of lashes and scarring can lead to inversion or eversion (entropion or ectropion) of the lid margins and prevent adequate lid closure. Scarring of the conjunctiva can impair the production of mucus and the function of the lacrimal gland ducts, thereby causing dryness of the eyes. X-ray radiation in a dose of 500–800 R directed toward the lens surface can cause cataract, sometimes with a delay of several months to a year before the opacities appear. Treatment for these injuries is the appropriate oculoplastic repair of lid deformities and scarring. Deficiencies of tears and mucus can be improved by the topical use of artificial tears and protection from evaporation by wearing protective glasses with side shields that seal to the face. Radiation cataracts can be surgically removed by the appropriate standard technique.

## Injuries Due to Ultraviolet Radiation

Ultraviolet radiation of wavelengths shorter than 300 nm (actinic rays) can damage the corneal epithelium. This is most commonly the result of exposure to the sun at high altitudes and in areas where shorter wavelengths are readily reflected from bright surfaces such as snow, water, and sand. Exposure to radiation generated by a welding arc can cause welding flash burn, a form of keratitis. After a latent period of several hours, the injured epithelial cells soften and slough, causing sudden onset of pain. Treatment of these injuries consists of applying antibiotic ointment and patches until the epithelial cells have had an opportunity to heal (see Injuries of the Corneal Epithelium, above).

Wavelengths of 300–400 nm are transmitted through the cornea, and about 80% are absorbed by the lens, where they may cause cataractous changes. Accidental exposure to an inadequately shielded dental instrument used to accelerate the hardening of plastic fillings has caused significant lens opacities in dental personnel. Epidemiologic studies suggest that exposure to solar radiation in these wavelengths near the equator is correlated with an increased incidence of cataracts. They also indicate that workers exposed to bright sunlight in occupations such as farming, truck driving, and construction work appear to have a higher incidence of cataract than those who work primarily indoors. Experimental studies have shown that these wavelengths cause changes in the lens protein, which lead to cataract formation in animals.

## CATARACT

Any opacity in the lens is called a cataract. Some degree of opacity is present in almost all lenses, and the significance of the changes depends solely on their effect on vision. Peripheral opacities, for example, that do not interfere with vision are of no clinical significance.

The lens is composed of lens protein arranged in an ordered pattern of cytoplasmic fibers produced by the lens epithelium. These cells continue to produce new fibers at a slow rate throughout life. The lens thus slowly increases in volume—mainly in thickness—pushing the iris forward.

Changes in the chemistry and hydration of the lens protein create various types of cataracts. These changes may be induced by a variety of agents, including near ultraviolet radiation of 300–400 nm. These wavelengths are absorbed by the central lens fibers, causing the brownish discoloration of lenticular nuclear sclerosis. Ocular inflammation and corticosteroids, both topical and systemic, produce typical posterior subcapsular cataracts.

### Types of Cataracts

**A. Senile Cataracts:** Age-related (senile) cataract is the most common type seen. Some degree of opacity is almost universal. The progress of change and the related reduction of vision is usually quite slow. Nuclear sclerosis—an increasing density in the central mass of protein—causes a myopic change that can be corrected by changing glasses for some years—in many instances restoring vision to near normal.

**B. Congenital Cataracts:** These can be unilateral or bilateral, and many are thought to be of genetic origin. Some are due to maternal rubella during the first trimester of pregnancy. If the opacity prevents a clear view of the ocular fundus, surgical removal at an early age—even 2 months—is indicated to aid in the development of useful vision.

**C. Traumatic Cataracts:** Contusion injuries can cause opacities that may appear right away or develop slowly over weeks or even months. Penetrating wounds can tear the lens capsule, allowing aqueous humor to soften lens protein and usually creating major opacities. These cataracts almost always need to be removed acutely—in many cases at the time of wound repair.

**D. Secondary Cataracts:** These changes result from inflammatory processes in the eye (uveitis) and usually begin by producing opacities just inside the posterior lens capsule. Similar changes occur in association with retinitis pigmentosa, glaucoma, and, rarely, retinal detachments.

**E. Cataracts Associated With Systemic Dis-**

**eases:** These are usually bilateral and may appear in patients with myotonia dystrophica, hypoparathyroidism, diabetes mellitus, and Down's syndrome and in many other less common conditions.

**F. Toxic Cataracts:** Lens opacities are reported following exposure to or ingestion of numerous chemicals. They are described at some length in Grant's Toxicology of the Eye. The most common cause at the present seems to be prolonged use of corticosteroids, either topical or systemic. At least 2 years of moderate to high doses is usually necessary to produce cataract.

## Treatment

There is no effective medical treatment for cataract. Surgical removal usually results in significant improvement of vision in about 90% of patients. The results depend on whether other ocular changes are present such as macular scars or optic nerve changes. Indications for surgery depend almost entirely on the needs of the individual patient to improve vision. Of course, a rapidly swelling acute traumatic cataract needs early surgery.

There are two commonly used methods of cataract extraction. The lens may be removed totally in its capsule—the intracapsular technique. Extracapsular extraction removes all of the lens protein out of the lens capsular bag, leaving behind all of the capsule except for a portion of the anterior capsule removed along with the lens epithelium.

The presence of the intact posterior capsule facilitates implantation of an intraocular lens behind the iris. This lens replaces the optical power of the patient's own lens.

Complications of surgery are hemorrhage from the corneoscleral wound, infection, retinal detachment, and even damage to the macula from prolonged exposure to the light of the operating microscope.

## Prognosis

The results of cataract surgery are generally excellent. Significant visual improvement is reported in nearly 90% of cases following extraction of agerelated cataracts. The reduced expectations in eyes with injuries are due to unpredictable intraocular complications such as retinal scarring and macular damage.

## Injuries Due to Visible Radiation (Light)

Visible light has a spectrum of 400–750 nm. If the wavelengths of this spectrum penetrate fully to the retina, they can cause thermal, mechanical, or photic injuries.

**Thermal injuries** are produced by light intense enough to increase the temperature in the retina by 10 to 20 °C. Lasers used in therapy can cause this type of injury. The light is absorbed by the retinal pigment epithelium, where its energy is converted to heat, and the heat causes photocoagulation of retinal tissue.

**Mechanical injuries** can be produced by exposure to laser energy from a Q-switched or mode-locked laser, which produces sonic shock waves that disrupt retinal tissue.

**Photic injuries** are caused by prolonged exposure to intense light, which produces varying degrees of cellular damage in the retinal macula without a significant increase in the temperature of the tissue (usually no more than 1–2 °C). Recent studies have shown photic injuries not to be burns in the literal sense but damage from the light itself. Sun gazing is the most common cause of this type of injury, but prolonged unprotected exposure to a welding arc can also damage the retinal macula. When the initial retinal edema clears, there is usually some scarring that leads to a permanent decrease in visual acuity. The intensity of light, length of exposure, and age of the exposed individual are all important factors. The older the individual, the more sensitive the retina appears to be to photic injuries. Anyone who has had cataract surgery is much more vulnerable because filtration of light by the lens is impaired. In photic injuries caused by exposure to welding sources or other excessively bright light, treatment with systemic corticosteroids may be tried. A large initial dose of 60–100 mg of prednisone is rapidly tapered over a period of 10–14 days. This may reduce the acute edema or inflammatory response, but it is not always effective.

Wavelengths of 500–750 nm are most useful for vision and appear not to cause photic damage to the retina at exposures most commonly encountered. However, repeated exposure to bright sunlight by working outdoors for 3–4 hours each day can cause prolongation of the dark adaptation response, thereby reducing night vision.

## Injuries Due to Infrared Radiation

Wavelengths greater than 750 nm in the infrared spectrum can produce lens changes. Glassblower's cataract is an example of a heat injury that damages the anterior lens capsule. Denser cataractous changes can occur in unprotected workers who observe glowing masses of glass or iron for many hours a day.

## EFFECTS OF VIDEO DISPLAY TERMINAL USE

In recent years, employees who spend 6–8 hours a day looking at video display terminals have complained of eyestrain, headache, and general fatigue. The brightness of the light from such terminals is not great enough to produce any ocular injury. Posture, accommodative fatigue, and the early changes of presbyopia may contribute to feelings of eyestrain and physical stress.

Measures to alleviate these problems associated with video display terminal use are discussed in Chapter 6.

## REFERENCES

Albert DM, Jakobiec EA: *Principles and Practice of Ophthalmology.* Saunders, 1994.

Catania LJ: *Primary Care of the Anterior Segment,* 2nd ed. Appleton & Lange, 1995.

Duane TD (editor): *Clinical Ophthalmology.* Lippincott-Raven, 1995.

Fraunfelder FT: *Drug-Induced Ocular Side Effects,* 4th ed. Williams & Wilkins, 1994.

Grant WM: *Toxicology of the Eye,* 4th ed. Thomas, 1993.

Vaughan D, et al: *General Ophthalmology,* 14th ed. Appleton & Lange, 1995.

Webb LA: *Eye Emergencies—Diagnosis and Management.* Butterworth-Heinemann, 1995.

# 10

# Facial Injuries

*Kelvin C. Lee, MD, & Andrew H. Murr, MD*

Despite the widespread use of personal protective devices and mechanical safeguards, injuries of the face occur with alarming frequency in the workplace. The severity of a facial injury is usually directly correlated with the type, direction, and energy of the injuring force. Superficial abrasions or lacerations are commonly associated with low-energy forces and are usually preventable by use of appropriate protective devices. More severe injuries are commonly associated with equipment failure or improper use of high-speed or pressurized machinery. For example, the disruption of an air compressor or high-speed saw can result in dispersion of heavy particles at high energy, and the improper use of a sandblaster can result in penetration of the skin and eyes by small particles. Chainsaws and other cutting tools can cause deep lacerations if protective gear is not used or if improper technique is employed. Not only do these occupational injuries of the face have the potential for severe physical deformity and disability, but major facial scars have long-lasting psychologic effects on the worker.

## COMPREHENSIVE EARLY MANAGEMENT OF TRAUMATIC INJURIES

When encountering a patient with significant facial injury, the general principles used in the initial evaluation of patients with traumatic injuries should be applied. In localized injuries this may involve a cursory review of systems, while in more severe injuries a comprehensive assessment may require multiple radiographic studies and subspecialty consultations.

Steps for the initial management of traumatic injuries are as follows:

**A.   Stabilize the Airway:** The airway may be obstructed by blood, debris, loose dentures, teeth, or foreign bodies. An attempt should be made to remove these obstructions by suction or by direct instrumentation. The airway may be secured by positional changes if the patient is mobile. If a significant force has been delivered to the head and neck region by the trauma, cervical spine injury must be assumed until proven otherwise. In patients with such trauma, cervical manipulation should be minimized. In most cases, gentle extension of the head with neck flexion will maximize the patient's upper airway. In the event positional changes are not adequate, a forward thrust of the tongue, either by direct traction on the tongue or by forward traction of the symphysis or angles of the mandible, may be adequate to open the airway. If the airway cannot be satisfactorily maintained, endotracheal intubation or tracheotomy should be attempted.

**B.   Control Massive Hemorrhage:** Massive hemorrhage is ordinarily best controlled by the application of packing or pressure. Careful clamping of bleeding vessels should be undertaken only if packing or pressure does not suffice. Clamping of bleeding vessels with small hemostats should be avoided in injuries along the distribution of the facial nerve, except in an ideal environment such as the operating room (Figure 10–1).

**C.   Rule Out Cardiopulmonary Injury:** Early assessment of the patient's pulmonary and cardiac function is essential before attention to specific aspects of any maxillofacial trauma. The potential need for ventilatory support or fluid resuscitation should be evaluated soon after encountering the patient.

**D.   Rule Out Fracture of the Cervical Spine:** In all trauma involving a significant force striking the head and neck the stability of the cervical spine needs to be evaluated prior to manipulation of the head and neck. The head should be stabilized with sandbags or kept in a neutral position with a cervical collar until a cervical fracture is ruled out. In most cases this would require radiographic imaging of the cervical spine or examination by a spine specialist.

**E.   Rule Out or Treat Any Major Neurologic, Thoracoabdominal, and Orthopedic Injuries:** In cases of dramatic injuries to the face, the focus of attention too easily falls to the obvious site of injury. The patient's overall condition must not be jeopardized by undue attention to the maxillofacial region. A systematic review of the patient injuries is needed

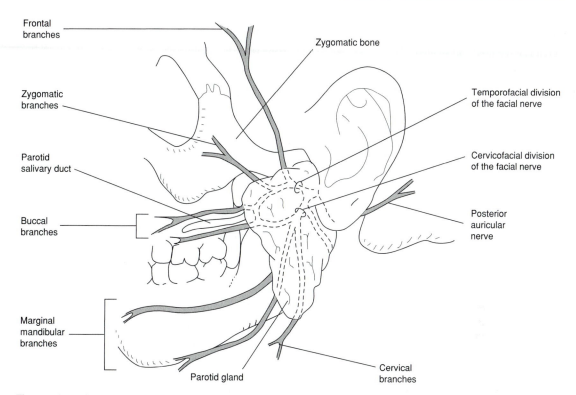

**Figure 10–1.** Course and distribution of the facial nerve branches after exiting the skull. Note association of buccal branch of the nerve with the parotid salivary duct. (Redrawn and reproduced, with permission, from Fonseca RJ, Walker RV: *Oral and Maxillofacial Trauma*. Saunders, 1991.)

including careful examination for neurological injury, and injury to the chest, abdomen, and/or extremities.

Only after completing the steps outlined above should a detailed and thorough evaluation of a facial injury be initiated.

## MANAGEMENT OF SOFT TISSUE INJURIES

Soft tissue may be damaged by blunt trauma or penetrating injury. The degree of damage is usually related to the amount of energy applied to the soft tissue and can vary dramatically with the etiologic agent. High-velocity, penetrating materials, such as those from an explosion, frequently cause more massive soft tissue injury than is immediately apparent due to late tissue necrosis. Continuing assessment is essential in such injuries because further debridement or repair may be needed as the true extent of destruction becomes apparent.

### Diagnostic Considerations

In any soft tissue injury of the face an assessment for the involvement of certain vital deeper structures is essential.

**A. Facial Nerve Injury:** The patient may complain of difficulty in moving parts of the face. All important facial motions must be evaluated. Ask the patient to wrinkle the forehead, close the eyes tightly, smile, and purse the lips. Failure to perform any of these movements in an otherwise cooperative patient suggests transection of the nerve. The nerve should be evaluated throughout its entire course to determine the site of injury. The presence of facial swelling can mask a regional facial nerve palsy. The clinician should be suspicious of an injury if a laceration or penetrating trauma crosses the usual course of the facial nerve (Figure 10–1). If complete hemifacial paralysis is noted, the injury to the nerve can be central, within the temporal bone or soon after the nerve exits the stylomastoid foramen. A central or temporal bone injury is initially evaluated by computed tomography (CT) scanning or magnetic resonance imaging (MRI). In certain cases, electrodiagnostic testing may be useful to evaluate the integrity of the facial nerve. Most peripheral nerve injuries in association with a laceration or penetrating trauma requires direct exploration and repair of the nerve at the site of injury.

**B. Medial Canthus Injury:** A laceration that involves the medial canthal area may involve the lacrimal drainage system. With such injuries, the integrity of the ducts must be assured by direct cannulation. Lacerations through this drainage system should be repaired and stented.

**C. Parotid Duct Injury:** By massaging the parotid gland, saliva can be obtained through the caruncle located opposite the second maxillary molar (Stenson's duct). Blood in the saliva flowing through this caruncle is a sign of injury to the parotid duct. Significant injury to this duct requires exploration and repair with stenting. Injury to the parotid duct is usually accompanied by injury to its anatomic companion the buccal branch of the facial nerve. With such duct injuries particular attention to facial nerve function is warranted.

## Treatment

**A. Care of Lacerations:** The major goal of treatment of lacerations is to convert a contaminated wound into one that is as clean as a surgical incision. Sterile technique should be used in all cases.

**1. Control of hemorrhage**–Hemorrhage should be controlled by persistent pressure and/or packing. If this is not adequate, careful clamping of vessels with suture ligation or cautery can be used. Special attention to the regions involving the facial nerve, parotid duct, and lacrimal system is needed to avoid inadvertent injury to these important structures with hemostatic measures. If such an injury is of concern, formal exploration in the operating room should be considered.

**2. Anesthesia**–Sensory and motor function of the nerves of the face and neck must be assessed prior to induction of local or general anesthesia. An anesthetic should be administered before the wound is cleaned. Local anesthesia is best achieved by infiltration of a solution such as 1% lidocaine with 1:100,000 epinephrine. In certain cases regional anesthesia using field blocks of specific nerves can also be used for facial wound repairs.

**3. Wound cleaning and preparation for repair**–After larger foreign bodies are mechanically removed from the wound, it is irrigated with copious amounts of normal saline solution to remove occult debris and bacteria. This can be done by using a blunt needle on a large syringe (eg, a 19-gauge blunt needle on a 60-mL syringe) and forcefully irrigating the complete depth of the wound. In almost every case, primary closure of facial lacerations is recommended. Because the blood supply to the face is excellent, only obviously necrotic tissue should be removed. The wound is sharply debrided so that macerated edges are excised. This measure may require excision of some normal skin. Even a millimeter of debridement provides more viable uninjured tissue for closure. Debridement makes undermining of wound edges a requirement so that the tissue can be advanced to achieve closure. The edges are undermined in a plane between the dermis and subcutaneous tissue to a distance of 1–2 cm horizontally

from the wound edge. No attempt should be made to straighten lacerations unless the laceration can be made to lie completely within or parallel to resting skin tension lines (Figure 10–2). These skin lines are similar to the lines of aging and are ordinarily directed in a perpendicular direction to the pull of facial muscles. A jagged laceration is eventually less apparent than one that is straight but crosses resting skin tension lines. Prior to wound closure, hemostasis must be meticulous.

**4. Wound closure**–Subcutaneous tissues are closed with absorbable suture of a suitable size, such as 3-0 or 4-0 chromic gut sutures. The skin is closed next with a subcuticular stitch of similar size. The needle enters the dermis and exits between the epidermis and dermis on one side, and it then enters between the epidermis and dermis on the opposite side and exits the dermis on that side. The knot is then tied. This technique results in the knot being placed below the surface and therefore not protruding between the skin edges. The wound should already be precisely approximated following closure of the subcuticular layer. The cuticular layer is then sutured with 5-0 or 6-0 monofilament nylon to achieve final closure. There should be no tension on the wound edges, and the cuticular stitch should not be used to close defects of more than 1 mm of skin. Larger de-

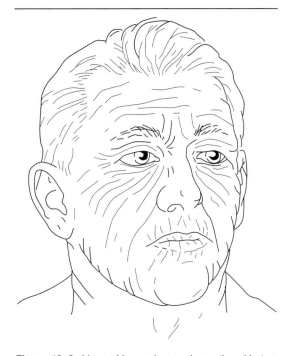

**Figure 10–2.** Lines of Langerhan or the resting skin tension lines. Repair of lacerations should attempt to parallel these lines when possible. (Redrawn and reproduced, with permission, from Fonseca RJ, Walker RV: *Oral and Maxillofacial Trauma.* Saunders, 1991.)

fects require placement of more subcuticular sutures to remove all tension from the edges of the skin.

**5. Wound dressings and follow-up care–** The wound is dressed with an antibiotic ointment, and a tetanus toxoid booster should be given if appropriate. Thereafter, the wound is cleaned three times daily with a sterile saline solution or hydrogen peroxide. Antibiotic ointment is then applied to help loosen eschars and facilitate epithelialization.

After the cuticular sutures have been in place for about 3–5 days, they are removed. Wound edges are treated with a substance that promotes adhesion, such as tincture of benzoin, and adhesive strips are applied in a crisscross fashion to the wound edges. These strips should be maintained for at least 5 days, after which time tissue strength begins to develop as a result of the maturation of tissue collagen.

**B. Special Considerations:**

**1. Special structures–**Nose, eyebrow, and mouth injuries require special attention in their repair because of their unique anatomy.

**a. Nasal injuries.** The anterior two thirds of the nose is supported by several cartilaginous structures that can be lacerated along with the nasal skin in an injury. The complex relationship of these cartilages and the need to evaluate the soft tissues within the nasal passages often requires evaluation by a specialist to obtain an optimal reconstruction of this structure. In simple lacerations with minimal cartilage damage, repair should include reapproximation of the cartilage by suture repair of the perichondrium with absorbable sutures. In some cases a figure eight or simple suture through the cartilage will be needed to maintain good position. The skin should be repaired as described above.

**b. Eyebrow injuries.** A laceration through the eye brow requires special care to minimize injury to the hair follicles that may be exposed by the injury. Hair follicle injury from overzealous hemostastic measures or debridement may leave a large part of the eyebrow permanently devoid of hair. Minimal debridement or undermining of tissues should be performed in this region. Primary repair should focus on realigning the hair line as accurately as possible with the first cuticular sutures.

**c. Mouth injuries.** Lacerations or penetrating injuries through the skin and extend through the buccal mucosa or lips can be more difficult to repair. With full thickness lacerations of the mouth, preparation of the wound is similar to other soft tissue injuries. With most of these injuries, the repair of the subcutaneous tissues including orbicularis oris should first be performed with simple interrupted absorbable 3-0 or 4-0 sutures. Oral mucosa is then repaired with simple interrupted 4-0 chromic gut sutures up to the transition of oral mucosa to the vermillion. The skin laceration should then be repaired with subcuticular and the cuticular sutures as previously described, focusing on reapproximating

the vermillion border as accurately as possible. Even a small discrepency of this border will be obvious to the casual observer when it is healed. After this is completed the remainder of the vermillion is closed with 4-0 absorbable subcuticular interrupted sutures followed by epidermal closure using 5-0 nylon sutures in a simple interrupted fashion.

**2. Delayed treatment–**Unlike other locations, because of it's exceptional blood supply, the delayed treatment of facial lacerations is similar to acute repairs in the absense of infection. If infection occurs, sutures are removed, the wound is opened, and wet-to-dry dressings are applied. When the wound has been cleansed of all purulent material and healthy granulation tissue is present, the above steps are used to reclose the wound.

**3. Care of abrasions–**Abrasive injuries can cause partial-thickness to full-thickness loss of the epidermis. A full-thickness loss of skin results in an anesthetic area similar to that of a third-degree burn.

**a. Anesthesia.** Anesthesia of a large abraded area can be achieved by local infiltration of an anesthetic solution such as lidocaine with epinephrine, by topical application of an anesthetic gel such as 4% lidocaine jelly, or by field block of specific nerves.

**b. Wound cleaning and repair.** After adequate anesthesia has been achieved, the wound is cleaned by irrigation. Scrubbing with a soft scrub brush may be required to remove small embedded particles, but scrubbing should be undertaken carefully to avoid causing further injury. Small areas of full thickness avulsion of less than 3 cm in diameter can usually be treated by the mobilization of adjacent tissue or by the rotation or advancement of local flaps. Larger areas of avulsion may require delayed skin grafting. To obtain the best color and texture match, the type of skin grafts and appropriate donor sites are chosen based on the location of the tissue loss. In addition, an attempt to preserve the facial aesthetic units with the use of flaps and skin grafting will help to maximize the benefit of the facial repair (Figure 10–3).

**c. Wound dressings and follow-up care.** Partial thickness abrasions are cleaned and covered with antibiotic ointment 2–3 times daily. For larger wounds a semiocclusive dressing may be used to protect this region. These dressing should be changed as recommended by the manufacturer of the dressing. No treatment is needed for pigmentary changes that occasionally occur after injury, since the pigment usually reverts to normal within 6–12 months.

**C. Care of Skin Penetrated by Small Foreign Bodies:** Certain injuries may result in skin penetration of multiple small foriegn bodies. Common examples include asphalt from a road burn or sand particles from a sandblast injury. These foreign bodies individually do not pose much of a problem, but they must be removed or they can result in a permanent tattoo.

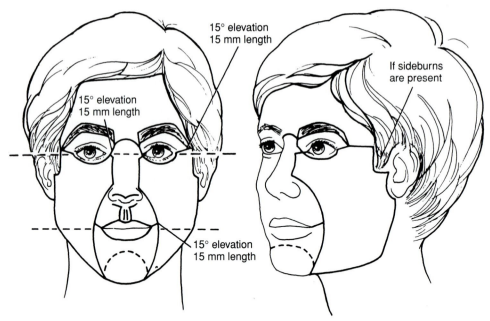

**Figure 10–3.** The facial aesthetic units should be preserved when possible. Laceration repair or reconstruction with flaps should be designed to spare these regions. (Redrawn and reproduced, with permission, from Thomas JR, Holt GR. *Facial Scars: Incision, Revision and Camouflage.* Mosby, 1989.)

**1. Wound cleaning and repair**–Sparsely placed foreign bodies can usually be removed mechanically with a fine forceps. Magnification provided by a loupe or microscope is frequently necessary to achieve adequate removal. In certain cases, an orthopedic debrider may be used to mobilize these particles. Diffusely placed small foreign bodies, such as sand particles, may require removal by dermabrasion. Dermabrasion should be continued only to the depth necessary to remove the particles without causing a full-thickness injury. It is sometimes preferable to perform dermabrasion in a symmetric fashion so that the resulting pattern will be less noticeable.

**2. Wound dressings and follow-up care**– Care of these types of injuries following their cleaning and repair is the same as that described for partial-thickness abrasions.

**D. Care of Scarred Facial Tissue.** Scarring that results from facial injuries may require secondary revision. Assessment of need for scar revision should be made only after the signs of acute inflammation have resolved, which usually requires 6–12 months. In this time period dramatic improvement of scar appearance often occurs as the wound matures. It is usually best to delay reconstructive measures, such as Z-plasty, running W-plasty, and geometric broken-line closures, until the scar revision stage of treatment. On occasion a facial scar can be so dramatic that early revision is indicated since the eventual need for scar revision even after expected wound maturation is clear. Proceeding with early reconstruc-

tive measures in these select cases will markedly improve patient morale.

## MANAGEMENT OF FACIAL FRACTURES

In the evaluation of the patient with facial injuries the likelihood of a facial fracture can be determined by knowing the type and focus of force received in the facial injury, and an understanding of the amount of force required to fracture the facial bones. The vulnerability of these facial bones vary considerably from the nasal bone, which requires minimal force to fracture, to the various skullbase fractures or Lefort fractures, which require a major blow to the mid face to occur.

Most facial fractures can be diagnosed on the basis of physical symptoms and signs alone. A hematoma points to a specific site of injury. Facial deformities secondary to depression of facial bone structures and impairment of sensory and motor functions of adjacent nerve structures are significant signs of a facial fracture.

General examination should include (1) assessment of facial symmetry and extraocular motility; (2) palpation of the orbital rims, frontozygomatic areas, zygomatic arches, and mandible; (3) evaluation of the dental occlusion; (4) determination of the stability and configuration of the nasal dorsum; and (5) evaluation of the three major cutaneous branches of the trigeminal nerve, particularly the infraorbital branch.

# 1. NASAL FRACTURES

Because of its prominent location and delicate construction, the nasal bones are the most commonly fractured structure in the facial skeleton. Fortunately, fracture of the nasal bone without displacement is without consequence to the patient and usually does not require repair.

## Clinical Findings

The most common finding in patients with nasal fratures is point tenderness over the nasal bones. Epistaxis may frequently be present following the injury. In more severe cases, the nasal dorsum is obviously deviated to one side or collapsed, and crepitation may be noted. Injury to the internal nasal structures will also frequently be evident. Inspection of the nasal vault may show an impaired airway on one side of the nasal septum with a corresponding concavity on the other side suggesting a traumatic septal deviation. With nasal trauma, hematomas can form between the septal cartiledge and the perichrondrium devascularizing the septum. If not treated, they will result in septal cartilage destruction. Thus, it is critical to examine every patient with significant nasal trauma for a septal hematoma. They appear as symmetric nasal septal convexities that are bluish in color and are slightly soft to palpation.

Lateral soft tissue x-rays will usually confirm the diagnosis of nasal bone fracture.

## Treatment & Prognosis

The presence of post-traumatic swelling can make assessment of the degree of nasal fracture displacement difficult. Often the decision to perform a reduction of the nasal fracture will be delayed until 3–5 days after the date of injury to allow soft tissue swelling to regress. After 7–10 days, the nasal bones will have started to heal, so that closed reduction becomes increasingly difficult. Nondisplaced nasal fractures do not require treatment, but a small splint may be helpful for comfort.

The nasal bone is not a weight bearing structure, thus closed reduction of a fracture without fixation is indicated for significantly displaced nasal fractures. Some surgeons prefer to wait until swelling has subsided, since they feel that more precise realignment of the nasal dorsum can be achieved at that time. However, performing closed reduction as soon as possible, preferably in the first 12 hours, rehabilitates the patient more rapidly and is likely to produce better results, since healing in the displaced position has not begun. The use of closed reduction corrects the majority of gross abnormalities that result from the nasal injury. Definitive repair of any nasal deformity due to nasal bone fractures may require an open reduction and repair, which is usually performed at least 6 months after the date of injury.

Dislocation of the nasal septum should be ad-dressed at the time of the repair of nasal fracture. In more severe cases, immediate or delayed septoplasty may be required to re-establish an adequate nasal airway.

Septal hematomas require immediate treatment to prevent infection and secondary necrosis of the septal cartilage. Treatment consists of draining the hematoma and using nasal packing to reapproximate the septal mucosa to the septal cartilage.

A 7- to 10-day period of disability is expected after reduction of a nasal fracture. A nasal splint is worn for approximately 7 days. Pressure or further injury to the nose must be avoided for at least 3 months following a nasal fracture.

# 2. MANDIBULAR FRACTURES

Mandibular fractures usually occur from direct trauma to the jaw. Given the prominent location of the mandible, it is the second most common type of facial fracture. The majority of cases involves at least two fractures of this arch shaped bone. The most frequent site of fracture is the region just below the condylar process (Figure 10–4).

## Clinical Findings

Swelling and tenderness in the soft tissue overlying the fracture sites, and pain with mastication are the most common signs of a mandibular fracture. Displacement of fracture fragments frequently results from the pull of the muscles of mastication causing malocclusion. Other symptoms and signs of a mandibular fracture may include a step-off deformity, instability of the dental arch, hypoesthesia of the mental nerve, foul-smelling breath, trismus, or deviation of the jaw on opening. In certain cases of bilateral mandibular fractures, mobility of the anterior segment may allow collapse of the base of the tongue into the airway resulting in airway obstruction. Anterior traction will immediately correct this problem, but these patients will require airway protection until the mandibular fractures are stabilized. In addition, particular attention should be paid to the patient's dentition. Fractured, chipped, or loosened teeth should be noted. Any avulsed teeth should be located, since they may have been aspirated. Chest x-rays should be performed if the teeth cannot be found immediately.

Plain mandibular radiographs or panorex dental imaging will confirm the presence of the mandibular fractures and display the degree of displacement.

## Treatment & Prognosis

The treatment approach for a mandibular fracture depends on the location, the number of fractures, and the availability of stable dentition. Single nondisplaced subcondylar fractures can be successfully managed with soft diet alone or a short period of in-

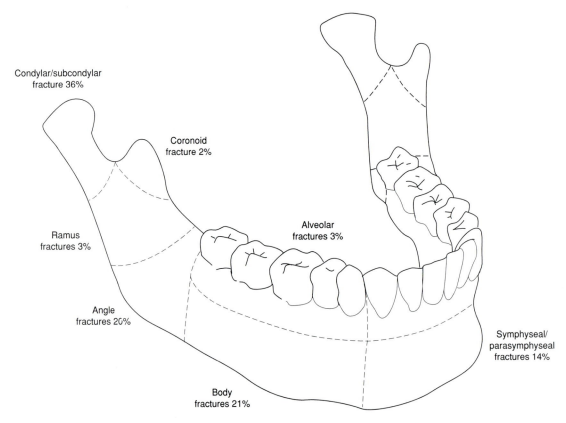

**Figure 10–4.** The frequency of fracture of various mandibular regions is represented. Mandibular fractures occur most frequently at the subcondylar, angle, and body of the mandible. (Redrawn and reproduced, with permission, from Mathog RH: *Maxillofacial Trauma*. Williams & Wilkins, 1994.)

termaxillary fixation (IMF). Traditionally, definitive treatment of other mandibular fractures consists of closed reduction followed by IMF for 4–6 weeks. IMF relies on sufficient dentition to maintain good fixation after centric occlusion has been achieved. Open reduction and internal fixation using compression plating has allowed effective management of many types of fractures and are particularly useful for those patients with little or no dentition. It has also offered an alternative technique that allows more rapid bone healing and earlier mobilization of the mandible compared with IMF alone.

Chipped teeth require temporary coverage of pulp and dentin at the time of fracture therapy. Definitive repair of damaged teeth can be done later. Avulsed teeth should be replanted within the first 2 hours of avulsion. They can be stabilized to adjacent teeth during the period of intermaxillary fixation to allow them to heal.

The prognosis for return to function of the mandible following proper treatment is excellent. Subcondylar fractures that remain displaced may cause temporomandibular joint pain on chewing and ultimately result in abnormal mobility of the joint.

The period of disability after mandibular fractures is usually 4–6 weeks. If intermaxillary fixation is used, it may be maintained for 6 weeks. In these patients, return to active heavy labor may not be possible for 6–8 weeks. If rigid internal fixation techniques are used, return to active heavy labor can be earlier. Return to work requires individualization based upon the type of injury, the type of repair, the job description, and other associated injuries.

### 3. MAXILLARY (LE FORT) FRACTURES

Maxillary fractures are classified as Le Fort I, II, and III fractures (Figure 10–5). These are uncommon fractures that usually require a very significant force striking the midface. The most common cause of these fractures is high speed motor vehicle accidents. A Le Fort I fracture is a horizontal fracture of the palate and does not involve the orbits. A Le Fort II fracture traverses through the lateral buttress of the maxilla, the infraorbital rim, the orbital floor, the medial wall of the orbit, and the perpendicular plate of the ethmoid bone. A Le Fort III fracture has the char-

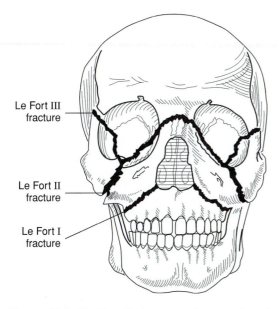

**Figure 10–5.** Maxillary fractures usually occur in patterns described by Le Fort. Le Fort Fractures I–III are represented and extend into the skull base through the pterygoid plates. (Redrawn and reproduced, with permission, from Bailey BJ: *Head & Neck Surgery—Otolaryngology.* Lippincott, 1993. Original illustration by Anthony Pazos.)

acteristics of a Le Fort II fracture with the addition of frontozygomatic fractures and is known as craniofacial disjunction. All of these fractures extend posteriorly to the pterygoid plates.

### Clinical Findings

In patients with maxillary fractures, the mid face is usually displaced posteriorly and inferiorly. This results in malocclusion with the molar teeth meeting prematurely and the incisor teeth meeting with an open bite called apertognathia. In most patients, the entire mid face appears to be flattened, and patients frequently present with epistaxis along with facial pain. The level of mobility in the mid face depends on the type of fracture. To test for mobility, the forehead is stabilized by the palm of one hand, and the opposite thumb and forefinger are used to grasp the incisor teeth or palate. An attempt is then made to manipulate the palate. In Le Fort I fractures, only the palate is mobile. In Le Fort II and III fractures, findings may include mobility of the nasal dorsum and anterior malar faces. These patients may also have hypoesthesia of the infraorbital nerve, a nasal fracture, and cerebrospinal fluid rhinorrhea resulting from an associated fracture of the cribriform plate or anterior skullbase. More severe cases may have concurrent mandibular fractures, nasoethmoid complex fractures, or both. In patients with significant displacement of their maxillary fractures, the posterior

displacement can impinge on the patient's airway and they may require airway protection until definitive repair of the fractures takes place. In these patients with significant midface fractures, no tubes of any sort should be passed nasally since the skullbase in these patients can be penetrated with instrumentation resulting in significant morbidity. Early ophthalmologic consultation to rule out globe injury is indicated given the degree of force required to produce these fractures and their involvement of the bony orbital walls.

Standard Waters and Caldwell x-ray views of the face are sufficient to diagnose these fractures, but fine cut CT scans are essential to define the exact extent of the injury and to accurately assess the status of the orbital floor.

### Treatment & Prognosis

Management of maxillary fractures includes reduction of the midface and restoration of normal occlusion followed by fixation. For best rsults, surgical intervention should occur in the period 3–7 days after the traumatic injury. In extreme cases when the patient is unstable due to other associated injuries, repair can be delayed up to 14 days. The repair of maxillary fractures usually requires intranasal manipulations and the use of intermaxillary fixation, thus a tracheotomy is indicated to maintain the airway perioperatively. In most cases, closed reduction is initially performed using specialized forceps for grasping and mobilizing the midface to restore its normal position. Normal occlusion is assured by the application of intermaxillary fixation. This step is followed by direct exposure of key points of the fracture, verification of reduction, and rigid fixation using metal plates. Rigid fixation usually allows immediate removal of IMF.

Most CSF leaks associated with maxillary fractures are self-limited and require no additional measures.

Recovery from the surgery usually requires 2–3 weeks. A further period of rehabilitation of 1–2 months following these severe maxillofacial injuries is often necessary. Other associated injuries, such as brain or orthopedic injuries commonly require more prolonged rehabilitation.

### 4. ZYGOMATIC FRACTURES

The zygoma is a prominent facial bone that forms the malar eminence, which gives projection to the cheek. This bone is frequently fractured by a direct blow to the cheekbone. This fracture was previously called the tripod fracture, but because more than three buttresses are fractured, it has been renamed the zygomatic complex fracture. The entire bone is usually dislocated posteriorly, inferiorly, and medially (Figure 10–6). With such an injury, prominence of

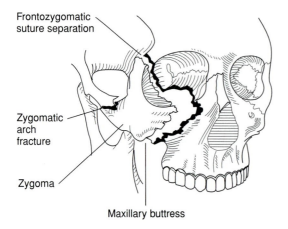

**Figure 10–6.** Fracture of the zygomatic complex usually results in medial, inferior, and posterior displacement. (Redrawn and reproduced, with permission, from Bailey BJ: *Head & Neck Surgery—Otolaryngology.* Lippincott, 1993. Original illustration by Anthony Pazos.)

the zygoma is lost, and this will result in an unsightly deformity if allowed to heal without reduction. In addition, the zygoma helps to form the orbital floor, thus untreated fractures with significant displacement may result in orbital complications.

### Clinical Findings

Symptoms and signs include pain over the malar area, hypoesthesia of the infraorbital nerve, step-off deformity of the infraorbital rim, flattening of the malar eminence and lateral subconjunctival hemorrhage. A downward slant of the palpebral fissure may occur due to inferior displacement of the attachment of the lateral tendon of the canthus. Limited extraocular motility suggests involvement of the orbital contents. However, muscle contusion or neuropraxia of the third cranial nerve as well as fracture of the orbital floor with entrapment of the inferior rectus muscle can result in diplopia. In some cases, the eye is displaced backward or recessed in the orbit as a result of a relative increase in the volume of the bony orbit. This complication is called enophthalmos and can result in significant long term diplopia if not corrected. The zygomatic arch may be displaced medially and impinge on the coronoid process, which can result in trismus or inadequate closure of the jaw.

Standard Caldwell, Waters, submentovertex, and lateral x-ray views should be obtained to screen for the presence of a zygomatic complex fracture. A Waters view will usually show infraorbital rim fractures and frontozygomatic suture separations, and it may also show fractures of the lateral maxillary sinus walls. An underpenetrated submentovertex ("bucket-handle") view will demonstrate a fracture of the zygomatic arch. If a fracture is found on plain x-rays, a CT scan of the mid face should be obtained to deter-

mine the degree of displacement present and to assist in the reconstructive effort. Direct coronal scans or coronal reconstructions are obtained to assess the integrity of the orbital floor.

### Treatment & Prognosis

Emergent treatment of zygomatic complex fractures is usually not required. In these patients with significant periorbital trauma, ophthalmologic consultation to rule out significant orbital injury should be obtained in the early phases of patient management. If needed, repair of the fracture should be performed between 3–7 days after the injury. Although zygomatic fractures that are minimally displaced require no treatment, those that are symptomatic or have more than a few millimeters of displacement should be treated by open reduction and fixation. Incisions are usually made sublabially onto the anterior face of the maxilla and over the frontozygomatic suture. The zygoma is placed in its normal position, and rigid plates are applied to maintain reduction.

The orbital floor must also be carefully evaluated, and significantly displaced fractures should be repaired through an infraorbital incision. If repairs are not made in cases where the bony orbital volume is significantly greater due to the floor fracture, enophthalmos may occur after the swelling associated with the injury subsides. This late post-traumatic enophthalmos is extremely difficult to repair. Reconstruction of the orbital floor may require the use of material such as bone or cartilage grafts to rebuild the floor and maintain the appropriate orbital volume.

The prognosis for return to full function after a zygomatic complex fracture is excellent. Swelling will usually be resolved by 2 weeks after the injury. Light work can be resumed at that time. Heavy labor is best delayed until 4 weeks after repair. The malar area should be protected from possible recurrent injury for 3 months after repair.

### 5. ORBITAL FLOOR ("BLOWOUT") FRACTURES

In certain cases an orbital floor can be fractured without the other facial bones being injured. Classically, this fracture results from a focused blow to the globe without significant impact to the infraorbital rim or the zygoma. The force is transmitted by the globe and fractures the weakest component of the bony orbit, the orbital floor.

### Clinical Findings

In orbital floor fractures, periorbital swelling and eye pain may be the only presenting complaints. Entrapment of the inferior rectus muscle in the floor fracture can occur and causes diplopia and fixation of the globe when the patient attempts to look upward. As with zygomatic complex fractures, if there is significant displacement of the orbital floor into the maxillary sinus, enophthalmos may result.

The Waters x-ray can usually demonstrate the orbital floor fracture. A teardrop deformity may appear beneath the orbital floor resulting from herniation of the orbital contents into the maxillary sinus below or hematoma formation in the mucosa of the sinus roof. As with zygomatic complex fractures, a CT scan is necessary to determine the exact extent of injury and the degree of displacement of the orbital floor.

## Treatment & Prognosis

As with any periorbital trauma, ophthalmologic consultation to rule out vision threatening orbital injury should be obtained as soon as possible. Surgical reconstruction of the orbital floor is required for entrapment of extraocular muscles, enophthalmos, or globe ptosis due to the size of the orbital floor defect. In questionable cases, repair may be delayed 10–14 days in order to obtain a more accurate assessment of the degree of deformity or impairment of function as the traumatic swelling recedes. An infraorbital incision is used to explore the orbital floor and repair it as needed. Grafting material is often needed to reestablish the orbital floor.

The prognosis for return to full function after an orbital floor fracture is excellent. Periorbital swelling has usually resolved by 2 weeks after the injury or surgery. Light work can be resumed at that time. Heavy labor is best delayed until at least 4 weeks after surgical repair.

## 6. NASOETHMOIDAL COMPLEX FRACTURES

With severe upper midface trauma, the entire nasal complex can be displaced posteriorly causing collapse of the nasal bones into the ethmoidal sinuses. This type of injury also destabilizes the medial canthal ligaments frequently resulting in posttraumatic telecanthus. In more severe cases, there may be an associated fracture of the anterior skull base and a potential for a cerebral spinal fluid leak.

### Clinical Findings

Common symptoms and signs of nasoethmoidal complex fractures include facial pain, anosmia, watery rhinorrhea, flattening of the nasal dorsum, and downward, lateral, and anterior displacement of the medial canthus. A torn cribriform plate can cause cerebrospinal fluid rhinorrhea. Disruption of the medial canthal area, with failure of apposition of the inferior lacrimal caruncle to the globe, may result in epiphora, the uncontrolled flow of tears.

Though plain x-rays may suggest an injury to this region, diagnosis requires a CT scan of the facial bones and paranasal sinuses.

## Treatment & Prognosis

Emergency reduction of nasoethmoidal complex fractures is only necessary in the rare event of uncontrolled bleeding or persistent cerebrospinal fluid rhinorrhea. Otherwise, treatment may be delayed until 5–7 days after injury; this will allow adequate resolution of edema so that the medial canthal area can be restored to its normal position. Direct wiring or rigid fixation with microplates of the nasal and lacrimal bones is necessary. Nasal packing may also be required to maintain the normal position of the nasal bones.

The prognosis for return to normal function after nasoethmoidal fractures is excellent. A significant number of patients have persistent slight widening of the intercanthal distance, which is not usually functionally significant. The period of disability is usually 6–8 weeks and is often not as long as the disability from other associated injuries.

## 7. FRONTAL SINUS FRACTURES

The frontal sinus bones are extremely strong compared to the other facial bones, thus fractures are relatively uncommon. Patients that have received sufficient force to fracture the frontal sinuses frequently have skull fractures and significant closed head injury. The clinician should be aware that these sinuses vary greatly in their development with 10% of the population having isolated unilateral development, 5% with rudimentary development, and 4% with no frontal sinuses on x-ray examination.

### Clinical Findings

A contusion or laceration over the glabella may be the sign of an underlying fracture of the frontal sinus. Other symptoms and signs include pain, cerebrospinal fluid rhinorrhea or bloody rhinorrhea, flattening of the glabella, and in some cases a step off along the fracture line. A subperiosteal hematoma or soft tissue swelling may obscure a depressed anterior table frontal sinus fracture during physical examination. These patients often display mental status changes due to concurrent intracranial injury. In one series reported by Ronrich et al, only 24% of patients with frontal sinus fractures was even conscious at presentation.

Caldwell x-ray views may reveal fractures of the frontal sinus, but more frequently suggest injury with sinus air fluid levels or sinus opacification. CT scans are essential for the definitive diagnosis of fractures of both the anterior and posterior sinus walls.

### Treatment & Prognosis

Emergency therapy is not ordinarily required. Surgical repair is indicated in patients with anterior or posterior wall fracture with significant displacement, frontonasal duct compromise, or persistent CSF leak.

If the fracture is severely comminuted, the entire sinus may be removed and the frontonasal ducts plugged with autogenous material. In cases with extensive posterior table fractures, neurosurgical assistance will be needed intraoperatively. Antedotal reports suggest that a mucocele can form many years following injury and may present as a brain abscess or as a mass with erosion of the frontal bones. Some authors advocate preventive treatment of these complications by obliteration of the frontal sinuses with fat.

The period of recuperation after treatment of frontal sinus fractures is usually 4–6 weeks. The period of disability is again usually more related to associated injuries than the frontal sinus injury.

## REFERENCES

Chu L, Gussack GS, Muller T: A treatment protocol for mandibular fractures. J Trauma 1994;36:48.

Gibson B: Management of Soft-Tissue Trauma. In: Bailey BJ (editor): *Head & Neck Surgery—Otolaryngology*. Lippincott, 1993.

Mathog RH: *Maxillofacial Trauma*. Williams & Wilkins, 1994.

Powers MP, Bertz J, Fonseca RJ: Management of soft-tissue injuries. In: Fonseca RJ, Walker RV (editors): *Oral and Maxillofacial Trauma*. Saunders, 1991.

Rohrich RJ, Hollier LH. Management of frontal sinus fractures. Clin Plast Surg 1992;19:219.

Stanley RB: Current approaches to Le Fort and zygomatic fractures. Fac Plast Surg Clin Noth Am 1995;3:97.

Stanley RB: Maxillary and periorbital fractures. In: Bailey BJ (editors): *Head & Neck Surgery—Otolaryngology*. Lippincott, 1993.

# Hearing Loss 11

David N. Schindler, MD, Robert K. Jackler, MD, & Scott T. Robinson, MPH, CIH, CSP

Occupational hearing loss may be partial or total; unilateral or bilateral; and conductive, sensorineural, or mixed (conductive and sensorineural). Conductive hearing loss results from dysfunction of the external or middle ear, which impairs the passage of sound vibrations to the inner ear.

In the workplace, hearing loss can be caused by blunt or penetrating head injuries, explosions, and thermal injuries such as slag burns sustained when a piece of welder's slag penetrates the eardrum. Sensory hearing loss results from deterioration of the cochlea, usually due to loss of hair cells from the organ of Corti. Among the many common causes of sensory hearing loss are continuous exposure to noise in excess of 85 dB, blunt head injury, and exposure to ototoxic substances.

## PHYSIOLOGY OF HEARING

Sound waves consist of alternating periods of compression and rarefaction within a medium such as air. The degree of this pressure variation has a correlation in the subjective awareness of loudness. Measurement of human hearing in terms of sound pressure level (SPL) in dynes/cm$^2$ is cumbersome because of the differing sensitivity of the ear at the various frequencies. For this reason, a scale (dBHL) allowing easy comparison among frequencies and individuals has been developed. This scale is a logarithmic measurement of human hearing that, through standardization, has defined 0 dBHL as the faintest sound that the *average* normal hearing young adult can detect. The human ear has a remarkable dynamic range of roughly 0–120 dB ($10^6$ SPL), which allows for detection of sound from the faintest noise to painful stimulation.

The frequency (or number of waves passing a point in a second) has a subjective correlate in pitch. The normal human cochlea is capable of detecting and encoding sound waves across the frequency range extending from approximately 20 Hz to 20,000 Hz. The most important range for human speech reception is between 500 Hz and 3000 Hz.

Because isolated pure tone waves seldom occur in nature, the cochlea is called on to analyze complex wave forms.

The adult external auditory canal has a resonant frequency of about 3200 Hz and can amplify sound pressures of 10–20 dB in mid frequencies.

There is considerable impedance to the passage of sound vibrations from air into the fluid-filled inner ear. To overcome this barrier, an impedance-matching mechanism known as the conducting system has evolved. This apparatus consists of the external auditory canal, tympanic membrane, and the three ossicles (malleus, incus, and stapes). The conducting system contributes approximately 45 dB toward normal hearing.

The transduction of mechanical energy to electrical potentials of sound energy takes place in the inner ear (cochlea) at the Organ of Corti. At the Organ of Corti, the stereocilia of the three rows of outer hair cells and the one row of inner hair cells oscillate against a tectorial membrane. The shearing action between the stereocilia and the tectorial membrane, caused by the traveling wave motion of the basement membrane, results in an electrochemical process in the hair cells.

As it travels from base to apex along the basilar membrane, the traveling wave reaches a peak amplitude that directly correlates with the frequency of the sound. Each point along the basilar membrane is frequency specific (tonotopically organized). The auditory nerve fibers innervated by the hair cells also carry frequency selectivity.

## EVALUATION OF HEARING

### Test of Spoken Word

The simplest form of hearing evaluation may be performed in a quiet room without any sophisticated equipment. The patient is asked to repeat spoken words of increasing intensity while competing noises (the crumpling of paper or the sounds from a Baranay noise box) are presented to the opposite ear. Test results may be expressed as the ability to hear a soft whisper, loud whisper, soft spoken voice, loud spoken voice, or shout.

## Tuning Fork Tests

Tuning fork tests should be performed with a 512-Hz tuning fork, because frequencies below this level will elicit a tactile response.

**A. Rinne Test:** In cases where the patient hears air conduction (tuning fork placed by the opening of the ear canal) better than via bone conduction (tuning fork placed on the mastoid bone), a *sensorineural* hearing loss or normal hearing is indicated. In cases where bone conduction is louder than air conduction, a *conductive* hearing loss is indicated.

**B. Weber Test:** When the tuning fork is placed on the forehead or front teeth, sound should lateralize toward a conductive loss and away from a sensorineural one.

## Pure Tone Audiometry

Sensitivity to pure tones are measured at 250, 500, 1000, 2000, 3000, 4000, and 8000 Hz for both air conduction (head phones) and bone conduction (bone oscillator). Thresholds of hearing are expressed in decibels, with the normal range at each frequency from 0–20 dB. Because loud signals may stimulate the opposite ear, masking the contra lateral ear with competing sound is necessary when asymmetry exist. When both air and bone conduction are decreased, a sensorineural hearing loss exists. Conductive losses are indicated by an "air-bone gap," in which the air conduction loss *exceeds* the bone conduction loss. Results may be presented numerically or shown graphically (Figures 11–1 to 11–5).

## Bekesy Audiometry

Pure tone thresholds may also be measured by Bekesy audiometry, in which the patient uses self-directed techniques that involve pressing and releasing a signal button. This procedure is used in some occupational screening programs, but it is generally not as reliable as are procedures that are administered by an audiologist.

## Speech Audiometry

Two routine tests are performed to assess speech reception and comprehension, which are the most important aspects of audition.

**A. Speech Reception Threshold:** The speech reception threshold (SRT) is the intensity (in decibels) at which the listener is able to repeat 50% of balanced two-syllable words known as spondee words (eg, baseball, playground, and airplane). The threshold is usually in close agreement (usually within 6–10 dB) with an average of the pure tone thresholds for frequencies between 500 and 3000 Hz. The normal range is between 0 and 20 dB, with losses of 20–40 dB termed "mild," 40–60 dB "mod-erate," 60–80 dB "severe," and greater than 80 dB "profound."

**B. Speech Discrimination Score:** In the speech discrimination score (SDS), monosyllabic words that are phonetically balanced are presented at intensities well above the threshold for speech reception (SRT plus 25–40 dB) in order to test speech comprehension. Results are expressed as a percentage of words correctly repeated. The normal range of SDS is 88–100%. Word lists are available for most languages. Significant depression of the SDS usually indicates socially significant disability.

## Impedance (Immittance) Audiometry

The mechanical aspects of the middle ear sound transformer system can be assessed by tympanometry and acoustic reflex testing.

**A. Tympanometry:** Tympanometry employs an acoustic probe to measure the impedance of the eardrum and ossicular chain. Reduced middle ear compliance usually indicates a partial vacuum due to auditory tube dysfunction, while noncompliance suggests either a tympanic membrane perforation or middle ear effusion. An increase in compliance suggests either laxity of the tympanic membrane or disruption of the ossicular chain.

**B. Acoustic Reflex Testing:** Contraction of the middle ear muscles in response to a loud noise results in a measurable rise of middle ear impedance. Interpretation of acoustic reflex testing may also yield information regarding the integrity of the auditory portion of the central nervous system. It is also an indirect measurement of recruitment (the abnormal sensitivity to loud sounds) that frequently accompanies sensorineural hearing loss.

## Evoked Response Audiometry (Brain Stem Audiometry)

In patients who demonstrate unilateral or asymmetric sensorineural hearing loss, retrocochlear lesions (lesions of the eighth cranial nerve, brain stem, or cortex) must be ruled out. Evoked potentials, which are typically elicited in response to clicking noises and recorded via scalp electrodes, provide information about the location of sensorineural lesions. For individuals with normal hearing, as well as most patients with cochlear hearing losses, a series of five electroencephalographic waves may be detected, representing the central auditory system from the eighth cranial nerve (wave 1) to the inferior colliculus (wave 5). The discovery of any significant delay or even a complete absence of response may indicate a cerebellopontine angle tumor (eg, acoustic neuroma) or a lesion of the brain stem. More definitive diagnosis of retrocochlear lesions requires computed tomographic (CT) scanning or magnetic resonance imaging (MRI).

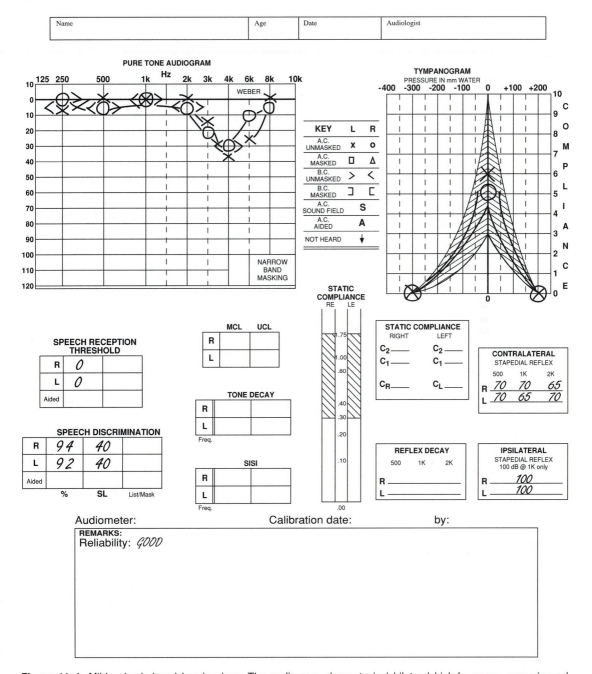

**Figure 11–1.** Mild noise-induced hearing loss. The audiogram shows typical bilateral high-frequency sensorineural hearing loss, which is most severe at 4000 Hz. Note the normal speech discrimination score.

## Stenger Test

This test is useful for detecting *feigned* unilateral hearing loss. The Stenger principle states that when two tones of the same frequency but of different loudness are presented to both ears simultaneously, only the louder tone will he heard. When the louder tone is presented to the ear with a feigned hearing loss, the patient stops responding because he or she perceives that all of the sound is coming from that side. Patients with true unilateral loss indicate that they continue to hear the sound in the opposite ear.

## Otoacoustic Emissions

A recent addition to the objective testing available

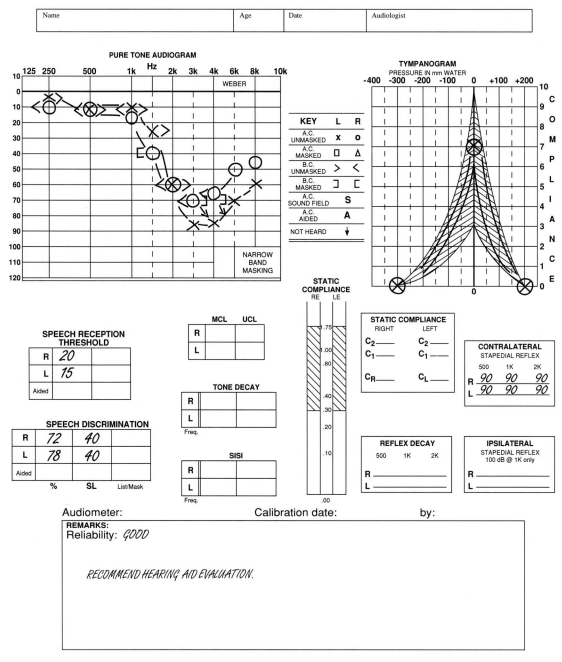

**Figure 11–2.** Noise-induced hearing loss. The audiogram shows moderate to severe high-frequency sensorineural hearing loss but preservation of the lower tones. Note the moderate decrease in the speech discrimination score.

to hearing professionals, for the evaluation of organic hearing loss, is the use of otoacoustic emissions (OAEs). When an external sound stimulus is received by the cochlea, the mechanical properties of the outer hair cells act in a manner in which a measurable sound is produced and emanated laterally through the middle ear to be recorded in the external auditory meatus. There are two types of evoked OAEs clinically used today. They are the Transient Evoked Otoacoustic Emissions (TEOAE) and the Distortion Product Otoacoustic Emissions (DPOAE). Individuals with hearing better than 35 dB (TEOAE) and 40 dB (DPOAE) will produce OAEs in 99% of instances, unless there is middle ear pathology. Thus,

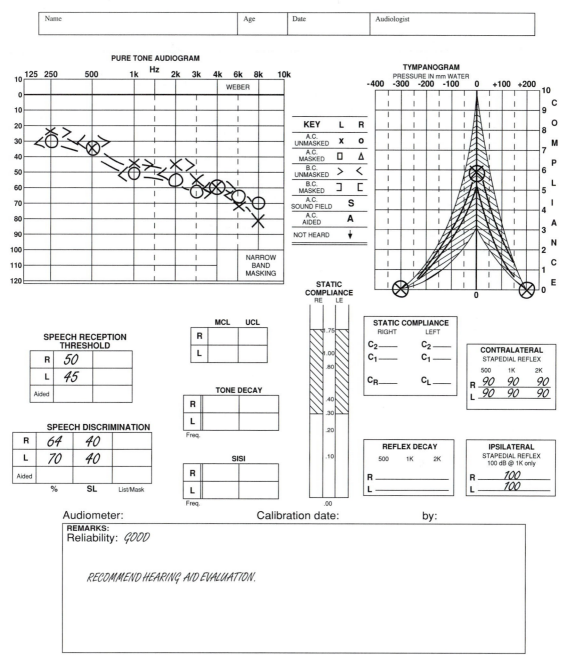

**Figure 11–3.** Presbycusis. The audiogram shows moderate to severe down-sloping sensorineural hearing loss. Note that the hearing threshold at 4000 Hz is better than at 8000 Hz, a pattern suggestive but not diagnostic of an aging change rather than exposure to noise.

if an individual generates OAEs, but does not admit to hearing, a nonorganic origin must be assumed. OAEs are rapid (30 seconds to 3 minutes) and frequency specific (from 1000 to 3000 Hz). Although OAEs do not determine threshold hearing per se, they are valid and reliable for a hearing impairment greater than a mild loss.

## DIFFERENTIAL DIAGNOSIS OF SENSORINUERAL HEARING LOSS

### Nonoccupational Hearing Loss

Before attempting to determine the extent of occupational hearing loss in a subject, the following

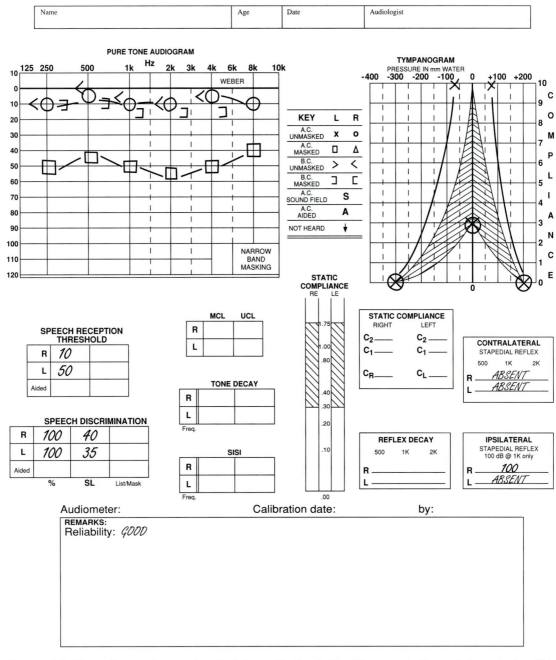

| Name | | Age | Date | Audiologist |
|---|---|---|---|---|

**PURE TONE AUDIOGRAM**

WEBER

NARROW BAND MASKING

**KEY**

| | L | R |
|---|---|---|
| A.C. UNMASKED | X | o |
| A.C. MASKED | □ | △ |
| B.C. UNMASKED | > | < |
| B.C. MASKED | ⊐ | ⊏ |
| A.C. SOUND FIELD | S | |
| A.C. AIDED | A | |
| NOT HEARD | ↓ | |

**TYMPANOGRAM**

PRESSURE IN mm WATER

**SPEECH RECEPTION THRESHOLD**

| | | |
|---|---|---|
| R | 10 | |
| L | 50 | |
| Aided | | |

**SPEECH DISCRIMINATION**

| | | | |
|---|---|---|---|
| R | 100 | 40 | |
| L | 100 | 35 | |
| Aided | | | |
| | % | SL | List/Mask |

**MCL   UCL**

| | | |
|---|---|---|
| R | | |
| L | | |

**TONE DECAY**

| | | |
|---|---|---|
| R | | |
| L | | |
| Freq. | | |

**SISI**

| | | |
|---|---|---|
| R | | |
| L | | |
| Freq. | | |

**STATIC COMPLIANCE**
RE    LE

**STATIC COMPLIANCE**

| | RIGHT | LEFT |
|---|---|---|
| $C_2$ — | | $C_2$ — |
| $C_1$ — | | $C_1$ — |
| $C_R$ — | | $C_L$ — |

**CONTRALATERAL STAPEDIAL REFLEX**

| | 500 | 1K | 2K |
|---|---|---|---|
| R | *ABSENT* | | |
| L | *ABSENT* | | |

**REFLEX DECAY**

| | 500 | 1K | 2K |
|---|---|---|---|
| R | | | |
| L | | | |

**IPSILATERAL STAPEDIAL REFLEX**
100 dB @ 1K only

| | |
|---|---|
| R | *100* |
| L | *ABSENT* |

Audiometer:                Calibration date:                by:

**REMARKS:**
Reliability: *GOOD*

**Figure 11–4.** The audiogram shows a disparity between the thresholds of bone conduction and air conduction. This "air-bone gap" represents the degree of hearing impairment due to dysfunction of the external or middle ear. The audiogram is typical of a left ossicular chain disruption.

nonoccupational hearing loss disorders must be ruled out first:

**A. Presbycusis:** Presbycusis is a slow and progressive deterioration of hearing that is associated with aging and not attributable to other causes (Figure 11–3). Presbycusis has been associated with a variety of inner ear pathologies including atrophy of the inner and outer hair cells and spiral ganglion in the basal turn of the cochlea. Other features that occur histologically include atrophy or degeneration of central auditory pathways and possibly mechanical changes in the cochlear duct affecting movement of the basement membrane. Usually the hearing loss is a gradual symmetrical progressive high frequency sen-

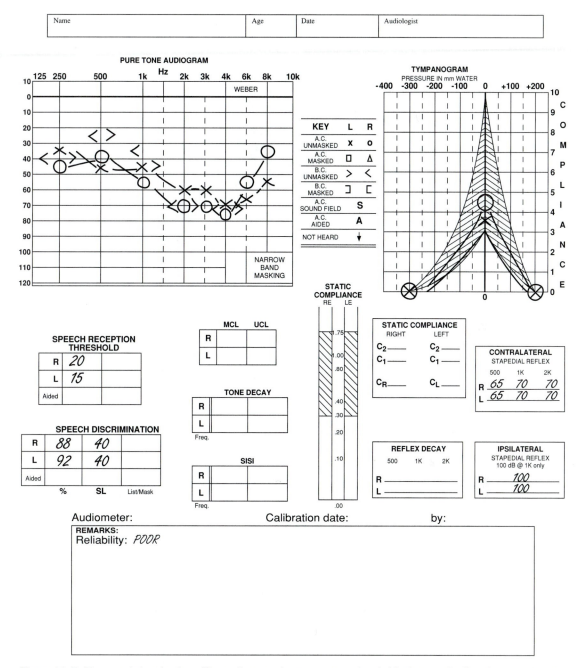

**Figure 11–5.** Nonorganic hearing loss. The audiogram shows pure tone thresholds that are significantly worse than the speech reception thresholds recorded on the same data.

sorineural associated with gradual deteriorating speech discrimination.

**B. Hereditary Hearing Impairment (HHI):** HHI is distinguished by a family history and early age at onset; however, there are delayed onset forms of HHI. HHI can be conductive, mixed, or sensorineural impairments. It may be associated with other physical findings that associate this impairment with a syndrome, or it can be nonsyndrome. Some HHIs are detected in early childhood particularly if they are associated with syndromes (eg, autosomal recessive Usher syndrome or x-linked Alport syndrome). However, many HHIs can be present in early or mid-adulthood and are nonsyndromes.

An example of a progressive partial penetrance autososomal dominant hearing loss that can be conductive, mixed, or sensorineural hearing loss is otosclerosis. Otosclerosis is a bony disease of the temporal bone that is characterized by bone reabsorption and spongy bone (otospongiosis) early in its process followed by depositing of denser bone (otosclerosis). The area of the anterior portion of the oval window is most common site of involvement. This process may fixate the foot plate of the stapes to the oval window and result in a conductive hearing loss. Involvement of the otic capsule in the area of the cochlea may result in a sensorineural hearing loss. The fixation of the foot plate may be surgically treated with a stapedectomy.

**C. Metabolic Disorders:** Progressive hearing loss may he related to diabetes mellitus, thyroid dysfunction, renal failure, autoimmune disease, hyperlipidemia, and hypercholesterolemia. These disorders may result in a sensorineural hearing loss that is bilateral, progressive, and high frequency.

In diabetes mellitus the pathology is varied involving primary neuropathy and/or small vessels disease.

Other metabolic disorders may involve pathology in the stria vascularis, which is important in maintaining the ion balance and the electrical potentials within the cochlea.

**D. Sudden Sensorineural Hearing Loss (SNHL):** This is differentiated by its sudden onset usually within 1 or 2 hours in the absence of precipitating factors. The hearing loss is almost always unilateral. The hearing loss in SNHL can be exhibited at low frequencies and improving in the high frequencies, flat, or high frequency with good low frequency hearing. The degree of hearing loss is unpredictable from mild to severe. Vertigo is present is some cases of SNHL and suggests a more severe insult.

The etiology of SNHL is unknown; speculation as to viral, vascular insult, or inner ear membrane rupture (Reisner's membrane, tectorial membrane) has been postulated. This disorder warrants a thorough evaluation in order to rule out any other known pathology.

The treatment of SNHL is debatable. The most common therapy includes no treatment or steroids. Vasodilators, anticoagulants, and diuretics have also been used in the treatment of some SNHL.

**E. Infectious Origin:** These include bacteria or virus infections including meningitis and encephalitis that may cause hearing loss.

Spirochete infections such as congenital or acquired syphilis and Lyme disease can result in hearing loss and vestibular dysfunction. The congenital syphilis sufferer may develop symptoms in infancy or later in life that may also be associated with vestibular symptoms similar to Meniere's syndrome; the hearing loss can be unilateral, but is usually bilateral. Late syphilis may present a slowly progressive sensorineural hearing loss and may also exhibit associated vestibular problems.

Mumps may cause a rather severe, most typically unilateral sensorineural hearing loss. Other childhood viral exanthams can also cause sensorineural hearing loss.

Congenital hearing loss can also be attributed to infectious origins such as rubella virus and cytomegalo virus.

**F. Central Nervous System Disease:** Cerebellopontine angle tumors, especially acoustic neuroma, may present progressive sensorineural hearing loss that is unilateral. This is in contrast to NIHL, where such hearing loss is usually bilateral. Patients with unilateral or asymmetric sensorineural hearing loss require further investigation to rule out these tumors. This investigation may require detailed audiometric studies and CT scan or MRI.

Demyelinating diseases (eg, multiple sclerosis) may present a sudden unilateral hearing loss that typically recovers to some degree.

**G. Meniere's Disease (Endolymphatic Hydrops):** Meniere's disease and its variants generally present a fluctuating low frequency or flat unilateral sensorineural hearing loss, fullness or pressure in the affected ear, tinnitus, and episodic disabling vertigo. In the early stages the hearing loss is usually low frequency sensorineural, but over time it may progress to a flat severe hearing loss. The etiology is unknown, however, histopathology reveals a hydropic dilation of the endolymphatic chambers of cochlea and membranous labyrinth.

**H. Nonorganic Hearing Loss:** Functional hearing loss for purposes of secondary gain is quite frequent. This may be seen in people with normal hearing or in those who embellish an existing organic hearing loss. With skillful audiometric techniques (as previously discussed), it is usually possible to distinguish organic from nonorganic hearing loss, but this may require referral to an audiologic center with considerable experience with this problem.

There are various indications of nonorganic hearing loss. Poor correlation between the speech reception thresholds and the average of the air conduction thresholds at 500, 1000, and 2000 Hz is the most common indication of functionality (Figure 11–5). The speech reception thresholds are generally within 6 dB of the average of the "speech frequencies." Test-retest variability is also suggestive. In cases of suspected unilateral functional hearing loss. the Stenger test is useful.

Evoked response audiometry, otoacoustic emissions tests, or both, may also be useful for objectively establishing hearing thresholds, in patients unable or unwilling to cooperate with conventional testing. Although this has gained widespread use in the testing of young children, it is not yet sufficiently reliable to provide accurate thresholds in the adult with functional hearing loss. Active research is progressing in this area.

# NOISE INDUCED HEARING LOSS

## Etiology & Pathogenesis

Noise-induced hearing loss (NIHL) results from trauma to the sensory epithelium of the cochlea. The sensory epithelium of the cochlea are comprised of one inner row of stereociliated hair cells and three outer rows of stereociliated hair cells supported by supporting cells (Hansen and Deiter cells). The most obvious injury is to the stereocilia of inner hair cells and outer hair cells hair cells (the electromechanical transducers of sound energy), which may become distorted or even disrupted under acoustically generated shearing forces of the tectorial membrane. All structures of the Organ of Corti can, however, be affected. Vascular, chemical, and metabolic changes occurring in the sensory cells cause loss of stereocilia stiffness possibly as the result of contraction of the rootlet structures that anchor the stereocilia to the cuticular plate at the top of the hair cell.

Initially the vascular, chemical, and metabolic changes are potentially reversible, and, given time, the hearing will recover. This is known as a temporary threshold shift (TTS). TTS can last for several hours. However, the condition in which continued noise exposure results in *permanent* loss of stereocilia with apparent fracture of the rootlet structures and destruction of the sensory cells, which are replaced by nonfunctioning scar tissue, is known as permanent threshold shift (PTS) and there is no recovery. The outer hair cells, which are important in tuning, are generally affected before the inner hair cells. A retrograde degeneration of cochlear nerve fibers occurs progressing centrally. Noise can involve other structures in the cochlea in the inner ear and has been noted histologically including vascular change in the area of the metabolically active stria vascularis. This results in a PTS. Because TTS may mimic PTS, individuals should be given audiometric tests after a recovery period of 12–24 hours following exposure to hazardous levels of noise. PTS may be caused by a brief exposure to extremely high intensity sounds, but it is more commonly caused by prolonged repetitive exposure to lower levels of hazardous noise.

Susceptibility to NIHL is highly variable. While some individuals are able to tolerate high noise levels for prolonged periods of time, others who are subjected to the same environment can rapidly lose hearing. Risk of permanent hearing impairment is related to the duration and intensity of exposure (Table 11–1) as well as genetic susceptibility to noise trauma.

Generally, prolonged exposure to sounds louder than 85 dBA is potentially injurious. It has been estimated that more than 20 million production workers in the United States are exposed to hazardous noise that could result in hearing loss. Continuous exposure to hazardous levels of noise tends to have its maximum effect in the high-frequency regions of the

**Table 11–1.** Relative intensity of common noises.

| Noise Level (dB) | Environmental Source | Human Speech |
|---|---|---|
| 140 | Air raid siren | . . . |
| 120 | Jet takeoff | . . . |
| 110 | Riveting machine | . . . |
| 100 | Pneumatic hammer | Shouting in ear |
| 90 | Subway train | Shouting at a distance of 2 ft |
| 80 | Vacuum cleaner | . . . |
| 70 | Freeway traffic | Loud conversation |
| 50 | Road traffic | Normal conversation |
| 30 | Library | Soft whisper |
| 20 | Broadcasting studio | . . . |
| 0 | Threshold of hearing | . . . |

cochlea. Noise-induced hearing loss is usually most severe around 4000 Hz, with downward extension toward the "speech frequencies" (500–3000 Hz) occurring only after prolonged or severe exposure. Interestingly, this tendency of noise-induced hearing loss to preferentially affect the high-frequency regions of the cochlea remains true regardless of the frequency of the injurious noise, and may be related to the resonance of the ear canal.

The biological effect of impulse noise is somewhat different from the effect of continuous noise. The inner ear is partially protected from the effects of continuous noise by the acoustic reflex. This reflex, which is triggered when the ear is subjected to noise louder than 90 dB, causes the middle ear muscles (the stapedius and tensor tympani) to contract and thereby stiffen the conductive system and make it more resistant to sound entry. Because this protective reflex is neurally mediated, it is delayed in onset for a period ranging from 25 to 150 ms depending on the intensity of the sound. High-intensity impulse noises (eg, gunshots) penetrate the cochlea before the acoustic reflex has been activated and thus are especially injurious. Impact noise exceeding 140 dB may cause immediate and irreversible hearing loss.

## Clinical Findings

Patients with NIHL frequently complain of gradual deterioration in hearing. The most common complaint is difficulty in comprehending speech, especially in the presence of competing background noise. Because patients with noise-induced hearing loss have a high-frequency bias to their hearing loss, they hear vowel sounds better than consonant sounds. This leads to a distortion of speech sounds when they are listening to people with higher pitched voices (eg, women and children). Background noise, which is usually low frequency in bias, masks the better-preserved portion of the hearing spectrum and further exacerbates the problems with speech comprehension.

Noise-induced hearing loss is frequently accompanied by tinnitus. Most often patients describe a high-frequency tonal sound (ringing), but the sound is sometimes lower in tone (buzzing, blowing, or hissing) or even nontonal (popping or clicking). This sensation may be intermittent or continuous and is usually exacerbated by further exposure to noise. Because tinnitus is usually most bothersome to patients when there is little ambient noise present, some of them complain of inability to fall asleep or to concentrate when in a quiet room.

On tuning fork examination, the patient hears air conduction better than bone conduction, which indicates a sensorineural hearing loss. When serial tuning forks from 512 to 4096 Hz are used, there is often a marked decrease in hearing in the higher frequencies. Formal audiometic examination usually reveals a bilateral, predominantly high-frequency sensorineural hearing loss with a maximum drop of the pure tone thresholds occurring at or around 4000 Hz on the pure tone audiogram (Figures 11–1 and 11–2).

The "4000 Hz notch," which frequently develops relatively early in the workers exposure to hazardous noise, will generally move laterally as further exposure continues; thus, lower and high frequencies become affected somewhat later if the exposure continues. Because the most important thresholds for comprehension of human speech are between 500 Hz and 3000 Hz, a significant decrease in speech discrimination threshold does not begin until frequencies of 3000 Hz and below are affected. The speech discrimination score is normal in the early stages of noise-induced hearing loss, but may deteriorate as the loss becomes more severe. Because of great variability, noise-induced hearing loss cannot always be eliminated or established by the shape of the audiogram.

Most frequently, the hearing loss in NIHL is bilateral although asymmetry can exist particularly when the source of the noise is lateralized (eg, rifle or shotgun firing).

Tinnitus (ringing or buzzing) may or may not be present. Tinnitus is a subjective complaint and measurements of tinnitus are based on the patient's ability to match the ringing in loudness and frequency. Often the tinnitus frequency matches the frequency of the hearing loss seen on the audiogram and is about 5 dB above that threshold in loudness. Tinnitus is frequently blocked out by ambient noise. Tinnitus in absence of hearing loss is probably not related to noise exposure.

## Prevention

The Occupational Safety and Health Administration (OSHA) regulates exposure to noise at or above an 8-hour time-weighted average (TWA) of 85 dBA. Historically, 85 dBA has been characterized as the approximate biological threshold above which permanent shifts in hearing are possible. The decision to make 85 dBA the regulated level of noise in the workplace was essentially a political one representing a compromise between the need for protection of susceptible workers and the efficiency and expense of the industrial process. OSHA has mandated that the presence of occupational noise at or above an 8-hour TWA exposure of 85 dBA is the threshold that triggers the need to implement a hearing conservation program.

A hearing conservation program (HCP) is the recognized method of preventing noise-induced hearing loss in the occupational environment. While there is a tendency to think of "hearing conservation" as the provision of audiometric tests and hearing protection, much more is required. An effective HCP integrates the following program elements:

1. Noise monitoring
2. Engineering controls
3. Administrative controls
4. Worker education
5. Selection and use of hearing protection devices (HPDs)
6. Periodic audiometric evaluations

Record keeping is also important, and OSHA has set record keeping requirements. HCP elements are briefly outlined below:

**A. Noise Monitoring:** If there is reason to believe that worker noise exposure will equal or exceed a TWA of 85 dBA, then noise monitoring is required. A sampling strategy must be designed to identify all workers who need to be included in the HCP. The noise present must be characterized in terms of frequency (predominantly high, predominantly low, or mixed), intensity (how loud is it), and type (continuous, intermittent, or impulse) using appropriate noise monitoring instrumentation. Anytime there is any change in production, process, equipment, or controls, all noise monitoring tests *must* be repeated.

**B. Engineering Controls:** The information collected during noise monitoring (particularly octave band analysis, which indicates the sound level at a selected frequencies) may be used to design engineering noise controls. Designers conceptualize possible engineering solutions in terms of the source (what is generating the noise), the path (the route[s] the generated noise may travel), and the receivers (the workers exposed to the noise). The noise controls may involve the use of enclosures (to isolate sources or receivers), barriers (to reduce acoustic energy along the path), or distance (to increase the path and ultimately reduce the acoustic energy at the receiver) to reduce worker noise exposure. In general, engineering controls are preferred but are not always feasible due to their costs in and limits in technology.

**C. Administrative Controls:** Administrative controls include (1) reducing the amount of time a given worker might be exposed to a noise source in order to prevent the TWA noise exposure from reaching 85 dBA, *and* (2) establishing purchasing guidelines to prevent introduction of equipment that would increase worker noise dose. While simple in principle, the implementation of administrative controls requires management's commitment and constant supervision, particularly in the absence of engineering or personal protection controls. In general, administrative controls are used as an adjunct to existing HCP noise control strategies rather than as an exclusive approach for controlling noise exposure.

**D. Worker Education:** Workers and management must understand the potentially harmful effects of noise in order to satisfy OSHA and most important to ensure that the HCP is successful. A good worker education program describes (1) program objectives, (2) existing noise hazards, (3) how hearing loss occurs, (4) purpose of audiometric testing, and (5) what workers can do to protect themselves. In addition, roles and responsibilities of the employer and the workers should be clearly stated. Training is required to be provided annually to all workers included in the HCP. Opportunities for maintaining awareness occur during periodic safety meetings, as well as during audiometric testing appointments when testing results are explained.

**E. Hearing Protection Devices:** Hearing protection devices (HPDs) are available in a variety of types from a number of manufacturers. There are three basic types of HPDs: (1) ear plugs or "aurals" (premolded, formable, and custom molded), (2) canal caps or "semiaurals" (with a band that compresses each end against the entrance of the ear canal), and (3) ear muffs or "circumaurals" (which surround the ear). Each of these types of devices has advantages and disadvantages that vary according to worker activity, equipment and facility noise characteristics, and the work environment (Figure 11–6). Selection of appropriate HPDs should include input from the industrial hygienist, the audiologist, the occupational medicine physician, and, of course, the workers who will use these devices. Although the HCP is triggered by the presence of noise levels equal to or greater than an 8-hour TWA of 85 dBA, HPDs must attenuate worker exposure to an 8-hour TWA at or below 90 dBA, the OSHA 8-hour permissible exposure level (PEL) for noise.

**F. Audiometric Evaluations:** Audiometric testing provides the only quantitative means of assessing the overall effectiveness of a hearing conservation program. A properly managed audiometric testing program supervised by a certified audiologist or physician who is trained and experienced in occupational hearing conservation will detect changes in response to environmental noise that might otherwise be overlooked. Results of audiometric testing must be shared with employees to ensure effectiveness. The overall results or trends noted in an audiometric testing program can be used to "fine tune" the HCP, ie, determining which types of HPDs to offer to employees or identifying where additional employee training is needed.

## Noise Reduction Ratings & Selection of Hearing Protection Devices

All hearing protection devices sold in the US are assigned a standardized value known as the noise reduction rating, or NRR. Manufacturers of HPDs are required by the Environmental Protection Agency to have various products tested in order to obtain an NRR prior to placing them on the market. While useful in making preliminary purchasing decisions, as-

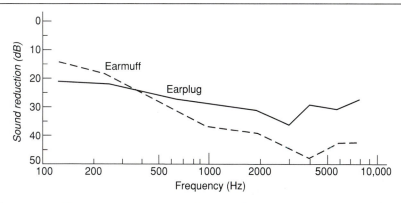

**Figure 11–6.** Comparison of the attenuation properties of a molded-type earplug and an earmuff protector. Note that the earplug offers greater attenuation of the lower frequencies, while the earmuff is better at the higher frequencies. (Reproduced, with permission, from Olishifski JB, Standard JJ: Industrial Noise. Chapter 9 in: *Fundamentals of Industrial Hygiene*, 4th ed. Plog BA [editor]. National Safety Council, 1996.)

signed NRRs must be viewed and applied cautiously. NRRs (listed in "dB") are based on laboratory attenuation data and achieved under ideal conditions. Actual noise reduction achieved under field conditions using any HPD will be much lower than the assigned NRR.

Adjustment of the assigned NRR may need to be made before a device is prescribed for field use. This is explained as follows:

**A. Weighting Scale Adjustment:** Depending on the monitoring method used to determine noise exposure, an initial adjustment to the NRR of a selected device may be necessary. For example:

If workplace noise levels are determined using the "C" scale (dBC) on the monitoring instrumentation, the assigned NRR may be subtracted directly from the actual measured TWA noise levels to determine the legal "adequacy" of the device selected relative to the 90 dBA criterion.

If workplace noise levels are determined using the "A" scale (dBA) on the monitoring instrumentation, the assigned NRR must be reduced by 7 dB before being subtracted from the actual measured TWA noise levels to determine the legal "adequacy" of the device selected relative to the 90 dBA criterion.

The "A" scale adjustment is necessary because this scale approximates the response of the human ear to speech frequencies and discounts much of the acoustic energy from the low and high frequencies that are present in the work environment. Since the "C" scale is essentially flat across the frequency spectrum, all of the acoustic energy present is integrated into the measurement, and no adjustment is necessary.

**B. 50% Derating:** In order to more accurately (and conservatively) predict the NRR of HPDs during actual use, a 50% derating of the assigned NRR (after weighting scale adjustment) should be applied to determine its "relative performance." As a typical example, if a device has an NRR of 21 and workplace noise measurements were made using the "A" scale, then the predicted field attenuation or "relative performance" of the device would be $(21 - 7) \div 2 = 7$ dBA. Such a device would be expected to provide protection (per the legal OSHA 90 dBA PEL) where 8-hour TWA noise levels up to 97 (90 + 7) dBA are present. As a worse case example, failure to make an adjustment for "A" scale noise measurements, along with a failure to apply a 50% derating, could lead an uninformed evaluator to falsely believe that the HPD would provide protection in environments with 8-hour TWA noise levels up to and including 111 (90 + 21) dBA. Workers in this situation would be at *increased risk* of sustaining a noise-induced hearing loss. *Remember:* the 50% derating of a HPD is not required by OSHA, but it does provide a conservative estimate of the likely field attenuation provided by a HPD.

**C. Combining HPDs:** Hearing protection devices may be combined (ie, wearing ear plugs and ear muffs) to provide more protection in high noise environments. However, the NRRs of the combined devices are not added together to determine the total noise reduction. Under such circumstances, OSHA advises its inspectors that 5 dB are to be added after the weighting scale adjustment is applied to the device with the higher NRR (OSHA does not require the 50% derating described above). This is a conservative approach to determining combined attenuation, and actual field attenuation (and protection) are probably higher.

**D. HPD Provision Versus HPD Enforcement:** For 8-hour TWA noise levels greater than or equal to 85 dBA (a 50% noise dose), but below 90 dBA (a 100% noise dose), the only requirement is that the HPDs be made available to the workers. For 8-hour TWA noise dose levels at or above 90 dBA, however, HPDs must be provided to workers and their proper use must be enforced by the employer. A suitable variety of HPDs must be provided. The weighting scale adjustment of the NRR must be applied, and it is advisable to apply a 50% derating of the adjusted NRR to ensure adequate protection of the worker.

## Treatment

There is no medical or surgical treatment available to reverse the effects of noise-induced hearing loss (NIHL). After the diagnosis has been established by otologic examination and performance of an audiometric test battery, the physician should counsel the patient on the likely consequences of continued exposure to excessive noise and should recommend techniques for avoidance of further noise-induced damage. Hearing amplification is reserved for those patients with socially impaired hearing. Hearing aids must be carefully fitted to optimally meet the needs of the individual with regard to frequency bias and gain. In bilateral hearing losses, bilateral amplification usually provides more satisfactory rehabilitation. Whether or not to try hearing amplification is the patient's decision. A reasonable criterion for referral to a professional for hearing aid evaluation is a speech reception threshold below 25 dB or a speech discrimination score of less than 80% when words are presented at a normal conversation level of 50 dBHL. There are also some instances in which hearing aids may be recommended that will assist the patient to hear in certain circumstances such as lectures or in group situations. In patients with high frequency hearing loss and relatively normal low frequency hearing, hearing aids are generally most helpful in those who have a significant hearing loss at 2000 Hz on the puretone audiogram. A borderline candidate may be an individual with normal hearing through 1500 Hz, a mild loss at 2000 Hz, and a moderate or greater loss at 3000 Hz and above.

The two basic hearing aids that are available are the analog hearing aid and the newer more expensive digitally programmable hearing aids. Before purchasing a hearing aid the patient should have a hearing aid evaluation (HAE) and a trial period with the patient wearing the hearing aids in various circumstances.

A patient's willingness to wear a hearing aid will depend on many factors, including cosmetic considerations and concerns about the ability to insert the hearing aid and to manipulate its controls. Numerous other clever instruments known as assistive listening devices are available to enhance comprehension in small or large groups (eg, at business meetings or conventions), with telephone use, and with various audio or visual media, such as television. Most of the these work wireless transmission of FM signals or infrared light beams. Aural rehabilitation classes designed to enhance the patient's ability to comprehend speech may also be helpful and are usually available in urban areas.

There is no cure for tinnitus resulting from noise induced hearing loss, although numerous amelioration measures are available. In the absence of further inner ear injury, tinnitus will gradually diminish, usually over a course of weeks to months. A subtle degree of tinnitus often persists and is especially obvious when the patient is in a quiet room. For the few patients who find this to be extremely troublesome, masking the tinnitus with music or some other form of pleasant sound is often helpful. In those with significant hearing loss, the most successful treatment may be appropriate hearing amplification. Modified hearing aids (tinnitus maskers) designed to produce masking noises have generally been of limited success. Use of biofeedback has helped some patients suppress their tinnitus. Psychiatric referral to manage associated depression is sometimes necessary.

## Prognosis

Hearing in patients with NIHL will generally stabilize if the patient is removed from the noxious stimulus. If not, hearing will continue to deteriorate and ultimately result in severe hearing impairment or, in extreme cases, total deafness. Although adequate noise protection is essential and should always be recommended, other factors may also play a role in the patient's prognosis. Presbycusis can add to the noise induced loss as the patient grows older, and preexisting noise-induced hearing loss will also cause the patient to be more susceptible to the adverse effects of ototoxic substances such as aminoglycoside antibiotic, loop diuretics, and antineoplastic agents used in the treatment of other disorders (see Ototoxic Hearing Loss, below).

## HEARING LOSS DUE TO PHYSICAL TRAUMA

### Etiology & Pathogenesis

A broad spectrum of injuries may cause trauma to the ears. Blunt head injury is by far the most common cause of traumatic hearing loss. A blow to the head creates a pressure wave in the skull that is transmitted through bone in a manner similar to the way a pressure wave in air is carried by the conducting mechanism of the ear. The cochlear injury observed following blunt head trauma closely resembles both histologically and audiologically that which is induced by high-intensity acoustic trauma. Motor vehicle accidents are the major cause of blunt head trauma and account for about 50% of temporal bone injuries. Penetrating injuries of the temporal bone are relatively rare, accounting for fewer than 10% of cases. Other occupational causes of ear injury include falls, explosions, and burns from caustic chemicals, open flames, or welder's slag that enters the ear canal.

### Examination & Treatment

In the conscious patient, hearing should be assessed immediately with a 512-Hz tuning fork. Even in an ear severely traumatized and filled with blood, sound will lateralize toward a conductive hearing loss and away from a sensorineural one. Complete audiometric examinations (see Evaluation of Hearing, above) can be performed after the patient has been stabilized. Patients should also be checked for signs of vestibular injury (nystagmus) and facial nerve trauma (paralysis).

**A. Injuries Causing Conductive Hearing Loss:**

**1.** Blunt head trauma without temporal bone fracture may cause hematotympanum: a collection of blood in the middle ear. If this is the sole injury, hearing usually recovers over several weeks.

**2.** Burns sustained when a piece of welder's slag penetrates the eardrum often heal poorly, and chronic infection often results.

**3.** A loud explosion with sound pressure levels exceeding 180 dB may cause rupture of the tympanic membrane.

**4.** Traumatic membrane perforations usually heal spontaneously if secondary infection does not develop (patients should be instructed, not to get the ear wet during the healing period), although hearing loss may persist.

Conductive hearing loss that persists more than 3 months after injury is usually due to a tympanic membrane perforation or disruption of the ossicular chain (Figure 11–4). These lesions are suitable for surgical repair, usually on a delayed basis. Repair is by grafting the tympanic membrane or by reconstructing the ossicular chain with homograft or prosthetic materials or both.

**B. Injuries Causing Sensorineural Hearing Loss:** Trauma to the inner ear most commonly results from blunt head injury. Labyrinthine concussion frequently occurs with transient vertigo, potentially permanent hearing loss, and tinnitus. Treatment is expectant with vestibular suppressants such as meclizine offering symptomatic relief of vertigo.

Trauma may also cause rupture of the round or oval window membranes, which can lead to leakage of inner ear fluids into the middle ear (perilymph fistula). Most perilymphatic fistulas heal spontaneously. Persistent perilymphatic leakage is difficult to diagnose and requires surgical treatment with autogenous material used to repair the defect. Most patients with surgically confirmed fistulas suffer recurrent episodes of vertigo and hearing loss, often temporally related to vigorous physical exercise.

**C. Injuries Causing Mixed Conductive and Sensorineural Hearing Loss:** Temporal bone injuries sometimes involve both the middle and inner ear, resulting in *mixed*, conductive, and sensorineural hearing loss. Fractures of the temporal bone tend to occur along lines that connect points of weakness in the skull base. Clinically, these fractures may be divided into two patterns: longitudinal and transverse. Longitudinal fractures are much more common (80% of cases) and usually result from a blow to the lateral aspect of the head. They frequently involve the structures of the middle ear but characteristically spare the inner ear resulting in a conductive or mixed hearing loss. Transverse fractures are less common (20% of cases) and usually result from a severe occipital blow. Serious intracranial injury frequently accompanies transverse fractures. Typically, they traverse the inner ear and cause total sensorineural hearing loss and labyrinthine death. Fractures through the inner ear are often accompanied by severe vertigo that lasts for weeks or even months.

Temporal bone fractures are recognized clinically by the presence of blood, cerebrospinal fluid, or both in the car canal or by the presence of blood in the middle ear behind an intact tympanic membrane. The ear canal should be carefully cleaned using, sterile suction to assess the integrity of the tympanic membrane. Under no circumstances should a recently traumatized ear be irrigated. Battle's sign (ecchymosis over the mastoid region) is occasionally seen. Definitive diagnosis requires high-resolution CT scanning to demonstrate the fracture lines.

## OTOTOXIC HEARING LOSS

### Etiology & Pathogenesis

Ototoxic hearing loss is frequently the result of exposure to substances that injure the cochlea. Most ototoxins injure hair cells either directly or through disruption of other cochlear homeostatic mechanisms. In the vast majority of cases, ototoxic hearing loss stems from the use of medications such as aminoglycoside antibiotics (eg, gentamicin), loop diuretics (eg, furosemide), antineoplastic agents (eg, cisplatin), and salicylates (eg, aspirin).

In industries with noise work environments, workers who are being treated with potentially ototoxic medications are at increased risk, since the combination of some ototoxic drug treatment and noise trauma can lead to a greater degree of hearing loss than either of these would produce by itself. Aspirin, however, is probably not associated with an increase likelihood of NIHL.

Patients with any type of preexisting sensorineural hearing loss, including NIHL, are considerably more susceptible to the ototoxic effects of medications.

Hearing loss may also result from exposure to ototoxic substances in the workplace. Heavy metals, including arsenic, cobalt, lead, lithium, mercury, and thorium, have documented ototoxic potential. Other chemicals that may be ototoxic include cyanide, benzene, aniline dyes, iodine, chlorophenothane, dimethyl sulfoxide, dinitrophenol, propylene glycol, methylmercury, potassium bromate, carbon disulfide, carbon monoxide, carbon tetrachloride, and such as industrial solvents styrene and toluene.

### Prevention

Audiometric evaluation is appropriate to identify and monitor ototoxic exposure. Identification of those at heightened risk of ototoxic hearing loss is important to avoid this complication. Persons with preexisting sensory hearing loss and compromised renal or hepatic function are at substantially increased risk.

Medicinal ototoxins should be administered in the lowest dose compatible with therapeutic efficacy. Serum peak and trough levels should be monitored to reduce the risk of excessive dosages. Simultaneous administration of multiple ototoxic drugs (eg, furosemide and an aminoglycoside antibiotic) should be avoided when possible to minimize synergistic effects.

## MEDICOLEGAL ISSUES

### Calculation of Percentage of Hearing Loss

Several methods for calculating the percentage of hearing loss are in widespread use. The current method recommended by the American Academy of Otolaryngology and Head and Neck Surgery (AAO) is as follows: (1) The average hearing threshold level at 500, 1000, 2000, and 3000 Hz is calculated for each ear. (2) The percentage of the impairment for each ear (the monaural loss) is calculated by multiplying the amount by which the above average exceeds 25 dBA (low fence) by 1.5 up to a maximum of 100%, which is reached at 92 dBA (high fence). (3) The hearing handicap (binaural assessment) should then be calculated by multiplying, the smaller percentage (better ear) by 5, adding this figure to the larger percentage (poorer ear), and dividing the total by 6.

The method recommended by the National Institute for Occupational Safety and Health (NIOSH) is the same as the AAO except that 500 Hz is not included in the calculation. This frequently yields a higher estimate of the percentage of hearing loss. This method was used by the US Department of Labor until February of 1986 when the AAO method was adopted.

For the above calculations to be valid, the audiometer employed must be checked daily and periodically calibrated by an independent agency. The booth used for testing must meet the standards of background noise levels established by the American National Standards Institute (ANSI) in 1977.

A note of caution is needed regarding the calculation of percentage of hearing loss based on older audiograms. Different standards for the measurement of hearing were in use prior to establishment of the current standard by the ANSI in 1969. From 1964 to 1969, the standard of the International Standards Organization (ISO) was used; this is essentially the same as the current ANSI standard, and no conversion is needed. However, from 1951 to 1964, the standard of the American Standards Association (ASA) was used, and audiograms obtained in this period *require* conversion for use in the above formula. To convert an audiogram from the ASA to the ANSI standard, add 14 dB at 500 Hz, 10 dB at 1000 Hz, 8.5 dB at 2000 Hz, 8.5 dB at 3000 Hz, 6 dB at 4000 Hz, and 9.5 dB at 6000 Hz. If the 3000-Hz threshold was not measured in older audiograms, a three-tone average of 500, 1000, and 2000 Hz may be substituted.

## Assessment of Impairment

As previously indicated, the normal range of speech reception threshold is between 0 and 20 dB, with losses of 20–40 dB termed "mild," 40–60 dB "moderate," 60–80 dB "severe," and greater than 80 dB "profound." Of course, the extent of disability suffered by the patient depends on many psychological, social, and work-related factors. Disability is a relative term. Assessment of the ability of an individual to do his or her job requires knowledge about the various duties performed by that individual. Some typical work-related issues for consideration include the amount of communication with coworkers and others that is required on the job, the type of communication (eg, in person or via the telephone), and the need to hear alerting signals or emergency warning alarms.

To meet the Social Security Administration's Guidelines for total disability due to hearing impairment, an individual must have either (1) an average hearing threshold of 90 dB or greater for the better hearing ear, based on both air and bone conduction at 500, 1000, and 2000 Hz or (2) a speech discrimination score of 40% or less in the better-hearing ear. In both cases, hearing must not be restorable by hearing amplification devices.

## Compensation for Occupational Hearing Loss

An example of how occupational hearing loss is compensated is provided by the statistics of the US Department of Labor. In the fiscal year 1995, there were 6704 claims. The total cost to the federal government was $35,023,844, and the average paid per claimant was $5,224. The Department of Labor treats aggravated or accelerated hearing losses in the same manner as losses entirely precipitated or proximally caused by the patient's employment. In other words the amount of pre-employment hearing loss is not subtracted when the percentage of loss is calculated. In contrast, local and state government regulations frequently take into account the level of preexisting hearing loss and use formulas to correct for the anticipated progression of presbycusis when calculating compensation awards.

The relationship between NIHL and presbycusis is very debatable at this time. Many studies have tried to address the issue of the worker exposed to hazardous noise for a long period of time and his "presumed" hearing loss based on his age (presbycusis). The International Standards Organization published a report in 1990 that attempts to quantitate that relationship. As with all large series, attempts to estimate hearing for individuals at certain age are also based on determining the median or averages of large populations at a given age. There is much debate whether epidemiological hearing loss data can be applied to individuals.

## REFERENCES

Axelsson A et al: (editors): *Scientific Basis of Noise-Induced Hearing Loss.* Thieme Medical, 1996.

Berger EH et al (editors): *Noise and Hearing Conservation Manual,* 5th ed. American Industrial Hygiene Association, 1996.

Dobie RA: *Medical-Legal Evaluation of Hearing Loss.* Van Nostrand Reinhold, 1993.

International Organization for Standardization: *ISO-1999: Acoustics: Determination of Occupational Noise Exposure and Estimation of Noise Induced Hearing Impair-*

*ment*. International Organization for Standardization, 1990.

Jackler RK, Brackman DE: *Neurotology*. Mosby, 1994

Morata T, Dunn D (editors): *Occupational Medicine: State of the Art Reviews*. Occupational Hearing Loss, Vol 10, No. 3, July–September 1995.

National Institute of Health: Consensus Statement: Consensus Development Conference on Noise and Hearing Loss. Vol 8, No. 1, January 1990.

Occupational Safety and Health Administration, Department of Labor, Occupational Noise Exposure: Hearing Conservation Amendment; Final Rule (29 CFR 1910.95).

Royster JD, Royster LH: *Hearing Conservation Programs: Practical Guidelines for Success*. Lewis Publishers, 1990.

Sataloff RT, Sataloff J: *Occupational Hearing Loss,* 2nd ed. Marcel Dekker, 1993.

# Injuries Due to Physical Hazards

**12**

*Richard Cohen, MD, MPH*

This chapter discusses health effects of occupational exposure to extreme temperatures (cold and heat), electricity, radiation, changes in atmospheric pressure, and vibration. Hearing loss associated with exposure to noise is covered in Chapter 11.

## HYPOTHERMIA
## (Cold Injury)

Cold injuries are classified as systemic or localized and as freezing (eg, frostbite) or nonfreezing (eg, immersion foot). Factors influencing the risk for these injuries include the atmospheric or water temperature, humidity, wind velocity, duration of exposure, type of protective equipment or clothing, type of work being performed and associated energy expenditure, and age and health status of the worker.

Workers at risk include both indoor and outdoor workers exposed to cold, such as meat packers and others who work with freezers, construction workers, warehouse personnel, divers, mail carriers, fire fighters, and road maintenance workers. The risk is increased if the employee is elderly; is intoxicated with drugs or alcohol; is receiving medications such as barbiturates, phenothiazines, or reserpine; or has adrenal insufficiency, diabetes, myxedema, any neurologic disease affecting hypothalamic or pituitary function or causing peripheral sensory impairment, or any cardiovascular disease causing diminished cardiac output.

### SYSTEMIC HYPOTHERMIA

#### Pathogenesis

Systemic hypothermia is reduction of the body's core temperature below 35 °C (95 °F). Hypothermia can occur at air temperatures up to 18.3 °C (65 °F) or in water up to 22.2 °C (72 °F).

When the body is exposed to cold environments, it has two types of normal physiologic reactions: (1) constriction of superficial blood vessels in the skin and subcutaneous tissue, resulting in heat conservation; and (2) increase in metabolic heat production through voluntary movement and by shivering. In cases of systemic hypothermia, physiologic functions are diminished. Oxygen consumption is decreased by about 7% per degree Celsius, myocardial repolarization is slowed, and ventricular fibrillation is a major hazard. In prolonged or slowly developing hypothermia (usually accompanied by physical exhaustion), hypoglycemia is probably due to glycogen depletion (hypoglycemia inhibits shivering).

#### Clinical Findings

The medical history should address the circumstances under which the patient was found, the probable duration of exposure, associated injuries or frostbite, preexisting medical conditions and problems with alcohol or drug abuse, and recent changes in the state of consciousness. Because body heat is lost more quickly when a person is wet, immersed in water, or exhausted, these factors should be considered.

The onset of hypothermia is often insidious, without any specific characteristics. With profound hypothermia, there is often diminished memory, a decrease or absence of shivering, and combativeness. Initial findings may include drowsiness, slurred speech, irritability, impaired coordination, general weakness and lethargy, recent diuresis, and puffy and cool skin and face.

Physical examination often reveals diminished neurologic reflexes, slow mental and muscular reactions, weak or nonpalpable pulse, arrhythmia, low blood pressure, and increased blood viscosity. Shivering and peripheral vasoconstriction begin with the core temperature at 35 °C. Heart and respiratory rates and blood pressure decrease with reduced temperature. With mild hypothermia (33–35 °C), there is extensive shivering which decreases as temperature subsides to 33 °C, wherein joint and muscle stiffness become more predominant.

Core temperature should be taken with a thermometer or thermocouple capable of measuring temperatures as low as 28 °C, and esophageal or deep rectal measurement (15 cm) is best. The temperature may range from 25 to 35 °C (77–95 °F). Below 35 °C, consciousness becomes dulled, causing disorientation, irrational thinking, forgetfulness, and hallucinations. Below 30 °C, semiconsciousness and confusion may occur. Nerve conduction is slowed, although the central nervous system is protected from ischemic damage. The respiratory rate falls to 7–12 per minute, and gastrointestinal motility slows or ceases. There may be hemoconcentration due to diuresis and loss of plasma volume. The latter occurs because of subcutaneous edema, which is accompanied by an elevation in corticosteroid levels. Loss of consciousness seldom occurs at temperatures above 28 °C.

Evaluation should also include a complete blood count; measurement of blood glucose, blood urea nitrogen, electrolytes, amylase, and alcohol and drug levels; urinalysis; urine volume; coagulation screen; sputum and blood cultures; thyroid function tests; arterial blood gas measurements with pH corrected for temperature (add 0.0147 pH unit for each degree under 37 °C); chest x-ray; and ECG. There may be evidence of metabolic acidosis, hypovolemia, elevation or depression of the blood glucose level, and renal failure. The ECG may show a pathognomonic J wave at the QRS–ST junction. The level of consciousness may worsen, and death may result from ventricular fibrillation or cardiac arrest.

## Prevention

The risk of hypothermia is directly related to the wind chill index, which includes both ambient temperature and wind velocity. Cold-stress threshold limit values (TLVs) are based on the wind velocity and temperature and are intended to prevent the core temperature from falling below 36 °C (Table 12–1). Ambient temperature is measured with a dry bulb thermometer; wind velocity is measured with a standard wind gauge. Work and break schedules should take into account the expected wind velocity and temperature and should follow the recommendations of the American Conference of Governmental Industrial Hygienists (ACGIH). Under high-risk weather conditions, workers should be under constant protective observation.

Hypothermia can be prevented by wearing clothing specially designed to resist wind and rain but also to allow water vapor generated by perspiration to escape. Overheating when strenuous work is required

**Table 12–1.** Threshold limit values work warm-up schedule for 4-hour shift.[1,2]

| Air Temp—Sunny Sky[3] °C (approx.) | °F (approx.) | No Noticeable Wind Max. Work Period (min) | No. of Breaks | 5 mph Wind Max. Work Period (min) | No. of Breaks | 10 mph Wind Max. Work Period (min) | No. of Breaks | 15 mph Wind Max. Work Period (min) | No. of Breaks | 20 mph Wind Max. Work Period (min) | No. of Breaks |
|---|---|---|---|---|---|---|---|---|---|---|---|
| −26 to −28 | −15 to −19 | (Norm. breaks) | 1 | (Norm. breaks) | 1 | 75 | 2 | 55 | 3 | 40 | 4 |
| −29 to −31 | −20 to −24 | (Norm. breaks) | 1 | 75 | 2 | 55 | 3 | 40 | 4 | 30 | 5 |
| −32 to −34 | −25 to −29 | 75 | 2 | 55 | 3 | 40 | 4 | 30 | 5 | Nonemergency work should cease | |
| −35 to −37 | −30 to −34 | 55 | 3 | 40 | 4 | 30 | 5 | Nonemergency work should cease | | | |
| −38 to −39 | −35 to −39 | 40 | 4 | 30 | 5 | Nonemergency work should cease | | | | | |
| −40 to −42 | −40 to −44 | 30 | 5 | Nonemergency work should cease | | | | | | | |
| −43 and below | −45 and below | Nonemergency work should cease | | | | | | | | | |

[1]Reproduced, with permission, from *American Conference of Governmental Industrial Hygienists TLV Booklet*, 1994–1995.
[2]Schedule applies to any 4-hour work period with moderate to heavy work activity, with warm-up periods of 10 minutes in a warm location and with an extended break (eg, lunch) in a warm location at the end of the 4-hour work period. For light-to-moderate work (limited physical movement), apply the schedule one step lower. For example, at −35 °C (−30 °F) with no noticeable wind (step 4), a worker at a job with little physical movement should have a maximum work period of 40 minutes with four breaks in a 4-hour period (step 5). TLVs apply only for workers in dry clothing.
[3]The following is suggested as a guide for estimating wind velocity if accurate information is not available: 5 mph, light flag moves; 10 mph, light flag fully extended; 15 mph, raises newspaper sheet; 20 mph, blowing and drifting snow. If only the wind chill cooling rate is available, a rough rule of thumb for applying it rather than the temperature and wind velocity factors given above would be: (1) special warm-up breaks should be initiated at a wind chill cooling rate of about 1750 W/m$^2$; (2) all nonemergency work should have ceased at or before a wind chill of 2250 W/m$^2$. In general, the warm-up schedule provided above slightly undercompensates for the wind at the higher temperatures, assuming acclimatization and clothing appropriate for winter work. On the other hand, the chart slightly overcompensates for the actual temperatures in the colder ranges because windy conditions rarely prevail at extremely low temperatures.

in extreme cold can be prevented by wearing a number of thin layers of clothing that can be removed or donned as necessary. Wet garments should be replaced as soon as possible with dry ones, and constrictive garments should not be worn.

Jobs should be designed so that workers remain relatively active when exposed to cold environments and provided with dry, wind-protected, heated shelters for tasks involving stationary work positions. Outdoor workers should have heated rest facilities and hot food and hot drinks available.

Workers exposed to the cold should be physically fit, without underlying vascular, metabolic, or neurologic diseases that place them at increased risk for hypothermia. They should be cautioned to avoid smoking and drug or alcohol use. New workers should be introduced into the work schedule slowly and instructed in the use of protective clothing, recognition of impending frostbite and early signs and symptoms of hypothermia, proper warming procedures, and first-aid treatment.

## Treatment & Prognosis

In cases of mild hypothermia (rectal temperatures > 33 °C), patients who are young and otherwise healthy should be treated by rewarming in a warm bed or bath or with warm packs and blankets and with oral rehydration with warmed fluids (caffeine-free and nonalcoholic). Mildly hypothermic elderly or debilitated patients should be treated conservatively, using an electric blanket heated to 37 °C. Patients with severe hypothermia (temperatures < 32 °C) should be treated more aggressively by experienced personnel, and cardiac rhythm and rate should be monitored. Because the risk of death due to ventricular fibrillation is high with severe hypothermia (< 32 °C), treatment methods that may trigger fibrillation (eg, central catheters, cannulas, or tubes) should be avoided unless their use is essential. If CPR is instituted, it should be continued until the patient has been rewarmed to at least 36 °C. Evaluation for and treatment of localized areas of trauma and frostbite should be undertaken.

Measures should be instituted to correct acid-base deficiencies, normalize the serum potassium and blood glucose levels, increase the blood volume, maintain cardiac output and blood pressure, and provide adequate ventilation. Adequate cardiovascular support, acid-base balance, arterial oxygenation, and intravascular volume should be established prior to rewarming to minimize the risk of organ infarction. Oxygen administration should begin prior to rewarming. Because most arrhythmias revert spontaneously to normal sinus rhythm as the patient rewarms, it is usually not necessary to give antiarrhythmic agents unless there is a preexisting cardiac condition. Ventricular arrhythmias, however, should be treated as in a euthermic patient. Blood volume expansion with 5% dextrose-normal saline solution, low-molecular-weight dextran, or albumin is recommended. Potassium-containing expanders should be avoided until the serum potassium levels have stabilized. Antibiotics should be given if infection is present. If myxedema is an underlying factor or if drug intoxication is present, appropriate treatment should be given. Localized areas of frostbite should be evaluated and managed as outlined below (see Hypothermia of the Extremities).

Use of steroids or antibiotics is not recommended unless otherwise clinically indicated. Core temperature should be monitored frequently during and after initial rewarming because of the potential for delayed, repeat hypothermia.

Although controversy exists concerning active external versus active internal rewarming methods for severe hypothermia, the latter is preferred. Treatment should increase in aggressiveness with decreasing core temperature, which in severe cases may call for both selected internal and external techniques.

**A. Active External Rewarming Methods:** Although relatively simple and generally available, active external warming methods may cause marked peripheral dilation that predisposes to ventricular fibrillation and hypovolemic shock. Either heated blankets or warm baths may be used for active external rewarming. Rewarming in a warm bath is best carried out in a tub of stirred water at 40–41 °C (104–107.6 °F), with a rate of rewarming of about 1–2 °C/h. It is easier, however, to monitor the patient and to carry out diagnostic and therapeutic procedures when heated blankets are used for active rewarming. Selective (external) thoracic rewarming has been recommended as a means of reducing the risk of peripheral vasodilation and resulting hypotension.

**B. Active Internal (Core) Rewarming Methods:** Internal rewarming is essential for patients with severe hypothermia; extracorporeal blood rewarming (venovenous, cardiopulmonary, or femoro-femoral bypass) is the treatment of choice. Repeated peritoneal dialysis may be employed with 2 L of warm (43 °C [109.4 °F]) potassium-free dialysate solution exchanged at intervals of 10–12 minutes until the core temperature is raised to about 35 °C (95 °F). Parenteral fluids should be warmed to 43 °C (109 °F) before administration. Heated, humidified air warmed to 42°C (107.6 °F) should be administered through a face mask or endotracheal tube. Warm colonic and gastrointestinal irrigations are of less value.

Passive rewarming (insulation from cold) is of value only for mildly hypothermic patients or as first-aid management on the scene. Hypothermia victims without vital signs should not be pronounced dead until they have been rewarmed to a core temperature of 36 °C and are found to be unresponsive to continued cardiopulmonary resuscitation at that temperature.

The prognosis is good for otherwise healthy patients but worsens with the presence of underlying predisposing problems or a delay in treatment.

## HYPOTHERMIA OF THE EXTREMITIES

The cheeks, nose, earlobes, fingers, toes, hands, and feet are the areas most likely to develop ice crystals within the tissue, resulting in localized hypothermic injury. As skin temperature falls below 25 °C, tissue metabolism slows, although oxygen demand increases if work continues. There may be tissue damage at 15 °C due to ischemia and thrombosis and at –3 °C due to actual freezing of the tissue.

Immersion foot (trench foot) is caused by a combination of cold temperature and exposure to water. This problem and chilblains (pernio) are nonfreezing injuries, whereas frostbite is a freezing injury. Predisposing factors for nonfreezing injuries include inadequate clothing and constricting garments. Those for frostbite include prior cold injuries, smoking, Raynaud's phenomenon, and collagen vascular disease.

### Clinical Findings

**A. Chilblains (Pernio):** Chilblains, also called acute pernio, consist of erythematous, pruritic skin lesions due to inflammation as a result of cold or dampness with cold. With prolonged exposure, this condition can progress to chronic pernio or "blue toes," characterized by erythematous, edematous, ulcerating lesions of the acral parts of the toes. Scarring, fibrosis, and atrophy can occur.

**B. Immersion Foot:** There are three clinical stages: an ischemic stage, a hyperemic stage, and a posthyperemic recovery stage.

Initially, feet are cold, numb, swollen, and waxy white or cyanotic. Two to 3 days following removal from the cold, hyperemia occurs, along with intense pain, additional swelling, redness, heat, blistering, hemorrhage, lymphangitis, ecchymoses, and in some cases sequelae such as cellulitis, gangrene, or thrombophlebitis. After 10–30 days, intense paresthesias sometimes occur and are accompanied by cold sensitivity and hyperhidrosis, which may persist for years.

Tropical immersion foot occurring at higher temperatures is similar but usually has less intense symptoms with faster recovery.

**C. Frostbite:** In frostbite, freezing of superficial tissues (skin, subcutaneous) usually causes symptoms of numbness, prickling, and itching; skin is gray-white and hard. In severe cases, there may be paresthesias and stiffness, as well as injury to deeper tissues—bone, muscle, and nerve. Skin is often white and edematous. Deep frostbite may be followed by ulceration, necrosis, or gangrene.

### Prevention

Prevention is the same as for systemic hypothermia (see above).

### Treatment

**A. Chilblains (Pernio) and Immersion Foot:**

Treatment includes elevating the extremities, gradually rewarming them by exposure to air at room temperature, and protecting pressure sites from trauma. Prazosin hydrochloride, 1 mg at bedtime, has been recommended for treatment and prophylaxis of pernio. Massage and immersion should be avoided. Antibiotics are given if infection develops.

**B. Frostbite:** At the site of exposure, extremities can be rewarmed by removing wet gloves, socks, and shoes; drying the extremities and covering them again with dry clothing; and either elevating them or placing them next to a warmer part of the body (eg, placing the hands in the armpits). *Caution:* Rewarming should not be attempted if refreezing is likely prior to definitive therapy.

In cases of severe frostbite, hospitalization is recommended until the extent of tissue damage has been determined. The patient should be evaluated and treated, if necessary, for systemic hypothermia (see above).

Rapid rewarming of the frostbitten parts of the body can be accomplished by placing them in a moving water bath heated to 40–42 °C (72–75.6 °F) and leaving them there until thawing is complete but no longer (often 30 minutes). Dry heat is not recommended, and external heat should be discontinued once normal temperature has been reached. The patient should remain in bed with the affected parts elevated and uncovered at room temperature. Frostbitten parts should not be exercised, rubbed, or exposed to pressure. Dressings and bandages should not be applied.

Infection can be treated with povidone-iodine soaks, water soaks, whirlpool therapy, systemic antibiotics, or a combination of these methods. Tetanus antitoxin or a tetanus toxoid booster may be indicated. Although anticoagulants have been recommended for prevention of thrombosis, their value has not been demonstrated (Figure 12–1).

Surgery should generally be avoided and amputation not considered until it is certain that the tissue is dead. Gangrenous and necrotic tissue should be treated by specialists.

Physical therapy can be instituted as healing progresses. The patient should be instructed to avoid exposure to the cold for several months and be advised of future hypersusceptibility to frostbite.

## DISORDERS DUE TO HEAT

Five medical disorders can result from excessive exposure to hot environments (in order of decreasing severity): heat stroke, heat exhaustion, heat cramps, heat syncope, and skin disorders. Among the many

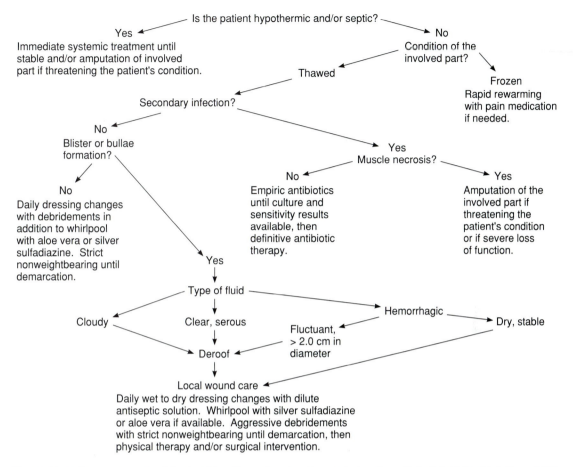

**Figure 12–1.** Treatment protocol for frostbite. (Reproduced, with permission, from Pulla RJ, Pickard LJ, Carnett TS: Frostbite: An overview with case presentations. J Foot Ankle Surg 1994;33:53.)

types of workers at risk are steel workers, oven and furnace operators, glassblowers, farmers, ranchers, fishermen, and construction workers.

A stable internal body temperature requires maintenance of a balance between heat production and loss, which the hypothalamus regulates by triggering changes in muscle tone, vascular tone, and sweat gland function. Production and evaporation of sweat are a major mechanism of heat removal. The transfer of heat from the skin to surrounding gas or liquid (convection) or between two solids in direct contact (conduction) may also occur, but this decreases in efficiency as ambient temperature increases. The passive transfer of heat via infrared rays from a warmer to a cooler object (radiation) accounts for 65% of body heat loss under normal conditions. Radiant heat loss also decreases as temperature increases up to 37.2 °C (99 °F), at which point heat transfer reverses. At normal temperatures, evaporation accounts for about 20% of body heat loss, but at excessive temperatures it becomes the most important means for heat dissipation. It, too, is limited as humidity increases and is ineffective at 100% relative humidity.

The scheduled and regulated exposure to heated environments of increasing intensity and duration (acclimatization) allows the body to adjust to heat by beginning to sweat at lower body temperatures, increasing the quantity of sweat produced, reducing the salt content of sweat, and increasing the plasma volume, cardiac output, and stroke volume while the heart rate decreases.

Health conditions that inhibit sweat production or evaporation and increase susceptibility to heat injury include obesity; skin disease; decreased cutaneous blood flow; dehydration; hypotension; cardiac disease resulting in reduced cardiac output; use of alcohol or medications that inhibit sweating, reduce cutaneous blood flow, or cause dehydration (eg, atropine, phenothiazines, tricyclic antidepressants, diuretics, laxatives, anticholinergics, antihistamines, monoamine oxidase inhibitors, vasoconstrictors, and beta blockers); and use of drugs that increase muscle activity and thereby increase the generation of body heat (eg, phencyclidine, LSD, amphetamines, cocaine, and lithium carbonate). Infections, cancer, malnutrition, and other medical conditions characterized by debilitation and poor physical condition can reduce the effectiveness of the sweating mechanism and circulatory response to heat. Age and sex also affect susceptibility to heat injury. Older people do not acclimatize as easily because of their reduced sweating efficiency, and women generally generate more internal heat than men when performing the same task.

## HEAT STROKE

Heat stroke is a life-threatening medical emergency due to thermal regulatory failure manifested by cerebral dysfunction with altered mental status, hyperpyrexia, abnormal vital signs, and, usually, hot, dry skin. Heat stroke becomes imminent as the core (rectal) temperature approaches 106 °F (41.1 °C). It is most apt to occur following excessive exposure to heat; it occurs in one of two forms: "classic" or "exertional." The classic form occurs under conditions of extreme heat among those with compromised heat dissipation capability (elderly individuals, infants, and chronically ill or debilitated patients). Exertional heat stroke results from strenuous exertion in hot en-

vironments, often in unacclimatized individuals. Morbidity or mortality can result from cerebral, cardiovascular, hepatic, or renal damage.

## Clinical Findings

Thermal regulatory failure is characterized by dizziness, weakness, nausea, vomiting, confusion, delirium, and visual disturbances; changes in mental status are its hallmark. Convulsions, collapse, or unconsciousness may occur. The skin is hot and initially covered with perspiration; later it dries. Blood pressure may be slightly elevated but becomes hypotensive. Core temperatures usually exceed 41 °C. As with heat exhaustion, hyperventilation can occur and lead to respiratory alkalosis and compensatory metabolic acidosis. There may also be abnormal bleeding, renal failure, or arrhythmias.

Laboratory evaluation may reveal an increase in leukocytes due to dehydration; decreased serum potassium, calcium, and phosphorus levels; increased blood urea nitrogen levels; hemoconcentration; decreased blood coagulation; and concentrated urine with proteinuria, tubular casts, and myoglobinuria. Thrombocytopenia, increased bleeding and clotting times, fibrinolysis, and consumptive coagulopathy may be present. Myocardial, liver, or renal damage may be reflected in laboratory tests (Table 12–2).

**Table 12–2.** Accidental hyperthermia—clinical differential.

|  | Heat Cramps | Heat Exhaustion | Heat Stroke |
|---|---|---|---|
| Pathophysiology | Salt deficiency | Volume/electrolyte depletion | Thermoregulatory failure |
| Symptoms | Painful muscle cramps/spasm<br>Weakness<br>Nausea<br>Vomiting | Weakness<br>Headache<br>Syncope<br>Nausea<br>Vomiting<br>Intense thirst (water depletion)<br>Fatigue<br>Muscle cramps (salt depletion)<br>Malaise | Irritability<br>Confusion<br>Prodromal heat exhaustion<br>Collapse<br>Severe/sustained physical<br>  exertion (exertional heat stroke)<br>Psychotic behavior |
| Objective Findings | Euthermia | Core temperature ≤ 38 °C<br>Profuse sweating<br>Orthostatic vital signs<br>Tachycardia<br>Hyperventilation<br>Tetany | Core temperature ≥ 40 °C<br>Altered mental status—bizarre behavior<br>Hot dry skin (classic heat stroke)<br>Moist skin (exertional heat stroke)<br>Coma<br>Seizure<br>Hypotension/shock<br>Tachycardia<br>Cyanosis<br>Rales |
| Laboratory | Elevated creatine phosphokinase (CPK), creatinuria | Oliguria | Hyperuricemia<br>CPK elevation<br>Dissemination intravascular coagulation<br>Respiratory alkalosis<br>Hypokalemia<br>Thrombocytopenia<br>Myoglobinuria<br>Hypoglycemia<br>Transaminase elevation |

## Prevention

ACGIH has developed an index of threshold limit values for exposure to heat in occupational settings. The values are based on a formula that includes the natural wet bulb temperature, shielded dry bulb temperature, and black globe temperature, which are measurements that account for effects due to solar radiant heat, air velocity, relative humidity, and ambient temperature. Exposure limits take into account the type of work-rest regimen and the work load, including body position, movement, and limb use. These determine the heat load or metabolic rate, which is then related to the index to arrive at a recommended exposure standard for workers in a particular situation. In the absence of wet bulb globe temperature (WBGT) data, Heat Index guidelines developed by the National Weather Service predict exposure risks according to ambient temperature and humidity (Figure 12–2). The standards are based on the assumption that workers are acclimatized and physically fit, are wearing appropriate clothing, and are supplied with adequate water and food. Occupational heat exposure can be minimized with engineering controls such as air conditioning/cooling or fans. Special cooled suits have been designed for hot environments.

For additional information on the thermal comfort zone, see Chapter 6 and Figure 6–9.

In occupations in which workers are exposed to excessive heat, medical evaluation is recommended to identify individuals at increased risk for heat disorders due to preexisting medical conditions or use of medications. Exposed workers should be trained to recognize early signs and symptoms of heat disorders and should be advised of the importance of proper attire, nutrition, and fluid intake. Employers should provide cool drinking water and make sure that there are shaded rest areas close to the work site. For workers unacclimatized to heat, balanced electrolyte solutions or 1% saline drinking water should be made available. Salt tablets are not recommended because their use may exacerbate or cause electrolyte imbalance. Organized athletic events should be man-

### Heat index

| Relative humidity (%) | 70° | 75° | 80° | 85° | 90° | 95° | 100° | 105° | 110° |
|---|---|---|---|---|---|---|---|---|---|
| 100 | 72° | 80° | 91° | 108° | | | | | |
| 90 | 71° | 79° | 88° | 102° | 122° | | | | |
| 80 | 71° | 78° | 86° | 97° | 113° | 136° | | | |
| 70 | 70° | 77° | 85° | 93° | 106° | 124° | 144° | | |
| 60 | 70° | 76° | 82° | 90° | 100° | 114° | 132° | 149° | |
| 50 | 69° | 75° | 81° | 88° | 96° | 107° | 120° | 135° | 150° |
| 40 | 68° | 74° | 79° | 86° | 93° | 101° | 110° | 123° | 137° |
| 30 | 67° | 73° | 78° | 84° | 90° | 96° | 104° | 113° | 123° |
| 20 | 66° | 72° | 77° | 82° | 87° | 93° | 99° | 105° | 112° |
| 10 | 65° | 70° | 75° | 80° | 85° | 90° | 95° | 100° | 105° |
| 0 | 64° | 69° | 73° | 78° | 83° | 87° | 91° | 95° | 99° |

Air temperature (°F)

| Heat index | Heat disorders possible with prolonged exposure and/or physical activity |
|---|---|
| 80° to 89° | Fatigue |
| 90° to 104° | Sunstroke, heat cramps and heat exhaustion |
| 105° to 129° | Sunstroke, heat cramps or heat exhaustion likely, and heat stroke possible |
| 130° or higher | Heatstroke/sunstroke highly likely |

NOTE: Direct sunshine increases the heat index by up to 15 °F

**Figure 12–2.** Heat index chart showing associated heat disorders. (Reproduced, with permission, from Bross MH, Nash BT, Carlton FB Jr: *Practical Therapeutics—Heat Emergencies. American Family Physician*, 1994.)

aged with attention to thermoregulation; the WBGT index should be monitored, water consumption should be encouraged, and medical care should be immediately accessible.

## Treatment

Treatment is aimed at rapid (within 1 hour) reduction of the core temperature and control of secondary effects. Evaporative cooling provides rapid and effective lowering of temperature and is easily accomplished in most emergency settings. Until medical care becomes available, the patient should be moved to a shady, cool place. Clothing should be removed and the entire body sprayed with cool water (15 °C); cooled or ambient air should be blown across the patient at high velocity (100 ft/min). The patient should be placed in the lateral recumbent position or supported in the hands-to-knees position to expose more skin surface to the air.

The cooling process should continue in the hospital with use of cool water or 70% isopropyl alcohol sponge baths. Other alternatives include use of cold, wet sheets accompanied by fanning.

Immersion in an ice-water bath has often been recommended but is no longer preferred both because it is often not feasible and because of its greater potential for complications of hypotension and shivering. Other treatment alternatives include ice packs (groin, axilla, neck) and iced gastric lavage, though these are much less effective than evaporative cooling. Treatment should continue until the core temperature drops to 39 °C. Because of the risks of hypoxia and aspiration, intubation should be considered and 100% oxygen administered until the patient is cooled. The temperature should continue to be monitored, though it usually remains stable after it has returned to normal. Chlorpromazine, 25–50 mg intravenously, can be used to control shivering and thus prevent an increase in heat. Aspirin should not be used as an antipyretic because of its effects on blood coagulation (Figure 12–3).

Patients should be monitored for hypovolemic and cardiogenic shock, either or both of which may occur. Attention should be paid to maintaining a patent airway, providing oxygen, correcting fluid and electrolyte imbalances, and supporting vital processes. Central venous or pulmonary artery wedge pressure should be assessed and intravenous fluids administered if indicated. If hypovolemic shock is suspected, 500–1000 mL of 5% dextrose in 1 N or 0.5 N saline solution may be given intravenously without overloading the circulation. Other medications appropriate for cardiovascular support should be considered. Corticosteroids have not been demonstrated to be of value.

Fluid output should be monitored through the use of an indwelling urinary catheter. Complications, including renal failure (due to rhabdomyolysis), hepatic failure, or cardiac failure, hypotension, elec-trolyte imbalance (hypokalemia), or coagulopathy (DIC), should be treated appropriately.

Because hypersensitivity to heat continues in some patients for prolonged periods following heat stroke, they should be advised to avoid reexposure to heat for at least 4 weeks.

## HEAT EXHAUSTION

In individuals performing strenuous work, prolonged exposure to heat and inadequate salt and water intake can cause heat exhaustion, dehydration, and sodium depletion or isotonic fluid loss with accompanying cardiovascular changes.

Symptoms and signs may include intense thirst, weakness, nausea, fatigue, headache, confusion, a core (rectal) temperature exceeding 38 °C (100.4 °F), increased pulse rate, and moist skin. Symptoms associated with both heat syncope and heat cramps (see below) may also be present. Hyperventilation sometimes occurs secondary to heat exhaustion and can lead to respiratory alkalosis. Progression to heat stroke is indicated by a rise in temperature or a decrease in sweating.

Treatment consists of placing the patient in a cool and shaded environment and providing hydration (1–2 L over 2–4 hours) and salt replenishment—orally if the patient is able to swallow. Physiologic saline or isotonic glucose solution should be administered intravenously in more severe cases. At least 24 hours' rest is recommended.

## HEAT CRAMPS

Heat cramps result from sodium depletion caused by replacement of sweat losses with water alone. They are usually characterized by slow and painful muscle contractions and severe muscle spasms that last from 1 to 3 minutes and involve the muscles employed in strenuous work.

The skin is moist and cool, and involved muscle groups feel like hard, stony lumps similar to billiard balls. The temperature may be normal or slightly increased, and blood tests may show low sodium levels and hemoconcentration. Because the thirst mechanism is intact, blood volume is not significantly diminished.

The patient should be moved to a cool environment and given a balanced salt solution or an oral saline solution consisting of 4 tsp of salt per gallon of water. Salt tablets are not recommended. Rest for 1–3 days with continued salt supplementation in the diet may be necessary before returning to work.

## HEAT SYNCOPE

In heat syncope, sudden unconsciousness results from cutaneous vasodilatation with consequent sys-

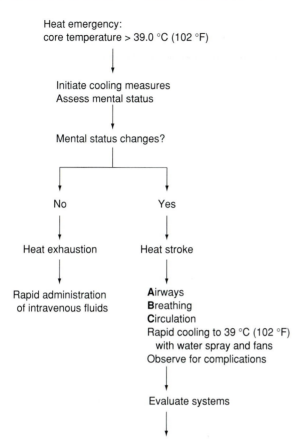

**Figure 12–3.** Algorithm for the management of heat emergencies. CT = computed tomographic; PA = pulmonary arterial; DIC = disseminated intravascular coagulation; $Po_2$ = partial pressure of oxygen; ARDS = adult respiratory distress syndrome; PEEP = positive end-expiratory pressure. (Reproduced, with permission, from Bross MH, Nash BT, Carlton FB Jr: *Practical Therapeutics—Heat Emergencies.* American Family Physician, 1994.)

temic and cerebral hypotension. Episodes commonly occur following strenuous work for at least 2 hours.

The skin is cool and moist and the pulse weak. Systolic blood pressure is usually under 100 mm Hg.

Treatment consists of recumbency, cooling, and liquids by mouth. Preexisting medical conditions should be monitored and treated if necessary.

## SKIN DISORDERS DUE TO HEAT

**Miliaria (heat rash)** is caused by sweat retention due to obstruction of the sweat gland duct. There are three forms, listed here in increasing order of severity: miliaria crystallina, miliaria rubra, and miliaria profunda. As the site of duct obstruction becomes deeper in the skin, the severity increases and presentation varies (eg, vesicles, erythema, desquamation, macules).

**Erythema ab igne** ("from fire") is characterized by the appearance of hyperkeratotic nodules following direct contact with heat that is insufficient to cause a burn.

**Intertrigo** results from excessive sweating and is often seen in obese individuals. Skin in the body folds (eg, the groin and axillas) is erythematous and macerated.

**Heat urticaria (cholinergic urticaria)** can be localized or generalized and is characterized by the presence of wheals with surrounding erythema ("hives").

Treatment for these disorders consists of reduction or removal of heat exposure, reduction of sweating, and control of symptoms. Antihistamines may help relieve pruritus in patients with urticaria. Corticosteroids are not beneficial.

## THERMAL BURNS[1]

### CLASSIFICATION

Thermal burns are classified by extent, depth, patient age, and associated illness or injury.

### Extent

The "rule of nines" (Figure 12–4) is useful for rapidly assessing the extent of a burn. Therefore, it is important to view the entire patient after cleaning soot to make an accurate assessment, both initially and on subsequent examinations. Only second- and

[1]This section was modified from that written by Brent RW Moelleken, MD, in Tierney LM Jr, McPhee SJ, Papadakis MA: *Current Medical Diagnosis & Treatment,* 35th ed. Appleton & Lange, 1996.

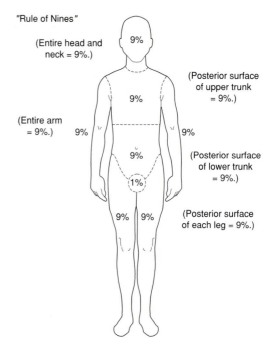

**Figure 12–4.** Estimation of body surface area in burns. (Reproduced, with permission, from Schroeder AS et al: *Current Medical Diagnosis & Treatment 1997.* Appleton & Lange, 1997.)

third-degree burns are included in calculating the total burn surface area (TBSA), since first-degree burns usually do not represent significant injury in terms of prognosis or fluid and electrolyte management. However, first- or second-degree burns may convert to deeper burns if treatment is delayed or infection/colonization occurs.

### Depth

Judgment of the depth of injury is difficult. The **first-degree burn** may be red or gray but will demonstrate excellent capillary refill. First-degree burns are not blistered initially. If the wound is blistered, this represents a partial-thickness injury to the dermis, or a **second-degree burn.** As the degree of burn is progressively deeper, there is a progressive loss of adnexal structures. The distinction between second- and third-degree burns is blurred. Deep second-degree burns are generally treated as full-thickness **(third-degree)** burns and excised and grafted early because of the excessively long time necessary for reepithelialization and the thin, poor quality of the resultant skin.

### Age of the Patient

As much as extent and depth of the burn, age of the victim plays a critical part. Even a relatively small burn in an elderly patient or infant may be fatal.

## Associated Injuries & Illnesses

An injury commonly associated with burns is smoke inhalation. Suspicion of inhalation injury is aroused when nasal hairs are singed, the mechanism of burn involves closed spaces, there is carbonaceous sputum, or the carboxyhemoglobin level exceeds 5% in non-smokers. This should lead the clinician to perform early intubation before airway edema supervenes, making endotracheal intubation difficult. The products of combustion, not heat, are responsible for lower airway injury. Burning plastic products produce both hydrochloric acid and hydrocyanic acid. Electrical injury that causes burns may also produce cardiac arrhythmias that require immediate attention. Electrical burns can produce significant deep-tissue necrosis, often distributed between entry and exit wounds. This is a frequent cause of rhabdomyolysis and unappreciated deep muscle necrosis. Premorbid physical and psychosocial disorders that complicate recovery from burn injury include cardiac or pulmonary disease, diabetes, alcoholism, drug abuse, and psychiatric illness.

## Special Burn Care Units & Facilities

The American Burn Association and the American College of Surgeons have recommended that major burns be treated in specialized burn care facilities. They also advocate that even moderately severe burns be treated in a specialized facility or hospital where personnel have expertise in burn care. The American Burn Association has classified burn injuries as follows (ABA classification):

**A.  Major Burn Injuries:**

1. Partial-thickness burns over more than 25% of body surface area in adults or 20% in children.
2. Full-thickness burns over more than 10% of surface area in any age group.
3. Deep burns involving the hands, face, eyes, ears, feet, or perineum.
4. Burns complicated by inhalation injury.
5. Electrical and chemical burns.
6. Burns complicated by fractures and other major trauma.
7. Burns in poor-risk patients (extremes of age or intercurrent disease).

**B.  Moderate Uncomplicated Burn Injuries:**

1. Partial-thickness burns over 15–25% of body surface area in adults or 10–20% of body surface area in children.
2. Full-thickness burns over 2–10% of body surface area.
3. Burns not involving the specific conditions listed above.

**C.  Minor Burn Injuries:**

1. Partial-thickness burns over less than 15% of body surface area in adults or 10% in children.

2. Full-thickness burns over less than 2% of body surface area.

## INITIAL MANAGEMENT

### Airway

The physician or emergency medical technician should proceed as with any other trauma, using standard Advanced Trauma Life Support (ATLS) guidelines. The first priority is to establish an airway, recognizing the frequent necessity to intubate a patient who may appear to be breathing normally but who has sustained an inhalation injury, then to evaluate the cervical spine and head injuries, and then to stabilize fractures. The burn wound itself has a lower priority. Nonetheless, fluid resuscitation by the Parkland formula may be instituted simultaneously with initial resuscitation. Endotracheal intubation should be considered for major burn cases, regardless of the area of the body involved, because generalized edema, including the soft tissues of the upper airway and perhaps the lungs as well, develops as fluid resuscitation proceeds. Tracheostomy is rarely indicated for the burn victim, unless dictated by other circumstances such as delay in endotracheal intubation and subsequent upper airway edema preventing cord visualization. Chest radiographs are typically normal initially but may show an ARDS picture in 24–48 hours with severe inhalation injury. Supplemental oxygen should be administered. Inhalation injuries should be followed by serial blood gas determination and bronchoscopy. The use of corticosteroids is contraindicated because of the potential for immunosuppression.

### History

As soon as possible, a detailed history of the circumstances of the injury, including locale, presence of closed-space injury, substances involved, and duration of exposure, should be obtained. Medications, previous medical history, especially cardiopulmonary problems, mental disturbances, confusion resulting from the injury, as the presence of an endotracheal tube may later prevent the recording of an accurate history.

### Vascular Access

All clothing and jewelry should be removed and an expedient physical examination performed to assess the extent of injury and associated injuries. Simultaneous with the above procedures, venous access must be sought, since the victim of a major burn may go into hypovolemic shock. A percutaneous, large-bore (14- or 16-gauge) intravenous line through nonburned skin is preferred. Subclavian lines are avoided in the emergency setting because of the risk of pneumothorax and subclavian laceration if they are placed in a volume-depleted patient. Femoral lines provide good temporary access during resuscitation. All lines placed while the patient is in the emergency department should be changed within 24 hours because of the high risk of unsterile placement. Distal saphenous cutdown is occasionally necessary. An arterial line may also be useful for monitoring mean arterial pressure and drawing blood. Swan-Ganz catheters may be necessary initially in severe burns or in patients with severe cardiopulmonary disease.

## FLUID RESUSCITATION

### Crystalloids

Generalized capillary leak results from burn injury over more than 25% of the total body surface area. This often necessitates replacement of a large volume of fluid. An intravenous line is recommended in the management of partial-thickness or full-thickness burns that cover more than 20% of total body surface area in the adult and 10% in the child.

There are many guidelines for fluid resuscitation. The Parkland formula is currently the most widely used in the United States. It relies on the use of lactated Ringer's injection. For adults and children, the fluid requirement in the first 24 hours is estimated as 4 mL/kg body weight per percent of body surface area burned. Deep electrical burns and inhalation injury increase this requirement. *Remember that a formula is only a guideline.* Adequacy of resuscitation is determined by clinical parameters, including urine output and specific gravity, blood pressure, and central venous or, if necessary, Swan-Ganz readings.

Half the calculated fluid is given in the first 8-hour period. The remaining fluid, divided into two equal parts, is delivered over the next 16 hours. An extremely large volume of fluid may be required. For example, an injury over 40% of the total body surface area in a 70-kg victim may require 13 L *in the first 24 hours.* The first 8-hour period is calculated from the hour of injury.

After 24 hours, capillary leaks have sealed in the majority of cases, and plasma volume may be restored with colloids (plasma or albumin).

A Foley catheter is essential for monitoring urinary output. *Diuretics have no part in this phase of patient management,* although the use of mannitol may be indicated in the resuscitation of an electrical burn victim to prevent myoglobin in the urine from precipitating in the kidneys.

### Escharotomy

As edema fluid accumulates, ischemia may develop under any constricting eschar of an extremity. Similarly, an eschar of the thorax or abdomen may limit respiratory excursion. Escharotomy incisions through the anesthetic eschar can save life and limb.

## THE BURN WOUND

Treatment of the burn wound is based on several principles: (1) Prevention or delay of infection by application of topical silver sulfadiazine or mafenide (Sulfamylon). (2) Protection from desiccation and further injury of those burned areas that will spontaneously reepithelialize in 7–10 days. (3) Excision and grafting of burned areas that cannot spontaneously reepithelialize during this period.

Regardless of the severity of the burn, prophylactic systemic antibiotics are usually not recommended.

### Wound Closure

The goal of therapy after fluid resuscitation is closure of the wound. Nature's own blister is the best cover to protect wounds that spontaneously epithelialize in 7–10 days (ie, superficial second-degree burns). Where the blister has been disrupted, silver sulfadiazine, human amnion, porcine heterografts (preferably fresh, or frozen and meshed), or collagen composite dressings (Biobrane) can substitute. Cadaver homografts can also serve this purpose if available.

Wounds that will not heal spontaneously in 7–10 days (ie, deep second-degree or third-degree burns) are best treated by excision and autograft; otherwise, granulation and infection may develop.

## PATIENT SUPPORT

During the wound closure phase, the patient must be supported in many ways, including adequate nutrition. Enteral feedings may begin once the ileus of the resuscitation period is relieved.

Pain plays a major role during the wound closure phase. The patient is more aware of pain during dressing changes and postsurgical periods. Hydrotherapy aids in dressing removal and joint range of motion, but it can be a source of wound contamination. Analgesics are essential, but overuse or under-use may be harmful.

## ELECTRICAL INJURIES

Electrical accidents comprise up to 4% of all fatal industrial accidents. Electricians, operators of high-power electric equipment and power generators, and maintenance personnel are at greatest risk for electric shock.

Physical contact with an energized electric circuit provides a pathway for electricity to traverse the body as it seeks a ground. Conductivity to the body is affected by skin moisture as well as moisture on contacting surfaces (eg, floors). Factors influencing the severity of electrical injury include the voltage (electrical force), amperage (current intensity), current type (alternating or direct current), duration of contact, area of contact, pathway of the current through the body, and amount of tissue resistance.

Electricity from alternating currents is more dangerous than that from direct currents. The alternating currents usually cause muscle tetanization and sweating, while the direct currents cause electrolytic changes in tissue. Most tissue damage is related to the heat produced by the electric current, and tissue resistance is largely influenced by the water content of the tissue. The vascular system and muscles are good conductors of electricity, while the bones, peripheral nerves, and dry skin have higher resistance.

A sudden exposure to intense electrical energy can cause not only tissue destruction and necrosis from heat and burning but also depolarization of electrically sensitive tissues such as nerve and heart. Alternating currents with voltages and frequencies as low as domestic circuits (100 V and 60 Hz) can produce ventricular fibrillation. High voltages (> 1000 V) can cause respiratory paralysis. Most shocks involving currents exceeding 10,000 V are of such magnitude that the electrical force knocks the victim away from the power source, which minimizes the electrical injury potential but often causes blunt trauma.

A tetanizing effect of voluntary muscles is greatest at frequencies between 15 and 150 cycles. Sustained grasp of the conductor does not usually occur at high voltages, because the circuit probably arcs before contact with the victim, who is thrown back instead. Current above 20 mA can cause sustained contraction of chest respiratory muscles; alternating currents above 30–40 mA can induce ventricular fibrillation, whereas direct current is more likely to cause asystole. Lightning injuries differ from high-voltage electric shock injuries in that lightning usually involves higher voltage, briefer duration of contact, asystole rather than ventricular fibrillation, nervous system injury, a shock wave characteristic, and multisystem pathologic involvement.

## Clinical Findings

Exposure to electric current can cause shock, flash burns, flame burns, or direct tissue necrosis. Surface wounds covering heat-induced tissue necrosis are usually round or oval and well-demarcated, and they may have a relatively innocuous yellow-brown appearance. A search must be made for both the entry and the exit wound to determine the electrical pathway through the body. Depending on the contact site and the pathway, there may be damage to nerves, muscles, or major organs such as the heart, brain, eye, kidney, or gastrointestinal tract. Technetium stannous pyrophosphate scintigraphy can identify areas of significant muscle damage.

In all cases, an ECG with a rhythm strip and a urine dipstick for blood and protein should be obtained, and the respiratory rhythm and rate should be checked. If organ, muscle, or nerve damage is suspected, appropriate diagnostic tests should be ordered such as urine myoglobin; creatine phosphokinase should be monitored for at least 24 hours if muscle symptoms occur or muscle injury is otherwise suspected. With muscle injury, the creatine phosphokinase level can be significantly elevated (> 1000) but the MB fraction will be below 3% if there is no cardiac muscle injury. Occult fractures may occur following muscle tetany or blunt trauma. Patients should be observed for several days, because some develop posttraumatic myositis with rhabdomyolysis.

Electrical injury causes increased vascular permeability, which may result in reduced intravascular volume and fluid extravasation in the area of internal injury. Hematocrit, plasma volume, and urine output should be monitored closely.

Acute- and delayed-onset central and peripheral nervous system complications are the most common sequelae of electrical injury. Cardiac complications usually consist of rhythm and conduction abnormalities, with rare infarction. Sepsis and psychiatric complications also occur.

## Prevention

Electrical injuries can be prevented in industrial settings by making sure that electrical workers are properly qualified and trained to follow safety procedures involving the installation, grounding, and disconnection of power sources. Particular attention should be given to work requiring equipment manipulation during "live" operation. Nonconducting tools and clothing should be used whenever possible. Barricades and warning signs should be placed around high-voltage areas, and procedures to exclude other employees from these areas should be strictly enforced.

Workers should be instructed in the proper measures to free a victim from contact with the electrical current. If possible, the power should be turned off. If not, a nonconducting object such as a rope, a broom or other wooden instrument, or an article of clothing can be used to pull the victim away from the current and protect the rescuer from injury. If necessary, cardiopulmonary resuscitation should be instituted until medical help arrives. Because the victim may have suffered spinal injury, extreme care must be taken during handling or transport.

## Treatment

First aid consists of freeing the victim from contact with the current. Power should be turned off and/or nonconductive devices should be used to separate the rescuer and victim from the current. The rescuer must be protected during this procedure. Smoldering clothes should be removed.

If major electrical injuries are suspected, the patient should be hospitalized and observed for secondary organ damage, impaired renal function, hemorrhage, acidosis, and myoglobinuria. Indications for hospitalization include significant arrhythmia or ECG change, large burn, loss of consciousness, pulmonary or cardiac symptoms, or evidence of significant deep tissue/organ damage. A tetanus booster or antitoxin should be administered if indicated.

Superficial tissue damage should be treated conservatively and the patient observed for sepsis, which is the most common cause of death in electric shock survivors. For severe burns, a topical antibiotic (eg, mafenide or silver sulfadiazine) is applied. If major soft tissue damage is suspected, surgical exploration, fasciotomy, or both must be considered.

Lactated Ringer's solution should be administered intravenously at a rate sufficient to maintain urine output between 50 and 100 mL/h. With major muscle necrosis, mannitol can enhance hemochrome excretion. Continuous monitoring and prompt correction of acid-base or electrolyte imbalance are necessary if rhabdomyolysis occurs.

---

# NONIONIZING RADIATION INJURIES

---

## INJURIES DUE TO RADIOFREQUENCY & MICROWAVE RADIATION

### Exposure

Injuries due to the thermal effects of acute exposure to high levels of radiofrequency (RF) and microwave radiation have been documented. Like other thermal injuries, these injuries are characterized by protein denaturation and tissue necrosis at the site of thermal exposure, with an accompanying inflammatory reaction and subsequent scar formation. Nonthermal effects of low-level exposure have been demonstrated in some laboratory studies, but their significance in humans is not clear.

RF radiation and microwave radiation consist of energy in wave form traveling in free space at the speed of light. The radiation is defined in terms of frequency and intensity, with the frequency portion of the electromagnetic spectrum extending from 0 to 1000 GHz (1 Hz equals 1 wave or cycle per second [cps]). Microwaves occupy only a portion of the frequency spectrum, ie, the portion between 300 MHz and 300 GHz (Figure 12–5).

RF radiation has insufficient energy to cause molecular ionization, but it does cause vibration and rotation of molecules, particularly molecules that have an asymmetric charge distribution or are polar in structure. It is composed of separate electric and magnetic field vectors, each perpendicular to the other and both perpendicular to the direction of the resultant electromagnetic wave (Figure 12–6). The electric field component is measured in volts per meter, the magnetic component in amperes per meter, and the resultant power density in watts per square meter.

Absorption of RF radiation is dependent upon the orientation of the body in relation to the direction of the electromagnetic wave. Radiation at frequencies below 15 MHz and above 25 GHz is poorly absorbed and unlikely to cause significant thermally induced damage. Factors affecting conduction of RF radiation within the body include the thickness, distribution, and water content of the various tissues. As the water content increases, energy absorption and thermal effects increase. RF radiation can be modulated according to amplitude (AM) and frequency (FM) and can be generated in pulsed or continuous form. Pulsed waves are considered more dangerous.

The risk of thermal injury increases with higher intensities of radiation and closer proximity to the radiation source. Other factors that affect human susceptibility to RF radiation injury include environmental humidity and temperature, grounding, reflecting medium, tissue vascularity, increased temperature sensitivity of tissues (eg, the testes), and lack of anatomic barriers to external radiation (eg, the eye).

Occupational exposures are likely in any workplace where employees are near equipment that generates RF radiation, particularly equipment for dielectric heating (used in sealing of plastics and drying of wood), physiotherapy, radio-communications, radiolocation, and maintenance of aerial transmitters and high-power electrical equipment (Table 12–3). Injuries have been documented for acute exposure to energy levels exceeding 10 mW/cm$^2$. In most cases, the levels were greater than 100 mW/cm$^2$. Most studies of RF radiation effects in animals and other biologic test systems have not demonstrated thermally-induced effects at energy levels below 10 mW/cm$^2$. In animal studies, thermally induced effects include superficial and deep tissue destruction, cataract, and testicular damage.

Generally, acute high-level or long-term low-level exposures are not thought to cause cancer, but there is evidence for carcinogenesis in association with exposure to extremely low frequency radiation, "magnetic fields," (< 200 Hz). Some studies have found an increased incidence of brain tumors, breast cancer (male), or leukemia in workers exposed to extremely low-frequency electromagnetic radiation. Similarly, teratogenicity is being questioned on the basis of findings of chromosomal breaks in power station workers, an increase in the incidence of neuroblastomas found in offspring of fathers exposed to electromagnetic radiation, and an increase in the incidence of anomalies found in offspring of male physical therapists. However, because of conflicting study results and confounding exposure, the questions of magnetic field–in-

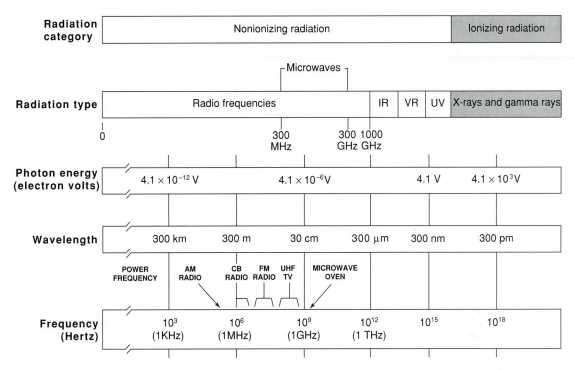

**Figure 12–5.** The electromagnetic radiation spectrum. IR = infrared radiation; VR = visible radiation (light); UV = ultraviolet light.

duced carcinogenicity or teratogenicity are not yet resolved. Although concern has been expressed concerning cataract formation following long-term low-level exposure, scientific evidence is lacking.

## Clinical Findings

Acute high-dose exposure is usually associated with a feeling of warmth on the exposed body part, followed by the feeling of hot or burning skin. The sensation of clicking or buzzing may also be present during the exposure. Other symptoms include irritability, headache or light-headedness, vertigo, pain at the site of exposure, watery eyes and a gritty eye sensation, dysphagia, anorexia, abdominal cramps,

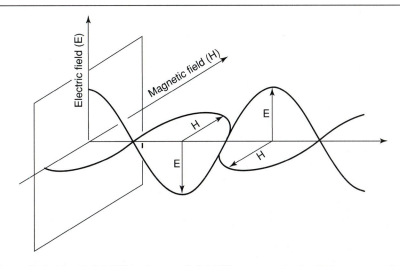

**Figure 12–6.** Electric field (E) and magnetic field (H) components of radiofrequency radiation.

**Table 12–3.** Occupational radiofrequency and microwave exposures.

| |
|---|
| Sealing and heating equipment |
|   Automotive trades |
|   Furniture and woodworking |
|   Glass fiber production |
|   Paper production |
|   Plastics manufacturing and fabrication |
|   Rubber product heating |
|   Textile manufacturing |
| Communication equipment source maintenance |
|   Radar |
|   Radio: AM, FM, CB |
|   Television: UHF and VHF |
|   Satellite |
|   Radio navigation |
| RF applications |
|   Microwave tube testing and aging |
|   RF laser |
|   RF welding |
|   Medical diathermy and healing promotion |
| Power transmission line workers |

and nausea. Localized thermally induced masses may appear within days after exposure and consist of interstitial edema and coagulation necrosis.

The exposed skin has a sunburned appearance, with erythema and slight induration. There may be vesiculation or bullae. Blood pressure may be increased, and creatine phosphokinase levels may be elevated. Hematologic values, electroencephalographic and brain scan findings, sedimentation rate, and electrolyte values are usually within normal limits.

Beyond the immediately evident thermal injury, no further structural injury would be anticipated. In one case report, essential hypertension developed 1–3 months following exposure and then resolved with treatment. Symptoms of posttraumatic stress disorder have occurred, with emotional lability and insomnia persisting for as long as 1 year.

## Differential Diagnosis

High-power equipment capable of generating RF and microwave radiation might also generate other forms of nonionizing radiation that should be considered. Chemical reactions due to heat sources in the workplace should be investigated, because thermal decomposition products of a heated hydrocarbon can cause the acute onset of similar symptoms, although blood pressure and creatine phosphokinase levels would not be expected to rise in such circumstances. Fear and anxiety resulting from the knowledge of a possibly damaging exposure may also cause many of the functional symptoms described above, although objective evidence of thermal injury and elevated creatine phosphokinase levels would not be expected.

## Prevention

Exposure assessment should include the following factors: the distance between the power source and exposed workers, the peak power density at the time of exposure, the frequency and type of radiation wave (pulsed or continuous), and the duration of exposure (in minutes).

Metal barriers around the energy source can be used to contain RF radiation. Intensity is proportional to $1/d^2$, where d is distance from the source. Accordingly, there is a rapid decrease in power density over distance, and specification of a "personnel not allowed" area can provide an effective barrier. Procedures to deenergize equipment are recommended when employees are working close to exposed sources. Protective clothing is generally not effective. Periodic environmental RF radiation measurements for equipment exposures are essential.

## Treatment & Prognosis

Treatment is the same as for other thermal injuries and includes immediately removing the worker from exposure, cooling the wound with saline soaks, cleaning and debriding tissue if necessary, and applying a topical antibiotic (eg, mafenide or silver sulfadiazine). Future exposure to radiation should be rigorously controlled to below recommended limits.

Thermal injuries usually heal without problems. If hypertension develops, it will usually resolve following a short course of antihypertensive therapy. Posttraumatic stress disorder and other psychological sequelae are generally responsive to short-term supportive psychotherapy.

## INJURIES DUE TO INFRARED RADIATION

Infrared radiation covers the portion of the electromagnetic spectrum between visible and RF radiation (Figure 12–5). It has wavelengths between 750 and 3 million nm and is composed of three spectral bands—A, B, and C—which begin at 750 nm, 1400 nm, and 3000 nm, respectively. Infrared radiation is given off from any object having a temperature greater than absolute zero. Occupational exposures—in addition to sunlight—include processes in which thermal energy from infrared radiation is used, such as heating and dehydrating processes, welding, glassmaking, and the drying and baking of coatings on consumer products.

Acute, high-intensity exposure to wavelengths shorter than 2000 nm can cause thermal damage to the cornea, iris, or lens. Thermal injury to the skin can also occur, but it is usually self-limited and results in an acute skin burn with increased pigmentation. Exposure to infrared radiation has been associated with cataract formation, particularly among glassblowers and furnace workers.

Injuries can be prevented by shielding heat sources, using protective eye and skin wear, and monitoring exposure levels. Threshold limit values for exposure intensity are frequency-dependent in the biologically active wavelength spectrum of 750–2000 nm. Wavelengths in this range cause molecular excitation and vibration, resulting in heat that is absorbed by tissues and can cause thermal injury. In contrast, wavelengths exceeding 2000 nm are absorbed by water and are not biologically active because of the high water content of tissues.

## INJURIES DUE TO VISIBLE RADIATION

Visible radiation (light) covers the portion of the electromagnetic spectrum between infrared and ultraviolet radiation (Figure 12–5) and the wavelengths between 400 and 750 nm. The eye is the most sensitive target organ, with damage resulting from structural, thermal, or photochemical light-induced reactions. Workers at risk are those with prolonged or repeated exposure to intense light sources, including sunlight, high-intensity lamps, lasers, flashbulbs, spotlights, and welding arcs. Extremely intense light sources such as lasers can also cause pressure-induced (mechanical) retinal damage.

The retina is the usual site of injury and is most sensitive to the wavelengths of 440–500 nm (blue light), which cause a destructive photochemical reaction. Blue light is responsible for solar retinitis (eclipse blindness) and may contribute to retinal aging and to senile macular degeneration, which can result in visual field defects. Because the lens normally filters out wavelengths between 320 and 500 nm, it provides some protection of the retina from blue light. Individuals with aphakia (absence of the lens), who are more susceptible to retinal damage, should be cautioned against looking into the midday sun and other intense light sources and urged to wear spectacle filters when working in bright environments.

Short bursts of high-intensity light can cause heat-induced flash blindness, in which the temporary visual loss and afterimage are due to bleaching of visual pigments. As the light intensity and exposure duration increase, the afterimage persists longer. With mild to moderate exposures, symptoms of flash blindness resolve quickly.

Insufficient lighting or reflected light (glare) can cause asthenopia (eyestrain), visual fatigue, headache, and eye irritation. These problems are more likely to occur in people over the age of 40 years. Symptoms are transient, and there is no indication that repeated episodes lead to ocular damage.

Contrast from surrounding light sources on areas of lesser intensity has led to complaints of asthenopia associated with video display terminal use. This can usually be corrected by decreasing surrounding light intensities, using antiglare filters, and adjusting the contrast of the light on the screen.

Treatment of eye injuries is discussed in Chapter 9. Measures to prevent injury in workers at risk include preemployment evaluations for individuals with aphakia or a history of light sensitivity and medical surveillance to detect changes in visual acuity or early signs of ocular damage; use of goggles or face shields by welders; proper illumination of the workplace to reduce glare (see Chapter 6); and use of filters on intense light sources to eliminate blue light wavelengths.

## INJURIES DUE TO ULTRAVIOLET RADIATION

Ultraviolet (UV) radiation covers the portion of the electromagnetic spectrum between visible radiation and ionizing radiation (Figure 12–5) and has wavelengths between 100 and 400 nm. The wavelengths are divided into 3 bands—A, B, and C—with the A and B bands representing the longer wavelengths and producing most of the biologic effects (Table 12–4). Wavelengths shorter than 200 nm are biologically inactive; they can exist only in a vacuum or an inert gas atmosphere and are absorbed over extremely short distances in air. Wavelengths of 200–290 nm are absorbed primarily in the stratum corneum of the skin or the cornea of the eye, while the longer wavelengths can affect the dermis, lens, iris, or retina.

Because UV radiation has relatively poor penetration, the only organs it affects are the eye and skin. Eye injury is caused by thermal action from pulsed or brief high-power exposures, and skin damage more commonly by photochemical reactions (including toxic and hypersensitivity reactions) from brief high or extended low-power exposures. The thermal effects of protein coagulation and tissue necrosis are rapid in onset. The effects of chronic exposure include accelerated aging of the skin, characterized by loss of elasticity, hyperpigmentation, wrinkling, and telangiectasia.

UV injuries occur in occupations involving drying and curing processes, arc welding, or use of lasers or germicidal UV lights (Table 12–5), but by far the greatest proportion of injuries result from occupations that expose workers to natural sunlight during the peak time of UV energy dissemination, 10 AM to 3 PM. Factors affecting the severity of injury include exposure duration, radiation intensity, distance from the radiation source, and orientation of the exposed individual relative to the source and its wave propagation plane.

**Table 12–4.** Ultraviolet light spectrum: UV-A and UV-B comparison.

| | UV-A | UV-B |
|---|---|---|
| Wavelength | 315–400 nm | 280–315 nm |
| Penetration | Air, water, glass, quartz through eye to retina | Air, quartz |
|   Physical | | Anterior chamber only |
|   Biological | | |
| Health effects | Skin and eye injury require greater energy than UV-B | Skin erythema at 280–315 nm |
| | | Peak carcinogenicity at 280–320 nm |
| | | Peak photokerotitis sensitivity at 270 nm |
| | | Cataract |
| Proportion of natural back-ground UV | 97% | 3% |

UV reflections from water and snow or their surrounding surfaces may increase exposure intensity.

## Clinical Findings & Treatment

### A. Photokeratoconjunctivitis (Welder's Flash):

**Table 12–5.** Workers potentially exposed to ultraviolet radiation.[1]

**Natural sunlight**

| | |
|---|---|
| Agricultural workers | Oil field workers |
| Brick masons | Open pit miners |
| Ranchers | Outdoor maintenance workers |
| Construction workers | Pipeline workers |
| Farmers | Police officers |
| Fishermen | Postal carriers |
| Gardeners | Railroad track workers |
| Greenskeepers | Road workers |
| Horticultural workers | Sailors |
| Landscapers | Ski instructors |
| Lifeguards | Sports professionals |
| Lumberjacks | Surveyors |
| Military personnel | |

**Arc welding ultraviolet**
Welders
Pipeline workers
Pipecutters
Maintenance workers

**Plasma torch ultraviolet**
Plasma torch operators

**Germicidal ultraviolet**
Physicians
Nurses
Laboratory technicians
Bacteriology laboratory personnel
Barbers
Cosmetologists
Kitchen workers

**Laser ultraviolet**
Laboratory workers

**Drying and curing processes**
Printers
Lithographers
Painters
Wood curers
Plastics workers

[1]Reproduced, with permission, from Adams RM: *Occupational Skin Disease*. Grune & Stratton, 1983.

Ocular exposure to UV wavelengths shorter than 315 nm (especially wavelengths of 270 nm, to which the eye is most sensitive) can cause photokeratoconjunctivitis. Symptoms occur 6–12 hours after exposure and include severe pain, photophobia, a sensation of a foreign body or sand in the eyes, and tearing. After a latency period that varies inversely with the severity of the exposure, conjunctivitis appears, sometimes accompanied by erythema and swelling of the eyelids and facial skin. Slit lamp examination may reveal diffuse punctate staining of both corneas.

Treatment consists of providing symptomatic relief, which may include ice packs, systemic analgesics, eye patches, and mild sedation. Local anesthetics should not be used because of the risk of further injury to the anesthetized eye.

Symptoms usually resolve within 48 hours. Permanent sequelae are rare, and the eye does not develop tolerance to repeated exposure.

**B. Cataracts:** Cataractogenesis has been attributed to both photochemical and thermal effects of intense exposure to UV wavelengths of 295–320 nm and usually appears within 24 hours. Cataract formation following repeated exposures to UV wavelengths longer than 324 nm has been reported but is not well-documented. Treatment is by cataract extraction and, usually, intraocular lens implantation.

**C. Other Eye Injuries:** The lens protects the retina from the effects of UV wavelengths shorter than 300 nm, but damage to the iris and retina is possible if individuals with aphakia are exposed to these wavelengths. In others, damage is possible with exposure to longer wavelengths or to high-power UV lasers. Treatment is supportive (Table 12–6).

Two lesions of the bulbar conjunctiva have been associated with repeated exposures to UV radiation: pterygium (a benign hyperplasia) and epidermoid carcinoma.

**D. Erythema:** Absorbed UV radiation reacts with photoactive substances present in the skin and 2–24 hours later causes erythema (sunburn), the most common acute UV effect. Erythema is most severe following exposure to wavelengths of 290–320 nm

**Table 12–6.** Eye injuries due to ultraviolet light.

| Location | UV Effect |
|---|---|
| Conjunctiva | Conjunctivitis |
| Sclera | Hyperemia |
| Cornea | Kerotitis |
| Cataracts | Lens |
| Aqueous | Toxic photochemicals |
| Vitreous | ? Degradation in aphakics |
| Retina | Chromophore damage in aphakics |

and may be accompanied by edema, blistering, desquamation, chills, fever, nausea, and, rarely, circulatory collapse.

Treatment of acute sunburn and any blistering that occurs is supportive and symptomatic and may include topical and mild systemic analgesics. Most symptoms subside within 48 hours. The resulting scaling, darkening of the skin (due to increased melanin production), and thickening of the stratum corneum provide increased protection against subsequent exposures.

**E. Photosensitivity Reactions:** Two types of acute photosensitivity reactions of the skin can occur following exposure to UV radiation: phototoxic (non-allergic) and photoallergic reactions.

**Phototoxic reactions** are much more common and frequently occur in association with use of medications such as griseofulvin, tetracycline, sulfonamides, thiazides, and preparations containing coal tar or psoralens. Phototoxicity may exaggerate or aggravate the effects of some systemic diseases, including lupus erythematosus, dermatomyositis, congenital erythropoietic porphyria, porphyria cutanea tarda symptomatica, pellagra, actinic reticuloid, herpes simplex, and pemphigus foliaceus. Photosensitivity reactions may be characterized by blisters, bullae, and other skin manifestations.

Exposure to UV wavelengths above 320 nm after skin contact with furocoumarin-producing plants such as celery can cause phytophotodermatitis. A mild phototoxic reaction causes pigmentary changes along the pattern of points of contact, while bullae may result from a more severe inflammatory reaction.

**Photoallergic reactions** to UV radiation occur in association with bacteriostatic agents and perfume ingredients, which cause skin irritation, erythema, and blistering.

Treatment of photosensitivity reactions depends on the particular underlying or associative cause and ranges from symptomatic care in mild cases to hospitalization and use of systemic corticosteroids in cases of severe reactions.

**F. Premalignant and Malignant Skin Lesions:** Premalignant lesions associated with chronic exposure to UV radiation include actinic keratosis, keratoacanthoma, and Hutchinson's melanosis. Malignant lesions associated with exposure are basal cell carcinoma (the most common), squamous cell carcinoma, and malignant melanoma. Hazardous UV wavelengths are thought to be between 256 and 320 nm. UV radiation also promotes carcinogenesis following exposure to some chemicals, including those found in tar and pitch.

Increased risk for premalignant and malignant lesions occurs in fair-skinned individuals and in those who have repeated sunburns or tan poorly. Patients with a history of xeroderma pigmentosum are at greater risk for malignant melanoma.

Patients should be referred to a dermatologist for definitive diagnosis and treatment. Premalignant lesions may be treated by removal or use of topical medication. Treatment of malignant lesions may involve simple excision, radiation, or major surgery.

### Prevention

Workplace exposure to UV radiation should be monitored on a routine basis. Figure 12–7 shows threshold limit values, based on wavelength and irradiance. Exposure intensities should be minimized if possible, and exposed individuals should be counseled concerning photosensitizing agents. Welders should be urged to wear goggles or face shields to protect their eyes.

Outdoor workers should be instructed to use sunscreen and protective clothing, and persons at increased risk because of preexisting medical conditions or excessive exposure should be examined periodically for the presence of premalignant or malignant lesions.

## IONIZING RADIATION INJURIES

The two most significant health responses to ionizing radiation are the acute radiation syndrome that follows a brief but massive exposure and the chronic effects that are due to a brief high-dose exposure or to high cumulative exposures. Approximately 100 significant radiation incidents have occurred since 1940 as a result of exposure to radioisotopes, x-ray generators and accelerators, radar generators, and similar sources of ionizing radiation. Because of the ubiquity of ionizing radiation in our environment, the effects of long-term low-dose exposures are more difficult to pinpoint, but clusters of illnesses have been found near nuclear test sites and in association with some occupations. Workers at risk, based on their history of exposures and resulting injury, in-

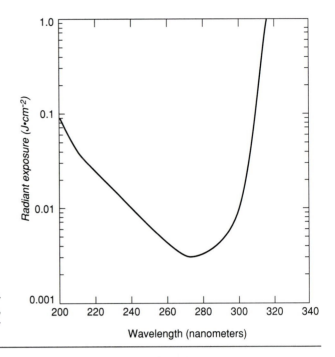

**Figure 12–7.** Threshold limit values (TLV) for ultraviolet radiation. (Reproduced, with permission, from *American Conference of Governmental Industrial Hygienists TLV Booklet,* 1995–1996.)

clude radiologists, uranium miners, radium dial painters, nuclear power plant operators, and military personnel. Other workers at risk, based on the potential for exposure, are listed in Table 12–7.

Ionizing radiation is emitted from radioactive atomic structures as energized particles (alpha, beta, proton, and neutron particles) that impart energy through collision with other structures or as high-energy electromagnetic x-rays or gamma rays. The different forms of ionizing radiation vary in natural source, energy, frequency, and penetrability, but they all share the ability to ionize incident materials and exist at the highest energies and frequencies of the electromagnetic spectrum (Figure 12–5). Dislocation of an electron from an incident atom and the resulting biomolecular chemical reactions and instability can cause tissue damage. A summary of the clinical effects of ionizing radiation is presented in Table 12–8.

External biologic exposure to x-rays, gamma rays, and proton and neutron radiation results in high absorption, whereas beta particles penetrate skin poorly and alpha particles do not penetrate at all. Internal exposure to alpha or beta particles by inhalation, implantation, or ingestion can result in serious acute or delayed injury. If radioactive contamination is suspected, decontamination procedures should be followed scrupulously during all phases of patient management.

As an emergency resource, the Oak Ridge Institute for Science and Education maintains 24-hour phone access to consultation regarding medical and health physics problems associated with radiation accidents [weekdays (615) 576-3131; evenings and weekends (423) 481-1000].

**Table 12–7.** Potential occupational exposures to ionizing radiation.

Aircraft workers
Atomic energy plant workers
Biologists
Cathode ray tube makers
Chemists
Dental workers
Drug makers and sterilizers
Electron microscope makers and operators
Electrostatic eliminator operators
Embalmers
Fire alarm makers
Food preservers and sterilizers
Gas mantle makers
High-voltage electron, x-ray, vacuum, radar, klystron or
    television tube makers, users, repairmen
Industrial radiographers and fluoroscopists
Inspectors using—and workers in proximity to—sealed
    gamma ray sources (cesium 137, cobalt 60, iridium 192)
    and x-rays
Liquid level gauge painters
Luminous dial painters
Military personnel
Oil well loggers
Ore assayers
Petroleum refinery workers
Physicians and nurses
Plasma torch operators
Plastics technicians
Prospectors
Radium refinery workers
Research workers, chemists, biologists, physicists
Thickness gauge operators
Thorium ore and alloy workers
Tile glazers
Uranium workers and miners
Veterinarians
X-ray aides and technicians
X-ray diffraction apparatus operators

**Table 12–8.** Summary of clinical effects of ionizing radiation dosages.

| | Subclinical Range | Therapeutic Range | | | Lethal Range | |
| --- | --- | --- | --- | --- | --- | --- |
| | 0–100 rem | 100–200 rem (Clinical Surveillance) | 200–600 rem (Therapy Effective) | 600–1000 rem (Therapy Promising) | 1000–5000 rem (Therapy Palliative) | >5000 rem (Therapy Palliative) |
| Incidence of vomiting | None | 5% at 100 rem 50% at 200 rem | 100% at 300 rem | 100% | 100% | 100% |
| Delay time for vomiting | . . . | 3 hr | 2 hr | 1 hr | 30 min | 30 min |
| Leading organ affected | None | Hematopoietic tissue | Hematopoietic tissue | Hematopoietic tissue | Gastrointestinal tract | Central nervous system |
| Characteristic signs and symptoms | None | Mild nausea and moderate leukopenia | Severe leukopenia, diarrhea, nausea, purpura, hemorrhage, and infection; hair loss above 300 rem | Severe leukopenia, purpura, hemorrhage, infection, prostration, coma | Diarrhea, fever, and disturbance of electrolyte balance | Convulsions, tremor, ataxia, and lethargy |
| Critical period postexposure | . . . | . . . | 4–6 wk | 4–6 wk | 5–14 days | 1–48 hr |
| Therapy required | Reassurance | Reassurance and hematologic surveillance | Blood transfusion, antibiotics, and hematopoietic growth factors | Blood transfusions, antibiotics, hematopoietic growth factors, and consider bone marrow transplant | Maintenance of electrolyte balance | Sedatives |
| Prognosis | Excellent | Excellent | Good | Guarded | Hopeless | Hopeless |
| Convalescent period | None | Several weeks | 1–12 mo | Long | . . . | . . . |
| Incidence of death | None | None | 0–80% | 80–100% | 90–100% | 90–100% |
| Time within which death occurs | . . . | . . . | 2 mo | 2 mo | 2 wk | 2 days |
| Cause of death | . . . | . . . | Hemorrhage and infection | Hemorrhage and infection | Circulatory collapse | Respiratory failure and brain edema |

## ACUTE RADIATION SYNDROME

Acute radiation syndrome is due to brief but heavy exposure of all or part of the body to ionizing radiation. The radiation disrupts chemical bonds, which causes molecular excitation and free radical formation. Highly reactive free radicals react with other essential molecules such as nucleic acids and enzymes, and this in turn disrupts cellular function. The clinical presentation and severity of illness are determined by the dosage, body distribution, and duration of exposure. Tissues with the most rapid cellular turnover are the most radiosensitive: reproductive, hematopoietic, and gastrointestinal tissues.

## Clinical Findings

Although symptoms are unlikely with exposure to doses under 100 cGy, abnormal laboratory findings may be seen at any dose over 25 cGy. For doses of 100–400 cGy, symptoms begin within 2–6 hours and may last up to 48 hours. For doses of 600–1000 cGy, symptoms begin within 2 hours and later merge into the illness phase. For those at Chernobyl who received over 600 cGy, headache, fever, and vomiting developed within the first half hour. Within 6 days, severe lymphopenia developed, followed by severe gastroenteritis, granulocytopenia, and thrombocytopenia. For those in the lowest exposure group (80–210 cGy), slight lymphopenia occurred within a few days, followed by mild granulocytopenia and thrombocytopenia at 4 weeks.

Doses of 1000–3000 cGy can cause immediate gastrointestinal symptoms and massive fluid, blood, and electrolyte loss resulting from denudation of the gastrointestinal mucosa. Doses exceeding 3000 cGy are lethal. They cause progressive neurologic incapacitation associated with ataxia, lethargy, tremor, and convulsions. Death is almost immediate with the highest doses.

Some patients with acute radiation syndrome pass through four phases: prodrome, latent phase, illness, and recovery.

**A. Prodrome:** Symptoms and signs may include anorexia, nausea, vomiting, diarrhea, intestinal cramps, salivation, dehydration, fatigue, apathy, prostration, arrhythmia, fever, respiratory distress, hyperexcitability, ataxia, headache, and hypotension. Gastrointestinal and central nervous system findings predominate.

**B. Latent Phase:** The prodrome is sometimes followed by a period of relative well-being prior to the onset of illness. In cases of exposure to higher doses of radiation, the latent period is shortened or eliminated and central nervous system or gastrointestinal effects predominate.

**C. Illness Phase:** Symptoms and signs in this phase may include fatigue, weakness, fever, diarrhea, anorexia, weight loss, hair loss, arrhythmia, ileus, ataxia, disorientation, convulsions, coma, and shock. Effects are primarily hematopoietic and due to inhibition of hematopoietic stem cells. There may be a sequential decrease in lymphocytes, granulocytes, platelets, and erythrocytes. Leukopenia and thrombocytopenia may occur with secondary infection, hemorrhagic diathesis, or anemia. Cardiovascular collapse, pericarditis, and myocarditis have been reported. With doses exceeding 200 cGy, there may be reproductive system effects, including sterility, aspermatogenesis, and cessation of menses. Fetal and embryo toxicity or death can also occur.

**D. Recovery Phase:** The prognosis for recovery from exposures of up to 600 cGy is good when appropriate therapy is given. For higher exposures, the prognosis worsens as the dose increases. Infection and sepsis are the major causes of morbidity and mortality in cases involving exposures below 1000 cGy, in which the major impact is hematopoietic.

## Prevention

Occupational exposure to ionizing radiation should be monitored. The technology varies with the type of radiation and the target site. Personal exposure measurement devices include film badges (x-rays, gamma, and beta) or nuclear emulsion monitors (x-rays, gamma, beta, and neutrons), thermoluminescent dosimeters (beta, gamma, and neutron), and ionization dosimeters. A scintillation counter can be used to measure some radioisotopes in urine specimens or in tissue from target organs (eg, urine tritium or $^{32}P$, thyroid scintillation scan for $^{125}I$). Environmental or area monitoring devices include the Geiger-Müller counter, ionization chamber, and scintillation detector. Where an exposure potential occurs, shielding with lead or other effective barrier can contain emissions.

To quantify risk from radiation exposure, a system of units has been created and revised many times. The International Commission on Radiological Units and Measurements (ICRU) has recommended that the older CGS units be replaced by the equivalent SI units, as shown in Table 12–9. Recommended external exposure limits are shown in Table 12–10. The basis for the limits is what is referred to as the "acceptable" risk. This is thought to be 1 in 10,000 per year for workers with occupational exposures and 1 in 10,000–1,000,000 per year for the general public, based on estimated radiation-induced fatal cancers and serious hereditary disorders. Exposures can be easily prevented through the use of lead or other high-density material, which can enclose the source and/or shield the work area (eg, lead blocks, cement, and leaded glass).

## Treatment

The patient should be decontaminated, hospitalized, and placed under the care of hematologists and infectious disease specialists. Vital signs, fluid and electrolyte balance, and hematopoietic, gastrointestinal, and central nervous system functions should be monitored closely.

If the granulocyte counts fall below 1000, prophylactic antibacterial agents, acyclovir, and antifungals have been recommended. If there is fever or suspected sepsis, antimicrobial agents by intravenous infusion should be started immediately. A combination of a semisynthetic penicillin and a third-generation cephalosporin or an aminoglycoside has been recommended, but the choice of agents should also depend on the endemic pathogens at the particular hospital. Antimicrobial therapy should be continued until the granulocyte count exceeds 500/μL or until the patient has been afebrile for 5 consecutive days without evidence of infection. Reverse isolation should be maintained.

Granulocyte, platelet, and red cell transfusions may be necessary. Lymphocytes should be obtained immediately for HLA typing. Transfusions are recommended if the platelet count falls below 20,000/μL, the granulocyte count below 200/μL, or the hematocrit below 25%. Hematopoietic growth factors (filgrastim, sargramostim) have been effective in accelerating hematopoietic recovery. Bone marrow transplants have been successful in combating intractable hemorrhage and infection. They should be considered for patients exposed to 600–2000 cGy, and the decision about whether to use

**Table 12–9.** Radiation units.

| Parameter | SI Units[1] | CGS Units[2] | Conversion |
|---|---|---|---|
| Activity = rate of decay (disintegration per second) | Becquerel (Bq) | Curie (Ci) | 1 Ci = $3.7 \times 10^{10}$ Bq.<br>1 Bq + = $2.703 \times 10^{-11}$ Ci. |
| Exposure (dose) = quantity of x-ray or gamma radiation at a given point | Coulomb (C)/kg of air | Roentgen (R) | 1 C/kg of air = 3876 R.<br>1 R = 258 MC/kg of air. |
| Dose rate = dose per unit of time (counts per minute) | Coulomb (C)/kg of air/hr | Roentgen (R)/hr | Same as above. |
| Absorbed dose = quantity of radiation absorbed per unit of mass | Gray (Gy)<br>Joules (J)/kg | Rad<br>Erg | 1 Gy = 1 J/kg.<br>1 Gy = 100 rads.<br>1 rad = 0.01 Gy.<br>1 rad = 100 ergs. |
| Dose equivalent = absorbed dose in terms of estimated biologic effect relative to an exposure of 1 roentgen of x-ray or gamma radiation | Sievert (Sv) | Rem | 1 Sv = 100 rem.<br>1 rem = 0.01 Sv. |

[1]SI = international system of units.
[2]CGS = centigram-gram-second system of units.

them should be made within a week following radiation exposure.

Patients should receive supportive therapy as necessary for control of nausea, dehydration, and other symptoms. Ondansetron hydrochloride, 8 mg orally two or three times daily, has been recommended for nausea; chlorpromazine 25–50 mg given deeply intramuscularly every 4–6 hours is an alternative.

**Table 12–10.** External radiation exposure limits.

| Groups and Body Parts Exposed | Radiation Limit |
|---|---|
| **Adults**<br>Whole body, head, trunk, arm above elbow, and leg above knee | 5 rem (0.05 Sv) per year[1]<br>**or**<br>3 rem (0.03 Sv) in any quarter |
| Hand, elbow, arm below elbow, foot, knee, and leg below knee | 50 rem (0.5 Sv) per year |
| Lens of eye | 15 rem (0.15 Sv) per year |
| Skin (10 cm) | 50 rem (0.5 Sv) per year |
| **Pregnant women** | 0.05 rem (0.5 Sv) per month while pregnant<br>**or**<br>0.5 rem (5 mSv) per pregnancy |
| **Minors** | 10% of annual limits for adults |

[1]Includes cumulative yearly (external) deep-dose equivalent and (internal) committed effective-dose equivalent.

## ACUTE LOCALIZED RADIATION INJURIES

Exposure of isolated skin and body parts to ionizing radiation will result in hair loss (doses above 300 cGy), erythema (above 600 cGy), dry desquamation (radionecrosis) (above 1000 cGy), and wet desquamation (above 2000 cGy). Pain and itching occur shortly after exposure and are followed by erythema and blister formation. In cases of severe localized burns, there may be tissue ischemia and necrosis.

Prevention is as for acute radiation syndrome (see above).

Treatment is conservative and should not include surgery unless that is dictated by secondary complications. To conserve joint motion and prevent contractures, splinting and physical therapy may be required during convalescence. Injuries should be followed closely, because the extent of tissue damage is often not readily apparent. Subsequent fibrosis, ulceration, infection, necrosis, or gangrene may occur and require surgery or more radical medical treatment.

## RADIONUCLIDE CONTAMINATION

Skin contamination with radionuclides is rarely life-threatening. Immediate decontamination measures consist of gently scrubbing the skin with soap and warm water and, if necessary, cutting the hair. Hair clippings, material removed by scrubbing, swabs of the nares and mouth, clothing, and personal effects should be saved for radioactivity analysis and dosage calculation.

For contaminated open wounds, gentle surgical debridement should be performed and wound irrigation considered. Depending on the type of radionuclide causing the injury, administration of a chelating agent may be indicated. For plutonium and alpha emitters, diethylenetriaminepentaacetic acid (DTPA) is effective and can be administered systemically as well as in the wound irrigation solution. Blocking agents may also be considered, as in the case of radioiodines. For further information, the reader is referred to Report 65 of the National Council on Radiation Protection and Measurements, which is listed in the references at the end of this chapter.

Uranium and its associated radon daughter emissions are associated with lung cancer and probably reproductive effects, nonmalignant pulmonary disease, and nephritis.

## DELAYED EFFECTS OF HIGH-DOSE RADIATION

Radiodermatitis often occurs in association with ionizing radiation therapy. The skin is dry, smooth, shiny, thin, pruritic, and sensitive, and there are signs of telangiectasia, atrophy, and diffuse pigmentation. The nails are brittle and striated.

Scarring in other tissues following high-dose exposure has led to endarteritis obliterans, intestinal stenosis, pulmonary fibrosis, and cataracts.

Various cancers related to localized organ radioactivity have been described. These include bone cancer from localized radioisotopes, thyroid cancer following childhood thymus irradiation, liver cancer associated with thorium dioxide, and lung cancer associated with radon decay products (radon daughters) in uranium miners. Leukemia has been reported in patients receiving radiotherapy for ankylosing spondylitis; malignant glioma has been reported following radiotherapy.

Other effects of high-dose exposure include premature aging, shortening of the life span, and teratogenic (central nervous system deficit, mental retardation, microcephaly) and reproductive abnormalities.

## EFFECTS OF LOW-DOSE RADIATION

Controversy continues over whether the risk for somatic and genetic disorders is significantly increased by cumulative low-dose exposures. The dose-response curve in the low-dose range cannot be determined at present, so most estimates of risk continue to be based on mathematical extrapolations from experiences with higher doses. Although developmental abnormalities have been associated with doses as low as 10 cGy and cancers associated with levels below 100 cGy, the practical relevance of low-

dose phenomena is extremely difficult to establish, not only because of inconsistencies in the literature but also because the cumulative average exposure for people in the United States is approximately 8–10 cGy per lifetime (Table 12–11). In other words, the practical medical significance of these low lifetime cumulative exposures is presently unclear and imprecise. The Beir V report indicated that the incidence/risk of radiation-induced cancer varies according to cancer type, cumulative dose, and age at exposure (child versus adult). It indicates a nonthreshold linear or linear quadratic relationship between dose and cancer incidence (Table 12–12).

## LASER INJURIES

The energy of the laser source is transformed through atomic excitation into a coherent, collimated, monochromatic beam of radiation. Lasers operate at one wavelength, usually in the ultraviolet, visible, or infrared portion of the electromagnetic spectrum. They may emit radiation in continuous or pulsed waves.

Most industrial exposures to laser radiation occur in the construction industry, where lasers are used to provide alignment and grade levels on projects such as dam construction, tunneling, dredging, floor installation, and pipe laying. In the manufacture of electronics, laser use is increasing for welding, burning, and alignment. Intense laser sources are used to cut hard metals and diamonds, and less intense thermal applications include medical treatment.

Biologic effects at low intensities are unlikely, although there is some variation with wavelength. Injuries have not been associated with repeated low-intensity exposures. At high intensities, thermal or pressure-induced damage to the skin or eyes can occur. These injuries are more likely with lasers that have a high-intensity beam outside the visible light spectrum, because the worker's proximity to the beam may not be apparent. Because of the thermal mechanism, any damage that occurs would be expected to be immediately manifested with the symptoms and signs of a corneal, retinal, or cutaneous burn. Exposure to UV lasers is more likely to cause corneal damage, while infrared and visible-light lasers are more likely to injure the retina because of their ocular penetration. Eye symptoms of accidental high-intensity laser exposure include photophobias or sudden visual flash followed by scotoma or shadow of unusual size and color. Visual acuity or fields may be reduced. Retinal changes including edema, coagulation, hemorrhage, and opaque vitreous can occur.

**Table 12–11.** Average annual effective dose equivalent of ionizing radiations to a member of the US population.[1]

| Source | Dose Equivalent[2] | | Effective Dose Equivalent | |
|---|---|---|---|---|
| | mSv | mrem | mSv | % |
| Natural | | | | |
|   Radon[3] | 24 | 2,400 | 2.0 | 55 |
|   Cosmic | 0.27 | 27 | 0.27 | 8.0 |
|   Terrestrial | 0.28 | 28 | 0.28 | 8.0 |
|   Internal | 0.39 | 39 | 0.39 | 11 |
|   Total natural | — | — | 3.0 | 82 |
| Artificial | | | | |
|   Medical | | | | |
|     X-ray diagnosis | 0.39 | 39 | 0.39 | 11 |
|     Nuclear medicine | 0.14 | 14 | 0.14 | 4.0 |
|     Consumer products | 0.10 | 10 | 0.10 | 3.0 |
|   Other | | | | |
|     Occupational | 0.009 | 0.9 | <0.01 | <0.3 |
|     Nuclear fuel cycle | <0.01 | <1.0 | <0.01 | <0.03 |
|     Fallout | <0.01 | <1.0 | <0.01 | <0.03 |
|     Miscellaneous[4] | <0.01 | <1.0 | <0.01 | <0.03 |
|   Total artificial | — | — | 0.63 | 18 |
| Total natural and | | | | |
|   artificial | — | — | 3.6 | 100 |

[1]Reproduced, with permission, from *Health Effects of Exposure to Low Levels of Ionizing Radiation,* BEIR V. National Academy Press, Washington, DC, 1990.
[2]To soft tissues.
[3]Dose equivalent to bronchi from radon daughter products. The assumed weighting factor for the effective dose equivalent relative to whole-body exposure is 0.08.
[4]Department of Energy facilities, smelters, transportation, etc.

Treatment for these laser injuries is the same as that for other thermal injuries.

To prevent injuries, exposure levels should be monitored. Threshold limit values for lasers have been established by the American Conference of Governmental Industrial Hygienists (ACGIH) and are based on intensity, wavelength, and exposure time. The American National Standards Institute (ANSI) has developed a classification for lasers by degree of hazard, with class 1 representing no risk and class 4 representing a severe hazard even from diffuse reflection. Evaluation of workers following laser exposures should include an assessment of exposure intensity, wavelength, duration, viewing angle, and ANSI laser hazard classification.

Individuals working in proximity to high-power lasers should be instructed in proper operating procedures and provided with protective eye wear designed for the specific wavelength of the laser. In some cases, the eye wear does not by itself offer sufficient protection, owing to possible laser reflections. Other devices, including shields, barriers, and, where possible, remote viewing equipment, should be used. Skin protection is also important when high-power lasers are used. If feasible, systems should be designed with the beam line totally enclosed and shielded.

Preplacement examinations are recommended for individuals who will work with class 3B and 4 lasers and should consist of, as a minimum, the medical history, tests for visual acuity (near and far) and refractive errors, slit lamp examination, ophthal-moscopy, and inspection of the outer eye and skin. Because pathologic effects have not been associated with long-term low-intensity exposures, periodic evaluation is not recommended for laser operators unless an acute high-intensity exposure occurs.

# ATMOSPHERIC PRESSURE DISORDERS (Dysbarism)

Sudden shift to an environment of lower ambient pressure, as occurs with rapid ascension to the surface from deep-sea diving or with loss of cabin pressure while flying at high altitudes, causes decompression sickness. Compression sickness can occur following movement to an environment of higher ambient pressure, but the only common example of this is barotitis.

## DECOMPRESSION SICKNESS (Caisson Disease)

Decompression sickness results from mechanical and physiologic effects of expanding gases and bubbles in blood and tissue. When the body is exposed to

**Table 12–12.** Cancer excess mortality by age at exposure and site
for 100,000 persons of each age exposed to 0.1 Sv (10 rem).[1]

| Age at Exposure | Total | Leukemia | Nonleukemia | Breast | Respiratory | Digestive | Other |
|---|---|---|---|---|---|---|---|
| **Men** | | | | | | | |
| 5 | 1276 | 111 | 1165 | — | 17 | 361 | 787 |
| 15 | 1144 | 109 | 1035 | — | 54 | 369 | 612 |
| 25 | 921 | 36 | 885 | — | 124 | 389 | 372 |
| 35 | 566 | 62 | 504 | — | 243 | 28 | 233 |
| 45 | 600 | 108 | 492 | — | 353 | 22 | 117 |
| 55 | 616 | 166 | 450 | — | 393 | 15 | 42 |
| 65 | 481 | 191 | 290 | — | 272 | 11 | 7 |
| 75 | 258 | 165 | 93 | — | 90 | 5 | — |
| 85 | 110 | 96 | 14 | — | 17 | — | — |
| Avg[2] | 770 | 110 | 660 | — | 190 | 170 | 300 |
| **Women** | | | | | | | |
| 5 | 1532 | 75 | 1457 | 129 | 48 | 655 | 625 |
| 15 | 1566 | 72 | 1494 | 295 | 70 | 653 | 476 |
| 25 | 1178 | 29 | 1149 | 52 | 125 | 679 | 293 |
| 35 | 557 | 46 | 511 | 43 | 208 | 73 | 187 |
| 45 | 541 | 73 | 468 | 20 | 277 | 71 | 100 |
| 55 | 505 | 117 | 388 | 6 | 273 | 64 | 45 |
| 65 | 386 | 146 | 240 | — | 172 | 52 | 16 |
| 75 | 227 | 127 | 100 | — | 72 | 26 | 3 |
| 85 | 90 | 73 | 17 | — | 15 | 4 | — |
| Avg | 810 | 80 | 730 | 70 | 150 | 290 | 220 |

[1]Reproduced, with permission, from *Health Effects of Exposure to Low Levels of Ionizing Radiation*, BEIR V. National Academy Press, Washington, DC, 1990.
[2]Averages are weighted for the age distribution in a stationary population having US mortality rates and have been rounded to the nearest 10.

an environment of higher than atmospheric gas pressure, as in tunneling or diving, it absorbs more of the inhaled gases than it does at sea level. Aided by its fat solubility, nitrogen concentrations increase in tissues, particularly those of the nervous system, bone marrow, and fat. Because the blood supply is poor in bone marrow and fat, nitrogen enters and leaves these tissues more slowly than oxygen or carbon dioxide does. As the surrounding pressure decreases (decompression), nitrogen expands and will form gas bubbles if there is insufficient time for its dissolution from tissues. Because oxygen and carbon dioxide have greater fluid solubility and move more easily between tissue compartments, their tendency for bubble formation is reduced. Remaining nitrogen gas bubbles are more symptomatic and destructive in less elastic structures or tissues (eg, joints, central nervous system).

Most cases of decompression sickness have occurred after rapid ascension from sea depths in excess of 9 m or after sudden pressure loss at altitudes in excess of 7000 m.

## Clinical Findings

A complete evaluation of the systems affected—as determined by the history and physical examination—should be performed with appropriate x-rays and other diagnostic procedures. Anyone exhibiting signs or symptoms of decompression sickness within 48 hours after a high-pressure exposure should be given a compression test in which 100% oxygen at 3 atm is administered for 20 minutes in a hyperbaric chamber.

There are three types of decompression sickness, as described below. The type and severity of symptoms will depend on the age, weight, and physical condition of the patient; the degree of physical exertion; the depth or altitude before decompression; and the rate and duration of decompression.

**A. Type 1 Decompression Sickness:** This type, which has the best prognosis, affects the limbs and skin. Acute pain, usually around a major joint, may be incapacitating and cause the patient to assume a stooped posture ("the bends"). Pain may begin immediately after decompression or up to 12 hours later and is sometimes accompanied by urticarial and bluish-red mottling and itching of the skin ("diver's lice").

**B. Type 2 Decompression Sickness:** Type 2 is more severe than type 1. Symptoms and signs of central and peripheral nerve damage may include vertigo, "pins and needles" paresthesias, hypesthesia, ataxic gait, hyperreflexia, Babinski's sign, paralysis or weakness of the limbs, headache, seizures, vomiting, visual loss or visual field defects, incontinence, impaired speech, tremor, and coma. Pulmonary manifestations ("the chokes") may include substernal pain, chest tightness, severe coughing, dyspnea, pulmonary edema, and shallow respirations. Cardiovascular findings include arrhythmia and hypertension.

Type 2 sickness, which is probably caused by gas bubbles in the central nervous system and spinal cord, may have significant sequelae, such as vascular obstruction and tissue infarction, which are sometimes accompanied by hemoconcentration, changes in osmotic pressure, or lipid emboli; hemorrhagic infarcts of the lungs; ulcers of the colon; multifocal degeneration of white matter; and hypercoagulation of blood.

Pulmonary barotrauma and gas expansion in other tissues can cause arterial gas embolism, which is the second leading cause of death in divers (drowning is first).

**C. Type 3 Decompression Sickness:** The third type is characterized by aseptic necrosis of bone (osteonecrosis), which frequently involves the head or shaft of the humerus and less often the lower end of the femur and the tibial head. Osteonecrosis usually occurs 6–60 months following decompression and is asymptomatic unless there is joint involvement, which can cause permanent impairment. X-ray examination may show bone sclerosis and mottling. Lesions are often symmetric.

Osteonecrosis may be the result of nitrogen bubbles obstructing the capillaries and has been reported in up to 50% of divers and underwater workers, although disability occurs in fewer than 3%.

An increased incidence of memory deficits, retrograde amnesia, emotional instability, and other neurologic and psychiatric symptoms has been observed in divers with a history of multiple episodes of decompression sickness.

### Prevention

Divers, underwater workers, and pilots should be screened to make sure they are in good physical condition—not overweight and with no other conditions imposing an increased risk for dysbarism, such as vascular disorders, hypercoagulopathy, obstructive airway disease, dehydration, or recent bone fractures. They and their crews should receive training and education in proper compression and decompression procedures and in recognizing symptoms and signs of decompression sickness.

### Treatment

**A. Types 1 and 2 Decompression Sickness:** The patient should be placed in a supine position or, if pulmonary or central nervous system symptoms are present, in Trendelenburg's position but tilted slightly to the left—theoretically, to reduce the risk of cerebral air embolism—at an angle of 10–15 degrees. For immediate first aid, 100% oxygen should be administered, and aspirin may be given for analgesia. The patient should be transported rapidly to an emergency facility that has a hyperbaric chamber for recompression and decompression. Information about the nearest

facility and advice about recompression can be obtained 24 hours a day by calling the National Diving Accident Network at (919) 684-8111.

In the hyperbaric chamber, the patient is placed in an atmosphere of raised pressure. The pressure is then reduced at a slow rate, with decompression pressures and schedules determined on the basis of the duration and pressure exposure of the inciting incident. Breathing 100% oxygen by mask alternating with breathing normal air should shorten the period of decompression. Some centers use oxygen-helium mixtures as an alternative to protocols requiring 100% oxygen in an effort to speed decompression without causing oxygen toxicity.

Corticosteroids, diuretics, or both can be used for cerebral or spinal edema. Volume depletion should be corrected with oral or parenteral fluids. In severe cases, anticoagulation with heparin or plasma volume expansion with low-molecular-weight dextran 40 has been effective. Diazepam has been used for treatment of confusional states and oxygen toxicity if oxygen is administered during treatment.

In cases of type 2 sickness, decompression may take several days. To prevent reemergence of symptoms, the patient should breathe air for 30 minutes and then breathe oxygen for 30 minutes and continue this procedure for up to 8 hours after decompression. Careful monitoring should be maintained to guard against oxygen toxicity of the lungs and central nervous system.

**B. Type 3 Decompression Sickness:** Osteonecrosis and sequelae due to chronic decompression sickness are treated in the same manner as these conditions due to other causes.

## COMPRESSION SICKNESS

When atmospheric pressure is increased, internal gases become compressed, usually with little effect. The only common form of compression sickness is barotitis. This can occur with descent of an aircraft from a high altitude, which causes a relative vacuum in the middle ear space if the auditory tube is already obstructed due to allergies or upper respiratory tract infection. Symptoms may include pain or a foggy feeling in the ears, dizziness, nausea, and vertigo. In more severe cases, the tympanic membrane may appear inflamed and retracted or ruptured.

Barotitis can be prevented in people at risk by avoiding high-pressure exposures or, for short exposures, by using decongestants. Barotitis is usually self-limiting but can be treated with decongestant nose drops, a nasal vasoconstrictor inhaler, or use of Valsalva's maneuver.

Types 1 and 2 decompression sickness also can occur with unpressurized descent from high altitude. Severity depends on the initial altitude and the rate of descent.

# DISORDERS DUE TO VIBRATION

Vibration occurs when mechanical energy from an oscillating source is transmitted to another structure. Every structure has its own natural vibration level, including the human body as a whole and each of its parts. When vibration of the same frequency is applied, resonance (amplification) of that vibration occurs, often with adverse effects. For example, at a frequency of 5 Hz, whole-body resonance occurs, and the body acts in concert with externally generated vibration and amplifies that effect.

## EFFECTS OF WHOLE-BODY VIBRATION

In the United States, approximately 7 million workers operate vehicles that expose them to the back-and-forth motion of whole-body vibration and place them at risk for associated injuries. Truck and bus drivers, heavy-equipment operators, miners, and others exposed to long-term whole-body vibration have been reported to have a higher incidence of musculoskeletal, neurologic, circulatory, and digestive system disorders than the general population. Low back pain, intervertebral disk damage, and spinal degeneration have been found frequently. European studies have found associated bony abnormalities (intervertebral osteochondrosis and calcification of intervertebral disks) and adverse reproductive effects (spontaneous abortion, congenital malformations, and menstrual changes). "Vibration sickness," characterized by gastrointestinal problems, decreased visual acuity, labyrinthine disorders, and intense musculoskeletal pain, has also been reported in these workers. Despite these reports, a relationship between exposure intensity or quantity and the disorders found in occupationally exposed groups has not been clearly defined. Although many questions remain unanswered regarding the effects of long-term whole-body vibration exposure, neurologic and spinal effects appear likely.

Although almost all clinical and experimental effects of whole-body vibration have occurred at frequencies less than 20 Hz, they have also been reported to occur at frequencies as high as 100 Hz, depending on other factors such as the amplitude, acceleration, duration, and direction (vertical or lateral) of the vibrating force. The International Organization for Standardization (ISO) has established guidelines for whole-body vertical vibration exposure times to various frequencies and accelerations, as shown in Figure 6–10 and discussed in Chapter 6 (ISO 2631, 1985). Not all investigators agree with existing exposure standards because of the many inconsistencies in the literature; however, prudence suggests that employers should try to minimize whole-body vibration exposures of their employees whenever possible by limiting the duration of exposure and choosing well-designed equipment that insulates workers from vibration.

## VIBRATION-INDUCED WHITEFINGER DISEASE (Hand Arm Vibration Syndrome—HAVS)

Vibration-induced whitefinger disease (HAVS) is the most common example of an occupational injury due to segmental vibration of the hands. In the United States, more than 1 million workers are estimated to have significant exposure to vibration from hand tools such as power saws, grinders, sanders, pneumatic drills, jackhammers, and other equipment used in construction, foundry work, machining, and mining. Although segmental vibration injury can occur with frequencies ranging from 5 to 1500 Hz, it usually occurs with frequencies of 125–300 Hz. Other factors affecting risk include the amplitude and acceleration of the equipment used and the duration of use. Cumulative trauma most often occurs with a work history of at least 2000 hours of exposure and usually over 8000 hours.

HAVS is characterized by spasms of the digital arteries (Raynaud's phenomenon) caused by vibration-induced damage of the peripheral nerve and vascular tissue, subcutaneous tissue, bones, and joints of the hands and fingers. The pathologic process may also involve arterial muscle wall hypertrophy; demyelinating peripheral neuropathy; excess connective tissue deposition in perivascular, perineural, and subcutaneous tissues; and microvascular occlusion. Attacks of vasospasm can last for minutes to hours and are more likely to occur with exposure to the cold and with strenuous physical exertion. The worker is often standing erect, with the hand held lower than the heart and maintained in a contracted position.

### Clinical Findings

Attacks in severe cases can last 15–60 minutes or as long as 2 hours. They are usually easily reversible if the individual is removed from vibration exposure. Early symptoms consist of tingling followed by numbness of the fingers. The fingers later begin to turn white in a cold environment or when cold objects are touched. Intermittent blanching often starts with the tip of one finger but progressively extends to other fingertips and eventually to the tips and bases of all fingers on the exposed hands. With increasing severity of disease, blanching or cyanosis of the fingers may extend into the summer season. Return of blood circulation (reactive hyperemia, or "red flush") following each episode is accompanied by redness and swelling, acute pain, throbbing, and paresthesias.

In more advanced cases, there may be degeneration of bone and cartilage, with resulting joint stiffness, restriction of motion, and arthralgia. Manual dexterity may decrease and clumsiness increase. With greater intensities of vibration, the period between exposure to vibration and the appearance of "whitefinger" is shorter.

Diagnosis is based on exposure history and response to cold. Specific diagnostic tests can include finger systolic pressure response to cold stress, finger temperature response to cold, vibrotactile sensitivity and perception threshold measurements, and other tests of localized vascular and neurologic function.

Diagnostic staging is based on the Stockhold Workshop Scales (1987), which consider both vascular and neurologic effects (Table 12–13).

### Differential Diagnosis

The diagnosis of HAVS is based on the occupational history of vibration exposures, the association of these exposures with episodes of Raynaud's phenomenon (digital vasospasms), and the exclusion of idiopathic Raynaud's disease and other causes of Raynaud's phenomenon, including trauma of the fingers and hands, frostbite, occlusive vascular disease, connective tissue disorders, neurogenic disorders, drug intoxication, and exposure to vinyl chloride monomer.

### Prevention

Segmental vibration can be prevented by using well-designed tools (Chapter 6), wearing gloves to minimize vibration and keep the hands warm, and following a work-rest schedule that prevents long periods of exposure to vibration. Workers should be instructed about the early symptoms and signs of HAVS and advised of factors that may place them at higher risk, such as the use of vasoactive drugs and cigarette smoking. Exposure limits developed by the

ACGIH rely on measurements of acceleration (of the tool) in each of three directional axes.

### Treatment

In most cases, symptoms and signs disappear when the worker is removed from exposure to vibration. In other cases, attacks can be reduced in severity or stopped by massaging, shaking, or swinging the hands or by placing them in warm water or warm air.

For more intractable episodes, nifedipine, 30–40 mg/d, is effective; thymoxamine is an alternative. For more severe cases, stanozolol or prostaglandin E may be useful. Biofeedback training has also been suggested. Surgical sympathectomy may be considered for irreversible cases. For medical or surgical therapy, the patient should be referred to the appropriate vascular specialist or hand surgeon.

## HIGH-PRESSURE INJECTION INJURIES

Use of pressurized tools and systems in manufacturing and service industries occasionally results in severe injection injury. Common types of materials injected include hydraulic fluid, paint and paint thinner, grease, and fuel. The nondominant hand is the most common injury location, but other sites such as the orbit have been reported.

### Pathogenesis

The extent of injury is determined by the type and amount of material injected, the anatomic location, and the velocity of injection. As an example of the effect of material type, paint and paint thinners often incite a large inflammatory response on a chemical basis and also have antibacterial properties. The amount of material injected determines the amount of localized tissue distention, which in turn determines the extent of vascular compromise. The site and velocity of injection affect the dispersion of the mate-

**Table 12–13.** Stockholm Workshop HAVS classification system for cold-induced peripheral vascular and sensorineural symptoms.[1]

| Stage[2] | Vascular Assessment | |
| | Grade | Description |
|---|---|---|
| 0 | — | No attacks |
| 1 | Mild | Occasional attacks affecting only the tips of one or more fingers |
| 2 | Moderate | Occasional attacks affecting distal and middle (rarely also proximal) phalanges of one or more fingers |
| 3 | Severe | Frequent attacks affecting all phalanges of most fingers |
| 4 | Very severe | As in stage 3, with trophic skin changes in the fingertips |

[1]Reproduced, with permission, from *American Conference of Governmental Industrial Hygienists TLV Booklet,* 1994–1995.
[2]Separate staging is made for each hand, eg, 2L(2)/1R(1) = stage 2 on left hand in two fingers: stage 1 on right hand in one finger.

rial injected along tissue layers as well as tissue penetration.

Pathologic response occurs in three stages. The first stage involves acute inflammation associated with vascular compromise as a result of tissue distention. Gangrene and/or infection often complicates the first stage. The second stage involves chemically induced inflammation and foreign body granuloma formation. The late stage involves tissue fibrosis and breakdown of skin overlying granulomas, resulting in ulceration and subcutaneous sinus formation.

## Clinical Findings

With the initial event, the patient may feel a momentary stinging sensation; numbness and swelling are the initial symptoms. In fact, the initial appearance of the injury often does not reflect the severity of the injury. Also present will be a small puncture wound, from which some of the injected material may be oozing. Pressure exerted around the puncture may increase the amount of oozing.

Within a few hours, throbbing pain and pallor or cyanosis may develop. The pain is sometimes described as a burning sensation.

Patients who do not seek immediate evaluation may present hours to several days later with leukocytosis and evidence of lymphangitis. Laboratory tests include x-ray for evidence of radiopaque materials such as metals or xeroradiography for grease. CT scanning has been used to demonstrate localized edema, gas pockets, and globe distortion involved in orbital injection injuries.

## Treatment

The goal of treatment is preservation of neurovascular structures. Aggressive decompression, debridement, and irrigation are recommended. Incision and debridement of devitalized tissues and removal of as much of the injected material should be done as soon as possible. Open debridement of all contaminated structures including tendon sheaths is recommended. Amputation may be required and is most frequent in injections involving paint or solvents. Pulsed-lavage irrigation, drainage, and open packing techniques have been used successfully. Delayed wound closure or closure by secondary intention is recommended.

Broad-spectrum antibiotic and tetanus prophylaxis, if indicated, should be provided. Early range-of-motion and intense physical therapy should be provided; twice-daily hand soaks in povidone-iodine and daily whirlpool treatments have been used successfully.

Initially, analgesics will be required, but local digital blocks should be avoided because of the risk of further vascular compromise. The value of steroid or dextran use has not been demonstrated for injection injuries, with the possible exception of steroids for high-pressure orbital injections, for which surgical debridement is more difficult or may not be appropriate.

## REFERENCES

### HYPOTHERMIA
### (Cold Injury)

Alaska Med 1993;35:4. [Entire issue.]

Danzl DF, Pozos RS: *Accidental Hypothermia,* N Engl J Med, 1994;331:1757.

Gentilello LM: *Advances in the Management of Hypothermia.* Surg Clin North Am, 1995;75:243.

Pulla RJ, Pickard LJ, Carnett TS: Frostbite: An overview with case presentations. J Foot Ankle Surg 1994;33:53.

Spittell JA Jr, Spittell PC: Chronic pernio: Another cause of blue toes. Int Angio 1992;11:46.

Weinberg AD: Hypothermia. Ann Emerg Med, 1993;22:370.

Wrenn K: Immersion foot—A problem of the homeless in the 1990s. Arch Intern Med 1991;151:785.

### DISORDERS DUE TO HEAT

Bross MH, Nash BT, Carlton FB Jr: Practical therapeutics—Heat emergencies. Am Fam Physician 1994;50:389.

Dessureault PC et al: Heat strain assessment for workers using an encapsulating garment and a self-contained breathing apparatus. Appl Occup Environ Hyg 1995;10:200.

Tek D, Olshaker JS: Heat illness. Emerg Med Clin North Am 1992;10:299.

*TLVs: Threshold Limit Values and Biological Exposure Indices for 1994–1995.* American Conference of Governmental Industrial Hygienists, pp 84–90.

Tom PA, Garmel GM, Auerbach PS: Environment-dependent sports emergencies. Med Clin North Am 1994;78:305.

### THERMAL BURNS

Fuller FW, Parish M, Nance FC: A review of the dosimetry of 1% silver sulfadiazine cream in burn wound treatment. J Burn Care Rehabil 1994;15:213.

Herndon DN, Zeigler ST: Bacterial translocation after thermal injury. Crit Care Med 1993;Feb; 21(2 suppl):550.

Hollinsed TC et al: Etiology and consequences of respiratory failure in thermally injured patients. Am J Surg 1993;166:592.

Milner SM et al: The Burns Calculator: a simple proposed guide for fluid resuscitation. Lancet 1993;342:1089.

Saffle JR et al: Multiple organ failure in patients with

thermal injury. Crit Care Med 1993; Nov; 21(11): 1673.

## ELECTRICAL INJURIES

Fish R: Electric shock. Part I: Physics and pathophysiology. J Emerg Med 1993;11:309.

Fish R: Electric shock. Part II: Nature and mechanisms of injury. J Emerg Med 1993;11:457.

Fontanarosa PB: Electrical shock and lightning strike. Ann Emerg Med 1993;22:378.

*Neurologic, Behavioral, Ophthalmologic and Related Aspects of Lightning and Electroshock Injuries.* Semin Neurol 1995;15(3–4):227–400.

## NONIONIZING RADIATION INJURIES

IEEE (ANSI): *Standard for Safety Levels with Respect to Human Exposure to Radio Frequency Electromagnetic Fields, 3 kHz to 300 Ghz,* C95.1-1991.

*Possible Health Effects of Exposure to Residential Electric and Magnetic Fields,* National Research Council, National Academy Press, Washington, DC, 1996.

Taylor HR et al: The long-term effects of visible light on the eye. Arch Ophthalmol 1992;110:99.

*TLVs and BEIs: Threshold Limit Values for Chemical Substances and Physical Agents. Biological Exposure Indices.* American Conference of Governmental Industrial Hygienists, 1996.

Yost MG: Occupational health effects of nonionizing radiation. Occup Med State of the Art Rev 1992;7:543.

Zigman S: Ocular light damage. Photochem Photobiol 1993;57:1060.

## IONIZING RADIATION INJURIES

Gale RP, Butturini A: Medical response to nuclear and radiation accidents. Occup Med State of the Art Rev 1991;6:581.

*Health Effects of Exposure to Low Levels of Ionizing Radiation: Beir V.* National Academy Press, Washington, DC, 1990.

IARC: Direct estimates of cancer mortality due to low doses of ionizing radiation: an international study. Lancet 1994;344:1039.

Limitation of Exposure to Ionizing Radiation: NCRP Report No. 116, National Council on Radiation Protection and Measurements, 1993.

Nussbaum RH, Kohnlein W: Inconsistencies and open questions regarding low-dose health effects of ionizing radiation. Environ Health Perspect 1994;102:656.

Shapiro J: *Radiation Protection: A Guide for Scientists and Physicians,* 3rd ed. Harvard University Press, 1991.

Vyas DR et al: Management of radiation accidents and exposures. Pediatr Emerg Care 1994;10:232.

## LASER INJURIES

*American National Standard for the Safe Use of Lasers.* ANSI No. Z136.1-1993. American National Standards Institute, 1993.

## ATMOSPHERIC PRESSURE DISORDERS (Dysbarism)

James PB: Dysbarism: The medical problems from high and low atmospheric pressure. J R Coll Physicians Lond 1993;27:1031.

Jerrard DA: Diving medicine. Emerg Med Clin North Am 1992;10:329.

Melamed Y et al: Medical problems associated with underwater diving. N Engl J Med 1992;326:30.

## DISORDERS DUE TO VIBRATION

Griffin NJ: *Measurement, Evaluation, and Assessment of Occupational Exposures to Hand-Transmitted Vibration.* Occup Environ Med 1997;54:73.

Pelmear PL, Taylor W: Hand-arm vibration syndrome: A clinical evaluation and prevention. J Occup Med 1991;33:1144.

Seidel H: Selected health risks caused by long-term, whole-body vibration. Am J Ind Med 1993;23:589.

*TLVs and BEIs: Threshold Limit Values for Chemical Substances and Physical Agents. Biological Exposure Indices.* American Conference of Governmental Industrial Hygienists, 1996, pp. 85–88.

## HIGH-PRESSURE INJECTION INJURIES

Hold JB et al: Hydraulic orbital injection injuries. Ophthalmology 1993;100:1475.

Pinto MR et al: High pressure injectin injuries of the hand: Review of twenty-five patients managed by open wound technique. J Hand Surg 1993;18A:125.

Proust AF: Special injuries of the hand. Emerg Med Clin North Am 1993;11:767.

# Section III.
# Occupational Illnesses

# Clinical Toxicology

# 13

*Jon Rosenberg, MD*

Toxicology is the study of physical and chemical agents and the injury they cause to living cells. All substances are potentially toxic. One of the objectives of clinical and experimental studies in toxicology is to define the capacity of substances to produce harmful effects (ie, toxicity), measure and analyze the doses at which toxicity occurs (ie, the dose-response relationship), and assess the probability that injury or illness will occur under specified conditions of use (ie, hazard and risk assessment).

A distinction is made between toxicity and hazard. An extremely toxic chemical that is in a sealed container on a shelf has inherent toxicity but presents little or no hazard. When the chemical is removed from the shelf and used by a worker in a closed space and without appropriate protection, the hazard becomes great. Thus, the manner of use affects how hazardous the substance will be in the workplace.

## TOXIC AGENTS & THEIR EFFECTS

### Classification of Toxic Agents

Toxic agents can be classified or described in terms of the following:

**A. Physical State of the Agent:** The different physical states of toxic agents, with some examples of each, are shown in Table 13–1. A metal such as lead may be harmless in solid form, moderately toxic as a dust, and extremely toxic as a fume.

**B. Chemical Structure of the Agent:** Chemical structure can determine toxicity. Often one but not another isomer of a compound possesses toxicity. For example, aromatic amines are carcinogenic when substituted in other than the para- positions. The stability of a substance and the presence of impurities, contaminants, or additives can also affect toxicity.

**C. Medium of the Agent:** The medium in which a toxic substance is found in part determines the population exposed and thus to some extent the hazard. Some toxic substances occur in a specific medium—eg, oxides of nitrogen in air (from vehicular exhaust), trihalomethanes in water (from chlorination), and nitrosamines in food (from nitrites). In the

United States, several governmental agencies, including the Environmental Protection Agency (EPA), Food and Drug Administration (FDA), and Occupational Safety and Health Administration (OSHA), have developed regulations regarding exposure to toxic substances in various media.

**D. Site of Injury by the Agent:** Toxic agents can be described in terms of their effects on target organs (hepatotoxins, nephrotoxins, etc).

**E. Mechanism of Action of the Agent:** Toxic agents are frequently categorized on the basis of their mechanism of action. Asphyxiants, for example, deprive tissues of oxygen. Simple asphyxiants (inert gases) act by diluting or displacing oxygen without causing other toxic effects. In contrast, chemical asphyxiants such as cyanide and carbon monoxide actively interfere with the delivery or utilization of oxygen—cyanide by inhibiting cytochrome oxidase and other enzymes necessary for cellular utilization of oxygen, and carbon monoxide by combining with hemoglobin to form carboxyhemoglobin, which decreases the oxygen-carrying capacity of the blood and inhibits release of oxygen to tissues.

**F. Clinical Effects of the Agent:**

**1. Onset of effects**–Toxic effects can be immediate, as occurs with some irritants that cause direct damage to tissues at the point of initial contact, usually resulting in inflammation; or delayed, as with chemical carcinogens.

**2. Reversibility of effects**–Whether or not the toxic effects of a substance are reversible depends on the capacity of damaged cells to regenerate or recover. For instance, brain and other nervous system cells have little capacity to regenerate, whereas liver and muscle cells are more likely to regenerate or recover after injury.

### Factors Affecting Clinical Response to a Toxic Agent

The following factors affect the dose-response relationship and the clinical response of humans to a toxic agent:

**A. Duration, Frequency, and Route of Exposure:** The severity of injury is usually related to the

**Table 13–1.** Physical states of toxic substances.

**Particulates**
  Dusts
    Nuisance
      Calcium carbonate
      Cellulose (paper fiber)
      Portland cement
      Silicon
    Fibrogenic
      Silica
      Coal dust
    Fibers
      Asbestos
      Mineral wool
    Fumes
      Metal
      Polymer (polytetrafluoroethylene decomposition
        products)
**Gases and vapors**
  Butane, methyl bromide, ethylene oxide (gas)
  Hexane, trichloroethylene, benzene (vapor)
**Liquids**
  Elemental mercury
**Solids**
  Plastics

duration and frequency of exposure. The route of exposure often determines toxicity. For example, ethylene glycol is toxic when ingested but poses little threat in the workplace except when sprayed or heated.

**B. Environmental Factors:** Toxicity is affected by atmospheric pressure, temperature, and humidity. For example, a concentration of carbon monoxide that has little effect at sea level can cause impairment of work capacity at an altitude of 5000 ft. Chemicals are more readily absorbed through skin that is injured or wet with perspiration and has increased blood flow in response to heat and humidity.

**C. Individual Factors:** Individual factors that determine "susceptibility" include racial and genetic background, age and maturity, sex, body weight, nutrition, life-style, immunologic and hormonal status, and presence of disease or stress. These factors are not independent of one another. For instance, genetic factors determine many of the other factors, and poor nutrition can affect immunologic status.

While much concern about the effect of age on individual susceptibility has focused on the fetus, the elderly also metabolize many chemicals less efficiently. As the work force ages, this may become an increasing concern.

The effect of nutritional deficiency on susceptibility to toxic agents has been of concern in developed countries primarily during war or famine, but it is relevant in developing countries as they industrialize. While toxicologic studies in animals readily demonstrate the effects of nutritional deficiency on susceptibility, the results of these studies are difficult to extrapolate to humans. The role of vitamins and minerals in chemical toxicity has been much debated.

There is controversy about the role of genetic factors and the development and use of genetic screening tests to identify individuals with increased susceptibility to toxic agents in the workplace. It is questioned whether such tests are accurate and whether job discrimination could result from their use as preemployment screening. Among the many genetic traits that might increase the risk of toxicity from exposure to chemicals or radiation, the most visible have been glucose-6-phosphate dehydrogenase (G6PD) deficiency, sickle cell anemia, and $\alpha_1$-antitrypsin deficiency.

G6PD deficiency is an X-linked recessive disorder that primarily affects American black males and Mediterranean Jews. Affected individuals are susceptible to hemolysis from many drugs. Although some chemicals—notably naphthalene and arsine—can cause hemolysis following overexposure, there is no evidence that workers exposed to workplace-acceptable concentrations of these chemicals are at increased risk. Screening for G6PD deficiency is thus not supported by solid evidence.

Similarly, there is no evidence that any of the 7–13% of American blacks with sickle cell trait are at increased risk of hypoxia when working as airplane pilots or of hemolysis when working with hemolytic agents, despite the fact that these "risks" have been cited to justify screening of individuals for these occupations.

Severe $\alpha_1$-antitrypsin deficiency, when present in the rare homozygous condition, can lead to early emphysema in the absence of environmental agents. The more common heterozygous condition, which affects 4–9% of the US population, may in combination with other factors place affected individuals at increased risk of developing emphysema from exposure to environmental agents.

## TOXICOKINETICS & TOXICODYNAMICS

Toxicokinetics is the study of the movement of toxic substances within the body (ie, their absorption, distribution, metabolism, and excretion) and the relationship between the dose that enters the body and the level of toxic substance found in the blood or other biologic sample. Toxicodynamics is the study of the relationship between the dose that enters the body and the measured response. The magnitude of a toxic response is usually related to the concentration of the toxic substance at its site of action.

### Bioavailability

The bioavailability of a toxic substance indicates the extent to which the agent reaches its site of action. If it is not in a "bioavailable form," as is the case with many orally ingested toxic substances that cause vomiting or diarrhea, it will be promptly removed. In other cases, some of the agent will be inactivated before it reaches the site of action. For example, when cyanide is taken orally, it is absorbed and passes to the liver, where the enzyme rhodanese may metabolize a portion of the ingested cyanide. On the other hand, if the cyanide in the form of gaseous hydrocyanic acid (HCN) is absorbed through the pulmonary circulation, it goes directly to the brain, where it may cause damage due to hypoxia.

## Cell Membrane Permeability & Cellular Barriers

Absorption, distribution, metabolism, and excretion all involve passage of toxic agents across cell membranes. Permeability is dependent upon a toxic substance's molecular size and shape, solubility at the site of absorption, degree of ionization, and relative lipid solubility.

The distribution of some toxic agents is altered by unique cellular barriers, eg, the blood-brain barrier, the blood-testis barrier, and the placenta, which may exclude toxic substances.

Many lipid-soluble toxic substances are stored in body fat. In an obese person with a fat content of 30–40%, this may form a stable reservoir for toxic substances, which may then be released slowly.

Bone is an important deep reservoir for many heavy metals (especially lead) and for radioactive materials, and the effects of these materials can persist long after they have left the circulation.

## Absorption

The rate of absorption is dependent on the concentration and solubility of the toxic agent. Agents in aqueous solution are absorbed more rapidly than those in oily suspension. Absorption is enhanced at sites that have increased blood flow or large absorptive surfaces (eg, the adult lung and gastrointestinal tract, whose surfaces are the size of a tennis court and a football field, respectively).

**A. Gastrointestinal Absorption:** The amount of absorption through the gastrointestinal tract is usually proportionate to the gastrointestinal surface area and its blood flow and depends on the physical state of the agent. Most toxic substances are absorbed in the small intestine. Therefore, agents that accelerate gastric emptying will increase the absorption rate, while factors that delay gastric emptying will decrease it. Some toxic substances may be affected by gastric juice; eg, the acidity of the stomach may release cyanide products and form hydrogen cyanide gas, which is even more toxic than the cyanide salt.

**B. Pulmonary Absorption:** The most common route of occupational exposure is pulmonary absorption. Gaseous and volatile toxic substances may be inhaled and absorbed through the pulmonary epithelium and mucous membranes in the respiratory tract. Access to the circulation is rapid because the surface area of the lungs is large and the blood flow is great.

The nasal hair, the cough reflex, and the mucociliary barrier help prevent dust particles and fumes from reaching the lung.

The solubility of gases affects their absorption. Highly water-soluble gases such as ammonia and sulfuric acid are absorbed in the upper airways and cause marked irritation there. This serves as a warning and limits the injury to the lung. Noxious gases of low water solubility such as nitrogen dioxide and phosgene, which have few early warning properties, reach the lungs and cause delayed injury there.

**C. Percutaneous Absorption:** Many toxic substances pass through the skin, intact or broken. The amount of skin absorption is generally proportionate to the surface area of contact and to the lipid solubility of the toxic agent. The epidermis acts as a lipid barrier, and the stratum corneum provides a protective barrier against noxious agents. The dermis, however, is freely permeable to many toxic substances.

Absorption is enhanced by toxic agents that increase the blood flow to the skin. It is also enhanced by use of occlusive skin coverings (eg, permeable clothes and industrial gloves) and topical application of fat-solubilizing vehicles. Hydrated skin is more permeable than dry skin. The thick skin on the palms of the hands and the soles of the feet is more resistant to absorption than is the thin skin on the face, neck, and scrotum. Burns, abrasions, dermatitis, and other injuries to the skin may alter its protective properties and allow absorption of larger quantities of the toxic substance.

**D. Ocular Absorption:** The eye is also a ready site of absorption. When chemicals enter the body through the conjunctiva, they bypass hepatic elimination and may cause severe systemic toxicity. This may occur when organophosphate pesticides are splashed into the eyes.

## Distribution

Toxic substances are transported via the blood to various portions of the body. Some are removed by the lymph, and some insoluble compounds are transported through tissues such as the lung via cells such as macrophages. Most toxic substances enter the bloodstream and are distributed into interstitial and cellular fluids. The pattern of distribution depends on the physiologic and physicochemical properties of the material. The initial phase of distribution usually reflects the cardiac output and regional blood flow. Lipid-soluble agents that penetrate membranes poorly are restricted in their distribution, and their potential sites of action are therefore limited. Exceptions are the blood-brain and blood-testis barriers, which limit the distribution of water-soluble but not lipid-soluble chemicals to these organs. Distribution may also be limited by the binding of toxic substances to plasma proteins. Toxic agents can accumulate in higher concentration in some tissues as a result of pH gradients, binding to special cellular proteins, or partitioning into lipids. Some agents accumulate in tissue reservoirs, and this may serve to prolong the toxic action, eg, lead may be stored for years in bone and may be released later.

## Metabolism

Toxic substances that are lipid-soluble may go through a series of metabolic conversions (biotransformation) to produce more polar (water-soluble) products and thereby enhance removal by urinary excretion. The most common site for biotransformation is the liver, but it can also occur in plasma, lung, or other tissue. Biotransformation may result in either a decrease (detoxification or inactivation) or an increase (activation) in the toxicity of a compound. Differences in the metabolism of toxic substances account for much of the observed differences between individuals and between animal species.

Biotransformation occurs in the liver by hydrolysis, oxidation, reduction, and conjugation. Microsomal enzymes play a key role in the process, and the activity of the microsomal enzyme system can be increased (induced) by many environmental and pharmacologic agents. Both normal individual differences in microsomal enzyme activity and susceptibility to induction are genetically determined and account for the marked variability in bioavailability of many toxic substances. Other factors that regulate key liver enzyme systems are hormones (which account for some sex-dependent differences) and disease states (eg, the presence of hepatitis, cirrhosis, or heart failure). Because the activity of many hepatic metabolizing systems is low in neonates—particularly premature neonates—they may be much more susceptible to toxic substances that are inactivated by liver metabolism. Inefficient metabolizing systems, an altered blood-brain barrier, and inadequate mechanisms of excretion combine to make the fetus and neonate sensitive to the toxic effects of many agents.

## Excretion

### A. Pathways and Mechanisms of Excretion:
Toxic substances are excreted either unchanged or as metabolites. Excretory organs other than the lungs eliminate polar (water-soluble) compounds more efficiently than they eliminate nonpolar (lipidsoluble) compounds. As discussed above, the latter must be metabolized to more polar compounds before they can be eliminated renally. The kidney is the primary organ of elimination for most polar compounds and their metabolites. Excretion of toxic substances in the urine involves glomerular filtration, active secretion, and passive tubular reabsorption. Alkalization or acidification of the urine may dramatically change excretion of some agents. When tubular urine is more alkaline, weak acids are excreted more rapidly because they are ionized and passive tubular reabsorp-

tion is decreased. In contrast, when tubular urine is made more acid, excretion of weak acid is reduced.

Many toxic substances metabolized by the liver are excreted first in the bile and later eliminated in the stool or reabsorbed into the blood and ultimately eliminated in the urine. Toxic substances can also be excreted in sweat, saliva, and breast milk, and there may be some minor removal in hair or skin.

### B. Clearance:
Clearance is the rate at which a toxic agent is excreted, divided by the average concentration of the agent in the plasma. Most toxic substances are eliminated as a linear function of concentration, ie, a constant fraction of the toxic material is eliminated over time (per unit of time). If the point of saturation is reached, the body will no longer be able to eliminate a constant fraction of the material but will instead eliminate a constant amount per unit of time. Under these circumstances, the clearance becomes quite variable. Note that clearance is a measure not of how much is being removed but rather of the volume of fluid that is freed of the toxic agent per unit of time.

### C. Volume of Distribution:
The volume of distribution is calculated by dividing the dose of the toxic substance administered by the concentration in the blood. This volume is not necessarily a physiologic volume; it is merely an estimate of the degree of distribution of the toxic agent in tissues. The volume of distribution for most toxic agents depends largely on pH factors, protein binding, partition coefficients, and regional differences in blood flow and binding to special tissues.

### D. Half-Time and Half-Life:
The time it takes for the plasma concentration of a substance to be reduced by 50% is the half-time. For substances that are eliminated as a linear function (ie, independent of concentration), the time it takes to eliminate 50% of the substance is the half-life. Calculation of half-life provides a means of estimating the dose that was absorbed. For a substance eliminated in linear fashion, about 90% of the amount in the body will be eliminated in 3.5 half-lives after the end of the period of exposure.

## TESTS OF TOXIC EFFECTS

Much of our information about the toxic effects of different agents comes from studying various strains and species of animals. Toxic substances frequently cause effects in animals, some immediately after administration and others after a prolonged period. Acute effects are sometimes qualitatively quite different from chronic effects. For example, the acute effect of benzene is central nervous system depression, while its chronic effects are aplastic anemia and leukemia.

Although tests in animals are the most common methods of identifying agents that cause toxicity, the results are difficult to extrapolate to humans, given the disparity among life spans (18–24 months for rodents versus 75 years for humans). In addition, different strains and species of animals may show both qualitative and quantitative differences in the pattern or intensity of response to a toxic agent. Even with the best statistical approaches and the best evidence of toxic responses in animals, there is no certain way of estimating the incidence of toxicity or determining the type of response to a toxic substance in a human population. Furthermore, there is no absolute certainty that safety factors for exposure to a toxic substance based on studies in animals would be valid for humans.

## Tests for Acute, Subacute, & Chronic Toxic Effects

Tests for acute effects are usually performed when there are no data available on the potential toxicity of a single exposure or a few exposures to a specific agent. An appropriate route of administration is chosen, and a specific end point (eg, death of the laboratory animal) is selected. The signs and symptoms before death are observed, and the animal is later examined for gross and histologic damage to tissues. In some cases, topical application of an agent is used to test for skin or eye injury.

Tests for subacute or sublethal effects of a specific agent are usually performed during a period of 21–90 days in animals, with the route of administration chosen on the basis of anticipated human exposure. Two different species of rodents are usually involved in each test.

Tests for chronic effects are performed in animals when long-term human exposure to a specific agent is anticipated or a long latency period between exposure and toxicity is expected. Rats and mice are usually exposed from a few weeks of age until their premature death or their sacrifice at the end of the expected lifetime. Short-term tests for genotoxicity, including mutagenicity, are used to prioritize agents for long-term testing or to provide supportive data for the results of long-term testing.

## Tests for Teratogenesis & Toxic Effects on Reproductive Organs

Teratologic tests involve exposing pregnant female animals to a specific agent at a critical time during pregnancy and then examining their offspring for malformations. Usually two or three species are used for comparison and controls. In reproductive studies, male and female animals are exposed to an agent and subsequently observed for reproductive failure or success. In cases of successful reproduction, the first- and second-generation offspring are also observed for their ability to reproduce. In cases of unsuccessful reproduction, male animals are often tested for sperm motility, count, and morphology.

## IDENTIFICATION OF THE MECHANISMS OF TOXICITY

The best approach to understanding the mechanisms of a toxic effect involves three essential considerations: (1) the time course of the concentration of the active forms of a toxic agent at its active sites, (2) the kinetics of interaction between the active forms of the toxic compound and its active sites, and (3) the kinetics of the sequence of events resulting from the interaction that occurs before toxicity has been manifested. These observations must then be validated against experimental evidence in animals or epidemiologic studies in humans.

A special task force on toxicologic assessment has suggested six questions whose answers would lead to the development of protocols that would effectively identify the mechanisms of toxicity: What is the manifestation of the toxicity? What element causes the toxicity? What factors govern the concentration of the toxic element at its active sites? What is the physical or chemical nature of the reaction of the toxic substance at its active sites? What subsequent events lead to the manifestation of toxicity? How can toxicity be modulated?

The answers to these six questions are not simple. For example, toxicologists are not certain about the significance of tumors in animal species in which the incidence of spontaneous liver tumor is high. It is important to understand whether toxic agents act without further biotransformation or by direct interaction with an essential cellular constituent that maintains the integrity of the cell. Even if the parent toxic substance does not cause injury, an active metabolite (eg, superoxide anion) may be detrimental to cell function.

The following types of research help identify the mechanisms of action of specific toxic agents: (1) studying the effects of a particular type of pretreatment on the toxin-metabolizing enzyme systems in various organs and tissues, (2) analyzing the effects of inhibitors or inducers on activation or detoxification pathways at potential sites of metabolism, (3) elucidating the nature of the substrate cell, (4) studying the influence of genetic and environmental factors that affect potential toxic target sites, (5) reviewing the age and sex differences in the enzymes and target systems affected by a given toxic agent, and (6) determining the manner in which a toxic effect can be modulated, eg, by alteration in diet or manipulation of hormones.

## TOXICOLOGIC RISK ASSESSMENT

### Steps in Risk Assessment

Risk assessment is the characterization of the potential adverse health effects of human exposure to hazardous substances. It can be divided into the following steps:

**Step 1. Hazard identification**–(a) Description of the population exposed to a substance (population at risk). (b) Determination of the adverse health effects that would be caused by that substance (eg, cancer and birth defects).

**Step 2. Dose-response assessment**–(a) Collection of epidemiologic and experimental dose-response data on the effects of the substance. (b) Identification of a "critical" dose-response relationship (discussed in detail below). (c) Quantitative expression of the dose-response relationship by mathematical extrapolation from high doses in animals to low doses in humans.

**Step 3. Exposure assessment**–Estimation of past, present, and future exposure levels of the population at risk and of actual doses received.

**Step 4. Risk characterization**–Estimation of the incidence of adverse health effects in the population predicted from the dose-response assessment (step 2) as applied to the exposure assessment (step 3).

## Uncertainties Inherent in Risk Assessment

There are a number of uncertainties inherent in risk assessment for toxic substances: (1) Human data are frequently lacking or are limited due to inability to detect low-incidence effects. Epidemiologic studies do not demonstrate causation or provide quantitative dose-response data, nor do they account for mixed and multiple exposures, a sufficient latency period for effects to be expressed, and differences between the populations studied. (2) Animal data are often of uncertain relevance to humans. A rational choice of the most appropriate species may not be possible. Toxicokinetic and toxicodynamic data are usually lacking. The route, frequency, and duration of exposure may be different from those of the human population. The doses are usually much higher, and the animals studied are genetically homogeneous and free of exposure to other toxic substances. (3) The mechanisms of action for effects are poorly understood. (4) The exposure of the population at risk may not be quantified, and calculation of doses may not be possible.

Because of these uncertainties, the practice of quantitative risk assessment is sometimes criticized for being "unscientific." However, since human exposure to toxic substances may result in medical and public health risks, risk assessment often provides the only basis for decisions on how to manage potential risks.

## Methods for Estimation of Risk

There are two basic methods for risk estimation, based on the presence or absence of a predicted threshold in the "critical" dose-response relationship identified in step 2.

**A. Threshold Method:** A threshold is generally assumed for all noncarcinogenic responses. Since human exposure is generally below the threshold for adverse effects in animals, estimated risk cannot be expressed as a numerical probability (eg, 1:1000). Risk is expressed instead as a safety factor. The safety factor is the ratio between the allowable daily intake (ADI) for humans and a threshold dose in animals.

An ADI is estimated by the steps outlined above. Following hazard identification (step 1), a "no-observed-adverse-effect level" (NOEL)—also called the "safe" level—is determined (step 2) from animal studies. Exposure assessment (step 3) is then performed. The NOEL in animals and the ADI in humans are converted into comparable doses (doses allowing for species differences and differences in route, frequency, and duration of exposure), and the NOEL is divided by the ADI to yield a safety factor (step 4). Calculations can also be made using the lowest dose that produced an effect, ie, the "minimum-observed-adverse-effect level" (MOEL), or "unsafe" level.

The size of the safety factor is an estimate of the probability of an effect occurring in the population, based on differences in sensitivity between an animal species and humans. A safety factor of 10 suggests human sensitivity 10 times that of animals. An additional factor of 10 (to yield 100) is used when there is human genetic variability and susceptibility due to other factors and exposures. An additional factor of 10 (to yield 1000) is used when the animal study was faulty in design or a NOEL was not determined and a MOEL was used instead.

**B. No-Threshold Method:** For carcinogens, the absence of a threshold is usually assumed, and quantitative risk estimation is controversial. Following hazard identification (step 1), step 2 consists of evaluating human epidemiologic studies and selecting the most appropriate animal study for extrapolation. This includes scrutiny of dose-response data for the tumor in a particular species, extrapolation from the high doses in the animal study to low doses in humans, and selection of a particular mathematic model. Depending on the model selected, resulting estimates of risk may differ by many orders of magnitude. Exposure assessment (step 3) is then performed. The risk to the population (step 4) is estimated by applying the dose-response model from step 2 to the doses calculated from exposure data in step 3. Several assumptions must be made to arrive at a single "best estimate" of risk or—more commonly—a range of estimates of risk.

## DOSE-RESPONSE CURVES

A dose-response relationship exists when changes in dose are followed by consistent changes in re-

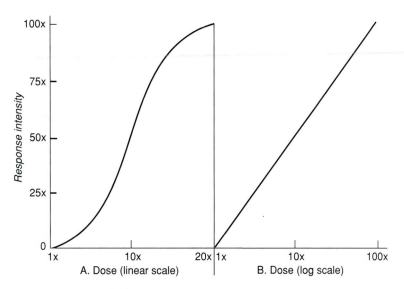

**Figure 13–1.** In these dose-response curves, A and B both show the intensity of the response to various doses in an individual. Because B uses a logarithmic scale, the curve is more linear.

sponse, as shown in dose-response curves. A variety of toxicologic phenomena can be demonstrated by these curves. Figure 13–1 shows the intensity of the response to various doses in an individual. Because Figure 13–1B is in a logarithmic scale, the shape of the curve is more linear. This makes it easier to determine values for specific points on the curve.

The frequency of a response in a population can be related to dose as a frequency distribution (as in Figure 13–2) or as a cumulative frequency (as in Figures 13–3 and 13–4).

In Figure 13–2, the existence of a threshold is indicated by the arrow at the point where the curve intersects the dose coordinate. Doses below this point do not produce a response. Individuals who exhibit the response at doses well below the average or the mean are considered hypersusceptible (H in Figure 13–2), while those who respond only to doses well above the average or the mean are considered resistant (R in Figure 13–2).

In Figure 13–3, cumulative frequency curves are used to compare two doses of the same toxic substance to the dose that is lethal to 50% of the population (LD50) and the dose that has an effect on 50% (ED50). The ED50 may, for example, represent an effect that is not harmful, such as odor. The ratio between comparable points on the curves (ie, the ratio of LD50 to ED50) will then represent the margin of safety for odor as a warning against the lethal effect.

In Figure 13–4, cumulative frequency curves are used to compare the doses at which the same toxic effect is elicited by 3 different toxic substances (A, B, and C). Substance A is clearly the most toxic, because at every dose level a greater percentage of the population exhibits the response to A than to B or C.

The LD50, the ED10, and the threshold for A are all lower than the corresponding values for B and C. The comparison between B and C is less clear and demonstrates the need to consider the entire dose-response curves rather than individual points when

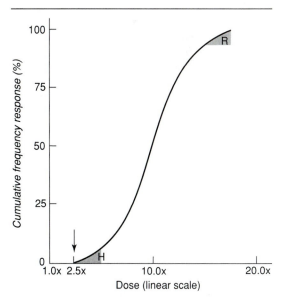

**Figure 13–2.** The existence of a threshold in this dose-response curve is indicated by the arrow. Doses below this point do not produce a response. Individuals who exhibit the response at doses well below the average or the mean are considered hypersusceptible (H), while those who respond only to doses well above the average or the mean are considered resistant (R).

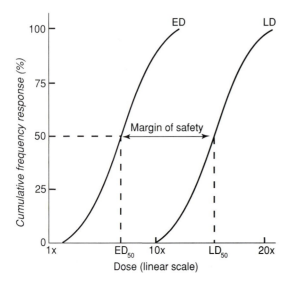

**Figure 13–3.** Dose-response curves comparing two doses of the same toxic substance. ED = effective dose; LD = lethal dose. The area between is the margin of safety.

comparing toxicities. Because the LD50 of B is lower than that of C, at this dose B is more toxic than C. However, because the ED10 of C is lower than that of B, at the lower dose C is more toxic than B. The shape of a dose-response curve is important for

assessing the hazard of a toxic substance. A substance that has a low threshold and shallow dose-response curve (such as C) may be more hazardous at low doses, while a substance that has a steep dose-response curve (such as B) may be more hazardous as the dose increases. Adequate assessment of the hazard of a toxic substance requires evaluation of dose-response data over a wide range of doses.

## DIAGNOSIS OF TOXIC EFFECTS

Different toxic substances often elicit similar clinical manifestations of toxicity. In some cases, the manifestations represent a response to more than one toxic agent or to a combination of toxic agents and naturally occurring causes. In general, the manifestations of acute toxicity due to high-dose exposures will be more specific than those of chronic toxicity or toxicity due to low-dose exposures.

For example, patients with acute poisoning caused by a high-dose exposure to organophosphate pesticides may present with involvement of the autonomic nervous system (nausea, vomiting, diarrhea, increased lacrimation and sweating, bronchorrhea, bronchoconstriction, blurred vision, small pupils, and bradycardia), the neuromuscular system (fasciculations, cramps, weakness, and hyporeflexia), and the central nervous system (confusion, hallucinations, and depressed consciousness). The presence of small

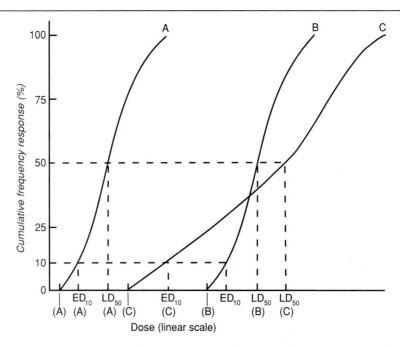

**Figure 13–4.** Dose–response curves comparing the doses at which the same toxic effect is elicited by three different toxic substances (A, B, and C).

pupils with the rest of these findings is diagnostic of organophosphate poisoning. Cholinesterase activity in blood or plasma is likely to be extremely low, confirming the diagnosis. The poisoning is likely to be accompanied by a clear history of overexposure, such as that caused by exposure to a leak or spill from pesticide spraying equipment or by deliberate or accidental ingestion. In contrast, patients with chronic or low-level exposures to organophosphate pesticides usually have poorly defined clinical manifestations, such as mild diarrhea, sweating, myalgias, and malaise (findings that are virtually indistinguishable from those of influenza), and cholinesterase activity levels may be normal. ("Toxidromes" for other substances are discussed under Clinical Findings in subsequent chapters.)

In some cases, the manifestations of toxicity due to high-dose exposure are totally different from those due to low-dose exposure. For example, benzidine causes methemoglobinemia at high doses and bladder cancer at low doses. There are relatively few compounds that cause methemoglobinemia, and most cases can be attributed to a specific toxic substance in the workplace or the environment. However, bladder cancer has a number of known causes in addition to exposure to benzidine, and this makes it difficult to attribute bladder cancer to low-dose toxic exposure. With chronic exposure to low doses, toxic agents are more likely to cause an increase in the incidence of disorders already present in the population than they are to cause a novel disorder.

Because of this nonspecificity of clinical manifestations, a systematic approach to diagnosis is necessary and should include a greater emphasis on the history (general, occupational, and environmental), as discussed in Chapter 2. A list of possible toxic agents should be generated from the exposure history and their toxicity reviewed. The results of physical examination and laboratory tests should be grouped according to findings related to each system or organ, and the findings should then be matched with findings due to specific toxic substances. A search for causes other than exposure to toxic agents should also be made, and additional diagnostic tests should be ordered as necessary to rule out these other causes. Although biologic measurements of specific toxic substances may be helpful on occasion (see Chapter 30), they are usually not available soon enough for use in cases of acute poisoning, and it is often too late to measure them in cases of chronic exposure.

## MANAGEMENT OF TOXIC EFFECTS

Management in most cases of toxicity consists of supportive care, symptomatic treatment, and removal from exposure to the toxic material. In cases of life-threatening toxicity, maintenance of cardiopulmonary function and fluid and electrolyte balance are usually indicated. Methods to enhance elimination, such as forced diuresis, hemodialysis, and hemoperfusion, have not been shown to be effective for treatment of poisoning due to most toxic agents of industrial origin.

There are only a few specific methods of treatment, or "antidotes." Chelating agents may reverse acute toxicity due to some metals (eg, lead, arsenic, and mercury), but they are less likely to affect subacute or chronic toxicity (see Chapter 27). Atropine and pralidoxime can be lifesaving in reversing the acute cholinesterase-inhibiting effects of organophosphate pesticides (see Chapter 32). In cases of acute cyanide or hydrogen sulfide poisoning, nitrites may be used to generate formation of cyanmethemoglobin or sulfmethemoglobin (see Chapter 33). Hydroxocobalamin (vitamin $B_{12a}$) is used in Europe and is currently being tested in the United States as an antidote for cyanide. Use of oxygen counters the effect and enhances the elimination of carbon monoxide (see Chapter 33).

## REFERENCES

Amdur MO, Doull J, Klaassen CD: *Casarett & Doull's Toxicology: The Basic Science of Poisons,* 5th ed. Pergamon Press, 1996.

Eaton DL, Robertson WO: Toxicology. In: *Textbook of Clinical Occupational and Environmental Medicine.* Rosenstock L, Cullen MR (editors). Saunders, 1994.

Ellenhorn MJ (editor): *Ellenhorn's Medical Toxicology: Diagnosis and Treatment of Human Poisoning.* Williams & Wilkins, 1997.

Goldfrank LR et al (editors): *Goldfrank's Toxicologic Emergencies,* 5th ed. Appleton & Lange, 1994.

Olson KR (editor): *Poisoning and Drug Overdose,* 2nd ed. Appleton & Lange, 1994.

Sullivan JB, Krieger GR (editors): *Clinical Principles of Environmental Health.* Williams & Wilkins, 1992.

# 14

# Clinical Immunology

*Richard S. Shames, MD, & Daniel C. Adelman, MD*

Immune hypersensitivity mechanisms play a part in many disorders of occupational medicine. In 1700, Bernardino Ramazzini, the founder of modern occupational medicine, reported that after repeated exposures to flour dust, bakers often developed respiratory problems—a disease now called baker's asthma. In the 20th century, many disorders of occupational medicine have been shown to be caused by immune reactions to environmental factors. Some of these include pigeon breeder's disease, farmer's lung, asthma induced by castor bean, nickel dermatitis, and poison oak dermatitis.

To understand the pathophysiology of these disorders, an appreciation of the underlying immune mechanisms is required. The purpose of this chapter is to review the primary immune response and the effector mechanisms, classify the major mechanisms responsible for immune hypersensitivity disorders found in occupational medicine, list some examples of these disorders, and conclude with a section on diagnosis and treatment of hypersensitivity diseases often seen in the practice of occupational medicine.

## OVERVIEW OF THE IMMUNE RESPONSE

The function of the immune system is to protect the host from invasion by foreign antigens by distinguishing "self" from "nonself." Such a system is necessary for survival in all living animals. A normal immune response relies on the careful coordination of a complex network of specialized cells, organs, and biological factors necessary for the recognition and subsequent elimination of foreign antigens. An abnormal, exaggerated immune response can cause hypersensitivity to foreign antigens with resultant tissue injury and the expression of a variety of clinical syndromes, which are often seen in the practice of occupational medicine.

The immune system consists of specific and nonspecific components that have distinct yet overlapping functions. The antibody-mediated and cell-mediated immune systems provide specificity and memory of previously encountered antigens. The nonspecific cellular component consists of phagocytic cells, whereas the complement proteins constitute the primary nonspecific plasma factors. Despite their lack of specificity, these components are essential because they are largely responsible for the natural immunity to a vast array of environmental microorganisms and foreign substances. Basic appreciation of the components and physiology of normal immunity are central to the understanding of the pathophysiology of hypersensitivity diseases of the immune system.

## IMMUNE RESPONSE

### Innate & Adaptive Immunity

Living organisms have two levels of response against external invasion: an **innate** system of natural immunity and an **adaptive** system, which is acquired. Innate immunity is present from birth and is nonspecific in its activity. The skin surface serves as the first line of defense of the innate immune system, whereas enzymes, the alternative complement system pathway, acute-phase proteins, natural killer cells, and certain cytokines provide additional layers of protection. Higher organisms have evolved the adaptive immune system, which is triggered by encounters with foreign agents that have evaded or penetrated the innate immune defenses. The adaptive immune system has **specificity** for individual foreign agents and **immunologic memory,** which allows for an intensified response upon subsequent encounter with the same or closely related agent. The introduction of a stimulus into the adaptive immune system triggers a complex sequence of events initiating the activation of lymphocytes, the production of antibodies and effector cells, and ultimately, the elimination of the inciting substance.

### Antigens & Immunogens

Foreign substances that can induce an immune response are called **antigens** or **immunogens.** Antigenicity implies that the substance has the ability to react with products of the adaptive immune system (ie, antibodies). Complex foreign agents possess distinct and multiple immunogenic components. Most immunogens are proteins, although pure carbohydrates may be immunogenic as well. The immune response to a particular immunogen may depend on the route of entry of the foreign substance. Blood-borne substances are normally removed by the spleen. Immunogens entering through the skin may provoke a local inflammatory response involving afferent lymphatic channels and regional lymph nodes. Entry of agents through mucosal surfaces (respiratory or gastrointestinal systems) stimulates the production of local antibodies. Activated lymphocytes are then carried to other lymphoid organs to amplify the initial response.

## Immune Response

The primary role of the immune system is to discriminate self from nonself and to eliminate the foreign substance. A complex network of specialized cells, organs, and biological factors is necessary for the recognition and subsequent elimination of foreign antigen. The major pathways of antigen elimination include the direct killing of target cells by a subset of T lymphocytes called **cytotoxic T lymphocytes (CTL)** (**cellular response**) and the elimination of antigen through **antibody-mediated** events arising from T and B lymphocyte interactions (**humoral response**). The series of events that embody the immune response include antigen processing and presentation, lymphocyte recognition and activation, cellular and/or humoral immune responses, and antigenic destruction or elimination (Figure 14–1).

**A. Antigen Processing and Presentation:** Most foreign immunogens are not recognized by the immune system in their native form and require capture and processing by specialized **antigen-presenting cells.** Antigen-presenting cells include macrophages, dendritic cells in lymphoid tissue. Langerhans cells in the skin, Kupffer cells in the liver, microglial cells in the nervous system, and B lymphocytes. Following encounter with immunogens, the antigen-presenting cells internalize the foreign substance by phagocytosis or pinocytosis, modify its parent structure, and display antigenic fragments of the native protein on its surface.

**B. T Lymphocyte Recognition and Activation:** The recognition of processed antigen by specialized T lymphocytes known as **helper T (CD4⁺) lymphocytes** constitutes the critical event in the immune response. The helper T lymphocytes orchestrate the many cells and biological signals that are necessary to carry out the immune response. Helper T lymphocytes recognize processed antigen displayed by antigen-presenting cells only in association with polymorphic cell surface proteins encoded by the **major histocompatibility gene complex (MHC).** The process of dual recognition is referred

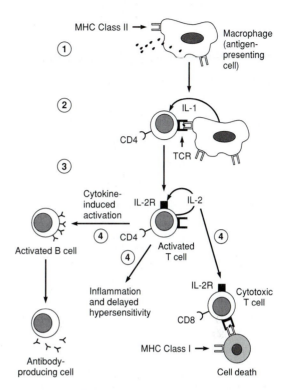

**Figure 14–1.** The normal immune response. ① Antigen processing and presentation by antigen-presenting cells. ② Recognition of antigen-MHC complex by CD4 T lymphocytes induces IL-1 secretion by antigen-presenting cells and subsequent cellular activation. ③ Activated T lymphocytes express IL-2 receptors and secrete IL-2, which upregulate IL-2 receptor expression in an autocrine fashion. ④ Activated CD4 T lymphocytes can stimulate CD8 cytotoxic T lymphocytes to mediate cellular cytotoxicity, B lymphocyte activation, and differentiation into antibody-producing plasma cells, which mediate humoral immunity or mediate delayed hypersensitivity and other inflammatory reactions. (Reproduced with permission from McPhee SJ et al [editors]. *Pathophysiology of Disease: An Introduction to Clinical Medicine.* Appleton & Lange, 1995.)

to as **MHC restriction.** Endogenously synthesized viral proteins are processed in association with **MHC class I** molecules, while exogenous foreign antigens that require an antibody-mediated response are expressed in association with **MHC class II** structures. All somatic cells express MHC class I, whereas only the specialized antigen-presenting cells can express MHC class II. Cytotoxic T lymphocytes expressing the surface protein **CD8** antigen recognize target cells bearing MHC class I complexed to antigen, while helper T lymphocytes expressing the **CD4** antigen recognize antigen in the context of MHC class II.

Helper T lymphocyte recognition of the antigen-MHC class II complex thereby activates the helper T lymphocytes. Two signals are required for activation of these cells: (1) binding of the antigen-specific **T lymphocyte receptor** to the antigen-MHC complex, and (2) release of **interleukin-1, (IL-1),** a soluble protein produced by the antigen-presenting cell. These two signals induce the expression of **IL-2** receptors on the surface of the CD4+ lymphocytes as well as the production of various cell growth and differentiation factors (**cytokines**) by the activated CD4+ T lymphocytes. The cytokine **IL-2,** produced and elaborated by activated CD4+ T lymphocytes, stimulates the growth of more cells expressing IL-2 receptors (**autocrine effect**), thus amplifying the initial response. Activated CD4+ T lymphocytes subsequently trigger the **effector cells** that mediate the cellular and humoral arms of the immune response.

**C. Activation of Cytotoxic T Lymphocytes (Cellular Immune Response):** Cytotoxic T lymphocytes (CD8+ T lymphocytes) eliminate target cells (virally infected cells, tumor cells, or foreign tissues), constituting the cellular immune response. Cytotoxic T lymphocytes differ from helper T lymphocytes in their expression of the surface antigen CD8 and by the recognition of MHC class I. Cytotoxic T lymphocytes become activated under the influence of two signals: (1) binding to the MHC class I-antigen complex and (2) following stimulation by IL-2 elaborated by helper T lymphocytes. Activated cytotoxic T lymphocytes then release substances called **cytotoxins,** which lead to the killing of infected target cells.

**D. Activation of B Lymphocytes (Humoral Immune Response):** Activated helper T cells may also induce the growth and differentiation of B lymphocytes, which mediate the **humoral** or **antibody-mediated response.** Release of cytokines with growth and differentiation activity by CD4+ T lymphocytes promotes the proliferation and terminal differentiation of B cells into high-rate antibody-producing cells, called **plasma cells,** which secrete antigen-specific antibody. B lymphocytes may also bind and internalize foreign antigen directly, process that antigen, and present it to CD4+ T lymphocytes. A pool of activated B lymphocytes may differentiate to form **memory cells,** which respond more rapidly and efficiently to subsequent encounters with identical or closely related antigenic structures.

**E. Antibody Structure and Function:** The primary function of mature B lymphocytes is to make antibodies. Antibodies are **immunoglobulins** directed toward specific antigens. Antibodies are proteins that combine specifically with antigens to initiate the humoral (antibody-mediated) immune response. Immunoglobulins serve a variety of secondary biological roles, including complement fixation, transplacental passage, and facilitation of phagocytosis **(opsonization),** all of which participate in host defense against disease. Circulating immunoglobulins have both a unique specificity for one particular antigenic structure and diversity to encounter a broad range of antigenic materials. This diversity arises from complex DNA rearrangements and RNA processing within B lymphocytes early in their ontogeny. All immunoglobulin molecules share a four-chain polypeptide structure consisting of two heavy and two light chains (Figure 14–2). Each chain includes an amino-terminal portion, containing the **variable (V) region,** and a carboxy-terminal portion containing four or five **constant (C) regions.** V regions are highly variable structures, which form the antigen-binding site, whereas the C domains support effector functions of the molecules. Digestion of an immunoglobulin molecule by the enzyme papain produces two antigen-binding F(ab[1]) fragments and the Fc (crystallizable) fragment. Pepsin digestion of the immunoglobulin molecule results in single F(ab)'$_2$ fragment joined by a disulfide bond.

There are five classes (**isotypes**) of immunoglobu-

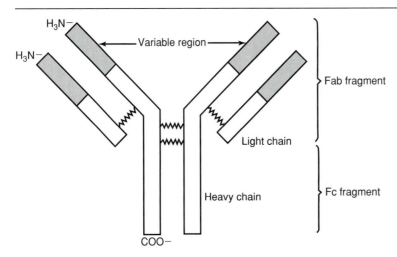

**Figure 14–2.** Structure of the immunoglobulin molecule. The immunoglobulin molecule is composed of two heavy and two light chains. The light chain and the amino (H$_3$N⁻) terminal half of the heavy chain make up Fab, the antibody-binding fragment of the molecule. The carboxyl (COO⁻) terminal halves of the heavy chains make up the Fc or crystalline half of the immunoglobulin molecule, which is responsible for the unique biological activities of a given immunoglobulin class. Interchain disulfide bonds (∿) bind the heavy and light chains.

lins, which are defined on the basis of differences in the C region of the heavy chains.

Table 14–1 summarizes many of the properties of the immunoglobulins.

IgG is the predominant immunoglobulin in serum. It has a molecular weight of 150,000. IgG antibodies are strong precipitins, and three subclasses—$IgG_1$, $IgG_2$, and $IgG_3$—can activate complement, qualities that make it operative in serum sickness and certain types of hypersensitivity pneumonitis (eg, bird breeder's disease).

IgA is the predominant immunoglobulin on mucous membrane surfaces. It exists predominantly as a monomer (MW 160,000) in serum and as a dimer or trimer (MW 390,000–550,000) on mucous membrane surfaces. When the dimer or trimer passes through the epithelial cells to a mucous membrane surface, it acquires a smaller molecule called secretory piece (MW 70,000) that stabilizes the molecule and prevents its degradation by proteolytic enzymes. IgA antibodies protect the host from foreign antigens on mucous membrane surfaces, but they do not fix complement by the classic pathway.

IgM is a pentamer (MW 900,000) that is found almost exclusively in the intravascular compartment. IgM antibodies are potent agglutinins and fix complement. They may mediate the trimellitic anhydride pulmonary anemia syndrome. IgD is a monomeric immunoglobulin (MW 180,000). Its biological function is unknown.

IgE is the heaviest immunoglobulin monomer (MW 190,000), with a normal concentration in serum varying from 20 to 100 IU, but the concentration may be 5 times normal or even higher in an atopic individual. The Fc portion of IgE binds to receptors on the surfaces of mast cells and basophils. IgE antibodies play an important role in immediate hypersensitivity reactions such as nasal allergy and allergic bronchial asthma in veterinarians, laboratory animal handlers, and enzyme detergent industry workers.

**F. Humoral Mechanisms of Antigen Elimination:** Antibodies can induce the elimination of foreign antigen through a number of different mechanisms. Binding of antibody to bacterial toxins or foreign venoms promotes elimination of these antigen-antibody complexes through the reticuloendothelial system. Antibodies can also coat bacterial surfaces, allowing clearance by macrophages in a process known as opsonization. Some classes of antibodies can complex with antigen and activate the complement system of cascading component activation, which culminates in lysis of the target cell. Finally, the major class of antibody, IgG, can bind to natural killer cells that subsequently complex with target cells and release cytotoxins (see the discussion of antibody-dependent cell-mediated cytotoxicity, below).

## MEDIATORS OF IMMEDIATE HYPERSENSITIVITY

Mediators of immediate hypersensitivity are chemicals generated or released by effector cells following activation. They have various biological activities and normally function in host defense, but they play a pathologic role in immune hypersensitivity. They exist in a preformed state in the granules of mast cells and basophils or are newly synthesized at the time of activation of these and some other nucleated cells (Tables 14–2 and 14–3). A number of stimuli activate mast cells and basophils, including the antigen bridging of two adjacent IgE molecules on the mast cell-basophil surface, anaphylatoxins (C3a, C4a, C5a), lectins (PHA, PWM), and drugs (morphine, codeine).

Preformed mediators include histamine, eosinophil and neutrophil chemoattractants, proteoglycans (heparin, chondroitin sulfate), and various proteolytic enzymes. Histamine is a bioactive amine that when re-

**Table 14–1.** Human immunoglobulin classes.

| Class | Mean Serum Conc. mg/dL | Molecular Weight | Sed. Coef. | Half-Life in Plasma (Days) | Biologic Function |
|---|---|---|---|---|---|
| IgG | 1200 | 150,000 | 7 | 23 | Fix complement<br>Cross placenta<br>Strongest precipitating capacity |
| IgA | 280 | 160,000<br>550,000 | 7, 10, 14 | 6 | Secretory antibody<br>Antiviral defense |
| IgM | 120 | 900,000 | 19 | 5 | Fix complement<br>Strongest agglutinating capacity |
| IgD | 3 | 180,000 | 7 | 3 | B lymphocyte surface receptor in newborn |
| IgE | 0.03 | 190,000 | 8 | 2.5 | Reaginic antibody |

**Table 14–2.** Mediators of immediate hypersentivity.[1]

**Vasoactive and smooth-muscle constricting mediators**
Preformed
    Histamine
Generated
    Arachodonic acid metabolites (PGD$_2$, LTC$_4$)
    PAF
    Adenosine
**Chemotactic mediators**
Eosinophil-directed
    Eosinophil chemotactic factor of anaphylaxis (ECFA)
    ECF oligopeptides
    PAF
Neutrophil-directed
    High-molecular-weight neutrophil chemotactic factor
    LTB$_4$
    PAF
**Enzymatic mediators**
Neutral proteases
    Tryptase
    Chymase
Lysosomal hydrolases
Other enzymes
    Superoxide dismutase
    Peroxidase

[1]Modified from Stites DP, Terr AI. *Basic & Clinical Immunology,* 7th ed. Appleton & Lange, 1991.

leased binds to H$_1$, H$_2$, and H$_3$ receptors on adjacent cells. Binding to H$_1$ receptors causes smooth muscle contraction, vasodilatation, increased vascular permeability, and stimulation of nasal mucous glands. Stimulation of H$_2$ receptors causes enhanced gastric acid secretion, mucus secretion, and leukocyte chemotaxis. Binding to H$_3$ receptors inhibits hista-

mine release and synthesis. Histamine is important in the pathogenesis of allergic rhinitis, allergic asthma, and anaphylaxis. Eosinophil and neutrophil chemoattractants have been observed in late asthmatic reactions, occurring 4–6 hours after antigen challenge.

Newly generated mediators include kinins, platelet-activating factor, and phospholipid-derived substances including leukotrienes and prostaglandins. Arachidonic acid, derived from the phospholipid bilayer of cells, is metabolized either by the lipoxygenase pathway to form leukotrienes (LT) or the cyclooxygenase pathway to form prostaglandins (PG) and thromboxanes (TXA$_2$ and TXB$_2$). Leukotrienes are generated by mast cells, granulocytes, macrophages, and basophils. LTB$_4$ is a potent chemoattractant for polymorphonuclear neutrophils. LTC$_4$, LTD$_4$, and LTE$_4$ constitute slow-reacting substance of anaphylaxis (SRS-A), which has a bronchial smooth muscle spasmogenic potency 100–1000 times that of histamine; leukotrienes are also important mediators in allergic rhinitis.

Prostaglandins are generated by almost all nucleated cells. The most important members are PGD$_2$, PGE$_2$, PGF$_2$, and PGI$_2$ (prostacyclin). Human mast cells produce large amounts of PGD$_2$, which causes vasodilatation, vascular permeability, and airway constriction. Activated polymorphonuclear neutrophils and macrophages generate PGF$_{2a}$, a bronchoconstrictor, and PGE$_2$, a bronchodilator. PGI$_2$ causes platelet disaggregation. TxA$_2$ causes platelet aggregation, bronchial constriction, and vasoconstriction.

Platelet-activating factor (PAF) is generated by

**Table 14–3.** Action of mediators in hypersensitivity reactions.

| | Bronchial Constriction | Chemotaxis | | Platelet Activation | Increased Vascular Permeability | Mucus Production | Pruritus |
|---|---|---|---|---|---|---|---|
| | | PMS | EOS | | | | |
| Histamine | X | X | X | | X | X (Nasal) | X |
| Leukotrienes C | X | | | | X | X | |
| D | X | | | | X | X | |
| E | X | | | | | X | |
| 5-HETE | | X | | | | | |
| PGD$_2$ | X | | | | X | | |
| TxA$_2$ | X | | | X | | | |
| Kallikrein | | | | | X | | |
| PAF | X | | X | X | | | |
| NCFA | | X | | | | | |
| ECFA | | X | X | | | | |

macrophages, neutrophils, eosinophils, and mast cells. It causes platelet aggregation, vasodilatation, increased vascular permeability, and bronchial smooth muscle contraction. PAF is the most potent eosinophil chemoattractant described. The kinins are vasoactive peptides formed in plasma when kallikrein—released by basophils and mast cells—digests plasma kininogen; they cause slow sustained contraction of bronchial and vascular smooth muscle, vascular permeability, secretion of mucus, and stimulation of pain fibers. Kinins may play a role in human anaphylaxis.

## EFFECTOR CELLS

A number of effector cells participate in immune hypersensitivity reactions. These include mast cells, basophils, polymorphonuclear neutrophils, eosinophils, macrophage-monocytes, platelets, and lymphocytes. Depending on the type of immune response, many or all play a part. The effector cells have membrane receptors for various chemoattractants and mediators (Table 14–3).

Mast cells are basophilic staining cells found chiefly in connective and subcutaneous tissue. They have prominent granules that are the source of many mediators of immediate hypersensitivity and have 30,000–200,000 cell surface membrane receptors for the Fc fragment of IgE. When an allergen molecule binds two adjacent mast cell surface-associated IgE antibodies, bridging between the two antibodies occurs. This perturbs the cell membrane surface, allows calcium to enter the cell, and activates enzyme systems that ultimately lead to the release of both preformed and newly generated mediators. Mast cells also have surface receptors for anaphylatoxins C3a, C4a, and C5a.

Basophils account for approximately 1% of circulating granulocytes. They possess a segmented nucleus and granules that are larger than those of mast cells. Like mast cells, they have cell membrane surface receptors for the Fc fragment of IgE and anaphylatoxins. On exposure to antigen, activation leading to the release of mediators occurs in a manner similar to mast cells. Basophils possess some but not all of the mediators found in mast cells. Absence of $PGD_2$ during late-phase reactions following antigen challenge implicates basophils as a potentially important source of mediators in allergic late-phase responses.

Neutrophils are granulocytes that phagocytose and destroy foreign antigens and microbial organisms. They are attracted to the site of antigen by chemotactic factors, including C5a, $LTB_4$, granulocyte colony-stimulating factor (G-CSF), granulocyte-macrophage colony-stimulating factor (GM-CSF), and PAF. They possess receptors for the Fc fragment of IgG and IgM antibodies (specific opsonins) and for C3b (nonspecific opsonin). Neutrophils are activated when they unite with C3b or with the Fc portion of IgG or IgM antibody bound to particles or cells. Smaller antigens are phagocytosed and destroyed by lysosomal enzymes. Particles too large to be phagocytosed are destroyed by locally released lysosomal enzymes. Neutrophils contain or generate a number of antimicrobial factors, including superoxides, which produce $H_2O_2$; myeloperoxidase, which catalyzes the production of hypochlorite; and proteolytic enzymes, including collagenase, elastase, and cathepsin B. Some or all of these factors may play a part in a number of hypersensitivity reactions, including the type I late asthmatic response, the type II cytotoxin reaction, and type III immune complex disease (see below).

Eosinophils play both a proactive and a modulating role in inflammation. They are attracted to the site of the antigen-antibody reactions by PAF, C5a, eosinophil chemotactic factor of anaphylaxis (ECFA), histamine, and $LTB_4$. They are important in the defense against parasites. When stimulated, they release major basic protein (MBP), eosinophil peroxidase, lysosomal hydrolases, and $LTC_4$. MBP destroys parasites, impairs ciliary beating, and causes exfoliation of respiratory epithelial cells; it may trigger histamine release from mast cells and basophils. It has been suggested that the eosinophils may play a modulating role in inflammation; they contain histaminase, which metabolizes histamine, and aryl sulfatase B, an enzyme that catabolizes various leukotrienes.

The tissue-fixed macrophages and the circulating monocytes are both phagocytes and antigen-processing cells. Monocytes are susceptible to chemoattraction by C5a. When they leave the circulation, they mature into macrophages. Both monocytes and macrophages contain receptors for C3b and the Fc portion of IgG. Activation of these cells occurs not only when these receptors are stimulated but also when they are exposed to various lymphokines and when they phagocytose antigen, silica, and asbestos. They contain aryl sulfatase, acid phosphatase, and β-glucuronidase and are able to produce $H_2O_2$. They produce and release leukotrienes, PAF, $PGE_2$, $PGF_2$, and many complement proteins. Besides their function as effector cells of hypersensitivity, they play a vital role in the primary immune response, ingesting, processing, and presenting foreign antigen in conjunction with class 2 antigens of the major histocompatibility complex (HLA D and HLA DR) to both CD4 (T helper-inducer) lymphocytes and B lymphocytes; they generate IL-1, which stimulates CD4 cells to produce IL-2 (Figure 14–1).

Human platelets play a vital role in the clotting sequence. They contain thromboxane and vasoactive amines. Thromboxane and PAF cause platelet aggregation and initiate the clotting sequence. Platelets produce many inflammatory mediators and cytokines and express surface receptors for immunoglobulin and autocoids, suggesting an active role in inflammatory processes. During antigen-induced acute airway reactions, there is evidence that platelet factor 4 (PF4) is released and stimulates mediator release from basophils.

Lymphocytes are responsible for the initial specific recognition of antigen. They are functionally and phenotypically divided into B and T lymphocytes. Structurally, B and T lymphocytes cannot be distinguished visually from each other under the microscope, although about 70–80% of circulating blood lymphocytes are T cells and 10–15% B cells; the remainder are referred to as null cells.

Null cells probably include a number of different cell types, including a group called natural killer (NK) cells. These cells appear distinct from other lymphocytes in that they are slightly larger, with a kidney-shaped nucleolus, and have a granular appearance. NK cells are capable of binding IgG because they have a membrane receptor for the IgG molecule (FcγR). Antibody-dependent cell-mediated cytotoxicity (ADCC) occurs when an organism or a cell is coated by antibody and undergoes NK cell-mediated destruction. Alternatively, NK cells can destroy virally infected cells or tumor cells without involvement of antibody. Other characteristics of NK cells include recognition of antigens without MHC restrictions, lack of immunologic memory, and regulation of activity by cytokines and arachidonic acid metabolites.

## COMPLEMENT

Activation of the classic complement pathway is initiated by the union of antigen with IgG or IgM antibody. Complement-fixing sites on the Fc region of these antibody molecules are exposed, allowing binding of the first component of the complement sequence, C1q. Other components of the complement sequence are subsequently bound, activated, and cleaved, eventually leading to cell lysis. Important by-products of the classic pathway include anaphylatoxins, the potent C3a and C5a and less potent C4a; C5a is chemotactic for PMNs and monocytes and causes activation and release of mediators from mast cells and basophils. C4b and C3b opsonize target cells, thus facilitating phagocytosis. Activation of the complement sequence by the alternative pathway is initiated by a number of agents, including lipopolysaccharides, trypsin-like molecules, aggregated IgA and IgG, and cobra venom. Activation does not require the presence of antigen-antibody complexes, nor does it utilize the early components of the complement sequence, C1, C4, and C2. It requires the presence of a different series of proteins, factors B and D and properdin, which facilitate activation, and factors H and I, which act as inactivators. Just as in the classic pathway, the important molecules—C3b,

C3a, and C5a—are generated. Ultimately, as a result of activation of the classic or alternative pathway, activation of the terminal complement sequence occurs, resulting in cell lysis.

## CLASSIFICATION OF IMMUNE HYPERSENSITIVITY DISORDERS

Gell and Coombs devised a classification scheme to define the basic immunopathologic mechanisms of hypersensitivity by four distinct types of reactions (Types I–IV) (Figure 14–3). Types I–III are all mediated by specific antibodies (humoral immune response) while type IV results from the actions of sensitized T lymphocytes (cell-mediated immune response). All defined mechanisms require an initial exposure to antigen (**sensitizing dose**), which induces a primary immune response (**sensitization**). Subsequent exposure to the same antigen (**challenge dose**) following a short lag period (usually at least 1 week) evokes the hypersensitivity response.

Elimination of foreign antigen by cellular or humoral processes is integrally linked to the inflammatory response, in which cellular messengers (cytokines) and antibodies trigger the recruitment of additional cells and the release of endogenous vasoactive and proinflammatory enzymatic substances (inflammatory mediators). Inflammation may have both positive and deleterious effects. Tight control of inflammatory mechanisms promotes efficient elimination of foreign substances and prevents uncontrolled lymphocyte activation and unregulated antibody production. However, inappropriate activation or dysregulation of the system can perpetuate inflammatory processes that lead to tissue damage and organ dysfunction. Inflammation is responsible for hypersensitivity reactions and for many of the clinical effects of autoimmunity.

### Type I: Anaphylactic or Immediate Hypersensitivity Reactions

These reactions represent an inflammatory response mediated by the interaction of antigen with specific IgE antibodies bound to mast cells and basophils and the subsequent release of inflammatory mediators that lead to tissue damage in specific target organs. Examples of type I reactions in the practice of occupational medicine include allergic rhinitis and asthma seen in bakers and animal handlers and systemic anaphylaxis in bee keepers and health care workers (latex allergy).

Initial exposure to antigen in a genetically predisposed host leads to the synthesis of antigen-specific IgE by mature B cells, constituting the **atopic** state. Induction of B lymphocytes to synthesize IgE requires two signals that are elaborated primarily by helper T (CD4+) lymphocytes: one that influences IgE isotype expression, and one that serves to acti-

A. TYPE I

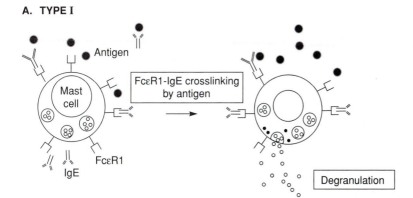

B. TYPE II

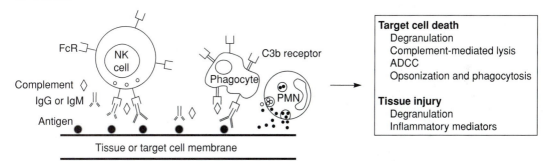

**Figure 14–3.** Hypersensitivity immune responses. (A) Type I reaction. Mast cells and basophils bind IgE via high-affinity Fc receptors (FcεR1). Antigen binding and crosslinking of FcεR1-IgE complexes induce cellular degranulation and release of inflammatory mediators. (B) Type II reaction. IgG or IgM antibodies against tissue or cellular antigens induces complement activation, which results in cell death and tissue injury.

vate B lymphocytes. Isotype switching is regulated by mitogens and cytokines. The cytokine **IL-4** is a critical factor for isotype switching to IgE and is sufficient to initiate germ line transcription of IgE. Additional B lymphocyte activation and differentiation factors are required for the expression of mature mRNA and subsequent IgE synthesis. In humans, a variety of secondary signals work in concert with IL-4 to promote IgE synthesis, including **IL-5** and **IL-6,** which promote terminal differentiation of the B lymphocyte into an antibody-producing plasma cell. In contrast, **interferon-γ (IFN-γ)** inhibits IL-4–dependent IgE synthesis in humans. Thus, an imbalance favoring IL-4 over IFN-γ may induce IgE formation.

Helper (CD4[+]) T lymphocytes play a central role in the induction of normal immune responses. In allergic inflammatory processes (type I reactions), T lymphocytes represent a source of both IL-4 and secondary signals necessary to drive the production of IgE by B lymphocytes. Two subsets of CD4[+] helper T lymphocytes, differing in their phenotypic patterns of cytokine synthesis and release, have been identi-

fied. TH1 cells elaborate **IL-2, IFN-γ, IL-3** and **GM-CSF** and are favored in cell-mediated immunity as well as in type IV delayed hypersensitivity reactions (see below). TH2 cells secrete **IL-3, IL-4, IL-5,** and **GM-CSF** and have been implicated in type I allergic and inflammatory responses. IL-3, together with other cytokines, induces mast cell differentiation and proliferation. IL-5 promotes activation and chemotaxis of eosinophils. GM-CSF drives the growth and differentiation of granulocytes, macrophages, and eosinophils. Activated T lymphocytes that release TH2-characteristic cytokines have been found at sites of inflammation in allergic airway disease and are believed to direct the immune response toward allergic inflammation.

Antigen-specific IgE binds to high-affinity **Fc receptors** on tissue mast cells and basophils as well as to low-affinity receptors on lymphocytes, macrophages, eosinophils, and platelets, thus sensitizing these cells for future allergen encounters. Upon reexposure to allergen, the sensitized individual can mount an accelerated immune response. Mast cells,

## C. TYPE III

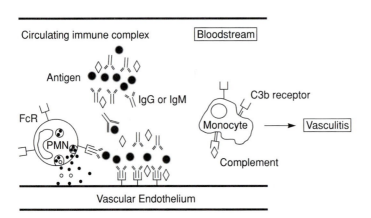

## D. TYPE IV

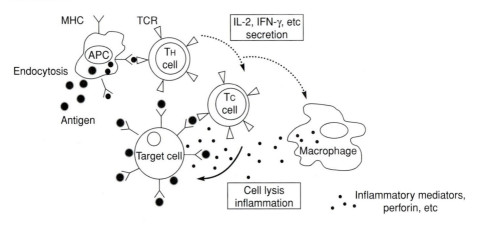

**Figure 14–3 (continued).** (C) Type III reaction. Circulating immune complexes composed of soluble antigen and IgG or IgM deposit on vascular endothelium of various tissues, which activates the complement cascade. PMN and other phagocytes are attracted to these sites of immune complex deposition via their Fc and C3b receptors and are induced to degranulate and phagocytose the complexes, resulting in local tissue injury and vasculitis. (D) Type IV reaction. Via their T cell receptors, helper T cells recognize target cell antigenic peptides bound to antigen-presenting cells. This T cell recognition results in the secretion of interleukin 2, interferon gamma, and other lymphokines that are required for the activation of tissue macrophages and cytotoxic T cells. Cytotoxic T cells recognize the same antigen bound to target cells and induce lysis by perforin and other molecules secreted by cytotoxic T cells. (From Shames R: *Pediatrics & Perinatology: The Scientific Basis,* 2nd ed. Gluckman & Heymann [editors]. In press.)

armed with antigen-specific IgE on their surfaces, can bind polyvalent allergen and can cross-link allergen (Figure 14–3). Bridging of cell-bound IgE requires that two IgE molecules be linked by multivalent antigen; a single Fab monomer is unable to induce the subsequent reaction. Binding of specific antigen initiates a physical approximation of surface IgE receptors triggering a sequence of biochemical events that results in the activation and degranulation of mast cells and basophils.

Activation of mast cells and basophils induces both the release of preformed mediators from cyto-plasmic granules (histamine, chemotactic factors and enzymes) and the synthesis and release of newly generated mediators (prostaglandins, leukotrienes, and platelet-activating factor). Mast cells and basophils also have the ability to synthesize and release proinflammatory cytokines, growth factors, and regulatory factors, which interact in complex networks.

The interaction of mediators with specific target organs and cells frequently induces a **biphasic** response: an early effect on blood vessels, smooth muscle, and secretory glands marked by vascular leakiness, smooth muscle constriction, and mucus hypersecretion and a late response characterized by mucosal edema and the influx of inflammatory cells. Early-phase events are mediated primarily by histamine, while late-phase events are induced by cytokines, preformed chemotactic mediators, arachidonic acid metabolites (leukotrienes), and platelet-activating factor.

The **early-phase response** occurs within minutes of an antigen exposure. Atopic individuals challenged intranasally with pollen allergen or with cold, dry air release vasoactive and smooth muscle-constrictive mediators, including histamine, TAME esterase, leukotrienes, $PGD_2$, kinins, and kininogens from mast cells and basophils. In allergic rhinitis, the early-phase response is marked grossly by erythema, localized edema, and pruritus that results largely from the interaction of histamine with target tissues of the upper airway. Histologically, the early response is characterized by vasodilatation, edema, and a mild cellular infiltrate of mostly granulocytes.

The **late-phase response** may either follow the early-phase response (**dual response**) or occur as an isolated event (**isolated late phase**). Late-phase reactions begin 2–4 hours after initial antigen exposure, reach maximal activity at 6–12 hours, and usually resolve within 12–24 hours. Mediators of the early-phase response except for $PGD_2$ reappear during the late-phase response in the absence of antigen rechallenge. The absence of $PGD_2$, an exclusive product of mast cell release, suggests that basophils and not mast cells are an important source of mediators in the late-phase response. The late-phase response is characterized grossly by erythema, induration, heat, burning, and itching and microscopically by an influx of primarily eosinophils and mononuclear cells. There is strong circumstantial evidence suggesting that eosinophils are important proinflammatory cells in allergic airway disease, particularly asthma. Eosinophils are frequently sampled from the nasal mucosa of patients with allergic rhinitis and from the sputum of asthmatics. Products of activated eosinophils such as major basic protein and eosinophilic cationic protein, which are destructive to airway epithelial tissue and predispose to persistent airway reactivity, have also been localized to the airways of patients with allergic disease. Epithelial disruption is a feature of patients with both atopic dermatitis and asthma. Inflammatory cells infiltrating tissues in the late response may further elaborate cytokines and histamine-releasing factors that may perpetuate the late-phase response, leading to a sustained hyperresponsiveness and disruption of the target tissue (eg, bronchi, skin, or nasal mucosa). Release of proinflammatory mediators and cytokines can thus precipitate a sustained inflammatory response resulting in localized edema, mucus secretion, epithelial disruption, and influx of eosinophils, neutrophils, and mononuclear cells. Late-phase reactivity has been found in disease states, including allergic rhinitis and conjunctivitis, asthma, food-sensitive atopic dermatitis, and anaphylaxis. It is possible that dual asthmatic responses seen in individuals with detergent worker's asthma, trimellitic anhydride asthma, and baker's asthma represent clinical examples of bronchial late-phase responses.

Immediate hypersensitivity can be demonstrated in vivo by a prick or intradermal skin test to specific antigen or in vitro by the radioallergosorbent test (RAST) or the enzyme-linked immunosorbent assay (ELISA). A positive skin test is marked by a pruritic wheal-and-flare reaction, which peaks at 20 minutes, confirming the presence of antigen-specific IgE bound to skin mast cells. In vitro tests measure antigen-specific IgE levels in the serum.

### Type II: Cytotoxic Reactions

In type II reactions, the antigen is a cell surface protein or antigenic substance that attaches to a cell surface protein (Figure 14–3). In transfusion reactions, the antigen is a protein on the cell membrane of the incompatible erythrocyte. In some type II hypersensitivity disorders, a low-molecular-weight substance—eg, trimellitic anhydride (TMA)—acting as a hapten attaches to a host cell surface protein that acts as a carrier. In the pulmonary disease-anemia syndrome that occurs in workers repeatedly exposed to high concentrations of volatile TMA, the chemical combines with an erythrocyte membrane protein or pulmonary basement cell membrane protein to form a complete antigen that in turn stimulates the formation of IgG or IgM antibody. On reexposure, cell surface-bound antigen-antibody union takes place, inducing a number of effects: (1) Opsonization of the target cells by IgG or IgM, which makes them more susceptible to phagocytosis by macrophages, monocytes, and polymorphonuclear leukocytes. These phagocytes are activated when their receptors for the Fc portion of IgG antibody attach to the antibody molecule on the surface of the target cell. They engulf the antigen and release lysozymal enzymes. (2) The target cell may be destroyed by NK cells, which have receptors for the Fc portion of IgG. (3) The union of antigen with antibody activates the complement cascade, generating C3b, an opsonin, which facilitates phagocytosis or activation of the terminal complement sequence, leading to cell lysis. The Coombs test is helpful in demonstrating IgG antibody on the surface of red cells and leukocytes.

### Type III: Immune Complex Reaction

Type III reactions depend on the union of soluble antigen with soluble IgG or IgM antibody and subsequent activation of the complement sequence (Figure 14–3). In one subtype, the Arthus reaction, an immune complex is formed locally; and in the other, serum sickness, circulating complexes are deposited in various tissues.

The **Arthus reaction** was first described in 1903 by Maurice Arthus, who intradermally injected bovine serum albumin into a previously sensitized rabbit. Induration and erythema were noted at the injection site in 2 hours, peaked at 6 hours, and resolved in 12–24 hours. In some instances, necrosis developed at the site. The type I LPR (see above) also peaks at 4–6 hours, but it is preceded by an immediate wheal and flare response and does not exhibit tissue necrosis. The Arthus reaction is the result of binding of localized but not fixed antigen to circulating antibody, forming an immune complex in situ. This reaction may be operative in hypersensitivity pneumonitis. An example is pigeon breeder's disease. The antigen, serum dried in pigeon excreta, is inhaled, sensitizing the host and leading to IgG and IgM antibody formation. On subsequent exposure to inhaled antigen, localized alveolar immune complex formation occurs. The complex activates the complement cascade, forming C4a, C3a, C5a, C4b, and C3b. C4b and C3b are opsonins, enhancing phagocytosis by polymorphonuclears, monocytes, and macrophages. C3a, C4a, and C5a are anaphylatoxins that stimulate mast cells and basophils to release histamine and other mediators which in turn cause vasodilatation and increased vascular permeability, facilitating the diffusion of other mediators and effector cells to the reaction site; C5a is also chemotactic for polymorphonuclear leukocytes and monocytes. PAF and thromboxane cause platelet aggregation and activation, leading to thrombus formation. PAF, $LTB_4$, and NCFA attract neutrophils, and ECFA attracts eosinophils to the site. The ingestion of immune complexes by polymorphonuclears causes activation of monocytes and macrophages and stimulates the release of lysosomal enzymes.

In **serum sickness,** or circulating immune complex disease, circulating antigen and IgG antibodies combine, forming immune complexes that in antigen excess form microprecipitates. These are filtered from the circulation at the postcapillary venule and activate the complement cascade. Just as in the Arthus reaction, the anaphylatoxins stimulate the release of mediators that induce increased vascular permeability, facilitating immune complex deposition. Examples of circulating immune complex disease include classic serum sickness, which occurs 8–13 days after injection of the foreign serum, and systemic lupus erythematosus, in which the antigen is host DNA. Clinical manifestations of serum sickness include generalized urticaria, polyserositis (arthritis, pleuritis, pericarditis), fever, and nephritis.

The presence of antibody in type III reactions may be demonstrated by the Ouchterlony gel diffusion technique (see below).

## Type IV: Cellular Immunity

Type IV delayed hypersensitivity reactions are not mediated by antibody but, rather, are mediated primarily by T lymphocytes (cell-mediated immunity). In contrast to type I reactions, which often occur within minutes of antigen challenge dose, type IV reactions require 24–72 hours to appear. Classic examples of type IV immunopathologic changes are the tuberculin skin test reactions and contact dermatitis.

Elimination of antigen by cell-mediated immunity generally involves two mechanisms. Specific T cells sensitized by their encounter with the antigen may become **cytotoxic** and directly destroy antigen-bearing cells or may be activated to secrete **lymphokines,** which drive the activation of mononuclear phagocytes. While both effector mechanisms may be important to the normal host defense, inappropriate activation or dysregulation of the system can result in immunologic tissue injury (type IV hypersensitivity). Cytotoxic T-lymphocytes (CTL) that induce necrosis of antigen-bearing cells represent an important immune system function in the elimination of tumor cells, virus-infected cells, or transplanted cells bearing foreign proteins. CTL arise from the antigen-driven activation and differentiation of resting mature small lymphocyte precursors. Activated CTL manufacture products linked to cytolytic effector activity, including a membrane pore-forming protein (**perforin** or **cytolysin**), IFN-γ, and tumor necrosis factor beta (**TNF-β,**). Killing of target cells by CTL requires direct cell-to-cell contact and proceeds sequentially by (1) adhesive interactions between CTL and target cell, (2) activation of CTL by antigen engagement of CTL receptors, (3) delivery of the lethal hit to target cells by poorly characterized mechanisms, and (4) programmed cell death of target cells. Target cell death ensues by changes in cell membrane permeability or apoptosis. The histologic appearance of T cell-mediated cytotoxicity is characterized by necrosis of affected cells and marked lymphocytic infiltration in affected tissues.

The second mechanism of cell-mediated immunity involves the secretion of cytokines (especially IFN-γ) by activated T cells that promotes the migration of mononuclear phagocytes into sites of antigen deposition and induces the activation and differentiation of macrophages (Figure 14–3). Activated macrophages have increased capacity and efficiency for killing microorganisms. Type IV injury may result from the uncontrolled activation of tissue macrophages.

Contact dermatitis is caused by a variety of agents, including Rhus antigens, latex, and nickel. In addition, type IV hypersensitivity may be important in the pathogenesis of hypersensitivity pneumonitis. Antigens derived from mold spores or thermophilic actinomycetes bind with sensitized T lymphocytes to initiate the reaction. Patch testing with standard antigen-impregnated patches is used to demonstrate delayed type contact sensitivity.

## NONIMMUNE ACTIVATION OF INFLAMMATORY REACTIONS

Inflammatory reactions can also be initiated by nonimmunologic activation of cellular and humoral effector mechanisms. Substances such as plant-derived lectins (concanavalin A from the jack bean, phytohemagglutinins from the red kidney bean, and pokeweed mitogen), gram-negative polysaccharides, pneumococcal polysaccharides, Epstein-Barr virus, trypsin, papain, silica, and asbestos act as pseudo-antigens, nonimmunologically activating lymphocytes, macrophages, mast cells, basophils, and, in some cases, the complement system.

Concanavalin A (Con A) and phytohemagglutinins (PHA) selectively stimulate nonsensitized T lymphocytes, whereas gram-negative polysaccharides stimulate B lymphocytes and macrophages, leading to immunoglobulin production and macrophage activation. The intradermal injection of Con A and PHA into nonsensitized guinea pigs leads to a response resembling delayed type hypersensitivity. Inhalation of these lectins produces prominent interstitial pneumonitis in previously nonexposed rabbits. A rabbit previously sensitized and then challenged with inhaled bovine serum albumin (BSA) does not react unless Con A or PHA is simultaneously administered. Thus, these lectins enhance antigen-antibody bonding and facilitate the formation of pathologic immune complexes.

Nonimmune activation of effector cells and mechanisms can also be induced by other agents. Products derived from fungi nonimmunologically activate T cells and macrophages in the lungs, resulting in interstitial pulmonary fibrosis. These agents stimulate lymphocytes to release cytokines, basophils and mast cells to release mediators, and macrophages to release IL-1. *Micropolyspora faeni,* a bacterium inducing farmer's lung, may activate B cells and macrophages, triggering immunelike reactions in the lung. It is possible that other pathogenic and environmental dusts induce nonimmunologic stimulation of the immune system. Silica and asbestos directly stimulate macrophages to release IL-1, which in turn stimulates fibroblast growth, collagen synthesis, and T and B cells. Patients with silicosis produce autoantibodies, immune complexes, antinuclear antibodies (ANA), and rheumatoid factor and exhibit hypergammaglobulinemia. Nonspecific activators functioning in concert with specific antigens may play an important role in the induction of immune hypersensitivity reactions observed in many occupational immune disorders.

## IMMUNE HYPERSENSITIVITY OCCUPATIONAL DISORDERS

The most common immune hypersensitivity occupational disorders include allergic asthma or rhinitis, hypersensitivity pneumonitis, and contact dermatitis. The reactions are dependent on the host, the duration, the degree and type of sensitization, and the antigen.

**Allergic asthma** and **allergic rhinitis** occur when sensitized workers inhale specific antigen. Occupational asthma is probably the most prevalent of the immunologically mediated occupational disorders of the airways and parenchyma in developed countries, although knowledge of its incidence is limited by the absence of a uniform definition of the disease and limited reporting schemes. Surveillance programs in the United Kingdom and in British Columbia, Canada, have indicated that occupational asthma accounts for 26 and 52% of all occupational lung disease, respectively. In the United States and Japan, an estimated 15% of newly diagnosed adult asthma is due to occupational exposure. Two categories of asthma in the workplace are occupational asthma and work-aggravated asthma. Occupational asthma is marked by variable airflow limitation, bronchial hyperresponsiveness, or both, as a result of conditions in a particular work environment. Work-aggravated asthma is defined as preexisting or concurrent asthma that is worsened by irritants or physical stimuli in the workplace. Expanded knowledge about these disorders has come from increased physician and patient awareness as well as from new technologies for studying the mechanisms. Sensitization may result from a broad array of natural or synthesized chemicals that may appear in a diverse range of materials and processes. The list of documented causal agents has expanded rapidly over the past 5–10 years and now numbers over 250 (Table 14–4).

In general, atopic patients are predisposed to sensitization to large-molecular-weight inhalants (proteins) such as animal danders, pollens, and house dust. There is no atopic predisposition to sensitization by low-molecular-weight chemicals such as toluene diisocyanate (TDI), TMA, or platinum salts. Exposure to high-molecular-weight antigens generally induces classic type I, IgE-mediated hypersensitivity reactions. Some low-molecular-weight compounds such as acid anhydrides and platinum salts act as haptens and induce specific IgE antibodies by combining with a cell surface or carrier protein, while others such as isocyanates do not appear to induce specific IgE antibody or agent-protein complexes. Specific inhalation challenges with relevant antigen may induce isolated early, isolated late, biphasic, or continuous asthmatic reactions. Isolated early reactions occur immediately after exposure, reach maximal intensity within 30 minutes, and end within 60–90 minutes. An isolated late-phase reaction occurs 4–6 hours after the challenge (often after a worker has returned home), reaches peak intensity within 8–10 hours, and ends after 24–48 hours. A biphasic reaction is characterized by an early response with spontaneous recovery followed by a late-

**Table 14–4.** Materials causally linked to rhinitis and asthma in the workplace.

| | Allergen | Occupational Point of Exposure |
|---|---|---|
| **Plant material** | Herbs | Food industry workers |
| | Buckwheat | Food industry workers |
| | Sesame seeds | Food industry workers |
| | Carob bean flour | Food industry workers |
| | Coffee beans | Coffee roasters |
| | Rose hips | Health food workers |
| | Wood dusts | Construction workers, carpenters |
| | Latex | Health care workers, laboratory workers, housekeepers (airborne dust from glove powder) |
| | Fodder | Dairy farmers |
| | Guar gum | Carpet manufacturers, pharmaceutical workers |
| | Grain dust | Bakers, millers |
| | Tobacco | Tobacco workers |
| | Cotton | Cotton workers |
| | Hops | Brewery workers |
| | Obeche (African maple) | Sauna builders |
| **Animal and insect products** | Grasshoppers | Laboratory workers |
| | Laboratory animals (rodents, rabbits, etc.) | Laboratory workers |
| | Midges | Laboratory workers |
| | Food mites | Food handlers (especially handling cheese, chorizo, salty ham) |
| | Animal danders | Veterinarians |
| | Red spider mites | Nursery workers |
| | Storage mites | Grain workers |
| | Live fish bait | Anglers |
| | Lactalbumin (dried cow's milk) | Confectioners |
| **Fungi and bacteria** | Library fungi | Librarians |
| | Lawn molds | Gardeners, lawn cutters |
| | Bacterial enzymes | Detergent workers, pharmaceutical workers |
| **Chemicals and enzymes** | α-Amylase | Bakery workers |
| | Chloramine T | Janitorial workers |
| | Acid anhydrides | Plastic manufacturers |
| | Epoxy resins | Epoxy manufacturers |
| | Diisocyanates | Polyurethane plastic and foam workers |
| | Platinum salts | Catalyst manufacturers |
| | Nickel, cobalt | Metal workers |
| | Reactive dyes | Dye manufacturers |

(*continued*)

**Table 14–4.** Materials causally linked to rhinitis and asthma in the workplace (continued).

|                     | Allergen                                 | Occupational Point of Exposure              |
|---------------------|------------------------------------------|---------------------------------------------|
|                     | Persulfates (permanent wave solution)    | Beauticians                                 |
|                     | Formaldehyde                             | Hospital workers, morticians                |
| **Metals**          | Stainless steel vapor                    | Welders                                     |
|                     | Cobalt                                   | Hard metal workers                          |
|                     | Platinum salts                           | Platinum refiners, catalyst manufacturers   |
|                     | Chromium                                 | Cement workers, tanners                     |
|                     | Nickel                                   | Metal plating workers                       |
| **Pharmaceuticals** | Corticotropin-releasing hormone          | Pharmaceutical workers                      |
|                     | Antibiotics (esp. penicillins)           | Health care providers                       |
|                     | Psyllium                                 | Health care providers                       |

phase reaction. Continuous asthmatic reactions occur without remission between early- and late-phase responses. In general, IgE-mediated reactions occur as isolated early-phase events or biphasic reactions, whereas IgE-independent reactions occur as isolated late-phase, biphasic, or atypical asthmatic reactions.

The true prevalence of occupational asthma is currently not known. Surveys among workers in high-risk occupations suggest that exposure is the most important risk factor for the development of occupational asthma. Atopy and concurrent smoking are risk factors for IgE-mediated hypersensitivities but do not appear to influence IgE-independent processes. Patients may develop occupational asthma early in the course of antigen exposure or may develop symptoms after 10 years of exposure.

Pathologic airway changes characterized by inflammatory cell infiltrates (primarily eosinophils), edema, hypertrophy of smooth muscle, subepithelial fibrosis, and obstruction of airway lumen by exudate or mucus are similar for patients with occupational asthma as for patients with other forms of asthma.

In principle, any agent that causes occupational asthma could also cause allergic rhinitis. Rhinitis has been reported in association with exposure to protein allergens including laboratory animal proteins, castor beans, and insect allergens, as well as with exposure to low-molecular-weight materials such as the isocyanates and anhydrides.

**Hypersensitivity pneumonitis** is a parenchymal pulmonary disease resulting from sensitization and subsequent exposure to a variety of inhalant organic dusts and related occupational antigens. Sensitization to bacterial products, small amounts of serum present in the excreta of animals, thermophilic actinomycetes (eg, *M faeni, T vulgaris,* and *Thermoactinomyces sacchari*), fungi, and vegetable proteins has produced hypersensitivity pneumonitis. Examples include pi-

geon breeder's disease, farmer's lung, humidifier lung, and bagassosis. Occupational agents demonstrated to induce hypersensitivity pneumonitis include the diisocyanates found in most polyurethane paints, foams, and coatings and epoxies in most plastics. Hypersensitivity pneumonitis due to plastics appears to have a more insidious course than does the classic farmer's lung. Prolonged treatment with systemic steroids may be required to clear inflammation and ventilatory impairment. The incidence varies with the type and frequency of antigen exposure and is not age-dependent. Sensitization is favored by the alveolar deposition of particulate antigen less than 5 µm in diameter.

In its acute form associated with short-term high-level exposure to antigen, the disease is characterized by fever, cough, dyspnea, and myalgias, which occur 4–12 hours after heavy exposure and remit within hours to days. The subacute or chronic form of the disease is associated with long-term, low-level antigen exposure and induces an insidious onset of symptoms and eventually an irreversible restrictive ventilatory impairment.

Possible immune mechanisms operative in hypersensitivity pneumonitis include (1) a type III Arthus reaction, in which specific antibody binds to antigen, forming immune complexes that in turn activate the complement system; (2) a type IV reaction, in which sensitized T cells bind to antigen and then release lymphokines; (3) nonspecific activation of immune hypersensitivity by lectins and lipopolysaccharide products of organic matter; and (4) any combination of the above.

There is evidence both to support and reject the concept that hypersensitivity pneumonitis is a type III reaction. Up to 90% of patients have antigen-specific precipitins in their serum. However, 50% of similarly exposed asymptomatic subjects also have precipitins to the same antigens, which suggests that the precipitins may merely be markers of antigen exposure. Passive transfer of serum from a rabbit with hypersensitivity pneumonitis to a nonsensitized rabbit and subsequent aerosol challenge with antigen has failed to induce the reaction, suggesting that a type III response may not be operative in this species.

Recent evidence suggests that a type IV or cell-mediated immune reaction to inhaled antigen may be important in hypersensitivity pneumonitis. Histopathologic study of the lesions reveals infiltration with neutrophils, lymphocytes, and macrophages; noncaseating granulomas, giant cells, and fibrosis may be present. Granuloma formation favors the diagnosis of cell-mediated immune reaction; however, this may also be induced by nonphagocytosed antigen-antibody complexes. The lymphocytes of sensitized patients release cytokines when exposed to specific antigen. Experimentally, lesions resembling alveolitis can be induced by first sensitizing rabbits using methods favoring a cell-mediated immune response and then challenging with inhaled antigen. Furthermore, when rabbits were passively sensitized by lymphocytes from sensitized rabbits and then challenged, typical lesions consistent with alveolitis developed. These studies favor a type IV response.

It is possible that nonimmune activation of effector mechanisms of hypersensitivity may be operative. Lipopolysaccharides found in the cell walls of certain bacteria and fungi may directly activate the alternative complement pathway, leading to the release of anaphylatoxins that are also chemotactic for phagocytes. Lipopolysaccharides stimulate lymphocytes to release cytokines, including lymphocytotoxins and macrophage activators, resulting in local tissue inflammation and necrosis. Although this mechanism may play a part in hypersensitivity pneumonitis, it probably is not a primary role; studies demonstrate that sensitization must take place before a reaction occurs. It may be that hypersensitivity pneumonitis is a combination of a type III and a type IV immune response, possibly enhanced by nonimmune activation of effector mechanisms.

Although the diagnosis used to rely on finding IgG antibodies against offending agents, efforts now focus on finding an intense alveolar lymphocytosis on bronchoalveolar lavage. Lavage fluid in hypersensitivity pneumonitis is marked by increased numbers of CD8$^+$ T cells, which often help distinguish the syndrome from sarcoidosis, in which CD4$^+$ T cells predominate, and idiopathic pulmonary fibrosis, which is characterized by a neutrophilic infiltration.

**Contact dermatitis** is a type IV reaction that usually occurs when low-molecular-weight (< MW 500) sensitizers acting as haptens first bind to proteins in the dermis to form a complete antigen. The complex in turn is recognized and bound by sensitized T cells

that release lymphokines, some of which activate macrophages. The most common agents are Rhus antigens, latex, and nickel. (See Type IV: Cellular Immunity.)

## ANTIGENS INDUCING OCCUPATIONAL IMMUNE HYPERSENSITIVITY DISORDERS

Antigens inducing occupational immune hypersensitivity disorders may be of animal, vegetable, or chemical origin. Table 14–4 lists and classifies reactions caused by a number of these agents. Immune hypersensitivity reactions occur when a sensitized worker encounters antigens in the work environment.

### Animal Products

Occupational exposure to animal products may cause a type I immediate response manifested by symptoms of acute or chronic asthma and rhinitis. Animal danders and excreta, insects, shellfish, and animal enzymes have all been shown to induce IgE antibodies and type I reactions. Cat dander and saliva and dog dander antigens may induce occupational allergies in veterinarians and animal handlers. Mouse urine and rabbit and guinea pig epithelia may sensitize laboratory workers and cause respiratory allergy. Of 5641 workers who were exposed to animals at 137 laboratory animal facilities in Japan, about one-quarter had one or more allergic symptoms related to laboratory animals, most commonly rhinitis. About 70% of workers developed symptoms during their first 3 years of exposure. The presence of atopy, the number of animal species handled, and the time spent in handling correlated significantly with the development of allergy. Bovine epithelial and urinary proteins have been demonstrated to cause asthma and rhinitis in farmers, as defined by immunologic tests and bronchial or nasal provocation. Insects including the red spider mite and other arthropods have induced occupational allergic disease in technicians and pest control workers.

Alcalase, derived from *B subtilis,* is used in the manufacture of detergents in Great Britain and was at one time so used in the United States. As a result of daily exposure, atopic workers are particularly predisposed to sensitization and the development of IgE-mediated type I respiratory symptoms.

### Vegetable Products

Castor bean, soy bean, and green coffee bean dust are potent antigens for some people, inducing a type I immediate response manifested as rhinitis and asthma. There are reports of patients living near castor bean processing plants who have developed severe asthma secondary to wind shifts resulting in inhalation of minute amounts of this dust. The inhalation of soybean dust released during the unloading of soybeans into a silo has caused outbreaks of asthma in Spain. Installing filters on silos to prevent airborne dissemination of allergenic soybean dust eliminated these outbreaks. It is estimated that 10% of workers handling green coffee beans develop IgE-mediated symptoms, especially oculorhinitis. The antigenic potency of the green coffee bean is destroyed by roasting. Workers who have an adverse immune response to green coffee dust are able to handle the roasted beans without difficulty.

An increasingly common problem and growing public health threat is hypersensitivity to natural rubber latex antigens derived from the commercial rubber tree *Hevea brasiliensis*. Between 1989 and 1993, the US Food and Drug Administration received more than 1100 reports of injury and 15 deaths associated with latex allergy. Latex is a complex intracellular product, the essential functional unit of which is the rubber particle, a spherical droplet of polyisoprene coated with a layer of protein, lipid, and phospholipid. Latex antigens coat the surface of a number of common products including gloves, catheters, balloons, and condoms. Immediate hypersensitivity reactions include systemic urticaria, rhinitis, conjunctivitis, bronchospasm, and anaphylaxis and may occur following cutaneous, percutaneous, mucosal, or parenteral contact. Aerosol transmission of antigen has also been reported. Workers at risk of latex allergy include health care workers and rubber industry workers. Risk factors for sensitization include increased exposure and atopy.

Five percent of workers in the Western United States cedar lumber industry develop asthma after a latent period of exposure that averages about 3–4 years. They exhibit bronchospasm to inhalation challenge with plicatic acid, a low-molecular-weight derivative of red cedar. Skin testing and RAST demonstrate IgE sensitivity in approximately 50% of affected workers, but positive results are also found in unaffected workers. Atopy does not predispose workers to sensitization. It is possible that some cases are due to IgE-mediated processes.

Colophony, a pine resin by-product (rosin) used as solder flux, has been shown to cause both immediate and dual respiratory reactions in sensitized workers. The reaction is probably IgE-mediated.

In the United States, the most common agent causing occupational dermatitis is the oil from plants of the genus *Rhus* (poison oak, poison ivy, and poison sumac). Poison oak is found west of the Rocky Mountains; poison ivy and poison sumac are found to the east. The active principle is pentadecylcatechol, a low-molecular-weight substance that binds to one of the skin proteins, forming a complete antigen. Studies reveal that over 90% of subjects are sensitized on exposure to these antigens. A subject will develop a type IV allergic contact dermatitis reaction 24–72 hours after challenge.

Respiratory symptoms secondary to exposure to flour dust occur in bakers. The mean annual incidence of occupational respiratory diseases among bakery workers over a 10-year period in Finland was reported to be 374 per 100,000 workers, compared with a rate of 31 per 100,000 workers in general. Affected workers may exhibit (1) an immediate or (2) an immediate followed by a late-onset reaction; both are probably IgE-mediated. There is a direct relation between duration of exposure and the percentage of bakers who exhibit skin test reactivity.

## Chemical Agents

Workers in industrial plants may be exposed to a wide variety of chemical agents. Two that have been extensively studied are the isocyanates and anhydrides. Isocyanates are used in the manufacture of pesticides, polyurethane foams, and synthetic varnishes. There are many case reports of obstructive airway problems related to TDI. These occur with equal frequency in atopic and nonatopic workers. The mechanism of obstructive airway disease has not been elucidated, but some hypotheses to explain the pathogenesis include the following:

(1) **An irritant effect:** Evidence opposed to this hypothesis includes the latent period observed in many cases and the fact that all workers are not affected.

(2) **Beta-adrenergic blockade:** In vitro studies demonstrate that TDI acts as a weak β-adrenergic blocking agent.

(3) **Immune hypersensitivity response:** This is suggested by the insidious onset of symptoms after a latency period of weeks to months, peripheral eosinophilia, and the induction of symptoms in sensitized workers on reexposure to minute quantities of the material. RAST and skin testing with a conjugate of a low-molecular-weight isocyanate with human serum albumin have demonstrated specific IgE antibodies and in some cases IgG antibodies; however, because the antibodies can be demonstrated in affected and nonaffected workers, they probably correlate with exposure and not with clinical disease.

TMA is used in the manufacture of plastics, epoxy resins, and paints. TMA dust or fumes have been associated with four clinical syndromes. In the **TMA immediate-type reaction,** the patient may have rhinitis, conjunctivitis, or asthma. The reaction requires a latent period of exposure before the onset of symptoms. IgE antibodies to trimellityl-human serum albumin (TMHSA) conjugates have been demonstrated. Although affected workers have no atopic predisposition, this is probably a type I reaction.

The **late reacting-systemic syndrome** ("TMA

flu") is characterized by cough, occasional wheezing, dyspnea, and systemic symptoms of malaise, chills, myalgia, and arthralgia. These reactions occur 4–6 hours after exposure to TMA. This may be a type III disorder in which immune complexes of IgG antibody and TMA protein conjugates are operative. Repeated exposure and a latent period of weeks to months are required before symptoms develop. IgG antibodies to TMHSA have been demonstrated.

The **pulmonary disease-anemia syndrome** develops after exposure to TMA fumes. It occurs after repeated high-dose exposure to the volatile fumes of TMA sprayed on heated metal surfaces to prevent corrosion. A Coombs-positive hemolytic anemia and respiratory failure are evident. This is an example of a type II cytotoxic reaction in which antibodies are directed toward TMA bound to erythrocytes and pulmonary basement membrane. High titers of IgG antibody to TMHSA and to a trimellityl-erythrocyte conjugate have been demonstrated.

The **irritant respiratory syndrome** occurs with the first high-dose exposure to TMA powder and fumes. Patients develop cough and dyspnea. Immune sensitization toward TMA conjugates has not been demonstrated.

Hexahydrophthalic anhydride (HHPA) is a component of some epoxy resin systems. A high fraction of HHPA-exposed workers display nasal symptoms, and some of them have specific serum antibodies. Eleven subjects, who were IgE sensitized against an HHPA-human serum albumin (HSA) conjugate and who reported work-related nasal symptoms, had a significant increase of nasal symptoms and a decrease of nasal inspiratory peak flow after HHPA-HSA nasal provocation. The symptoms were associated with the presence of specific serum IgE and significant increases in eosinophil and neutrophil counts and in levels of tryptase and albumin in nasal lavage fluid, suggesting an IgE-mediated syndrome. Nine subjects who were not sensitized but complained of work-related symptoms and 11 subjects who were not sensitized and had no symptoms displayed no changes in any of these parameters following challenge. Another study reported that risk factors for the development of immunologically mediated respiratory disease due to HHPA in 57 exposed workers included exposure level and the development of specific IgE or IgG antibodies.

Metallic salts are an important cause of immune hypersensitivity. After poison oak, nickel is the most common cause of contact dermatitis, a type IV reaction. There are reports of asthma, probably on a type I IgE basis, secondary to exposure to fumes of nickel and platinum salts. It is thought that these salts acting as haptens binding with body proteins cause the induction of IgE immune sensitivity and, on subsequent exposure, bronchial asthma.

## UNPROVEN & CONTROVERSIAL PRACTICES

Many patients complain of malaise and dysesthesia not associated with any measurable or demonstrable organ dysfunction. Practitioners of "clinical ecology" espouse the belief that many of these patients suffer from the controversial "syndrome of multiple chemical sensitivities." This syndrome is defined by clinical ecologists as an acquired disorder of recurrent symptoms involving multiple organ systems that is a response to exposure to a multitude of unrelated chemical compounds at doses below those generally regarded as safe in the general populace. Moreover, it is accepted by many of these practitioners that no single test of physiologic function correlates with symptoms. Disagreements between the traditional medical community and practitioners of clinical ecology center around the absence of any well-documented, controlled, reproducible studies that demonstrate that the dysesthesia is due to chemical exposures rather than to a misdiagnosed underlying disease (eg, endocrinopathy, cancer, collagen vascular disease) or an undiagnosed psychiatric disorder. Such misdiagnosis can lead to significant cost in unnecessary diagnostic studies, litigation, morbidity, and even mortality. A full discussion of the issues surrounding this controversial aspect of occupational medicine is fully discussed in Chapter 45. The following discussion will focus on the controversial procedures and practices often used in the diagnosis or treatment of the syndrome of "multiple chemical sensitivity."

Table 14–5 lists the unproven and inappropriate tests and therapies often used by practitioners of clinical ecology. An unproven test is one that lacks proven validity and has not be subjected to properly designed, placebo-controlled, randomized clinical trials. **Unproven procedures** are tests or therapies incapable of diagnosing or treating any disease. Some of the tests and therapies are modifications of valid tests and therapies for well-specified existing allergic or immunologic disorders. **Inappropriate procedures** are those technically capable of diagnosing or treating an illness but not necessarily the symptoms experienced by the patient. Proponents of the inappropriate use of these tests and therapies claim they are valid because they are used by "traditional" or "establishment" physicians. It is crucial that the physician specializing in occupational medicine try to educate such patients that any diagnostic test or therapy *can* be misused (eg, spinal radiographs to diagnose cardiac or gastrointestinal dis-

**Table 14–5.** Unproven and inappropriate tests and therapies.

| Test or Therapy | Unproven | Inappropriate |
|---|---|---|
| **I. Test** | | |
| Provocation neutralization | To determine nonspecific reactivity to an "offending" agent | |
| Applied kinesiology | To determine allergic reactivity to a food or chemical | |
| Cytotoxic leukocyte testing | To determine allergic reactivity to a food | |
| Electrodiagnosis | To determine allergic reactivity to a food | |
| Body/breath chemical analysis | To detect toxic chemicals in the body to account for symptoms | Diagnosis of "environmental" illness |
| Hair analysis | To detect toxic chemicals in the body to account for symptoms | Diagnosis of "environmental" illness |
| IgG antibodies, or circulating immune complexes | | Diagnosis of food allergy |
| Lymphocyte subsets, immunoglobulins, other immune system function tests | | Alleged "multiple chemical sensitivity" without signs or symptoms of immunodeficiency |
| Pulse rate changes | | Diagnosis of chemical, food, or alleged "food allergy" |
| Uncontrolled chamber challenges | | Responses to putative offending agents |
| **II. Therapy** | | |
| Neutralization therapy | To "neutralize" symptoms caused by intake of offending agent | |
| Rotation diets | To prevent "sensitization" to a given food | |
| Acupuncture | To relieve allergic symptoms | |
| Orthomolecular therapy | To correct presumed deficiency of vitamins and/or minerals; to cure certain diseases | |
| Homeopathic remedies | To prevent or cure disease | |
| Removal of mercury amalgam | To treat mercury-induced symptoms or fatigue, malaise, etc. | |
| Multiple food elimination diets/ chemical avoidance | To "boost" the immune response | "Boosting the immune system" |
| Anti-*Candida* therapy | | "Treatment" of alleged release of immunotoxins from normal *Candida albicans* body flora |
| Clinical ecology | | Symptoms allegedly arising from low-level exposure to organic and inorganic environmental chemicals (see Chapter 45) |
| Detoxification therapy | | Symptoms allegedly arising from low-level exposure to organic and inorganic environmental chemicals (see Chapter 45) |

ease, thyroid hormone therapy in euthyroid patients for the treatment of fatigue).

**Provocation-neutralization testing.** This test is supposed to determine the patient's sensitivity to a food, chemical, or allergen extract. In this procedure, a test dose of the putatively offending substance is administered orally, sublingually, or parenterally. Any and all subjective symptom responses occurring over a specified period are deemed a positive challenge. Subsequent challenges with the same substance are then administered at different doses until the patient's symptoms are "neutralized." One double-blind, placebo-controlled study failed to demonstrate different responses between the test foods and placebo responses in patients who previously, in an unblinded challenge, had responded positively to antigen and negatively to controls. There is no scientific validity to this test. Patients and their care providers must be cautious not to succumb to the power of suggestion.

**Applied kinesiology,** This test is supposed to determine a patient's allergic reactivity to a food or chemical. In this test, a technician subjectively tests the muscle strength of the upper extremities before and after placing against the patient's skin a sealed glass vial that contains an allergen. A positive reaction is demonstrated by a "weakening" of the skeletal musculature. There is no scientifically valid rationale for performing this test and no proof of its ability to determine allergic reactivity.

**Cytotoxic leukocyte testing.** This test is reputed to determine allergic reactivity to foods. An unstained drop of whole blood or buffy coat cells is placed on a microscope slide pre-coated with a food extract. Without specification of time, temperature, pH, or osmolarity, the slide is then examined under the microscope. Vacuolation, crenation, or any distortion of the cellular morphology represents a positive test for food allergy. There is no scientifically valid rationale for this test because allergic reactions to foods do not result in cytotoxicity. Moreover, double-blind controlled studies have not demonstrated reproducible results.

**Electrodiagnosis.** The theory behind this test is that an alleged allergic reaction will cause changes in electrical resistance in the skin. An extract of the impugned food is sealed in a glass container that is in contact with an aluminum plate and is inserted in a "circuit" between the skin and a galvanometer. Practitioners of electrodiagnosis claim that the measurement of electrical resistance on the skin surface is useful for the diagnosis of allergy. There are no data validating the effectiveness of this test procedure.

**Body, breath, and hair chemical analysis.** In these tests, practitioners believe that some chemicals that are "normal" constituents of the body or its metabolism are potentially harmful. These chemicals can be detected in the blood, breath samples, or hair specimens, and they provide evidence of exposures that may correlate with a symptom complex. From this, these practitioners infer causality. These tests are frequently reported at extraordinarily low levels (in parts per quadrillion) and are plagued by a multitude of false results; the most common source of error is contamination of the samples by improper handling or storage.

Body chemical analyses are examples not only of unproven procedures but also of **inappropriate tests.** Inappropriate tests are those that have clear diagnostic value for specific clinical conditions but have no value for the specific disorder they are being used to diagnose. Although hair and breath sample analyses are of no proven validity in the diagnosis of "environmental illness," these tests can be of significant clinical utility in the diagnosis of certain diseases in which the results have been previously validated. Thus, the commercial application of these tests not only is without validation but also is neither economically nor medically beneficial to patients.

Other examples of inappropriately utilized tests include the quantitative or qualitative measurement of serum immunoglobulins or circulating immune complexes for the diagnosis of food allergy; the assessment of lymphocyte subsets and other quantitative immunologic parameters in patients with symptoms of "environmental" or "ecologic" disease in the absence of symptoms or signs of autoimmune or immunodeficiency disease; the measurement of pulse rate changes as an indication of "allergic" reaction to a chemical, food, or other substance; the uncontrolled provocative challenge of patients without prespecified, objective end points, or the exposure to "irritant" doses of the alleged offending agent in a nonblinded, nonplacebo-controlled fashion.

**Neutralization therapy.** This is an unproven therapy in which a patient who has undergone provocation-neutralization testing then self administers (either subcutaneously or sublingually) each antigen at a concentration that "neutralized" the symptoms which were provoked by the provocation testing. Patients are advised to administer the antigen to either prevent or acutely treat symptoms. Patients responding will report that any symptom will respond to treatment, although there is no immunologic or physiologic basis of validity and any anecdotal responses can only be attributed to the nature of suggestion.

**Rotation diets.** The theory behind this unproven therapy is that the patient is intolerant (or allergic) to all foods and that eating a food frequently increases the patient's reactivity to that food. Patients on this diet rotate the foods consumed, not eating the same food more frequently than every 4–5 days. The rotation diet has not been demonstrated to be efficacious in controlled studies.

**Acupuncture.** This has a clearly accepted place as a therapeutic modality in the control of many forms of pains. Some practitioners however, have championed the use of acupuncture for the treatment of allergic symptoms. This therapy has not been scientifically scrutinized for efficacy in the treatment of allergic diseases.

**Orthomolecular therapy.** This therapy involves the supplemental administration of vitamins, minerals, enzymes, and amino acids in large quantities. Often, these supplements are given without objective rationale on the basis of the belief that they will correct any presumed deficiency or possibly cure certain disease (eg, cancer). Although there are no objective data to support the use of high doses of these supplements, practitioners often tout the merits of such therapies on the basis of "intuitive" reasoning.

**Mercury amalgam.** Many practitioners of clinical ecology and even some dentists claim that some patients develop an ill-defined hyperreactive state to the silver-mercury amalgam in dental fillings. Although this type of dental filling has been used for over a century, these practitioners claim that the mercury in the fillings is the cause of a wide variety of nonspecific medical and psychiatric symptoms. This unsubstantiated theory has led to the unnecessary removal of a large number of fillings. There is no scientific validity to the claims, although it is important to note that mercury salts do very rarely cause a contact dermatitis.

**Multiple food elimination diets or chemical avoidance diets.** These diets and avoidance measures are based on belief that the elimination of multiple foods will, by some undefined mechanism, "boost" the immune system. The selection of foods to be eliminated is based on the diagnosis of multiple food allergy by one of the unproven methods previously described. These diets are frequently recommended to patients allegedly suffering from the "syndrome of multiple chemical sensitivities." There are no scientifically derived data to substantiate the effectiveness of these diets.

*Candida* **hypersensitivity syndrome.** Treatment for the unsubstantiated syndrome involves the use of antifungal drugs to treat overgrowth of *Candida albicans,* a normal member of the human flora. The theory behind this treatment is that *Candida albicans* releases an "immunotoxin" that causes a multitude of symptoms. The diagnosis of the *Candida* hypersensitivity syndrome is based on responses to a questionnaire and the absence of physical or laboratory findings that define the syndrome. In addition to the use of oral or parenteral antifungal agents, patients are subjected to sugar-free, yeast-free rotation diets. There are no scientifically valid data to support the existence of the syndrome or the effectiveness of the proposed treatment regimen.

It is important for physicians specializing in occupational medicine to fully understand the basis and theories behind the unproven or inappropriate procedures and therapies used by many practitioners of clinical ecology so as to be able to inform patients about the validity and utility of the tests and treatments recommended. It is particularly important to recognize that a patient's perception of symptoms is that patient's reality, and every effort should be made to generate appropriate and effective diagnostic and treatment plans.

The California Medical Association Scientific Board Task Force on Clinical Ecology reviewed this subject in 1985, and their conclusion best summarizes the scientific knowledge to date: "No convincing evidence was found that patients treated by clinical ecologists have unique, recognizable syndromes, that the diagnostic tests employed are efficacious and reliable, or that the treatments used are effective."

# DIAGNOSIS OF HYPERSENSITIVITY DISEASES IN OCCUPATIONAL MEDICINE

From the standpoint of both the patient and the employer, it is important to establish an early diagnosis. Many obstructive pulmonary problems that are reversible with proper early management become fixed disabilities with prolonged exposure to offending agents. Diagnosis of occupational hypersensitivity diseases should include both the diagnosis of the hypersensitivity disease and the establishment of a relationship between the disease and the workplace. The requirements for establishing the relationship to work are generally more stringent for medical situations than for field epidemiologic surveys. Although it is often possible to demonstrate a pattern of symptoms and signs suggesting occupational illness, confirmatory tests for occupational hypersensitivity diseases are generally not available. Occupational hypersensitivity diseases should be suspected in a person exposed at work to agents known to cause occupational disease, although the failure to identify a known agent does not rule out the disorder. An occupational history regarding possible past and current exposures should be obtained, since early exposure to an agent may have induced chronic asthma.

## HISTORY & PHYSICAL EXAMINATION

The initial work-up should include a detailed history and physical examination and, when indicated, a complete chest film, and pulmonary function evaluation blood count, sputum or nasal smear for eosinophils, chest film, and pulmonary evaluation (Figure 14–4).

The type of symptoms, aggravating and relieving factors, their temporal relationship with the work environment, and the effects of vacation and weekends should be noted. A history of improvement of symptoms during weekends and holidays and a worsening on return to work suggests but does not confirm occupational hypersensitivity disease. Late-onset respiratory reactions may not occur until a patient has returned home from work. The personal or family history of atopy (hay fever, allergic asthma, or atopic dermatitis) should be investigated. If there is bronchospasm, it is important to review medications the patient is currently receiving, including beta-block-

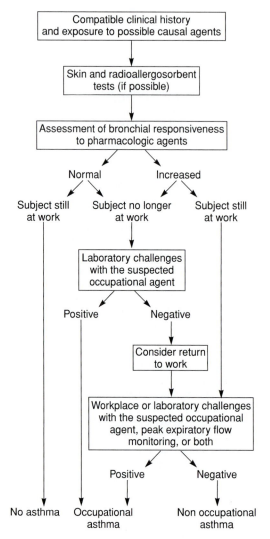

**Figure 14–4.** Algorithm for the clinical investigation of occupational asthma. (Reproduced with permission from Chan-Yeung M, Malo JL: Occupational Asthma. N Engl J Med 1995;333:107.)

ers, aspirin, and nonsteroidal anti-inflammatory drugs, all of which may induce bronchial asthma; acetylcholinesterase inhibitors may cause cough. The home environment should be reviewed, including any changes that have occurred, the presence of pets and molds, any recent moves, hobbies, and the use of tobacco by the patient or others in the household. Finally, a detailed occupational history should be elicited, including information regarding present and past employment. The assessment should include a detailed history of specific job duties and work processes for both the patient and coworkers. The frequency and intensity of exposures and peak concentrations of potential agents should be assessed. The investigator should review safety data sheets for

chemicals in the workplace, industrial hygiene data, and employee health records.

At times it is helpful—with the permission of the employer—to visit the work site.

Physical examination should include evaluation of the skin and the upper and lower respiratory tracts. Evidence of atopy should be sought, including the presence of allergic facies, cobblestoning of the conjunctiva, pale and boggy mucous membranes, posterior pharyngeal lymphoid plaques, expiratory wheezing, and signs of atopic dermatitis. Evidence of clubbing, increased anteroposterior diameter of the chest, and the location and quality of skin rashes should be noted. Other causes of the patient's symptoms must be ruled out.

## LABORATORY INVESTIGATION

The diagnosis of occupational disease should be confirmed by objective data.

A **complete blood count** demonstrating evidence of eosinophilia may aid in the diagnosis of atopy. The presence of eosinophilia on a stained smear of **sputum or nasal secretions** is consistent with asthma and allergic rhinitis, respectively. **Total serum IgE** level is often elevated in atopic patients, although this test is neither sensitive nor specific for establishing the diagnosis of atopy.

A baseline **posteroanterior and lateral x-ray of the chest** should be obtained in patients with pulmonary problems, noting increased anteroposterior chest diameter, flattening of the diaphragms, infiltrates, evidence of bronchiectasis, hyperaeration, and diffuse micronodularity.

**Pulmonary function studies** before and after bronchodilator administration should be obtained in the case of pulmonary disorders; at a minimum, they should include forced expiratory volume in 1 second ($FEV_1$), forced vital capacity (FVC), forced expiratory flow between 25% and 75% of FVC ($FEF_{25-75}$), and peak expiratory flow rate (PEFR). Complete pulmonary function tests including lung volumes and diffusion capacity (DLCO) determination may be helpful in ruling out a restrictive component of lung disease.

Measurements of blood gases may prove helpful (see Chapter 20).

Measurement of **bronchial hyperresponsiveness to pharmacologic agents** including methacholine or histamine is an important step in the diagnostic workup. Hypersensitivity to pharmacologic agents is helpful in establishing increased bronchial irritability in patients who present with an atypical history for asthma, eg, cough as a sole manifestation of lung disease. Asthmatics are up to 1000 times more sensitive than normal individuals to methacholine challenge. The absence of bronchial hyperresponsiveness after a person has worked for 2 weeks under normal working conditions virtually rules out the diagnosis of occupational asthma. The presence of bronchial hyperresponsiveness requires further testing to define the relationship of asthma to the workplace. Sensitization to antigen and pharmacologically induced bronchial hyperresponsiveness are associated with an 80% likelihood of immediate hypersensitivity to antigen in laboratory challenge.

## IMMUNOLOGIC TESTS

Based on the initial evaluation, specific immunologic tests may be ordered. These include immediate allergy skin tests, patch tests, in vitro tests for IgE antibody, Ouchterlony gel diffusion tests, and provocative challenge with specific antigens.

### Skin Tests
Epicutaneous (prick) and intradermal skin tests are helpful in establishing sensitivity to a number of inhalant protein antigens, including molds, house dusts, animal danders, feathers, pollens, and extracts of suspected large-molecular-weight antigens in the work environment. Standardized occupational allergens are not commercially available at present.

Low-molecular-weight materials usually do not give a positive immediate skin test response unless they are linked to a protein carrier such as human serum albumin. The initial wheal-and-flare reaction may be followed in 4–6 hours by an IgE-mediated late phase reaction evidenced by erythema, induration, pruritus, and tenderness at the skin test site.

### Patch Testing
Patch tests are useful in evaluating skin contact sensitivity (type IV delayed hypersensitivity). The test employs standard antigen-impregnated patches applied to the skin. They are removed after 24–48 hours. A positive reaction consists of erythema, induration, and in some cases vesiculation. In addition to antigens available in the standard antigen patch test kit obtained from the American Academy of Dermatology, suspected materials may be utilized from the work environment (see Chapter 18).

### In Vitro Antibody Tests
RAST and ELISA are in vitro procedures used to detect antigen-specific IgE antibody. In these tests, inert particles coated with antigen are incubated with serum. If specific antibody is present, it binds to antigen on the surface of the particles. The complex is washed, incubated with radiolabeled or enzyme-labeled anti-IgE, and then washed again. The amount of anti-IgE measured by radioactivity or enzyme activity determines the amount of specific IgE antibody attached to the antigen.

### Ouchterlony Gel Diffusion Test
This test is used to demonstrate IgG precipitating antibody to antigen. Suspected antigens and the patient's serum are placed in separate wells cut into a gel-coated plate. The antigen and serum diffuse toward one another. If sufficient antibody is present, precipitin lines composed of antigen-antibody complexes form at some intermediate point. This test is helpful in type III reactions.

### Inhalation Challenge Tests
These tests are conducted by exposing the worker to the suspected antigen. *Caution:* Inhalation challenge studies are not without risk. Sensitized patients are susceptible to late-onset asthmatic reactions that may develop up to 12 hours after the initial challenge. These reactions are often refractory to bronchodilator treatment.

The challenge may be performed in the work environment or in a hospital laboratory situation. The patient probably should be hospitalized and observed for 12–24 hours after a laboratory challenge.

**A. Work Challenge:** The patient is instructed to monitor and record peak expiratory flow for 2 weeks while at work and for an additional 2 weeks while away from work. There is good correlation with specific inhalation challenge; however, this method is subject to patient bias and effort. Combining measurement of peak flow with serial measurements of bronchial hyperresponsiveness does not appear to improve sensitivity or specificity. The use of computerized peak flow meters may improve accuracy but does not correct for patient effort. If initial peak flow monitoring is suggestive of occupational asthma, a technician may be sent to the workplace to monitor hourly spirometry during the workday.

**B. Laboratory Inhalation Challenge:** This can be obtained in three ways: (1) After the worker's condition is stabilized off work, baseline tests are obtained; the worker is placed in a closed environment and asked to transfer suspected antigen dust, mixed in lactose powder, back and forth between two trays. (2) In another variation, the subject, in a hospital setting, is exposed to various volatile agents (eg, solder, varnish) by actually working with the materials. In each of these challenges, pulmonary function tests are obtained immediately before and for several hours after exposure. (3) Aerosol inhalation challenge involves the administration of gradually increasing amounts of aerosolized suspected material while pulmonary function tests are monitored. A 20% or greater fall in $FEV_1$ is considered a positive response. False-negative inhalation challenge test results may occur if the incorrect agent or dose is used or if the patient has had an extended absence from work and has lost bronchial hyperresponsiveness.

## TREATMENT

The diagnosis of occupational hypersensitivity disease has considerable economic implications for the worker and his or her family, the employers, and government agencies. Complete removal of the worker from the workplace environment may be ideal but may place considerable economic hardships on all involved. An attempt may be made to retrain workers for other roles within the same company or with another employer, to reduce exposure by improving ventilation or providing a respirator, or to make changes in the workplace to abide by existing laws. Public health agencies should be enlisted to begin surveillance programs when index cases have

been identified. Patients who return to the same workplace require close medical monitoring and follow-up. Even after removal from the workplace, patients may continue to have chronic airway disease and require the use of medications. Experience with western red cedar (plicatic acid), TDI, and other low-molecular-weight substances reveals that at least half of the patients will continue to have persistent, even worsening asthma despite removal from the source of exposure. Duration of symptoms greater than 6 months before removal is a strong risk factor for progressive disease even after removal from the workplace. Worker impairment and disability should be evaluated to determine if appropriate compensation is available.

## REFERENCES

### GENERAL

Frank M et al (editors): *Samter's Immunologic Diseases,* 5th ed. Little, Brown, 1995.
Middleton E et al (editors): *Allergy, Principles and Practice,* 4th ed. Mosby, 1993.
Stites DP, Terr AI, Parslow TG: *Basic & Clinical Immunology,* 8th ed. Appleton & Lange, 1994.

### IMMUNE RESPONSE

Brodsky FM, Guagliardi LE: The cell biology of antigen processing and presentation. Annu Rev Immunol 1991;9:707.
Goodman JW: The immune response. In: *Basic & Clinical Immunology,* 8th ed. Stites DP, Terr AI, Parslow TG (editors). Appleton & Lange, 1994.
Podack ER, Kupfer A: T cell effector functions: Mechanisms for delivery of cytotoxicity and help. Annu Rev Immunol 1991;7:479.
Shames RS, Adelman DC: Disorders of the immune system. In: *Pathophysiology of Disease, An Introduction to Clinical Medicine.* McPhee SJ et al (editors). Appleton & Lange, 1995.

### IMMUNOGLOBULINS

Goodman JW, Parslow TG: Immunoglobulin proteins. In: *Basic & Clinical Immunology,* 8th ed. Stites DP, Terr AI, Parslow TG (editors). Appleton & Lange, 1994.
Rodgers JR, Rich RR: Molecular biology and immunology: An introduction. J Allergy Clin Immunol 1991; 88:535.
Vercelli DV, Geha RS: Regulation of IgE synthesis in humans: A tale of two signals. J Allergy Clin Immunol 1991;88:285.

### MEDIATORS OF IMMEDIATE HYPERSENSITIVITY

Holtzman MJ: Arachodonic acid metabolism. Am Rev Respir Dis 1991;143:188.
Romagnani S: Lymphokine production by human T

cells in disease states. Annu Rev Immunol 1994; 12:227.
Stevens RL, Austen KF: Recent advances in the cellular and molecular biology of mast cells. Immunol Today 1989;10:381.

### EFFECTOR CELLS OF IMMUNE HYPERSENSITIVITY

Gleich GJ, Adolphson CR, Keiferman KM: The biology of the eosinophilic leukocyte. Annu Rev Med 1993; 44:85.
Keller R: The macrophage response to infectious agents: Mechanisms of macrophage activation and tumor cell killing. Res Immunol 1993:144:271.
Ritz J: The role of natural killer cells in immune surveillance. N Engl J Med 1989;320:1748.
Stevens RL, Austen KF: Recent advances in the cellular and molecular biology of mast cells. Immunol Today 1989;10:381.

### COMPLEMENT

Frank MM: Complement and kinin. In: *Basic & Clinical Immunology,* 8th ed. Stites DP, Terr AI, Parslow TG (editors). Appleton & Lange, 1994.

### CLASSIFICATION OF IMMUNE HYPERSENSITIVITY DISORDERS

Barnes PJ: Pathophysiology of allergic inflammation. In: *Allergy, Principles and Practice,* 4th ed. Middleton E et al (editors). Mosby, 1993.
Engelfrie CP, Overbeeke MAM, von dern Borne AEG: Autoimmune hemolytic anemia. Semin Hematol 1992,29:3.
Frew AJ, Kay AB: Postgraduate course: Eosinophils and T-lymphocytes in late-phase allergic reactions. J Allergy Clin Immunol 1990;85:533.
Lawley TJ: Immune Complexes. In: *Samter's Immunologic Diseases* , 5th ed. Frank MM et al (editors). Little, Brown, 1994.

Lemanske RF: Late phase pulmonary reactions. J Asthma 1990;27:69.

Maibach HI, Dannaker CJ: Contact skin allergy. In: *Allergy, Principles and Practice,* 4th ed. Middleton E et al (editors). Mosby, 1993.

Waters AH: Autoimmune thrombocytopenia: Clinical aspects. Semin Hematol 1992;29:18.

**IMMUNE HYPERSENSITIVITY OCCUPATIONAL DISORDERS**

Chan-Yeung M, Malo JL: Occupational asthma. N Engl J Med 1995;333:107.

Cullen MR, Cherniack MG Rosenstock L: Occupational medicine. N Engl J Med 1990; 594:322.

Grammer LC: Occupational asthma. Immunol Allergy Clin North Am 1993;13:1.

Grammer LC et al: Risk factors for immunologically mediated respiratory disease from hexahydrophthalic anhydride. J Occup Med 1994;36:642.

Nilsson R et al: Asthma, rhinitis, and dermatitis in workers exposed to reactive dyes. Br J Ind Med 1993;50:65.

Reijula K, Patterson R: Occupational allergies in Finland in 1981–91. Allergy Proc 1994;15:163.

**ANTIGENS INDUCING OCCUPATIONAL IMMUNE HYPERSENSITIVITY DISORDERS**

Anto JM et al: Preventing asthma epidemics due to soybeans by dust-control measures. N Engl J Med 1993; 329:1760.

Aoyama K et al: Allergy to laboratory animals: An epidemiological study. Br J Ind Med 1992;49:41.

Lugo G et al: A new risk of occupational disease: Allergic asthma and rhinoconjunctivitis in persons working with beneficial arthropods. Preliminary data. Int Arch Occup Environ Health 1994;65:291.

Rasanen L et al: Comparison of immunologic tests in the diagnosis of occupational asthma and rhinitis. Allergy 1994;49:342.

Slater JE: Allergic reactions to natural rubber. Ann Allergy 1992;68:203.

**UNPROVEN & CONTROVERSIAL PRACTICES**

Jewett DL, Fein G, Greenberg MH: A double-blind study of symptom provocation to determine food sensitivity. N Engl J Med 1990;323:429.

**DIAGNOSIS OF HYPERSENSITIVITY DISEASES IN OCCUPATIONAL MEDICINE**

Bousquet J, Michel FB: In vivo methods for study of allergy: Skin tests, techniques and interpretation. In: *Allergy, Principles and Practice,* 4th ed. Middleton E et al (editors). Mosby, 1993.

Fish JE: In vivo methods for study of allergy: Mucosal tests, techniques and interpretation. In *Allergy, Principles and Practice,* 4th ed. Middleton E et al (editors). Mosby, 1993.

Grammer LC et al: Guidelines for the immunologic evaluation of occupational lung disease. J Allergy Clin Immunol 1989;84:805.

**TREATMENT & NATURAL HISTORY**

American Thoracic Society Ad Hoc Committee on Impairment/Disability Evaluation in Subjects with Asthma. Guidelines for the evaluation of impairment/disability in patients with asthma. Am Rev Respir Dis 1993;147:1056.

National Asthma Education Program: *Guidelines for the Diagnosis and Management of Asthma.* DHHS publication no. (NIH) 91-3042. Bethesda, Md: Public Health Service, 1991.

# 15

# Occupational Hematology

*Hope S. Rugo, MD, & Lloyd E. Damon, MD*

Occupationally related hematologic toxicity has occurred in cyclic fashion, historically associated with the development of the chemical industry and the advent of each World War. Common factors contributing to "epidemics" of toxicity have been the rapid introduction of many new chemicals and the exposure of large numbers of workers without adequate protection or education. As the toxicities of these agents gradually became known, regulation of their use was instituted, and exposure to some toxins such as radium has been eliminated. Hematologic toxins such as lead, benzene, arsenic, and arsine gas still exist; poisoning has still not been eliminated from the workplace; and worker education is still inadequate. As new chemicals are introduced and new products become available, it is important to be aware of potential mechanisms of toxicity so that the epidemic poisonings of the past will not be repeated.

Hematotoxicity has improved our understanding of hematologic pathophysiology, taught important pharmacologic lessons, and introduced the concept of individual susceptibility to specific toxic agents. Observation of individual variations in susceptibility to toxic agents was made by recognizing that chemicals with oxidative potential could cause cyanosis and a life-threatening hemolytic anemia in some individuals at exposure levels that had little effect on the population at large. The normal population will manifest similar toxicities, but only when exposed to much higher levels. It has therefore become important to identify workers with increased sensitivity to certain chemicals and place them in jobs with less risk of contact with these specific toxic substances.

Exposure to hematotoxins may affect blood cell survival (denaturation of hemoglobin and hemolysis), metabolism (porphyria), formation (aplasia), morphology and function (preleukemias and leukemias), or coagulation (thrombocytopenia).

# DISORDERS ASSOCIATED WITH SHORTENED RED BLOOD CELL SURVIVAL

## METHEMOGLOBINEMIA & HEMOLYSIS PRODUCED BY OXIDANT CHEMICALS

Methemoglobin is formed by the oxidation of ferrous ($Fe^{2+}$) hemoglobin to ferric ($Fe^{3+}$) hemoglobin. It was first recognized in the 1800s when coal tars were converted into individual chemicals that served as precursors for many products ranging from explosives to synthetic dyes and perfumes. Overexposure to these chemicals—which included anilines, nitrobenzenes, and quinones—was common, and little was known about their potential toxicity. Workers in these plants came to be known as "blue workers" or suffered from "blue lip" owing to the chronic cyanosis from toxic methemoglobinemia that developed in almost all of them. Gradually it was recognized that oxidation of hemoglobin was toxic to red blood cells and could be followed by an acute and life-threatening hemolysis known as Heinz body anemia. Heinz bodies are red blood cell inclusions that represent precipitated hemoglobin and are classically seen in individuals with a deficiency of glucose-6-phosphate dehydrogenase (G6PD) after exposure to an oxidant stress. Normal individuals exposed to large amounts of oxidant chemicals will develop methemoglobinemia and occasionally Heinz body hemolytic anemia. It is not understood why some chemicals may cause methemoglobinemia, hemolysis, or both, but the disorders are certainly related to individual susceptibility. Oxidative chemicals are common in industry, and it is important to know what toxic agents have been implicated, to recognize the presenting signs and symptoms, and to be able to provide appropriate treatment when it is needed.

Despite the understanding of this phenomenon

which developed in the 19th century, as new compounds were developed for each World War—eg, aniline and other coal tar derivatives, new cycles of toxicity were again seen. As new chemicals continue to be synthesized, awareness of their toxicity is necessary to avoid similar outbreaks of poisoning characterized by cyanosis and hemolysis. An understanding of the pathophysiology of this phenomenon is essential to correctly handle this medical emergency; it will also help in understanding the myriad of therapeutic agents that may cause oxidative hemolysis in a susceptible individual.

## Pathophysiology of Oxidant Hemolysis

Hemoglobin is unique in its ability to combine reversibly with oxygen without oxidizing its iron moiety. The small amount of oxidized hemoglobin or methemoglobin produced is readily reduced by an efficient enzyme system linked to energy provided by glucose metabolism via the Embden-Meyerhof pathway (Figure 15–1).

Methemoglobin is dangerous because of its inability to bind oxygen and because it increases the oxygen affinity of the remaining heme groups in hemoglobin tetramer, thereby decreasing oxygen delivery to the tissues. Oxidation results in denaturation of hemoglobin with the formation of precipitated hemoglobin (Heinz bodies) within the red cell. The presence of Heinz bodies alters the surface membrane of the red cell, causing increased rigidity and leakage. Macrophages in the reticuloendothelial system of the spleen and liver (the "extravascular" compartment) sense the altered red cell surface and pit out Heinz bodies via partial phagocytosis (extravascular hemolysis). Since the red cell surface is unable to reseal and form a spherocyte (as in autoimmune hemolysis), the red cell remains intact as a cell with a piece missing, the so-called bite, or blister, cell. Heinz bodies may also be formed from a second form of denatured hemoglobin, sulfhemoglobin. Unlike methemoglobin, sulfhemoglobin is irreversibly associated with the heme moiety.

The development of methemoglobinemia or oxidative hemolysis in an individual exposed to an oxidant stress is dependent on the route of exposure, the specific chemicals involved, the dose and duration of exposure, and, most importantly, individual susceptibility. Inborn structural abnormalities (unstable hemoglobins)—or, much more commonly, disorders of normal reducing capabilities such as the X-linked deficiency of the oxidation-reduction enzyme G6PD—cause some individuals to be much more susceptible to oxidant stress than others. There are many varieties of both of these abnormalities. Recognition of these high-risk individuals in the workplace is important to reduce their chance of particularly toxic exposures.

The normal individual has less than 1% circulating methemoglobin. Ninety-five percent of methemoglobin formed daily by the auto-oxidation of hemoglobin is reduced by $NADH_2$ generated by the dehydrogenation of phosphotriose by phosphotriose dehydrogenase. This reaction is catalyzed by NADH methemoglobin reductase (NADH cytochrome $b_5$ reductase). A rare inborn deficiency of NADH methemoglobin reductase results in congenital cyanosis due to methemoglobinemia (Figure 15–2).

An alternative methemoglobin reduction pathway exists, though it is a slow enzymatic reduction that is not physiologically functional without the presence of a redox cofactor, which may serve here as an electron carrier intermediate. In this reaction, NADPH from the first two steps of the hexose monophosphate shunt converts methemoglobin to reduced hemoglobin. Deficiency of the enzyme that catalyzes this reaction, NADPH methemoglobin reductase, does not result in methemoglobinemia or cyanosis. The formation of NADPH is dependent on G6PD. The presence of a redox agent such as methylene blue, which is used to treat toxic and congenital methemoglobinemia, can precipitate a hemolytic crisis in an individual with G6PD deficiency because of its own oxidative potential. In normal individuals, the administration of a redox agent may dramatically increase the rate of reduction of hemoglobin so that it greatly exceeds that of the NADH-methemoglobin reductase reaction (Figure 15–3). This is the rationale for the effectiveness of methylene blue in toxic methemoglobinemia.

Two other pathways exist, but they reduce methemoglobin only to a small extent. Glutathione is responsible for conversion of less than 7–10% of ferrihemoglobin to ferrohemoglobin, and ascorbic acid in

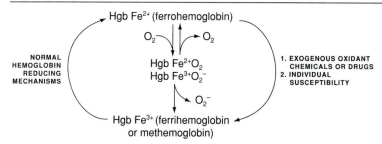

**Figure 15–1.** Oxidation of hemoglobin by the Embden-Meyerhof pathway.

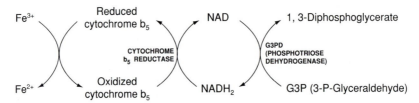

**Figure 15–2.** Reduction of hemoglobin by NADH methemoglobin reductase (NADH cytochrome $b_5$ reductase).

pharmacologic amounts will reduce oxidized hemoglobin. Because of the high redox potential of ascorbic acid, however, the rate of reduction is very slow, making it less effective in therapy. In physiologic concentrations, the contribution of ascorbic acid to methemoglobin reduction is insignificant.

## 1. ANILINE

Historically, most work-related episodes of methemoglobinemia and hemolytic anemia have been due to exposure to aromatic nitro and amino compounds. These compounds have been used most extensively as intermediates in the synthesis of aniline dyes; they are used also as accelerators and antioxidants in the rubber industry and in the production of pesticides, plastics, paints, and varnishes. Table 15–1 lists chemicals that have been associated with methemoglobinemia and their industrial uses. Many medicinal drugs are oxidants and can cause methemoglobinemia but will not be discussed here.

The clinical presentation of methemoglobinemia is exemplified by aniline toxicity. Aniline, used in the manufacture of dyes and in the rubber industry, is the most common and best-described aromatic amine. It is fat-soluble and readily penetrates the intact skin even through clothing. The vapor form may also gain entry to the body through the lungs. Ingestion is rare in the industrial setting but causes serious toxicity when it does occur. Aniline is converted by hepatic microsomes to phenylhydroxylamine, which behaves as a catalyst in mediating hemoglobin oxidation. Hepatic clearance of phenylhydroxylamine is slow because its oxidized form, nitrosobenzene, is rapidly converted back to phenylhydroxylamine. Another clearance pathway gradually eliminates the amine from the body.

## Clinical Presentation

Acute exposure is usually associated with spills or improper usage. Symptoms vary depending on the concentration of methemoglobin (Table 15–2). Most cases are mild and transient and present as asymptomatic blueness of the lips and nail beds. In more severe cases, the patient will appear deeply cyanotic. Freshly drawn blood appears dark maroon-brown and does not become red after exposure to air. Laboratory results reveal hypoxia and may indicate hemolysis with an elevated reticulocyte count and variable degree of anemia. Examination of the peripheral blood smear shows evidence of reticulocytosis (polychromasia, possibly nucleated red cells) and may show bite or blistered red cells.

In chronic methemoglobinemia, polycythemia may be seen in response to chronic hypoxia. Hemolytic Heinz body anemia may or may not accompany methemoglobin formation, or may follow resolution of cyanosis. Heinz bodies are easily detected by examining the peripheral blood smear stained by a supravital stain but will not be evident on a smear stained with Wright's stain. Blood methemoglobin levels should be monitored closely. Methemoglobin is measured in the laboratory as a characteristic spectrophotometric absorption band.

## Prevention

The most important safeguard in preventing oxidative hemolysis is to minimize atmospheric and cutaneous exposure to potentially oxidizing chemicals such as coal tar products. The identification of susceptible individuals such as those with G6PD deficiency may help to avoid significant toxicity in high-risk job situations. Screening for G6PD deficiency must be done before a hemolytic episode or 1–2 months after the hemolysis has resolved. Young red blood cells, particularly reticulocytes, have normal

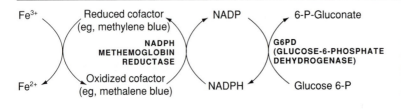

**Figure 15–3.** Reduction of hemoglobin by NADPH methemoglobin reductase can be accelerated by a redox agent such as methylene blue.

**Table 15–1.** Chemicals associated with methemoglobinemia or oxidative hemolysis.

| Chemical | Use |
|---|---|
| Aniline | Rubber, dyestuffs; production of MDI (methylene bisphenyl isocyanate) |
| Nitroaniline | Dyes |
| Toluidine | Dyes, organic chemicals |
| p-Chloroaniline | Dyes, pharmaceuticals, pesticides |
| o-Toluidine | Laboratory analytic reagent, production of trypan blue stain, chlorine test kits, test tapes, curing agent for urethan resins |
| Naphthalene | Fumigants used in clothing industry |
| Paradichlorobenzene | Fumigants used in clothing industry |
| Nitrates | Soil fertilizers |
| Trinitrotoluene | Explosives |

G6PD levels in most G6PD-deficient individuals. During an acute hemolytic episode, older red blood cells are destroyed and replaced by young red blood cells. The result of a G6PD deficiency screen will be normal in that acute setting. Biological monitoring in the workplace may be done by measuring methemoglobin levels and reticulocyte counts (see Chapter 38).

## Treatment

Treatment is dependent on rapid recognition of the problem. It is important to obtain as complete an exposure history as possible, since it will guide treatment. The most important aspect of therapy is to ensure removal of the offending agent. Because of the fat-soluble nature of these compounds, it is essential that clothing be removed and the patient washed thoroughly. For mild intoxication (< 20% blood methemoglobin), observation should be sufficient to watch for progression of symptoms. For moderate to severe intoxication (> 30% blood methemoglobin), 100% oxygen by mask is given to saturate the remaining hemoglobin and the antidote, methylene blue, is administered. Care must be exercised in using methylene blue to avoid increasing methemo-

**Table 15–2.** Symptoms of methemoglobinemia.

| % Methemoglobinemia | Symptoms |
|---|---|
| 10–30 | Cyanosis, mild fatigue, tachycardia |
| 30–50 | Weakness, breathlessness, headache, exercise intolerance |
| 50–70 | Altered consciousness |
| >70–80 | Coma, death |

globin from the oxidative potential of methylene blue itself.

For initial management, methylene blue should be given intravenously as a 1% solution at a dose of 1–2 mg/kg over 10 minutes. The maximal effect should be seen within 1 hour. If no response is evident by this time, administration of methylene blue may be repeated and exchange transfusion considered—though its role in methemoglobinemia has not been well defined. A patient who does not respond to methylene blue may have G6PD deficiency, and further administration could exacerbate hemolysis without altering hypoxia.

If the patient is better after 1 hour, administration of methylene blue may be repeated at hourly intervals, either in intravenous form in the patient with altered consciousness or orally (50–100 mg) in an awake patient. Repeat doses should be given for symptoms, not solely on the basis of the methemoglobin level.

Ascorbic acid may be given in conjunction with the oral dose of methylene blue at a dose of 300–400 mg orally, though its role for this purpose remains controversial. Its onset of action is slow and its potential for urine acidification may potentiate renal toxicity in patients who are actively hemolyzing.

## 2. CHLORATE SALTS

Chlorate salts, used primarily in pesticides and herbicides, cause an unusual form of methemoglobinemia and hemolysis that is unresponsive to methylene blue. Hemolytic anemia has also been seen in uremic patients undergoing hemodialysis when the water supply was found to be contaminated with oxidant compounds made up of chlorine and ammonia termed chloramines. The denaturation of hemoglobin caused by chlorates is thought to be due to their direct oxidizing capacity and their ability to inhibit the hexose monophosphate shunt.

Treatment for poisoning with chlorates is supportive, since there is no specific antidote. Exchange transfusion has been advocated for severe toxicity.

## HEMOLYSIS ASSOCIATED WITH EXPOSURE TO HEAVY METALS

After methemoglobinemia and oxidative hemolysis, transitional elements and heavy metals are the most important causes of work-related hemolytic anemia. These agents include arsenic, lead, mercury, copper, and others. The mechanism of hemolysis is not known, but it is thought to be related to the affinity of these directly cytolytic metals to thiol groups such as are found on the surfaces of red blood cells and in the cysteine residues of hemoglobin. When the sulfhydryl-binding metals are exposed to red cells, the red cell membrane becomes permeable and takes on solute and water. This causes the red cell to swell and ultimately burst while in the vascular circuit (intravascular hemolysis).

## 1. ARSINE

The most dramatic example of acute metal-induced hemolysis is that caused by arsine. Arsine is a volatile, colorless, nonirritating gas at room temperature (boiling point $-62$ °C). It is usually produced accidentally by the action of acid on a metal contaminated with arsenic. However, arsine gas is now also used extensively in the growth and preparation of crystals and conducting devices in the semiconductor industry.

The toxicity of arsine may be best demonstrated by a case of two near fatalities reported in 1979 by Parish et al. Two workers at a chemical manufacturing plant were cleaning a floor drain that had become clogged during a clean-up operation. Although the company had discontinued production of arsenical herbicides more than 5 years previously, a steel tank used to mix the chemicals had been left on a loading platform, where it collected rainwater. In attempting to open the drain, the two workers emptied water from the tank onto the floor with a drain cleaner containing sodium hydroxide, sodium nitrate, and aluminum chips. They then spent 2–3 hours working to unclog the drain, noting that the drain bubbled and gave off a sewerlike odor. By the next morning, both workers were hospitalized with acute hemolytic anemia.

Exposure was documented by the presence of arsenic in the drain as well as the blood and urine of both patients. Each patient required multiple-unit exchange transfusions and fluid replacement; recovery took nearly a month for both. One patient remains on chronic dialysis.

Arsine gas was formed in this incident by the action of arsenic trioxide present in the storage tank and contaminated drain with hydrogen:

$$6H_2 + A_2O_3 \longrightarrow 2AsH_3 + 3H_2O$$

(Arsenic trioxide)  (Arsine)

Hydrogen was formed by the combination of sodium hydroxide and aluminum. Antimony may also be present with arsenic and under the same conditions can form stibine, a gas with toxicity similar to that of arsine. The toxicity of arsine here and in other reports is heightened by the fact that arsine is 2.5 times denser than air. This is particularly important in smelting and refinery work, where toxicity is likely to occur when workers are cleaning out large tanks containing acids and metal compounds.

The potential for arsine gas formation and exposure exists in a wide range of occupations and may be combined with exposure to stibine. Most occupational exposure occurs in the smelting, refining, and chemical industries. The respiratory tract is the most important portal of entry.

Chronic arsine poisoning has been described in workers at a zinc smelting plant and in workers engaged in the cyanide extraction of gold. These patients may be anemic, with chronic low-level hemolysis.

### Clinical Presentation

**A. Symptoms and Signs:** Many manifestations of acute arsine poisoning are due to acute and massive intravascular hemolysis. Appearance of symptoms may be delayed for 2–24 hours after exposure. Symptoms include nausea and vomiting, abdominal cramping, headache, malaise, and dyspnea. Patients will often be alarmed by the presence of tea-colored urine not associated with pain on urination, causing them to seek medical attention. Physical examination may reveal a peculiar garlicky odor of arsine, fever, tachycardia, tachypnea, and hypotension. Later in the course of hemolysis, the patient may appear jaundiced, and there is often generalized nonspecific abdominal tenderness.

**B. Laboratory Findings:** The earliest laboratory finding may be hemoglobinuria. This occurs when the amount of free plasma hemoglobin exceeds normal haptoglobin binding and renal proximal tubular reabsorption. Accordingly, plasma haptoglobin levels fall and free hemoglobin levels may be very high (> 2000 mg/dL have been reported; normal, < 1 mg/dL). The plasma may be brownish-red from the presence of methemalbumin (oxidized hemoglobin bound to albumin). Although anemia may not be present on the first blood count, evaluation of the peripheral smear will reveal red cell fragmentation with marked poikilocytosis, basophilic stippling, and polychromasia. As the hematocrit falls, reticulocytosis develops. Total bilirubin is elevated, reflecting a rise primarily in the unconjugated or indirect form. When hemolysis is brisk, disseminated intravascular coagulation may occur, manifest as a low (or falling) fibrinogen level, a prolonged prothrombin time (due to circulating fibrin split products), and the presence of schistocytes and thrombocytopenia. Renal function is often affected to various degrees, with an early rise in serum creatinine. This may be due both to precipitated hemoglobin casts, causing renal tubular obstruction, and to direct toxicity of arsine on the renal tubular and interstitial cells.

Arsenic levels in blood and urine are useful as indicators of exposure rather than as guidelines for therapy.

### Treatment

Initial therapy should include vigorous hydration to ensure adequate renal perfusion. For severe hemolysis with plasma hemoglobin levels greater than

400–500 mg/dL, exchange transfusion has been advocated. Repeated exchange is indicated for increasing levels of hemoglobin.

Renal function may be preserved with hydration. However, should renal failure develop, acute hemodialysis may be required. All patients must be monitored closely until all evidence of hemolysis has resolved and renal function has stabilized. Some patients may be left with renal insufficiency or chronic failure requiring dialysis or transplantation. All survivors of acute arsine poisoning must be evaluated regularly for at least 1 year to watch for residual renal dysfunction.

In chronic arsine poisoning, reduction of exposure or removal from exposure is the most important treatment.

## 2. LEAD

Lead will be more fully discussed with porphyria, below. In addition to the suppression of erythropoiesis and heme synthesis described there, hemolytic anemia may be seen. Severe acute intravascular hemolysis is rare and is usually seen only with very high atmospheric exposure, as in power sanding and use of a blow torch. The anemia of chronic lead toxicity is enhanced by shortened red cell survival as well as by inhibition of hemoglobin synthesis.

It has been suggested that the pathogenesis of lead-induced hemolysis is related to its marked inhibition of pyrimidine-5' nucleotidase. The hereditary homozygous deficiency of this enzyme is marked by basophilic stippling of erythrocytes, chronic hemolysis, and intraerythrocytic accumulations of pyrimidine-containing nucleotides. These nucleotides perhaps compete with adenine nucleotides in binding to the active site of kinases in the glycolytic pathway, thereby altering red cell membrane stability. Because lead causes an acquired deficiency of this enzyme and the clinical findings are similar, severe toxicity has been likened to this hereditary disease.

## 3. COPPER

Copper sulfate is used in India in the whitewashing and leather industry. Toxicity is primarily due to accidental ingestion and suicide attempts and results in intravascular hemolysis, methemoglobinemia, renal failure, and often death.

Hemolysis has also been caused by hemodialysis with water contaminated by copper piping. In vitro data suggest that multiple mechanisms are involved, including inhibition of glycolysis, oxidation of NADPH, and inhibition of G6PD.

No specific treatment exists other than supportive therapy, with transfusions and hemodialysis as indicated.

## THE PORPHYRIAS

The porphyrias are a group of disorders characterized by abnormalities in the heme biosynthetic pathway (Figure 15–4) that result in the abnormal accumulation of heme precursors. Although these are genetic disorders (inherited or sporadic) of enzymatic activity, acquired porphyria has been described following exposure to various toxins. Heme biosynthesis occurs chiefly in the liver and bone marrow and to a certain extent in nervous tissue. The rate-limiting step in heme biosynthesis is the synthesis of δ-aminolevulinic acid (ALA) from glycine and succinyl-CoA via δ-aminolevulinic acid synthetase. This step is under negative feedback control by heme. Clinically, symptomatic porphyria can occur either as a result of inadequate enzymatic function along any step in heme biosynthesis or as a result of inappropriate overstimulation of δ-aminolevulinic acid synthetase, usually in the setting of decreased heme concentration.

The clinical syndromes of porphyria are characterized by neurotoxicity or cutaneous photosensitivity (both may occur). Neurotoxicity—typically abdominal colic, constipation, autonomic dysfunction, sensorimotor neuropathy, and psychiatric problems—is considered the result of direct toxic effects of the urine-soluble heme precursors, δ-aminolevulinic acid and porphobilinogen, on nervous tissue. Neurotoxicity may also be the result of heme deficiency interrupting nervous tissue homeostasis. Cutaneous photosensitivity is manifested as repetitive vesiculation, scarring, and deformity, with hypertrichosis of sun-exposed areas of the skin. This is the result of the relatively urine-insoluble heme precursors—uroporphyrin III, coproporphyrin III, and protoporphyrin IX—fluorescing in the skin following absorption of 400-nm wavelength electromagnetic radiation. These fluorescing porphyrias can also cause discoloration of teeth and occasionally hemolysis of erythrocytes in which porphyrins accumulate.

A number of industrial and environmental toxins have induced **toxic porphyrias** similar to porphyria cutanea tarda in people heavily exposed to the agents (Table 15–3). These toxins usually cause liver injury and deranged hepatic heme synthesis. Although the exact metabolic effects of these agents are not entirely understood, unregulated stimulation of δ-aminolevulinic acid synthetase is usually demonstrable.

## 1. HEXACHLOROBENZENE

In an outbreak of acquired porphyria in Turkey between 1955 and 1958, over 4000 people developed a cutaneous porphyria syndrome resembling congenital erythropoietic porphyria about 6 months following ingestion of wheat containing a fungicide, hexa-

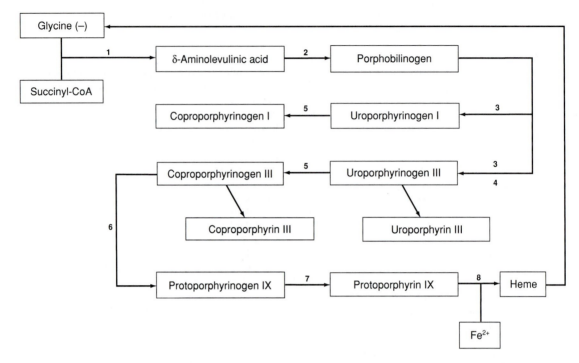

**Figure 15–4.** The heme biosynthetic pathway. Heme is a feedback inhibitor of enzyme (1) δ-aminolevulinic acid synthetase. Other enzymes are (2) δ-aminolevulinic acid dehydrase, (3) uroporphyrinogen I synthase, (4) uroporphyrinogen III cosynthase, (5) uroporphyrinogen decarboxylase, (6) coproporphyrinogen oxidase, (7) protoporphyrinogen oxidase, and (8) ferrochelatase.

chlorobenzene. The wheat was intended for planting and contained 2 kg of 10% hexachlorobenzene per 1000 kg of wheat to control a fungus, *Telletia tritici.* Affected people demonstrated cutaneous photosensitivity with skin hyperpigmentation, hypertrichosis, bullae, weakness, and hepatomegaly, a condition termed kara yara, or "black sore." Porphyrinuria was nearly universal, with the urine being pigmented red or brown. The mortality rate was 10%. Breast-fed infants under 2 years of age had a 95% mortality rate when ingesting mother's milk contaminated with the fungicide. These infants developed weakness, convulsions, and cutaneous annular erythema, a condition termed pembe yara, or "pink sore." Excess porphyrins could not be detected in the urine of these infants. This is compatible with animal models of hexachlorobenzene-induced porphyria. Infant rats and mice die of neurologic toxicity from hexachlorobenzene without porphyrinuria, while adult rats and rabbits develop cutaneous photosensitivity and porphyrinuria following prolonged exposure to the chemical.

A follow-up study was performed between 1977 and 1983 in which 204 patients who previously suffered from hexachlorobenzene porphyria were examined. The mean age of these individuals was 32 years, and the mean time from hexachlorobenzene exposure was 7 years. The mean duration of cutaneous porphyria symptoms was 2.4 years. At the time of study, 71% of people had hyperpigmentation and 47% had hypertrichosis. Residual scarring on sun-exposed areas of the skin was evident in 87%. Other features included perioral scarring, small hands, arthritis, short stature, weakness, paresthesias, and myotonia. Seventeen patients still had red urine and demonstrated porphyrinuria (especially uroporphyrinuria). Hexachlorobenzene was measurable in 56 samples of human milk obtained from porphyric

**Table 15–3.** Toxic substances associated with acquired porphyria in humans.

| Toxin | Use |
| --- | --- |
| Hexachlorobenzene | Fungicide |
| 2,4-Dichlorophenol | Herbicide |
| 2,4,5-Trichlorophenol | Herbicide |
| 2,3,7,8-Tetrachlorodibenzo-*p*-dioxin | Herbicide contaminant |
| *o*-Benzyl-*p*-chlorophenol | Cleanser and disinfectant |
| 2-Benzyl-4, 6-dichlorophenol | Commercial disinfectant |
| Vinyl chloride | Plastics |
| Lead | Paint compounds |
| Aluminum | Phosphorus binder |

mothers at a mean value of 0.51 ppm (versus 0.07 ppm in control).

The Turkish experience was the first associating exposure to an industrial chemical with acquired porphyria in humans. Not only were the symptomatic attack and mortality rates significant, but also the biochemical lesion persisted for decades in many survivors. The exact mechanism by which hexachlorobenzene induces porphyria remains to be elucidated. Most liver mitochondria of animals made porphyric by exposure to chlorinated benzenes, such as hexachlorobenzene, demonstrated increased activity of δ-aminolevulinic acid synthetase, the enzyme that controls the rate of porphyrin production. With the exception of mice made porphyric with diethyl-1, 4,-dihydro-2,4,6-trimethylpyridine-3,5-dicarboxylate, animal porphyric livers have demonstrated an increased production of heme. Heme normally inhibits the activity of δ-aminolevulinic acid synthetase. This suggests that porphyrinogenic compounds are somehow interfering with the repressor signal of heme on δ-aminolevulinic acid synthetase. Other theories suggest that porphyrinogenic compounds induce δ-aminolevulinic acid synthetase by altering the intracellular oxidation state through action on the electron transport chain, thus stimulating succinyl-CoA production, depressing intracellular ATP levels, or both. In any event, the net result is overproduction of porphyrins mediated by unregulated δ-aminolevulinic acid synthetase activity.

The role of iron overload in the pathogenesis of hexachlorobenzene-induced porphyria has been examined. The suggestion that iron might be involved was based on the observation that 80% of patients with porphyria cutanea tarda—a disease associated with reduced hepatic uroporphyrinogen decarboxylase activity—have increased liver iron stores and increased levels of uroporphyrin I. Further, decreasing hepatic iron stores by phlebotomy in patients with porphyria cutanea tarda often induces disease remission and a decrease in urinary uroporphyrin I excretion. In a porcine and human liver model, ferrous iron was found to markedly inhibit uroporphyrinogen III cosynthetase activity, enhance total porphyrin production, and greatly overproduce uroporphyrin I. In rats made porphyric with hexachlorobenzene, iron overload results in decreased production of liver heme, cytochrome P-450, and cytochrome $b_5$ and an absence of uroporphyrinogen decarboxylase activity. In addition, the NAD: NADH ratio was over twofold higher in siderotic rats made porphyric with hexachlorobenzene compared to nonsiderotic rats. Furthermore, phlebotomized iron-deficient mice were protected from the porphyrinogenic effect of 2,3,7,8-tetrachlorodibenzo-p-dioxin.

Most authorities believe that iron plays a permissive rather than a causative role in porphyrias. This is based on the facts that not all patients with porphyria cutanea tarda are iron-overloaded, that porphyria cutanea tarda is rare in patients with hemochromatosis, and that phlebotomy does not correct the biochemical lesion in patients with porphyria cutanea tarda. In addition, rats made porphyric by hexachlorobenzene did not require iron overload for porphyria to develop, although the porphyria was worsened by iron overload. Thus, it remains unsettled whether iron overload is permissive or etiologic in patients exposed to porphyrinogenic toxins.

## 2. HERBICIDES

A number of herbicides have been clearly associated with symptomatic porphyria. Bleiberg and colleagues reported on 29 patients exposed to 2,4-dichlorophenol and 2,4,5-trichlorophenol at a manufacturing plant. All 29 patients exhibited chloracne, 13 had hyperpigmentation, 11 had hirsutism, and 5 had skin fragility. Eleven patients had increased excretion of urine porphyrins (uroporphyrin and coproporphyrin). Thus, these patients had developed an acquired porphyria cutanea tarda-like syndrome after variable exposure to these herbicides. A follow-up study of 73 workers at this same herbicide plant 6 years later found no people with the porphyric syndrome and only one with persistent uroporphyrinuria. The authors of the follow-up study hypothesized that the decrease in the syndrome was due to improved personal safety habits of the workers and decreased exposure to the chemicals. An alternative explanation is that the true porphyrinogenic agent is perhaps 2,3,7,8-tetrachlorodibenzo-p-dioxin, a by-product of 2,4,5-trichlorophenol, and that this contaminant had been effectively eliminated from the chemical stores at the factory. The contaminant was strongly implicated in an outbreak of acquired porphyria cutanea tarda, chloracne, and polyneuropathy in 80 industrial workers producing herbicides in Czechoslovakia.

## 3. DISINFECTANTS

The commercial disinfectants o-benzyl-p-chlorophenol and 2-benzyl-4,6-dichlorophenol have been implicated as a cause of acquired porphyria cutanea tarda in one woman exposed to these compounds.

## 4. ALUMINUM

A porphyria cutanea tarda-like syndrome has been described in patients with chronic renal failure being maintained on regular hemodialysis. Plasma and urine uroporphyrins are increased in these patients, whereas plasma and urine coproporphyrins are often low. Since aluminum is known to inhibit some heme synthetic enzymes and since many chronic renal failure patients on hemodialysis are aluminum-overloaded, aluminum has been implicated, but without proof, as the cause of porphyria in these patients.

## 5. VINYL CHLORIDE

Vinyl chloride is a known hepatotoxin used in the production of plastics. A study of 46 persons working in a polyvinyl chloride production plant revealed significantly elevated urinary coproporphyrin levels compared with normal controls. Exposure periods ranged from 2 to 21 years. The pathogenesis of coproporphyrinuria involves inhibition of coproporphyrinogen oxidase, inhibition of uroporphyrinogen decarboxylase, and perhaps induction of δ-aminolevulinic acid synthetase. Persons with excess urinary coproporphyrin production also manifested thrombocytopenia, splenomegaly, esophageal varices, sclerodermalike skin changes, Raynaud's syndrome, and acro-osteolysis.

## 6. LEAD

Lead intoxication (blood lead level > 60 μg/dL in adults; > 25 μg/dL in children) causes symptoms and signs remarkably similar to those associated with acute intermittent porphyria. The classic acute intermittent porphyria triad is abdominal pain, constipation, and vomiting—all representing the neurotoxic effects of excess δ-aminolevulinic acid and porphobilinogen. This triad is seen with equal frequency in lead intoxication. Other shared characteristics include neuromuscular pains, paresis or paralysis, paresthesias, diarrhea, and seizures. The major differences between the two diseases are (1) an increase in neuropsychiatric signs in acute intermittent porphyria compared with lead intoxication and (2) anemia, which is present in lead intoxication but virtually absent in porphyria. The anemia of lead poisoning is a characteristic microcytic anemia with basophilic stippling of erythrocytes and sideroblasts in the bone marrow.

The biochemical features of lead poisoning demonstrate why these two diseases are clinically so similar. Patients with lead intoxication have markedly elevated urinary δ-aminolevulinic acid levels, as in acute intermittent porphyria. Mild lead poisoning (preanemia stage) is associated with normal porphobilinogen excretion, but once anemia occurs, excess urinary porphobilinogen becomes demonstrable. Although mild elevations of urine coproporphyrins and uroporphyrin I are present, fecal uroporphyrin and coproporphyrin are normal in patients with lead poisoning. These alterations in porphyrins are present only in patients with inorganic lead intoxication, not in patients with organic lead intoxication. Excess accumulation of protoporphyrin IX has also been found in erythrocytes of lead-intoxicated patients.

Lead poisoning is associated with greatly diminished activity of δ-aminolevulinic acid dehydrase in the brain, liver, kidney, and bone marrow. δ-Aminolevulinic acid dehydrase is polymorphic, and this may result in different levels of sensitivity to lead exposure in different individuals depending on the particular form of the enzyme that is inherited. Lead also blocks the incorporation of iron into protoporphyrin IX by depressing the activity of ferrochelatase, an event most closely linked with the production of anemia and elevation of free erythrocyte protoporphyrin IX levels. Coproporphyrinogen oxidase activity has also been shown to be depressed by lead. Thus, the effect of lead on heme synthesis disruption occurs at multiple steps in the synthetic pathway, all of which occur in the mitochondrion.

## TREATMENT OF TOXIC PORPHYRIAS

Since there is often no effective means of eliminating toxic environmental or industrial substances once they are incorporated into tissues, exposure to porphyrinogenic compounds must be avoided. Although no prospective data are available to support the use of phlebotomy for this purpose, this therapy may be of benefit in patients with toxic porphyria whose disease complex resembles porphyria cutanea tarda and in whom evidence of iron overload can be demonstrated. Patients with acute intermittent porphyria occasionally respond to high-dose carbohydrate infusions (400 g of dextrose/d) or hematin infusions (3 mg/kg intravenously every 12 hours for 10–12 doses). However, the use of hematin infusions in toxic porphyria may not be of benefit since, as in the case of hexachlorobenzene, the toxic agent may be interrupting the negative feedback signal by heme on δ-aminolevulinic acid synthetase.

For lead intoxication, prevention is again the best treatment. Unlike all other toxic porphyrias, specific therapy for lead intoxication is available with lead chelators (see Chapter 27).

## DISORDERS ASSOCIATED WITH DECREASED OXYGEN SATURATION

## CARBON MONOXIDE POISONING

Carbon monoxide is an odorless, colorless, nonirritating gas produced by the incomplete combustion of organic materials, particularly hydrocarbons. The workers at greatest risk are automobile mechanics (automobile exhaust systems), fire fighters, and chemical workers exposed to methylene chloride (converted to carbon monoxide through in vivo metabolism).

Carbon monoxide binds to hemoglobin, forming carboxyhemoglobin, which decreases hemoglobin oxygen saturation and shifts the oxygen-hemoglobin dissociation curve to the left. Hemoglobin has an affinity for carbon monoxide 210 times greater than that for oxygen. Carbon monoxide also increases the stability of the hemoglobin-oxygen combination, thus inhibiting oxygen delivery to the tissues. In addition, carbon monoxide binds to the cytochrome oxidase chain, interfering with cellular respiration. These properties of carbon monoxide result in chemical asphyxiation.

### Clinical Findings

Symptoms include general malaise, headache, nausea, dyspnea, vomiting, and alteration in mental status at high levels. Severe exposure may cause coma, seizures, arrhythmias, and death. Symptoms of anoxia may be prominent without cyanosis due to the cherry-red color of carboxyhemoglobin.

Laboratory findings at chronic low levels may show polycythemia; at higher levels, hypoxia is seen. Carboxyhemoglobin levels should be measured; a level under 6% may cause impairment in vision and time discrimination; at 40–60% alterations in mental status and death may be seen. Blood carboxyhemoglobin levels can be significantly elevated both after intense exposures of short duration and after chronic low-level exposure.

### Treatment & Prevention

Treatment is dependent on the degree of carboxyhemoglobin. At low levels, removal from the source of exposure is sufficient. At higher levels, the treatment of choice is inspiration of 100% oxygen. Oxygen markedly decreases the half-life of carboxyhemoglobin from 5–6 hours at room air to 90 minutes at 100% inspired oxygen by dilutional displacement of the carbon monoxide. Severe toxicity, including mental status aberrations, may call for hyperbaric oxygen therapy, which decreases the half-life of carboxyhemoglobin further to 23 minutes at 3 atmospheres.

Prevention depends on adequate ventilation, with venting of combustion devices to the outside air.

# DISORDERS AFFECTING BLOOD CELL FORMATION & MORPHOLOGY

Premalignant and malignant hematologic diseases have been linked to a variety of occupational exposures. Because the determination of cause and effect is very difficult to verify when the latency period is long and the exposure history is poorly documented, other methods for ascertaining this link have been explored. Cytogenetic study consists of examining the somatic chromosomes of hematologic cells in metaphase.

### CYTOGENETICS

The chromosomal analysis of hematologic disorders is an important mechanism for classification and as a guide to prognosis and therapy. Cytogenetic analysis serves two purposes in occupational hematology: (1) to screen populations at risk for toxic exposure so that cryptic toxic agents can be identified; and (2) in individual cases, to identify diseases that might have been caused by exposure to mutagenic agents.

Abnormalities in chromosomes can be used as a marker for exposure to noxious environmental agents. Through extensive epidemiologic study, certain abnormalities have been associated with specific diseases and prognostic categories. Toxic agents that have been shown to be associated with chromosomal abnormalities in vivo have been linked to the development of cancers and leukemias.

Cytogenetic analysis for hematologic disorders is best done by direct examination of cells obtained from bone marrow. Since these cells are continuously proliferating, it is relatively easy to examine those undergoing mitosis when the chromosomes are visible microscopically. High-resolution banding techniques are used to precisely identify deletions, translocations, inversions, and other structural chromosomal abnormalities.

Cells obtained from peripheral blood require artificial stimulation by a mitogen such as phytohemagglutinin and culture for 2–3 days to obtain enough cells in mitosis for analysis. Artifactual aberrations may be induced in cells that are manipulated after removal from the patient before fixing for analysis. The resulting risk of falsely abnormal evaluations increases the necessity and importance of well matched and multiple controls.

### Screening & Prevention

Cytogenetic analysis has been used as a screening tool to monitor industrial populations for early exposure to mutagenic chemicals and to identify possible mutagens. In this way, workers at risk might be removed from potentially dangerous conditions when the effects are still reversible. Peripheral blood lymphocytes rather than bone marrow must be used for obvious reasons of worker comfort, time, and cost.

The problem with using cytogenetics for monitoring is the relative insensitivity of the method to low levels of exposure. The only known dose-response relationship for exposure and somatic chromosome aberrations has been described with ionizing radiation. In a recent study of workers exposed to low levels (below exposure limits) of chemicals in a petrochemical plant in the Netherlands, cytogenetic monitoring by chromosomal banding techniques was carried out from 1976 to 1981. Results of these studies, published in 1988, found no increase in the frequencies of chromosome aberrations in the exposed populations compared with control populations. They concluded that the examination of peripheral blood lymphocytes for chromosomal aberrations is not sufficiently sensitive for routine monitoring of cytogenetics in workers exposed to low levels of the compounds.

A second technique that has been evaluated in monitoring is sister chromatid exchange, a method of evaluating symmetric intrachromosomal rearrangements of DNA. Although this technique is faster and cheaper than cytogenetic analysis, the presence of exchanges does not necessarily correlate with the incidence of chromosomal aberrations or the development of disease.

Further progress in methods to detect induced DNA damage is needed for cytogenetic analysis to be an adequate screening tool for large populations. With the advent of molecular biological techniques, this should be possible in the future on a population-wide scale. At present, although individual health consequences cannot be estimated by population screening methods, abnormal chromosomal or cytogenetic findings are clearly an adverse sign when correlated with specific exposure risk data.

### Relationship of Cytogenetic Abnormalities to Specific Diseases

Cytogenetic study provides a means of relating chromosomal aberrations in the bone marrow of a patient with preleukemia or leukemia to exposure to mutagenic agents. The population benefited includes workers exposed to industrial agents and radiation as well as patients previously treated with chemotherapeutic agents or radiation. Many studies have suggested that this population has a much higher incidence of chromosomal abnormalities than a similar nonexposed group with the same diseases. In a summary of three retrospective studies of patients with de novo acute nonlymphocytic leukemia, individuals were grouped as nonexposed and exposed on the basis of occupation. Individuals who worked with insecticides, chemicals and solvents, metals or minerals, petroleum products, and ionizing radiation were considered exposed, whereas students, white-collar workers, and housewives were classified as nonexposed. Sixty-eight of 236 patients (29%) were found to be in the exposed group. Fifty-one of the 68 (75%) in the exposed group had abnormal karyotypes, versus only 60 of 168 (36%) in the nonexposed group. In addition to this generalized increase in chromosomal aberrations, abnormalities in chromosomes 5 and 7 were observed in 37% of the exposed and in 12% of the nonexposed individuals.

These specific chromosomal abnormalities have also correlated positively with the development of leukemia after exposure to therapeutic mutagens (chemotherapy or radiation) used to treat other cancers. Specifically, a loss of the entire chromosome or of part of the long arm of either or both of these chromosomes has been seen. Although these chromosome abnormalities may occur in the absence of exposure to mutagens, patients with leukemias or preleukemic conditions with deletions involving chromosomes 5 or 7 should arouse a suspicion of prior exposure to chemical carcinogens or radiation, and this history should be vigorously sought. The prognosis for patients with abnormalities of chromosomes 5 or 7—or with multiple cytogenetic abnormalities when associated with prior exposure to mutagenic agents—is poor compared with that of patients with a normal chromosome analysis.

Clearly the greatest usefulness of cytogenetics is in the area of prevention and developing better techniques to assess future pathologic consequences of exposure at a time when effects may still be reversible. As more sensitive techniques are developed, they may also serve as a guideline for determining the threshold limit values for potential mutagens.

## WORK-RELATED APLASTIC ANEMIA AND HEMATOLOGIC CANCERS

Hematologic cancers are discussed in detail in the chapter on occupational cancers (Chapter 17). In this section, we will discuss only diseases not covered in that chapter: aplastic anemia, myelodysplasia, and multiple myeloma.

### 1. APLASTIC ANEMIA

Aplastic anemia, or medullary aplasia, is an acquired abnormality of the pluripotential hematopoietic stem cells resulting in pancytopenia. The average incidence of fatal aplastic anemia per year in the United States is about 2 per million and rises with age to an annual age-specific mortality rate of about

10 per million in people over age 65. Approximately 50% of cases of aplastic anemia in North America and Western Europe are idiopathic; most of the remainder are termed secondary aplastic anemias and may be caused by drugs, chemicals, radiation, infection, and immunologic mechanisms. A small percentage of cases are due to hereditary diseases.

The largest category of secondary aplastic anemia is due to therapeutic drugs; probably only a small fraction are due to environmental and occupational causes. The drug most commonly implicated is chloramphenicol; others include acetazolamide, phenylbutazone, phenytoin, and sulfonamides—and there are many others. This section will discuss only occupation-related cases of aplastic anemia.

Many cases of aplastic anemia develop after the occurrence of dysplastic morphologic changes in hematologic cells with associated chromosomal abnormalities. The incidence of acute nonlymphocytic leukemia in patients with aplastic anemia who survive 2 years after diagnosis is about 5–10%; in patients with preceding dysplasia, the incidence may be higher. Chemicals that are capable of inducing bone marrow damage must be assumed to be potential leukemogens. It is difficult to link specific chemicals to the development of aplastic anemia because of the absence of a specific test for exposure and the frequency of multiple or unknown exposures. Only three agents have been firmly established as a cause of aplastic anemia on a dose-dependent basis. These include benzene, ionizing radiation, and cytotoxic drugs such as antimetabolites and alkylating agents. Benzene and ionizing radiation are discussed at greater length in Chapter 17.

## Benzene

Benzene was first described as a cause of fatal aplastic anemia in 1897. Early unregulated exposure to benzene—used widely as a solvent in the production of many products, including fabrics and pesticides—led to many cases of acute and chronic toxicity. Workers now at greatest risk of exposure are those involved in rubber manufacturing, shoemaking, petroleum and chemical production, printing, and steelworking.

Before 1950, benzene was the single most common cause of toxic aplastic anemia. With chronic doses of over 100 ppm, isolated cytopenias and aplastic anemia were common. The cytopenias usually resolved after termination of exposure; even with persistent exposure, spontaneous remissions have been described. At exposures of 100 ppm or higher, some workers will develop fatal aplastic anemia. Great variation in susceptibility to exposure has been seen, with evidence of poisoning sometimes appearing only after weeks or years. Cases of cytopenia have also been seen several years after exposure has been terminated; these cases are less likely to resolve with time and may be part of a preleukemic syn-

drome. In severe chronic poisoning, decreased red cell survival with hemolysis has been reported.

Toxicity is directly related to the amount and duration of exposure, although again there is individual variation in susceptibility. The current US exposure limit is 1 ppm. The diagnosis is made by examination of the bone marrow after an abnormal complete blood count is reported. The bone marrow will reveal hypocellularity with fatty replacement, though islands of hypercellularity may be seen. Although cytogenetic abnormalities have been associated with benzene exposure, specific chromosome changes have not. The initial prognosis in benzene-related aplastic anemia is better than that for idiopathic aplastic anemia; up to 40% may recover completely after removal from the source of exposure. If hypocellularity persists for more than several months, recovery is not likely to occur. Exposure has been associated with the development of acute nonlymphocytic leukemia, chronic myelogenous leukemia, and multiple myeloma—either de novo or in workers who have recovered from a bout of aplastic anemia—and in cases of irreversible aplastic anemia.

Treatment is supportive (ie, with transfusions and such growth factors as erythropoietin, granulocyte colony-stimulating factor, and granulocyte-macrophage colony-stimulating factor). Drugs such as androgens to stimulate hematopoiesis have not been used extensively in benzene-induced aplastic anemia but should be tried when no other treatment option exists (such as bone marrow transplantation or colony-stimulating factors). Allogeneic bone marrow transplantation is the only known cure for irreversible aplastic anemia and is hampered by donor availability, the age of the patient, and the toxicity of the transplant regimen.

## Ionizing Radiation

Ionizing radiation has also been associated with aplastic anemia in a dose-dependent manner. Internal exposure to absorbed alpha particles associated with aplastic anemia was most strikingly demonstrated in the radium watch dial workers who ingested radium by wetting their paintbrushes on their tongues. External exposure to radiation is much more common and may be in the form of whole-body exposure to a large dose, as in a nuclear accident or therapeutic radiation, or long-term exposure to small amounts, as may occur in the practice of radiology as a medical specialty.

Data from patients radiated for ankylosing spondylitis and from the survivors of the atomic bombing of Hiroshima and Nagasaki suggest that the risk of aplastic anemia is increased until 3–5 years after exposure, after which there is a marked decline in incidence. The most important late disturbance following irradiation of the bone marrow is leukemia. The ability to recover from a single dose of penetrating radiation is dependent on the fraction of surviving stem cells. Chromosomal aberrations are associated with exposure to ionizing radiation and rise in a linear manner as a function of the dose of radiation absorbed. The presence of these aberrations, including an increase in the number of sister chromatid exchanges, may signify excessive exposure but is not predictive of aplastic anemia or leukemia.

Strict regulation of exposure and monitoring with badges has virtually eliminated aplastic anemia due to radiation except in cases of accidental overexposure. In this case, treatment again is primarily supportive. Recovery may be seen after a prolonged period of aplastic anemia lasting 3–6 weeks and may be predicted from the known total dose of radiation. If recovery does not occur, permanent injury to the stem cell population has resulted in chronic cellular hypoplasia or dysplasia or in leukemia. Treatment may then include bone marrow transplantation if a donor is available. Trials to study the use of hematopoietic growth factors in treating aplastic anemia are now going forward.

### Other Chemicals

Aplastic anemia has been reported following exposure to a variety of other chemicals listed in Table 15–4. Toxicities often resolve completely with cessation of exposure. Again, individual susceptibility plays an important role, though it is poorly understood.

Two chemicals in particular deserve mention here. The aplastic anemia associated with **trinitrotoluene** may be accompanied by methemoglobinemia, oxidative hemolysis, liver damage, and dermatitis.

The incidence of overexposure to **arsenic** has declined with its decreasing use during the past 3 decades. Fewer than 10 cases of poisoning are now reported annually in the United States. If arsenic-induced aplastic anemia or pancytopenia is suspected, laboratory confirmation of the exposure (see Chapter 27) should be obtained. Complete spontaneous recovery is usually seen if the patient is removed from the source of exposure within a few days to weeks.

## 2. MYELODYSPLASTIC SYNDROMES

Both benzene and ionizing radiation have also been implicated in the development of myelodysplasia. Myelodysplasia or preleukemia is a group of five syndromes classified by the morphology of the bone marrow and peripheral blood. These syndromes are linked by the presence of bizarre hematopoietic morphology and the tendency to transform into acute leukemia. Most patients with myelodysplasia do not develop leukemia, though specific syndromes associated with exposure to both occupational chemicals and cytotoxic drugs have a high incidence of progression to frank leukemia. The median survival from these diseases is less than 12 months, and all patients develop leukemias or succumb to complications related to cytopenias. Two syndromes—classified as refractory anemia with excess blasts (RAEB) or RAEB in transformation—are associated with an increase in chromosomal aberrations. Exposure and treatment-related myelodysplasia is specifically associated with a high incidence of deletions involving chromosomes 5 and 7.

Myelodysplastic syndromes are more common in men than in women, and 85% of patients are over 40 years of age at the time of diagnosis. Laboratory features of RAEB include cytopenias of various degrees and often an increase in mean corpuscular volume. The marrow reveals dysplasia in all three cell lines (granulocyte/erythroid/megakaryocyte [platelet-forming]) and various degrees of cellularity, usually hypercellular. There is an abnormal increase in the percentage of blast cells.

Several treatment options are available, though they are far from ideal. Allogeneic bone marrow transplantation is the only known cure and is primarily limited here by patient age, since most will not be eligible even if a donor exists. Transfusions and treatment of infections may be aided by the use of hematopoietic growth factors currently under clinical investigation. An experimental antimetabolic chemotherapeutic agent, 5-azacytidine (5-AZA) is showing some promise. Approximately 40% of patients treated with 5-AZA (75 mg/m$^2$/d for 1 week, either subcutaneously or as a continuous infusion, on a monthly schedule) demonstrate a reduction in transfusion needs (including transfusion independence) and an improvement in blood counts and sense of well-being.

**Table 15–4.** Chemicals reported to cause aplastic anemia in an occupational setting.

| Chemical | Use |
|---|---|
| Benzene | Intermediate in the synthesis of fabrics, pesticides, rubber. Solvent for glues, varnishes, inks, paints. Octant booster for gasoline. |
| Trinitrotoluene (TNT) | Production of explosives |
| Hexachloroclyclohexane (lindane) Pentachlorophenol Chlorophenothane (DDT) | Pesticide |
| Arsenic | Manufacture of glass, paint, enamels, weed killers, tanning agents, pesticides |
| Ethylene glycol monomethyl or monobutyl ether | Production of paints, lacquers, dyes, inks, cleaning agents |

### 3. MULTIPLE MYELOMA

Multiple myeloma is a chronic leukemia of differentiated B cells (termed plasma cells), which accounts for 15% of all hematologic cancers. It is characterized by anemia, painful lytic and osteopenic bone disease, monoclonal immunoglobulin production (in serum or urine or both), hypogammaglobulinemia, and short survival. Patients may also have hypercalcemia, renal failure, or neuropathy. Treatment involves chemotherapy (with such agents as melphalan, vincristine, vinblastine, doxorubicin, cyclophosphamide, or carmustine) and corticosteroids with the goal of alleviating bone pain, correcting complications of the disease, and prolonging life. Although generally considered incurable, with survival rates of 2–6 years depending on the stage of disease at presentation, there is emerging evidence that one quarter of young patients with multiple myeloma may be cured by allogeneic bone marrow transplantation. Autologous bone marrow transplantation soon after diagnosis appears to improve both disease-free and overall survival. This less toxic form of therapy is available to a wider range of patients up to age 70.

The peak incidence of multiple myeloma is between ages 55 and 65, and fewer than 2% of cases occur before the age of 40. Multiple myeloma is equally common in men and women but almost twice as common in blacks as in whites. The incidence of multiple myeloma has been increasing over the last 3 decades in North American and European men, but this rise has not been noted in the stable study populations in Minnesota and Sweden and may simply reflect an increase in our ability to diagnose the disease. The rise in incidence has aroused concern that myeloma might be associated with environmental or occupational factors.

Although no definitive link has been made between occupational exposure and the risk of multiple myeloma, many epidemiologic studies suggest an association. Exposure to petroleum products, organic solvents, heavy metals, pesticides, and asbestos has been implicated, but most studies are small and can only be used as a basis for hypotheses. Workers thought to be at risk include agricultural workers, chemicals workers, miners, smelters, stokers, and furniture workers in the early part of this century.

A study published in 1987 reviewed mortality and exposure data in a cohort of rubber manufacturers in the United States occupationally exposed to benzene. The analysis found that there was a statistically significant excess of deaths from multiple myeloma in workers exposed to low levels of benzene and that the latency period was over 20 years. A strong positive exposure-response relationship between benzene and leukemia was also found. Benzene is metabolized through a complex series of enzymatic steps that result in the production of oxygen radicals. These oxygen radicals have radiomimetic effects, which damage DNA and can induce hematopoietic cancer. Most, but not all, occupational studies have linked benzene exposure to an excessive risk of the development of multiple myeloma.

An important association between high-dose radiation exposure and multiple myeloma has been observed in cohorts of controls and survivors of the atomic bombings in Hiroshima and Nagasaki for the period of 1950 to 1976. The relative risk for persons with an estimated air-dose exposure of 100 cGy or more was over 4 times higher than that of controls. This excess risk became apparent about 20 years after exposure. An association has also been proposed—but not confirmed—between the risk of multiple myeloma and exposure to low-dose radiation. At present, except in the case of high-dose radiation, there are insufficient data upon which to base a firm conclusion about the relationship between exposure to ionizing radiation and the risk of developing multiple myeloma. Further large-scale incidence studies on this topic are needed.

## TOXIC THROMBOCYTOPENIA

Unlike thrombocytopenia associated with toxicant-induced aplastic anemia, isolated toxic thrombocytopenia is a rare event. A number of toxic exposures have been reported that resulted in isolated thrombocytopenia (Table 15–5). Two cases of isolated thrombocytopenia were described in 1963 in individuals exposed to the polymerizing agent **toluene diisocyanate**. In both, thrombocytopenia developed 14–22 days following a significant exposure that also induced bronchospasm. These patients developed thrombocytopenic bleeding with nadir platelet counts

**Table 15–5.** Toxic agents associated with isolated thrombocytopenia.

| Toxic Agent | Use | Mechanism |
| --- | --- | --- |
| Toluene diisocyanate | Polymerizing agent | Immune |
| 2, 2-Dichlorovinyl dimethylphosphate<br>Dieldrin<br>Pyrethrin<br>Lethane<br>Hexachlorocyclohexane (lindane)<br>Chlorophenothane (DDT) | Insecticide | Megakaryocyte hypoplasia |
| Turpentine | Organic solvent | Immune |
| Vinyl chloride | Plastics | Liver insufficiency with hypersplenism |

of 6000/μL and 30,000/μL. Bone marrow samples in both cases showed increased megakaryocytes. The pathophysiologic defect was enhanced peripheral platelet destruction, presumably on an immune basis (immune thrombocytopenic purpura). One patient responded transiently to corticosteroid therapy and then completely to splenectomy; the second patient had resolution of thrombocytopenia without any therapy.

Two more cases of toxin-induced immune thrombocytopenic purpura were described in 1969. Two children with significant **turpentine** exposure (one respiratory and cutaneous exposure, the second ingestion) developed petechiae and severe thrombocytopenia with increased bone marrow megakaryocytes. Both responded fully to corticosteroid therapy.

**Insecticides** can cause a selective megakaryocyte aplasia in people with significant inhalation or ingestion exposure. Isolated thrombocytopenia has been reported after exposure to 2,2-dichlorovinyl dimethyl phosphate, dieldrin, pyrethrin, lethane, hexachlorocyclohexane (lindane), and chlorophenothane (DDT). These patients demonstrated absent or decreased bone marrow megakaryocytes. Some megakaryocytes were vacuolated. Most patients received corticosteroids and responded with full platelet recovery.

A third form of toxic thrombocytopenia was described in 1984. Forty-six people exposed to vinyl chloride with evidence of toxic coproporphyrinuria also had thrombocytopenia. Although these patients were not described in detail, they appeared to have significant vinyl chloride liver toxicity, with esophageal varices and splenomegaly. The likely pathophysiologic mechanism of thrombocytopenia was thus enhanced peripheral platelet consumption due to hypersplenism, although there were insufficient data presented to rule out an immune or megakaryocyte toxic mechanism.

Normal hemostasis is dependent not only on the quantity of platelets present but also on their ability to aggregate appropriately under physiologic stimulation. Qualitative disturbances in platelet function as a result of various occupational and environmental substances have been described. Some (but not all) pesticides, such as p,p'-DDE (2,2-bis-(p-chlorophrenyl)-1,1-dichloroethylene) and Arochlor 1242 (a chlorinated biphenyl that is 42% chlorine), inhibit platelet aggregation in a dose-dependent manner. They do this by inhibiting platelet cyclooxygenase activity (an aspirin-like effect). Exposures to these substances could cause mucocutaneous bleeding in susceptible individuals. On the other hand, some environmental substances (methyl mercury, cadmium, and triethyl lead) induce platelet aggregation and could result in hypercoagulation. These qualitative platelet disturbances have not yet been reported in humans subject to occupational exposure and remain theoretical risks.

# OCCUPATIONAL EXPOSURE TO ANTICANCER DRUGS

Oncology nurses and pharmacists who prepare and administer chemotherapy to patients on a regular basis are at risk for exposure to potentially mutagenic agents. Data from a variety of sources are available on the mutagenic potential of many anticancer drugs. Epidemiologic studies have linked certain drugs (and radiation) to the development of secondary cancers; analytic in vitro methods of assessing mutagenicity have offered confirmational evidence.

There are several obvious problems in assessing the risk to nurses. First is the low and intermittent exposure rate relative to the patients who receive these drugs therapeutically and who serve as in vivo models for the effects of heavy exposure. This limits the usefulness of epidemiologic data such as exposure rates and disease incidence when attempting to assess individual risks. Second, the methods for detecting exposure are often contradictory and may be cumbersome in time relative to work. For example, it may be difficult for nurses to obtain urine 6 hours after the end of a shift.

Methods for assessing risk include measuring blood and urine levels of drug, urine mutagenicity assays, cytogenetic monitoring and sister chromatid exchange studies, and environmental monitoring. Blood and urine levels may be difficult to interpret when drugs are rapidly metabolized. Studies evaluating oncology nurses versus control populations of other nurses or non-health care workers have been published with both positive and negative results using all of the above methods. Clearly a combination of monitoring tools is required.

In addition to the above studies, which assess potential risk, the effect on human reproduction in terms of spontaneous abortion and teratogenic effects has also been examined. Again, the results are inconclusive but suggest an increase in both effects with frequent exposure. Information on safety practices is not available.

The agents most commonly implicated in mutagenic potential are those that are also implicated as causes of secondary cancers in patients receiving therapeutic drugs such as alkylating agents. Clearly, any cytotoxic drug should be handled with great care and with the goal of absolutely minimum exposure to personnel. This can be accomplished by worker education, gloves and protective clothing, laminar hoods for preparing drugs, and proper waste disposal. Periodic atmospheric checks and biological monitoring can improve hygienic standards, but conclusions regarding the long-term health effects based on these results are not possible.

# REFERENCES

## GENERAL

Hoffman R et al (editors): *Hematology: Basic Principles and Practice,* 2nd ed. Churchill Livingstone, 1995.

Rosenstock L, Cullen MR (editors): *Textbook of Clinical Occupational and Environmental Medicine.* Saunders, 1994.

Sauter D, Goldfrank L: Hematologic aspects of toxicology. Hematol Oncol Clin North Am 1987;1:335.

Zenc C, Dickerson OB, Horvath (editors): *Occupational Medicine,* 3rd ed. Mosby, 1994.

## METHEMOGLOBINEMIA & OXIDATIVE HEMOLYSIS

Fairbanks VF: Blue gods, blue oil, and blue people. Mayo Clin Proc 1994;69:89.

French CL et al: Potency ranking of methemoglobin-forming agents. J Appl Toxicol 1995;15:167.

Giardina B et al: The multiple functions of hemoglobin. Crit Rev Biochem Mol Biol 1995;30:165.

Khan MF et al: Hematopoietic toxicity of linoleic acid anilide: Importance of aniline. Fundam Appl Toxicol 1995;25:224.

Mansouri A, Lurie AA: Concise review: Methemoglobinemia. Am J Hematol 1993;42:7.

Nross BC, Ayebo AD, Fuortes LJ: Methemoglobinemia. Nitrate toxicity in rural America. Am Fam Phys 1992;46:183.

Steffen C, Wetzel E: Chlorate poisoning: Mechanisms of toxicity. Toxicology 1993;84:217.

## ARSINE

Hatlelid KM, Brailsford C, Carter DE: Reactions of arsine with hemoglobin. J Toxicol Environ Health 1996;47:135.

Klimecki WT, Carter DE: Arsine toxicity: Chemical and mechanistic implications. J Toxicol Environ Health 1995;46:399.

## LEAD

Goyer RA: Lead toxicity: From overt to subclinical to subtle health effects. Environ Health Perspect 1990; 86:177.

Osterode W: Hemorheology in occupational lead exposure. Scand J Work Environ Health 1996;22(5):369.

Ward JH: Hematologic effects of occupational hazards. In: Rom WN (editor): Environmental and Occupational Medicine, 3rd ed. Lippincott-Raven, 1997.

## TOXIC PORPHYRIA

Calvert GM et al: Evaluation of porphyria cutanea tarda in US workers exposed to 2,3,7,8-tetrachlorodibenzo-*p*-dioxin. Am J Ind Med 1994;25:559.

Jung D et al: Porphyrin studies in TCDD-exposed workers. Arch Toxicol 1994;68:595.

Meola T, Lim HW: The porphyrias. Dermatol Clin 1993;11:583.

## CARBON MONOXIDE

Penney DG: Acute carbon monoxide poisoning: Animal models: A review. Toxicology. 1990;62:123.

Schusterman D et al: Methylene chloride intoxication in a furniture refinisher. A comparison of exposure estimates utilizing workplace air sampling and blood carboxyhemoglobin measurements. J Occup Med 1990; 32:451.

## CYTOGENETICS

deJong G, vanSittert NJ, Natarajan AT: Cytogenetic monitoring of industrial populations potentially exposed to genotoxic chemicals and of control populations. Mutat Res 1988;204:451.

Scarpato R et al: Cytogenetic monitoring of occupational exposure to pesticides: Characterization of GSTM1, GSTT1 and NAT2 genotypes. Environ Mol Mutagen 1996;27:263.

## APLASTIC ANEMIA

Fleming LE, Timmeny H: Aplastic anemia and pesticides. An etiologic association? J Occup Med 1993; 35:1106.

Goiget M, Baumelu E, Mary JY: A case-control study of aplastic anemia: Occupational exposures. The French Cooperative Group for Epidemiologic Study of Aplastic Anemia. Int J Epidemiol 1995;24:993.

Young NS, Alter BP: *Aplastic Anemia: Acquired and Inherited.* Saunders, 1994.

## MYELODYSPLASIA

Boultwood J, Fidler C: Chromosomal deletions in myelodysplasia. Leuk Lymphoma 1995;17:71.

Ciccone G et al: Myeloid leukemias and myelodysplastic syndromes: Chemical exposure, histologic subtype and cytogenetics in a case control study. Cancer Genet Cytogenet 1993;68:135.

West RR et al: Occupational and environmental exposures and myelodysplasia: A case-control study. Leuk Res 1995;19:127.

## MULTIPLE MYELOMA

Hansen ES: A mortality study of Danish stokers. Br J Ind Med 1992;49:48.

Infante PF: State of the science on the carcinogenicity of gasoline with particular reference to cohort mortality study results. Environ Health Perspect 1993;101(6 suppl):105.

Wong O: Risk of acute myeloid leukemia and multiple myeloma in workers exposed to benzene. Occup Environ Med 1995;52:380.

Yardley-Jones A, Anderson D, Parke DV: The toxicity of benzene and its metabolism and molecular pathology in human risk assessment. Br J Ind Med 1991; 48:437.

## TOXIC THROMBOCYTOPENIA

Lundholm CE, Bartonek M: A study of the effects of p,p′-DDE and other related chlorinated hydrocarbons on inhibition of platelet aggregation. Arch Toxicol 1991;65:570.

## RISK TO HEALTH PROFESSIONALS

Karelova J et al: Chromosome and sister-chromatid exchange analysis in peripheral lymphocytes, and mutagenicity of urine in anesthesiology personnel. Int Arch Occup Environ Health 1992;64:303.

# Occupational Infections

# 16

*Richard Cohen, MD, MPH*

Occupational infections are those human diseases caused by work-associated exposure to microbial agents, including bacteria, viruses, fungi, and parasites (helminths, protozoa). An infection is distinguished as occupational by some aspect of the work that involves contact with a biologically active organism. Occupational infection can occur following contact with infected persons, as in the case of health care workers; with infected animal or human tissue, secretions, or excretions, as in laboratory workers; with asymptomatic or unknown contagious humans, as happens during business travel; or with infected animals, as in agriculture. This chapter highlights tuberculosis, hepatitis B and acquired immunodeficiency syndrome (AIDS), travel-related infections, and brucellosis as examples of the four types of exposure.

The etiology, pathogenesis, clinical findings, diagnosis, and treatment of occupational and nonoccupational infections are the same except for practical differences related to identification of the source of exposure, epidemiologic control, and prevention. This chapter will focus on the occupational aspects of microbial exposures and relevant strategies for prevention.

Table 16–1 lists the more frequent occupational infections according to agent, source, exposed occupations, and preventive measures. The references at the end of the chapter are selected as those most useful for practitioners engaged in diagnosis, treatment, and prevention of occupational infectious disease.

## INFECTIONS DUE TO EXPOSURE TO INFECTED HUMANS OR THEIR TISSUES

Health care and clinical laboratory workers are at increased risk of infection by organisms whose natural hosts are humans, as in the case of hepatitis, rubella, AIDS, tuberculosis, and staphylococcal disease. Some infections may be transmitted through close personal contact with infected patients. Exposure and infection due to almost any of the viruses, bacteria, fungi, and parasites pathogenic for humans can result from direct contact with the organism in culture or in human tissue. Tuberculosis is an example of a relatively common occupational infection resulting from repeated close contact with infected patients; and type B hepatitis exemplifies a serious and relatively frequent infection resulting from manipulation of infected human blood and inoculation by infectious virus particles.

## TUBERCULOSIS

*Mycobacterium tuberculosis* usually infects the lungs, with resulting pneumonia or granuloma formation, and may have other systemic effects also. Medical house staff have 2–3 times the tuberculosis infection rate of nonmedical personnel, and laboratory workers exposed to *M tuberculosis* have 3 times the incidence of nonexposed workers. Other high-prevalence work environments include most health care settings (especially hospitals, long-term care facilities, and dialysis centers), refugee/immigration centers, homeless shelters, substance abuse treatment centers, and correctional institutions.

Tubercle bacilli may be present in gastric fluid, cerebrospinal fluid, urine, sputum, and tissue specimens harboring active lesions. Infectious patients disseminate the organism when coughing, sneezing, or talking by expelling small infectious droplets that may remain suspended in air for several hours and inhaled by susceptible persons. After an incubation period of 4–12 weeks, infection usually remains subclinical and dormant without development of active disease, but the purified protein derivative (PPD) skin test will become positive. However, the organism may be activated at any time, resulting in acute severe pulmonary or other systemic disease. The risk of development of clinical disease following infection is higher in selected age groups (infancy, ages 16–21), in states of undernutrition, in certain immunopathologic states (eg, AIDS), in certain genetic groups (persons with HLA-Bw 15 histocompatibility antigen), and in persons with some coexisting dis-

**Table 16–1.** Occupational infections.

| Disease | Agent | Target Organ | Occupational Source | Exposed Occupations | Preventive Measures |
|---------|-------|--------------|---------------------|---------------------|---------------------|
| **Bacteria** | | | | | |
| Anthrax | *Bacillus anthracis* | Skin, lung, systemic | Dust (spores) on imported wool, goat hair, hides (goat, horse, cattle, sheep) | Weavers; goat hair, wool, or hide handlers; butchers, veterinarians, agricultural workers | Immunization |
| Brucellosis | *Brucella abortus, B suis, B melitensis, B canis* | Systemic | Blood, urine, vaginal discharges, milk, secretions, and tissues from cattle, swine, sheep, and caribou | Packing and slaughterhouse employees, livestock producers, veterinarians, hunters | Personal hygiene; serologic identification of infected animals; livestock vaccine |
| Erysipeloid | *Erysipelothrix rhusiopathiae (insidiosa)* | Skin | Fish, shellfish, meat, poultry | Fishermen, meat and poultry workers, veterinarians | Personal hygiene, gloves |
| Leptospirosis | *Leptospira interrogans* | Liver, kidney, brain, systemic | Urine or tissue of domestic or wild animals or rodent excreta; contaminated water | Field agricultural workers, abattoir workers, farmers, sewer workers, veterinarians, miners, fishermen | Personal hygiene, boots, gloves; animal immunization; identification of contaminated water supplies; doxycycline prophylaxis |
| Listeriosis | *Listeria monocytogenes* | Meninges, brain, systemic | Infected fetuses | Farmers, veterinarians | Pasteurization, proper handling of aborted fetuses |
| Plague | *Yersinia pestis* | Lung, systemic | Fleas from infected rats, squirrels, prairie dogs | Hunters, trappers, field workers, laboratory workers | Immunization |
| Tetanus | *Clostridium tetani* | Nervous system | Soil, skin puncture by unclean sharp object | Construction workers, gardeners, farmers | Immunization |
| Tuberculosis | *Mycobacterium tuberculosis* | Lung, systemic | Infected patient or nonhuman primate | Patient care workers, laboratory workers, primate handlers | PPD skin testing followed by prophylaxis for positive reactors |
| Tularemia | *Francisella tularensis* | Ulcerating papule, systemic | Blood, tissue, secretions, or bites of infected animals or arthropods | Hunters, forestry workers, farmers, veterinarians, trappers | Personal hygiene, gloves, immunization, insect control |
| **Fungi** | | | | | |
| Candidiasis | *Candida albicans* | Skin | Frequent skin trauma in a wet environment | Cannery workers, dishwashers, poultry processors | Skin protection, keeping dry |
| Coccidioidomycosis | *Coccidioides immitis* | Lung, meninges | Spores in soil in certain ecologic zones | Farm workers, archeologists, excavation workers, construction workers | Dust control (where practical) |
| Dermatophytoses, ringworm, athlete's foot | *Microsporum, Trichophyton, Epidermophyton* | Skin | Animals, hot humid environments, farmers | Animal handlers, ranchers, athletes | Personal hygiene, keeping dry |
| Histoplasmosis | *Histoplasma capsulatum* | Lung, systemic | Soil contaminated with fowl droppings | Farmers, poultry producers, rural demolition workers | Dust control, environmental sanitation; formaldehyde spraying of contaminated surfaces |
| Sporotrichosis | *Sporothrix schenki* | Skin, lymphatics | Thorns, splinters | Farmers, horticulturists | Gloves |

Table 16–1. Occupational infections (continued).

| Disease | Agent | Target Organ | Occupational Source | Exposed Occupations | Preventive Measures |
|---------|-------|--------------|---------------------|---------------------|---------------------|
| **Protozoa and helminths** | | | | | |
| Echinococcosis | *Echinococcus granulosus, E multiocularis* | CNS, lung, liver | Feces of infected dog, fox, other canids | Ranchers, sheepherders, veterinarians | Personal hygiene |
| Hookworm | *Ancylostoma duodenale, Necator americanus* | Small intestine | Larvae in human feces that penetrate intact skin | Barefoot farmers, excavators, sewer workers, recreation workers | Sanitary disposal of human feces; use of shoes, boots, gloves |
| Toxoplasmosis | *Toxoplasma gondii* | Reticuloendothelial system, eye | Cat feces | Laboratory workers, veterinarians, cat handlers | Personal hygiene |
| **Rickettsiae and chlamydiae** | | | | | |
| Ornithosis | *Chlamydia psittaci* | Lung, systemic | Discharges or excreta of infected domestic birds (parrots, pigeons, parakeets, etc) | Bird handlers, pet shop workers, zoo attendants, poultry workers | Identification and treatment of infected birds |
| Q fever | *Coxiella burnetii* | Systemic, liver, lung, brain | Placental tissue, birth fluids, or excreta from infected animals (cattle, sheep, goats, wild animals) | Laboratory workers, rendering plant and slaughterhouse workers, farmers, ranchers | Personal hygiene, immunization |
| Rocky Mountain spotted fever | *Rickettsia rickettsii* | Systemic, skin | Ticks from infected rodents, dogs | Ranchers, farmers, foresters, rangers, lumberjacks, hunters | Tick avoidance |
| **Viruses** | | | | | |
| Encephalitis (St. Louis, equine) | *Arbovirus* | CNS | Laboratory virus cultures, infected arthropods | Virus laboratory workers | Adherence to biologic safety practices, immunization, insecticides |
| Hepatitis A | Hepatitis A virus | Liver | Sewage, contaminated food | Sewer workers, travelers to endemic areas | Personal hygiene, immunization, and careful food and drink selection |
| Hepatitis B | Hepatitis B virus | Liver | Accidental inoculation with infected human blood and blood products | Oral surgeons, dentists, phlebotomists, dialysis workers, clinical laboratory workers, patient care workers | Personal hygiene, immunization |
| Newcastle disease | Paramyxovirus | Eyes | Poultry | Poultry handlers, veterinarians, animal laboratory workers | Personal hygiene |
| Rabies | Rabies virus | CNS | Wild animals (skunk, fox, bat, raccoon); rarely, domestic animals | Laboratory workers, veterinarians, trappers, hunters; persons who handle wild or unidentified animals | Immunization of human contacts and of certain animal species (dog, cat) |
| Rubella | Rubella virus | Fetus, systemic | Infected humans | Health care workers | Immunization |
| AIDS | HIV | Immune system | Body fluids of infected humans | Health care workers | Universal body substance precautions |

CNS = central nervous system; HIV = human immunodeficiency virus.

eases (silicosis, end-stage renal disease, malnutrition, leukemia, lymphoma, upper gastrointestinal tract carcinoma, diabetes).

PPD is a chemical fractionation product of tubercle bacilli culture filtrate. Intradermal injection of 5 tuberculin units of PPD in a patient with subclinical or clinical tuberculous infection results in a delayed hypersensitivity reaction manifested by induration at the site of injection within 48–72 hours. A minimum of 5 mm of induration is required for a test to be "positive" or "reactive" in close contacts of infectious patients or persons with known or suspected HIV infection. A reaction of 10 mm or more is considered positive in other high-prevalence (>5%), high-risk occupational groups (above) or high-risk groups including immigrants from high prevalence areas, alcoholics, intravenous drug users, immunosuppressed persons, and those with other disease states mentioned above. In persons with no risk factors in areas of low prevalence, induration of 15 mm or more is required for a "positive" reaction (Table 16–2). The PPD test may be negative in the presence of overwhelming tuberculosis, measles, Hodgkin's disease, sarcoidosis, or immunosuppressive states. The test will usually revert to negative following elimination of viable tubercle bacilli. If the initial test is negative in individuals with suspected reduced immune response or in those who will be screened annually because of occupational or other risk, it should be repeated. PPD tests are likely to be reactive for extended periods following BCG vaccination. However, prior BCG vaccination is not a contraindication to skin testing.

PPD skin testing is an accepted method for screening high-risk populations for primary infection. Persons having a reactive test are at risk of developing active clinical infection at any time (lifelong) following the primary infection owing to reactivation of the primary infection as long as viable tubercle bacilli remain in the body.

Diagnosis and treatment of clinically active disease follows established microbiologic and antibiotic protocols, with treatment variations depending on the antibiotic resistance of the specific strain.

## Prevention & Control

PPD testing can identify persons whose tests are reactive, indicating primary infection. Serial testing (biennial or more frequently) can identify recently infected individuals whose tests have become reactive ("converters") within the past 2 years. Occupational candidates for periodic PPD testing include those having contact with suspected or known infected pa-

**Table 16–2.** Summary of interpretation of PPD tuberculin skin test results.[1]

1. An induration of ≥5 mm is classified as positive in:
   Persons who have HIV infection or risk factors for HIV infection but unknown HIV status
   Persons who have had recent close contact[2] with persons who have active tuberculosis (TB)
   Persons who have fibrotic chest radiographs (consistent with healed TB)
2. An induration of ≥10 mm is classified as positive in all persons who do not meet any of the criteria above but who have other risk factors for TB:
   High-risk groups
   Injecting drug users known to be HIV seronegative
   Persons who have other medical conditions that reportedly increase the risk for progressing from latent TB infection to active TB (eg, silicosis; gastrectomy or jejuno-ileal bypass; being ≥10% below ideal body weight; chronic renal failure with renal dialysis; diabetes mellitus; high-dose corticosteroid or other immunosuppressive therapy; some hematologic disorders, including cancers such as leukemias and lymphomas; and other cancers)
   Children ≤4 years of age or infants, children, and adolescents exposed to adults in high-risk categories
   High-prevalence groups
   Foreign-born persons recently arrived within the past 5 years from countries in Asia, Africa, the Caribbean, and Latin America that have high prevalence of TB
   Persons from medically underserved, low-income populations
   Residents and employees of long-term-care facilities (eg, correctional institutions and nursing homes)
   Persons from high-risk populations in their communities, as determined by local public health authorities
3. An induration of ≥15 mm is classified as positive in persons who do not meet any of the above criteria.
4. Recent converters are defined on the basis of both size of induration and age of the person being tested:
   ≥10-mm increase within a 2-year period is classified as a recent conversion for persons ≤35 years of age
   ≥15-mm increase within a 2-year period is classified as a recent conversion for persons ≥35 years of age
5. PPD skin test results in health-care workers (HCWs):
   In general, the recommendations in sections 1, 2, and 3 of this table should be followed when interpreting skin test results in HCWs. However, the prevalence of TB in the facility should be considered when choosing the appropriate cut point for defining a positive PPD reaction. In facilities where there is essentially no risk for exposure to *M tuberculosis* (ie, minimal) or very low risk facilities, an induration ≥15 mm may be a suitable cut point for HCWs who have no other risk factors. In facilities where TB patients receive care, the cut point for HCWs with no other risk factors may be ≥10 mm
   A recent conversion in an HCW should be defined generally as a ≥10-mm increase in size of induration within a 2-year period. For HCWs who work in facilities where exposure to TB is very unlikely (eg, minimal-risk facilities), an increase of ≥15 mm within a 2-year period may be more appropriate for defining a recent conversion because of the lower positive predictive value of the test in such groups

[1]From Centers for Disease Control: Screening for Tuberculosis and Tuberculosis Infection in High-Risk Populations, Morbid Mortal Weekly Rep 1995;**44(RR-11):**24, Table 1.
[2]Recent close contact implies either household or social contact or unprotected occupational exposure similar in intensity and duration to household contact.

tients, persons working with potentially infected primates or cattle (veterinarians, zoo keepers, primate handlers), and all others working in the higher-risk environments mentioned above.

Recent asymptomatic "converters" or others recently discovered to be tuberculin-reactive ("reactors")—whose date of conversion is unknown and who are least likely to develop complications due to antibiotic therapy—should receive drug treatment according to protocols recommended by the Centers for Disease Control and Prevention or local health departments.

Isoniazid prophylaxis is recommended for persons found to have a positive PPD who fall into any of the following categories: newly infected persons, including recent converters (within 2 years); household contacts of active cases; persons with an abnormal chest x-ray consistent with clinical tuberculosis and inadequate past antituberculous therapy or prior active disease with inadequate past therapy; persons whose reactivation may have public health consequences (eg, schoolteachers); patients with AIDS (or persons with antibodies to human immunodeficiency virus [HIV]), silicosis, insulin-dependent diabetes mellitus, hematologic or reticuloendothelial cancer, prior gastrectomy, chronic undernutrition, ileal bypass, renal failure requiring dialysis, or a history of prolonged use of glucocorticoid or immunosuppressive therapy, as well as intravenous drug users; and all reactors younger than age 35 with none of the above risk factors.

Before starting isoniazid prophylaxis, a chest x-ray should be taken on all skin test reactors. Any abnormalities found should be thoroughly evaluated for evidence of clinically active disease.

If adequate prior prophylaxis or therapy for active disease has been completed or if the patient has had previous adverse reactions to isoniazid or acute liver disease due to any cause, isoniazid prophylaxis should not be given. Patients at increased risk of chronic liver disease should be identified and closely monitored for isoniazid hepatic effects.

Preventive therapy for adults is with isoniazid, 300 mg orally in a single dose daily for 6 months or more depending on risk status and PPD reaction size (Table 16–3). Following completion of therapy, if no adverse reactions to isoniazid have occurred, no further follow-up or x-rays are necessary. Rifampin is recommended for prophylactic management of patients suspected of having isoniazid-resistant tubercle bacilli.

Persons for whom prophylactic antibiotic therapy is contraindicated should receive surveillance chest x-rays if they become symptomatic. Persons having known contact with an infectious patient for whom PPD status has not been previously documented should be PPD-tested immediately and then again 8–12 weeks after the infectious contact. If conversion occurs, physical examination and chest x-ray should occur to rule out acute clinical infection.

Attenuated tubercle bacilli—particularly BCG—have been used in many countries as a vaccine. In the United States, use of BCG is rarely indicated.

## HEPATITIS B

Before the availability of an effective vaccine, hepatitis B was the most frequent laboratory-associated infection. The virus can be transmitted in blood, semen, cerebrospinal fluid, saliva, and urine. Transmission

**Table 16–3.** Criteria for determining need for preventive therapy for persons with positive tuberculin reactions, by category and age group.[1]

| Category | Age Group (yr) | |
|---|---|---|
| | **<35** | **≥35** |
| **With risk factor[2]** | Treat at all ages if reaction to 5 TU of PPD if ≥10 mm (or ≥5 mm and patient is recent contact, HIV-infected, or has radiographic evidence of old TB) | |
| **No risk factor** | | |
| High-incidence group[3] | Treat if PPD ≥10 mm | Do not treat |
| Low-incidence group | Treat if PPD ≥15 mm[4] | Do not treat |

[1]From Centers for Disease Control: Screening for tuberculosis and tuberculous infection in high-risk populations and the use of preventive therapy for tuberculosis infection in the United States. *Morbid Mortal Weekly Rep* 1990;**39(RR–8):**1.
[2]Risk factors include HIV infection, recent contact with infectious person, recent skin test conversion, abnormal chest x-ray, intravenous drug abuse, and certain medical risk factors (see text).
[3]High-incidence groups include foreign-born persons, medically underserved low-income populations, and residents of long-term care facilities.
[4]Lower or higher cut points may be used for identifying positive reactions, depending upon the relative prevalence of *M tuberculosis* infection and nonspecific cross-reactivity in the population.

usually occurs by exposure of mucous membranes or broken skin to infected blood or blood products.

The marker for viral infection is the surface antigen (HBsAg). HBsAg is present during clinical infection in most patients for approximately 4 weeks prior to the appearance of clinical disease and for approximately 8–10 weeks following the onset of clinical hepatitis. Between 6 and 10% of acutely infected adults will carry the virus beyond 12 weeks and are classified as chronic carriers, remaining infectious until the surface antigen disappears.

Persons at increased risk include workers at institutions for the mentally retarded, health care workers having frequent blood contact (eg, phlebotomists, laboratory workers, surgical and emergency personnel, blood gas technicians, blood bank personnel, nurses, dialysis and oncology unit nurses, pathologists, dentists), and other workers having frequent potential for percutaneous inoculation with infected blood or saliva such as mortuary staff. The virus may remain viable in dried blood or blood components for several days, making contaminated health care equipment potentially infectious if parenteral inoculation occurs.

The incubation period is from 50 to 180 days (average, 60 to 90 days). The disease has an insidious onset, usually with a gradual and prolonged rise in serum alanine aminotransferase (ALT; formerly SGPT). ALT values may range between 500 and 2000 IU/L and are usually higher than serum aspartate transaminase levels (AST; formerly SGOT). Aminotransaminase levels may remain elevated for up to 6 months or more after clinical illness disappears. Findings on history and physical examination are indistinguishable from those associated with other forms of hepatitis. Microbial, biliary, alcoholic, drug-induced, and toxic causes of hepatitis may present with identical findings and must be ruled out.

Serologic testing for the surface (s), core (c), and "e" antigens and their respective antibodies allows prompt characterization of the stage and infectivity of hepatitis B. When this is combined with serologic testing for other types of hepatitis, it assists in definitive diagnosis of type B versus non-type B hepatitis. Table 16–4 illustrates that once the patient is negative for all antigens and antibodies except for antibodies to the surface and core antigens, the disease is no longer communicable and the patient is immune to further type B infection. It also demonstrates the potential value of serologic testing as part of surveillance for asymptomatic infection and subsequent immunity.

Treatment is as for any other form of hepatitis and is for the most part supportive. Alcohol and other hepatotoxins should be avoided during convalescence.

## Prevention

Because exposure to patients, patients' body fluids, contaminated glassware, and other contaminated equipment such as needles may provide an opportunity for mucous membrane or parenteral inoculation, strict infection control procedures should be developed for risk situations such as phlebotomy, dentistry, and hemodialysis. Splash control, rigid containment of sharp instruments (eg, contaminated needles), and use of gloves are required whenever contact is likely with biological fluids such as semen, saliva, or blood, as with surgery, including dental surgery. Hygienic and safety procedures should be clearly defined and rigidly enforced. Laboratory personnel handling such fluids should consider all human specimens potentially infected with type B virus and handle them accordingly.

In its regulation, Occupational Exposure to Bloodborne Pathogens 29 CFR 1910.1030, the Occupational Safety and Health Administration (OSHA) now requires employers and workers to use universal precautions when handling all potentially infected material. It also requires physical and procedural barriers, training, labeling, disposal, and other actions designed to prevent such occupational infections.

Workers at increased risk for hepatitis B infection should receive hepatitis B vaccine. Some recommend screening vaccine candidates by testing for surface antigen antibody; if it is present, vaccination is unnecessary. The vaccine confers immunity in 90% of vaccinees, and for this reason some experts recommend serologic testing for surface antigen antibody following vaccine administration to verify an immunologic response. The vaccine is produced by recombinant DNA technology without using human cells or plasma.

For persons not vaccinated, hepatitis B immune globulin and/or vaccine should be administered as postexposure prophylaxis immediately following inoculation with suspected contaminated fluids. The schedule and dosage of administration vary depending on the victim's vaccination status and the source's infectivity (Table 16–5).

Exposure surveillance as a measure of hygiene and containment practices can identify asymptomatic previously infected individuals. The combination of testing for the surface antigen, the core antibody, and the surface antigen antibody should identify all such individuals. Almost all past asymptomatic cases can also be identified by testing for the surface antigen antibody alone.

Because hepatitis B is also transmitted through sexual and other intimate social contact, questions often arise about how employees in non-health care industries who develop the disease through such contact should be treated in the workplace. Other than the means of transmission mentioned above, there is no evidence that a chronic surface antigen carrier or a person acutely ill with type B hepatitis will serve as a source of infection to coworkers in the absence of parenteral or intimate contact. Restrictions on contact with type B hepatitis-infected workers are therefore not appropriate in most work situations.

For updated information on transmission, diagnosis, and prevention, the Centers for Disease Control and Prevention has an automated hepatitis information hotline at (404) 332-4555.

**Table 16–4.** Representative serologic patterns in viral hepatitis.[1]

| Serologic Markers (+, present; −, absent) | | | | | Interpretation |
|---|---|---|---|---|---|
| HBsAg | HBeAg | Anti-HBc | Anti-Hbe | Anti-Hbs | |
| + | − | − | − | − | Incubation period or early hepatitis B: Infective. |
| + | + | + | − | − | Acute hepatitis B or chronic carrier: Infective. |
| + | − | + | + | − | Resolving acute hepatitis or chronic carrier: Low infectivity. |
| − | + | + | − | − | Acute hepatitis in "window" period or low-grade chronic carrier: Infective. |
| − | − | + | + | − | Convalescence from acute hepatitis: Low infectivity. |
| − | − | + | + | + | Recent recovery from acute hepatitis: Not infective; immune. |
| − | − | + | − | + | Post recovery from hepatitis: Not infective; immune. |
| − | − | − | − | + | Past subclinical infection or active-passive immunzation: Not infective, immune. |

[1]Reproduced, with permission, from Mandell HN: *Laboratory Medicine in Clinical Practice.* John Wright, 1983.

Types C and non-A, non-B viral hepatitis are being diagnosed more frequently because of the availability of serologic testing for types A, B, and C. Transmission is mostly transfusion-related, but workers with type B exposure risks are probably at analogous but lesser risk for types C and non-A, non-B hepatitis; preventive measures are as for type B.

## ACQUIRED IMMUNODEFICIENCY SYNDROME (AIDS)

There is great anxiety among workers concerning potential contact with AIDS patients in the workplace. Fortunately, the virus is not transmitted through casual nonintimate workplace contact or social encounters such as eating in restaurants or using public transportation or bathroom facilities. Other than infants delivered from AIDS-infected mothers, more than 98% of all new patients or have the known risk factors of male homosexuality, parenteral drug abuse, medical treatment with blood or blood products, or sexual contact with an AIDS-infected person.

### Transmission

Human immunodeficiency virus (HIV) has been isolated from blood, semen, saliva, tears, urine, cerebrospinal fluid, solid tissue, and cervical secretions and is likely to be present in other bodily fluids, secretions, or tissues from infected humans. Potential routes

**Table 16–5.** Recommendations for hepatitis B prophylaxis following percutaneous or permucosal exposure.[1]

| Exposed Person | Treatment When Source Is: | | |
|---|---|---|---|
| | HBsAg-Positive | HBsAG-Negative | Not Tested or Unknown |
| **Unvaccinated** | HBIG × 1[2] and initiate HB vaccine | Initiate HB vaccine | Initiate HB vaccine |
| **Previously vaccinated** Known responder | Test exposed for anti-HBs 1. If adequate,[3] no treatment 2. If inadequate, HB vaccine booster dose | No treatment | No treatment |
| Known nonresponder | HBIG × 2 or HBIG × 1 plus 1 dose HB vaccine | No treatment | If known high-risk source, may treat as if source were HBsAG-positive |
| Response unknown | Test exposed for anti-HBs 1. If inadequate,[3] HBIG × 1 plus HB vaccine booster dose 2. If adequate, no treatment | No treatment | Test exposed for anti-HBs 1. If inadequate,[3] HB vaccine booster dose 2. If adequate, no treatment |

[1]From Centers for Disease Control: Protection against viral hepatitis: Recommendations of the Immunization Practices Advisory Committee (ACIP). *Morbid Mortal Weekly Rep* 1990;**39(RR–2)**:1.
[2]HBIG dose, 0.06 ml/kg IM.
[3]Adequate anti-HBs is ≥10 SRU by RIA or positive by EIA.

of infection include percutaneous or parenteral inoculation and direct contact of cuts, scratches, abrasions, or mucosal surfaces with material containing live virus. Possible transmission may therefore occur through parenteral inoculation, through needle sticks, broken glass, or sharps contaminated with HIV, or through spillage of infected material onto abraded skin or mucous membranes. Neither ingestion nor inhalation has been shown to be a mode of transmission. Like hepatitis B virus, HIV is a "blood-borne pathogen," but given identical exposure circumstances, HIV is transmitted much less frequently than is hepatitis B virus. The concentration of virus is higher in blood, serum, cerebrospinal fluid, and semen and much lower in AIDS patients' saliva, tears, urine, breast milk, amniotic fluid, and vaginal secretions.

It follows that transmission is most likely to occur as the result of sexual contact with an infected partner, by parenteral exposure to infected blood or blood products, and by perinatal exposure of offspring of infected mothers. Casual contact, fomites (coffee cups, drinking fountains, telephone receivers, insects, etc) have not been shown to be mechanisms or circumstances of transmission.

### Risk of Occupational Infection

The following occupational groups are at potential risk of contact with HIV-infected body fluids: blood bank technologists, dialysis technicians, emergency room personnel, morticians, dentists, medical technicians, surgeons, laboratory workers, and prostitutes. Multiple studies of health care workers have been published in which the presence of antibody to HIV or evidence of clinical AIDS infection was investigated in association with needle sticks, parenteral or splash exposures to known infected material, or laboratory work with concentrated virus in culture. These and other studies consistently show that the incidence of AIDS infection following such contact with material known to be infected with HIV is consistently less than 1% and usually less than 0.5%. AIDS infection of prostitutes is occurring at increasing rates and is clearly related to both sexual activity and parenteral drug abuse.

Because HIV has been found in saliva, there has been concern that cardiopulmonary resuscitation (CPR) and first aid activities place those providers at increased risk for AIDS. To date, the risk appears to be quite low: No cases of HIV infection have been reported as a result of mouth-to-mouth CPR or the provision of first aid services. Nevertheless, many public safety organizations (police, fire fighters, paramedics) now routinely use special patient masks for providing mouth-to-mouth CPR.

In work situations other than those described above, AIDS has not been shown to be transmitted. Workers sharing the same work environment as a coworker infected with AIDS have not been found at risk in environments such as schools, offices, factories, and construction sites. AIDS has not been transmitted via food; a food service worker infected with HIV does not place restaurant customers at increased risk of HIV infection.

Personal service workers are defined as individuals whose occupations involve close personal contact with clients: hair dressers, barbers, cosmetologists, manicurists, massage parlor personnel, or persons who perform tattooing, ear piercing, or acupuncture. There is no evidence of transmission of AIDS between personal service workers and their clients, but sensible precautions in disinfection of instruments should be observed.

### Legal & Social Issues

Major AIDS-related issues for many workers involve fear of contagion, AIDS testing, confidentiality, civil rights, and insurance benefits.

Fear and panic among workers resulting from misinformation concerning HIV transmission can be a disruptive force in a work environment when it becomes known that a fellow worker is an AIDS victim. Other than in the few "personal service" occupations mentioned above, AIDS does not present a risk of transmission in the normal course of employment. Many people do not understand this and do not want to be near an AIDS victim. The employer, on the other hand, cannot banish the AIDS patient from the workplace in these situations, since there is no public health risk to other employees—the only basis for employment restriction would be physical or mental incapacity to perform the requirements of the job.

Coworkers who refuse to work with the AIDS victim may continue to do so until they have been educated concerning the disease and its transmission. Educational material is available from CDC and commercial sources that will provide information for employees so that the employer can then require employees, once educated, to continue their work alongside the AIDS-infected coworker.

Some employers have considered AIDS testing for prospective employees. There is no medical justification for such testing, since AIDS transmission does not occur in work activities other than those mentioned above. In some states, eg, California, statutes prohibit preemployment AIDS testing and impose restrictions on release of information concerning the diagnosis of AIDS.

As with other personal medical conditions, the employer is also bound to honor the confidentiality and privacy rights of its employees. Because there is no public health risk to coworkers in most employment situations, the employer has no obligation to release information regarding a diagnosis of AIDS in a given worker. The employer may do so only with the worker's written consent and even then would be well advised to withhold such information, since it serves no purpose and is likely to result in unnecessary disruption.

AIDS has been designated in some courts as a protected handicap, meaning that the employer cannot refuse to hire an AIDS-infected patient simply because he or she has AIDS. In order to justify denial of employment, the AIDS victim must be so debilitated as to be unable to perform the physical or mental requirements of the job and the employer must show an inability to make a reasonable job accommodation.

## Prevention

For occupational health professionals, employer-sponsored first aid workers, and public safety personnel who may provide medical services to HIV-infected individuals, reasonable steps should be taken to avoid skin, parenteral, or mucous membrane contact with potentially infected blood, plasma, or secretions. Hands or skin should be washed immediately and carefully if blood contact occurs. Mucous membranes—including the eyes and mouth—should be protected by eyeglasses, masks, or face shields during procedures that could generate splashes or aerosols of infected blood or secretions (suctioning, endoscopy). Contaminated surfaces should be disinfected with 5% sodium hypochlorite.

Personal service workers who work with needles or other instruments that can penetrate intact skin should follow precautions indicated for health care workers and practice aseptic technique and sterilization of instruments. All personal service workers should be educated concerning transmission of blood-borne infections, including AIDS and hepatitis B.

If a health care or other worker experiences parenteral or mucous membrane exposure to blood or other potentially infected bodily fluids, the likelihood of HIV infection should be determined for the source patient. If possible, the source patient should undergo serologic testing for HIV infection. If the source patient has serologic or other evidence of HIV infection or refuses to submit to testing, the exposed worker should be evaluated clinically and serologically for HIV infection as soon as possible after the event. If the result is negative, the worker should be retested at 6, 12, and 26 weeks following exposure. If the source patient is seronegative, has no AIDS risk factors, and has no other evidence of HIV infection, the risk of infection is less than 0.01%; additional follow-up can be considered.

Postexposure prophylaxis with antibiotics is recommended based on exposure type and source material (Table 16–6).

Pregnant health care workers should be educated regarding the possibility of transmission of HIV to newborns. Because of the increased risk of cytomegalovirus infection among AIDS patients, care of AIDS patients by pregnant women may be contraindicated.

Additional recommendations concerning general workplace exposures—including those of health care workers, precautions during invasive procedures, and precautions for laboratory workers—are updated periodically in *Morbidity and Mortality Weekly Reports*. Workplace requirements relevant to occupational exposure are detailed in OSHA's Bloodborne Pathogen regulation (see above).

## TRAVEL-ASSOCIATED INFECTIOUS DISEASES

International travel is a necessary part of work for thousands of workers. It often involves travel to distant and sometimes rural locales having endemic pathogens never established or long since eradicated at the traveler's point of origin. From a workers' compensation standpoint, any illness or injury that occurs as a result of work that would not have occurred at that time due to nonoccupational activities is usually considered work-related. For example, salmonellosis or malaria developing following travel to an area where these disorders are endemic is attributable to work-related presence in the area.

Travel-related infection therefore could include the whole range of human pathogens, depending upon the agents endemic to the area being visited and opportunities by the traveler for exposure. Water purification, waste sanitation, food preparation, vector control, recreational activities during travel, and personal hygiene of the traveler influence exposure potential.

Commonly encountered travel-related diseases include traveler's diarrhea (from infection with *Salmonella, Shigella, Giardia, Entamoeba histolytica,* pathogenic *Escherichia coli,* and selected viral agents), hepatitis A, yellow fever, typhoid fever, cholera, and malaria. Other diseases that have been virtually eliminated from countries with effective childhood vaccination programs—the prime example is poliomyelitis—may be endemic in underdeveloped areas, placing the nonimmunized person at particular risk for these diseases.

## Prevention

Public health authorities should be consulted to determine what vaccinations are recommended or required and what diseases are endemic in areas to be visited. The traveler's routine immunization status should be maintained in accordance with the recommendations of the Immunization Practice Advisory Committee (ACIP) for persons living in the United States (diphtheria, tetanus, measles, mumps, rubella, hepatitis B, and poliomyelitis). Effective vaccines are available for cholera, yellow fever, typhoid fever, rabies, hepatitis A, hepatitis B, plague, and meningococcal meningitis. Prophylactic immunoglobulin (gamma globulin) is an effective alternative to hepatitis A vaccine for travel lasting less than 3 months. The CDC maintains a 24-hour automated FAX information line with current travel and immunization recommendations at (404) 332-4555. This information is also available through the Internet by selecting "Travelers' Health" on the CDC home page (http://www.cdc.gov/).

Malarial prophylaxis is strongly recommended for visits to areas of endemic infection, particularly to rural areas in tropical developing countries. Prophylaxis of chloroquine-sensitive strains of all species

**Table 16–6.** Provisional Public Health Service recommendations for chemoprophylaxis after occupational exposure to HIV, by type of exposure and source material—1996.

| Type of Exposure | Source Material[1] | Antiretroviral Prophylaxis[2] | Antiretroviral Regimen[3] |
|---|---|---|---|
| Percutaneous | Blood[4] | | |
| | Highest risk | Recommend | ZDV plus 3TC plus IDV |
| | Increased risk | Recommend | ZDV plus 3TC, ± IDV[5] |
| | No increased risk | Offer | ZDV plus 3TC |
| | Fluid containing visible blood, other potentially infectious fluid[6], or tissue | Offer | ZDV plus 3TC |
| | Other body fluid (e.g., urine) | Not offer | |
| Mucous membrane | Blood | Offer | ZDV plus 3TC, ± IDV[5] |
| | Fluid containing visible blood, other potentially infectious fluid[6], or tissue | Offer | ZDV, ± 3TC |
| | Other body fluid (e.g., urine) | Not offer | |
| Skin, increased risk[7] | Blood | Offer | ZDV plus 3TC, ± IDV[5] |
| | Fluid containing visible blood, other potentially infectious fluid[6], or tissue | Offer | ZDV, ± 3TC |
| | Other body fluid (e.g., urine) | Not offer | |

[1]Any exposure to concentrated HIV (e.g., in a research laboratory or production facility) is treated as percutaneous exposure to blood with highest risk.

[2]*Recommend*—Postexposure prophylaxis (PEP) should be recommended to the exposed worker with counseling (see text). *Offer*—PEP should be offered to the exposed worker with counseling (see text). *Not offer*—PEP should not be offered because these are not occupational exposures to HIV (*1*).

[3]Regimens: zidovudine (ZDV), 200 mg three times a day; lamivudine (3TC), 150 mg two times a day; indinavir (IDV), 800 mg three times a day (if IDV is not available, saquinavir may be used, 600 mg three times a day). Prophylaxis is given for 4 weeks. For full prescribing information, see package inserts.

[4]*Highest risk*—BOTH larger volume of blood (e.g., deep injury with large diameter hollow needle previously in source patient's vein or artery, especially involving an injection of source-patient's blood) AND blood containing a high titer of HIV (e.g., source with acute retroviral illness or end-stage AIDS; viral load measurement may be considered, but its use in relation to PEP has not been evaluated). *Increased risk*—EITHER exposure to larger volume of blood OR blood with a high titer of HIV. *No increased risk*—NEITHER exposure to larger volume of blood NOR blood with a high titer of HIV (e.g., solid suture needle injury from source patient with asymptomatic HIV infection).

[5]Possible toxicity of additional drug may not be warranted (see text).

[6]Includes semen; vaginal secretions; cerebrospinal, synovial, pleural, peritoneal, pericardial, and amniotic fluids.

[7]For skin, risk is increased for exposures involving a high titer of HIV, prolonged contact, an extensive area, or an area in which skin integrity is visibly compromised. For skin exposures without increased risk, the risk for drug toxicity outweighs the benefit of PEP.

Reproduced from Morbid Mortal Weekly Report, 1996;**45:**471.

consists of taking 500 mg of chloroquine phosphate orally once weekly beginning 1–2 weeks before arrival and continuing for every week during travel and for 4 weeks after leaving a malaria-endemic area. In certain areas of Asia, South America, and Africa, chloroquine-resistant strains of *Plasmodium falciparum* are prevalent. For travel to these areas, mefloquine or doxycycline should be considered, depending on the patient's personal medical history, drug sensitivity, length of stay, and other factors in accordance with the CDC recommendations.

The CDC Malaria Prevention Information System at (404) 332-4555 can provide updated guidelines for treatment and prophylaxis 24 hours a day.

Antibiotic prophylaxis of traveler's diarrhea is recommended less frequently now because of the effectiveness of prompt treatment (Table 16–7) and concerns about the development of resistant strains.

Should diarrhea develop, empiric treatment regimens include rehydration, antimotility agents (unless dysentery is suspected), and antibiotics (Table 16–8).

Other general protective measures include insect repellents where insect vectors may transmit disease (malaria, yellow fever, dengue, filariasis, leishmaniasis, trypanosomiasis, and hemorrhagic fevers). Use of light-colored and protective clothing and mosquito

netting, avoidance of being outdoors between dusk and dawn, and avoidance of scented cosmetics may be helpful. The traveler should take care not to eat or drink contaminated food or water and should avoid uncooked foods. Swimming in contaminated waters and walking with inadequately protected feet should be avoided where possible.

Jong and Southworth have recommended items for inclusion in a traveler's personal medical kit that should be tailored to the particular destination and its endemic risks (Table 16–9).

# INFECTIONS TRANSMITTED FROM ANIMALS TO HUMANS: ZOONOSES

Zoonoses are defined as diseases that infect both humans and animals. Occupations involving contact with infected animals, their infected secretions or tissues, or contact with arthropod vectors from infected animals can result in work-related zoonotic disease.

**Table 16–7.** Summary of the recommended measures for preventing traveler's diarrhea.[1]

1. Food and water precautions should be followed.
2. Consider antibiotic prophylaxis if the trip is to be less than 2 wks and one or more of the following are present:
   Patient has potentially reduced gastric acidity
   Patient is elderly
   Patient is receiving chronic histamine $H_2$-receptor antagonist therapy
   Patient has had gastric surgery
   Patient has a chronic illness, such as diabetes, renal disease, cancer, or an immunosuppressive disorder (eg, AIDS)
   Patient is taking a critially important trip or a trip that would be severely affected if the traveler's diarrhea occurred
3. If prophylactic therapy is selected, one of the following may be used in adult patients:
   Ciprofloxacin (Cipro), one 500-mg tablet or two 250-mg tablets per day
   Norfloxacin (Noroxin), one 400-mg tablet per day
   Trimethoprim-sulfamethoxazole, double strength (Bactrim DS, Cotrim DS, Septra DS), one tablet per day
   Bismuth subsalicylate (Pepto-Bismol), two tablets four times daily

[1]Reproduced, with permission, from Heck JE, Cohen MB: Traveler's diarrhea. *Am Fam Physician* 1993;**48**:793.

Such occupations include animal laboratory workers, veterinarians, farmers, breeders, dairy workers, hunters, wildlife workers, hide and wool handlers, slaughterhouse (abattoir) workers, ranchers, rendering plant workers, pet shop workers, taxidermists, zoo attendants, agricultural workers, sewer workers, miners, military personnel, and butchers. Although these diseases are relatively rare, some of the more common occupational zoonoses in the United States include tularemia, Rocky Mountain spotted fever,

**Table 16–8.** Empiric therapy for adults with traveler's diarrhea.[1]

**Fluid and electrolyte replacement**
Oral rehydration solution, if available; if appropriate solutions are not available, the adult traveler with diarrhea should drink fruit juice, caffeine-free soft drinks, or bottled water, and should eat salted crackers
**Antibiotics[2]**
Ciprofloxacin (Cipro), one 500-mg tablet or two 250-mg tablets twice daily for 3 days
*or*
Trimethoprim-sulfamethoxazole, double strength (Bactrim DS, Cotrim DS, Septra DS), one tablet twice daily for 3 days
**Antimotility medications**
Loperamide (Imodium), two 2-mg tablets after the first loose stool, then one tablet after each loose stool, for a maximum of 16 mg in 24 hours
*or*
Diphenoxylate with atropine (Lomotil), two 2.5-mg tablets four times daily for loose stools

[1]Reproduced, with permission, from Heck JE, Cohen MB: Traveler's diarrhea. *Am Fam Physician* 1993;**48**:793.
[2]Antibiotics may be used in combination with antimotility medications.

**Table 16–9.** Traveler's personal medical kit (nonprescription items).[1]

Acetaminophen (Tylenol) or aspirin tablets: for general relief or minor aches and pains or headache.
Antibiotic ointment for minor skin/wound infection.
Decongestant and antihistamine capsules: for nasal congestion and allergic rhinitis.
Glucose and electrolyte powdered mix: to be mixed in safe water for fluid replacement and rehydration during severe diarrhea.
Itch stick or hydrocortisone cream for relief of itching due to insect bites.
Insect repellent liquid: for topical application.
Insect repellent spray: for use in unscreened rooms and other areas.
Sunscreen lotion (eg, PreSun 8): for protection against sunburn.
Povidone-iodine liquid: for cleansing of minor cuts and abrasions.
Water purification cup: for purification of unsanitary water.
Water purification tablets: iodine-based tablets will kill microorganisms that chlorine-based tablets will not.
Bandages: Band-Aids, 2 × 2 sterile gauze pads, roll of surgical tape.
Case or box, metal or plastic: the smallest size that will accommodate contents of the medical kit.
Dust mask for use in desert areas.
Moleskin blister protection for poorly fitting shoes.
Oral thermometer.
Safety pins.
Scissors or sterile razor blade, penknife, Swiss army knife.

[1]Adapted from Jong EC, Southworth M: Recommendations for patients traveling. *West J Med* 1983;**138**:746.

Lyme disease, brucellosis, leptospirosis, plague, psittacosis, and rabies. Brucellosis is discussed below as an example of one of the more common occupational zoonotic infections in the United States.

## BRUCELLOSIS

Brucellosis in humans (undulant fever, Malta fever) is caused by several gram-negative bacteria of the genus *Brucella*. The species varies with the animal host, as follows: *Brucella melitensis,* goats and sheep; *Brucella suis,* swine; *Brucella abortus,* cattle; and *Brucella canis,* dogs. More than 75 cases of brucellosis were reported in 1990 in the United States, approximately half transmitted by occupational exposure.

Most cases occur in abattoir workers and the remainder in veterinarians, livestock industry workers, and laboratory workers. The disease is more common in animals from rural underdeveloped countries.

### Pathogenesis & Clinical Findings

Occupational brucellosis occurs as a result of mucous membrane or skin contact with infected animal tissues. Aborted placental and fetal membrane tissues from cattle, swine, sheep, and goats are well-documented sources of human exposure. The incubation period is from 1 to 6 weeks. The onset is insidious, with fever, sweats, malaise, aches, and weakness. The fever has a characteristic pattern, often rising in the afternoon and falling during the night ("undulant fever"). The infection is systemic and may result in gastric, intestinal, neurologic, hepatic, or musculoskeletal involvement. There is usually an initial septicemic phase, following which a more chronic stage may develop characterized by low-grade fever, malaise, and in some cases psychoneurotic symptoms.

### Diagnosis & Treatment

Diagnosis is aided by both culture and serologic techniques. Treatment will vary with organism sensitivity, but brucellae are often sensitive to tetracyclines or ampicillin. More resistant species may require combined therapy with streptomycin and trimethoprim-sulfamethoxazole. Prolonged treatment is often necessary.

### Prevention

Identification and treatment or slaughter of infected animals combined with effective immunization of susceptible animals can eliminate disease in livestock populations. Diagnosis is by serologic testing. Personal hygiene and protective precautions should be observed in handling potentially infected animal tissues or secretions, particularly those resulting from abortion.

Immunization of humans is still experimental.

## OCCUPATIONAL IMMUNIZATION, PROPHYLAXIS, & BIOLOGICAL SURVEILLANCE

Recommended occupational immunizations are listed in Table 16–10. In addition, laboratory workers at risk of contact with live organisms and travelers to areas of endemic infection should be considered for appropriate immunization, prophylaxis, or surveillance if the technology is available. Preparations are available for protection against diphtheria, pertussis, tetanus, measles, mumps, rubella, smallpox, yellow fever, poliomyelitis, hepatitis A, hepatitis B, influenza, rabies, cholera, pneumococcal pneumonia, meningococcal disease (certain serotypes), plague, typhoid fever, tuberculosis, Q fever, adenovirus infection, anthrax, pertussis, and *Haemophilus influenzae* infection. In addition, many unlicensed or experimental vaccines are available through the CDC (eg, for various anthropod-borne viruses).

Skin testing can be useful in surveillance of tuberculosis and some mycoses (coccidioidomycosis, histoplasmosis, blastomycosis). Skin tests may also detect prior infection with mumps and vaccinia.

Serologic testing for evidence of subclinical infec-

**Table 16–10.** Occupational preexposure immunization and prophylaxis for susceptible (unvaccinated) adults.[1]

| | Immunization or Prophylaxis | Source or Clue to Exposure |
|---|---|---|
| Rubella | Vaccine, 0.5 mL SC | Indicated for those in contact with pregnant or infected patients |
| Hepatitis A | Vaccine, 1 mL IM at 0 and 6–12 months[2] | Travel to endemic area |
| Hepatitis B | Vaccine, 1 mL IM at 0, 1, and 6 months | Handling blood or other human fluid |
| Measles | Vaccine, 0.5 mL SC | Contact with infected patients |
| Poliomyelitis | Vaccine (Sabin), 0.5 mL at 0 and 2 months and again at 8–14 months | Contact with infected patients or laboratory culture |
| Smallpox | Contact CDC for vaccine and directions | Laboratory culture |
| Plague | Vaccine, 1 mL at 0 month, 0.2 mL at 1 and 6 months | Laboratory culture, infected animals |
| Rabies | Vaccine and prophylaxis; dosage varies with vaccine type | Laboratory culture, infected animals |
| Tetanus | Toxoid, 0.5 mL. Give 1 dose stat and at 6–8 weeks, 1 year, and every 10 years | Infected patients; contaminated (dirty) objects and materials |
| Influenza | Vaccine (dose varies with vaccine type) If vaccine unavailable, give amantadine, 100 mg orally twice daily | Infected patients |

[1]For travelers or microbiology laboratory workers, many additional vaccines, toxoids, immune globulins, and antitoxins are available and may be indicated depending on diseases endemic to the area visited or organisms present in the laboratory (see *Morbid Mortal Weekly Rep* 1994; **43[RR–1]:**1).
[2]Immune globulin 0.02 mL/kg IM is an alternative.

**Table 16–11.** Approach to suspected communicable disease outbreak.[1]

I. **Verify reported case:**
  A. Review type and result of laboratory confirmation (serology, culture, etc).
  B. Review clinical presentation with patient or treating physician.
  C. If diagnosis unclear, perform laboratory determination based on clinical impression.
  D. Report suspected outbreak to public health authorities.
  E. Treat and isolate source case or material in accordance with clinical and public health guidelines.
II. **If the diagnosis or etiology remains unclear, collect, analyze, and summarize:**
  A. Available laboratory data.
  B. Symptoms and signs from each suspected case.
  C. Stool, blood, urine, or other appropriate fluid or tissue for further laboratory evaluation as suggested by the clinical findings.
  D. Samples for microbiologic analysis of nonhuman materials (food, animals, waste, etc) that may be sources.
  E. Epidemiologic and exposure data from a similar but clinically unaffected (control) group. Compare the case and control group for differences in rates of exposure to the various suspected microbially contaminated sources.
III. **Identify susceptibles with potential exposure to source case or substance:**
  A. Review usual host, period of communicability, and mode of transmission and period of communicability.
  B. Interview source case, family, or custodian of source material (eg, cook, farmer) to determine range of activity, travel, social interaction, or vector association during communicable period.
  C. Identify all susceptible persons or animals within source case or material's range of activity during communicable period who could have had sufficient contact with infectious case, material, or vector for disease transmission. Public agency assistance may be necessary.
IV. **Identify secondary cases:**
  A. Evaluate individuals identified in III, above, for evidence of infection and communicability.
  B. Continue steps III and IV.A until perimeter of outbreak is defined.
V. **Institute control measures:** Follow recommended actions appropriate to the suspected causal agent (see Benenson reference) for concurrent disinfection, isolation, investigation, or immunization of contacts, quarantine, hygiene, treatment, and work practices.
VI. **Prevention:** Institute appropriate preventive measures (eg, immunization, work practices, serologic, and other biologic surveillance).

[1]Adapted from Last JM (editor): *Maxcy Rosenau's Preventive Medicine and Public Health,* 12th ed. Appleton & Lange, 1996.

tion in selected high-risk populations should be carefully considered but may be of value for the following diseases: brucellosis, chlamydial infections, leptospirosis, plague, tularemia, salmonellosis, toxoplasmosis, some parasitic diseases (amebiasis, trichinosis), most occupational viral diseases (hepatitis A and B, herpes simplex, influenza, rabies, infectious mononucleosis), mycoplasmal pneumonia, and some rickettsioses.

As with the administration of any surveillance test or therapeutic agent, disease prevalence, occupational exposure risk, contraindications, and side effects from the prophylactic agent should all be considered before administration of any immunologic agent or use of any biological surveillance test. MMR, for example, should not be given within 3 months before or during pregnancy. Yellow fever and oral polio vaccine should not be given during pregnancy unless there is a substantial risk of exposure.

Guidelines for investigation and control of a communicable disease or common source outbreak are presented in Table 16–11.

## Exposure Evaluation

Investigation of human or animal sources of infectious agents can use serologic or other clinical microbiologic techniques. Environmental exposure evaluation associated with inanimate sources such as contaminated ventilation systems or centrifuges is more esoteric. However, technologies exist for collection and measurement of airborne bacteria and viruses. A knowledgeable industrial hygienist can select the appropriate instrumentation and sampling strategy based on the presumed biological characteristics of the organism, air velocity, sampler efficiency, anticipated concentration, "particle" size, sampler physical requirements, and the study objective.

## REFERENCES

### GENERAL

**Hotline/Internet**

Centers for Disease Control Internet Access (http://www.cdc.gov/) or Automated (phone) Information Service (404) 332-4555 (current information on travel recommendations, immunization, injury pre-

vention, and infectious disease [AIDS, hepatitis, influenza, malaria, etc]).

**Others**

Benenson AS (editor): *Communicable Diseases Manual,* 16th ed. American Public Health Association, 1995.
Centers for Disease Control: *Health Information for In-*

*ternational Travel. MMWR* Supplement, published annually.

Centers for Disease Control: *Morbidity and Mortality Weekly Report.* Available through the Massachusetts Medical Society, CSPO Box 9120, Waltham, MA 02254-9120.

Centers for Disease Control/National Institute of Health: *Biosafety in Microbiological and Biomedical Laboratories.* US Government Printing Office, 1993.

Last JM (editor): *Maxcey-Rosenau Public Health & Preventive Medicine,* 13th ed. Appleton & Lange, 1996.

*The Medical Letter on Drugs and Therapeutics.* Published bimonthly. The Medical Letter, Inc.

## TUBERCULOSIS

Centers for Disease Control: Screening for tuberculosis and tuberculous infection in high-risk populations and the use of preventive therapy for tuberculous infection in the United States. MMWR 1990;39(RR-8):1.

Centers for Disease Control and Prevention: Guidelines for preventing the transmission of *Mycobacterium tuberculosis* in health-care facilities, 1994. MMWR 1994;43(RR-13):1.

Huebner RE, Schein MF, Bass JB Jr., *The Tuberculin Skin Test,* Clinical Infectious Diseases 1993;17:968–975.

Salpeter S: Tuberculosis chemoprophylaxis. West J Med 1992;157:421.

*Screening for Tuberculosis and Tuberculosis Infection in High Risk Populations.* MMWR 1995;44(RR-11):19–34.

Stead WW: Managment of health care workers after inadvertent exposure to tuberculosis: A guide for the use of preventive therapy. Ann Intern Med 1995;122:906.

## HEPATITIS B

Centers for Disease Control: Protection against viral hepatitis: Recommendations of the Immunization Practices Advisory Committee (ACIP). MMWR 1990;39(RR-2):1.

Occupational Exposure to Bloodborne Pathogens 29 CFR 1910.1030, US Government Printing Office.

Ramos-Soriano AG, Schwarz KB: Recent advances in the hepatitides. Pediatric Gastroenterology, Part I. Gastroenterol Clin North Am 1994;23:753.

## AIDS

Centers for Disease Control: 1988 Agent summary statement for human immunodeficiency virus and report on laboratory-acquired infection with human immunodeficiency virus. MMWR (April 1) 1988; 37(Suppl S-4):1.

Centers for Disease Control: Guidelines for prevention of transmission of human immunodeficiency virus and hepatitis B virus to health-care and public-safety workers. MMWR 1989;38(S-6):1.

Centers for Disease Control: Recommendations for preventing transmission of human immunodeficiency virus and hepatitis B virus to patients during exposure-prone invasive procedures. MMWR 1991;40 (RR-8):1.

Centers for Disease Control: Recommendations for prevention of HIV transmission in health-care settings. MMWR (Aug 21) 1987;36(Suppl 2S):1.

Centers for Disease Control: Update: *Provisional Public Health Service Recommendations for Chemoprophylaxis After Occupational Exposure to HIV.* MMWR 1996;45:468.

Centers for Disease Control: Update: Universal precautions for prevention of transmission of human immunodeficiency virus, hepatitis B virus, and other bloodborne pathogens in health care settings. MMWR 1988;37:377.

Coates TJ, Lo B: Counseling patients seropositive for human immunodeficiency virus: An approach for medical practice. West J Med 1990;153:629.

Gerberding JL: Management of occupational exposure to blood-borne illness. N Engl J Med 1995;332:444.

### AIDS HotLine

Centers for Disease Control: 1-800-342-AIDS.

## TRAVEL-RELATED INFECTIONS

Heck JE, Cohen MB: Traveler's diarrhea. Am Fam Physician 1993;48:793.

Shepherd SM, Talbot-Stern JK: Evaluation of the traveler: An introduction to emporiatrics for the emergency physician. Emerg Med Clin North Am 1991;9:273.

## BRUCELLOSIS

Radolf JD: Southwestern International Medicine Conference: Brucellosis: Don't let it get your goat! Am J Med Sci 1994;307:64.

Trout D et al: Outbreak of brucellosis at a United States pork packing plant. J Occup Environ Med 1995;37:697.

## IMMUNIZATION & PROPHYLAXIS: BIOLOGICAL SURVEILLANCE

Adult immunization: Recommendations of the Immunization Practices Advisory Committee (ACIP). MMWR (Jan 28) 1994;RR-1.

## EXPOSURE EVALUATION

American Industrial Hygiene Association: *Biosafety Reference Manual,* 2nd ed. American Industrial Hygiene Association, 1995.

# Occupational Cancer

# 17

Hope S. Rugo, MD, & Michael L. Fischman, MD, MPH

It is estimated that one of every two or three individuals in the industrialized world will develop some type of cancer during their lifetimes. The majority of cancers in adults are thought to be due to a combination of factors, including environmental exposure and lifestyle. Approximately 2–8% of all human cancers are thought to be due to occupational exposure to carcinogens; however, the risks within an occupationally exposed population are much higher.

The identification of occupational carcinogens is important, at least in part because most occupational cancers are completely preventable with appropriate personnel practices and strict protective legislation. In this chapter, the fundamental properties of occupational carcinogenesis will be reviewed. Investigative methods used to identify possible carcinogens, general and specific strategies for prevention, and clinical presentations of well-described occupational cancers will be covered in detail. A modified version of the International Agency of Research on Cancer's classification of occupational carcinogens is included in table form.

## CARCINOGENESIS: FUNDAMENTAL PROPERTIES

Evidence suggests that cancers arise from a single abnormal cell. After progressing through a number of stages, this cell then replicates itself through repeated divisions to form a large clone of tumor cells. The initial stage in development of the abnormal cell appears to result from an alteration or mutation in the genetic material, deoxyribonucleic acid (DNA). This alteration may occur spontaneously or may be caused by exogenous factors, such as exposure to carcinogenic chemicals or radiation. Whether a tumor develops from this altered cell may depend on a variety of factors, such as the ability of the cell to repair the damage, the presence of other endogenous or exogenous agents that foster or inhibit tumor development, and the effectiveness of the immune system.

## Stages in Tumor Development

A variety of evidence indicates that cells must undergo multiple heritable changes before a cancer cell develops. Early animal studies suggested that tumor development involved at least two distinct stages: initiation and promotion. The classic example of this phenomenon is the mouse skin tumor model. A small dose of a carcinogen, known as the initiator (typically a polycyclic aromatic hydrocarbon [PAH]) is applied to the skin. Though large doses of such substances alone can readily induce skin tumors, observation of the animals has revealed that the smaller dose alone does not. However, subsequent application of certain substances, known as promoters (eg, croton oil) results in tumor development following a low dose of the PAH.

Application of the promoter alone or prior to administration of the initiator does not result in skin tumors. Similar stages have been demonstrated in the development of tumors in other organs, such as mouse liver and lung and rat trachea. For example, ingestion of a small quantity of various nitrosamines (initiators) followed by regular ingestion of polychlorinated biphenyls (promoters) results in production of liver tumors in mice.

From a functional point of view, it now appears helpful to view carcinogenesis as a three stage process—initiation, promotion, and progression. Initiation is thought to result from an irreversible change in the genetic material (DNA) of the cell, arising from interaction with a carcinogen that is a necessary, but not sufficient, condition for tumor development. It is this somatic mutation that sets the stage for tumor development, the basis for the somatic mutation theory of carcinogenesis.

On the other hand, promotion consists of those processes subsequent to initiation that facilitate tumor development, presumably by stimulating proliferation of the altered cell. The mechanisms of promotion, sometimes referred to as epigenetic mechanisms (as opposed to the genotoxic or mutational effects of initiators), are incompletely understood. Promotion does not result from binding to and alteration of DNA. In the case of the mouse skin tumor model, croton oil appears to interact with membrane receptors to affect cellular growth and differentiation. As promotion typically yields a benign tumor or group of preneoplastic cells, progression involves those additional heritable changes necessary for the development of a malignant tumor.

The model of carcinogenesis that emerges is referred to as the multi-step or multi-stage model. Barrett indicates that evidence supports the occurrence of 3–10 mutational or genetic changes in common adult human cancers, such as colorectal cancer.

While it is clearly simplistic to do so, carcinogens are often divided into initiating agents, known as initiators, genotoxic (DNA-reactive) or "early stage" carcinogens; and promoting agents, known as promoters, or epigenetic or "late stage" carcinogens. The distinguishing features of initiating and promoting agents are listed in Table 17–1. Some agents (eg, cigarette smoke) that seem to possess both initiating and promoting properties are termed "complete carcinogens." Given the complexity of the multi-stage model and increasing experimental evidence that tends to blur the distinction between these categories, the value of categorizing agents is probably limited.

The mechanism by which a carcinogen-induced alteration in DNA could lead to initiation and ultimately to tumor development was obscure until recently, when the role of two types of genes, proto-oncogenes and tumor-suppressor genes, was discovered. Proto-oncogenes contain DNA sequences, which, when altered by a mutational event into an oncogene, stimulate transformation and proliferation of an altered potentially neoplastic cell. There are a number of proto-oncogenes in normal human and animal cells that are responsible for normal cellular differentiation and maturation. Similarly, a genetic change in one or more tumor-suppressor genes, which appear to be negative regulators of cell growth, results in inactivation of the gene, thereby allowing unfettered growth of the altered cells. The observation that tumors develop only after activation of one or more oncogenes and inactivation of one or more tumor suppressor genes provides a mechanistic explanation for the multistep model of carcinogenesis.

There are a number of mechanisms by which these genes have been found to be altered—point mutations, chromosome translocation or rearrangement, gene amplification, and the induction of numerical chromosome changes (aneuploidy), each of which theoretically could be induced by a chemical exposure. For example, point mutations in *ras* proto-oncogenes (so called because they were originally identified in rat sarcomas) have been observed at codons 12, 13, and 61 in human and rodent tumors. Like other genes, the *ras* gene codes for a protein product, a 21,000-MW protein known as p21. It is felt that this protein product from the activated oncogene, differing by only one amino acid from the normal protein, is the direct cell-transforming agent, and confers malignant potential to the cell.

For most toxic effects, the persistence or progression of damage requires the continued presence of the offending chemical agent. For cancer initiators, however, a single exposure may induce genetic damage in the cell sufficient to result in tumor development years after exposure has ceased.

## Induction-Latency Period

Both experimental animal models of cancer and the study of human cancers with known causes have revealed the existence of a significant interval between first exposure to the responsible agent and the first manifestation of the tumor. This interval is correctly referred to as the induction-latency period or the incubation period, but conventionally is often referred to simply as the latency period. As noted by Barrett, the requirement for multiple heritable changes in the cell may account, in part, for the prolonged latency interval.

For humans, the length of the induction-latency

**Table 17–1.** Distinctions between initiators and promoters of carcinogenesis.

| Initiators | Promoters |
|---|---|
| Genotoxic. | Not genotoxic; epigenetic mechanism. |
| Carcinogenic alone. | Not carcinogenic alone; active only after initiator exposure. |
| Generally yield electrophilic compounds; highly reactive (often form free radicals). | Not electrophilic. |
| Covalently bind to nucleophiles (eg, DNA), leading to irreversible alteration in genetic material. | Generally do not bind to nor alter DNA; often act by induction of cellular proliferation; effects may be reversible. |
| Generally active in short-term tests (mutagenic). | Not active in short-term tests. |
| Existence of threshold dose cannot be verified. | Threshold probably exists. |
| Single exposure may be sufficient to induce subsequent cancer. | Repeated exposures required. |

period varies from a minimum of 4–6 years for radiation-induced leukemias to perhaps 40 or more years for some cases of asbestos-induced mesothelioma. For most tumors, however, the interval is about 12–25 years. Obviously, this long period of time may obscure the relationship between a remote exposure and a newly found tumor.

## THE QUESTION OF THRESHOLDS

With most toxic effects, there are doses or exposures below which no adverse effects occur. If this threshold dose is not exceeded, there are no consequences to the health of the animal or human. With carcinogens, it is much more difficult to determine if such a threshold exists. If no threshold exists, there is no dose (other than zero) at which the risk of cancer is nil.

There is controversy about the existence of threshold doses for carcinogenic agents. An understanding of the arguments on both sides is useful, particularly when trying to comprehend the basis for policies and regulations.

Given that a single alteration (mutation) in DNA in one cell may set the stage for tumor development, it is at least theoretically possible that exposure of the cell to only one molecule of a carcinogen will ultimately lead to tumor formation. Though the probability of tumor formation may increase with increasing frequency and magnitude of exposure to the carcinogen, a single small exposure may be sufficient. For example, in the mouse skin tumor model described above, a single exposure to a polycyclic aromatic hydrocarbon is capable of inducing a tumor.

On the other hand, a number of arguments have been advanced against the concept that there are no thresholds for carcinogens. Even if one acknowledges that a single molecule may induce a tumorigenic change in a cell, the likelihood that the molecule will reach its target cell is lowered with small doses. The agent may react with other cellular nucleophiles, such as proteins or noncritical segments of DNA. If the carcinogen is subject to rapid metabolic deactivation, as in a "first-pass" effect in the liver after ingestion, the ability of a small dose to contact the susceptible cell is reduced. DNA repair mechanisms (eg, excision of altered DNA nucleotides) may allow repair of an induced mutation before a clone of tumor cells results. There is some evidence both in humans and in animals that immunologic mechanisms may be capable of destroying transformed cells before a tumor develops. Finally, cancer induction by a number of agents appears to require a preceding pathologic effect on the tissue (eg, cellular hyperplasia or necrosis). For example, alcohol and probably some chlorinated hydrocarbon solvents, if administered in high doses, will initially induce liver damage and cirrhosis, following which there is a higher risk of liver tumor development. Since there is a threshold for the initial toxic effects below which no damage occurs, there is also a threshold for the secondary tumor formation. If any of these phenomena pertain for a given carcinogen, there will be a threshold dose below which no carcinogenic effect will occur.

The controversy regarding thresholds persists, although the more conventional viewpoint is that there are no demonstrable thresholds or safe levels for carcinogens. Ames and Gold challenge this view on several grounds. They argue that the findings of animal bioassays at very high doses may well be due to mitogenesis leading to mutagenesis (ie, cellular proliferation stimulated by injury ultimately leads to carcinogenicity). Similarly, historical outbreaks of occupational cancer have occurred with exposure at uncontrolled high levels, where mitogenesis might occur. Because mitogenesis does not occur at the much lower doses to which humans are generally exposed, the carcinogenic stimulus will not be present. On the other hand, Benigni and Andreoli found a poor correlation between toxicity and carcinogenicity for known carcinogens in their analysis (and reported similar findings by other authors), suggesting that carcinogenicity is not likely due simply to the secondary effects of cytotoxicity. Ames and Gold also note the very high rate of spontaneous mutation in human and animal cells induced by endogenous oxidants; such damage is almost fully eliminated by DNA repair mechanisms. Presumably, the impact of low levels of exogenous mutagens or toxins will be minimal in relation to the high rate of spontaneous endogenous mutations and as a result of effective DNA repair mechanisms.

Unfortunately, these arguments are not generally susceptible to experimental verification for individual carcinogens, because of limitations in the methodology and analysis of human and animal studies. Moreover, as stated by David Rall (cited in Huff): "But the issue is not thresholds or no thresholds; it is one of adding a new carcinogen to a pool of present carcinogens."

### Dose-Response Relationships

Although thresholds may or may not exist, there is strong evidence for a dose-response effect for most carcinogens that have been adequately studied. In other words, larger doses result in a higher incidence and mortality rate of tumors in an exposed population than do smaller doses. Both animal experimental studies and human epidemiologic reports support this concept.

Such studies have revealed very large differences—10 million-fold or more—in the relative potency of carcinogens. For example, in long-term animal studies, a daily dose of less than 1 μg/d of aflatoxin induced tumors in 50% of exposed animals, while an equipotent dose of trichloroethylene was greater than 1 g/d.

Although dose-response curves for some carcinogens are known, data points represent relatively high doses. We would like to know the behavior of such curves in the range of typical human exposures. We cannot predict the shape of the curve at low doses from the high dose data—for example, at low doses, is the curve linear, concave, or convex, or is there a threshold? Some possible models for low-dose extrapolation are illustrated in Figure 17–1. Again, the conventional view is that there is linearity at low doses.

## INVESTIGATIVE METHODS IN THE ASSESSMENT OF CHEMICAL CARCINOGENICITY

Evidence to support the carcinogenicity of a chemical for humans may be derived from four types of studies: human epidemiologic studies, experimental studies in animals, a variety of short-term tests, and analysis of structural similarities to known carcinogens.

Epidemiologic studies potentially provide the strongest evidence for human carcinogenicity, precisely because they are conducted on human subjects. However, such studies are subject to a number of limitations that reduce their ability to detect and confirm carcinogenic effects.

Well-conducted animal bioassays can provide strong support for carcinogenicity in the animal species tested. However, the implications for humans are less clear than with epidemiologic studies.

The role of short-term assays (eg, for bacterial mutation) is not fully defined, because the significance for human risk of positive results is unknown. Currently, at least, further study of the chemical in animal bioassays would be warranted.

Structural similarity of a chemical to known carcinogens may also suggest the need for further study in short-term or animal tests. Though the presence of such similarity has, in fact, predicted the carcinogenicity of previously untested compounds, the overall utility of structural analysis has not been established.

## EPIDEMIOLOGIC STUDIES

Epidemiologic studies have the potential for providing the strongest evidence for human carcinogenicity, because the subjects studied are human. Though case reports and descriptive epidemiologic studies may provide suggestive evidence for human carcinogenicity, evidence for causality of an association can only be derived from analytic epidemiologic studies, or, in other words, cohort or case-control studies. The nature and design of such studies are

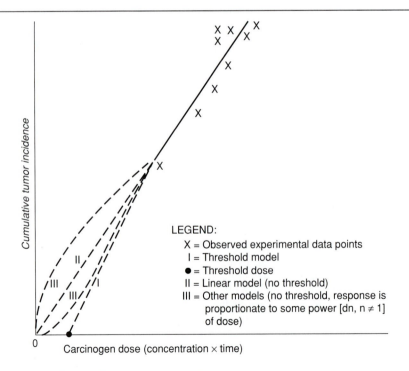

**Figure 17–1.** Carcinogenesis: Possible dose-response models.

discussed in the Appendix. When they are well-conducted and yield positive results, they provide strong evidence in support of carcinogenicity.

A number of criteria, originally proposed in a similar form by Sir Austin Bradford Hill, have been used to help decide whether a positive association in epidemiologic studies indicates causality. The most important are strength, consistency, biological gradient, biological plausibility, and temporality:

1. The **strength** of an association is the magnitude of the relative risk in the exposed group compared to that of the control group. Strong associations are more likely to be causal because it is less likely that biases (eg, the confounding effects of smoking) would account for the association without being very obvious.
2. **Consistency** of an association is the extent to which it is reported from multiple studies conducted under different circumstances.
3. The **biological gradient** of an association is the degree to which it exhibits a dose-response relationship (ie, the observation that higher doses result in a higher frequency of adverse effects).
4. The **biological plausibility** of a study is based on the assessment that it makes sense in light of what is known about the mechanism of production of the adverse effect.
5. A study's **temporality** rests on the conclusion or observation that the cause (ie, exposure) preceded the effect in time.

Despite the utility of these criteria in making assessments of causality, only one of them, temporality, is absolutely required. A weak association not consistently reported that does not exhibit a dose-response effect and does not (as yet) fully make sense may nevertheless be causal. Furthermore, fulfillment of some of the criteria may occur when the association is in fact due to chance or bias.

However. if most of the criteria are met, the likelihood that an association is causal is certainly high. The International Agency for Research on Cancer (IARC), in the preamble to its recent monographs, has established similar criteria for the designation of an agent as a carcinogen.

## Limitations of Epidemiologic Studies

Failure to demonstrate a positive association in an epidemiologic study does not always indicate that there is no association between the agent and the effect studied. In some cases, a "false-negative" epidemiologic study may result because of a variety of shortcomings. Some of these limitations include difficulties in identifying exposures and effects, difficulties in choosing appropriate study (exposed) and control populations, inadequate duration of follow-up

given long induction-latency periods, and the relative lack of sensitivity of epidemiologic methods.

The existence of all of these limitations accounts for the consensus among scientists that negative epidemiologic studies do not provide proof of noncarcinogenicity of an agent. Such negative data are generally outweighed by the finding of positive results in animal experimental studies. Greater credence may be given to a negative study if the subjects studied had a sufficiently long period of exposure (an average of 15 or more years), if they were followed long enough to observe an effect (25 or more years), and if the number of exposed subjects was large enough so that an excess risk as small as 50% for the particular tumors studied could be detected.

## ANIMAL BIOASSAYS

### Design

Experimental studies in animals involve the administration of a test chemical to a group of animals followed by observation for the development of tumors. Procedures for such studies are now standardized and accepted by most of the sponsoring or evaluating institutions (eg, the National Toxicology Program [NTP] and IARC). The basic requirements are listed in Table l7–2. In brief, protocols include at least 50 animals of each sex with two species in each of two dosage groups and incorporate thorough pathologic examination and proper statistical analysis of results. Animals are dosed throughout their lifetimes at the maximal tolerated dose (MTD) and one-half the maximal tolerated dose.

### Interpretation

Results from well-executed animal bioassays can yield clear evidence to support the carcinogenicity of a compound to the tested animal. In Supplement 4 to its Monograph series, the IARC, an independent scientific institution within the World Health Organization (WHO), laid out criteria for the "assessment of evidence of carcinogenicity from studies in experi-

**Table 17–2.** IARC requirements for animal bioassays.

1. Two species of animals (generally mice and rats), both males and females.
2. Sufficient numbers of animals in each test group and concurrent control group (at least 50 per sex).
3. Duration of dose administration and observation must extend over most of the animal's life expectancy (typically 2 years for rats and mice).
4. Treated groups tested at 2 or ideally 3 different doses—at a higher dose (near the maximum tolerated dose, MTD) and at a lower dose.
5. Outcome determined from adequate pathologic examination of animals.
6. Proper statistical analysis of data.

mental animals." There are four categories, based on the following criteria: sufficient evidence, limited evidence, inadequate evidence, and no data. The first three are described below.

i. *Sufficient evidence* of carcinogenicity, which indicates that there is an increased incidence of malignant tumors: (a) in multiple species or strains; or (b) in multiple experiments (preferably with different routes of administration or using different dose levels); or (c) to an unusual degree with regard to incidence, site, or type of tumor, or age at onset. Additional evidence may be provided by data on dose-response effects, as well as information from short-term tests or on chemical structure.

ii. *Limited evidence* of carcinogenicity, which means that the data suggest a carcinogenic effect but are limited because: (a) the studies involve a single species, strain, or experiment; or (b) the experiments are restricted by inadequate dosage levels, inadequate duration of exposure to the agent, inadequate period of follow-up, poor survival, too few animals, or inadequate reporting; or (c) the neoplasms produced often occur spontaneously and, in the past, have been difficult to classify as malignant by histological criteria alone (eg, lung and liver tumors in mice).

iii. *Inadequate evidence*, which indicates that because of major qualitative or quantitative limitations, the studies cannot be interpreted as showing either the presence or absence of a carcinogenic effect; or that within the limits of the tests used, the chemical is not carcinogenic.

## Correlation With Human Effects

Animal bioassay results have served as good predictors of human carcinogenicity. Nearly one third of agents now known to be human carcinogens were first discovered to be carcinogenic in animals. In attempting to extrapolate data from animal research to conclusions about cancer risks in humans, the important issues to be considered are (1) whether all chemicals that have been shown to cause cancer in animals are also capable of causing cancer in humans, and vice versa; and (2) from a quantitative viewpoint, whether humans are equally susceptible to the carcinogenic effects of equivalent doses of known animal carcinogens.

With no clear exceptions, the available evidence suggests that, qualitatively, there is a good correlation between animal and human results. Until recently, it had not been possible to demonstrate in animals the carcinogenicity of arsenic, a known human skin and lung carcinogen. Arsenic was for that reason cited as an instance in which there was a discrepancy between human and animal studies, which then raised a question about the adequacy of animal bioas-

says to be sensitive predictors of human carcinogenicity. However, in the view of IARC, there is now limited evidence of carcinogenicity of arsenic compounds (arsenic trioxide, calcium arsenate) in laboratory animals, based on intratracheal instillation experiments in rats and hamsters. Thus, all known human carcinogens for which adequate animal studies have been conducted have virtually always shown sufficient evidence of carcinogenicity in some tested animals.

The issue of the specificity of animal testing as a predictor of human carcinogenicity is more difficult to resolve. Because of limitations inherent in epidemiologic studies (discussed above), it is unlikely that clear-cut evidence for human carcinogenicity can be derived for many chemicals proved to be carcinogenic in animals. Nevertheless, for the limited number of compounds for which there are adequate data in both humans and animals, most authors concur that there are no substances proved to be carcinogenic in animals that have been proved to be noncarcinogenic in humans.

Though there appears to be a good qualitative correlation between animal and human carcinogenicity, the target site at which cancers develop may be different for rodents and humans. For example, benzidine produces liver tumors in rats, hamsters, and mice but produces bladder tumors in humans and dogs. Nevertheless, for all known human carcinogens, at least one site of cancer in humans matched a site in at least one animal species tested.

The second major issue in the use of animal bioassays is the degree to which the susceptibility of humans to carcinogenic effects parallels the dose-response patterns in animals. The data base that permits comparison of the sensitivity of humans relative to that of animals is quite limited. For the limited numbers of substances for which there are quantitative data in both humans and animals, it appears that the sensitivity of humans, on a total dose per body weight basis, is roughly similar to that of animals.

## Limitations of Animal Bioassays

There are a number of difficult issues in the analysis of animal experimental studies that may limit their utility in human cancer risk assessment. Because of the small number of animals studied, the bioassays are relatively insensitive in detection of carcinogenicity. The agent under study must cause a 15% increase in the incidence of tumors in order for a statistically significant excess of tumors to be detected in a bioassay of standard size. A lower excess risk will not be demonstrable, particularly if there is any background rate of tumor development in untreated animals.

In a necessary attempt to increase the sensitivity of animal experiments, high dose levels approaching the maximal tolerated dose are chosen. These doses are well above the human exposure levels in occupational or environmental settings. Moreover, the incidence of tumors greatly exceeds that experienced in any human population. In some cases, only an increased incidence of types of tumors not observed in humans are found. For risk quantification, the high doses add an additional difficulty, because predictions must be made based on extrapolation to the much lower doses experienced by humans. The mathematical models used for extrapolation are controversial and unproved and thus add more uncertainty to risk estimates.

Certain factors will at least theoretically affect the likelihood that the animal bioassay results will be a good predictor of the human response. The use of high doses, well above human exposure levels, may result in false-positive results if carcinogenicity occurs only secondary to a primary toxic pathologic alteration. If high doses overwhelm metabolic detoxifying mechanisms that normally would prevent exposure of the susceptible organ, false-positive results might occur. If metabolic processes acting in the animal studied and in humans for the particular chemical differ substantially, the possibility of both false-positives and false-negatives exists if the carcinogenic metabolite is produced only in the animal or only in humans, respectively. For most chemicals, evidence regarding comparative pharmacodynamics in humans and animals does not yet exist.

Since agents are often administered to animals by a route that is different from the one reported for human exposures, such as ingestion or intraperitoneal injection, it is at least theoretically possible that the outcome in the animal will differ from the effect in humans. However, there is no evidence to substantiate such a discrepancy in outcome based on differences in route of administration. Finally, there is some controversy about the classification of an agent as a potential carcinogen in the rare circumstance where experimental results indicate an increased frequency of benign tumors only.

## SHORT-TERM TESTS

### Types of Assays

A variety of assays have been designed that provide evidence of mutagenicity, or the ability to induce chromosomal damage by chemicals, without a long period of observation or follow-up, as is required in epidemiologic studies or animal bioassays. These short-term tests are therefore much quicker and less expensive to perform. End-points that have been assessed include gene mutation, induction of DNA damage and repair, DNA binding, chromosomal aberrations, sister chromatid exchange, or neoplastic transformation of mammalian cells. The tests ultimately rely upon the fact that most carcinogens covalently bind to DNA and thereby induce DNA damage.

The best-studied and most commonly performed short-term test is the Ames test, which utilizes a mutant strain of *Salmonella typhimurium* that is deficient in the enzymes required to synthesize histidine and will not grow unless histidine is added to the growth medium. The chemical to be tested, along with a liver microsomal enzyme fraction from rodents or humans that can metabolically activate "procarcinogens," is added to the bacterial culture. Bacterial colonies that subsequently grow and can be counted indicate the occurrence of a reversion mutation to the wild strain, thus reflecting the mutagenic activity of the agent studied. Similar mutagenic testing is possible in cultured mammalian cells in vitro.

Tests for DNA repair can demonstrate that DNA damage has occurred following exposure to a chemical. Chromosomal aberrations in mammalian cells may be detected by cytogenetic tests that assess changes in the morphologic structure of chromosomes. Such tests can be performed on animal or human cells, including human lymphocytes. Morphologic changes that may occur include chromosomal translocations and the formation of micronuclei.

Testing for sister chromatid exchange is a more sophisticated form of cytogenetic investigation based on differential staining of sister chromatids or and allowing for detection of the interchange of genetic material between chromatids. Such changes are more subtle than gross structural chromosomal aberrations. Again, tests for sister chromatid exchanges may be performed on animal or human cells.

Finally, tests for neoplastic transformation of mammalian cells in culture assess the ability of chemicals to alter growth characteristics of such cells toward neoplasia. Such altered cells can produce tumors when injected into the animal. A variety of other short-term tests are being or have been developed.

### Interpretation & Limitations

The predictive value of short-term tests for the carcinogenicity of a chemical to humans is unclear. The correlation between results in short-term assays and human or animal study results is imperfect. No single short-term test is capable of detecting all chemicals positive in animal bioassays. As a result, a battery of such tests has been routinely performed on a chemical to be tested. Unfortunately, a recent study for a large number of chemicals comparing the results of animal bioassays and a battery of four commonly used short-term tests failed to demonstrate any advantage of a battery of tests over the Ames test used alone in predicting the results of the bioassays. The concordance of any of the in vitro tests with the animal bioassay results was approximately 60%. A number of compounds were identified as mutagenic in the short-term tests that were noncarcinogenic in animal bioassays. The low specificity of the Ames test for detecting carcinogenicity (ie, the high number of false positives among noncarcinogens) demonstrates the inability to correctly predict animal carcinogenicity on the basis of short-term test results. While most genotoxic carcinogens are positive in short-term tests, these in vitro tests are not generally able to permit detection of chemicals that induce cancers by nongenotoxic or epigenetic mechanisms (ie, they are not sensitive to the effects of promoting agents).

Some of these tests (eg, tests for sister chromatid exchanges and measurement of DNA adducts) can be performed on cells (typically lymphocytes) taken from humans exposed occupationally or environmentally to suspected carcinogens. For example, testing for sister chromatid exchanges has been performed on ethylene oxide workers. An increased frequency of sister chromatid exchanges has been found in some of these workers. Though this merits further study, the clinical significance of these findings for the workers is unknown. The contribution of other factors, such as cigarette smoking, that have been shown to increase sister chromatid exchange frequency is also unclear. At this time, no predictions can be made based on results of such testing in workers. Thus, use of these tests should be limited to well-designed research studies.

Given the current state of knowledge, most authorities state that positive results in short-term tests on previously untested materials warrant further study in animal bioassays and further scrutiny in human exposure situations. Similarly, positive results on these tests provide corroboration for positive findings in animal bioassays, particularly when the animal results provide only limited or suggestive evidence of carcinogenicity. On the other hand, isolated positive short-term assay results do not constitute sufficient evidence to force immediate regulatory action.

## THE ROLE OF MOLECULAR BIOLOGY IN THE STUDY OF OCCUPATIONAL CANCER

Some recent developments in biochemistry and molecular biology offer the promise of detecting variations in susceptibility to chemically induced cancers and understanding the mechanisms and etiology of occupational cancer. Vainio and Husgafvel-Pursiainen term this development molecular epidemiology, because of the combination of epidemiologic study and molecular biology methodology. In some cases, these methods appear to simultaneously allow the assessment of exposure and possible early health effects.

Most carcinogenic chemicals are metabolized to the active carcinogenic metabolite by Phase I enzymes, primarily multiple enzymes in the cytochrome P450 monooxygenase class. Variations in the activity of these enzymes, which may be genetically or environ-

mentally determined, may result in differences in susceptibility to chemical carcinogenesis. For example, an isoform of one such enzyme, CYP1A1, has been associated with an increased risk for lung cancer in smokers. This enzyme catalyzes the oxidation of polycyclic aromatic hydrocarbons (PAHs) to reactive metabolites such as epoxides. Other genetically determined variants in Phase II enzymes, such as glutathione S-transferase and N-acetyltransferase, appear to play a role in lung cancer associated with PAHs and bladder cancer associated with exposure to aromatic amines (in slow acetylators), respectively. As the relationship between isoenzyme patterns and risk for cancer induction becomes clearer, from epidemiologic studies, it may be possible to better predict individual cancer risk associated with chemical exposure. However, because so many factors contribute to chemical carcinogenesis, the predictive value of such tests may be limited. Their use would also raise some ethical implications.

Another promising tool is the measurement of levels of specific carcinogens covalently bound to DNA or proteins, referred to as DNA or protein adducts. Binding to DNA may lead to DNA damage. Protein adducts (to albumin or hemoglobin) serve as a surrogate for DNA binding. Adducts present a better potential method of quantifying dose, in particular the internal dose at the site of toxicity/carcinogenicity, than older available methods, such as air monitoring or measuring blood levels of an agent. Application of these methods has included measurement of PAH-DNA adducts in smokers and lung cancer patients and of hemoglobin adducts of aromatic amines in smokers and occupationally exposed groups. Epidemiologic studies may ultimately show that adduct levels are a good predictor of cancer risk, possibly allowing classification of cohorts into high and low risk groups.

The abnormal protein products coded for by oncogenes or altered tumor suppressor genes can be identified in the serum and urine. For example, Nuorva et al demonstrated p53 protein accumulation in lung cancers of patients exposed to cigarette smoke and asbestos. Accumulation occurred more often in those exposed to asbestos compared to individuals who were unexposed. Moreover, there was a significant association between p53 accumulation and the measured asbestos content of the lung tissue. Similarly, patients with strongly p53-positive tumors were heavier smokers. Husgafvel-Pursiainen et al reported the results of a study of radon-exposed uranium miners who had developed lung cancers, in which over half of the patients had an identical G to T transversion at codon 249 of the p53 gene. It is possible that these proteins may be useful as preclinical response indicators in premalignant and early malignant lesions in occupationally exposed cohorts, with a role in early detection. To the extent that exposure-specific mutations can be identified, these mutations and the resulting protein products could serve as a marker for specific occupationally induced cancers. Considerable additional information from epidemiologic and pathologic studies will be necessary before these measurements can be readily applied in clinical situations.

## IMPLICATIONS FOR REGULATORY ACTION & PREVENTIVE MEDICINE

When a sufficient body of evidence supporting carcinogenicity exists, corrective action to protect public and worker health must proceed, even if there is some remaining uncertainty in the conclusions. Convincingly positive results from a well-conducted epidemiologic study merit immediate action. Sufficient evidence of carcinogenicity in animal bioassays, as defined by IARC, should also prompt immediate attempts to reduce worker exposure as much as possible. The finding of limited evidence in animal bioassays or positive results in short-term tests should, at the very least, serve as a stimulus for further study of the suspect chemical. When the results in different tests are contradictory, results suggesting carcinogenicity generally outweigh the negative evidence. Given the limited sensitivity of epidemiologic methods, this axiom seems particularly applicable when positive animal studies are analyzed alongside negative epidemiologic studies.

Based on analysis of epidemiologic and animal studies then available, the IARC issued, in 1987, several lists of chemicals with different degrees of evidence for human carcinogenicity. Since that time, several additional agents have been added to the lists based upon new evidence. There are 22 industrial chemicals, groups of chemicals, or mixtures in Group 1 that have been shown to cause human cancer, including beryllium, cadmium, ethylene oxide, strong inorganic acid mists containing sulfuric acid, and wood dust, all of which have been added since 1987. Along with several additional carcinogenic hazards not reviewed by IARC or that are environmental hazards, these are listed in Table 17–3. Table 17–4 lists some of the industrial processes that have been causally associated with cancer in humans. There are 27 industrial or environmental chemicals in group 2A, for which there is sufficient animal evidence, but limited or inadequate human evidence, of carcinogenicity (probably carcinogenic to humans). These chemicals are listed in Table 17–5. There are over 100 agents in group 2B, for which there is less compelling evidence to suggest possible human carcinogenicity. Some of these agents are listed in Table 17–6. More comprehensive lists are available in the excellent review by Boffetta et al. There were an additional 147 substances in 1987 for which there was sufficient evidence of animal carcinogenicity, but for which there was either inadequate or nonexistent epidemiologic data. IARC concluded that, "In the absence of adequate data on humans it is reasonable, for practical purposes, to regard chemicals for which there is sufficient evidence of carcinogenicity in animals as if they presented a carcinogenic risk to humans."

In analyzing the IARC data, Bartsch and Malaveille assessed the concordance between results indicating genotoxicity in short-term tests and the human and animal carcinogenicity data. The short-term tests measured DNA damage, mutations, and/or chromosomal effects; sufficient evidence of genotoxicity required effects in mammalian cells in vitro or in vivo. Overall, roughly 80–90% of the agents in each of the groups 1, 2A, and 2B showed sufficient or limited evidence of genotoxicity. The authors conclude that it is likely that genotoxic carcinogens and perhaps other genotoxic compounds contribute more to the burden of cancer in man than do nongenotoxic carcinogens, suggesting that a reduction in exposure to these agents should be a high public health/occupational health priority.

The nature of the appropriate response by government to evidence for carcinogenicity of a chemical is controversial. Given the uncertainty about the existence of thresholds and the shape of the dose-response curve at low doses, it is not possible to establish clearly "safe" doses for carcinogens. Ideally, human exposure to known carcinogens should be reduced to nil. In practice, political, economic, social, and technical factors constrain the power of regulators to adopt such stringent standards.

Of course, industry health and safety staff and managers have the opportunity to go further than the regulations require in using information regarding carcinogenicity when making decisions about chemical use and control. For example, choosing to avoid the use of chemicals in groups 1 and 2A (or those with evidence that might place them in these categories) and to use agents in group 2B only with very tight controls when there are no viable alternatives could lead to reductions in the risk of occupational cancer. Alternatively, use of these agents only with very tight controls (enclosure, local exhaust ventilation, etc) that completely prevent exposure could have a similar beneficial effect. Obviously, factors that affect the likelihood of exposure (eg, volatility or potential for skin absorption) would influence the ease with which these materials could be safely controlled. Pressure of chemical users upon chemical manufacturers to study suspect chemicals and to develop safe alternatives to potential carcinogens could be another effective approach. Secondly, proper hazard communication should inform workers of potential carcinogens and provide them with the training and tools to prevent exposure.

Some assistance in policy development can be derived from quantitative risk assessment methodology. Mathematical models have been designed that allow

**Table 17–3.** Occupational exposures causally associated with human cancer (Group 1).[1]

| Occupational Exposure | Cancer Site |
| --- | --- |
| 4-Aminobiphenyl | Bladder |
| Arsenic and arsenic compounds[2] | Lung, skin, liver(?), angiosarcoma |
| Asbestos | Pleura and peritoneum (mesothelioma), lung, larynx(?), gastrointestinal tract, kidney |
| Benzene | Leukemia (ANLL) |
| Benzidine | Bladder |
| Beryllium | Lung |
| Bis(chloromethyl) ether[3] | Lung (mainly oat cell) |
| Cadmium and cadmium compounds | Lung |
| Chromium compounds, hexavalent[2] | Lung |
| Coal tar pitches | Skin, scrotum, lung, bladder |
| Coal tars | Skin, scrotum, lung, bladder(?) |
| Ethylene oxide | Leukemia |
| Ionizing radiation | Leukemia, skin, other |
| Mineral oils, untreated and mildly treated | Skin, scrotum, lung(?) |
| Mustard gas | Lung |
| β-Naphthalamine | Bladder |
| Nickel and nickel compounds (oxide[?], sulfide) | Lung, nasal sinuses |
| Radium | Bone (sarcomas) |
| Radon | Lung |
| Shale oils | Skin, scrotum |
| Solar radiation | Skin |
| Soots, tars, and oils[2] | Skin, lung, bladder(?) |
| Strong inorganic acids containing sulfuric acid | Lung |
| Talc containing asbestiform fibers | Lung, mesothelioma(?) |
| Vinyl chloride | Liver (angiosarcoma), brain(?), lung |

[1]Sources: International Agency for Research on Cancer; Boffetta et al.
[2]The compounds responsible for the carcinogenic effect in humans cannot be specified.
[3]And technical grade chloromethyl methyl ether, which contains 1–8% bis(chloromethyl) ether.

for the extrapolation from high-dose studies to lower-dose exposures, providing an estimate of the excess risk or excess number of cases that might be seen in a given population as a result of these exposures. Though there is considerable uncertainty in such estimates, it can provide an approximate upper limit on the excess risk attributable to these exposures. Recent developments in the use of physiologically-based pharmacokinetic (PBPK) models for the estimation of dose at the target site (through the use of pharmacokinetic data regarding absorption, distribution, and metabolism of agents) will likely improve the accuracy of quantitative risk assessments for can-

cer. Such risk assessments can help to place hazards from various chemicals in the occupational environment into proper perspective by allowing comparison of the risk estimate against the risk from other known hazards. These risk comparisons may allow regulators or decision-makers to prioritize exposure problems for the purpose of allocating scarce resources for clean-up or problem resolution.

Ames et al (1987) have developed an approach for risk comparisons called the human exposure/rodent potency (HERP) percentage. The HERP compares the human exposure (daily lifetime dose in milligrams per kilogram) to the rodent TD50, the daily

Table 17–4. Selected industrial processes causally associated with human cancer.

| Industrial Process | Possible or Probable Agent | Cancer Site |
|---|---|---|
| Aluminum production | Polycyclic aromatic hydrocarbons | Lung, bladder |
| Auramine manufacture | Auramine | Bladder |
| Boot and shoe manufacture and repair (certain occupations) | Benzene | Leukemia |
| Coal gasification | Polycyclic aromatic hydrocarbons | Lung, bladder, skin, scrotum |
| Coke production | Polycyclic aromatic hydrocarbons | Lung, kidney(?) |
| Furniture manufacture | Wood dust | Nasal cavity (mainly adenocarcinoma) |
| Iron and steel founding | Polycyclic aromatic hydrocarbons(?), silica, metal fumes | Lung |
| Isopropyl alcohol manufacture (strong acid process) | Diisopropyl sulfate, isopropyl oils | Paranasal sinuses, larynx(?) |
| Magenta, manufacture of | Magenta(?), precursors(?) (eg, orthotoluidine) | Bladder |
| Nickel refining | Nickel oxides, nickel subsulfide | Nasal cavity, lung, larynx(?) |
| Rubber industry | Aromatic amines, solvents(?) | Bladder, leukemia (lymphatic), stomach(?), lung, skin, colon, prostate, lymphoma |
| Underground hematite mining (with exposure to radon) | Radon(?) | Lung |

dose in milligrams per kilogram to halve the percentage of tumor-free animals by the end of a standard lifetime (as determined from animal bioassays). The lower the HERP percentage, the lower the possible hazard from average human exposures. Using this index, it is possible to compare the hazard of a variety of natural and synthetic carcinogens. Such comparisons frequently demonstrated a greater apparent hazard from natural carcinogens (eg, aflatoxin as a contaminant in peanut butter or hydrazines in raw mushrooms) than from better-publicized alleged hazards such as PCBs in the diet or trichloroethylene in contaminated well water. The priority setting that such an index facilitates may permit policy makers to focus attention and regulation on the most significant exposure problems.

While exposure to known or suspected carcinogens has clearly declined in the United States and other economically developed countries due to both regulation and industry measures, it is likely that exposures to workers in developing countries are increasing in frequency and, in some cases, intensity. Where measurements exist in developing countries, it has generally been found that exposure levels in given industries to carcinogens tend to be considerably higher than in developed countries (and generally above regulatory standards in developed countries). The transfer of hazardous industries to developing countries will likely further increase car-

cinogen exposure. There is little health data with regard to the consequences of these exposures. Recognizing the inability of many developing countries to effectively regulate these hazards, it is incumbent upon industrial concerns from developed nations to attempt to control these hazards for workers in developing countries.

## Medical Surveillance

The proper role of medical surveillance in workers currently or previously exposed to known or suspected carcinogens is unclear. Surveillance of populations at high risk of cancer is only effective if the screening test is sensitive and easy to perform, if it detects premalignant abnormalities or tumors at an early stage in their development, and if there is an effective intervention that reduces morbidity and mortality when applied to such "early" tumors. For certain tumors not associated with chemical exposures (eg, cervical cancer) screening techniques and effective therapy for early lesions have had a significant impact upon the disease. There is some evidence that a small group of workers at high risk of bladder tumors as a result of prior exposure to aromatic amines used in dyestuff manufacturing can benefit from early detection by the use of urine cytology and cystoscopy as screening tools. For the remainder of occupational cancers, including asbestos-associated

**Table 17–5.** Selected probable occupational carcinogens
(Group 2A)–limited evidence of human carcinogenicity.[1]

| Occupational Exposure | Suspected Human Cancer Site |
|---|---|
| Acrylonitrile | Lung |
| 2-Amino-3-methylimidazo (4,5-*f*)quinoline (IQ) | |
| Benz*(a)*anthracene | |
| Benzidine-based dyes | Bladder(?) |
| Benzo*(a)*pyrene | Lung, skin, bladder |
| 1,3-Butadiene | Leukemia, lymphoma |
| *p*-Chloro-*o*-toluidine | Bladder |
| Creosotes | Skin, scrotum |
| Dibenz(*a,h*)anthracene | |
| Diesel engine exhaust | |
| Diethyl sulfate | Larynx |
| Dimethylcarbamoyl chloride | |
| Dimethyl sulfate | Lung(?) |
| Epichlorhydrin | Respiratory tract |
| Ethylene dibromide | |
| Formaldehyde | Nasopharynx |
| 4,4′-Methylene-bis(2-chloroaniline) (MOCA) | Bladder |
| N-Nitrosodimethylamine | |
| Polychlorinated biphenyls | Liver |
| Silica (crystalline) | Lung |
| Styrene oxide | |
| Tetrachloroethylene | Esophagus, lymphoma |
| Trichloroethylene | Liver, lymphoma |
| 1,2,3-Trichloropropane | |
| Tris(2,3-dibromopropyl) phosphate | |
| Vinyl bromide | |
| Vinyl fluoride | |

[1]Sources: International Agency for Research on Cancer; Boffetta et al.

bronchogenic carcinoma, there is virtually no evidence that screening and early detection reduce mortality rates.

Nevertheless, properly collected medical surveillance data—particularly when combined with industrial hygiene data collection—may prove quite useful in future epidemiologic studies and in the refinement of our knowledge regarding human dose-response phenomena. If medical surveillance is to be performed, the protocol should be designed for each agent of concern based on the presumed target site

from prior human and animal studies and the availability of screening tools. In practice, some form of medical surveillance is required by OSHA standards for asbestos, arsenic, benzene, and a variety of other carcinogens as listed in Table 17–7.

## Implications for Clinical Practice

The practice of occupational medicine often requires an assessment as to whether a cancer in an exposed worker is causally related to work or to exposure. Such an assessment may occur informally in

**Table 17–6.** Selected possible occupational carcinogens (Group 2B)—inadequate evidence of human carcinogenicity.[1]

| Occupational Exposure | Cancer Site | |
| --- | --- | --- |
| | Animal | Human |
| Acetaldehyde | Nasal mucosa, larynx | |
| Acrylamide | thyroid, adrenal, mammary gland, skin | |
| Antimony trioxide | Lung | |
| β-Butyrolactone | | |
| Carbon tetrachloride | Liver | |
| Ceramic fibers | Lung | |
| Chloroform | Liver, kidney | |
| Chlorophenols and phenoxyacetic acid herbicides | | Soft tissue sarcoma(?) and lymphoma(?) |
| Chlorophenothane (DDT) | Liver, lung, lymphoma | |
| 1,2-Dibromo-3-chloropropane (DBCP) | Nasal cavity, lung, stomach | |
| p-Dichlorobenzene | Liver, kidney | |
| 1,2-Dichloroethane | | |
| Dichloromethane | Lung, liver | |
| Diesel fuel, marine | | |
| Di(2-ethylhoxyl)phthalate | | |
| Dimethylformamide | | Testicular(?) |
| 1,4-Dioxane | Liver, nasal cavity | |
| Ethyl acrylate | Forestomach | |
| Ethylene thiourea | Thyroid | |
| Gasoline | Kidney | Leukemia(?), (related to benzene[?]) |
| Glasswool | Lung | |
| Hexachlorocyclohexanes | Liver | Leukemia(?) |
| Hydrazine | Lung, liver, mammary gland, nose | |
| Lead compounds, inorganic | Kidney | |
| Nickel, metallic | | |
| Phenylglycidyl ether | | |
| Polybrominated biphenyls (PBBs) | Liver | |
| Rockwool | Lung | Lung |
| Slagwool | | Lung |
| Styrene | Lung | |
| 2,3,7,8-Tetrachlorodibenzo-p-dioxin (TCDD) | Liver, lung, other | Soft tissue sarcoma(?), lymphoma(?) |
| Tetrachloroethylene | Liver, leukemias | |
| Toluene diisocyanates | | |
| o-Toluidine | vascular tumors | Bladder tumors(?) |
| Welding fumes | | Lung(?), (related to nickel, chromium[?]) |

[1] Sources: International Agency for Research on Cancer; Boffetta et al; Enterline.

**Table 17–7.** Carcinogens for which medical surveillance is required.

2-Acetylaminofluorene
Acrylonitrile
4-Aminodiphenyl
Arsenic (inorganic)
Asbestos
Benzidine (and its salts)
Bis(chloromethyl) ether
Coke oven emissions
1,2-Dibromo-3-chloropropane
3,3′-Dichlorobenzidine (and its salts)
4-Dimethylaminoazobenzene
Ethyleneimine
Ethylene dibromide
Ethylene oxide
4,4′-Methyelene-bis(2-chloroaniline)
Methyl chloromethyl ether
α-Naphthylamine
β-Naphthylamine
4-Nitrobiphenyl
N-Nitrosodimethylamine
β-Propiolactone
Vinyl chloride

Source: Subchapter 7, General Industry Safety Orders, of title 8, Industrial Relations, California Administrative Code, 1986.

discussion with a concerned affected employee or more formally in the setting of a workers' compensation claim or toxic tort case. Unfortunately, neither the principles of carcinogenesis nor the investigative methods for assessing the carcinogenicity of a particular chemical were designed to be used in, and cannot be directly applied to, the assessment of an individual case.

Some of the same factors used in the assessment of the work-relatedness of any illness, largely derived from the medical and occupational history and medical, employment, and exposure records, are important in the assessment of a possible occupational cancer. Obtaining such information may be complicated by the long time elapsed since exposures began and the absence of industrial hygiene or exposure records. Nevertheless, one needs to assess the nature of the agents involved, the intensity, setting and control of the exposures, and the timing and duration of the exposures. Potential sources for this information include the individual, coworkers and managers, material safety data sheets or other sources of chemical use information, and, if available, industrial hygiene data. Knowledge of the presence or absence of other symptoms that may be due to exposure, used in conjunction with dose-response information, could be helpful. For some industries, there may be contemporaneous published exposure-assessment information. From these sources, it is usually possible to get a qualitative sense of the intensity, timing, and duration of exposures.

The medical history and medical records provide information about the cancer site and cell type and the presence of any other risk factors for the cancer.

Physical examination is not very helpful, though it may provide evidence of findings suggestive of other conditions associated with the exposure or other risk factors.

Literature review can provide the descriptive epidemiology of the tumor type, including age, sex, and racial patterns of incidence, as well as information regarding nonoccupational risk factors for the tumor type. Literature searches can identify any relevant epidemiologic studies, which may be chemical-specific or job- or process-specific. In addition, there are a number of published occupational mortality studies that can provide some information about mortality due to cancers at certain sites in occupational groups. Because these are not formal epidemiologic studies and provide no correction for confounding factors, the results must be viewed with caution. Literature searches can also identify animal experimental studies of specific chemicals, from which tumor site, type, frequency, and dose response can be determined.

Synthesis of this information first involves assessment of the quality of the epidemiologic and animal experimental evidence, using the criteria discussed above. For example, one would give less weight to a small excess of a particular cancer in an occupational group if the number of observed cases were small and information regarding potential confounders were unavailable, particularly if the excess had not been observed in other studies. Similarly, one would assess the quality of data regarding other nonoccupational risk factors. One needs to assess the overall significance of the exposure, relative to exposure-response information in the literature. For example, one-time exposures are much less likely to be of etiologic importance than regular, long-term exposures.

Assessing the duration of a presumed latency period can be helpful. As there is a consensus that exposure-related solid tumors in humans require a minimum of 10–12 years latency, it is unlikely that tumors that develop within a few years of initial exposure to the suspect agent are causally related to that exposure. Although cohort studies of workers exposed to known carcinogens will occasionally demonstrate the occurrence of some cases with a shorter interval since first exposure, these tumors could be related to the background incidence in the general population. In these situations, no statistically significant excess of tumors is demonstrable compared to the reference population for the subcohort with less than about 10 years latency.

Finally, if an individual with cancer had experienced only very low-level or short duration exposures to a known or suspect carcinogen relative to the high doses in cohorts that had been demonstrated to have an increased risk for cancer, the cancer is not likely to be exposure-related. With the rare exception of sentinel tumors, such as mesotheliomas, which almost universally stem from asbestos exposure, there is nothing about the appearance or behavior of a tumor that allows a differentiation between work-related and spontaneous tumors. If the dose is low and the incidence of the tumor in the general unexposed population is relatively high, it is more likely that the occurrence of the tumor reflects the background incidence of the tumor or the effect of more prevalent risk factors present in the general population (eg, smoking). Empirically, the data regarding human carcinogenicity, or an increased risk of cancer, from chemical exposures uniformly implicate high dose exposures. While some evaluators may try to invoke the no-threshold model or the "one molecule" or "one fiber" theory to attribute a cancer in an individual to low-level exposures, it is clear that the intent of the no-threshold linear model was to attempt to predict risk for carcinogenicity in exposed populations at low doses, not to provide post hoc determinations of causation in individual cases. At most, information indicating exposure to "one molecule," or, in other words, a very low dose, could raise the possibility of a connection between the exposure and the cancer. It would not prove that there is a causal connection in either the scientific or medical-legal arena. Since the standard of proof in workers' compensation and toxic tort cases is reasonable medical probability (ie, that the exposure or employment more likely than not caused the medical condition), a statement that a connection is possible is not sufficient to establish causation.

In the absence of markers on tumors that establish their chemical origins or a scientific consensus on an approach to establishing causation in individual cases, one logical method involves the use of the epidemiologic concept of attributable proportion—the rate in the exposed population minus the rate in the unexposed population divided by the rate in the exposed population. Assuming that epidemiologic data are available that establish an index of mortality (eg, SMR, SMOR) for groups exposed to different cumulative doses of a carcinogen relative to an unexposed reference population and assuming that some information is available regarding cumulative dose for the affected individual, it will be possible to estimate a relative risk for the individual related to his/her exposure. If the relative risk estimate were two, then 50% of the cancers observed would likely be due to the exposure, while the other 50% would be due to the background incidence of the tumor. When the relative risk estimate exceeds two and there is a high degree of confidence in the epidemiologic data and the comparability of the individual's exposures, a tumor in that individual is more likely than not related to the exposure. Conversely, when the relative risk estimate is less than or equal to two, it is not probable that the cancer is exposure-related. As an example, consider a hypothetical population of service station workers who have been exposed to benzene (in gasoline) for a working lifetime at a time-weighted average concentration of 0.1 ppm. Rinsky et al, using epidemiologic data and risk assessment methodology, determined that the odds ratio for leukemia at this cumulative exposure level was 1.05. At this level of exposure, it is not likely that a leukemia occurring in a member of this population is work-related. In fact, fewer than 5% of leukemias in this population would be exposure-related, the remainder being due to the background incidence of leukemia in the general population. Proper use of this approach requires that the individual be roughly comparable to an exposed group in the epidemiologic study in terms of exposure level and confounding factors. Further, the assessment is only as good as the quality of the epidemiologic data used. Along these lines, there must be strong scientific evidence of a causal association between the exposure or occupation and the cancer, which means, as above, that the association must be strong, consistent across different populations, and so forth. The demographic features, latency period, and nonoccupational risk factors in the affected individual need to be factored into the assessment of causation. Guidotti provides an excellent discussion of this approach in a recent article about cancer risk in firefighters.

Possible clusters of cancer in a working population pose somewhat different challenges to the occupational physician in investigation and risk communication. In that clusters are groups of like or similar illnesses aggregated in space and time, the first challenge is to confirm that there is indeed a cluster. A commonly encountered scenario involves the recognition by a group of workers that several individuals have had cancer. Investigation by interview of the affected individuals or by review of medical records often establishes that the individuals have distinctly different types of tumors, which are etiologically unrelated (eg, breast cancer, Hodgkin's disease, and lung cancer); in other words, there is no cluster of like events. Alternatively, the individuals may not have shared the same space for very long, or one may have had cancer prior to joining the group. If initial investigation does reveal that a true cluster may exist, it may be helpful to confirm that the observed incidence exceeds what would have been expected in a population of comparable size and demographics (ie, that the apparent clustering did not occur by chance). This assessment requires appropriate statistical methods and cancer incidence data. In parallel with these activities, it would be reasonable to perform an appropriate exposure assessment of the work area, to look for potential sources of exposure to carcinogens or other hazardous chemical or physical agents. Since there are a number of published investigations of clusters where no plausible responsible environmental factor could be identified, a failure to determine an environmental cause after a thorough investigation should not be surprising. Caldwell reported the results of the investigation of 108 space-time cancer clusters performed by the Centers for Disease

Control from 1961 to 1983. No clear-cut environmental causative explanations were identified in any of these investigations. In these circumstances, presentation of the investigation results, good communication skills, and patience may help to ease unnecessary concerns in the work force.

## CARCINOGENESIS REFERENCES

Ames B, Gold L: Too many rodent carcinogens: Mitogenesis increases mutagenesis. Science 1990;249:970.

Ames BN, Magaw R, Gold LS: Ranking possible carcinogenic hazards. Science 1987;236:271.

Barrett JC: Mechanisms of multistep carcinogenesis and carcinogen risk assessment. Environ Health Perspect 1993;100:9.

Bartsch H, Malaveille C: Prevalence of genotoxic chemicals among animal and human carcinogens evaluated in the IARC monograph series. Cell Biol Toxicol 1989;5:115.

Benigni R, Andreoli C: Rodent carcinogenicity and toxicity, in vitro mutagenicity, and their physical chemical determinants. Mut Res 1993;297:281.

Boffetta P et al: Current perspectives on occupational cancer risks. Int J Occup Environ Health 1995;1:315.

Caldwell G: Twenty-two years of cancer cluster investigations at the Centers for Disease Control. Am J Epidemiol 1990;132(Suppl 1):S43.

Enterline P: Carcinogenic effects of man-made vitreous fibers. Annu Rev Publ Health 1991;12:459.

Fung VA, Barrett JC, Huff J: The carcinogenesis bioassay in perspective: Applications in identifying human cancer hazards. Environ Health Perspect 1995;103:680.

Guidotti T: Occupational mortality among firefighters: Assessing the association. J Occup Environ Med 1995;37:1348.

Hemminki K: DNA and protein adducts. Toxicology 1995;101:41.

Hirvonen A: Genetic factors in individual responses to environmental exposures. J Occup Environ Med 1995;37:37.

Huff J: Chemicals and cancer in humans: First evidence in experimental animals. Environ Health Perspect 1993;100:201.

Husgafvel-Pursiainen K et al: p53 and *ras* gene mutations in lung cancer: Implications for smoking and occupational exposures. J Occup Environ Med 1995;37:69.

International Agency for Research on Cancer: Overall Evaluations of Carcinogenicity: An Updating of IARC Monographs Volumes 1–42 IARC Monographs (Suppl 7), WHO/IARC, 1987.

Krewski D et al: Applications of physiologic pharmacokinetic modeling in carcinogenic risk assessment. Environ Health Perspect 1994;102(Suppl 11):37.

McMahon G: The genetics of human cancer: Implications for ecotoxicology. Environ Health Perspect 1994;102 (Suppl 12):75.

Nuorva K: p53 protein accumulation in lung carcinomas of patients exposed to asbestos and tobacco smoke. Am J Respir Crit Care Med 1994;150:528.

Pearce N et al: Occupational exposures to carcinogens in developing countries. Ann Acad Med Singapore 1994;23:684.

Rannung A et al: Genetic polymorphism of cytochromes P450 1A1, 2D6 and 2E1: Regulation and Toxicological Significance. J Occup Environ Med 1995;37:25.

Ruder AM: Epidemiology of occupational carcinogens and mutagens. Occup Med 1996;11(3):487.

Shubik P: Chemical carcinogens and human cancer. Cancer Lett 1995;93:3.

Sinclair WK: Radiation protection recommendations on dose limits: The role of the NCRP and the ICRP and future developments. Int J Rad Oncol Biol Phys 1995;31:387.

Tennant RW et al: Prediction of chemical carcinogenicity in rodents from in vitro genetic toxicity assays. Science 1987;236:933.

Vainio H, Husgafvel-Pursiainen K: Elimination of environmental factors or elimination of individuals: Biomarkers and prevention. J Occup Environ Med 1995;37:12.

# CLINICAL PRESENTATIONS

## LUNG CANCER

### Essentials of Diagnosis

- Asbestos, radon, chloromethylether, polycylic aromatic hydrocarbons (PAHs), chromium, nickel, inorganic arsenic exposure.
- Cigarette smoking or exposure to cigarette smoke.
- Cough, hemoptysis, dyspnea, weight loss.
- Mass lesion, pulmonary infiltrate, hilar or mediastinal adenopathy on chest x-ray.
- Diagnosis usually made with one or more of the following: sputum cytology, bronchoscopy with brushings and biopsy, transthoracic needle biopsy. Thoracotomy rarely required.

### Occupations at Risk

- Asbestos.
  - Asbestos miners.
  - Textile manufacturing.
  - Insulation and filter material production.
  - Shipyard workers.
- Radon.
  - Uranium mining.
  - Domestic exposure.
- Chloromethyl ethers.
  - Chemical production workers.
- PAHs.
  - Coke oven workers.
  - Rubber workers.
  - Roofers.
  - Aluminum reduction workers.
- Chromium.
  - Chromate production.

- Nickel.
  - Nickel mining, refining.
- Arsenic.
  - Arsenical pesticide production and use.
  - Copper, lead, zinc smelting.

## General Considerations

Lung cancer is the leading cause of cancer deaths in the United States and its incidence continues to rise, particularly in women. It is estimated that 99,000 men and 78,000 women will develop lung cancer and 160,000 will die of this disease in 1996. Fatality rates remain high; lung cancer currently accounts for almost 30% of all cancer deaths.

## Etiology

Cigarette smoking is the most important and most preventable risk factor for cancer of the lung. More than 80% of lung cancer deaths are attributable to cigarette smoking. Although its relative importance may decline if recent trends toward reduced cigarette consumption and the use of cigarettes with decreased tar and nicotine continue, the increasing incidence of lung cancer in women correlates with an increase in the smoking habit. The proportion of risks attributable to exposures in the workplace is significant; however, estimates vary widely, ranging from 4% to 40%. The association of lung cancer with exposure to asbestos, radon, chloromethyl ethers, PAHs, nickel, chromium, and inorganic arsenic appears to be independent of cigarette smoking. However, the effects of some known occupational carcinogens are greatly enhanced by smoking (eg, asbestos, radon). Occupations with a high smoking prevalence have an increased risk of cancer. This includes restaurant wait staff, cashiers, orderlies, drivers, construction workers, watchmen, and others where smoking prevalence may be higher than 40%. In addition, it appears that high levels of environmental tobacco smoke, such as is found in restaurants and bars, may significantly increase the risk of lung cancer in employees.

**A. Asbestos:** Asbestos is the substance generally considered to pose the greatest carcinogenic threat in the workplace. Asbestos-related lung cancer was first reported in 1934, but perhaps the most striking data were presented in 1947 when Britain's Chief Factory Inspector reported that lung cancer was found in 31 (13.2%) of 235 men with asbestosis who died between 1924 and 1946. However, it was not until separate epidemiologic studies were published in 1955 by Doll and also by Breslow that asbestos exposure was indeed recognized as being associated with cancer of the lung. Since then, many studies have documented the increase in lung cancer in workers with previous asbestos exposure, including a landmark study by Selikoff in which he followed 17,800 asbestos workers from 1967 to 1976 and found 486 deaths due to lung cancer (against an expected 105.6 deaths).

Asbestos is a fibrous silicate composed of various types. The minerals are divided into two classes: serpentine (chrysotile) and amphiboles (amosite, crocidolite, anthophyllite, and tremolite). The three most common commercial forms are chrysotile, amosite, and crocidolite; however, 90% of the asbestos used in the United States is chrysotile. Although crocidolite is thought to be the most carcinogenic mineral, all of the three commonly used forms of asbestos have been associated with an increased risk of cancer. It is of interest to note that within the chrysotile industry, low rates of lung cancer are reported in occupations such as mining and yet some of the highest rates are found in the textile industry. This is thought to be due to the higher carcinogenic potential of the very long chrysotile fibers used in the textile industry rather than the shorter fibers found in mines. Long, thin fibers are more likely to be inhaled and therefore result in pulmonary disease. Exposures are usually to mixed forms of asbestos.

Lung cancer is a major asbestos-related disease, accounting for 20% of all deaths in asbestos-exposed cohorts and up to 4% of all lung cancer is attributable to asbestos exposure. A latency period of approximately 20 years has been noted before the majority of lung cancer cases are seen. Although a dose-response relationship between asbestos exposure and lung cancer has now been established, increased risk is seen even after short but intense exposures. Asbestos exposure was shown in Selikoff's study to increase the risk of lung cancer fivefold. Other investigators have found the risk not to be this high. For example, individuals who worked in shipyards during the 1940s have been found to have a risk of lung cancer up to 1.7 times what would have been expected. These risks can be contrasted with the 25-fold increase of lung cancer risk in persons who have been heavy smokers of cigarettes for 20 years. Several studies have also shown evidence that cigarette smokers also exposed to asbestos have an even greater increased risk of developing cancer of the lung, suggesting an initiator effect of cigarette smoke followed by a promotor effect from asbestos exposure.

**B. Radon:** Radon exposure is known to increase the risk of lung cancer. This carcinogenic effect was discovered when increased mortality rates from lung cancer were identified in uranium miners. Excesses in pulmonary disease were noted as early as 1879 in the uranium mining towns of Europe, with some cases of tuberculosis and silicosis, but much of it lung cancer. Large-scale mining of uranium began in the United States in 1948 because of the need for uranium to make nuclear weapons. By the 1960s, 20% of deaths in uranium miners in the United States were due to lung disease. Excessive lung cancer in uranium miners is independent of cigarette smoking, though exposure to both is synergistic.

Ores containing uranium include all of its decay products, which form a series of radionuclides, of which one is the inert gas radon. Radon diffuses out of the rock into the mine atmosphere, where it decays into radioisotopes of polonium, bismuth, and lead—termed radon daughters. These radionuclides are found in the air and are then inhaled as free ions or as attachments to dust particles. Epidemiologic studies of workers in US uranium mines have demonstrated that the risk of lung cancer is proportionate to the cumulative radon daughter exposure. Increased risk of lung cancer has also been found in fluorspar miners, iron ore (hematite) miners, and hard rock miners. Data from animal models support the carcinogenic effect of radon; respiratory tumors can be induced by inhaled radon daughter products.

Data from animal models support the carcinogenic effects of radon; respiratory tumors can be induced by inhaled radon daughter products. Domestic radon exposure has been an issue of concern since 1984, when high radon levels were discovered in homes built on the Reading Prong geologic formation in Pennsylvania. The risk of lung cancer from low-level radon exposure has been extrapolated from studies of mine workers to the general population, but appears to be very low.

**C. Chloromethyl Ethers:** Exposure to multiple chemical substances can cause an increase in lung cancers in exposed workers. Among the most important of these are the chloromethyl ethers, which include chloromethyl methyl ether (CMME) and bis (chloromethyl) ether (BCME). Chloromethyl ethers are produced in order to chloromethylate other organic chemicals in the manufacture of ion exchange resins, bactericides, pesticides, dispersing agents, water repellents, solvents for industrial polymerization reactions, and flame-proofing agents. The potential for chloromethyl ethers to cause cancer was first suspected in humans in 1962. In Philadelphia, a cluster of three cases of small cell lung cancer occurred among approximately 45 men working in a single building of a large chemical plant. A large proportion of tumors occurred in young men and nonsmokers. Numerous other studies have confirmed these findings, with increased risk seen in workers with prolonged or intense exposure. Unlike other chemical carcinogens, which can cause a variety of cancers, the chloromethyl ethers are primarily associated with the induction of small cell lung cancer. Inhalation studies in animals have shown that the chloromethyl ethers produce bronchial epithelial metaplasia and atypia, and both carcinogens are active alkylating agents. BCME is a more potent carcinogen than CMME.

**D. Polycyclic Aromatic Hydrocarbons:** PAHs, formed from the incomplete combustion of coal tar, pitch, oil, and coke, have long been recognized as carcinogens. The first description implicating PAHs in the induction of cancer was in 1775 when Sir Percival Pott reported an increased risk of scrotal cancer in chimney sweeps due to dermal exposure to soot. Epidemiologic evidence linking PAHs to lung cancer was provided in 1936, when a study of exposed workers in a coal carbonization plant in Japan revealed a marked increase in the rate of lung cancer.

Exposures to PAHs linked to an increased risk of lung cancer have been found in coke oven workers, roofers, printers, and truckers. Rubber plant workers and those employed in asphalt production, coal gasification, and aluminum reduction facilities are also at risk. The best described occupational group are coke oven workers, where direct exposure to the coke ovens results in increased rates of lung cancer. A clear dose-response relationship has been described based on proximity of work to the ovens.

**E. Other Chemicals:**

**1. Arsenic–**Exposure to inorganic arsenic has been shown to increase the risk of lung cancer; the first cases of arsenic-induced lung cancer were reported in 1930. Arsenic exposure in copper smelting, fur handling, sheep-dip compound manufacturing, and arsenical pesticide production and use has resulted in increased rates of lung cancer. Long latency periods of approximately 25 years are seen after exposure before the development of cancer. Arsenic is thought to act as a late-stage promoter of cancer and may interfere with DNA repair mechanisms. A dose-response relationship in exposed workers has been described, as has an increase in the risk of arsenic-induced lung cancer in cigarette smokers.

**2. Chromium–**Increased rates of lung cancer have been reported in industries that use chromate, including chromate production, chrome plating, chrome alloy production, and others. Other lung carcinogens used in the electroplating industry, such as nickel and PAHs, may confound this relationship. The greatest risk of lung cancer appears to be present in occupations involving chromate production, in which all lung cancer types are increased.

**3. Nickel–**Exposure to nickel in mining, refining, and subsulfide roasting facilities has been associated with increased rates of lung and nasal cancer. Soluble forms of nickel appear to be more potent carcinogens, with no increased risk seen after exposure to nickel alloys and pure nickel dust.

**4. Mustard Gas–**Studies of Japanese and German workers in factories that manufactured mustard gas during World War II have shown an excess of respiratory cancers. This is consistent with finding that mustard gas can produce lung tumors in laboratory animals. There may be a higher rate of squamous cell cancer of the lung in humans.

**5. Probable Lung Carcinogens–**Incomplete data exists regarding the risk of lung cancer associated with exposure to acrylonitrile (textile fiber, rubber workers), beryllium (production of beryllium alloys, aerospace industry), cadmium (cadmium and other metal smelters, manufacturers of batteries, plastics, dye, and pigments), vinyl chloride (plastics production), formaldehyde (production of formaldehyde resins, molding, apparel), and inorganic acid mists containing sulfuric acid (metal production/processing).

## Pathology

The four major types of lung cancer are squamous cell (epidermoid) carcinoma, adenocarcinoma, large cell carcinoma, and small cell (oat cell) carcinoma. All histologic types of lung cancer are linked to cigarette smoking. There is no one cell type that is pathognomonic of an occupationally related lung cancer. A notable exception is workers exposed to CMME or BCME, who are much more likely to develop the relatively uncommon small cell histology. Although early work suggested that the peripheral distribution of asbestos fibers was associated with a higher incidence of adenocarcinomas in this region, this has not been found in recent, more thorough studies. It appears that lung cancers in asbestos-exposed persons occur equally throughout the lung and all pathologic types are seen.

## Clinical Findings

**A. Symptoms and Signs:** The findings in patients with lung cancer may arise secondary to local tumor growth, invasion of nearby structures, regional growth of nodal metastases, or paraneoplastic syndromes. The primary tumor often causes cough, hemoptysis, wheezing, dyspnea, or pneumonitis secondary to obstruction. Tumor spread may cause tracheal obstruction or esophageal compression; and superior vena cava syndrome may result from compression of vascular structures. The peripheral nervous system may be involved, with recurrent laryngeal nerve paralysis (causing hoarseness), sympathetic nerve involvement (Horner's syndrome), or phrenic nerve paralysis. Nonspecific symptoms such as weight loss, anorexia, and fatigue may be evident.

**B. Laboratory Findings:** In approximately 60% of cases, a positive diagnosis can be made on the basis of sputum cytologic examination. Using flexible fiberoptic bronchoscopy, it is possible to visualize approximately 65% of lesions in lung cancer patients, with biopsy and brushings true-positive in approximately 90% of these. Transthoracic fine needle aspiration biopsy with fluoroscopic guidance is useful for peripheral lesions that cannot be reached with the bronchoscope. If these less invasive diagnostic procedures fail to lead to diagnosis, exploratory thoracotomy may be required.

**C. Imaging:** The chest x-ray is the most important tool for the diagnosis of lung cancer. Findings are related to the tumor cell type, with variation as to central or peripheral location of tumor mass, and existence of regional spread. Squamous cell cancers are more often located centrally, with associated hilar adenopathy. Adenocarcinoma presents more commonly as a peripheral nodule with pleural and chest wall involvement, and large cell carcinoma is seen as a large peripheral mass with associated pneumonitis. A central lesion with atelectasis and both hilar and mediastinal adenopathy are common features of small cell carcinoma. The extent of disease may be defined more accurately by computer tomographic imaging of the chest.

## Prevention

Complete avoidance of exposure to the carcinogen is the ultimate goal, but this is not always possible. The most effective method of reducing the mortality rate for lung cancer is primary prevention. This includes identification of etiologic agents in the workplace, adherence to strict workplace standards, and worker education. Since tobacco use is known to increase the incidence of lung cancer in occupationally exposed groups, aggressive anti-smoking campaigns in the workplace are critically important.

Medical monitoring in the workplace has been attempted as a method of secondary prevention to aid in early detection. Serial chest x-rays and sputum cytologic examinations are now recommended by NIOSH and OSHA in high-risk occupational groups. The main problem with this approach is that there is no evidence that early detection improves the prognosis for persons with lung cancer. Thus far, serial chest x-rays have been more useful than sputum cytologic examinations in detecting lung cancer. However, sputum cytology may reveal signs of mucosal damage, such as atypia, that could identify individuals at increased risk and lead to decreased exposure.

Chemoprevention of lung cancer is under investigation, with only preliminary results available.

## Treatment & Prognosis

Therapy of occupational lung cancers is no different from treatment for each of the specific cell types of lung cancer that may be seen. Surgical resection is currently the best hope for cure in non-small cell cancer. Unfortunately, most patients do not qualify for a curative surgical procedure, and these patients are treated with palliative chemotherapy or radiotherapy in an attempt to improve survival, since cures at this stage are rare. Survival is related to both cell type and stage of disease, with squamous cell cancers having the best prognosis. In general, even in patients with localized disease, long-term survival is the exception rather than the rule. Overall, 5-year survival ranges from 10–13%. Small cell carcinoma has traditionally had the worst prognosis, with early and widespread metastases, although there have been some encouraging results with chemotherapy in limited disease.

## MESOTHELIOMA

### Essentials of Diagnosis
- Asbestos exposure, including trivial contact.
- Persistent gnawing chest pain, dyspnea, dry cough, weight loss.
- Findings consistent with pleural effusion, pleural friction rub on physical examination.
- Chest x-ray and CT scan showing extensive pleural effusions, thick pleural rind lining the chest wall.
- Diagnosis by open thoracotomy with multiple biopsies.

### Occupations at Risk
- Asbestos.
  - Asbestos miners.
  - Textile manufacturing.
  - Insulation and filter material production.
  - Construction workers.
  - Welders, plumbers, electricians.
  - Roofers.
  - Shipyard workers.

### General Considerations
Mesothelioma was not accepted as a pathologic entity until about 50 years ago, when Klemperer and Rahn advocated general use of the term mesothelioma for primary pleural tumors originating from the surface lining cells, or the mesothelium. This tumor is uncommon, accounting for only a small fraction of deaths due to cancer, but it and other asbestos-related diseases have been of great interest to occupational health physicians, public health professionals, biomedical researchers, and personal injury attorneys.

The first case reports of mesothelioma associated with asbestos were published in the 1940s, but the problem received scant attention until 1960, when Wagner reported diffuse pleural mesothelioma associated with asbestos exposure in the western Cape Province of South Africa. The incidence of mesothelioma is increasing, with an annual incidence for adults in North America of approximately 12 cases per million for white men and 2–3 cases per million for women. In Canada, England, and Italy, areas of heavy occupational asbestos use, rates vary from 2.3 to 21.4 cases per million.

### Etiology
Diffuse mesotheliomas of the peritoneum and pleura are considered "signal tumors," or pathognomonic of exposure to asbestos. Since the early report of Wagner, many additional reports and cohort mortality studies have clearly implicated asbestos as the etiologic factor in occupational mesothelioma. Evidence is lacking for any causal relationship between asbestos exposure and the development of solitary or localized mesothelioma.

The most convincing evidence of an association between asbestos and mesothelioma was brought out in Selikoff's report and indicated that 8% of 17,800 asbestos insulation workers in the United States and Canada followed from 1967 to 1976 died from malignant mesothelioma. Selikoff and others have shown that a dose-response relationship exists between the risk of developing mesothelioma and the intensity and length of asbestos exposure.

The latency period from asbestos exposure to the diagnosis of mesothelioma is 30 years or more. Higher quantitative asbestos fiber content of dried lung has been found in patients with mesothelioma. Further evidence of the etiologic role of asbestos has been shown in experimental animals, in which intrapleural injection with asbestos fibers causes mesothelioma histologically identical to human tumors.

Epidemiologic data show that variable levels of exposure to asbestos can result in mesothelioma, despite the known dose-response relationship. In one study of 168 patients with mesothelioma in England and South Africa, one-third of cases were associated with occupational exposure intensive enough to cause asbestosis or lung cancer. Another third were asbestos-related only by trivial contact at work or in the home environment (eg, exposure of wives washing their husbands' contaminated work clothes). The remaining third had no history of contact with asbestos.

The major value of studies done to date has been to identify segments of the population at risk, but reports of patients with mesothelioma who do not have a history of occupational or paraoccupational exposure to asbestos raises other questions. The proportion of patients with no exposure history ranges from 0% to 87% in various studies. The long latency period from exposure to disease results in problems with forgotten or unknown exposures. In addition, the variety of occupations associated with asbestos exposure leads to problems with overlooked exposures. Exposure occurs in the milling, mining, and transportation of raw asbestos and in the manufacture of asbestos cement pipe, friction materials, textiles, and roofing materials. Construction workers, plumbers, welders, and electricians are all exposed; and shipyard tradesmen can be "innocent bystanders" when they are exposed to airborne asbestos fibers. There is also evidence that nonasbestos agents can induce malignant mesotheliomas, and substances such as nickel, beryllium, silica dust, and zeolite fibers have been studied in this regard. Cigarette smoking does not increase the risk of malignant mesothelioma. Unlike lung cancer, there is no evidence for synergy between cigarette smoking and asbestos exposure in the development of this tumor.

### Pathogenesis
All types of asbestos are capable of causing mesothelioma, though there is some evidence that crocidolite may be the most potent carcinogen. Very

few mesotheliomas have been associated with the chrysotile fiber alone. The mechanisms of induction are unknown. Cancer development is apparently related not to chemical composition but to physical properties (ie, fiber size and dimension). In work done in rats, long thin fibers of a variety of types have proved carcinogenic, whereas short fibers and those with a relatively broad diameter have failed to produce mesothelioma. Inhaled fibers are expectorated or swallowed. Short fibers are cleared more readily than long fibers. Fibers that remain accumulate in the lower lung, adjacent to the pleura. These findings are consistent with epidemiologic observations documenting the relatively common occurrence of tumors in populations exposed to grades of crocidolite consisting chiefly of long, thin fibers and the rarity of tumors in persons exposed to amosite and anthophyllite. The location of mesothelioma is related to the type of asbestos fiber, as well. Chrysotile has been associated with pleural, but not peritoneal, tumors in Canadian miners, although this association may be related at least in part to contamination of the asbestos with tremolite, an uncommon fiber, rather than the chrysotile. Peritoneal mesothelioma has been shown to occur only in individuals exposed to amphibole asbestos, and the pathogenesis is thought to be similar to tumor in the pleural cavity. Fibers of asbestos are transported in lymphatics to the abdomen, and asbestos is also transported across the mucosa of the gut after ingestion.

The mechanism of malignant transformation of mesothelial tissue is obscure. Mesothelial cells phagocytose asbestos and proliferate when exposed to asbestos in vitro. The activated mesothelial cells then release cytokines, which mediate an inflammatory and fibrotic reaction. Proto-oncogenes, such as platelet-derived growth factor, are unregulated in alveolar macrophages and result in mesothelial cell proliferation. It is of interest that malignant transformation has not been documented after exposure of cultured mesothelial cells to asbestos.

## Pathology

One of the major areas of difficulty in the study of mesothelioma has been distinguishing its pathologic features. Many tumors metastasize and spread to the mesothelial lining of the chest and abdomen: this has led to misdiagnosis of mesothelioma as a metastatic tumor. Confusion also exists due to the tumor's diverse microscopic appearance.

Two types of mesothelioma have been described: benign solitary and diffuse malignant mesothelioma. The benign solitary type remains localized, though it may become large and compress neighboring thoracic structures. This tumor has not been associated with asbestos exposure; it is a benign tumor arising from fibroblasts and other connective tissue elements in the areolar submesothelial cell layers of the pleura and is not occupational in origin. By contrast, diffuse

malignant mesothelioma arises from either the pluripotential mesenchymal cell or the primitive submesothelial mesenchymal cell, which retains the ability to form epithelial or connective tissue elements.

Malignant mesothelioma is a diffuse lesion that spreads widely in the pleural space and is usually associated with extensive pleural effusion and direct invasion of thoracic structures. On gross examination, numerous tumor nodules may be noted, and in advanced cases, the tumor has a hard, woody consistency. Microscopically, malignant mesotheliomas consist of three histologic types: an epithelial type that may resemble metastatic adenocarcinoma, a mesenchymal type, and a mixed type. Histochemical techniques using acid mucopolysaccharide with colloidal iron or alcian blue stains can detect epithelial cells. This staining can be removed from the tissue with hyaluronidase, a helpful finding characteristic of mesothelioma that can help distinguish it from adenocarcinoma. Studies with the electron microscope have defined certain characteristic features that are also helpful in differentiating the tumor from metastatic disease.

### Clinical Findings

**A. Symptoms:** Symptoms in diffuse mesothelioma may be entirely absent or minimal at the time of onset of the disease. Disease progression results in the most common symptom of a persistent gnawing chest pain on the involved side, which may radiate to the shoulder and arm. In most patients, pain becomes the most incapacitating symptom. Dyspnea on exertion, dry cough (occasionally hemoptysis), and increasing weight loss are frequent accompanying symptoms. Some patients have low-grade fever, which can result in an incorrect diagnosis of chronic infection. A minority of patients have paraneoplastic syndromes such as hypertrophic pulmonary osteoarthropathy, syncopal attacks from hypoglycemia, or generalized anasarca from massive involvement of the pericardium or obstruction of the inferior and superior venae cavae.

**B. Signs:** Physical findings vary with the stage of disease. Most patients present with pleural effusion. Local tumor growth may depress the diaphragm and displace the liver or spleen, giving the impression of hepatomegaly or splenomegaly. In advanced disease, there may be obvious enlargement of the affected hemithorax, with bulging of the intercostal spaces and displacement of the trachea and mediastinum to the unaffected side. After removal of pleural fluid, a pericardial or pleuropericardial rub may be heard. Advanced signs may also include fever, arthralgias, supraclavicular and axillary node enlargement, subcutaneous nodules in the chest wall, and clubbing. Encroachment on the mediastinal structures may lead to neuropathic signs such as vocal cord paralysis or Horner's syndrome. Congestion and edema may develop in the upper trunk or lower limbs secondary to compression of the superior or inferior vena cavae.

**C. Laboratory Findings:** Although patients may have the syndrome of inappropriate antidiuretic hormone secretion with hyponatremia, most have normal blood chemistries. Elevation of lactate dehydrogenase may occur as a nonspecific finding.

**D. Imaging:** X-ray studies of the chest most commonly show unilateral pleural effusion. After thoracentesis, the pleura may show thickening or nodularity, seen usually at the bases. CT scanning, which is the most sensitive test for evaluating the pleural surface, may show thickened tumor along the chest wall, and late in the disease tomograms or an overpenetrated film will show compressed lung surrounded on all sides by a tumor 2–3 cm thick. Extrapleural extension can result in soft tissue masses or radiologic evidence of rib destruction. Signs of asbestos such as interstitial pulmonary fibrosis, pleural plaques, and calcification are valuable findings when present.

**E. Special Examinations:**

**1. Sputum Cytology**–Microscopic examination of sputum rarely shows malignant cells unless the tumor has invaded lung parenchyma. Asbestos bodies may be seen.

**2. Thoracentesis**–The considerable force necessary to enter the pleural space with a thoracentesis needle may be a clue to the presence of pleural mesothelioma. Pleural fluid is serosanguineous or hemorrhagic in 30–50% of cases, but is commonly straw-colored. Cytologic examination of pleural fluid is useful in one-half to two-thirds of cases; however, distinguishing malignant mesothelioma from metastatic adenocarcinoma or benign inflammatory conditions is often difficult. The pleural fluid often contains a mixture of normal mesothelial cells, differentiated and undifferentiated malignant mesothelial cells, and a varying number of lymphocytes, histiocytes, and polymorphonuclear leukocytes. The diagnostic value of cytologic tests is limited. Mesothelial hyperplasia is not uncommon in benign pleural effusions and can easily be mistaken for malignant cells.

**3. Thoracotomy and Thoracoscopy**–Because of the limitations of pleural fluid cytologic examination, biopsy confirmation is required. An open thoracotomy with multiple biopsies from different pleural areas is generally required for diagnosis. Thoracoscopy with biopsy of pleural masses can be a less invasive and effective technique as well.

## Differential Diagnosis

The major disorders that must be differentiated from mesothelioma are inflammatory pleurisy, primary lung cancer, and metastatic adenocarcinoma or sarcoma. Inflammatory pleurisy is suggested by the associated clinical picture and by typical findings in the analysis of sputum and pleural fluid. In primary lung cancer, the more prominent symptoms of cough, the less common presence of severe chest pain, the presence of parenchymal tumors, and the absence of pleural abnormalities after thoracentesis help to differentiate between these two types of cancer. Primary tumors of the pancreas, gastrointestinal tract, or ovary should be excluded, since these tumors can metastasize to the pleural or peritoneal space and mimic mesothelioma.

## Prevention

Regulations governing asbestos exposure have been difficult to develop. Morbidity and mortality data have been used to look retrospectively at members of occupational groups with varying exposures in the remote past or over a lifetime. The difficulties are compounded by the long latency period of asbestosis and asbestos-related cancers, especially mesothelioma. Setting permissible limits requires establishment of dose-response relationships, with subsequent determination of an acceptable level of risk. The difficulty is that all industrial processes, fiber types, and asbestos-related diseases have dissimilar dose-response relationships. Although the exposures to asbestos that lead to mesothelioma are less intense and of shorter duration than those exposures that lead to asbestosis or lung cancer, most standards are now based on preventing asbestosis.

Control of asbestos dust in industry has become progressively more rigorous during the last 40 years. Recommendations for levels of asbestos in the air of occupational settings were first established in the 1940s, but it was not until 1970 that federal regulations began as a result of the passage of the Occupational Safety and Health Act and the Clean Air Act. Initial standards were based on the light microscopic count of fibers of a length of 5 μm, collected by mechanical means. A concentration of 5 fibers\mL of air averaged over an 8-hour period was considered acceptable, with stipulation for transient excesses above that concentration. In 1986, the exposure standard of 2 fibers/mL was lowered by OSHA to 0.2 fibers/mL. Allowable exposure varies with the different mineral fibers.

## Treatment

**A. Surgical Measures:** Surgery has been used with some success as the primary method of treatment in pleural mesotheliomas. Even with tumors with extensive infiltration of adjoining viscera, partial surgical resection has led to an apparent increase in longevity. Subtotal pleurectomy with decortication is the accepted procedure. More radical surgeries such as pleuropneumonectomy may be appropriate for selected patients. Postoperative adjuvant chemotherapy and radiation therapy are sometimes used, but there are no studies to support their use. Surgical resection of all visible disease is believed to be the treatment of choice. Surgical excision has no role in the management of peritoneal mesothelioma unless the tumor is localized.

**B. External Radiotherapy:** Radiation therapy has clearly been shown to be of benefit in controlling pain and pleural effusion in mesothelioma. Although antitumor efficacy has been noted using high-dose radiation, this modality is relatively ineffective in altering the dismal survival statistics for this disease.

**C. Instillation of Radioactive Compounds:** Because colloidal gold has an affinity for serosal lining cells, instillation of radioactive colloidal gold into the pleural space has been attempted. Responses with apparent long-term survival have been reported, with no significant toxicity. Therapy must be given early in the disease, before the pleural cavity is obliterated by tumor. Radioactive phosphate in conjunction with abdominal irradiation has been used for peritoneal mesothelioma, and the small number of patients treated in this fashion have had increased lengths of survival.

**D. Chemotherapy:** There has been no systematic study of the role of cytotoxic drugs in mesothelioma, but there are well-documented reports of definite antitumor effects in some patients. Doxorubicin has been demonstrated to induce tumor regression and perhaps to prolong the survival of responding patients. Single-agent doxorubicin therapy has therefore become the standard therapy for patients with unresectable disease, but no patient has been cured with chemotherapy.

Other reported active antitumor agents include methotrexate and alkylating agents such as cyclophosphamide, mechlorethamine, and thiotepa. There are few studies using combination chemotherapy, but regimens containing doxorubicin appear to be most effective.

## Course & Prognosis

Approximately 75% of patients die within one year after diagnosis, with an average survival after diagnosis of 8–10 months. Several factors correlate with improved survival in mesothelioma. Patients whose tumors are in the pleura survive twice as long as those with peritoneal tumor; survival is longer for patients with epithelial types than for those with mixed or fibrosarcomatous types; and survival is longer for patients younger than 65, those who respond well to chemotherapy, and those able to undergo surgical resection.

## CANCER OF THE NASAL CAVITY & SINUSES

## Essentials of Diagnosis

- Presenting symptoms are unilateral nasal obstruction, nonhealing ulcer, and occasional bleeding.
- More frequent in men than women (2:1).
- Usually squamous cell histology.

## Occupations at Risk

- Wood and other dusts.
  - Furniture workers.
  - Boot and shoe manufacturing.
  - Textile manufacturing.
- Nickel.
  - Nickel refinery workers.
- Chromium.
  - Chromate pigment manufacturing.
  - Metal plating workers.
- Isopropyl alcohol, formaldehyde.
  - Laboratory workers.
  - Other industries.

Cancers of the nasal cavity and sinuses are relatively rare, and account for less than 10 cases per million in the United States per year. This disease is very uncommon in workers under 50, and rates increase with age. Evidence suggests a fairly steady or slightly declining incidence over the years. About one-half of all sinonasal tumors are squamous cell and 10% are adenocarcinomas. Both of these histologies have been linked to occupational exposures. Other histologic types include lymphoma, adenoid cystic carcinoma, and melanoma.

## Etiology

Many different occupational exposures have been linked to cancer of the nasal cavity and paranasal sinuses. These include wood dust, nickel, chromium, mustard gas, and cutting oils. Employment in several industries has also been associated with these cancers, including furniture and shoe manufacturing and coal mining. Furnacemen in the gas, coke, and chemical industries, furnacemen in foundries, and textile workers have also been shown to be at increased risk. The process of manufacturing isopropyl alcohol has been associated with this form of cancer and is considered to be due to the dimethyl sulfate used during the process.

**A. Wood and Other Organic Dusts:** The earliest report that linked cancer of the nose to exposure to wood dust was in 1965, when a laryngologist in England observed an unusually high incidence of cancer of the nasal cavity and sinuses among workers in the furniture industry. Fifteen of the 20 reported cases were involved in the production of wooden chairs. Woodworkers without carcinoma were also examined, and many exhibited chronic hypertrophic rhinitis, dry atrophic nasal mucosa, or nasal polyps. Since this first report, many studies have shown an increased incidence of carcinoma of the sinonasal area in persons exposed to wood dust. Adenocarcinoma of the ethmoids and middle turbinates are the most frequent cell types encountered in these workers. The exact substance in wood dust responsible for carcinogenesis has not been identified.

An excess of both adenocarcinomas and squamous carcinomas of the nasal sinuses has also been observed among workers in the boot and shoe industry. As in the case of woodworkers, the specific etiologic agent in boot and shoe manufacture is unknown. Dusts involved in the textile industry and flour dusts in bakeries and flour mills have also been associated with the development of sinonasal cancers.

**B. Nickel:** Both nasal cancer and lung cancer have been linked to occupational nickel exposure. Most studies have been done on nickel refinery workers exposed to complex particulates (insoluble nickel sulfide dust, nickel oxides, and soluble nickel sulfate, nitrate, or chloride) and gaseous nickel carbonyl. The mean latency period between exposure and diagnosis of cancer in refinery workers is 20–30 years.

The earliest report of an increased risk of sinonasal carcinoma in nickel refinery workers was in 1932 when 10 cases were described in Wales, where a nickel carbonyl process was employed. Studies confirming these findings have subsequently been done in Canada, Norway, Germany, Japan, and the USSR. Clearly, nickel and nickel carbonyl are carcinogenic under experimental conditions, yet epidemiologic evidence points away from the nickel carbonyl process and incriminates exposure to dust from the preliminary processes. Neoplasms in nickel workers occur most frequently in the nose and the ethmoid sinuses, and are usually of the squamous or anaplastic cell type.

**C. Other Occupational Exposures:** Tumors of the nasal epithelium and mastoid air cells have been noted in women exposed to radium used for painting dials of watches and in radon chemists. Workers involved in the manufacture of hydrocarbon gas have been noted to have excess cases of cancer of the paranasal sinuses. Chromium is known to cause ulceration and perforation of the nasal septum, and there is an excess risk of sinonasal cancer in workers involved in manufacturing chromate pigments. Mustard gas, isopropyl alcohol, cutting oils, and formaldehyde have also been linked to excess cancers of the nasal cavity and paranasal sinuses.

### Clinical Findings

The earliest symptoms of nasal cavity neoplasms are a low-grade chronic infection, associated with discharge, obstruction, and minor intermittent bleeding. The patient often complains of "sinus trouble" and may have been inappropriately treated with antibiotics for prolonged periods before the true diagnosis was known. Subsequent symptoms depend on the pattern of local growth. Maxillary sinus tumors develop silently when they are confined to the sinus, producing symptoms only with extension outside the walls. With extension into the oral cavity, pain may be referred to the upper teeth. Nasal obstruction and bleeding are common complaints, along with "sinus pain" or "fullness" of the involved antrum. Observation and palpation of the face may reveal a mass. Ethmoid sinus carcinoma presents initially with mild to moderate sinus aching or pain. A painless mass may present along the inner canthus, and with invasion of the medial orbit, diplopia develops.

### Diagnosis & Treatment

In all cases, the patient should receive careful inspection and palpation of the facial structures, with attention to the eye and especially the extraocular movements. The nasal and orbital cavities should be examined closely. A fiberoptic nasoscope is a useful aid in visualizing the posterior and superior nasal cavities and the nasopharynx. Sinoscopy of the maxillary antrum may also be required. Helpful radiologic studies include facial bone or sinus x-ray series and CT scan of the involved areas. Identification of the site of tumor origin is important in determining the treatment plan.

Tumor in the nasal cavity is usually biopsied with a punch forceps. Biopsy of tumor in the maxillary antrum is usually approached with a Caldwell-Luc procedure, which is an incision through the gingivobuccal sulcus opposite the premolars. Biopsy of ethmoid tumors is usually taken from the extension into the nasal cavity. An undiagnosed orbital mass may also be biopsied secondary to incomplete examination of other areas. Frontal sinuses are approached by supraorbital incision and osteotomy.

Surgical therapy is usually indicated because of the frequency of osseous involvement; it involves resection of all gross disease. Any desire for wide margins is tempered by the reluctance to mutilate, and reconstructive and cosmetic surgery using prosthetic devices is often necessary. Radiation therapy is nearly always necessary because the resection margins are often narrow and the neoplasm is frequently of high grade. Chemotherapy is reserved for advanced disease. The prognosis is better for nasal cavity cancers, because they tend to be diagnosed at an early stage. The 5-year survival rate is approximately 30–40% for tumors of the maxillary and ethmoid sinuses and dismal for frontal and sphenoid sinus carcinomas.

## CANCER OF THE LARYNX

### Essentials of Diagnosis

- Hoarseness is an early presenting symptom.
- Cigarette smoking and alcohol abuse are the primary etiologic factors.
- Much more frequent in men than women (4.5:1), usually middle aged or older.
- Usually squamous cell histology.

### Occupations at Risk

- Asbestos.
  - Asbestos miners.
  - Textile manufacturing.
  - Insulation and filter material production.
  - Shipyard workers.

Cancer of the larynx is much more common than sinonasal cancer, representing about 2% of the total cancer risk in the United States. In most areas of the world, there is evidence that cancer of the larynx is increasing in men and, in more developed countries, also among women.

### Etiology

Cancer of the larynx appears to be primarily related to cigarette smoking. Alcohol is less important in the causation of laryngeal cancer than in other tumors of the head and neck. Occupational exposure to asbestos has been suggested as a risk factor for development of this disease, with one retrospective study finding asbestos to be a more important risk factor than either tobacco or alcohol. Most other studies do not support this contention, however. Asbestos exposure in miners, shipyard workers, asbestos product manufacturers, and insulators has been associated with high rates of laryngeal cancers. Epidemiologic studies have also linked laryngeal cancer to "strong acid" manufacturing of ethanol and isopropanol, as well as workplace exposures to wood dust, mustard gas, nickel, and cutting oils. The risk from these agents has not been clearly established.

Laryngeal cancer is primarily a disease of older workers—the median age is usually in the sixth or seventh decade. At the time of diagnosis, approximately 60% are localized, 30% show regional spread, and 10% have distant metastases. Laryngeal tumors in the United States are classified into three groups according to anatomic site of origin, with 40% supraglottic, 59% glottic, and 1% subglottic cancers. Nearly all are squamous cell carcinomas.

### Clinical Findings

Symptoms of laryngeal carcinoma vary depending on the site of involvement. Any patient who complains of persistent hoarseness, difficulty in swallowing, pain on swallowing, a "lump in the throat," or a change in voice quality should be examined promptly by indirect laryngoscopy. Any limitation of motion or rigidity should be noted, and direct laryngoscopy with biopsy of suspicious lesions is necessary. Lateral soft tissue radiographs of the neck and CT scanning are also useful, especially to delineate extent of disease.

### Treatment

The treatment plan must include preservation of the patient's life and voice. There has been an increasing tendency to use more limited surgical procedures plus radiation therapy, or radiation therapy alone. For failures of conservative therapy or deeply infiltrative tumors, total laryngectomy is required, necessitating tracheostomy and loss of normal voice. Because of the early symptom of hoarseness, true vocal cord tumors are detected early and carry the best

prognosis; localized disease in this area has a 90% 5-year survival rate.

## BLADDER CANCER

### Essentials of Diagnosis

- Cigarette smoking is the most important etiologic factor.
- α- and β-Naphthylamine, benzidine exposure.
- Presenting complaints of hematuria and vesical irritability.
- Diagnosis by urine cytologic examination and cystoscopy.

### Occupations at Risk

- α,β-Naphthylamine.
  - Textile workers (dye/pigment manufacturing).
- 4-Aminobiphenyl.
  - Tire and rubber manufacturing.
- Benzidine.
  - Dye/pigment manufacturing.
- Chlornaphazine.
  - Leather workers.
- 4-Chloro-o-toluidine.
  - Bootblacks.
  - Textile workers.
- o-Toluidine.
  - Painters.
- 4,4'-Methylene bis (2-chloroaniline).
  - Truck drivers.
  - Rubber manufacturing.
- Methylene dianiline.
  - Drill press operators.
- Benzidine-derived azo dyes.
  - Chemical workers.
- Phenacetin-containing compounds.
  - Petroleum workers.
  - Hairdressers.

### General Considerations

Bladder cancer accounts for about 2% of all malignant tumors, with a steady increase in incidence. It is projected that 52,900 new cases will be diagnosed in the United States in 1996 and 11,700 people will die of this disease. The male-to-female ratio is 3:1, but the increased incidence in men is probably secondary to the relationship between bladder cancer and smoking. The incidence of bladder cancer increases with age, with a peak incidence in the seventh decade. The incidence of urinary tract neoplasms is higher in industrialized countries than in the underdeveloped regions and higher in rural than in urban areas.

### Etiology

Cigarette smoking is the most important known preventable cause of bladder cancer, with as many as

60% of cases attributed to this common habit. The roles of coffee drinking and the use of artificial sweeteners have also been the objects of scrutiny. Occupations have long been suspect, and it is believed that 20% of all bladder cancers are due to work exposures. The increasing incidence of bladder cancer despite a decrease in smoking in the United States suggests an important role for other environmental factors. Exposure to water contaminated with pesticides and other chemicals may increase the risk of bladder cancer.

As early as 1895, Rehn, a Swiss urologist, described a high incidence of bladder tumors among aniline dye workers. Large-scale production of aromatic amines as dye intermediates was started in the United States during World War I, and by 1934 the first occupational bladder cancers in the United States were described. Twenty-five cases of bladder tumor were reported in workers exposed to β-naphthylamine or benzidine and two cases in workers exposed to α-naphthylamine. Several years later, 58 additional cases were reported from the same plant. In addition, β-naphthylamine was reported to induce urinary bladder tumors in dogs and subcutaneous injections of benzidine was shown to induce carcinomas in rats. During the next three decades, several studies both in the United States and Great Britain showed an increase in urinary bladder tumors in workers exposed to these chemicals. The latency period between exposure and cancer was quite variable, with a mean of 20 years.

Occupational categories with a confirmed or strongly suspected increased risk for bladder cancer are dyestuff and chemical manufacturing, pigment and paint manufacturing, cable manufacturing, textile manufacturing (dyeing), leather working, roofing and other activities involving handling of coal tar, the coal tar industry, electrical workers, hairdressers, mechanics, metal workers, cobblers, and rubber workers. Recently, benzidine-derived dyes—Direct Blue 6, Direct Black 38, and Direct Brown 95—have been reported to cause cancers resulting from occupational exposures. NIOSH concluded in 1979 that all benzidine-derived dyes should be recognized as potential human carcinogens, and since then virtually all companies in the United States have stopped their manufacture.

### Pathogenesis

Most occupation-related urinary tract tumors are thought to be caused by contact with carcinogens in the urine. Because of the concentrating ability of the kidney, the bladder is exposed to higher concentrations of these materials than other body tissues. In addition, this exposure occurs over prolonged periods of time in certain areas of the urinary tract, most notably the bladder trigone area. Most of the proved urinary carcinogens are aromatic amines, which may be inhaled, ingested, or absorbed through the skin.

Aromatic amines must be conjugated to sulfates or glucuronic acid in the liver before they can exert their carcinogenic effects. After transport to the kidneys, the conjugated amines are exposed in the urine to the enzyme β-glucuronidase and the optimal pH for its activity, with the result that there is enhanced splitting of the conjugated form and heavy exposure of urinary tract epithelium to hydroxylated carcinogens.

### Pathology

Other less common work-related urologic neoplasms include tumors of the renal pelvis, ureter, and urethra—all with the same histologic and etiologic features as bladder tumors. Thus, all four types are usually considered together as "lower urinary tract cancers" for epidemiologic purposes. Over 90% of urothelial tumors are of the transitional cell type, approximately 6–8% are squamous cell, and 2% are adenocarcinoma. The tumors may be papillary or flat, in situ or invasive, and are graded according to degree of cellular atypia, nuclear abnormalities, and number of mitotic figures.

Multiple genetic changes have been associated with bladder cancer, such as expression of the *ras* and *myc* proto-oncogenes. Mutation of the tumor suppressor gene p53 is correlated with an increased risk of disease progression. Mutation of the retinoblastoma (RB) gene with resulting decreased expression of the RB protein is associated with higher-grade tumors invading muscle.

### Clinical Findings

The most common presenting symptom of bladder cancer is hematuria, which occurs in 80% of patients and is usually painless, gross, and intermittent. More than 20% of patients have vesical irritability alone, with increased frequency, dysuria, urgency, and nocturia. In advanced cases, patients present with symptoms secondary to lymphatic or venous occlusion, such as leg edema.

Urinalysis generally shows red blood cells, and bleeding can be severe enough to cause anemia. Uremia can occur if the bladder tumor has obstructed the ureters as they enter the bladder.

The diagnosis of bladder cancer may be made on the basis of urinary cytologic examination, which has been proposed as a screening tool. Up to 75% of patients with bladder cancer have abnormal urine cytology. Most patients undergo excretory urography, which is useful in ruling out upper tract disease, and may show a filling defect in the bladder. Definitive diagnosis relies on cystoscopy and transurethral biopsy of the suspicious areas.

Bladder carcinoma that has invaded the muscular wall is potentially lethal and may metastasize even before urinary symptoms bring the patient to a physician. Bladder cancer generally spreads by local extension, through lymphatics, or by hematogenous dissemination. Clinical sites of metastatic disease include the pelvic lymph nodes, lungs, bones, and liver (in decreasing order of occurrence). Once the diagnosis has been confirmed by biopsy, a chest x-ray, radionuclide bone scan, and liver and renal function studies should be done. CT scans are extremely useful in staging. Current staging depends on depth of involvement, nodal involvement, and the presence or absence of distant metastases.

## Prevention

Prevention of exposure to known carcinogens is the most effective means of preventing occupational urinary tract cancer. On an immediate basis, personal protective equipment can be used, and ultimately the recommended means of control is by engineering methods aimed at zero exposure levels.

One appealing means of control is screening, and the use of urinary cytologic examinations has been suggested for this purpose in addition to urinalysis to look for microscopic hematuria. Estimates are of 75% sensitivity and 99.9% specificity for the urine cytology test, which would be used to screen only certain occupations at risk.

Immunocytology is under investigation and may improve the sensitivity of urine cytology. Screening of high-risk patients may result in a significant reduction of the stage of disease at diagnosis, with improved long-term survival. In addition, early detection of disease may be an indicator of inadequate primary prevention and could result in the incorporation of better local control measures.

## Treatment

Therapy varies with the stage of cancer, although initial treatment for nonmetastatic disease is surgical. Carcinoma in situ is treated with transurethral resection of the malignant areas, occasionally followed by intravesical immunotherapy or chemotherapy. Superficial disease is managed by transurethral resection and fulguration but is associated with a high incidence of recurrence. This high-risk disease may be treated with intravesical therapy with improved recurrence rates. Bacillus Calmette-Guerin (BCG) is used as immunotherapy, and thiotepa, mitomycin C, and doxorubicin have all been shown to be effective agents when instilled intravesically in the postoperative setting.

Carefully selected patients with bladder carcinoma may undergo partial cystectomy, but invasive disease usually requires radical cystectomy. The current role of preoperative radiation therapy is controversial. Chemotherapy is reserved for metastatic disease, with cisplatin and methotrexate being the most efficacious single agents. Doxorubicin and vinblastine also demonstrate antitumor activity. Combination chemotherapy is more efficacious, but also more toxic than treatment with single agents.

## Prognosis

Prognosis varies with the stage of the disease. Patients with superficial disease who are appropriately treated should have excellent 5-year survival, since disease becomes invasive in only one-third of these patients. The 5-year survival rate in patients with documented muscle invasion ranges from 40% to 50%. With local spread of disease in the pelvis, 10–17% of patients survive 5 years, and there are few long-term survivors once visceral metastases have occurred.

## LIVER CANCER: HEPATIC ANGIOSARCOMA

### Essentials of Diagnosis

- Major exposure to vinyl chloride.
- Right upper quadrant abdominal pain, weight loss.
- Hepatomegaly on physical examination.
- Diagnosis by hepatic arteriogram and open liver biopsy.

### Occupations at Risk

- Vinyl chloride.
  - Polyvinyl chloride production.
- Arsenic.
  - Arsenical pesticide production and use.
  - Copper, lead, zinc smelting.
  - Wine makers (contamination of drinking water).

### General Considerations

Angiosarcoma is a rare tumor with strong epidemiologic links to vinyl chloride and arsenic exposure. Thorotrast (thorium dioxide) exposure was the main nonoccupational risk factor when this agent was used as a radiographic contrast agent from about 1930 to 1955. It occurs most commonly in middle-aged men, with a male-to-female ratio of 4:1. The mean age at presentation is 53. Characteristic features of the disease include a long period of asymptomatic laboratory abnormalities, difficulty in diagnosis, and poor response to treatment.

### Etiology

Vinyl chloride is the raw material with which the common plastic polyvinyl chloride is made, and, as is true of many other industrial products, was initially thought to be harmless. In 1974, a cluster of cases of angiosarcoma of the liver in men were reported by an alert physician in Louisville, Kentucky. The men were all workers at a local industrial plant that polymerized vinyl chloride. By 1981, 10 cases of hepatic angiosarcoma were identified among 1855 employees over 35 years of age, with no other cases of angiosarcoma identified in the Louisville area. In one review of 20 patients with angiosarcoma of the liver after vinyl chloride exposure, the mean time from first exposure to development of tumor was 19 years, with a range of 11–37 years. In addition to the Louisville experience, cancer in other patients from plants elsewhere producing vinyl chloride has been noted. Similar hepatic lesions in experimental animals exposed to high concentrations of vinyl chloride have also been observed.

Although the evidence is not as striking, angiosarcoma of the liver has also been associated with arsenical pesticides, arsenic-contaminated wine, and Fowler's solution used medicinally. Methylhydrazine, urethan, diethylnitrosamine, and dimethylnitrosamine have induced angiosarcoma in laboratory animals, but there is no evidence to date that any of these have caused human angiosarcomas.

**Pathophysiology**

The carcinogenicity of the vinyl chloride monomer is related to the metabolic formation of reactive metabolites. There is an enhanced positive mutagenic response in certain strains of *Salmonella typhimurium* exposed to vinyl chloride monomer metabolized by microsomal enzymes or liver homogenates. Vinyl chloride is deactivated by conjugation with the hepatic nonprotein sulfhydryl compounds glutathione and cystine. It is hoped that further knowledge of the metabolism and pharmacokinetics of the vinyl chloride molecule will provide a scientific basis for guidelines concerning tolerable levels of exposure.

The two distinctive hepatic lesions seen after exposure to vinyl chloride are a peculiar hepatic fibrosis and angiosarcoma. The hepatic fibrosis is characterized by three features: a nonspecific portal fibrosis, capsular and subcapsular fibrosis in a nodular form (the most characteristic lesion), and focal intralobular accumulation of connective tissue fibers. In addition to this pattern of fibrosis apparent in all specimens, a focal irregular sinusoidal dilatation is also seen. A spectrum of changes occurs with increasing degrees of atypia and proliferation of sinusoidal cells, culminating in progressive multicentric, infiltrative angiosarcoma. The neoplasm is hemorrhagic and cystic and replaces most of the normal tissue. Microscopic examination shows that the angiosarcoma is multicentric, with several structural patterns, including sinusoidal, papillary, and cavernous. Hepatic angiosarcomas caused by Thorotrast and inorganic arsenicals have shown many of the histologic features observed in the evolution of the hepatic angiosarcoma in the vinyl chloride workers.

**Clinical Findings**

**A. Symptoms and Signs:** The symptoms of hepatic angiosarcoma are nonspecific, and some patients may be asymptomatic. Abdominal pain is the most common symptom, usually in the right upper quadrant. Fatigue, weakness, and weight loss are

seen in 25–50% of patients. Physical examination reveals hepatomegaly with ascites, jaundice, and splenomegaly, which is seen less often. Other less common physical findings include abdominal mass, tenderness, spider angiomas, and cachexia.

**B. Laboratory Findings:** A mild anemia is commonly present in these patients, and target cells and schistocytes are occasionally seen. Leukocytosis and thrombocytopenia are seen in about half of the patients. Other abnormalities include prolonged prothrombin time, elevated fibrin split products, and hypofibrinogenemia.

Almost all patients have some abnormality of liver function testing. Most common is elevation of serum alkaline phosphatase. Many patients also exhibit elevated serum AST (SGOT), total serum bilirubin, serum LDH, and serum ALT (SGPT), with decreased serum albumin. Tests for alpha-fetoprotein, carcinoembryonic antigen, and hepatitis B antigen are negative.

**C. Imaging:** Routine abdominal x-rays and gastrointestinal contrast studies are usually normal. Occasionally, a mass lesion can be seen pushing aside the stomach; esophageal varices are common. Chest x-rays will often show abnormalities at or near the right hemidiaphragm, including elevation of the diaphragm, a right pleural effusion, atelectasis, or pleural masses. Radionuclide liver scans are abnormal in most patients, but the findings can range from distinct filling defects to nonspecific nonhomogeneous uptake (which can be confused with cirrhosis and splenomegaly). Hepatic arteriograms are the most helpful diagnostic tool, usually demonstrating normal-sized hepatic arteries that may be displaced by tumor, peripheral tumor stain, puddling during the middle of the arterial phase, and a central area of hypovascularity. Hepatic ultrasound may also demonstrate a hepatic mass.

**D. Special Examinations:** Definitive diagnosis of angiosarcoma is best made by thoracoscopic liver biopsy. Closed biopsy can be complicated by hemorrhage from this vascular tumor. Because of the difficulty in making the diagnosis and rapid clinical deterioration, over 50% of hepatic angiosarcomas are diagnosed only after death.

**E. Screening Tests:** Employees at risk of exposure should receive periodic testing consisting of history and physical examination, complete blood count, liver function tests, and liver-spleen scan. Patients with hepatomegaly or splenomegaly should be evaluated with upper gastrointestinal x-rays, hepatic angiography, and liver biopsy. Those with abnormal liver scans or liver function test abnormalities that persist on retesting at three weeks should undergo a full work-up with hepatic angiography and liver biopsy.

These tests are generally accepted in high-risk populations, but of note are serious drawbacks in using biochemical screening with liver function tests.

The principal anatomic lesion in vinyl chloride-associated liver disease is fibrosis with relative sparing of the hepatocyte, so tests of hepatocellular function may be normal. Indocyanine green hepatic uptake is discussed in Chapter 22.

## Prevention

Preventive measures for angiosarcoma include stringent limitations for employee exposure to vinyl chloride. The current United States occupational standard is one ppm averaged over any 8-hour period or 5 ppm averaged over 15 minutes or less. Tighter seals on polymerization vats and protective respirators for workers cleaning the vats are also recommended.

## Treatment

Partial hepatectomy with intent to cure is possible in only a very limited number of patients because of extensive fibrosis in the uninvolved liver. Hepatic radiation has not been evaluated in a controlled trial. Chemotherapy with doxorubicin, cyclophosphamide, and fluorouracil have resulted in some temporary tumor regression. Recent studies have suggested that liver transplantation early in the course of the disease may be curative.

## Course & Progress

Major complications occurring prior to terminal events are common in these patients and include congestive heart failure secondary to arteriovenous shunts, hemolytic anemia, peripheral platelet destruction, hepatic failure, and hemoperitoneum. The major cause of death is irreversible rapidly progressive hepatic failure. Overall survival is usually measured in months, with the median survival approximately 6 months and only a small percentage of patients surviving 2 years.

## SKIN CANCER
## (Nonmelanomatous)

### Essentials of Diagnosis
- Major risk is ultraviolet radiation.
- Skin findings: crusting, ulceration, easy bleeding, changing pigmented lesion.
- Fair complexion at increased risk.

### Occupations at Risk
- Ultraviolet radiation.
  - Outdoor workers.
- PAHs.
  - Coal tar workers (fuel production).
  - Electrode production.
  - Pigment industry workers.
  - Roofers.
  - Shale oil workers, tool setters, etc (mineral oils).
- Arsenic.
  - Arsenical pesticide production and use.
  - Copper, lead, zinc smelting.
  - Sheep dip manufacturers (contamination of drinking water).
- Ionizing radiation.
  - Uranium miners.
  - Health workers.

### General Considerations

Neoplastic diseases of the skin are commonly divided into melanoma and nonmelanomatous skin cancer, which consists mainly of basal cell and squamous cell carcinoma. Nonmelanomatous skin cancer (NMSC) is currently the most common form of cancer in the caucasian population of the United States, accounting for one-third of all diagnosed cases of cancer. Although the dominant risk factor for nonmelanomatous skin cancer (ultraviolet light) has been established, epidemiologic study of skin cancer has been limited. Nonmelanomatous skin cancer has an excellent prognosis, with 96–99% cure rates, making death certificate reviews useless.

There is an incorrect perception that skin cancer other than melanoma is a trivial disease. In addition, patients are rarely hospitalized, with the result that they are commonly not included in cancer registries. Because of failure to register or record skin cancers, much of the data on incidence are from surveys conducted many years ago. It is projected that more than 80,000 Americans will develop NMSC each year. Basal cell cancer is more than three times as common as squamous cell cancer.

### Etiology

The primary causes of skin cancer in industry include ultraviolet radiation (UV), PAHs, arsenic, and ionizing radiation. The information presented below primarily refers to NMSC. An increased risk of melanoma has been associated with UV light exposure. Limited evidence exists linking melanomatous skin cancer to exposures to chemicals such as PAHs.

**A. UV Radiation:** Clearly, the major risk factor for skin cancer in lightly pigmented persons is radiation from the sun. The experiment of nature in which different intensities of UV radiation occur at different global latitudes has provided the opportunity for many epidemiologic studies to show an increased incidence of nonmelanomatous skin cancer in Caucasians at latitudes closer to the equator. The earliest realization that excess sun exposure leads to skin cancer was made on the basis of occupation in 1890, when Unna described changes of the skin of sailors, including skin cancer that resulted from prolonged exposure to the weather.

There are approximately 4.8 million outdoor workers in the United States, with certain occupations at greater risk, such as those in agriculture and professional sports. Another estimated 300,000 workers are exposed to industrial radiation sources (eg, welding arcs, germicides, and printing processors). The carcinogenic hazard of industrial radiation, which includes wavelengths shorter than that of the sun, is not yet understood. In experimental animals, the most carcinogenic wavelength is in the 290–300 nm range (sunlight does not include wavelengths less than 290 nm); 254 nm is less carcinogenic, but wavelengths as low as 230 nm will still produce skin cancers.

The actual carcinogenic spectrum for humans is unknown. It is also notable that in experimental animals, a variety of foreign substances, including phototoxic chemicals (eg, coal tar), chemical carcinogens (eg, benzo[a]pyrene), and nonspecific irritants (eg, xylene) under suitable conditions augment UV carcinogenesis.

**B. PAHs:** Although chemical carcinogenesis of the skin does not seem to be nearly as frequent a cause of NMSC as UV radiation, it was described over a century earlier. Percival Pott described the increased incidence of scrotal cancer in chimney sweeps in 1775, but it was not until the 1940s that a polycyclic aromatic hydrocarbon, benzo(a)pyrene, was shown to be a constituent of soot. These hydrocarbons have the ability to induce skin cancers in laboratory animals, and mixtures of them are found in coal tar, pitch, asphalt, soot, creosotes, anthracenes, paraffin waxes, and lubricating and cutting oils. Exposures to mineral oil have been linked to skin and scrotal cancers among shale oil workers, jute processors, tool setters, mule spinners, wax pressmen, metal workers exposed to poorly refined cutting oils, and machine operators using lubricating oils. Latent periods between exposure to polycyclic aromatic hydrocarbons and skin cancer vary from about 20 years (coal tar) to 50 years or more (mineral oil).

**C. Arsenic:** Arsenic has been shown to cause cancer in experimental animals and is a well-recognized human carcinogen. Skin tumors associated with arsenic occur following ingestion, injection, or inhalation, as well as from skin contact. Medicinal inorganic arsenicals and arsenic in drinking water are the sources most commonly implicated. Recent detailed studies in Taiwan established that use of well water with high arsenic concentrations resulted in skin cancer, with a dose-response relationship. An estimated 1.5 million workers in the United States are exposed to inorganic arsenic in such diverse trades as copper and lead smelting, the metallurgical industry, sheep dip manufacturing, and the production and use of pesticides; however, skin tumors attributed to occupational arsenic exposure are very uncommon. It is thought that some of the cases cited in the literature of agricultural workers with arsenic-induced skin cancers may be the result of other carcinogenic influences, such as sunlight and tars. The simultaneous presence of arsenical hyperkeratoses or hyperpigmentation, which occurs at lower exposure levels, strongly implicates arsenic as the etiologic agent in an individual with NMSC. In addition, cancers tend to be multiple and occur in younger patients than those attributable to UV light.

**D. Ionizing Radiation:** Ionizing radiation is as carcinogenic for skin as it is for many other tissues. Roentgen radiation-induced skin carcinoma was first reported in 1902, shortly after the discovery of x-rays, in those who worked the machines. There was a definite excess in skin cancer deaths among radiologists in the period from 1920 to 1939, and an excess risk has also been found for uranium miners. Patients receiving radiation for acne, tinea capitis, and facial hair in the past had an increased risk of invasive skin cancers. The latent period for radiation-induced skin cancers varies inversely with the dose, with the overall range from 7 weeks to 56 years (average, 25–30 years), and the skin cancers often occur in areas with chronic radiation dermatitis. Although epidemiologic studies do not give reliable data on dose-response relationships, the risk from exposures under 1000 cGy appears to be small, and skin cancer may be induced by dose-equivalents of 3000 cGy. There are now strict controls on industrial and occupational exposure to ionizing radiation, and currently it appears that ionizing radiation is not responsible for much cutaneous carcinogenesis.

**E. Other Factors:** Other risk factors for the development of NMSC include chewing tobacco or betel nuts, where squamous cell cancer of the lip and oral cavity have been described. Chronic irritation or inflammation is thought to induce these cancers. Patients with either primary or secondary (long-term immunosuppressive therapy) immunodeficiencies are at increased risk for skin cancer. Several genetically inherited syndromes such as xeroderma pigmentosum and albinism are associated with increase susceptibility to skin cancers.

## Pathophysiology

Work by Rous in 1941 and Berenblum in 1964 elucidated the two-stage theory of carcinogenesis. Berenblum found that a single application of a potent carcinogen such as benzo(a)pyrene applied in a quantity insufficient to cause tumors allowed tumor development after subsequent application of croton oil, which by itself produced no tumors at all. He theorized that the production of a tumor was initiated by the carcinogen, but that its subsequent development could be promoted nonspecifically. It appears that initiation is permanent and irreversible, but promotion, up to a point, is reversible.

UV light fits into this theory of chemical carcinogenesis in that it appears to be both an initiator and a promoter for carcinoma of the skin. Two major effects of UV radiation on the skin that seem likely to be responsible for the carcinogenic effects are photochemical alteration of the DNA and alterations in immunity. Certain immunologic defects, both in skin and in lymphocytes, can be induced by UV radiation. Exposure to UV light depletes the dermis of Langerhans cells and renders it unable to be sensitized to potent allergens. Alterations at the level of DNA are also thought to be responsible for ionizing radiation-induced skin cancers.

## Pathology

The histologic types of skin lesions associated with sun exposure include solar keratoses, basal cell epitheliomas, squamous cell carcinomas, keratoacanthomas, and malignant melanomas. Solar keratoses contain morphologically cancerous cells, but they are considered premalignant, since invasion is limited to the most superficial part of the dermis. About 13% of all solar keratoses develop into squamous cell carcinomas, but these are rarely aggressive. The estimated incidence of metastases from all sun-induced squamous cell carcinomas is 0.5% or less. Almost all squamous cell carcinomas in Caucasians occur in highly sun-exposed areas, but 40% of basal cell epitheliomas occur on shaded areas of the head and neck.

Regardless of the source of exposure, certain features are common in all cases of arsenic-induced skin cancers. Punctate keratoses of the palms and soles and hyperpigmentation are frequently seen. The skin tumors are of several types. Squamous carcinomas arise either from normal skin or from keratoses. Basal cell epitheliomas, including multiple superficial squamous cell and basal cell epitheliomas, as well as areas of intraepidermal carcinoma (Bowen's disease), have been described. Multiple tumors are the rule, most of which are found on unexposed areas. Cancer of the scrotum, which is seen following topical exposure to PAHs, is rare.

Early radiation workers with heavy exposure from uncalibrated machines developed predominantly squamous cell carcinomas, found mainly on the hands and feet and occasionally on the face. More recently, basal cell cancers have been described following repeated occupational exposures.

Radiation-related tumors usually arise in areas of chronic radiation dermatitis, and whether they can occur on clinically normal skin is a matter of dispute. Radiation-induced malignant melanoma and sweat gland tumors have rarely been described.

## Clinical Findings

Basal cell epithelioma frequently presents as a nodular or nodular-ulcerative lesion on the skin of the head and neck, and only 10% of the time on the skin of the trunk. It is much less common on the upper extremities and very uncommon on the lower extremities. The lesion is generally smooth, shiny, and translucent, with telangiectatic vessels just beneath the surface. It is usually not painful or tender, even with ulceration, except when crusting or bleeding is seen with minor trauma. Basal cell carcinomas rarely metastasize, but can invade widely and deeply, extending through the subcutaneous tissue to involve

neurovascular structures and occasionally erode into bone.

Squamous cell carcinoma presents first in a premalignant stage characterized by actinic keratosis, a rough, reddened plaque on sun-exposed skin. There is then an in situ stage, which appears as a well-demarcated, slightly raised erythematous plaque with more substance and scaling than actinic keratosis. Squamous cell cancers arising in sun-exposed areas of the body tend to be on the most highly irradiated areas, such as the tip of the nose, the forehead, the tips of the helices of the ears, the lower lip, or the backs of the hands. Metastases are more common than from basal cell cancer, and squamous cell cancers on mucosal membranes metastasize more frequently than do those found on the skin surface.

## Prevention

The most important step in prevention of occupation-related skin cancers is avoidance of ultraviolet light. This is especially true for workers who are more susceptible to UV light, such as those with fair complexions or with certain hereditary diseases (eg, albinism and xeroderma pigmentosum).

Protective clothing, such as wide brimmed hats and long sleeves, is the most effective barrier to UV radiation exposure in outdoor workers. Sunscreens that provide protection in the UVA and UVB spectrum should be used daily. The effectiveness of sunscreens in preventing carcinoma is unknown, though their effectiveness for avoidance of erythema has been proved. Periodic examinations are recommended to detect the presence of malignant and premalignant skin lesions.

The incidence of scrotal cancer is now rare because of preventive measures. If possible, a noncarcinogenic material should be substituted for a carcinogenic one. The efficacy of this approach was clearly demonstrated in Britain in 1953 when noncarcinogenic oil use became obligatory in the mule-spinning industry, with a steady fall in the number of reported cases of scrotal carcinoma. Good personal hygiene should include compulsory showering and changing of clothes when entering and leaving the plant, as well as washing of exposed skin after leaving contaminated areas. Isolated or closed-system operations, protective clothing, and employee education are also critical in avoidance of skin cancer induced by polycyclic aromatic hydrocarbons.

Currently, the maximum allowable dose equivalent of ionizing radiation for occupational exposure to the skin is 30 rems in any year, except that forearms and hands are allowed 75 rems in any year (because there is little red marrow in the forearms and hands). These recommendations are mainly based on avoidance of hematologic disease and may need to be revised in order to prevent skin cancer. Exposure can be further limited by the use of shielding devices such as lead gloves and aprons.

## Treatment

Biopsy is necessary in all cases of suspected skin carcinoma. For small skin cancers not located in areas where primary closure would be difficult, excisional biopsy should be done. If an incisional biopsy is done, it is imperative that an adequate amount of tissue be obtained from the involved area.

Actinic keratoses may be excised or removed superficially with a scalpel, followed by cautery or fulguration. One to 5 percent fluorouracil may be used topically, followed by excision of persistent lesions.

Squamous cell carcinoma should be treated with excision, but radiation is an alternative. Mohs' technique of micrographic surgery to remove skin carcinomas results in the highest cure rate. Basal cell carcinoma is treated with excision, curettage, and electrodesiccation, by irradiation, or with Mohs' technique. Cryosurgery may be used, but is associated with a large number of recurrences.

## HEMATOLOGIC CANCERS

### Essentials of Diagnosis

- Radiation, benzene exposure.
- Presenting complaints of weakness, malaise, anorexia, fever, and easy bruisability.
- Pallor, hepatosplenomegaly, lymph node enlargement on physical examination.
- Leukocytosis or leukopenia, with immature white cells in peripheral blood and bone marrow.
- Anemia, thrombocytopenia.

### Occupations at Risk

- Radiation.
  - Health workers.
  - Military personnel.
  - Nuclear power plant workers.
- Benzene.
  - Petrochemical and refinery workers.
  - Rubber workers.

### General Considerations

The two major forms of leukemia that have been linked to occupation are acute nonlymphocytic leukemia (ANLL), including myelodysplasia or preleukemia, and chronic myelogenous leukemia (CML). Multiple myeloma is covered in Chapter 15. The acute leukemias are malignant diseases of the blood-forming organs characterized by a proliferation of immature blood cell progenitors in the bone marrow and other tissues. Together with replacement of the normal marrow with leukemic cells, there is a diminished production of normal erythrocytes, granulocytes, and platelets. Acute leukemias are classified morphologically by reference to the predominant cell line involved as lymphocytic and nonlymphocytic forms. Non lymphocytic leukemias are further classified as de novo (no underlying cause known and without preexisting myelodysplasia) or secondary (known cause such as chemical exposure or preexisting myelodysplasia or chronic leukemia). The acute leukemias, taken collectively, are relatively common diseases, with a projected incidence in the United States of 28,000 new cases in 1996. The annual incidence of ANLL is constant from birth throughout the first 10 years at about 10 cases per million. The incidence peaks in late adolescence, remains at 15 per million to age 55, and then rises to 50 per million at age 75. Eighty percent of all adult acute leukemias are of the nonlymphocytic variety, and unlike acute lymphoblastic leukemia, ANLL has been reported as a complication of chemical exposures and irradiation.

Chronic leukemias are classified as lymphocytic and myelogenous; only chronic myelogenous leukemia has been reported as an industrial disease. Chronic myelogenous leukemia is a neoplastic disease resulting from the development of an abnormal hematopoietic stem cell. There is excessive growth of the blood cell progenitors in the marrow, which initially function as normal hematopoietic cells. The leukemic cells gradually undergo further malignant transformation, with loss of ability to differentiate in the later stages of the disease, with the resulting development of acute leukemia and death. In the early stages of the disease, large numbers of mature and immature granulocytic cells accumulate in the blood, and extramedullary hematopoiesis produces gross enlargement of the liver and spleen. Chronic myelogenous leukemia accounts for about 20% of all deaths from leukemia in the western world, with an incidence that, unlike other forms of leukemia, has not recently been increasing. Although rare cases are reported in infants, most patients with CML are aged 25–60 years, with a median age of about 45.

### Etiology

The cause of human leukemia is unknown. As in the case of most other cancers, it is probable that no single factor is responsible. Most cases are thought to result from the interaction of host susceptibility factors, chemical or physical injury to chromosomes, and, in animals and presumably in humans, incorporation of genetic information of viral origin into susceptible stem cells.

**A. Radiation:** Radiation remains the most conclusively identified leukemogenic factor in human beings. The earliest evidence began to accumulate soon after the discovery of x-rays, which were used mainly in the medical workplace; thus, radiologists, radiation therapists, and radiation technicians were all at risk. Several studies showed an excess risk of leukemia among radiologists (approximately nine times that of other physicians) during the years 1930–1950, with a latency period of about 18 years. With the institution of dose limits, careful monitoring, and adequate shielding since that time, this excess risk has decreased significantly and should be eliminated.

The data from Hiroshima and Nagasaki atomic bomb survivors leave little doubt that the incidence of leukemia is increased following exposure to mixed gamma and neutron radiation and that the response is dose-dependent. The risk of leukemia is increased in populations exposed to ionizing radiation at doses as low as 50–100 cGy. Between 100 cGy and 500 cGy, there is a linear correlation between dose and leukemia incidence. The data suggest that the risk of leukemia is increased at a rate of 1–2 cases per million population per year per centigray. Maximal risk occurs approximately 4–7 years after exposure, and an increased risk has been seen in Japanese people as long as 14 years after exposure.

Whole-body exposure to radiation in single doses results in suppression of marrow growth, and a single whole-body dose of over 400 cGy is usually fatal in humans. In sublethal exposure, cytopenias may occur, which gradually recover but indicate significant damage to the marrow precursor elements. Patients are then at risk to develop leukemia with a delay between exposure and disease of 8–18 years. Following radiation exposure, both acute and chronic myelogenous leukemia may occur. In the atomic bomb survivors, chronic lymphocytic leukemia has not been seen. The specific rates per 100,000 for people within 1500 meters of the hypocenter are 8.1 for acute nonlymphocytic leukemia, 25.6 for chronic myelogenous leukemia, and 21.7 for acute lymphocytic leukemia.

Workers at risk secondary to exposure to ionizing radiation include military personnel in the vicinity of nuclear tests, uranium miners, and workers in nuclear power plants. Approximately 250,000 troops are estimated to have been present at multiple detonations of nuclear devices carried out by the United States from 1945 to 1976. In 1976, over 3000 men exposed at the 1957 nuclear test explosion "Smoky" were studied, and a significant excess of leukemia was discovered. A review of death certificates of former workers at the Portsmouth Naval Shipyard in Portsmouth, New Hampshire (where nuclear submarines are repaired and refueled), revealed an observed-to-expected ratio of leukemia deaths of 5.62 among former nuclear workers.

**B. Benzene:** Certain chemicals (eg, chemotherapeutic agents) are known to be toxic to marrow cells, and many of these also possess leukemogenic potential. Occupational evidence of leukemogenicity is strongest for benzene, where recent epidemiologic studies have shown significant increases in leukemia in workers with past exposure to benzene. Benzene has been known for almost a century to be a powerful bone marrow poison, leading to aplastic or hypoplastic anemia. It is now widely believed that any chemical capable of inducing bone marrow damage must be assumed to be a potential leukemogen. Over

the past few decades, evidence has been accumulating that benzene produces not only aplastic anemia but also leukemia, and that the fatal cases of leukemia outnumber those of true aplastic anemia. In 1928, Delore and Borgomano described the first case of acute leukemia in a worker from a plant with such heavy exposure to benzene that none the employees could work for more than two months without becoming ill. In 1932, Lignac produced several cases of leukemia in white rats given benzene in olive oil, but many subsequent animal studies were inconclusive. Only in the last few years have investigators shown that benzene can systematically induce cancers in rats.

Benzene is a cyclic hydrocarbon obtained in distillation of petroleum and coal tar. It is used widely in chemical synthesis in many industries, in the manufacture of explosives, and in the production of cosmetics, soaps, perfumes, drugs, and dyes. Benzene was once used in the dry cleaning industry, but that is no longer the case. In addition, nearly 2% of unleaded gasoline is benzene.

An estimated 2 million workers in the United States have exposure to benzene. One of the most recent studies in workers exposed to benzene in the manufacture of rubber showed a nearly 6-fold greater incidence of death from leukemia than would be expected. Workers exposed for 5 years or more had a 21-fold increased risk of death from leukemia. Many other studies, including several undertaken in the shoe manufacturing industry, have shown an increase in the risk of leukemia in workers with exposure to benzene. Although many studies have suggested a link between benzene exposure and an increased risk of CML, no definitive data exist.

**C. Other Chemicals:** Chemicals other than benzene are suspected of causing leukemia, but the epidemiologic data in this area are incomplete. Ethylene oxide exposure has been associated with an increased risk of leukemia. This chemical is used as a sterilant and in chemical processing. An increase in leukemia in chemists in Norway has been described, and an increase in marrow chromosome breakage has been noted in patients with leukemia who have histories suggesting occupational exposure to carcinogens. Indirect evidence of leukemogenicity of organic hydrocarbons comes from a study that showed an increased incidence of leukemia in Nebraska farmers, thought to be secondary to exposure to chemicals used on the farm. The data linking exposure to electromagnetic fields with an increased risk of leukemia remain unclear. Treatment with a variety of chemotherapeutic agents has been associated with an increased risk of leukemia within 2–5 years of initiation of chemotherapy. This can occur after very short-term exposure. There is a known synergistic interaction of radiation therapy and treatment with alkylating chemotherapeutic drugs for underlying malignancies such as Hodgkin's disease, resulting in a significant increase in the risk of subsequent leukemia.

## Pathophysiology

**A. Ionizing Radiation:** The effects of radiation on human tissue depend on multiple factors, such as type of radiation, dose of radiation, length of exposure, body part exposed, and oxygen content of the exposed tissue. Damage secondary to radiation is greatest in rapidly dividing cells such as bone marrow stem cells, epithelial cells, and gamete-forming cells. The mechanism of radiation-induced injury at the cellular level involves direct and indirect damage to nucleic acids and proteins. DNA is a radiosensitive target, with even minor molecular damage resulting in profound effects on the cell and the organism. Radiation-induced molecular damage may be so severe that the cell no longer functions, and cell death results. Cells exposed to radiation may survive with no effects (if only a small number of nonessential molecules are affected) or may survive with altered structure and function. If the alteration is within the DNA, clinical disease may not appear until after a latency period. Cancer induction appears to depend upon an interaction of defective cellular repair and damage to the cell's regulator genes.

**B. Benzene:** Benzene toxicity may present as an acute illness or as a chronic disease developing up to 30 years after exposure. Chronic or recurrent exposure to concentrations of benzene exceeding 100 ppm (320 mg/m$^3$) leads to a very high incidence of cytopenias. When the exposure ends, there is usually spontaneous remission. Among workers who have been exposed to atmospheric concentrations of benzene in excess of 300 ppm for at least one year, as many as 20% will acquire pancytopenia or aplastic anemia. The chronic form of illness is related to the effect of benzene on the bone marrow, where benzene appears to exert a colchicine-like effect, blocking mitosis of the marrow proliferative cells. This then results in mutagenic effects that play a role in the subsequent development of leukemia. Aplastic anemia generally occurs in subjects while they are still exposed to high concentrations of benzene; leukemia may occur at the same time or shortly after cessation of exposure. Leukemia often develops in subjects with benzene-induced hyporegenerative anemia or long-standing pancytopenia and represents the acute terminal stage of the disease. Approximately one patient in 60 with benzene-induced pancytopenia or aplastic anemia and one patient in 10 with unremitting, progressive marrow failure who survive beyond one year will develop acute nonlymphocytic leukemia.

## Clinical Findings

**A. Symptoms and Signs:**

**1. Radiation–**As noted above, 300–400 cGy of whole body radiation is lethal in humans. Sublethal exposures will cause symptoms of nausea and vomiting, after which bone marrow suppression occurs. Thrombocytopenia, anemia, and neutropenia will develop, with their attendant symptoms. The development of leukemia occurs after a delay of 8–18 years after the onset of exposure. Most patients with early stage CML are asymptomatic. Occasionally, patients will present with fatigue, fevers, anorexia due to massive splenomegaly, or retinal hemorrhages. When the disease progresses, symptoms are identical to acute leukemia. Physical examination reveals splenomegaly in the majority of cases. The symptoms of acute leukemia, which may also develop after radiation exposure, are described below.

**2. Benzene–**Acute exposure to benzene may result in headache, dizziness, and vertigo. Chronically, there is inhibition of marrow cell proliferation, and symptoms appear as pancytopenia develops. A decrease in hematocrit results in pallor, shortness of breath, and weakness. Thrombocytopenia leads to the appearance of petechiae and purpura. Infections and painful mouth sores can occur secondary to a decrease in the number of neutrophils. Leukemia may present with general complaints such as fever, weakness, malaise, anorexia, bone pain, and easy bruisability. Physical findings such as hepatosplenomegaly, enlarged lymph nodes, swollen gums, skin nodules, and ecchymoses are seen. Occasionally, gum bleeding after dental procedures or major ecchymoses after minor trauma may be the major presenting complaint.

**B. Laboratory Findings:** Most cases of CML present with the well-recognized hematologic characteristics of peripheral myeloid leukocytosis, thrombocytosis, anemia, and basophilia. Granulocytic leukocytosis is the fundamental abnormality, averaging 200,000/μL, with a range of 15,000–600,000/μL at diagnosis. The bone marrow is hypercellular, with granulocytic hyperplasia and, often, increased numbers of megakaryocytes. The presence of the Philadelphia chromosome [t(9;22)] on chromosomal analysis or the bcr/abl translocation on polymerase chain reaction is diagnostic.

Patients with benzene toxicity usually present with pancytopenia, but any combination of anemia, thrombocytopenia, or leukopenia may occur. The anemia is usually normochromic and normocytic, with normal red cell morphology. The reticulocyte count is inappropriately low and parameters of hemolysis such as bilirubin and LDH will be normal. White cell morphology is also initially normal, with a decrease in neutrophils and an increase in the percentage of lymphocytes.

Evaluation of the blood counts in acute leukemia usually reveals a marked decrease in at least two cell lines. Leukocytosis with circulating blasts found on evaluation of the peripheral blood smear is common, but leukopenia may also been seen. Circulating blast cells may contain Auer rods or peroxidase stain-positive granules. The bone marrow may be hyper- or hypocellular, with more than 30% leukemic blast forms. Secondary leukemias may develop slowly, beginning as myelodysplasia, with a gradually increasing blast count in the bone marrow and markedly abnormal growth of the myeloid, erythroid, and platelet precursor cells. Secondary leukemias are often associated with chromosomal abnormalities such as loss of all or part of chromosome 5 or 7, which is unusual in de novo disease.

## Prevention

**A. Radiation:** X-rays were discovered by Roentgen in 1895, and by 1902 the basic principles of radiation protection had already been elaborated: to minimize dose by reducing the time of exposure and by using shielding and distance. Since 1928, the International Council on Radiation Protection (ICRP) and the National Council on Radiation Protection have defined acceptable levels of radiation exposure for workers. The concept of dose equivalent or "rem" (Roentgen equivalent man) is used because the same amounts of absorbed radiation energy can produce different levels of damage, depending on the type of radiation present. Acceptable exposures for different organs vary, with a maximum permissible dose ranging from 5 rems of whole body exposure to 30 rems of skin or bone exposure.

**B. Benzene:** Regulated standards of benzene began in 1926, and in 1974, NIOSH published a recommended standard based on the evidence for hematologic changes: 10 ppm as an 8-hour time-weighted average (TWA), with a ceiling limit of 25 ppm. In 1977, OSHA issued an emergency standard decreasing the acceptable 8-hour TWA exposure to one ppm after a study showing excess deaths due to leukemia in benzene-exposed workers, but these recommendations as a permanent standard have not been upheld. This remains an area of controversy, in that with current allowable levels the lifetime incidence of excess leukemia for exposed workers is estimated to be from 1.4% to 15.2%. Periodic hematologic screening is believed to be mandatory in populations exposed to increased atmospheric levels of benzene, with both removal from the work environment and further hematologic testing indicated for any aberrations found.

## Treatment & Prognosis

With excess exposure or signs of toxicity in workers exposed to either radiation or benzene, removal from the offending environment is the first priority. Benzene-induced aplastic anemia is treated like any pancytopenia (ie, with supportive care in the form of transfusions, infection precautions, etc). The outcome is similar to that of other aplastic anemias, with a 5-year survival rate of 30%. One-half of deaths occur in the first six months. Bone marrow transplantation is the only known cure for severe aplastic anemia. Immunosuppressive therapy is not effective for toxin-induced aplasia.

There have been recent major advances in the treatment of acute leukemias with the use of combination chemotherapy and bone marrow transplantation. ANLL is most successfully treated with an induction protocol consisting of daunorubicin and cytarabine, resulting in a 60% complete response in adults. This is followed by repeated courses of consolidation chemotherapy or bone marrow transplantation. For de novo ANLL, a 45–60% long-term disease-free survival is seen following aggressive therapy. Unfortunately, secondary ANLL has a poor prognosis, with median survivals of 1–2 years and no cures obtained from chemotherapy alone. Bone marrow transplantation is the only curative option and is limited by patient age and donor availability. The median survival for CML is 3–5 years from the date of diagnosis. Treatment is initially aimed at controlling leukocytosis and thrombocytosis and results in improved symptoms. Hydroxyurea is the agent of choice. Aggressive treatment with alpha interferon early in the course of disease has been shown to result in cytogenetic remissions (loss of the Philadelphia chromosome) and improved long-term survival. Bone marrow transplantation is the only known cure for CML and, like ANLL, is limited by patient age and donor availability. The transformation of CML to acute leukemia (blast phase CML) is associated with survivals of six months or less.

## OTHER CANCERS

Many other cancers have been reported to be associated with specific occupational or environmental exposures. However, the majority of these associations are casual and are not supported with sufficient epidemiologic or animal data. An increased incidence of renal cell cancer has been reported in some workers. PAHs and other organic solvents, asbestos, cadmium, and lead salts have all been investigated as possible etiologic agents. Cancers of the gastrointestinal tract may be increased in workers exposed to asbestos (gastric, colon) and coal dust (gastric). Cancer of the thyroid has been definitely associated with exposure to ionizing radiation, as has cancer of the salivary glands. Outdoor workers have an increased risk of cancer of the lip resulting from exposure to ultraviolet radiation. The association of exposure to electromagnetic fields with brain and other neoplasms remains unclear.

# REFERENCES

## GENERAL

Bang KM: Epidemiology of occupational cancer. Occup Med 1996;11(3):467.

DeVita VT, Hellman S, Rosenberg S (editors): *Cancer: Principles and Practice of Oncology,* 4th ed. Lippincott, 1993.

Huuskonen MS: Screening for occupational cancer. Scand J Work Environ Health 1992;18(Suppl 1):110.

Rom WN (editor): *Environmental and Occupational Medicine,* 3rd ed. Lippincott–Raven, 1997.

Rosenstock L, Cullen MR (editors): *Textbook of Clinical Occupational and Environmental Medicine.* Saunders, 1994.

Ruder AM: Epidemiology of occupational carcinogens and mutagens. Occup Med 1996;11(3):487.

Stellman JM, Stellman SD: Cancer and the workplace. CA Cancer J Clin 1996;46:70.

Zenz C, Dickerson OB, Horvath EP (editors): *Occupational Medicine,* 3rd ed. Mosby, 1994.

## RESPIRATORY CANCERS

Coultas DB, Samet JM: Occupational lung cancer. Clin Chest Med 1992;13:341.

Dement DM, Brown DP: Lung cancer mortality among asbestos textile workers: A review and update. Ann Occup Hygiene 1994;38:525.

Demers PA et al: Wood dust and sino-nasal cancer: Pooled reanalysis of twelve case-control studies. Am J Ind Med 1995;28:151.

Hyers TM, Ohar JM, Crim C: Clinical controversies in asbestos-induced lung diseases. Semin Diagn Pathol 1992;9:97.

Fusco V et al: Malignant pleural mesothelioma. Multivariate analysis of prognostic factors on 113 patients. Anticancer Res 1993;13:683.

Langard S: Prevention of lung cancer through the use of knowledge on asbestos and other work-related causes—Norwegian experiences. Scand J Work Environ Health 1994;20:100

Maier H et al: Risk factors of cancer of the larynx: Results of the Heidelberg case-control study. Otolaryngol Head Neck Surg 1992;107:577

Morgan LG, Usher V: Health problems associated with nickel refining and use. Ann Occup Hygiene 1994; 38:189.

Nylander LA, Dement JM: Carcinogenic effects of wood dust: Review and discussion. Am J Ind Med 1993; 24:619.

Peterson GM: Epidemiology, screening, and prevention of lung cancer. Curr Opin Oncol 1994;6:156.

Siegel M: Involuntary smoking in the restaurant workplace. A review of employee exposure and health effects. JAMA 1993;270:490.

Spirtas R et al: Malignant mesothelioma: Attributable risk of asbestos exposure. Occup Environ Med 1994; 51:804.

Stayner LT, Dankovic DA, Lemen RA: Occupational exposure to asbestos and cancer risk: A review of the amphibole hypothesis. Amer J Public Health 1996; 86(2):179.

Vogelzang NJ: Malignant mesothelioma: Diagnostic and management strategies for 1992. Semin Oncol 1992;19:64.

## BLADDER CANCER

Choi BC, Connolly JG, Zhou RH: Application of urinary mutagen testing to detect workplace hazardous exposure and bladder cancer. Mut Res 1995;341:207.

Lamm DL, Torti FM: Bladder cancer 1996. CA Cancer J Clin 1996;46:93.

Risch A et al: Slow N-acetylation genotype is a susceptibility factor in occupational and smoking related bladder cancer. Hum Mol Gen 1995;4:231.

Schulte P et al: Bladder cancer screening in high risk groups. J Occup Med 1990;32:787-945.

Siemiatycki J et al: Occupational risk factors for bladder cancer: Results from a case-control study in Montreal, Quebec, Canada. Am J Epidemiol 1994;140: 1061.

Zhang ZF et al: Tobacco smoking, occupation, and p53 nuclear overexpression in early stage bladder cancer. Cancer Epidemiol, Biomarkers Prevent 1994;3:19.

## LIVER CANCER: HEPATIC ANGIOSARCOMA

Laplanche A et al: Exposure to vinyl chloride monomer: Results of a cohort study after a seven year follow-up. The French VCM group. Br J Ind Med 1992;49: 134.

Moreno-Gonzalez E et al: Orthotopic liver transplantation for primary liver tumors. J Surg Oncol 1993; 3(Suppl):74.

Neshiwat LF et al: Hepatic angiosarcoma. Am J Med 1992;93:219.

## SKIN CANCER

Adams RM (editor): *Occupational Skin Disease.* 3rd ed. Saunders, 1988.

Kricker A, Armstrong BK, English DR: Sun exposure and non-melanotic skin cancer. Cancer Causes Contr 1994;5:367.

Pion IA et al: Occupation and the risk of malignant melanoma. Cancer 1995;75:637.

Streetly A, Markowe H: Changing trends in the epidemiology of malignant melanoma: Gender differences and their implications for public health. Int J Epidemiol 1995;24:897.

## HEMATOLOGIC CANCERS

Ciccone G et al: Myeloid leukemias and myelodysplastic syndromes: Chemical exposure, histologic subtypes and cytogenetics in a case-control study. Cancer Genet Cytogenet 1993;68:135.

Levine EG, Bloomfield CD: Leukemias and myelodysplastic syndromes secondary to drug, radiation, and environmental exposure. Semin Oncol 1992;19:47.

Paustenbach DJ, Bass RD, Price P: Benzene toxicity and risk assessment, 1972–1992: Implications for future regulation. Environ Health Perspect 1993;101(Suppl 6):177.

Preston DL et al: Cancer incidence in atomic bomb survivors. Part III. Leukemia, lymphoma and multiple
myeloma, 1950–1987. Rad Res 1994;139:129.

Richardson S et al: Occupational risk factors for acute
leukaemia: A case-control study. Int J Epidemiol
1992;21:1063.

Snyder R, Kalf GF: A perspective on benzene leukemo-
genesis. Crit Rev Toxicol 1994;24:177.

Taylor JA et al: *ras* oncogene activation and occupational exposures in acute myeloid leukemia. J Natl
Cancer Inst 1992;84:1626.

Wong O: Risk of acute myeloid leukemia and multiple
myeloma in worker exposed to benzene. Occup Environ Med 1995;52:380.

# 18

# Occupational Skin Disorders

*Robert M. Adams, MD*

Although human skin has the ability to withstand many of the assaults of a frequently hostile environment, the skin is the most commonly injured organ in industry today. Skin disorders comprise more than 35% of all occupationally related diseases, affecting annually approximately one worker per thousand in the private sector. Numerous cases are never reported, however, and the hardship and financial loss to workers and employers alike is very substantial. Most occupational skin disease results from contact with a chemical substance, of which there are more than 90,000 in the environment today. Under certain conditions, all of them can irritate the skin, and about 2000 or so are now recognized as contact allergens. In addition, workers bring to their work pre-existing diseases, as well as physical, mental, and hereditary traits, almost any of which can be aggravated to one degree or another by work.

## CONTACT DERMATITIS

### Irritant Contact Dermatitis

Irritant contact dermatitis is a polymorphous process with a complex pathophysiology, a varied natural history, and divergent clinical appearance. This contrasts with allergic contact dermatitis, in which a specific chemical is the central cause. Many factors come into play to induce irritant reactions, acting singly or in concert. These include the intrinsic nature of the substance, the environment, and the individual (Table 18–1). Irritant dermatitis is also the most common form of occupational skin disease, and in the US accounts for nearly 80% of all occupational dermatitis. Statistics from other countries, where patch testing is more routinely performed, report irritant dermatitis at rates of approximately 50%. The real incidence is probably somewhere in between.

Irritant dermatitis has been conveniently divided into two types: immediate and delayed. **Immediate irritant dermatitis** results from a single contact with a strong chemical substance, causing an acute, toxic reaction similar to a burn. Erythema, blistering, and ulceration occur at the site almost immediately after contact. Also termed **absolute** irritants, these substances are intrinsically damaging to the skin, are often corrosive, and rapidly injure any person's skin almost immediately. Examples are strong alkalis, acids, certain metallic substances and their salts, and many organic compounds. The chief determinants are the intrinsic nature of the chemical, the concentration of the chemical, and the duration of contact. Almost every person will respond with a similar reaction to contact with these substances, given identical exposure conditions.

The majority of chemicals, however, damage the skin only after multiple contacts, often repeated or prolonged, which results in **delayed irritant dermatitis**. Erythema, increasing dryness and thickening, patchy hyperkeratosis with itching, and painful fissuring are characteristic signs. There is great individual variation in this response, even under identical exposure conditions. Atopics, for example, are most likely to develop dermatitis after only brief and sometimes minimal exposure. Soaps, detergents, mild acids and alkalis, etc, are the most common causes. Friction, occlusion, minor lacerations, excessive environmental heat or cold, and low relative humidity are among the important contributing factors. Because there are similarities in appearance, delayed onset irritant dermatitis is often confused with allergic contact dermatitis.

From contact with certain oils, greases, tars, etc, a **pustular** and **acneiform irritant dermatitis** may result (Table 18–2). Repeated rubbing and friction in many individuals produces a thickened, scaling, sharply demarcated plaque resembling psoriasis, known as **lichen simplex**. Polyhalogenated biphenyls and related chemicals may induce **chloracne** (Table 18–3). Excessive sweating, especially under occlusion, and ultraviolet and infrared radiation may cause **miliaria**. Irritation may also result in **hyperpigmentation or hypopigmentation, alopecia, urticaria**, and in the case of certain chemicals introduced into the skin, **granulomas**.

Anatomic differences in exposure site are important. Irritation is usually greater in areas where the skin is thin, such as dorsa of the hands, between the

**Table 18–1.** Factors contributing to cutaneous irritation.[1]

**Factors related to the substance**
Chemical nature of the substance
  pH
  Solubility in water and fats
  Detergent action
Physical state
  Gas
  Volatile liquid
  Heavy liquid
  Semisolid
  Solid
Concentration
  Amount
  Contact with skin

**Host factors**
Surface area affected
Region of skin
Length of exposure
Presence or absence of occlusion
Dryness
Sweating
Pigmentation
Presence of hair
Sebaceous activity
Concurrent and preexisting skin disease
Pruritogenic threshold

**General host factors**
Age
Sex
Race
Genetic background

**Environmental factors**
Temperature
  Heat
  Cold
Humidity and moisture
  Friction
  Pressure
  Occlusion
  Lacerations

[1]From: Adams RM: *Occupational Skin Disease,* 3rd ed. W.B. Saunders Company, 1998.

**Table 18–2.** Examples of environmental acne in the workplace.

| Type | Occupation |
|---|---|
| Cosmetic acne | Actors, models, cosmetologists |
| Acne mechanica | Auto and truck mechanics, athletes, telephone operators |
| Ultraviolet acne | Models<br>Lifeguards |
| Oil acne | Machinists<br>Auto mechanics<br>Fry cooks<br>Roofers<br>Petroleum refinery workers, rubber workers<br>Highway pavers |

induced lesions are occasionally seen and can be recognized by their bizarre shapes and locations with an inconsistent and suspicious history of occurence.

### Phototoxic Reactions

A nonimmunologic phototoxic eruption may result from contact with certain chemicals, often the juice of a plant with simultaneous exposure to natural or artificial light. Vesicle and bullae formation are characteristic of these reactions, often accompanied by minimal erythema and followed by hyperpigmentation. The most common causes are the polycyclic aromatic hydrocarbons in tar and creosote and furocoumarins (psoralens) found in certain plants (Table 18–4). Phototoxic reactions may follow contact with raw celery and simultaneous exposure to the ultraviolet (UV) emissions of grocery store check-out counters. Numerous systemic drugs may also cause these reactions.

## SPECIFIC TYPES OF CUTANEOUS IRRITATION

### Hydrofluoric Acid Burns

Hydrofluoric acid (HF) readily penetrates intact skin, dissociating into free hydrogen and free fluo-

fingers, volar forearms, inner thighs, and dorsum of the feet. Irritant dermatitis from airborne substances develops most commonly on regions most heavily exposed: face, hands, and arms. Dusts and volatile chemicals are the most frequent causes, but depending on the occupational situation, many other environmental and occupational irritants may cause airborne irritation.

The diagnosis of irritant contact dermatitis is often made by exclusion of allergic contact dermatitis. Patch testing is often necessary to rule out allergic contact dermatitis, but it should be emphasized that testing should be avoided with irritants, except in nonirritating concentrations.

The most common predisposing factor in the development of irritant dermatitis in the workplace is atopy, which is inherited in varying degrees by from 15% to 20% of the population. Dry skin and advancing age are also important predisposing factors. Self-

**Table 18–3.** Chloracne-producing chemicals.

Polyhalogenated naphthalenes
Polyhalogenated biphenyls
Polyhalogenated dibenzofurans
Contaminants of polychlorophenol compounds,
  especially the herbicide 4,5-T
  2,3,7,8-Tetrachlorodibenzo-p-dioxin
  Tetrachlorodibenzofuran
Contaminants of 3,4-dichloroaniline and related herbicides
Others
  DDT (crude trichlorobenzene)

**Table 18–4.** Selected phototoxic drugs and chemicals.[1]

**Coal tars and related products**
  Acridine
  Anthracene
  Coal tar
  Creosote

**Furocoumarins**
  Psoralen
  8-Methoxypsoralen
  4,5,8-Trimethylpsoralen

**Aminobenzoic acid derivative**
  Amyl-ortho-dimethylaminobenzoic acid

**Dyes**
  Disperse Blue 35

**Drugs and pharmaceuticals**
  Sulfonamides
  Phenothiazines
  Sulfonylureas
  Tetracyclines
  Thiazides

[1]From Epstein JH, Ormsby A, Adams RM: Occupational Skin Cancer, in Adams RM (editor): *Occupational Skin Disease,* 2nd ed. Saunders, 1990, p 186.

ride ions. The fluoride ion is responsible for most of the tissue destruction. The typical signs and symptoms of an acute HF injury are usually delayed for several hours after contact. If the concentration of the HF is 50–70%, for example, there may be enough hydrogen ions to produce immediate burning and a warning of exposure. However, the concentrations of HF employed are usually much lower, often 15–20%, and the typical signs and symptoms of injury after exposure are delayed, often for several hours. When the symptoms emerge, there is a deep, throbbing, excruciating pain. At this stage, however, there may be an absence of visible signs of injury. The area becomes erythematous and swollen, and, as the tissue injury progresses, pallor and blistering of the skin occur, followed by tissue necrosis. Because fluoride ions have a marked affinity for bone, extensive demineralization may occur. HF burns cause marked tissue destruction, including the loss of parts of or entire digits.

Management of HF burns is covered in Chapter 28.

## Cement Burns

Severe burns can result from contact with wet cement, because of its high alkalinity due to the presence of calcium oxide and hydroxide. The burns usually result from workers kneeling in wet cement or spilling it into boots or gloves. Because of its alkalinity and weight, wet cement is especially irritating. Workers frequently delay removing contaminated boots and gloves in order to finish a job before the concrete hardens. Initially there is burning and ery-

thema, but ulceration is delayed several hours, and later becomes deep and necrotic. Healing is very slow, sometimes requiring several weeks and ultimately leaving disfiguring scars.

## Fibrous Glass Dermatitis

Commercially produced since the 1930s, fibrous glass is available in two forms: wool fiberglass and textile fiberglass. The former is used chiefly for insulation, acoustical panels, and ceiling boards in construction. Textile fiberglass is made into yarns or processed into short fibers for reinforcement of plastics, rubber, paper, and other materials. Binders are used on wool fiberglass, most commonly thermosetting phenol-formaldehyde-type resins. The sizing agent for textile fiberglass varies, but once the sizing agent is cured, the risk of allergic contact dermatitis is diminished. Almost all fiberglass manufactured today has a diameter of more than 4.5 μm, which can readily penetrate the sweat glands and cause irritation. The sizing agents and binders are completely cured before use and rarely cause dermatitis.

Contact with fibrous glass produces irritation, with itching and prickling of the skin, especially in skin folds and areas where clothing rubs. Often there is itching without objective findings. A maculopapular rash may be present, usually obscured by excoriations. When widespread, the rash is occasionally incorrectly diagnosed as scabies.

Application of a piece of scotch tape to the skin and then to a microscopic slide will, on examination, disclose the uniform, rod-like fibers of glass.

The symptoms usually subside after a few days. Allergic sensitization is not a factor, and because many workers develop "hardening," they are able to return to work and continue without recurrence. Atopics and those with dermographism, however, are usually unable to tolerate continued contact and must change jobs.

## Pigmentary Changes

Chemical agents may induce either increased or decreased pigmentation, and sometimes both in the same patient. Melanosis denotes hyperpigmentation, where as leukoderma refers to loss of pigment. Inflammation usually precedes the color change, but sometimes it is barely apparent. Trauma, especially when repeated, can increase pigmentation, especially in dark-skinned persons. Repeated friction, chemical and thermal burns, and exposure to UV light may also cause skin darkening, as will coal tar, pitch, asphalt, creosote and other tar and petroleum derivatives. Psoralens, found in certain plants, induce phytophotodermatitis with contact, which is followed by hyperpigmentation.

Occupational leukoderma resembles idiopathic vitiligo and differentiation is difficult and at times impossible. However, to be considered work-induced, the initial site of leukoderma should be the site of re-

**Table 18–5.** Chemicals causing leukoderma.[1]

Hydroquinone
Monobenzylether of hydroquinone
Monomethylether of hydroquinone
para-tertiary Butyl phenol
para-tertiary Butyl catechol
para-tertiary Amylphenol
para-Isopropyl catechol
para-Methyl catechol
para-Octylphenol
para-Nonylphenol
para-Phenylphenol
para-Cresol

[1]From Gellin GA: Pigmentary changes, in Adams RM (editor): *Occupational Skin Disease,* 2nd ed. Saunders, 1990, p 24.

peated contact with a known depigmenting chemical (Table 18–5), usually the hands and forearms. From continued contact, depigmentation may spread to distant body sites not in direct contact with the chemical.

Chemical leukoderma is reversible if exposure is discontinued soon after onset; if not, it may be permanent. Topical and oral psoralen ultraviolet A (PUVA) has been used to induce repigmentation, but acral lesions, especially on the hands, are often refractory to treatment.

## Allergic Contact Dermatitis

Although somewhat less frequent than irritant dermatitis, allergic contact dermatitis is perhaps of greater importance, as ordinary protective measures usually are ineffective, and many patients must change jobs or learn a new trade. By contrast, workers with irritant dermatitis can often return to work, provided they use protective measures such as gloves and if the workplace is made less hazardous.

Allergic contact dermatitis is an immunologic reaction classified as a type IV, delayed, or cell-mediated hypersensitivity. This distinguishes it from type I reactions, which are immediate and antibody-mediated. Although most contact allergens produce sensitization in only a small percentage of exposed persons, there is great variation among individuals dependent on numerous factors, not the least of which is the nature of the allergen itself. The allergen in poison ivy or oak, for example, will sensitize nearly 70% of exposed persons, whereas *p*-phenylenediamine, the allergen in permanent hair dyes and widely used by both women and men, sensitizes a relatively small percentage of persons who repeatedly come into contact with it.

Sensitization requires at least 4 days to develop. Many workers, however, repeatedly contact an allergen in their work for months and even years before developing sensitivity. The precipitating cause of sensitization can be even a minor episode of irritant dermatitis, for example, or even increased frequency of contact with greater pressure and sweating at the site. Once allergic sensitization is fully operative, the dermatitis begins within 24–48 hours after contact. A pruritic, erythematous rash develops rapidly, followed by papule-formation and blistering. Itching is always a prominent symptom. The dermatitis originates at the site of contact with the allergen, but new lesions may appear at distant, seemingly unrelated sites, usually because of inadvertent transfer of the allergen by the hands. After several days, a subacute and chronic stage evolves, characterized by thickened, fissured skin that occasionally erupts into more acute dermatitis on re-exposure to the allergen or with aggravation by contact with irritating substances.

There is considerable variation in the intensity of reaction depending on the body area affected. The mucous membranes usually are not affected, and the hair-bearing scalp is usually less involved than the adjacent skin. The palms and soles may be less affected than the dorsal and interdigital areas. The eyelids and periorbital skin are especially sensitive areas, while reaction almost never occurs on the vault of the axillae.

Allergic contact dermatitis must be differentiated from atopic dermatitis, psoriasis, so-called pustular eruptions of the palms and soles, herpes simplex and zoster, idiopathic vesicular reactions to *Trichophyton* infections of the feet, dyshidrotic and nummular eczemas, and drug eruptions, and, as stated above, irritant contact dermatitis.

**Photoallergic reactions** are immunologically based. They are less common than phototoxic reactions and develop only in individuals previously sensitized by simultaneous exposure to a photosensitizing chemical and appropriate UV radiation. The biological process is similar to allergic contact dermatitis, except that UV converts the chemical to a complete allergen. The radiation is usually in the UVA spectrum, although it may extend into the UVB.

Photoallergic reactions appear suddenly with an acute eczematous eruption, later becoming lichenoid and thickened on the face, neck, dorsum of the hands, and exposed arms, often extending to other areas. The diagnosis is suggested by the distribution and character of the eruption, but confirmation requires careful questioning and photopatch testing. Sparing of skin under the chin and upper eyelids is strongly suggestive of a photo eruption. Some causes of photoallergic reactions are provided in Table 18–6.

**A. Diagnosis:** The key to diagnosis of allergic contact dermatitis is diagnostic patch testing, a valuable tool that has been used since the mid-1890s. Among its unique and valuable features, the opportunity to select the site of application and the ability to use only a minute concentration of test substance, confining it to a small area of skin, are most important. Because the organ tested is the same as affected

**Table 18–6.** Selected causes of photoallergic reactions.[1]

**Halogenated salicylanilides and related compounds**
   Tetrachlorosalicylanilide
   3,4,5-tribromosalicylanilide
   4,5-dibromosalicylanilide
   Bithionol
   Hexachlorophene
   Dichlorophene
   Fentichlor
   Jadit (Buclosamide)
   Bromochlorosalicylanilide

**Sulfanilamide**

**Phenothiazines**
   Chlorpromazine
   Promethazine

**4,6-dichlorophenolphenol**

**Diphenhydramine**

**Quinoxaline 1,4-di-N-oxide**

**Fragrances**
   Musk ambrette
   6-Methylcoumarin

**Optical brighteners (stilbenes)**

**Sunscreens**
   PABA esters
   Digalloyl trioleate

**Plants of the *Compositae* family**

**Photosensitivity component in allergic reactions**
   Hexavalent chromium
   Lichens

[1]From Epstein JH, Ormsby A, Adams RM: Occupational Skin Cancer, in Adams RM (editor): *Occupational Skin Disease,* 2nd ed. Saunders, 1990, p 1189.

with the disease, and because the same mechanism for production of the disease is used, the patch test remains one of the most direct and valuable of all methods of medical testing.

Standarized procedures in patch testing are very important. Most important are the concentration of the allergen and type and characterstics of the vehicle. During the past couple of decades there has been standardization of patch testing, and today concentrations and vehicles are nearly identical throughout the world.

Two methods are currently in use worldwide. The older is the Finn Chamber, which employs an aluminum cup, 8 mm in diameter, fixed to a strip of Scanpor tape, a finely meshed paper tape with a polyacrylate adhesive. The allergens are squeezed into the cups, covering slightly more than half its diameter, and fixed to the skin with Scanpor tape. A new method, called the TRUE Test, manufactured by Pharmacia in Sweden and sold in the United States by Glaxo Pharmaceuticals, is a convenient "ready-to-use" strip of tape upon which a measured amount of allergen is incorporated in a thin hydrophilic gel film printed on a polyester patch measuring $9 \times 9$ mm. The patches contain 24 different allergens, are mounted on strips of acrylic tape protected by a plastic sheet, and are packaged in airtight envelopes. The thin sheet of plastic is removed, and the strips are placed on the skin. On contact with skin moisture, the dry film dissolves into the gel and the allergen is released onto the skin. This method permits rapid application and avoids the ever-present hazard of mistakes in application.

The upper back is the favored site of application. Any hair must be removed, using an electric rather than a safety razor to minimize damage to the keratin layer. The patches are left on the skin for 48 hours and then removed, and the sites are identified with a fluorescent inked pen, for example. Reading is done at 72 or 96 hours after application, and occasionally at 1 week. When a fluorescent pen has been used to delineate the allergens, a hand-held black light will identify the sites. A single reading at 48 hours will miss approximately 35% of positive results. Patch test interpretation codes are shown in Table 18–7.

Interpretation is the most difficult aspect of patch testing. Irritant reactions show varied patterns such as fine wrinkling, erythematous follicular papules, petechiae, pustules, and sometimes large bullae. Such reactions rarely occur when using commercially prepared allergens. A classic positive patch test reaction consists of erythema, mild edema, and small, closely set vesicles.

A description of the commonly used 24 allergens present in the new TRUE Test and additional allergens for detecting vehicle and preservative allergy are shown in Table 18–8.

Adverse reactions are rare. The most common are increased pigmentation at the site of a positive reaction, persistence of a reaction (especially with a positive reaction to gold), a mild flare of the original dermatitis with brisk reactions, the development of psoriasis in a positive test site (rare), active sensitiza-

**Table 18–7.** Patch test interpretation codes.

| 1 | + | = | Weak reaction, nonvesicular, with erythema, mild infiltration |
|---|---|---|---|
| 2 | + | = | Strong reaction, erythema, edema, vesicles |
| 3 | + | = | Extreme reaction, spreadin, bullous, even ulcerative |
| 4 | | = | Doubtful, faint erythema only |
| 5 | | = | Irritant reaction |
| 6 | | = | Negative |
| 7 | | = | Excited skin reaction |
| 8 | | = | Not tested |

**Table 18–8.** Standard and vehicle preservative allergens.

## Standard allergens (TRUE Test)

1. **Nickel sulfate 0.2 mg/cm$^2$**
   Found in many alloys, jewelry, pigments, dentures, orthopedic appliances, scissors, razors, eyeglass frames, eating utensils, etc. One of the most common sensitizers, found in more than 10% of all women.

2. **Wool alcohols 1.00 mg/cm$^2$**
   Derived from lanolin. In numerous cosmetics, topical medications such as creams, lotions, ointments, and soaps. Wool alcohols are weak allergens, but because lanolin is so widely used, reactions are common.

3. **Neomycin sulfate 0.23 mg/cm$^2$**
   Common allergen of the aminoglycoside class, found in topical antibiotics, first-aid creams, eardrops, and nosedrops. The patch test reaction may be somewhat delayed, to 4–5 days, so reading should be done at 7 days when possible.

4. **Potassium dichromate 0.023 mg/cm$^2$**
   This is the hexavalent form of chromium responsible for nearly all chromium contact allergy. It is found in cement in minute amounts, tanning solutions for leather, safety matches, electroplating solutions, many anticorrosives, paints, glues, pigments, and some detergents, and is used in photography.

5. **Caine mix 0.63 mg/cm$^2$**
   Topical anesthetics. Contains three anesthetics used for topical application: benzocaine, dibucaine hydrochloride, and tetracaine hydrochloride. Often used in dentistry, but also widely found and used in topical preparations to reduce itching, pain, and stinging. Widely used in hemorrhoidal preparations, and cough syrups. Because it is used on inflamed skin, sensitization is fairly common.

6. **Fragrance mix 0.43 mg/cm$^2$**
   Present in many toiletries, soaps, after-shave lotions, shampoos, scented household products, and in many industrial products such as cutting fluids. Contains alpha amyl cinnamic alcohol, cinnamic aldehyde, cinnamic alcohol, oakmoss absolute, hydroxycitronellal, eugenol, isoeugenol, and geraniol.

7. **Colophony 0.85 mg/cm$^2$**
   Colophony is more commonly known as "rosin" in the United States. It is used by string players, and violinists especially are likely to develop allergy. Baseball players and bowlers also use it. It is derived from several conifer species. It is found in cosmetics, adhesives, lacquers, varnishes, soldering fluxes, paper, and many other industrial products. The exact allergen is not known but is probably present in the resin acid fraction.

8. **Epoxy resin 0.05 mg/cm$^2$**
   Basic, two-part epoxy adhesives are widely used. This epoxy is based on the low-molecular weight (340) epoxy based on bisphenol A and epichlorhydrin. The resin is a sensitizer only when uncured or incompletely cured.

9. **Quinoline mix 0.19 mg/cm$^2$**
   Contains clioquinol and chlorquinaldol—antimicrobials found in certain medicated creams, ointments, and bandages, and veterinary products.

10. **Balsam of Peru 0.80 mg/cm$^2$**
    A flavoring agent for drinks and tobacco, as well as a fixative and fragrance in perfumes. Also found in many topical medications, dental agents, etc. The chief allergens are esters of cinnamic and benzoic acid and vannilin. Cross reactions occur with colophony (rosin) and balsam of Tolu, the cinnamates, benzoates, styrax, and tincture of benzoin. Probably also some photosensitization, but of the toxic type.

11. **Ethylenediamine dihyrochloride 0.05 mg/cm$^2$**
    This is used as an emulsifier and stabilizer in certain topical medications, eyedrops, some industrial solvents, curing agents for certain plastics, and anticorrosion agents.

12. **Cobalt dichloride 0.02 mg/cm$^2$**
    In some paints, cement, metal, metal-plated objects. Often co-reactive with nickel, but this is not cross-sensitivity.

13. **p-tert Butylphenol formaldehyde resin 0.04 mg/cm$^2$**
    A resin formed by condensation between p-tert-butylphenol and formaldehyde. In leather finishes—especially shoes—fabrics, rockwood, furniture, and paper, as well as in certain glues.

14. **Paraben mix 1 mg/cm$^2$**
    Five different parabens are present: methyl, ethyl, propyl, butyl, and benzyl parahydroxybenzoates. They are the most common preservatives used throughout the world, present in numerous creams and cosmetics, and in some industrial oils, fats, and glues. Weak allergens.

15. **Carba mix 0.25 mg/cm$^2$**
    Used as accelerators in rubber, rubber glues, vinyl, and some pesticides.

16. **Black rubber mix 0.075 mg/cm$^2$**
    In rubber, and may cross-react with hair dyes.

17. **Cl$^+$ Me$^-$ Isothiazolinone 0.0040 mg/cm$^2$ (Kathon CG)**
    Found in cosmetics and skin care products, in some medications, in household cleaning products, and in certain industrial fluids and greases.

*(continued)*

**Table 18–8.** Standard and vehicle preservative allergens. (continued)

18. **Quaternium 15 0.1 mg/cm$^2$**
    Common preservative in cosmetics and in some household cleaners and polishes.

19. **Mercaptobenzothiazole 0.075 mg/cm$^2$**
    Rubber, adhesives, coolants.

20. **p-Phenylenediamine (PPD) 0.090 mg/cm$^2$**
    Hair dyes, some inks, photodevelopers, and textile dyes.

21. **Formaldehyde 0.18 mg/cm$^2$**
    Released by Quaternium 15, and occasionally by imidazolidinyl urea. Used widely in formulation of plastics, resins for clothing, glues, adhesives.

22. **Mercapto mix 0.075 mg/cm$^2$**
    Rubber, glues, coolants, and other industrial products.

23. **Thimerosal 0.0080 mg/cm$^2$**
    Preservative in contact lens solutions, in certain cosmetics, nose and ear drops, and injectables. Source often not found.

24. **Thiuram mix 0.025 mg/cm$^2$**
    Common rubber allergen, also in adhesives, certain pesticides, and medications (Antabuse).

**Recommended additional allergens**

1. **Benzophenone-3 1% (2-hydroxy-3-methoxybenzophenone)**
   Sunscreens.

2. **Bronopol 0.5% (2-Bromo-2-nitropropane-1,3-diol)**
   Preservative commonly used in certain cosmetics, coolants, shampoos, hair preparations, barrier creams, and industrial hand cleaners.

3. **p-Chloro-m-cresol 1%**
   Antimicrobial, especially effective against fungi, found in topical antiseptics, pharmaceuticals, shampoos, baby cosmetics, and coolants.

4. **Diazolidinyl urea 1% (Germall II)**
   Preservative used in numerous cosmetics, especially creams, lotions, shampoos, and hair products.

5. **DMDM Hydantoin 1%**
   A preservative that acts as a formaldehyde donor, found in cosmetics, especially shampoos, skin care products, hair conditioners, soaps, leave-on cosmetics, etc.

6. **Propylene glycol 10% aq**
   A widely used pharmaceutical and cosmetic base vehicle. Also used in food as a solvent for coloring and flavoring agents. Prevents growth of fungi and is useful in medications as a humectant. May also be found in industrial coolants.

7. **Captan 0.25%**
   A fungicide used on fruits, vegetables, and numerous plants. It is also used in paints, soaps, and certain shampoos as a bacteriostat. May also be used in seed treatments against molds.

8. **p-Chloro-m-Xylenol 1%**
   A common antimicrobial used in cosmetics, protective creams, coolants, hair conditioners, deodorant soaps, etc.

9. **Chlorhexidine digluconate 0.5%**
   An antimicrobial agent in cosmetics and pharmaceuticals, surgical soaps, anticaries solutions in dentistry, and toothpaste. May also be a photosensitizer.

10. **Ammoniated Mercury 1%**
    Once widely used as an antibacterial agent, it is now used for patch testing to detect mercury sensitivity.

11. **Glutaraldehyde 1%**
    An antimicrobial widely used in medicine and dentistry. It is especially common in cold sterilization in dental offices and also for sterilizing endoscopic instruments. It is also an excellent tanning agent for leather and is used as a hardener for photographic gelatin.

12. **Imidazolidinyl urea 2%**
    A currently popular preservative for cosmetics, especially creams, lotions, hair conditioners, shampoos, and deodorants. Releases a small amount of formaldehyde.

13. **BHA 2% (Butyl hydroxyanisole, butyl methoxy phenol)**
    A common antioxidant for fats and oils, is found in food packaging, and is used as a preservative for medications.

14. **BHT 2% (Butyl hydroxytoluene)**
    A widely used preservative, antioxidant in food products, animal feeds, plastics, rubber, and jet fuels. Also found in aviation gasoline.

15. **Sorbitan sesquioleate 20%**
    Emulsifier and stabilizer in foods, cosmetics, drugs, textiles; also found in plastics and agricultural chemicals.

tion (very rare), and anaphylactoid reactions (exceedingly rare).

In determining the relevance of positive reactions, we should keep in mind that the test is a template of allergic contact sensitization developed over a person's lifetime. Thus, the relevance of each positive reaction must be determined. This can be accomplished only with extensive knowledge of commercial and industrial materials and their ingredients. Information can be obtained from a variety of sources, including standard textbooks, manufacturers, and Material Safety Data Sheets.

**B. Treatment:** Treatment of contact dermatitis depends upon the stage of the disease. Acute, vesicular eruptions are treated with wet dressings for the first 24–36 hours, using Burow's solution, followed by a corticosteroid lotion. When the eruption begins to dry, corticosteroid creams can be used, accompanied by internal antihistamines for itching. Oral antibiotic therapy is indicated when secondary infection is suspected or likely to develop. Topical antibiotic and antihistamine preparations should be avoided, however, because of risk of sensitization.

## Contact Urticaria

Contact urticaria develops within minutes to an hour or so following contact with a substance. Because of the mounting number of cases, especially due to exposures to natural rubber latex, interest in and knowledge of this reaction has greatly increased during the last 15 years. The two main types are nonallergic and allergic.

**A. Nonallergic Contact Urticaria:** Given sufficient provocation, nearly all exposed individuals will develop a reaction. Previous sensitization is not necessary. Gardeners may develop reactions from contact with nettles and other plants, caterpillar hair, and moths and other insects; cooks from cinnamic acid and aldehyde, sodium benzoate, sorbic acid, fruits, vegetables, fish and meat; and medical and related personnel from alcohols, balsam of Peru, DMSO, and other substances.

**B. Allergic Contact Urticaria:** Allergic contact urticaria is most commonly caused by latex in natural rubber, especially gloves, which has become a major problem for medicodental personnel, kitchen and dairy workers, pharmacists, semiconductor workers, and others who must wear gloves throughout the workday. The reactions range from mild erythema with itching at the site of contact, to severe anaphylactic reactions sometimes resulting in death. They are type I immediate hypersensitivity reactions, are IgE mediated, and appear to be more common in atopics. The cause is natural latex from the sap of the tree *Hevea brasiliensiis*, a *cis*-1,4 polyisoprene, the precursor of the rubber molecule. It has been estimated that there are 50 or 60 different proteins in latex that provoke the allergic response. The chief symptoms are itching, redness, and wheal and flare

formation at the site of contact. The symptoms usually appear 10–60 mintues after contact and, when mild, disappear without treatment in 2–3 hours. Severe reactions progress rapidly and include generalized urticaria, swelling of the face and lips, asthma, collapse, and death. Natural latex gloves most commonly cause these reactions, but condoms, urinary catheters, elastic bandages, adhesive tape, wound drains, dental dams, hemodialysis equipment, balloons, pacifiers, barium enema tips, and countless other latex-based rubber products have been implicated. Because of cross-reactions, avocados, water chestnuts, kiwi, papaya, and bananas may also provoke reactions in sensitive persons. It should be remembered that airborne contamination by rubber glove powder may also induce symptoms in very sensitive patients.

Skin prick testing is the most common diagnostic method for this condition. A standardized test material should be used, and testing should be performed only if resuscitation measures are readily available. "Use" tests with a glove or a single finger of a glove should be performed, but not in patients with a history of anaphylaxis or when the results of skin prick test or the latex RAST (Pharmacia, Sweden) are positive. It should be remembered, however, that the RAST is only 60–65% sensitive.

The Federal Drug Administration plans to prohibit the labeling of latex-containing medical products as "hypoallergenic" and to require the statement, "This product contains natural rubber latex" on all latex-containing products that are directly or indirectly in contact with the body.

The mechanism resulting in reactions to ammonium persulfate, used by hairdressers to achieve a platinum blond effect on clients, is uncertain. The reaction is immediate and can be very severe, with erythema, swelling of the lips and face, marked itching, urticaria and wheezing, severe respiratory difficulty, and sometimes syncope. Hairdressers should be made aware of this alarming reaction in clients.

## BIOLOGICAL CAUSES

### Bacterial Diseases

**A. Staphylococcal and Streptococcal Infections:** Infection of minor lacerations, abrasions, burns, and puncture wounds account for most staphylococcal and streptococcal infections. A work relationship is not always easy to establish, however, and many cases are unreported. Nevertheless, these infections are common in certain occupations, especially agricultural and construction workers, butchers, meat packers, and slaughterhouse workers. The history should clarify whether a work relationship is likely, although frequently in worker compensation cases the patient's statements must be accepted as valid.

Furunculosis is common among auto and truck repair persons, especially in dirty jobs such as tire repair. Paronychia may be seen in persons working in close contact with infected persons, such as nurses, hairdressers, and manicurists.

Atopic dermatitis patients are especially likely to experience skin colonization with staphylococci. In a high percentage of atopics, *Staphylococcus aureus* can be cultured from their eczematous skin, which often has been made worse by heavy and prolonged application of corticosteroid creams and ointments. Daily oral antibiotics should be a part of the long-term treatment of these patients. Employment of persons with active atopic dermatitis in food service industries and hospital patient care should be restricted.

**B. Cutaneous TBC—Typical Mycobacterial Infections:** Infection with tubercle bacilli is covered in Chapter 16. A classic example of tuberculosis of the skin acquired through inoculation of *M tuberculosis hominis* is seen in pathologists ("prosector's wart") and morgue attendants ("necrogenic wart" or "anatomic tubercle"). Surgeons are also at risk for such granulomatous infections. Veterinarians, farmers, and butchers may acquire infection with *M tuberculosis var bovis*, which at one time was a common cause of disease in livestock in the United States, but beginning in the middle 1930s bovine tuberculosis became exceedingly rare. In some countries, however, the disease is still fairly common. In the United States and other parts of the world, as a result of movement of populations and the increasing prevalence of Human Immunosuppressant Virus (HIV), the incidence of infection with human strains of tuberculosis has greatly increased. Between 1985 and 1991, 39,000 more cases occurred in the United States than expected, and drug resistance, especially in those with HIV infection, has seriously compounded the problem.

The typical skin lesions are slowly progressive, warty, hyperkeratotic plaques, which, if left untreated, eventually regress after many months or years, leaving disfiguring scars. Demonstration of organisms either directly or from cultures is often difficult.

**C. Atypical Mycobacterial Infections:** Atypical mycobacterial infections are most commonly caused by infection with *M marinum*. This infection is usually acquired from exposure to infected fish, especially in aquariums and fish tanks, by persons who clean these tanks. Swimming pools become contaminated with this organism, and attendants and pool cleaners are also at risk. Treatment with rifampin (RMP) and ethambutol are usually effective.

As in other mycobacterial skin infections, the clinical picture consists of granulomatous papules and nodules that ulcerate and exude a clear, thin serum. Not infrequently, a pattern resembling sporotrichosis develops, with nodules and papules ascending the arm (or leg) along the course of regional lymphatics. Persons with acquired immunodeficiency syndrome

(AIDS) are at special risk for developing these infections. Other atypical mycobacteria include *M ulcerans, M fortuitum, M avion, M intracellulare, M kansasii,* and *M chelonae.*

**D. Tularemia:** The organism causing this disease, *Francisella tularensis,* is a gram-negative pleomorphic coccal bacillus transmitted by fleas, ticks, and deerflies harbored by rabbits, deer, squirrels, skunks, muskrats, rodents, and numerous other wild animals. The organism penetrates unbroken skin. Most cases of tularemia in the United States are transmitted by infected rabbits, and many cases result from skinning the animals. The onset of infection is manifested by an ulcer at the site of inoculation, followed by marked enlargement of regional lymph nodes. In many cases severe consitutional symptoms develop, with headaches, chills, fever, and aching of muscles and joints. A generalized, maculopapular, hemorrhagic eruption appears during the course of the febrile illness. Those at greatest risk are recreational hunters, but also at risk are veterinarians, farmers, butchers, foresters, fur handlers, and laboratory workers, as well as surgeons and autopsy personnel. Because of the high degree of infectiousness, great caution should be used in handling infected tissues and excreta. Treatment with streptomycin, gentimycin, tetracycline, and chloramphenicol is usually effective.

**E. Brucellosis (Malta Fever, Undulant Fever):** Brucellosis, caused by one of several Brucella organisms, is still observed in some rural areas, affecting farmers, veterinarians, slaughterhouse workers, meat packers and inspectors, and livestock workers. The disease has an abrupt onset, with chills, fever, headache, and extreme weakness. A maculopapular rash occurs, which may become petechial. A chronic form of the disease was common in the past, with a recalcitrant ulcer at the site of inoculation and abscesses in internal organs. Treatment with tetracycline, when started early, is curative. Streptomycin is useful for more serious cases.

**F. Anthrax:** Anthrax, caused by the spore-forming bacterium *Bacillus anthracis,* produces a "malignant" pustule at the site of inoculation and elaborates a highly toxic endotoxin, which is lethal to infected animals. A vegetative form of the organism may remain dormant in soil for many years. Infection in humans is usually through the skin, but has also resulted from ingestion of contaminated meat. A pulmonary form of the disease, caused by inhalation of the spores, is often rapidly fatal if not promptly treated.

Occupational infection is usually caused by importation of contaminated animal products and occurs chiefly in agricultural workers, stock farmers, slaughterhouse workers, butchers, and those employed in bone and bone meal processing. Workers handling imported goat hair, wool, and hides from endemic regions are at special risk. These include longshoremen, freight handlers, warehouse workers, and employees of processing industries where the hides are treated for sale. Anthrax responds to treatment with penicillin and tetracycline.

**G. Erysipeloid:** This acute, slowly evolving skin infection is almost always occupational in origin. Caused by inoculation of the gram-positive bacillus *Erysipelothrix rhusiopathiae*, usually through a penetrating hand wound, the disease begins with a characteristic raised, purplish-red indurated maculopapular lesion, with burning and itching. Regional lymphadenopathy does not occur. The disease is self-limiting, usually clearing within 3 or 4 weeks.

Butchers and fish handlers are at most risk ("fish-handlers' disease"). Turkeys and chickens may also carry the organism. Benzathine penicillin and erythromycin are curative.

## Viral Diseases

**A. Herpes Simplex:** This is by far the most frequent viral infection of occupational origin. Caused by the herpes simplex virus, also known as herpes virus hominis (HSV), workers at greatest risk include dentists and dental assistants, physicians and nurses, and respiratory technicians. The consistent wearing of disposable gloves, masks, and safety glasses will reduce infection in these workers.

**B. Viral Warts:** Meat handlers, especially butchers and slaughterhouse workers, are at greatest risk for development of the common wart, caused by the **human papilloma virus (HPV)**, of which there are at least 35 types. These warts are most numerous on the hands and fingers of these workers, and minor cuts and abrasions inoculate the virus. *Mollusca contagiosa* infections occur in wrestlers, boxers, and other sportsmen.

**C. Orf (Contagious Ecthyma):** Endemic in sheep and goats, orf is caused by infection with a parapox virus, usually involving the mouth and nose of infected animals. Mostly farmers and veterinarians are affected with this relatively mild, self-limited disease, including children of farmers who feed the newborn animals. Usually only one or two lesions are present, almost always on fingers, and may be associated with mild fever, lymphangitis, and regional lymphadenopathy. An erythema multiforme-like rash may also occur. Treatment is symptomatic; antibiotics are used for complications, which are rare.

## Fungal Infections

**A. Candida:** Infection with *Candida*, chiefly *Candida albicans*, is the most common occupationally related fungal disease. The organism is ubiquitous, and proliferation is favored by moisture, occlusion, and irritation. Drug-resistant strains have appeared recently. Most occupationally acquired candidal infections are on the hands, especially in the paronychial areas and interdigital spaces. Occupations in which prolonged wearing of rubber gloves is

required, such as dentistry, medicine, and technical work in clean rooms in the semiconductor industry, show the highest incidence of this condition. Diabetics and neutropenic, immunocompromised patients are especially at risk.

**B. Dermatophytes:** Dermatophytic infections are also exceedingly common. *Trichophyton verrucosum* is an animal fungus that readily infects farmers and cattle tenders. The lesions are often quite inflammatory and may resemble pyoderma. Farmers, milkers, cattle tenders, veterinarians, and tannery workers, especially hide sorters, are at risk. *T rubrum* and *T mentagrophytes* are examples of fungi that cause tinea infections in the general population, especially tinea manum and tinea pedis. *Microsporum canis* frequently infects small animals and causes infection in pet shop workers, veterinarians, and personnel in contact with laboratory animals. *M gypseum* is a rare fungus found in soil, causing occasional infection in agricultural workers.

Physicians are often requested to decide whether a *trichophyton* infection is work-related or not, especially *T rubrum* and *T mentagrophytes* infections in the hands and nails. Onychomycosis is extremely common, and most of those affected do not seek medical attention. Workers engaged in repetitive hand activities, however, especially where there is sweating and pressure, or repetitive nail trauma in the case of onychomycosis, may believe their work to be the primary cause of the infection. Each case must be studied individually, but most often the work cannot be considered a primary cause.

**C. Coccidioidomycosis (San Joaquin or Valley Fever):** Inhalation of dust containing spores of the fungus *Coccidioides immitis* is responsible for most cases of this disease, which is endemic to arid and semiarid regions of the southwestern United States and northern Mexico. The usual infection is a self-limited, influenza-like respiratory illness in which hypersensitivity reactions such as erythema nodosum, erythema multiforme, and urticaria may occur. In a small number of persons, especially immunosuppressed patients, a severe form of the disease may develop, with multiple, cutaneous abscesses in internal organs, especially bones, viscera, and the central nervous system. Culture of skin biopsies usually yields the fungus, but finding the spherules microscopically in biopsy specimens is sometimes difficult. The fatality rate of the disseminated form is 55–60%. An inoculation type of local granulomatous lesion may also rarely occur.

Persons at greatest risk are migrant workers, farmers, construction workers, military personnel, highway construction crews, baseball players, and laboratory workers. Epidemics of the disease occur in hot, dusty summers. Treatment of the disseminated type is with amphotericin B or ketoconazole.

**D. Sporotrichosis:** This fungal disease is most often acquired by persons who work with soil, such as nursery, agricultural, and forestry workers. Veterinarians and miners are also at risk. The etiologic agent is the dimorphic fungus *Sporothrix schenckii*, which has a worldwide distribution. There are two clinical manifestions. A fixed type, restricted to the site of inoculation, may be nodular, ulcerative, or verrucous. The more common, and classic form, of the disease is a relatively nontender, subcutaneous nodule that appears at the site of inoculation of the fungus. The nodule slowly enlarges and later ulcerates, followed by the appearance of secondary lesions ("nodular lymphangitis") along the lymphatics draining the initial site. The cutaneous forms of the disease are chronic, indolent, and rarely fatal. Treatment with potassium iodide saturated solution for a prolonged period of time is effective. In disseminated disease, which is fatal in approximately 30% of cases, intravenous administration of amphotericin B is indicated. Itraconazole has also been recommended for treatment of both forms.

Other possible causes of nodular lymphangitis should be kept in mind. These include *Mycobacterium marinum, Norandia brasiliensis, Leishmania brasiliensis, Coccidioides immitis*, and *Francisella tularensis*.

**E. Blastomycosis (Gilchrist's Disease):** This is an infectious disease primarily of the lungs, but occasionally hematogenous dissemination occurs, usually to the skin. The disease is caused by a thick-walled budding yeast, *Blastomyces dermatitidis*, occurring most commonly in the Southeastern United States, but also in Africa, India, and Israel. After an episode of bronchopneumonia, the skin is involved through hematogenous spread; also the prostate, epididymis, testis, bone, and subcutaneous tissue are affected. In immunocompromised persons there is a 30–40% fatality rate. The skin lesion is characteristic, with a verrucous pustule, a serpiginous border, and central clearing.

Occupational sources of this infection include farming, forestry, construction, and workers using heavy earth-moving equipment. Amphotericin B is the drug of choice, which usually results in rapid clearing.

**F. Chromomycosis (Chromoblastomycosis):** Chromomycosis is a deep mycosis beginning at the site of a puncture wound or other trauma with implantation of one or more of five soil-inhabiting fungi—*Phialophora verucosa, Fonsecaea pedrosoi, F compactum, F dermatitidis*, and *Cladosporium carrionii*. The initial lesion is a papule that rapidly becomes a warty tumor ("mossy foot"), gradually spreading to form a plaque, with central scarring. Considerable induration of the skin occurs, and the fistulas resemble those seen in mycetoma. The legs are most often affected. Potassium hydroxide preparations of skin scrapings may show pigmented muriform bodies ("copper pennies"), which are pathognomonic for chromomycosis. The organism can easily be isolated on culture. Treatment with itroconazole

has been recommended. The occupations associated with risk of chromomycosis are mostly agricultural workers in tropical and subtropical climates.

## PARASITIC DISEASES

### Protozoa

**A. Cutaneous Leishmaniasis:** Most parasitic diseases, such as amebiasis, giardiasis, and malaria, present general rather than cutaneous health problems. An exception is cutaneous leishmaniasis, caused by *Leishmania tropica* (Oriental sore, bouton d'orient), found in the Middle East, and *L brasiliensis* (American leishmaniasis, Uta), endemic to Central and South America. The disease is transmitted by a tiny sandfly that thrives in warm climates and is endemic in persons working in tropical forests in southeastern Mexico, Columbia, and Venezuela. The disease manifests as cutaneous ulcers, with metastatic mucocutaneous lesions known as espundia. When the ulcers are localized to the face they are known as chiclero ulcers (Mexico). Sodium antimony gluconate is the treatment of choice.

**B. Helminths:** Penetration of the cercariae of schistosomes into the papillary dermis induces a highly pruritic papular eruption termed **swimmer's itch**. Urticaria often accompanies the rash and may be widespread. Migratory birds are usually the definitive hosts, with salt water mollusks serving as intermediate hosts. The condition lasts for 2 or 3 weeks, often with secondary infection of excoriated lesions. Skin divers, lifeguards, dock workers, and workers who maintain lakes and ponds (eg, at golf courses) may be affected. Treatment is symptomatic.

**Larva migrans (creeping eruption)** occurs in subtropical and tropical regions where people work in and on moist soil infected with hookworm larvae. Dogs, cats, cattle, and occasionally human feces carry the larvae, and humans are the final host. Characteristic of the disease is the appearance of a thread-like, red or flesh-colored, circuitous, slightly raised line, often on the feet, legs, back, or buttocks, caused by movement of the larva in the epidermis. Humans are infected with the larvae of *Ancylostoma braziliense* and *Necator americanus*, the ova of which are deposited in the soil. Topical application of an oral 10% suspension of thiabendazole to affected areas four times daily for 7–10 days is usually curative. Agricultural workers, lifeguards, shoreline fishermen, ditch diggers, and sewer workers are at greatest risk.

Other nematode diseases that are occasionally occupational include trichinosis, dracunulosis, filariasis, loiasis, enterobiasis, strongyloidiasis, and toxocariasis.

### Arthropods

Bees, wasps, ants, moths, flies, mosquitos, fleas, and blister beetles are among the most common cause of occupationally related arthropod diseases. Mites, ticks, spiders, and scorpions are also included in this group. Milipedes and centipedes may induce severe skin reactions caused by their toxins or allergenic products. Outdoor workers, food handlers, and entomologists are most frequently affected. Chicken farmers are exposed to chicken mites. Mites infect grain in food processing plants, and dock workers and restaurant workers are also affected.

**A. Scabies:** Epidemics of **scabies** have occurred in nursing homes, hospitals, and residential facilities for the aged. The disease is highly contagious and spreads rapidly. It is often initiated by an infected employee, who transmits the mite to patients. They, in turn, spread the disease to other personnel. The scabicide of choice is permethrin, but treatment of the more severe types of scabies (ie, Norwegian scabies) is difficult and may require repeated treatment with other scabicides such as lindane and precipitated sulfur. Immunosuppressed persons are at greatest risk.

**B. Lyme Disease:** Lyme disease is an important inflammatory disease that follows tick-induced erythema chronicum migrans (ECM) weeks or months after inoculation. ECM begins with a small erythematous macule, usually on an extremity, which enlarges with central clearing. The lesion sometimes reaches a diameter of 50 cm, and smaller satellite lesions are often present. In nearly half the patients, a type of arthritis occurs within weeks or months of the ECM, and there may be associated neurologic abnormalities as well as myocardial conduction alterations, serum cryoprecipitants, elevated serum immunoglobulin M (IgM) levels, and an increased sedimentation rate. Elevated serum IgM and later IgG appears within weeks of infection as well as circulating cryoprecipitates and other immune complexes. Erythema chronicum migrans is an important diagnostic marker for this disease. The ticks *Ixodes dammini, I pacificus* (in the United States), and *I ricinus* (in Europe) transmit the spirochete *Borrelia burgdorferi*, which is responsible for the disease. There is no evidence as yet that any relationship exists between Lyme disease and carpal tunnel syndrome, but in some cases localized scleroderma appears to be linked to *Borrelia* infection. Tick bites are common in outdoor workers, loggers, wilderness construction workers, guides, and ranchers.

Besides Lyme disease, other major tick-borne diseases in the US are relapsing fever, tularemia, Rocky Mountain spotted fever, ehrlichiosis, Colorado tick fever, babesiosis, and tick paralysis.

## PHYSICAL CAUSES

### Mechanical Trauma

Intermittent friction of low intensity will induce lichenification (thickening) of the skin. With greater pressure, corns and calluses appear. After minor trauma, calluses frequently develop painful fissures, which may become infected. After years of repeated frictional hand trauma during work, permanent calluses may result, leading to disability and early retirement. Calluses also represent the effects of a particular occupation. At one time they were very common and clearly indicated the worker's occupation. With increasing automation and less frequent manual operation of tools and better protective clothing, occupational marks are less frequent and have almost disappeared from many industries.

### Heat

**A. Burns:** arising from the occupation are common and exhibit characteristic occupational patterns. The resulting scarring and pigmentary changes are of chief concern to dermatologists, who rarely treat acute burns. Hypopigmentation is especially susceptible to actinic damage, and scars and the hyperpigmentation are often disfiguring.

**B. Miliaria:** caused by sweat retention, is often seen in the work environment and frequently is misdiagnosed as contact dermatitis. The eruption can be extensive, accompanied by burning and itching. The most superficial form, *miliaria crystallina*, is due to poral closure and rupture of the ducts within the upper level of the epidermis. The condition commonly occurs on the palms and in intertriginous areas, with asymptomatic desquamation of the surface. When the closure occurs deeper in the epidermis, vesiculation, with marked pruritus, results. Termed **miliaria rubra**, or prickly heat, it is the type most likely to be confused with contact dermatitis. If poral obstruction extends deeper in the epidermis and into the upper dermis, the condition is known as **miliaria profunda**, resulting in deep-seated, asymptomatic vesicles. This condition is caused by prolonged exposure to a hot environment and often follows an extended period of miliaria rubra. Heat exhaustion and collapse may be sequellae.

**C. Intertrigo:** is a macerated, erythematous eruption in body folds, resulting from excessive sweating, especially in obese workers. Secondary bacterial and candidal infections are common. The interdigital space between the third and fourth fingers is a common site in workers whose hands are continuously wet, especially from rubber gloves. Medical and dental personnel, bartenders, cannery workers, cooks, swimming instructors, and housekeepers are especially predisposed to this condition.

Overheating, especially in conjunction with physical exercise, may result in heat-induced urticaria, and rarely anaphylaxis. Acne vulgaris and rosacea are aggravated by prolonged exposure to heat, especially from ovens, steam, open furnaces, and heat torches. Herpes simplex may be triggered by intense heat, especially sunburn and UVB exposure.

## Cold

**A.   Frostbite:** In frostbite there is progressive vasoconstriction, causing impairment of circulation. In superficial frostbite, only the skin and superficial dermis are involved. Redness, transient anaesthesia, and superficial bullae are seen. In more severe cases, deep tissue destruction occurs, often with gangrene and loss of a limb. As the temperature falls, the affected area becomes numb, and the initial redness is replaced by a white, waxy appearance, with blistering and later areas of necrosis. The area ultimately becomes pain free, and the cold discomfort disappears. At this stage it is not possible to accurately estimate future tissue loss; several weeks may be necessary. Long-term effects, even for relatively minor degrees of frostbite, include Raynaud-like changes, with paresthesias and hyperhidrosis. Squamous cell carcinoma may develop in old, healed scars.

Treatment consists of slow rewarming in a whirlpool or waterbath, a painful procedure requiring adequate relief. Infection must be treated vigorously.

Persons at greatest risk are military personnel, utility maintenance personnel, sailors, fishermen, firefighters, mail delivery persons, rescue personnel, arctic laboratory workers, and many others.

**B.   Chilblains (Perniosis):** This mild form of cold injury, although certainly an abnormal reaction to cold, is in fact less common in very cold climates, where homes are usually well-heated and warm clothing is worn. Northern United States and Europe are areas where this condition is frequently seen. The lesions are reddish blue, swollen, boggy discolorations with bullae and ulcerations. The fingers, toes, heels, lower legs, nose, and ears are especially affected. Genetic factors with vasomotor instability are often found to be important background features. Treatment is symptomatic. The calcium channel blockers, such as nifedipine, have been recommended.

## Vibration Syndrome

That a connection exists between the vibration of hand-held tools and Raynaud's phenomenon has been known since the early part of this century. The popular names are "dead fingers" and "white fingers," and clinically the condition is a type of Raynaud's phenomenon. Operation of heavy vibrating tools such as jackhammers, especially in cold weather, produces vasospasm of the digital arteries, causing episodic pallor, cyanosis, and erythema of fingers. Chain saws, hand-held grinders, riveting hammers, and other pneumatic tools have also been associated with this condition. Tingling and numbness, blanching of the tips of one or more fingers, and clumsiness of fingers and hands occur. The symptoms may be indistinguishable from other forms of Raynaud's phenomenon, but asymmetry is usually observed. Occupational disability seldom results, and most workers continue at their jobs. Vibration fre-

quencies between 30 and 300 Hertz are most likely responsible.

**A.   Acro-osteolysis (Vinyl Chloride Disease):** A serious form of Raynaud's phenomenon occurs from exposure to vinyl chloride monomer in workers cleaning reactor tanks used for polymerization. In addition to Raynaud's phenomenon, lytic lesions occur in bones, especially the fingers, hence the name acro-osteolysis. Sclerodermatous skin changes are also seen. With engineering modifications during manufacture and better protective measures, the condition has nearly disappeared.

## Ionizing Radiation

Numerous industrial processes utilize ionizing radiation, including the curing of plastics, sterilization of food and drugs, testing metals and other materials, medical and dental radiography, therapy with radioisotopes, and operation of high-powered electronic equipment. Although ionizing radiation is widely used, exposure is much less now than several decades ago, chiefly because of better construction and shielding of the x-ray equipment.

Occupational exposure to ionizing radiation may be acute or chronic and is usually localized. In **acute radiodermatitis**, often resulting from a single accidental exposure to 1000 Roentgens or more, erythema, edema, and blanching of the skin rapidly occur, reaching a peak at about 48 hours. Anorexia, nausea, vomiting, and other systemic symptoms also occur. There follows a latent period of apparent recovery, lasting a few days, after which the skin again becomes erythematous, with purplish ecchymotic areas that become vesicular and bullous. Pain is intense, usually requiring narcotics. A repair stage follows, and as re-epithelialization takes place, the skin becomes atrophic, hairless, and lacks functioning sebaceous glands. With large single doses, ulceration usually follows, but often is delayed for 2 or 3 months. Healing is very slow, and an atrophic, disfiguring scar is left.

**Chronic radiodermatitis** results from exposures to smaller doses of ionizing radiation (300–800 R) received daily or weekly over a long period of time, to a total dose of 5000–6000 R. The skin becomes red and eczematous, with burning and hyperesthesia. Often the epidermis sloughs, and regrowth occurs slowly over a period of 4–6 weeks. Hair is also lost, often permanently, and the sebaceous glands cease activity. The skin becomes hypopigmented and atrophic, with multiple telangiectasias. The systemic effects of irradiation are described in Chapter 12.

**A.   Video Display Terminals (VDTs):** Measurements of radiation emissions from VDTs have consistently shown nondetectable levels or levels that are consistent with background. As with many electrical devices, there is an increase in static magnetic energy very close to the terminal, but these levels have never been associated with adverse health effects. The ergonomics of the work are important, however, as tendonitis of the hands and forearms, neck strain, back pain, etc are work-related disorders that may result from disharmony between the position of the operator and the structure and function of the work station.

## OCCUPATIONAL ACNE

### Oil Acne

A better term is oil folliculitis, a common condition resulting from heavy exposure to oil, especially under oil-soaked clothing. The arms and thighs are usually affected with numerous comedones—which are often black—and pustules, furuncles, and sometimes carbuncles. This condition was once very common, especially in oil fields and refineries, but with improved engineering and less heavy contact with oils, it is seen much less frequently today. Many cases are never reported, because most workers know that with better hygiene the condition improves. The most common sources today are insoluble cutting oils in machinists and greases and lubricating oils in mechanics. Also, workers handling heavy tar distillates and coal tar pitch may develop this form of acne. Melanosis and photosensitivity also occur. Roofers, oil well drillers, coke oven workers, petroleum refiners, rubber workers, textile mill workers, and road pavers are commonly affected.

Other forms of environmental acne include **acne cosmetica** in actresses, actors, and cosmetologists; **acne mechanica** from local pressure, friction, rubbing, squeezing, and stretching, as in the wearers of heavy clothing and helmits. **Tropical acne** is common in hot, moist climates. During World War II, thousands of military personnel were evacuated from the South Pacific because of this condition. The so-called **"McDonald's" acne** results from contact with the grease and fat of frying hamburgers (Table 18–2). Nonoccupational sources of environmental acne should also be considered. These include acne from medications such as corticosteroids, testosterone and progresterone, isoniazid, diphenylhydrantoin, and iodides and bromides.

Treatment of oil folliculitis consists of oil-impervious aprons and environmental measures to limit exposure. Gloves cannot usually be worn by machinists and mechanics because of the danger of catching them in the machinery. Modernization of cutting machines with automation and special guards decreases skin contact.

### Chloracne

Chloracne is a rare condition with multiple, closed comedones and pale yellow cysts on the skin from cutaneous and systemic exposure to chloracne producting chemicals. These include polyhalogenated naphthalenes, polyhalogenated diphenyls, polyhalo-genated dibenzofuranes, contaminants of poly-chlorophenol compounds, and 3,4-dichloroaniline and related herbicides (Table 18–3). Other body areas affected are the cheeks, forehead, and neck. The shoulders, chest, back, buttocks, and abdomen may also be involved. The genitalia are especially affected, while the nose is often spared, except in systemic exposure. In addition, there may be hypertrichosis, hyperpigmentation, and increased skin fragility suggesting porphyria cutanea tarda, which is a frequent systemic complication. Conjunctivitis, swelling, and discharge from swollen meibomian glands of the eyelids are also seen, as well as a brownish pigmentation of the nails. Peripheral neuritis and hepatotoxicity may occur, which suggest systemic toxicity.

Although treatment of chloracne is often unsatisfactory, oral antibiotics, acne surgery, and occasionally dermabrasion may be helpful. Oral isotretinoin should be tried. However, the majority of cases clear within 1–2 years following cessation of exposure.

## OCCUPATIONAL SKIN CANCER

Approximately 400,000 new cases of nonmelanoma skin cancer occur in the United States each year, comprising about 30–40% of all cancers reported annually. Malignant melanoma accounts for another 18,000 or so cases. How many of these cancers are induced by the workplace is disputed, but most observers agree that it is a significant number. The most common causes of skin cancers in the work environment are (1) ultraviolet light, (2) polycylic aromatic hydrocarbons, (3) arsenic, (4) ionizing radiation, and (5) trauma. (For more information on occupational cancers see Chapter 17.)

### Ultraviolet Light

Sunlight is the most common cause of skin cancer, but workers seldom consider sunlight from the workplace as contributing to their actinically damaged skin and skin cancer. The most common skin cancers are squamous cell and basal cell carcinomas. Precursors of these are actinic keratoses and keratoacanthomas. Not only are basal cell and squamous cell carcinomas related to prolonged exposure to sunlight, but they may also be initiated by tar and oils, mechanical trauma, and burns. The primary carcinogenic action spectrum of sunlight is in the UVB range (290–320 nm). UVC (100–228 nm) and UVA (320–400 nm) rays are also photocarcinogenic; UVA rays appear to accelerate UVB-induced malignancy. UVC rays are not present in sunlight reaching the earth but are found in welding arcs and germicidal lamps.

The evidence for the skin carcinogenicity of UVB and UVA is overwhelming. Such cancers occur much more frequently in outdoor workers, as well as in persons with fair skin, light hair and eye color, and in those who tan poorly and burn easily. In addition to the time spent in sunlight, the ultraviolet radiation received by an outdoor worker depends on the latitude, season, time of day, altitude, and weather. Artificial sources of carcinogenic UV radiation include welding arcs; germicidal lamps; devices for curing and drying printing ink, plastics, and paint; UV lasers, mercury vapor lamps, and medical UV therapy machines. Radiometers are currently available and can measure the amount of UV a worker is receiving.

The evidence of a relationship between sunlight exposure and malignant melanoma is not as overwhelming. Epidemiologic studies in countries where there is a large blond-fair-skinned population, as in Australia, have shown a higher incidence of melanomas of the head, face, and neck in outdoor workers, which contrasts with office workers, in whom melanomas are more commonly found on the covered parts of the trunk and limbs. Lentigo maligna are almost always present on exposed, sun-damaged skin and become invasive after a variable period of time. Persons with xeroderma pigmentosa, a hereditary disease, are extremely sensitive to the carcinogenic effects of sunlight; a frequent cause of death in these individuals is malignant melanoma, often occurring at a young age.

## Polycyclic Aromatic Hydrocarbons

For nearly 250 years, coal tar products and certain petroleum oils have been considered potential causes of cutaneous cancers in individuals who work in certain industries. In this century, the relationship became firmly established, not only from experimental animal studies but also from numerous epidemiologic surveys. Polycyclic aromatic hydrocarbons, such as those found in soot and carbon black, coal tar, pitch and tarry products, creosote oil, and certain oils, account for the majority of cutaneous tumors. Photosensitization develops initially, with recurring erythema and intense burning of the exposed skin. After repeated episodes, poikilodermatous changes appear, especially on the exposed skin of the face, neck, and hands. Keratotic papillomas (tar warts) then develop, which later may become squamous cell carcinomas, basal cell carcinomas, and keratoacanthomas. Polycyclic aromatic hydrocarbons and UVB appear to act synergistically to induce malignant change.

## Arsenic

Although final experimental proof of carcinogenicity is lacking, epidemiologic studies since the late 1940s have strongly linked inorganic arsenic exposure to squamous cell cancers of skin and lungs. Arsenic keratoses, characteristic of chronic arsenicalism, are multiple yellow, punctate keratoses distributed symmetrically on the palms and soles. Squamous cell carcinomas and especially multiple lesions of intraepidermal squamous cell carcinoma (Bowen's disease) may develop from these keratoses. Basal cell carcinomas also occur from arsenic exposure, and they are often multiple, superficial, and pigmented.

Occupational arsenic exposure occurs in ceramic enamel workers, copper smelters, fireworks makers, gold refiners, hide preservers, carpenters (removing old wallpaper), semiconductor workers, taxidermists, and others. Arsenic as an insecticide is rarely used today; it is still employed, however, as a rodenticide.

## Ionizing Radiation

(*See "Physical Causes" section above.*)

## Trauma

Malignancies resulting from burn scars and other trauma have been reported since early in the last century. The Kangri cancers in India and the Kairo cancer in Japan are well known examples. In 1863, Virchow proposed a theory for carcinogensis based on repeated trauma; nevertheless, cancer arising from a single trauma has remained a controversial subject even today. However, litigation alleging that malignant tumors were caused by a single injury has been increasing in the United States since the 1950s, especially in worker compensation hearings. Because the etiology of cancer is still unclear, the courts have generally accepted a relationship with trauma if the evidence shows a greater than 50% probability a cancer was caused by a specific trauma.

## WORK-UP & DIAGNOSIS OF PATIENTS

The work-up and diagnosis of patients with work-related skin disease requires considerably more time than for a general dermatologic work-up. Making a premature diagnosis before studying all the evidence should be resisted, because an incorrect diagnosis can have long-lasting and severely detrimental effects. Review of the medical records, patch testing, fungal and bacterial cultures, biopsy, and other diagnostic measures as well as plant visits are often necessary to reach a correct diagnosis. Diagnosis of an endogenous or consititutional eczema or dermatitis as primary cause can be difficult for many workers to accept. Yet atopic eczema, although inherited, often has onset for the first time in adult life when precipitated by work activities, and aggravation is often considered work-related. Many other constitutional diseases can be considered similarly.

A brief outline of a typical evaluation of a work-related illness in seen in Table 18–9. The following 24 headings can serve as a form for recording the results of the work-up. The text under each heading de-

**Table 18–9.** Outline for dermatology examinations of workers' compensation patients.

| | |
|---|---|
| 1. History | 13. Discussion |
| 2. Job description | 14. Disability status |
| 3. Current treatment | 15. Factors of disability |
| 4. Present complaints |     Subjective |
| 5. Medical history |     Objective |
| 6. Family history | 16. Apportionment |
| 7. Social history | 17. Future medical care |
| 8. Personal data | 18. Vocational rehabilitation |
| 9. Medical record review |     Work restrictions |
| 10. Physical examination | 19. Disclosures |
| 11. Diagnosis | 20. Signature |
| 12. Support for diagnosis | |

tails the information that should be gathered and recorded.

## History of Injury & Current Complaints

It is important to learn exactly which anatomic skin site was first affected. Because the diagnosis is usually contact dermatitis, the eruption should begin at the site of contact with the offending agent(s). Spreading then takes place, especially in the case of allergic sensitization. The date of the initial appearance of the dermatitis is important, because often a change in workplace ergonomics and contact with new substances, or even greater contact with long-used substances, can precipitate dermatitis. Itching is important, as irritant contact dermatitis and especially allergic contact dermatitis are almost always pruritic. If improvement occurs away from work and aggravation regularly takes place on resumption of the same work, a work relationship is almost always found, and worker compensation courts will often accept this even without other evidence. Over-the-counter medicines and home remedies often contain contact allergens that can sometimes be the sole cause.

**A. Job History:** A description of the job as provided by the patient is often more accurate than the official job title. Not infrequently the worker has performed the same job for a long period of time before onset of dermatitis. This suggests a new process or contactant introduced into the workplace or home environment.

**B. Prior Employment:** The nature of previous jobs and dermatitis, as well as previous exposure to irritants and potential sensitizers, is important.

**C. Off-Work Activities:** The 40-hour work week occupies only about one-third of the week, leaving sufficient opportunity for other part-time jobs, hobbies, and house and garden work.

**D. Past Medical History:** Although 15–20% of the population has a family or personal history of atopy, it is an often overlooked cause of recurrent dermatitis, especially among hairdressers, kitchen helpers, medical-dental personnel, auto and truck repairpersons, etc. Persons even with mild atopy may

develop a major work-related hand dermatitis at the time of first employment following repeated contact with irritants. Psoriasis also can be precipitated by trauma, especially repeated intense friction and pressure on the hands.

**E. Family History:** A family history of atopy is the most important. Psoriasis, although irregularly inherited, may also be a background family condition.

**F. Habits:** Nonwork activities should be explored during the taking of the history, including habitual traumatic activities such as picking and digging the skin, especially with wooden or metal articles used for scratching and rubbing.

**G. Review of Systems:** A general review of body systems should be done.

## Review of Medical Records

Often voluminous, the records must be thoroughly examined to supplement the history as provided by the patient.

## Examination

Examination should not be limited to the part affected, as the presence of dermatitis elsewhere, as well as other skin conditions, can change an initial impression. This is especially true when psoriasis, tinea infections, lichen planus, etc are found.

**A. Special Studies:** Patch testing is the most important special study and should include not only suspected specific allergens but also a standard series of common allergens.

**B. Diagnosis:** The specific diagnosis should be recorded here, with an opinion regarding a work relationship.

**C. Summary:** This should be a brief summary of the findings, with an explanation of the conclusions. Nonmedical terms should be used as much as possible.

## Temporary & Total Disability

The disability status, total or partial, is described here. In most cases of hand dermatitis, the disability is temporary, but because of the manual nature of most work, total disability is also possible.

## Permanent & Stationary Status

Once the dermatitis has reached a plateau and no further improvement is anticipated, permanent and stationary (P and S) status is reported. This does not mean, however, that treatment cannot be resumed, should a recurrence cause a worsening of symptoms.

## Objective Findings

A brief review of the objective findings is recorded here.

## Subjective Findings

A review of the patient's complaints and a description of any impairment is provided here.

## Work Restrictions

Work restrictions, if any, can be recorded here.

## Loss of Pre-Injury Capacity

For purposes of permanent disability rating, one should describe any loss of preinjury capacity, as may occur with contact allergy.

## Causation & Apportionment

If any aspect of the impairment is related to a previous employment or any preexisting disability, this is explained here, estimating the percentage of impairment associated with each.

## Future Medical Treatment

An estimation of type and duration of future medical treatment is described here.

## Vocational Rehabilitation

Once a permanent and stationary state is reached, vocational rehabilitation must be considered. It is important to offer guidance to vocational rehabilitation personnel in job selection for disabled workers.

## Compliance Statement
## (Required in Caifornia)

In California, a compliance statement is required by law: "I declare that I personally took the history, performed the physical examination, supervised the patch testing and read the results, prepared and typed this report and read it for accuracy. I further declare under penalty of Statute 139.3 that I have not offered, delivered, received, or accepted any rebate, fund, commission, preference, patronage, dividend, discount or other consideration, whether in the form of money or otherwise, as compensation or inducement for any referred examination or evaluation."

## Signature, Date, & Place

## Patch Testing

The most important diagnostic test for occupational skin disease is the patch test. This is especially true because nearly 90% of occupational disease is contact dermatitis. Because irritant and allergic dermatitis resemble each other so closely, differentiation can be made only by patch testing, which will not only reveal the specific cause of a work-related dermatitis but, when negative after testing all possible allergens in the patient's work, will effectively rule out allergic contact dermatitis as a cause. Unfortunately the test is often performed badly or incompletely, if at all. Patch testing should be done by experienced physicians according to accepted methods with nonirritating concentrations of test substances, preferably chemicals obtained commercially from manufacturers of patch test materials.

A list and description of common contact allergens is present in Table 18–8.

## Additional Diagnostic Tests

Fungal, bacterial, and viral smears and cultures, biopsies, and prick testing if contact urticaria is suspected are sometimes required. Plant visits are an essential and integral part of the evaluation, often providing information vastly different from that learned during the patient's evaluation.

## TREATMENT

The treatment of occupational skin disease depends on the cause and differs in no essential feature from treatment of nonoccupational disease. Because in many cases a specific cause is not found, and recurrences continue to afflict the patient, treatment with corticosteroids often continues for prolonged period of time, leading to atrophy of skin and systemic complications. Although recovery may occur rapidly following treatment, the skin retains a nonspecific hypersensitivity for several weeks and for this reason, resumption of work should not be precipitous, even when the patient and/or employer are pressuring the physician.

## PREVENTION

Measures to lower the incidence of work-related dermatitis in the workplace include (1) identification of potential irritants and allergens in the workplace (utilization of MSDS), (2) engineering controls and/or chemical substitution to prevent recurrence, (3) personal protective measures, (4) insistance on personal and environmental hygiene, (5) educational efforts to promote awareness of potential irritants and allergens both at work and home, (6) motivational techniques to assure safe work practices, and (7) preemployement and periodic health screening.

### Skin Cleaners

These should be available and designed for the use intended: heavy-duty cleansers for mechanics and others working with grease and oils; mild bar or liquid soaps for workers in less dirty occupations. Industrial cleansers often contain harsh abrasives, and potentially allergenic antibacterial agents.

Waterless hand cleaners remove industrial dirt without water and can be of value in worksites without convenient washing facilities. Most are based on relatively nonirritating detergents and are removed from the skin with towels, wastepapers, or rags. When repeatedly used, they may contain a large number of irritants from the worksite.

## Protective Clothing

Protective clothing is available for almost every work situation and exposure. It must be selected with consideration of the type of work and exposures and must be inspected regularly for holes and tears. It should be remembered that certain allergens, such as methyl and ethyl methacrylate, glyceryl monothioglycolate, paraphenylenediamine, and others, readily pass through rubber gloves. Not infrequently, workers wear gloves to protect an active dermatitis; the occlusion can aggravate an existing eruption, and contact with rubber can lead to allergic sensitization to ingredients of the gloves.

## Barrier Creams

Barrier creams have been termed invisible gloves. As substitutes for protective clothing, they are almost useless and have been greatly overrated. The only effective barrier cream is a sun protective cream, which should be worn in sufficient strength (a sun protection factor of 15 or more) by all outdoor workers, especially those with fair skin.

## Plant Surveys

An often neglected part of the study of patients with occupational skin disorders is a survey of the conditions at the plant. The visit should not focus exclusively on the patient's work site, but the entire plant or at least a whole section should be visited. With a knowledgeable person as tour guide, the various worksites can be walked through. The incidence of dermatitis in the past, the presence of engineering controls, protective measures (especially protective clothing), and the general environment of the plant should be checked, including the general temperature and relative humidity. Safety Data Sheets should be available to the workers, and if there is a research and development section, further information can be obtained. Examination of workers should be conducted in private, giving the worker opportunity to openly discuss the working conditions, perceived attitudes of management, etc. A detailed written report is required.

## REFERENCES

### GENERAL

Adams RM (editor): *Occupational Skin Disease*. 3rd ed. W.B. Saunders, 1998.
Adams RM: Occupational dermatoses and disorders due to chemical agents. In: Fitzpatrick TB et al: *Dermatology in General Medicine*. Vol 1. McGraw-Hill, 1993.
Guin JD (editor): *Practical Contact Dermatitis*. McGraw-Hill, 1995.
Marks JG Jr, DeLeo VA: *Contact and Occupational Dermatology*. Mosby Year Book, 1992.
Rietschel RL, Fowler JF Jr: *Fisher's Contact Dermatitis*. Williams & Wilkins, 1995.
Rycroft RJG et al (editors): *Textbook of Contact Dermatitis*. Springer-Verlag, 1992.

### IRRITANT CONTACT DERMATITIS

Bjorkner BE: Industrial airborne dermatoses. Dermatol Clin 1994;12:501.
Elsner P: Irritant Dermatitis in the workplace. Dermatol Clin 1994;12:461.
Frosch PJ: Cutaneous irritation. Pages 28–61 in: Rycroft RJG et al (editors): *Textbook of Contact Dermatitis*. Springer-Verlag, 1992.
Jackson EM, Goldner R: *Irritant Contact Dermatitis*. Marcel Dekker, 1990.

### HYDROFLUORIC ACID BURNS

Kirkpatrick JJ, Enion DS, Burd DA: Hydrofluoric acid burns: A review. Burns 1995;21:483.

Sheridan RL et al: Emergency management of major hydrofluoric acid exposures. Burns 1995;21:62.

### PIGMENT ALTERATIONS

Gellin GA: Pigmentary changes. Pages 21–25 in: Adams RM (Editor): *Occupational Skin Disease*, 2nd ed. Saunders, 1990.

### ALLERGIC CONTACT DERMATITIS

Adams RM: Allergic contact dermatitis. Pages 26–31 in: Adams RM (editor): *Occupational Skin Disease*, 2nd ed. Saunders, 1990.
Belsito DV: Allergic contact dermatitis. Pages 1531–1542 in: Fitzpatrick TB et al: *Dermatology in General Medicine*. Vol 1. McGraw-Hill, 1993.

### PATCH TESTING

Andersen KE, Burrows D, White IR: Allergens from the standard series. Pages 416–456 in: Rycroft RJG et al (editors): *Textbook of Contact Dermatitis*, 2nd ed. Springer-Verlag, 1995.
Cronin E: Some practical supplementary trays for special occupations. Semin Dermatol 1986;5:243.
Fischer T, Maibach HI: Easier patch testing with True test. J Am Acad Dermatol 1989;20:447.
Fischer T, Maibach HI: Improved, but not perfect, patch testing. Am J Cont Derm 1990;1:73.
Rietschel R et al: The case for patch test readings beyond day 2. J Am Acad Dermatol 1988;18:42.
Wahlberg JE: Patch testing. Pages 239–268 in: Rycroft

RJG et al (editors): *Textbook of Contact Dermatitis.* Springer-Verlag, 1992.

## CONTACT URTICARIA

Hamann CP, Kick SA: Allergies associated with medical gloves. Dermatol Clin 1994;12:547.

Lahti A: Immediate Contact Reactions. Pages 62–74 in: Rycroft RJG et al (editors): *Textbook of Contact Dermatitis.* Springer-Verlag, 1992.

Turjanmaa K: Update on occupational natural rubber latex allergy. Dermatol Clin 1994;12:561.

## BIOLOGICAL CAUSES

Ancona, AA: Biologic causes. Pages 89–112 in: Adams RM (editor): *Occupational Skin Disease.* Saunders, 1990.

## PHYSICAL CAUSES

Kanerva L: Physical causes of occupational skin disease. Pages 41–65 in: Adams RM (editor): *Occupational Skin Disease.* Saunders, 1990.

## VIBRATION SYNDROME

Kanerva L: Physical causes of occupational skin disease. Page 63 in: Adams RM (editor): *Occupational Skin Disease.* Saunders, 1990.

Wasserman DE: Occupational vibration. In: Rom WN (editor): *Environmental and Occupational Medicine,* 3rd ed. Lippincott–Raven, 1997.

## CHLORACNE

Bond GG et al: Incidence of chloracne among chemical workers potentially exposed to chlorinated dioxins. J Occup Med 1989;31:771.

Coenraads P-J et al: Chloracne. Dermatol Clin 1994; 12:569.

## OCCUPATIONAL SKIN CANCER

Epstein JH, Ormsby A, Adams RM: Occupational Skin Cancer. Pages 136–159 in: Adams RM (editor): *Occupational Skin Disease,* 2nd ed. Saunders, 1990.

Green A, Battistutta D: Incidence and determinants of skin cancer in a high-risk Australian population. Int J Ca 1990;46:356.

## DIAGNOSIS

Freeman S: Diagnosis and differential diagnosis. Pages 194–214 in: Adams RM (editor): *Occupational Skin Disease,* 2nd ed. Saunders, 1990.

Marrakchi S, Maibach HI: What is occupational contact dermatitis? Occupational Dermatoses 1994;12:477.

## ATOPY IN OCCUPATION

Rystedt I: The role of atopy in occupational skin disease. Pages 215–222 in: Adams RM (editor), *Occupational Skin Disease,* 2nd ed. Saunders, 1990.

## WORKERS' COMPENSATION

Adams RM: The dermatologist and workers' compensation. Dermatol Clin 1994;12:583.

US Chamber of Commerce: Analysis of Workers' Compensation Laws—1996 Edition. US Chamber of Commerce.

## PREVENTION, REHABILITATION, & TREATMENT

Mansdorf SZ, Lubs PL: Role of the industrial hygienist: Evaluation and management of occupational skin disease. Dermatol Clin 1994;12:591.

Mansdorf SZ: Guidelines for the selection of gloves for the workplace. Dermatol Clin 1994;12:597.

# Upper Respiratory Tract Disorders

# 19

*Dennis Shusterman, MD, MPH*

The respiratory tract, with of its limited defense mechanisms and high degree of exposure to the environment, is one of the most vulnerable organ systems to chemical pollutants. As the initial portal of entry for airborne contaminants, the upper airway, including the nasal cavity, pharynx, and larynx, is the first line of defense—as well as target—for these pollutants. In addition to toxicologic agents, the upper respiratory tract can react to antigenic stimuli, allergic rhinitis occurring with (or without) asthma in some individuals. This chapter describes the spectrum of upper respiratory tract health effects associated with workplace (and environmental) chemical exposures, as well as allergic syndromes unique to workplace settings.

## ANATOMY & PHYSIOLOGY

### Functions of the Upper Airway

The upper respiratory tract, extending from the nares to the larynx (Figure 19–1), performs several essential physiological functions, including air conditioning, filtering, microbial defense, sensation, and phonation. During the fraction of a second that inspired air travels through the upper airway, its temperature is raised (or occasionally, lowered) to near body temperature, and its relative humidity is brought to between 75 and 80%. Particulate matter greater than 5–10 μm in diameter is captured on the surface of the nasal turbinates by a mechanism known as *impaction*. The majority of impacted material—captured in the mucous blanket—is transported via ciliary action until it empties into the nasopharynx and is then swallowed (a smaller fraction being transported anteriorly to the nasal vestibule). The high surface area of the turbinates and the high water content of nasal mucus further provide a "scrubbing" mechanism for water-soluble air pollutants. In terms of microbial defense, nasal secretions contain both nonspecific antimicrobial factors (lysozyme and lactoferrin) and specific factors (secretory and nonsecretory IgA); these substances are important in the host defense against viral and bacterial infections carried by the airborne route.

The sensory functions of the upper airway are twofold: odor and irritant perception (Figure 19–2). Odor perception, mediated by cranial nerve I, the olfactory nerve, not only conveys quality to life—augmenting the primary tastes in the appreciation of food, for example—but also has a safety function. Individuals lacking odor perception (anosmics) cannot distinguish fresh from spoiled food, tell that a gas pilot light has gone out in their kitchen, or sense that a respirator filter has saturated with a vapor against which they were to be protected. Upper respiratory tract irritant perception (conveyed by cranial nerve V, the trigeminal nerve) is also protective, in that nose and throat (as well as eye) irritation will trigger escape behavior during an industrial mishap, thus helping the exposed individual protect the lower respiratory tract against serious chemical injury. With lower-level exposures, however, eye, nose, and throat irritation may be the primary health end points of concern, and, as noted below, may be difficult to distinguish from allergy symptoms in some individuals.

### Acute Response Mechanisms in the Upper Airway

**A. Allergy:** Like all mucous membranes, the mucosa of the upper respiratory tract is equipped with mast cells, bearing on their surface receptors for the $F_C$ fragments of IgE molecules. In sensitized individuals, IgE molecules encountering the proper antigen can cross-link at adjacent $F_c$ receptor sites and initiate mast cell degranulation. (In addition to antigen-mediated activation, mast cells can degranulate in response to plant lectins, bee venom, and systemically-administered opiates.) Mast cell degranulation immediately releases such preformed mediators as histamine, heparin, tryptase, and leukocyte chemotactic factors; leukotrienes, prostaglandins, and cytokines are released on a delayed basis. The effects of these mediators include glandular secretion (rhinorrhea), chemotaxis (inflammation), and vasodilation (congestion). Note, airflow limitation occurs in the

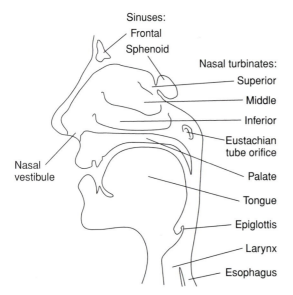

**Figure 19–1.** Anatomy of the upper respiratory tract. (Adapted with permission from: Proctor DF: The upper airways. Pages 113–118 in: *Rhinitis,* 2nd ed. Settipane G [editor]. Oceanside, 1991.)

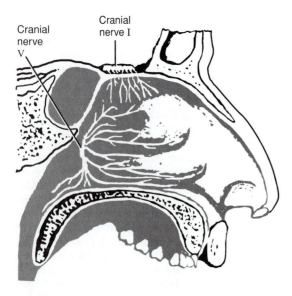

**Figure 19–2.** Innervation of the nasal cavity (simplified). "Cr. N. I" = first cranial (olfactory) nerve; "Cr. N. V" = fifth cranial (trigeminal) nerve. (Source: Shusterman D. Critical review: The health significance of environmental odor pollution. Arch Environ Health 1992;**47**:76; reproduced with permission.)

upper respiratory tract due to venous pooling and/or extravasation of plasma, not via smooth muscle contraction as in the lower tract. This produces engorgement of the nasal mucosa and thereby encroaches on the airway.

**B. Neurogenic Reflexes:** Of perhaps equal importance with reference to occupational and environmental exposures are the various neurogenic reflexes that can be triggered by chemical irritant exposures. Stimulation of trigeminal nerve afferents—which are sensitive to low pH, some endogenous inflammatory mediators (such as bradykinin), and chemical irritants (the prototype being capsaicin)—results in two major types of reflex response: (1) parasympathetic reflexes, carried by the facial nerve (cranial nerve VII) and (2) axon reflexes, consisting of neuropeptides release from *afferent* branches of the trigeminal nerve. A familiar example of a parasympathetic response is so-called "gustatory rhinitis," a copious, watery rhinorrhea that occurs with the ingestion of spicy foods. The axon reflex, on the other hand, is of more theoretical than proven importance in the upper airway response to chemical irritants. A postulated pathophysiologic scheme including both allergic and neurogenic mechanisms appears in Figure 19–3.

## OCCUPATIONAL/ ENVIRONMENTAL CONDITIONS

### Occupational Allergic Rhinitis

An estimated 20% of the population suffers from allergic rhinitis, and another 5% suffers from various forms of nonallergic rhinitis. Typically, these individuals experience either seasonal pollinosis or—if allergic to common indoor allergens—perennial symptoms of sneezing, rhinorrhea, and nasal congestion. Workplace allergens producing allergic rhinoconjunctivitis may either be commonly encountered allergens, exposure to which may be incidental to the work environment (eg, grass pollen exposure in a landscaper), or may be unusual agents encountered only in industrial environments (eg, trimellitic anhydride exposure in a plastics worker). Initial sensitization may occur either in the workplace or outside, with the latter scenario being more likely with common environmental allergens. Thus, as is the case with asthma, occupational allergic rhinitis may either be work-*induced* or work-*exacerbated*. Representative agents producing occupational allergic rhinitis appear in Table 19–1; the reader will immediately recognize these same agents can produce occupational asthma (and, indeed, many sensitized individuals suffer from both conditions).

Additional—and unanticipated—consequences may accrue from the diagnosis of allergic rhinitis. Limited data exist linking variations in nasal congestion, as measured by nasal airway resistance, in rhinitics and

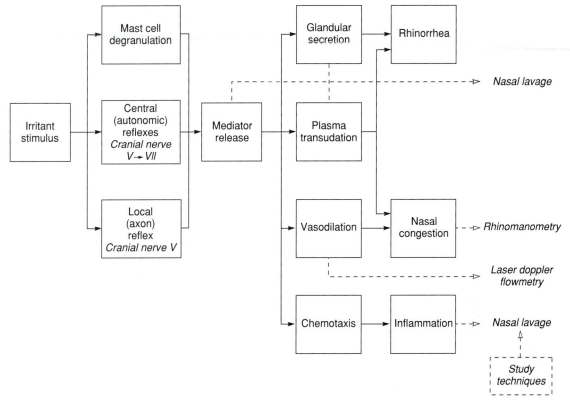

**Figure 19–3.** Potential mechanisms responsible for the acute nasal response to irritants; applicable study techniques appear on the right.

variations in severity of obstructive sleep apnea symptoms. In addition, high-grade nasal obstruction predisposes to oral breathing, thus bypassing some of the microbial defenses normally operative during nasal breathing, and in some occupational contexts

potentially rendering the worker more susceptible to selected airborne pathogens.

**A. Diagnosis and Management:** Allergic rhinitis is characterized by sneezing, itching, rhinorrhea, and congestion, with or without associated eye and chest symptoms. Nonoccupational symptoms occurring during a portion of the year (typically from pollens) characterize "seasonal allergic rhinitis," in contrast to "perennial allergic rhinitis" (with symptoms occurring year-round, in response to such indoor allergens as dust mite, cat dander, cockroach, or mold spores). Occupational allergic rhinitis may exhibit either of the above temporal features, although perennial is somewhat more common. Superimposed on variations across the calendar year may be variation across the work week, with "ratcheting" of symptoms on successive work days and improvement on weekends and vacations. Importantly, individuals with occupational allergic rhinitis may be sensitized to both workplace and nonworkplace antigens and may also react to irritants, further complicating the diagnostic picture.

The diagnosis of occupational allergic rhinitis is based upon the history, physical examination, with a pale, boggy nasal mucosa being typical, and labora-

**Table 19–1.** Agents associated with occupational allergic rhinitis.

**High molecular weight compounds (proteins)**

Animal antigens (animal handlers, farmers, veterinarians)
Green coffee bean and castor bean (dock workers)
Proteolytic enzymes (detergent workers, cosmetologists)
Grains/contaminants (bakers, farmers, grain handlers)
Insect antigens (various occupations)
Gum arabic/gum acacia (printers)
Psyllium (health care workers)
Latex (health care workers)

**Low molecular weight compounds**

Diisocyanates (polyurethanes → painters, boat builders, etc)
Acid anhydrides (plastics → painters, fabricators, etc)
Colophony (rosin core solder → electronics workers)
Plicatic acid (western red cedar → saw mill workers)
Antibiotics (health care workers)

tory testing. The latter may include a complete blood count and/or nasal smear demonstrating eosinophilia, increased serum total IgE, and the in vitro RAST (radioallergosorbent testing) or ELISA (enzyme-linked immunosorbent assay) finding of work antigen-specific IgE. Skin prick testing, with saline and histamine controls, is considered by many clinicians to be the "gold standard" of allergy testing. If neither an in vitro system or an allergy testing extract is available for a suspected occupational allergen, response to allergen avoidance and/or therapy may provide the best clue to the specific diagnosis. Nasal inspiratory peak flow measurements (see below) may provide objective validation of cross-shift symptoms and can be employed during adjacent periods of allergen avoidance and normal work routine to help establish an occupational etiology.

As alluded to above, allergen avoidance should be an important component of therapy, both for the control of nasal symptoms and to prevent the progression of incipient occupational asthma. Whether engineering controls or personal protective equipment can sufficiently control antigen exposure levels must be answered on a case-by-case basis; some individuals may require reassignment, particularly if chest symptoms are coincident. A particularly frustrating situation presents itself in health care settings, where latex-sensitive individuals with respiratory allergies are not only prevented from wearing latex gloves, but frequently cannot work near others wearing such gloves (the powder on the gloves serves as a carrier for the latex antigen).

Mainstays of medical therapy for allergic rhinitis include systemic antihistamines, nasal steroids, and the mast cell stabilizer, cromolyn sodium; newer inhaled medications are either pending or newly released at the time of writing (ie, antihistamines and cholinergic blockers). Of the antihistamines, terfenadine, loratidine, and astemizole are nonsedating alternatives that may allow one to control symptoms while simultaneously staying productive and alert. Because of potentially serious drug interactions, terfenadine and astemizole should not be prescribed with some antibiotics (erythromycin, azithromycin, or clarithromycin) or antifungals (ketoconozole or itraconazole). Of the nasal topical steroids, aqueous-based formulations tend to be less irritating than alcohol-based; patients should be instructed that as much as 2 weeks of therapy may be necessary before an optimal response is observed from either topical steroids or cromolyn sodium. Nasal topical decongestants are to be avoided except for very brief control of acute symptoms, the possibility of tachyphylaxis and rebound ("rhinitis medicamentosa") being ever-present. The efficacy of desensitization ("allergy shots") has been better evaluated for common aeroallergens than for specific occupational sensitizers.

## Occupational Irritant Rhinitis

The eyes, nose, and throat are sensitive to chemical irritants (including gases, vapors, dusts, and smokes), with mucous membrane irritation giving rise to the most commonly reported symptoms in problem work environments. Subtypes of chemical irritants in office or home air include combustion products (from tobacco smoke and malfunctioning appliances) and volatile organic compounds or "VOCs" (from cleaning products, office supplies and machines, and building materials and furnishings). Industrial environments may present workers with an even wider range of airborne irritants, with the majority of both threshold limit values (TLV) and permissible exposure limits (PEL) being based upon the irritancy of the compound in question. Extreme forms of industrial irritant rhinitis occur in electroplaters and others exposed to chromic acid, who may develop nasal mucosal ulcerations and even septal perforation. Finally, exposure to photochemical air pollution can also produce objective inflammatory changes in the upper airway. Pathophysiologically, it is believed that the most important determinant of a compound's initial site of irritancy is its water solubility (Figure 19–4).

**A. Diagnosis and Management:** Since irritant-associated symptoms—such as nasal congestion and rhinorrhea—may mimic an allergic response, the treating health professional may be faced with a diagnostic challenge in determining responsible etiologic agents and pathophysiologic processes. The report of predominantly irritant symptoms rather than itching or sneezing, a high symptom prevalence rate among co-workers, and dramatic improvement at night and on weekends supports a diagnosis of irri-

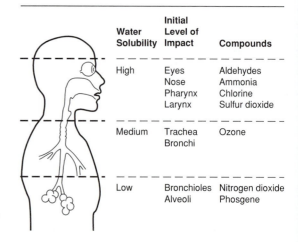

| Water Solubility | Initial Level of Impact | Compounds |
|---|---|---|
| High | Eyes Nose Pharynx Larynx | Aldehydes Ammonia Chlorine Sulfur dioxide |
| Medium | Trachea Bronchi | Ozone |
| Low | Bronchioles Alveoli | Nitrogen dioxide Phosgene |

**Figure 19–4.** Water solubility of pollutants and initial site of irritation. (Adapted from: United States Department of Health and Human Services: The Health Consequences of Involuntary Smoking. Surgeon General's Office, 1996.)

tant rhinitis. Similarly, erythema of the mucous membranes—particularly punctate erosion of the nasal mucosa—supports an irritant process, although the finding is neither sensitive nor specific. In irritant rhinitis the laboratory workup is essentially "negative," including a lack of systemic eosinophilia, a normal total serum IgE, the predominance of neutrophils on nasal smear, and—when applicable—a lack of skin test (or in vitro) reactivity to identified workplace allergens. Air monitoring data may be of assistance in industrial settings but are more often a source of frustration in the investigation of so-called "problem buildings," since symptoms may be reported in settings in which levels of VOCs are low relative to current occupational exposure limits. The role of complex mixtures in explaining such discrepancies is explored below, under the heading of "Research Studies."

Treatment for occupational irritant rhinitis consists of reduction of exposure, nonspecific supportive measures (eg, saline nasal lavage), and occasionally topical steroids. Patients troubled by prominent reflex symptoms (eg, congestion and rhinorrhea) may benefit from the topical cholinergic blocker, ipratropium bromide. In atopic patients, control of intercurrent allergic rhinitis—whether occupational or nonoccupational—may also decrease reactivity to chemical irritants, although this issue has not been well-studied.

## Occupational "Vasomotor" Rhinitis

Vasomotor rhinitis—a subcategory of nonallergic rhinitis—is a term that is sometimes used to describe augmented nasal reactivity to nonspecific physical stimuli. Symptoms of rhinorrhea tend to predominate. Relevant physical stimuli include low humidity, extremes in—or rapid changes of—temperature, and excessive air motion. Possibly linked to this diagnosis are "gustatory rhinitis" (rhinorrhea in response to the ingestion of spicy foods) and "bright light rhinitis" (self-explanatory). Guidelines for temperature and humidity control in indoor air have been promulgated by the American Society of Heating, Refrigerating, and Air-Conditioning Engineers (ASHRAE) and by the Occupational Safety and Health Administration (OSHA); these parameters should be assessed as part of any "problem building" investigation.

**A. Diagnosis and Management:** Although no routine diagnostic tests characterize this condition, methacholine or histamine have sometimes been used, in titrated doses, to document nonspecific nasal reactivity in this—or other—rhinitis syndromes (see "Diagnostic Techniques," below). Treatment of vasomotor rhinitis may include environmental intervention, nonspecific topical measures (eg, saline lavage), or use of the topical anticholinergic agent, ipratropium bromide. Decongestant nasal sprays should

be used with caution because of potential tachyphylaxis and rebound.

## Other (Nonoccupational) Rhinitis Syndromes

Along with the rhinitis syndromes reviewed above—which may have occupational, nonoccupational, or mixed inciting factors—there are a number of other rhinitides that have not been linked with environmental exposures. These diagnoses are listed here for the sake of completeness in differential diagnosis:

- Nonallergic rhinitis with eosinophilia ("NARES") syndrome
- Endocrine rhinitis
- Wegener's granulomatosis
- Nasal polyposis
- Immotile cilia/Kartagener's syndrome
- Cystic fibrosis

## Paranasal Sinus Disease

Active smokers are at higher risk for developing acute (and chronic) sinusitis than are nonsmokers. Evidence for a link between sinusitis and environmental tobacco smoke exposure, on the other hand, is equivocal at this time. Relatively few studies have examined the endpoint of sinusitis and occupational exposures. Surveys of furriers, spice workers, vegetable picklers, hemp workers, and grain and flour workers all include increased prevalence rates for sinusitis, but these studies are based upon self-report only and should therefore be viewed as preliminary. Pathophysiologically, the causal sequence for an occupationally-induced (or exacerbated) sinusitis may include initial allergic or irritant rhinitis, ciliastasis (with impaired clearance of pathogenic organisms), mucous membrane swelling (with occlusion of sinus ostia and impaired drainage), and finally, infection. Clinically, a worker who recounts a story of apparent occupational rhinitis followed by sinusitis may well be describing a work-related condition. Cases refractory to antibiotic treatment should be revisited from the standpoint of allergen avoidance, irritant avoidance, or both.

Inflammation in the upper and lower respiratory tracts appears to be linked, in that active sinusitis apparently augments nonspecific bronchial reactivity in asthmatics. Postulated mechanisms include up-regulation of neurogenic responses and aspiration of biochemical-mediator laden nasal secretions into the lower respiratory tract. Another link between the upper and lower respiratory tracts occurs in the clinical triad of nasal polyposis, asthma, and aspirin sensitivity, although no occupational connection is known to exist with this syndrome.

A variety of occupations and imputed exposures have been linked with the development of malignant neoplasms of the paranasal sinuses; these appear in

**Table 19–2.** Agents and processes associated with sino-nasal cancer.

Wood dust
Leather dust
Nickel refining
Chromates ($Cr^{6+}$)
Cigarette smoking
Mustard gas manufacturing
Isopropanol manufacturing (strong acid method)
Welding, flame cutting, and brazing(?)

Table 19–2. The strongest (and most consistent) findings pertain to leather- and wood-workers, although nickel refining, chrome refining and plating, and formaldehyde-exposed workers have also been found to be at risk in some studies.

## Laryngeal Pathology

Symptoms referable to phonation—typically, "hoarseness"—can also occur in work settings. Temporary and reversible hoarseness may occur either from exposure to inhaled chemical irritants or due to overuse of the voice. Although overuse is most widely recognized in lecturers and singers, it also occurs among industrial employees who need to communicate (shout) in noisy environments. The most ominous condition heralded by hoarseness—squamous cell carcinoma of the larynx—has been associated with a number of occupations/exposures; these appear in Table 19–3.

At least two other occupational/environmental conditions deserve mention. Laryngeal strictures may occur after a smoke inhalation injury—resulting either from the initial chemical/thermal insult or secondary to prolonged intubation. Finally, laryngeal papillomatosis has been described in a physician whose apparent exposure was human papillomavirus aerosolized during laser surgery; this occurred despite the use of a conventional smoke extractor and paper mask during the procedures.

## Otitis Media in Children

An increased incidence of otitis media with effusion (OME) has been reported among children exposed to environmental tobacco smoke (ETS), typically in the home. The highest risk appears to occur at approximately 18 months of age, although measurable excesses occur from at least ages 6 months to

**Table 19–3.** Agents and processes associated with laryngeal cancer.

Asbestos
Cigarette smoking
Ethanol consumption
Formaldehyde(?)
Leather and textile workers(?)
Gasoline, diesel oil, mineral oil(?)

3 years. Postulated mechanisms center on eustachian tube dysfunction, with ETS-associated irritants producing ciliastasis and mucous membrane congestion, resulting in impaired pressure equalization, middle ear effusion, reduced drainage of middle ear secretions, and finally, infection. Because of the strength and consistency of this finding, the workup of recurrent otitis media in young children should always include questions about parental smoking.

## Sensory (Olfactory) Alterations

Both temporary and long-lasting alterations in olfactory function have been reported among workers exposed to a variety of industrial chemicals. Chemically-induced olfactory dysfunction may include (1) **quantitative defects**, including *hyposmia* (reduced odor acuity) and *anosmia* (absent odor perception); and (2) **qualitative defects**, including *olfactory agnosia* (decreased ability to identify odors) and various *dysosmias*—distorted odor perception—including *aliosmias* (unpleasant sensations from normally pleasant odorants) and *parosmias* (phantom odors). Occupational groups and exposures for which defects in odor detection or identification have been identified have included alkaline battery workers and braziers (cadmium ± nickel exposure), tank cleaners (hydrocarbon exposure), paint formulators (solvent ± acrylic acid exposure), and chemical plant workers (ammonia and sulfuric acid exposures); other groups have been studied less systematically. Toxicologically, hydrogen sulfide is well-known to produce acute and reversible "olfactory paralysis" upon exposure at levels in excess of approximately 50 parts per million; the various mercaptans may share this property. Among patients with hyposmia or anosmia as a group, nasal obstruction is the most common etiology. Chemical irritant exposures may cause hyposmia via inflammation and consequent nasal obstruction or may produce direct damage to the olfactory epithelium itself.

Experimentally, at least one study has shown the olfactory equivalent of a "temporary threshold shift" (reversible olfactory deficit) after several hours of controlled exposure to either toluene or xylene; subjects recovered olfactory acuity within about 2 hours of cessation of exposure. Since the deficit was evident for the test odorant closely related to the experimental exposure (toluene), but not for a test compound unrelated to the exposure (phenyl-methyl carbinol), this phenomenon might be thought of as an extension of the familiar process of *adaptation*, in which odors lose their intensity during continuous exposure.

Of importance in the differential diagnosis, causes of olfactory impairment not directly related to chemical exposures include head trauma, chronic nasal obstruction (of whatever etiology), postinfectious inflammation, neurodegenerative and endocrine disorders, hepatic and renal disease, neoplasms, various drugs, ionizing radiation, congenital defects (eg, Kallmann's syndrome), and selected psychiatric conditions.

## DIAGNOSTIC TECHNIQUES

A number of different diagnostic techniques may be useful in study of nasal responses to environmental agents; these have been classified here as "routine," "semi-routine," and "experimental" methods.

### Routine Methods

Several techniques that are routine in otolaryngologic and allergy practice may contribute to the diagnostic workup of patients with upper airway conditions of suspected occupational or environmental origin.

**A. Allergy Skin Testing:** Often called "skin prick testing," allergy skin testing is the most commonly applied diagnostic test in allergy specialty practices. In vitro allergy tests (RAST and ELISA) provide analogous (but not necessarily equivalent) data to skin testing and require less time and technical expertise on the part of the treating physician. Both techniques are used to identify antigen-specific IgE in clinically significant concentrations. Skin prick testing results in an acute skin reaction, with the size of a wheal being compared to saline and histamine controls, whereas the in vitro assays provide a quantitative estimate of allergen-specific IgE. Because of limited numbers of affected individuals, some occupational allergens may not be readily available as either skin test antigens or in vitro reagents.

**B. Nasal Cytology:** Nasal smears for cytologic analysis are used to provide information regarding the inflammatory cells in nasal mucus and/or the superficial mucosal layers. Various staining techniques are used to distinguish among cell types. Typically, eosinophils predominate in allergic inflammation, whereas lymphocytes and neutrophils predominate with viral and bacterial infections, respectively. Based upon both experimental and field studies of air pollutant effects, one would expect neutrophils to predominate in nasal smears taken from individuals with irritant rhinitis.

**C. Impedance Tympanometry:** This test is used to document middle ear pathology, including eustachian tube dysfunction and middle ear effusions. The technique is based upon the premise that tympanic membrane impedance is increased (and sound energy conduction is decreased) if tympanic membrane mobility is restricted in any way and that the changes in sound conduction that occur with changes in externally-applied pressure reveal the state of pressurization of the middle ear. Functionally, impedance tympanograms are classified as types A (normal), B (otitis media with effusion), and C

(eustachian tube dysfunction). Impedance tympanometry is a valuable screening tool in children because it is objective, minimally invasive, and does not require a high degree of cooperation by the child being tested.

**D. Nasal Endoscopy:** Nasal endoscopy—particularly utilizing a flexible scope—is a procedure that could potentially be mastered by most primary care (including occupational medicine) clinicians. With an external diameter of less than 3.5 mm, the flexible nasopharyngoscope is generally well-tolerated and permits the examiner to directly visualize nasal, pharyngeal, and glottic structures with relative ease. Identification of nasal polyps, purulent secretions per sinus ostia, lymphoid hyperplasia, neoplasms, vocal cord pathology, and other pathologic conditions becomes relatively straightforward using the flexible nasopharyngoscope. The examination requires use of both a topical anesthetic and a vasoconstrictor for optimal visualization and patient comfort. Some otolaryngologists prefer the use of rigid nasal endoscopes because of their superior optics; multiple instruments (with varying view angles) may then be needed in order to provide an adequate field of view.

### Semi-Routine Methods

In addition to routine techniques, there are several study methods that, in experienced hands, may prove valuable in diagnosing occupational or environmental upper airway conditions. These include:

- Nasal peak flow measurement
- Rhinomanometry
- Acoustic rhinometry
- Psychophysical testing
- Mucociliary clearance tests.

**A. Nasal Peak Flow Measurement:** Nasal inspiratory peak flow measurement is not considered "routine," not because of any technical difficulty involved, but because the technique and equipment are not well-known. One readily available commercial unit consists of a Wright mini peak-flow meter mounted "backwards" within a transparent plastic cylinder, with an anesthesia mask mounted at the outlet of the flow meter (Figure 19–5). A stainless steel rod allows patients to reset the sliding pointer, which would otherwise be inaccessible within the plastic sleeve. To take a measurement, the patient breathes out maximally (to residual volume), places the mask over his or her nose and mouth, and then inhales forcefully through the nose to total lung capacity. Three replicate measures are usually taken, with the highest value being "counted." A diary of nasal peak flow measurements (along with nasal symptom ratings) can be kept, with the patient recording peak flow before, during, and after a work shift, preferably over at least one work week and adjacent weekends (Figure 19–6). Interpretation of

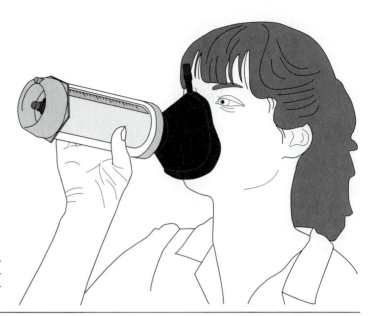

**Figure 19–5.** Commercial nasal peak inspiratory flow meter. (Source: Clement-Clark Corporation, Columbus, OH; reproduced with permission.)

these data is very similar to the process of interpreting peak expiratory flow data in the diagnosis of occupational asthma, although no consensus standards exist for "significant" work-related decrements in peak flow. Inevitably, issues of trust arise in cases involving medical/legal issues; instructions should consequently be explicit with respect to technique, but not with respect to expected data patterns.

**B. Rhinomanometry:** Rhinomanometry, the measurement of nasal airway resistance, was first described using modified pulmonary function equipment in the mid-1960s. Basically, the technique in-

Name _____     ID No. _____

| Date | Time | Nasal Peak Flow | | | Please rate any symptoms (0–5)* | | | | | Notes |
|------|------|---|---|---|------|------|------|------|------|------|
| | | 1 | 2 | 3 | Nasal Congestion | Nasal Irritation | Runny Nose | Postnasal Drip | Headache | |
| | | | | | | | | | | |
| | | | | | | | | | | |
| | | | | | | | | | | |
| | | | | | | | | | | |
| | | | | | | | | | | |
| | | | | | | | | | | |
| | | | | | | | | | | |
| | | | | | | | | | | |
| | | | | | | | | | | |
| | | | | | | | | | | |
| | | | | | | | | | | |
| | | | | | | | | | | |

* Symptom rating: 0=None; 1=Slight; 2=Moderate; 3=Strong; 4=Very strong; 5=Overpowering.

**Figure 19–6.** Sample format for nasal symptom/nasal peak inspiratory flow rate diary.

volves measuring two pressure differentials—one across a precision flow resistor, or pneumotachometer ("flow"), and the other between the nasopharynx and anterior nares ("pressure"). Usually, the individual being tested wears a face mask (eg, anesthesia mask) during testing, and the pressure within the mask is taken as anterior nasal pressure. Nasopharyngeal pressure, in turn, is measured in one of two ways. In "anterior" rhinomanometry, one nostril at a time is occluded with a pressure tap, and the subject breathes slowly through the opposite nostril. In "posterior" rhinomanometry, the subject holds a flexible tube between the tongue and hard palate, and breathes slowly through both nostrils.

The two approaches to rhinomanometry have differing strengths, weaknesses, and anatomical/patient cooperation requirements. Anterior rhinomanometry is particularly useful for documenting fixed anatomical pathology that may be unilateral in distribution (eg, deviated septum or polyposis). Posterior rhinomanometry gives a more stable estimate of total nasal airway resistance than the anterior technique and is therefore of particular utility in documenting the response of the nose to challenge agents (allergens or irritants). In anterior rhinomanometry, the pressure at the anterior nares on the occluded side can be taken as equal to nasopharyngeal pressure as long as flow is zero between the two points (the nares is indeed sealed), the nasal cavity on the occluded side is at least partially patent, and there is no septal perforation. The zero-flow requirement is also relevant in posterior rhinomanometry (ie, the oral pressure tap is taken to be at the same pressure as the nasopharynx as long as the lips are tightly sealed). Although the other (anatomical) requirements do not pertain to the posterior technique, patient cooperation is sometimes problematic, with an estimated 15–20% of subjects being unable to produce usable curves without extensive coaching. Anterior rhinomanometry, on the other hand, requires minimal subject preparation.

Measurement conventions for rhinomanometry specify a location from which a line is drawn to the graphical origin (0 pressure, 0 flow) in order to estimate a slope that defines "nasal airway resistance" (NAR = pressure/flow). Alternatives include (1) the intersection of the pressure-flow tracing with a line of constant pressure (normally, 150 Pa for anterior rhinomanometry and 75 Pa for posterior rhinomanometry); (2) the intersection of the pressure-flow tracing with an ellipse connecting specified pressure and flow intercepts (the "Broms" method); and (3) the point at which the pressure-flow tracing crosses a line of constant flow (eg, 150 cc/sec). Of these, the first two conventions have been favored. A single posterior rhinomanometry tracing interpreted utilizing various measurement conventions is illustrated in Figure 19–7.

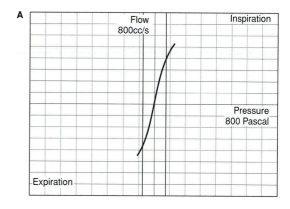

NAR = 211 Pa / L / sec

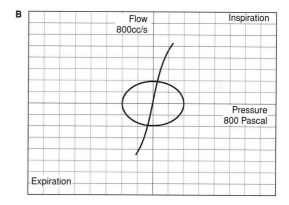

NAR = 190 Pa / L / sec

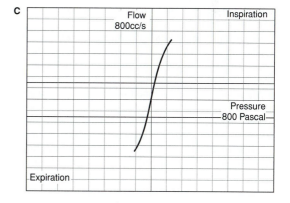

NAR = 143 Pa / L / sec

**Figure 19–7.** A single posterior rhinomanometry tracing interpreted utilizing: *(A)* the pressure-cutoff method (75 Pa); *(B)* the "Broms" method (200 "units"); and *(C)* the flow-cutoff method (150 cc/sec). Note that the different methods yield different nasal airway resistance (NAR) values.

Factors influencing nasal airway resistance include chronic anatomical changes (see above), short-term physiologic changes (the so-called "nasal cycle," in which the two sides of the nose alternately congest and decongest during the day), and reversible pathophysiologic processes (allergen- or irritant-induced vasodilatation or plasma extravasation, producing engorgement of the turbinates and encroachment on the airway). Other factors known to influence NAR include exercise (decreases) and recumbency (increases). NAR has been used as the endpoint for various pharmacologic challenge protocols, notably the use of serially increasing concentrations of histamine or methacholine designed to specify the concentration necessary to induce a predetermined percent increase in NAR. Using this method, allergic rhinitics studied in and out of season show systematic differences in nonspecific nasal reactivity (greater during allergy season). This information is analogous to that provided by a bronchial methacholine challenge test and may be of equal utility in diagnosing occupational allergic or irritant rhinitis.

**C. Acoustic Rhinometry:** Acoustic rhinometry is another technique designed to measure nasal airway patency. The apparatus consists of a tube with an acoustic pulse generator (and microphone) at one end and a nasal speculum at the other; the instrument alternately sends and receives sound pulses. By measuring the intensity of reflected sound waves at various time intervals from the initial pulse, an acoustic rhinometer produces a map of total nasal cross-sectional area as a function of distance from the nares. The relationship between cross-sectional area and nasal airway resistance, however, is a complex one, rendering the physiologic and symptomatic interpretation of acoustic rhinometry even more difficult than is the case with rhinomanometry.

**D. Psychophysical Testing:** Psychophysical testing of olfaction focuses on one of a number of endpoints. *Qualitative odor testing* utilizes panels of test odorants to assess odor identification ability. Typically, such tests are administered as a multiple-choice task, in order to prevent the patient's personal experiential background from having undue influence on testing results. One commercially available qualitative test, the University of Pennsylvania Smell Identification Test (UPSIT), takes the form of "scratch-n-sniff" panels on a paper or cardboard base, for ease of administration; the test has been well-standardized with adequate population norms. *Qualitative odor testing* takes two general forms: threshold and supra-threshold. Threshold testing usually involves a forced-choice discrimination task using an ascending (or, occasionally, descending) series of squeeze bottles with matching blanks. The concentration of the test odorant (usually dissolved in water or mineral oil) varies geometrically rather than arithmetically, in accordance with the so-called Weber-Fechner law (which states that the perceived

intensity of a stimulus varies with the log of its intensity). A threshold so obtained is an *olfactory detection threshold*. At least one commercial vendor (Olfacto Labs, El Cerrito, Calif) markets a variety of test odorants in pre-diluted bottles; again, the clinical utility of these test sets is predicated upon their population standardization. A *hybrid qualitative-quantitative test* is the determination of the so-called *olfactory identification threshold* of a familiar odorant. Olfactory stimuli above threshold can also be quantitatively rated using a variety of systems, some of which allow for comparisons of the so-called *psychophysical function* (steepness of the rating response vs stimulus strength curve) between subjects.

**E. Mucociliary Clearance Tests:** Mucociliary clearance tests include both invasive and noninvasive procedures. Perhaps the best standardized test is the observation of ciliary beat frequency in vitro. This method is often employed as a screening step (prior to electron microscopic examination of biopsy specimens) in the diagnosis of disorders involving ultrastructural abnormalities in epithelial cilia (eg, primary ciliary dyskinesia, with or without full-blown Kartagener's syndrome). Specimens are typically obtained either by scraping or biopsy of the inferior turbinate; ciliary beat frequency is normally in the 9–15 Hz range. In addition to frequency, trained observers can note the degree of spatial coordination of adjacent ciliary units, an important component of intact function. Although ciliary beat frequency is a relatively objective and reproducible measure, its relationship to particle clearance and clinical symptoms is less constant, as noted below.

Another method of documenting mucociliary clearance involves tracking—radiographically—the movement of objects placed in the nasal cavity, typically on the superior surface of the inferior turbinate. The object in question may be a radio-opaque disk or spherule (in which case imaging is by serial plain films), or a radiotagged particle that is tracked with a gamma camera. An obvious drawback of this technique is the exposure of patients (or experimental subjects) to small doses of ionizing radiation.

The so-called *saccharine test* is the least intrusive measure of nasal mucociliary dysfunction currently in use. In this procedure, a small drop of saccharine solution is placed on the anterior portion of the inferior turbinate and the time interval before the subject *tastes* the saccharine is recorded. A prolonged test—defined as greater than 30 minutes—indicates impaired mucociliary function. The major drawback of the saccharine test lies in its lack of cross-test correlation with other mucociliary clearance measures.

Mucociliary clearance is important because of its essential function in microbial defense. Patients with impaired mucus formation (cystic fibrosis) or impaired ciliary function (primary ciliary dyskinesia) experience repeated episodes of bronchitis, otitis, and sinusitis, with ultimate cardiopulmonary complications (bronchiectasis and cor pulmonale) being a distinct likelihood. Environmental factors that have been noted to impair mucociliary clearance include viral infection, antigen challenge, cigarette smoke, and sulfur dioxide (see below).

## Experimental Methods

**A. Nasal Mucosal Blood Flow:** Nasal mucosal blood flow is significant physiologically, since engorgement of submucosal venous sinusoids produces reversible thickening of the nasal mucosa and a consequent decrease in airway cross-sectional area and increase in airway resistance. This parameter can be documented noninvasively by the use of laser Doppler flowmetry, enabling investigators to measure flow rate (per unit volume of tissue), mean RBC velocity, and tissue blood volume percent. The technique works on the principle that coherent light reflected from moving blood elements is shifted in frequency relative to incident (and reflected) light. A drawback of this technique is the requirement that a fiberoptic probe remain in relatively constant approximation to the mucosa, severely restricting an experimental subject's movement during provocation testing. Consistent with this limitation, provocation tests to date have focused on rapidly acting (pharmacologic or antigenic) stimuli. Notwithstanding these limitations, this technique could be adapted for irritant inhalation challenge tests in the future, particularly with such rapidly acting agents as environmental tobacco smoke.

**B. Nasal Lavage:** Nasal lavage is a technique used in experimental studies for examining the effect of allergens (or irritants) on inflammatory cell recruitment and biochemical mediators. Several specific techniques have been developed, including the use of aerosol sprays with either forced expulsion of lavage fluid or drainage under suction (Figure 19–8). Another set of techniques involves the introduction of several cc of warmed, physiologic saline via syringe and nasal "olive" (plug), with subsequent withdrawal of the lavage fluid directly into the syringe. Potential parameters examined in nasal lavage fluid include (1) cell count and differential and (2) concentrations of biochemical mediators (eg, histamine, tryptase, neuropeptides, cytokines, and leukotrienes) and markers of plasma transudation, glandular secretion (eg, albumin, lactoferrin, lysozyme), or both. Depending on the response patterns of these various markers, it may be possible to distinguish between allergic (mast cell-mediated) and neurogenic (parasympathetic and/or neuropeptide-mediated) response mechanisms to various provocation stimuli.

**C. Chemosensory Evoked Responses:** Chemosensory evoked responses include responses to olfactory nerve stimulation ("olfactory evoked potentials") and responses to trigeminal nerve stimulation ("chemosomatosensory evoked potentials"). As is the case with other sensory evoked responses, special

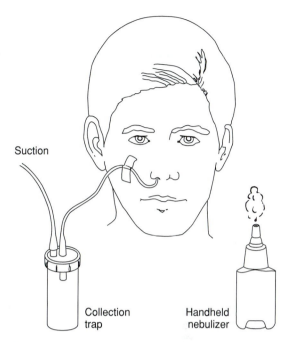

**Figure 19–8.** Nasal lavage technique utilizing aerosolized saline and catheter connected to suction. (Source: Raphael G, et al. How and why the nose runs. J Allergy Clin Immunol 1991;**87:**457; reproduced with permission.)

stimulus-delivery devices must be constructed to allow sharply demarcated pulsed stimuli to be presented to the target site (the nose). Electroencephalographic differentiation of these stimuli involve differing spatial patterns of recording potentials, with olfactory evoked potentials being more apparent in the parieto-central area, and chemosomatosensory (or trigeminal) evoked potentials being stronger in the vertex. These techniques are of considerable theoretical importance, although, to date, their clinical applications have been explored to only a limited degree.

**D. Irritant-Induced Mucosal Potentials:** Irritant-induced mucosal potentials consist of negative voltage spikes that occur transiently with the onset of nasal irritant stimuli. Recording of these potentials requires the placement of a salt bridge in contact with the nasal septum, with the insertion of a reference electrode subcutaeously (normally in the forearm). Interestingly, capsaicin desensitization—a method of reducing one's symptomatic response to irritant stimuli—simultaneously decreases this electrophysiologic response. This technique represents an important advance in recording technology, although its invasiveness may limit its use to research applications.

## Controlled Exposure Studies of Upper Airway Irritants

A number of study techniques, listed above under

**Table 19–4.** Controlled exposure studies of upper respiratory tract irritants.

| Pollutant | Rhino- manometry | Nasal Lavage | Mucociliary Clearance | Mucosal Blood Flow |
|---|---|---|---|---|
| Ozone | Blocks exercise decongestion of non-allergics | ↑ PMNs (+ eosinophils in allergic rhinitis) | | |
| Sulfur dioxide | ↑ /nc NAR | | ↓ Clearance | |
| ETS | ↑ NAR* | nc histamine albumin, kinins | ↓ Clearance | |
| VOCs | | ↑ PMNs | | |
| Carbonless copy paper | ↑ NAR | | | |
| Ammonia | ↑ NAR | | | |
| Capsaicin | nc NAR | nc histamine albumin, kinins; sl. ↑ TAME | | ↑ Blood flow |

↑ = Increased  NAR = Nasal airway resistance
↓ = Decreased  TAME = [tosyl-L-arginine methyl ester] esterase activity
"nc" = No change  * = Historically ETS-sensitive subjects only

either "semi-routine" or "experimental," have been applied to the study of the upper airway response to chemical irritants under controlled circumstances. These studies appear in condensed form in Table 19–4. These studies are important because of their ability to isolate the effects of single exposures, in contrast to the multiple exposures in most work situations. In addition, some of these studies were structured to elucidate response mechanisms (eg, allergic vs neurogenic). Pathophysiologically, the most important findings to date have come from studies of environmental tobacco smoke (ETS) exposure:

1. Approximately 25–30% of the general public report reacting to ETS with nasal symptoms, including congestion, rhinorrhea, postnasal drip, and sinus headache. Individuals with a history of allergic rhinitis are more likely than those without such a history to report nasal reactivity to ETS (and other air pollutants).

2. On average, individuals reporting more pronounced nasal reactivity to ETS do, indeed, respond to ETS challenge with greater increases in nasal airway resistance than do subjects who report that ETS does not bother them.

3. Despite the similarity of ETS-induced nasal symptoms to classical allergy, neither nasal lavage studies nor allergy skin testing support the notion that the acute response to ETS in most individuals is allergically mediated.

4. Alternative response mechanisms to nasal irritants may include the two neurogenic pathways: central (parasympathetic) and local (axon) reflexes. The clinical implications of these pathways in air pollution situations has been largely unexplored.

# REFERENCES

## GENERAL

Bascom R, Raford P: Upper airway disorders. Pages 315–328 in: Rosenstock L, Cullen MR (editors): *Textbook of Clinical Occupational and Environmenal Medicine.* Saunders, 1994.

Leopold DA: Nasal toxicity: End points of concern in humans. Inhalation Toxicol 1994;6(Suppl):23.

Settipane GA: *Rhinitis,* 2nd ed. Oceanside Publications, 1991.

Witek TJ: The nose as target for adverse effects from the environment: Applying advances in nasal physiologic measures and mechanisms. Am J Indust Med 1993; 24:649.

## PATHOPHYSIOLOGY

Raphael GD, Baraniuk JN, Kaliner MA: How and why the nose runs. J Allergy Clin Immunol 1991;87: 457.

Silver WL: Neural and pharmacological basis for nasal irritation. Ann N Y Acad Sci 1992;641:152.

Widdicombe J: Nasal pathophysiology. Respir Med 1990;84(Suppl A):3.

## ALLERGIC RHINITIS

Eggleston PA et al: Occupational challenge studies with laboratory workers allergic to rats. J Allergy Clin Immunol 1990;86:63.

Jaeger D et al: Latex-specific proteins causing immediate-type cutaneous, nasal, bronchial, and systemic reactions. J Allergy Clin Immunol 1992;89:759.

Niinimaki A et al: Papain-induced allergic rhinoconjunctivitis in a cosmetologist. J Allergy Clin Immunol 1993;92:492.

Schwartz H, Arnold J, Strohl K: Occupational allergic rhinitis reaction to psyllium. J Occup Med 1989;31: 624.

## IRRITANT RHINITIS

Bascom R: Air pollution. Pages 32–45 in: Mygind N, Naclerio RM (editors): *Allergic and Non-allergic Rhinitis*. Munksgaard, 1993.

Bascom R: The upper respiratory tract: Mucous membrane irritation. Environ Health Perspect 1991;95:39.

Calderon-Garciduenas L et al: Histopathologic changes of the nasal mucosa in southwest Metropolitan Mexico City inhabitants. Am J Pathol 1992;140:225.

Cometto-Muniz JE, Cain WS: Sensory irritation: Relation to indoor air pollution. Ann N Y Acad Sci 1992; 641:137.

Frischer T et al: Ambient ozone causes upper airways inflammation in children. Am Rev Respir Dis 1993; 148:961.

Holmstrom M, Rosen G, Wilhelmsson B: Symptoms, airway physiology and histology of workers exposed to medium-density fiber board. Scand J Work Environ Health 1991;17:409.

Skoner DP, Hodgson MJ, Doyle WJ: Laser-printer rhinitis [letter]. N Engl J Med 1990;322:1323.

Theander C, Bende M: Nasal hyperreactivity to newspapers. Clin Exp Allergy 1989;19:57.

## SINUS PATHOLOGY

Brugman SM et al: Increased lower airways responsiveness associated with sinusitis in a rabbit model. Am Rev Respir Dis 1993;147:314.

Comba P et al: A case-control study of cancer of the nose and paranasal sinuses and occupational exposures. Am J Indust Med 1992;22:511.

Fukuda K, Shibata A: Exposure-response relationships between woodworking, smoking or passive smoking, and squamous cell neoplasms of the maxillary sinus. Cancer Causes Control 1990;1:165.

Leopold DA: Pollution: the nose and sinuses. Otolaryngol Head Neck Surg 1992;106:713.

Lund VJ: Toxicity of nasal respiratory mucosa in humans. Inhalation Toxicol 1994;6(Suppl):277-287.

## LARYNGEAL PATHOLOGY

Ahrens W et al: Alcohol, smoking, and occupational factors in cancer of the larynx: A case-control study. Am J Indust Med 1991;20:477.

Hallmo P, Naess O: Laryngeal papillomatosis with human papillomavirus DNA contracted by a laser surgeon. Eur Arch Otorhinolaryngol 1991;248:425.

Sataloff RT: Vocal aging: Medical considerations in professional voice users. Med Problems Perform Art 1992;7:17.

Smith AH, Handley MA, Wood R: Epidemiological evidence indicates asbestos causes laryngeal cancer. J Occup Med 1990;32:499.

Wortley P et al: A case-control study of occupational risk factors for laryngeal cancer. Br J Indust Med 1992;49:837.

## OTITIS MEDIA

Etzel RA et al: Passive smoking and middle ear effusion among children in day care. Pediatrics 1992;90:228.

Strachan DP, Jarvis MJ, Feyerabend C: Passive smoking, salivary cotinine concentrations, and middle ear effusion in 7 year old children. BMJ 1989;298:1549.

US Department of Health and Human Services: *The Health Consequences of Involuntary Smoking*. Surgeon General's Office, 1996.

## OLFACTORY DISORDERS

Cometto-Muniz JE, Cain W: Influence of airborne contaminants on olfaction and the common chemical sense. Pages 765–785 in: Getchell T et al (editors): *Smell and Taste in Health and Disease*. Raven Press, 1991.

Fortier I, Ferraris J, Mergler D: Measurement precision of an olfactory perception threshold test for use in field studies. Am J Indust Med 1991;20:495.

Mergler D, Beauvais B: Olfactory threshold shift following controlled 7-hour exposure to toluene and/or xylene. Neurotoxicology, 1992;13:211

Schwartz BS et al: Solvent-associated decrements in olfactory function in paint manufacturing workers. Am J Ind Med 1990;18:697.

Shusterman D, Sheedy J: Occupational and environmental disorders of the special senses. Occup Med 1992: 7:515.

Snow JB et al: Categorization of chemosensory disorders. Pages 445–447 in: Getchell T et al (editors): *Smell and Taste in Health and Disease*. Raven Press, 1991.

## DIAGNOSTIC TECHNIQUES

Ahman M: Nasal peak flow rate records in work related nasal blockage. Acta Otolaryngol (Stockh) 1992;112: 839.

Dias MA et al: Upper airway diagnostic methods. Pages 67–89 in: Harber P, Schenker M, Balmes J (editors): *Occupational and Environmental Respiratory Disease*. Mosby-Yearbook, 1995.

Druce HM et al: Measurement of multiple microcirculatory parameters in human nasal mucosa using laser-Doppler velocimetry. Microvasc Res 1989;38: 175.

Graham DE, Koren HS: Biomarkers of inflammation in ozone-exposed humans: Comparison of the nasal and bronchalveolar lavage. Am Rev Respir Dis 1990;142: 152.

## CONTROLLED EXPOSURE STUDIES

Bascom R et al: Effect of ozone inhalation on the response to nasal challenge with antigen of allergic subjects. Am Rev Respir Dis 1990;142:594.

Bascom R, Kagey-Sobotka A, Proud D: Effect of intranasal capsaicin on symptoms and mediator release. J Pharmacol Exp Ther 1991;259:1323.

Bascom R et al: Upper respiratory tract environmental tobacco smoke sensitivity. Am Rev Respir Dis 1991; 143:1304.

Koren H, Graham D, Devlin R: Exposure of humans to a volatile organic mixture: Inflammatory response. Arch Environ Health 1992;47:39.

Koren H, Hatch GE, Graham DE: Nasal lavage as a tool in assessing acute inflammation in response to inhaled pollutants. Toxicol 1990;60:15.

Lacroix JS et al: Improvement of symptoms of non-allergic chronic rhinitis by local treatment with capsaicin. Clin Exper Allergy 1991; 21:595.

Nadarajah J et al: Sidestream tobacco smoke (SS) alters regional nasal mucociliary clearance: comparison of sensitive and nonsensitive subjects. Am Rev Respir Dis 1993;147:A216.

Rajakulasingam K et al: Nasal effects of bradykinin and capsaicin: influence on plasma protein leakage and role of sensory neurons. J Appl Physiol 1992;72:1418.

Willes S et al: Differential responses to ozone in allergic and non-allergic subjects. Am Rev Respir Dis 1991; 143:A91.

Willes S, Fitzgerald T, Bascom R: Nasal inhalation challenge studies with sidestream tobacco smoke. Arch Environ Health 1992;47:223.

# Occupational Lung Diseases

# 20

*John R. Balmes, MD, & Cornelius H. Scannell, MD, Bch, BAO, MPH*

The respiratory tract is often the site of injury from occupational exposures. The widespread use of potentially toxic materials in the environment poses a major threat to both the airways and lung parenchyma. The respiratory tract has a limited number of ways to respond to injury. Acute responses include rhinosinusitis, laryngitis, upper airway obstruction, bronchitis, bronchoconstriction, alveolitis, and pulmonary edema. Chronic responses include asthma, bronchitis, parenchymal fibrosis, pleural fibrosis, and cancer. Early recognition and appropriate treatment of occupational lung diseases by physicians can significantly reduce both morbidity and mortality and greatly impact patient outcome. This chapter will focus on common occupational lung diseases and on how to diagnose and manage them.

## ANATOMY

The respiratory tract is anatomically divided into (1) upper airways, (2) lower airways, and (3) the lung parenchyma. The upper airways consist of the oronasal passages and the larynx, and the lower airways refer to the conducting airways below the larynx (ie, the tracheobronchial tree). The pulmonary parenchyma is primarily made up of terminal respiratory units that contain the alveoli and supporting interstitium. This anatomical division of the respiratory tract relates to important protective functions. Although increased work is required, humans tend to favor nasal over oral breathing. Nasally inspired air passes two acute bends before it reaches the relatively straight pharyngolaryngeal path. The anatomical arrangement of the nasal passages with the turbinates provides a large mucosal surface area that allows warming, humidification, and filtration of inspired air.

The trachea begins at the lower border of the cricoid cartilage, distal to the vocal cords. The trachea, bronchi, and larger bronchioles form the conducting portion of the lower respiratory tract. The gas-exchanging portion is composed of the many terminal respiratory units that each begin with a respiratory bronchiole, include alveolar ducts, and terminate in alveoli. The airway lining as far as the terminal bronchiole consists of epithelial cells, which are of pseudostratified columnar and ciliated type. Interspersed are the mucus-secreting goblet cells. The terminal respiratory unit is composed of a number of different cell types, including type 1 and type 2 alveolar epithelial cells, alveolar macrophages, pulmonary capillary endothelial cells, fibroblasts, and lymphocytes in the intra-alveolar septa.

The site of deposition of inhaled materials is dependent on water-solubility for gases, and particle size for solids (Table 20–1). Water-soluble gases and particles with a diameter in excess of 10 μm tend to get deposited in the upper airways, while insoluble gases and larger particles penetrate to the lower airways. Subsequent respiratory injury is dependent on both the site of toxin deposition, and on the type of cell/structure damaged.

## EVALUATION OF PATIENTS WITH OCCUPATIONAL LUNG DISEASE

A careful evaluation can successfully identify and diagnose occupational lung disease in most cases. The following four areas of approach are recommended: (1) detailed history, including occupational and environmental exposures; (2) thorough physical examination; (3) appropriate imaging studies; and (4) pulmonary function testing.

### History

A detailed history of both the patient's complaints and environmental/occupational exposures is essential. Work practices should be extensively explored with attention to types and duration of exposures, whether appropriate environmental controls are present, and if respiratory protective gear is used. Material Safety Data Sheets (MSDS) should also be reviewed, if available. These documents profile the important health, safety, and toxicologic properties of the product's ingredients and under federal law

**Table 20–1.** Site of respiratory tract deposition and effect.

| Water Solubility | Examples | Site of Injury |
|---|---|---|
| High | Ammonia, formaldehyde | Upper airway |
| Moderate | Chlorine, sulfur dioxide | Lower airways |
| Low | Nitrogen oxides, phosgene | Lung parenchyma |
| **Particle size (aerodynamic diameter)** | | |
| >10 μm | Dust from earth's crust | Upper airway |
| 2.5–6 μm | Some fire smoke particles | Lower airways |
| <2.5 μm | Metal fumes, asbestos fibers | Lung parenchyma |

must be furnished by the employer to the worker or his/her health care provider on request.

If available, actual industrial hygiene data on the level of exposure and the agent to which the patient was exposed should be obtained. The history should include the condition of the patient's home, any hobbies, and social habits because exposures outside of the workplace that contribute to or cause the lung injury may be discovered.

## Physical Examination

Occupational lung diseases do not present with specific clinical findings. It is difficult, for example, to distinguish asbestosis from idiopathic pulmonary fibrosis or chronic beryllium disease from sarcoidosis. Only in the context of the exposure history will the correct diagnosis be made. A physician suspecting the presence of an occupational lung disease should, nonetheless, perform a complete physical examination rather than focus narrowly on findings suggested by the exposure history. Relevant nonoccupational disease may otherwise be missed.

The physical examination may be helpful if abnormal, but it is in general insensitive for detection of mild respiratory tract injury. The vital signs and the level of respiratory distress, if any, should be assessed. The presence of cyanosis and finger clubbing should be noted. Examination of the skin and eyes can yield signs of irritation and inflammation. Oropharyngeal and nasal areas should be inspected for inflammation, ulcers, and polyps. The presence of wheezing, rhonchi, or both, is evidence of airways disease, and crackles are suggestive of the presence of parenchymal disease. Examination of the cardiovascular system for evidence of left ventricular failure is important when crackles are heard. The presence of isolated right ventricular failure suggests the possibility of cor pulmonale as a result of chronic severe lung disease with hypoxemia.

## Imaging Studies

A chest radiograph should be part of the work up when lung disease is suspected. However, normal radiographic findings do not exclude significant damage to the lung. Immediately after toxic inhalational injury, the chest radiograph is frequently normal. On the other hand, dramatically abnormal chest radiographs can be seen in individuals without significant lung injury who are exposed chronically to iron oxide or tin oxide. Abnormalities on the chest radiograph do not necessarily correlate with the degree of pulmonary impairment or disability. These are better assessed by pulmonary function testing and arterial blood gas determination.

With dust-exposed persons, chest films should be interpreted according to the International Labour Office (ILO) classification for pneumoconiosis, in addition to the routine interpretation. The purpose of the ILO classification is to provide a standardized, descriptive coding system for the appearance and extent of radiographic change caused by pneumoconiosis. The classification scheme consists of a glossary of terms and a set of 22 standard radiographs that demonstrate various degrees of pleural and parenchymal change due to pneumoconiosis. The worker's posteroanterior chest film is scored in comparison to the standard films. In the United States, a certification process for readers using the ILO classification has been developed under the auspices of the National institute for Occupational Safety and Health (NIOSH). By NIOSH parlance, an "A reader" has taken the American College of Radiology (ACR) pneumoconiosis course but has not passed the certification examination. A "B reader" has taken the ACR course and passed the examination.

Computed tomography (CT) is a radiographic technique that scans axial cross-sections and produces tomographic slices of the organ(s) scanned. Conventional computerized tomography of the chest is better able to detect abnormalities of the pleura and the mediastinal structures than is plain chest radiography, in large part because it is more sensitive to differences in density. When performed after the administration of intravenous contrast medium, CT scanning is considered to be the imaging study of choice for evaluation of the pulmonary hila.

High-resolution CT (HRCT) scanning incorporates thin collimation (1–2 mm as opposed to 10 mm in conventional CT) with high spatial-frequency reconstruction algorithms that sharpen interfaces between adjacent structures. Studies suggest that HRCT is more sensitive than either conventional CT or chest radiography for assessing the presence, character, and severity of a number of diffuse lung processes such as emphysema and interstitial lung disease.

## Pulmonary Function Testing

Pulmonary function testing is used to detect and quantitate abnormal lung function. Measurement of lung volumes and diffusing capacity, gas exchange analysis, and exercise testing need to be performed in a well-equipped pulmonary function laboratory, but spirometry can and should be done in most evaluating centers. There are two different types of spirometers, volume- and flow-sensing devices. Modern computerized versions of both types of spirometers can produce exhaled volume-time and expiratory flow-volume curves. There are advantages and disadvantages to each type of spirometer. Whether a volume- or flow-sensing device is chosen, the best spirometers have comparable accuracy and precision. Performance requirements for spirometers of either type were described in a 1987 American Thoracic Society (ATS) statement.

The most valuable of all pulmonary function parameters are those obtained from spirometry, namely forced expiratory volume in 1 second ($FEV_1$), forced vital capacity (FVC), and the $FEV_1$/FVC ratio. These parameters provide the best method of detecting the presence and severity of airway obstruction as well as the most reliable assessment of overall respiratory impairment. The forced expiratory flow from 25–75% of vital capacity ($FEF_{25-75}$) and the shape of the expiratory flow-volume curve are more sensitive indicators of mild airway obstruction. A simple portable spirometer can be used to obtain the necessary measurements. Lack of patient cooperation, poor testing methods, and unreliable equipment can produce misleading results. The 1987 ATS statement contains criteria for the performance of spirometry, and NIOSH oversees courses for spirometry technicians that leads to their certification. Results of spirometry can be compared to predicted values from reference populations (adjusted for age, height, and sex) and expressed as a percentage of the predicted value. The presence of obstructive, restrictive, or mixed ventilatory impairment can then be determined from the comparison of observed with predicted values. Because the commonly used reference populations consist entirely of Caucasians, there can be problems using predicted values to evaluate patients of non-Caucasian background. Typically, a 10–15% lowering of the predicted value is done to correct for the generally smaller lungs of non-Caucasians.

Another commonly used single-breath test that reflects the degree of airway obstruction is the peak expiratory flow rate (PEFR). Portable instruments such as the mini-Wright peak-flow meter can be used for its measurement. The major limitation of the PEFR is that patient self-recording of measurements is usually done and thus there is a potential for malingering. Despite this limitation, the test is useful in detecting changes in airway obstruction over time. Serial peak flow measurements are especially valuable in the diagnosis of occupational asthma to document delayed responses after the workshift is over.

Because FVC can be reduced due to disease processes that either restrict airflow into or obstruct airflow from the lungs, differentiation of restrictive from obstructive processes often requires measurement of static lung volumes, ie, total lung capacity (TLC), functional residual capacity (FRC), and residual volume (RV). These lung volumes are measured by inert gas dilution or body plethysmography. Restrictive lung diseases cause a reduction in TLC and other lung volumes, while obstructive diseases may result in hyperinflation and air trapping, ie, increased TLC and RV/TLC ratio.

The diffusing capacity of the lung for carbon monoxide ($DL_{CO}$) is a test of gas exchange in which the amount of inhaled carbon monoxide absorbed per unit time is measured. The $DL_{CO}$ is closely correlated with the capacity of the lungs to absorb oxygen. A reduced $DL_{CO}$ is a nonspecific finding; obstructive, restrictive, or vascular diseases can all cause reductions. Nevertheless, the $DL_{CO}$ is often used in combination with other clinical evidence to support a specific diagnosis or to assess respiratory impairment.

## Bronchoprovocation Tests

Bronchoprovocation tests are useful in the diagnosis of occupational asthma. Pulmonary function responses to inhaled histamine and methacholine are relatively easy to measure and give an indication of the presence and degree of nonspecific hyperresponsiveness of the airways. A measure of airway obstruction such as $FEV_1$ is obtained repeatedly after progressively increasing doses of histamine or methacholine to generate a dose-response curve. The test is usually terminated after a 20% fall in $FEV_1$. Patients with asthma typically respond with such a change in lung function after a relatively low cumulative dose of methacholine. Nonspecific challenge testing as described above is relatively inexpensive and can be performed on an outpatient basis.

Inhalation challenges testing with specific allergens thought to be causing occupational asthma can also be performed. Bronchoconstriction may occur early (within 30 minutes), late (in 4–8 hours), or in with a dual response (Figure 20–1). The occurrence of any of these responses after inhaled allergen is specific and diagnostic of occupational asthma. Unfortunately, specific inhalation challenge tests are both expensive and potentially hazardous. These tests should only be performed at specialized centers.

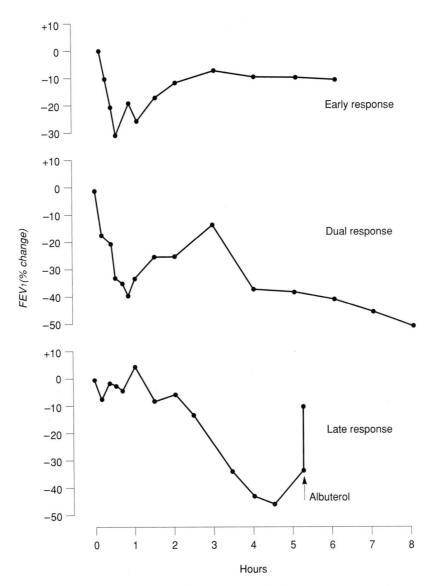

**Figure 20–1.** Potential responses to inhaltion of allergen in sensitized workers with asthma. (From Harber P, Schenker M, Balmes J: *Occupational and Environmental Respiratory Disease.* Mosby, 1996.)

## TOXIC INHALATION INJURY

Short-term exposures to high concentrations of noxious gases, fumes, or mists are generally due to industrial or transportation accidents or fires. Inhalation injury from high-intensity exposures can result in severe respiratory impairment or death. The effects of inhaled irritants are also discussed in the chapter on Gases and Other Inhalants (see Chapter 33).

The site of injury depends on the physical and chemical properties of the inhaled agent. As discussed above, the site of deposition of an inhaled gas is determined primarily by water solubility. Other important factors are the duration of exposure and

the minute ventilation of the victim. The concentration of an inhaled water-soluble gas such as ammonia is greatly reduced by the time it reaches the trachea due to the efficient scrubbing mechanisms of the moist surfaces of the nose and throat. In contrast, a relatively water-insoluble gas such as phosgene is not well-absorbed by the upper airways and thus may penetrate to the alveoli. The effects of inhalational exposure to toxic materials can range from transient, mild irritation of the mucous membranes of the upper airways to fatal adult respiratory distress syndrome (ARDS) (Table 20–2).

The adverse respiratory effects are dependent on the concentration of the substances inhaled. Low-dose ex-

**Table 20–2.** Potential effects of inhaled irritants.

| Site of Injury | Acute Effects | Chronic Effects |
|---|---|---|
| Eye, nose, sinuses, oropharynx | Irritation, inflammation | Corneal scarring, nasal polyps |
| Upper airway | Laryngeal edema, upper airway obstruction | Laryngeal polyps |
| Lower airways | Tracheobronchitis, bronchorrhea, decreased mucociliary clearance | Asthma, bronchiectasis |
| Lung parenchyma | Pneumonitis, pulmonary edema/adult respiratory distress syndrome | Pulmonary fibrosis, bronchiolitis obliterans |

posure to a water-soluble agent like ammonia or chlorine usually produces local irritation of conjunctival membranes and the upper airway. Moderate exposure to such an agent can result in hoarseness, cough, and bronchospasm. Acute high-level exposure can cause adult respiratory distress syndrome. Due to poor water solubility, certain agents such as phosgene and oxides of nitrogen are only mildly irritating to the upper respiratory tract. Once inhaled and deposited in the lower respiratory tract, however, these agents are highly irritating to the pulmonary parenchyma and may cause tissue necrosis. Long-term sequelae from toxic inhalation injury include bronchiectasis, bronchiolitis obliterans, and persistent asthma (see the discussion of irritant-induced asthma below).

## Evaluation

Details about the exposure should in most cases establish the causative chemical. The more serious exposures generally occur after major spillages due to industrial or transportation accidents or fires. Early effects are dependent on the level of exposure and may range from mild conjunctival and upper respiratory membrane irritation in low-dose exposures to life-threatening laryngeal or pulmonary edema in high-dose exposures.

The initial focus of the physical examination must be on the airway. If the nose and throat are badly burned or if there is hoarseness or stridor, chemical laryngitis should be suspected. The presence of early wheezing suggests that the exposure was relatively heavy. Spirometry or peak flow measurements may demonstrate airway obstruction relatively early after exposure.

The chest radiograph will usually be normal immediately post-exposure. Chemical pneumonitis and pulmonary edema (ARDS) may develop within 4–8 hours of heavy exposure. Arterial blood gas measurements may show hypoxemia prior to radiographic evidence of parenchymal injury. Because of the relative lack of immediate signs and frequent delayed reactions to poorly water-soluble agents such as phosgene and oxides of nitrogen, patients exposed to significant concentrations of these agents should be observed for a minimum of 24 hours.

## Management

Management of toxic inhalation injury should include immediate decontamination of exposed cutaneous and conjunctival areas by irrigation with water. If facial cutaneous burns are noted, direct laryngoscopy or fiberoptic bronchoscopy is recommended by some to assess for the presence of laryngeal edema. If present, endotracheal intubation should be considered. However, it is by no means clear as to who will develop life threatening upper airway obstruction. A conservative approach of careful clinical monitoring of the victim in an intensive care unit may be appropriate. If bronchoscopy is performed, evidence of significant inhalation injury includes erythema, edema, ulceration, and/or hemorrhage of the airway mucosa. If particulate material was inhaled, it may be visualized on the airway mucosa.

Simple spirometry or peak expiratory flow rate measurements to detect early airway obstruction are often quite useful. Flow-volume loops have been used both to diagnose upper airway obstruction and as a more sensitive detector of early lower airway obstruction than simple spirometry or peak expiratory flow rates. Supplemental oxygen should be administered if there is any sign of respiratory distress. Wheezing should be treated with inhaled bronchodilator. Serial periodic clinical examinations, spirometry or peak flow measurements, chest radiographs, and arterial blood gases are useful in monitoring progression of disease. There is no evidence to support the use of prophylactic antibiotics or the immediate use of corticosteroids in exposed patients.

Vigorous bronchial hygiene measures are required in those who develop severe tracheobronchitis. Drainage of mucus plugs and respiratory secretions should be encouraged by postural drainage, chest physical therapy, deep inspiratory maneuvers, and adequate hydration. If intubated, frequent suctioning of the airways should be performed to remove any adherent soot that may contain irritant and corrosive chemicals. Some authors recommend fiberoptic bronchoscopy to lavage off this adherent material.

Patients who develop pulmonary edema/ARDS require intensive care unit management including mechanical ventilatory assistance. However, if such patients can be supported through the acute phase of the disease process they may recover with no significant loss of lung function.

Controversy exists, however, about the potential for long-term pulmonary sequelae after toxic inhalation injury. For example, there are well-documented reports of persisting airway obstruction, nonspecific airway hyperresponsiveness, and sequential reduction in residual volume following acute chlorine gas exposure. Until this controversy is resolved, it would seem prudent to follow exposed individuals with periodic clinical examinations and pulmonary function testing for the development of any persistent respiratory impairment. Although there is no controlled experimental evidence to support the practice, a trial of corticosteroids can be considered in a patient who is not recovering promptly. Such a trial may be especially beneficial in a patient with bronchiolitis obliterans following inhalation injury.

## OCCUPATIONAL ASTHMA

Asthma is characterized by airway obstruction that is reversible (but not completely so in some patients) either spontaneously or with treatment, airway inflammation, and increased airway responsiveness to a variety of stimuli. In occupational asthma, there is variable airways obstruction and/or airway hyperresponsiveness due to workplace exposure(s). Work-related variable airway obstruction can be caused by several mechanisms, including type I-immune reactions, pharmacologic effects, inflammatory processes, and direct airway irritation. Over 200 agents in the workplace have been shown to cause asthma and the list is growing as new materials and processes are introduced. Work-aggravated asthma occurs when workplace exposures lead to exacerba-

tions of preexisting nonoccupational asthma. In the United States, asthma occurs in about 5% of the general population, and at least 3% of these cases are occupational in origin. Work-related asthma (ie, both occupational asthma and work-aggravated asthma) has been estimated to be 15% of all asthma.

There are two major types of occupational asthma. **Sensitizer-induced asthma** is characterized by a variable time during which "sensitization" to an agent present in the work site takes place. **Irritant-induced asthma** occurs without a latent period after substantial exposure to an irritating dust, mist, vapor, or fume. **Reactive airways dysfunction syndrome (RADS)** is a term used by some to describe irritant-induced asthma caused by a short-term, high-intensity exposure.

Sensitizing agents known to cause occupational asthma can be divided into high-molecular weight (>1000 daltons) and low-molecular-weight compounds (Table 20–3). High-molecular-weight compounds tend to cause occupational asthma via type I, immunoglobulin E-mediated (IgE-mediated) reactions, whereas the mechanism(s) of low-molecular-weight compounds is currently unknown. Sensitizer-induced asthma is characterized by specific responsiveness to the etiologic agent. The mechanism of irritant-induced asthma is also unknown, but there is no clinical evidence of sensitization. Irritant-induced asthma involves persistent nonspecific airway hyperresponsiveness but not specific responsiveness to an etiologic agent. While there is no doubt that irritant-induced asthma can be caused by a single intense exposure (ie, RADS), it appears that lower-level exposure over a longer duration of time (months to years) can also cause the disease.

### Pathophysiology

Airway inflammation is now recognized as the

**Table 20–3.** Some agents causing occupational asthma.

| Mechanism | Examples |
|---|---|
| **Without "sensitization"** | |
| Anticholinesterase effect | Organophosphate pesticide (agricultural workers) |
| Endotoxin effects | Cotton dust (textile workers) |
| Airway inflammation | Acids, ammonia, chlorine (custodial workers, paper manufacturing workers) |
| Airway irritation | Dusts, fumes, mists, vapors, cold (construction workers, chemical workers) |
| **With "sensitization"** | |
| High-molecular-weight agents | |
| IgE-mediated (complete allergens) | Animal and plant proteins (laboratory workers, bakers) |
| Low-molecular-weight agents | |
| IgE-mediated (haptens) | Antibiotics, metals (pharmaceutical workers, metal plating workers) |
| Mechanism undefined | Acid anhydrides, diisocyanates, plicatic acid (epoxy plastics and paints, polyurethane foams and paints, western red cedar products) |

paramount feature of asthma. Asthmatic airways are characterized by (1) infiltration with inflammatory cells, especially eosinophils; (2) edema; and (3) loss of epithelial integrity. Airway obstruction in asthma is believed to be the result of changes associated with airway inflammation. Airway inflammation is also believed to play an important role in the genesis of airway hyperresponsiveness.

Most of the research on mechanisms that mediate airway inflammation in asthma has focused on high-molecular-weight allergen-induced responses. In a previously sensitized individual, inhalation of specific allergen allows interaction of the allergen with airway cells (mast cells and alveolar macrophages)

that have specific antibodies (usually IgE) on the cell surface. This interaction initiates a series of redundant amplifying events that lead to airway inflammation. These events include mast cell secretion of mediators, lymphocyte interaction, and eosinophil recruitment to the airways. The generation and release of various cytokines from alveolar macrophages, mast cells, sensitized lymphocytes, and bronchial epithelial cells are central to the inflammatory process (Figure 20–2). Cytokine networking, with both enhancing and inhibitory feedback loops, is responsible for inflammatory cell targeting to the bronchial epithelium, activation of infiltrating cells, and potential amplification of epithelial injury. Adhesion mole-

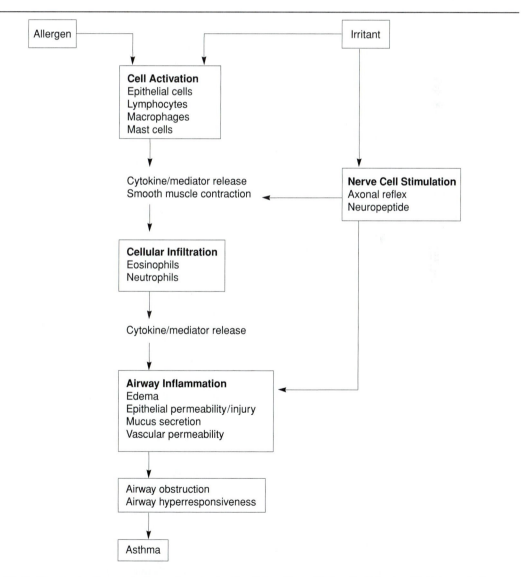

**Figure 20–2.** Proposed pathways in the pathogenesis of asthma. (From Harber P, Schenker M, Balmes J: *Occupational and Environmental Respiratory Disease*. Mosby, 1996.)

cules also play critical roles in the amplification of the inflammatory process. The expression of various adhesion molecules is upregulated during the inflammatory cascade, and these molecules are essential for cell movement, cell attachment to the extracellular matrix and other cells, and possibly cell activation. As noted above, the mechanism of low-molecular-weight sensitizer-induced asthma is not well understood, although bronchial biopsy studies of affected workers have clearly demonstrated that airway inflammation is present.

Inhalation of the specific etiologic agent in a worker with sensitizer-induced asthma will often trigger rapid-onset but self-limited bronchoconstriction, called the early response (Figure 20–1). In many sensitized workers, a delayed reaction will occur 4–8 hours later, called the late response. The late response is characterized by airway inflammation, persistent airway obstruction, and airway hyperresponsiveness. In some workers there is a dual response, and in others, only an isolated late response (Figure 20–1). Mast cell degranulation and release of mediators such as histamine are believed to be responsible for the early response. The role of the mast cell in the genesis of the late response is more controversial, but the release of chemoattractant substances such as leukotrienes and cytokines (ie, interleukin (IL)-3, IL-4, and IL-5) may be involved in the influx of neutrophils and eosinophils into the airway epithelium. The eosinophil can release proteins (eg, major basic protein, eosinophilic cationic protein, eosinophil-derived neurotoxin, and enzymes), lipid mediators, and oxygen radicals that can cause epithelial injury. There is increasing evidence that lymphocytes, especially a CD4+ subset known as $TH_2$ cells, are involved in the release of cytokines that may activate both mast cells (IL-3 and IL-4) and eosinophils (IL-5). In IgE-mediated allergic asthma, $TH_2$ cells may be responsible for the maintenance of chronic airway inflammation.

Although the mechanisms by which airway inflammation occurs in irritant-induced asthma are not well understood, neurogenic pathways may be involved (Figure 20–2). The axonal reflex involving C-fiber stimulation and the release of neuropeptides have been implicated in models of irritant-induced airway inflammation. With high-level irritant exposure, direct chemical injury can lead to an inflammatory response. The important unanswered question is what causes this response to persist in certain individuals.

As the sensitizer or irritant-induced airway inflammatory process proceeds, mucosal edema, mucus secretion, and vascular and epithelial permeability all increase, leading to a reduction of the caliber of the airway lumen and resultant airflow obstruction (Figure 20–3). The level of airway obstruction in patients with asthma is a marker of the severity of disease. With mild asthma, there may be no evidence of ob-

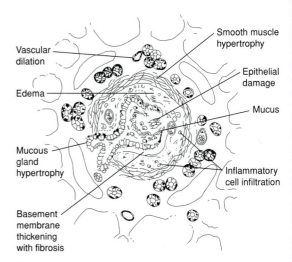

**Figure 20–3.** Morphologic changes in asthma. (Adapted from National Asthma Education Program Expert Panel: Guidelines for the diagnosis and management of asthma, NIH Pub No 91-3042A, 1991, National, Heart, Lung and Blood Institute.)

struction between acute exacerbations, but nonspecific airway hyperresponsiveness is likely to be present. With more severe asthma, there is increased airway hyperresponsiveness and airway obstruction is present between attacks.

Two other mechanisms by which variable airway obstruction due to workplace exposure can occur are reflex and pharmacologic bronchoconstriction. In reflex bronchoconstriction, neuroreceptors in the airway are stimulated by agents such as cold air, dusts, mists, vapos, and fumes. The reaction does not involve immunologic mechanisms and does not lead to airway inflammation. In most cases, the patient has a history of preexisting nonoccupational asthma with nonspecific airway hyperesponsiveness so that this is the primary mechanism of work-aggravated asthma. Pharmacologic bronchoconstriction occurs when an agent in the workplace causes the direct release of mediators (eg, cotton dust in textile mills) or a direct effect on the autonomic regulation of bronchomotor tone (eg, organophosphate pesticides inhibit cholinesterase).

## Diagnosis

The diagnosis of occupational asthma is made by confirming the diagnosis of asthma and by establishing a relationship between asthma and the work environment. The diagnosis of asthma should only be made when both intermittent respiratory symptoms and physiologic evidence of reversible or variable airways obstruction are present. The relationship between asthma and workplace exposure may fit any of the following patterns: (1) symptoms occur only at work; (2) symptoms improve on weekends or vacations; (3) symptoms occur regularly after the work-shift; (4) symptoms progressively increase over the course of the work week; and (5) symptoms improve after a change in the work environment.

At least one of the symptoms of wheezing, shortness of breath, cough, and chest tightness should occur while the worker is at or within 4–8 hours of his/her leaving the workplace. Often the worker's symptoms improve during days off work or while away from his/her usual job. With persistent exposure, the symptoms may become chronic and lose an obvious relationship to the workplace. Concomitant eye and upper respiratory tract symptoms may also be noted. The diagnosis of occupational asthma should also be considered when there is a history of recurrent episodes of work-related "bronchitis" characterized by cough and sputum production in an otherwise healthy individual. While high-molecular-weight sensitizers typically cause early or dual responses, the low-molecular-weight sensitizers tend to induce isolated late responses that may occur hours after the workshift is over.

The evaluation for possible occupational asthma requires a detailed history of the work environment. As noted above, attention should be given to the agents to which the worker is exposed, the type of ventilation in the workplace, whether respiratory protective equipment is used, and, if possible, the level of exposure (ie, whether it is high or low or if accidental exposure through spills ever occurs). A helpful clue to a significant problem in a workplace is the presence of other workers with episodic respiratory symptoms.

The detection of wheezing on chest auscultation is helpful, but the physical examination is frequently normal in asthmatic patients not currently suffering from an exacerbation.

Chest radiographs are normal in most individuals with asthma because the disease involves the airways rather than the lung parenchyma. Hyperinflation and flattening of the diaphragms, indicating air trapping may be seen during exacerbations. Fleeting infiltrates indicating mucus plugging and bronchial wall thickening reflecting chronic inflammation may also be noted.

As noted previously, spirometry for measurement of $FEV_1$ and FVC is the most reliable method for assessing airway obstruction. However, because asthmatic patients typically have reversible airway obstruction, they may have normal lung function during intervals between acute attacks. The response to inhaled bronchodilator administration has been used as a measure of airway hyperresponsiveness. A 12% improvement in $FEV_1$ after inhaled bronchodilator is how the ATS defines a significant improvement indicative of hyperresponsive airways. Across-work-shift spirometry, when available, can provide objective evidence of occupational asthma. A greater than 10% fall in $FEV_1$ across a workshift is suggestive of an asthmatic response.

Serial recording of PEFR over a period of weeks to months is often the best way to document the work-relatedness of asthma. The worker records his/her PEFR at least four times while awake as well as respiratory symptoms and medication use. When interpreting the worker's log, attention should be given to any work-related pattern of change. A 20% or greater diurnal variability in PEFR has been considered evidence of an asthmatic response (Figure 20–4). The major advantage of serial PEFR measurement over spirometry is the ability to detect late responses that occur after the workshift ends.

Methacholine or histamine challenge can demonstrate the presence of nonspecific airway hyperresponsiveness in a worker suspected to have occupational asthma who has normal spirometry. Such testing can be particularly valuable if it demonstrates an increase in airway responsiveness on returning to work or a decrease when away from work. Specific inhalational challenge testing, ie, challenging the patient with the suspected agent at levels and under conditions that mimic workplace conditions, can be done for medicolegal purposes or to determine the precise etiology in a complex exposure scenario. However, specific challenge testing is time-consuming, potentially dangerous, and usually should be reserved for evaluation of patients in whom there is diagnostic uncertainty.

Allergy skin tests with common aeroallergens can be used to establish whether or not the worker is atopic. Atopy is a risk factor for high-molecular-weight sensitizer-induced asthma. When high-molecular-weight compounds are responsible for occupational asthma, skin tests with the appropriate extracts

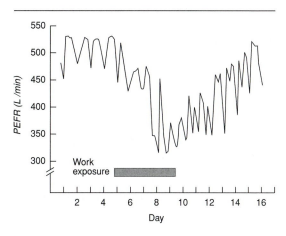

**Figure 20–4.** Serial peak expiratory flow rates (PEFR) during a 16-day period in a worker with occupational asthma before, during, and after 1 week of exposure to the inciting agent. (From Fine JM, Balmes JR: Clin Chest Med 1988;**9:**577, with permission.)

may help identify the etiologic agent. Extracts of materials such as flour, animal proteins, and coffee will give positive skin tests in specifically sensitized individuals. Skin testing may also be helpful for a few low-molecular-weight compounds such as platinum salts. IgE antibodies assayed by the radioallergosorbent test (RAST) or by enzyme-linked immunoabsorbent assay (ELISA) may confirm exposure to allergens such as flour, animal proteins, acid anhydrides, plicatic acid, or isocyanates. However, the presence of positive skin reactions and/or specific antibodies is not always correlated with the presence of occupational asthma.

## Treatment

Acute asthma attacks requiring emergency management should be treated with supplemental oxygen, beta-agonists, corticosteroids, and if infection is suspected, antibiotics. Hospitalization should be considered in the more severe cases because of the potential for respiratory failure.

Once the diagnosis of occupational asthma is made, the primary intervention is to reduce or eliminate the worker's exposure to the offending agent. This may be achieved through modifications in the workplace. It may be possible to substitute the offending agent with another safer one. Improved local exhaust ventilation and enclosure of specific processes may also be helpful. With irritant-induced asthma, the use of personal protective equipment may lower exposures to levels that do not induce bronchospasm. Workers who are allowed to continue in the job should have regular follow-up visits including monitoring of their lung function and nonspecific airway responsiveness. With sensitizer-induced asthma, however, the worker should be precluded from further exposure to the sensitizing agent. It may be necessary to completely remove the worker from the workplace as even exposure to minute quantities of the offending agent may induce bronchospasm. If a worker is required to leave the workplace (eg, a baker with flour-induced asthma), he/she should be considered 100% impaired on a permanent basis for the job that caused the illness and for other jobs with exposure to the same causative agent.

In addition to reduction or elimination of exposure to any specific offending agent, the worker should also avoid exposure to other materials/processes that may exacerbate his/her asthma such as irritating dusts, mists, vapors, etc. Cessation of smoking and avoidance of exposure to environmental tobacco smoke are also essential.

## Prevention

Prevention of further occupational asthma should be considered in all workplaces where cases are diagnosed. This can primarily be achieved through environmental control of processes known to involve exposure to potential sensitizers and irritants. Protection of workers by the use of appropriate ventilation systems, respiratory protective equipment, and worker education about appropriate procedures should be recommended. Avoidance of high-intensity exposures from leaks and spills that may initiate the development of occupational asthma is essential. Medical surveillance for early detection of cases can also contribute to reducing the burden of impairment/disability due to occupational asthma.

## Severity of Disease

Once occupational asthma has been diagnosed, an attempt should be made to classify the degree of impairment/disability. An approach to the evaluation of impairment in patients with asthma was recently promulgated by the ATS. Asthma is a dynamic disease that does not generally result in a static level of impairment. The criteria used for impairment rating are degree of post-bronchodilator airway obstruction by spirometry, measurement of airway responsiveness, and medication requirements. Assessment of impairment/disability should be done only after optimization of therapy and whenever the worker's condition changes substantially, whether for better or worse.

## Natural History

Multiple follow up studies of workers with occupational asthma caused by such diverse agents as diisocyanates, snow crab, and western red cedar showed persistence of symptoms and the presence of nonspecific airway hyperresponsiveness for periods up to 6 years after removal from the offending agent. Factors that affect the long-term prognosis of the patient with occupational asthma are the total duration of exposure, the duration of exposure after the onset of symptoms, and the severity of asthma at the time of diagnosis. Those who do poorly have a delayed diagnosis, lower lung function values, and greater nonspecific airway hyperresponsiveness, hence the importance of early diagnosis and early removal from future exposure to the etiologic agent.

## Specific Agents

**A. Diisocyanates:** Chemicals of the diisocyanate group are widely used in the manufacture of polyurethane surface coatings, insulation materials, car upholstery, and furniture. The most commonly used diisocyanate is toluene diisocyanate (TDI). Because of its high vapor pressure, the less volatile agent methylene diphenyl diisocyanate (MDI) is used in some production processes. Other diisocyanates such as hexamethylene diisocyanate (HDI), naphthylene diisocyanate (NDI), isophorone diisocyanate (IPDI) also have commercial uses. These chemicals are all highly reactive due to the presence of –N–C–O groups, which easily react with biological molecules and are potent irritants to the respiratory tract. Upper respiratory tract inflammation occurs in almost everyone exposed to TDI levels of 0.5 ppm or more.

Five major patterns of airway response to TDI have been described in humans: (1) occupational asthma of the sensitizer-type, which occurs in 5–10% of exposed workers weeks to months after the onset of exposure; (2) chemical bronchitis; (3) acute, but asymptomatic, deterioration of respiratory function during a workshift; (4) chronic deterioration of respiratory function associated with chronic exposure to low doses; and (5) persistent asthma or RADS after exposure to high doses.

**B. Vegetable Dusts, Including Cotton (Byssinosis), Flax, Hemp, and Jute:** Byssinosis occurs in certain workers in the cotton textile industry. The characteristic symptoms are chest tightness, cough, and dyspnea 1–2 hours after the patient returns to work after several days off. The symptoms usually resolve overnight and on subsequent days become milder until by the end of the work week the worker may become asymptomatic. The prevalence of byssinosis is higher in workers with longer duration of exposure and with greater respirable dust exposure, such as during opening bales and carding, and lowest in those with a shorter exposure history and with lesser dust exposure.

The mechanism underlying byssinosis remains unclear. Cotton dust extracts are capable of causing direct release of histamine and contain endotoxins that can induce a number of inflammatory responses.

**C. Metal Salts:** Complex salts of platinum used in electroplating, platinum refinery operations, manufacture of fluorescent screens, and jewelry-making are known to cause occupational asthma. Specific IgE antibodies to platinum salts conjugated to human serum albumin have been found in sensitized workers by RAST. Rhinitis and urticaria frequently accompany asthma, and this triad is sometimes called "platinosis." Nickel, vanadium, chromium, and cobalt are other metals known to cause occupational asthma.

**D. Acid Anhydrides:** Epoxy resins often contain acid anhydrides as curing or hardening agents. Phthalic anhydride, trimellitic anhydride (TMA), and tetrachlorophthalic anhydride (TCPA) are several of the more commonly used acid anhydrides. Occupational asthma occurs in a small percentage of exposed workers. The serum of affected workers typically contains specific IgE antibodies against acid anhydride-protein conjugates.

Trimellitic anhydride exposure can give rise to four clinical syndromes: (1) symptoms of immediate airway irritation; (2) immediate rhinitis and asthma; (3) late asthma with systemic symptoms of fever and malaise; and (4) infiltrative lung disease (hemorrhagic alveolitis) with hemoptysis and anemia.

**E. Wood Dusts:** A wide variety of wood dusts are known to cause rhinitis and asthma. Western red cedar is the best studied. This wood contains the low-molecular-weight compound, plicatic acid, which is believed to be responsible for causing asthma through an unclear mechanism. Western red cedar asthma falls under the category of low-molecular-weight, sensitizer-induced asthma and clinically is much like diisocyanate asthma. There is often a long period between onset of exposure and onset of symptoms, and asthma only develops in a small proportion of exposed subjects. A small dose of plicatic acid can induce a severe asthmatic attack in a sensitized individual, and many workers continue to have persistent asthma years after cessation of exposure.

# HYPERSENSITIVITY PNEUMONITIS

Hypersensitivity pneumonitis, also known as extrinsic allergic alveolitis, refers to an immunologically-mediated inflammatory disease of the lung parenchyma that is induced by inhalation of organic dusts that contain a variety of etiologic agents (eg, bacteria, fungi, amoebae, animal proteins, and several low-molecular-weight chemicals). Although there are many different antigens capable of causing hypersensitivity pneumonitis (Table 20–4), the basic clinical and pathologic findings are similar regardless of the nature of the inhaled dust. The nature of the inhaled antigen, the exposure conditions, and the nature of the host immune response all contribute to the risk for the disease. Hypersensitivity pneumonitis is characterized initially by a lymphocytic alveolitis and granulomatous pneumonitis, with improvement or complete resolution if antigen exposure is terminated early. Continued antigen exposure may lead to progressive interstitial fibrosis.

The pathogenesis of hypersensitivity pneumonitis involves repeated inhalational exposure to the antigen, sensitization of the exposed individual, and immunologically-mediated damage to the lung. The inflammatory response that results in hypersensitivity pneumonitis appears to involve a combination of humoral, immune-complex-mediated (type III) and cell-mediated (type IV) immune reactions to the inhaled antigen. In the presence of excess antigen, immune complexes may be deposited in the lungs. These complexes activate complement, leading to an influx of neutrophils. The local immune response later shifts to a T lymphocyte-predominant alveolitis, with a differential cell count in bronchoalveolar lavage (BAL) fluid of up to 70% lymphocytes. Examination of BAL lymphocyte subpopulations in patients with hypersensitivity pneumonitis often has revealed a predominance of CD8+ suppressor/cytoxic cells. The peripheral blood and BAL T lymphocytes from patients with hypersensitivity pneumonitis will proliferate and undergo blastogenic transformation with cytokine generation when exposed in vitro to antigen. Animal models also support the role of cell-mediated immunity in the disease. Passive transfer of

**Table 20–4.** Some agents causing hypersensitivity pneumonitis.

| Antigen | Exposure | Syndrome |
|---|---|---|
| **Bacteria** | | |
| *Faenia rectivirgula* | Moldy hay | Farmer's lung |
| *Thermoactinomycetes vulgaris* | Moldy grain, compost | Grain worker's lung, Mushroom worker's lung |
| *Thermoactinomycetes sacchari* | Moldy sugar cane fiber | Bagassosis |
| *Thermoactinomycetes candidus* | Heated water reservoirs | Humidifier lung |
| *Bacillus subtilus* | Detergent | Detergent worker's lung |
| **Fungi** | | |
| *Aspergillus clavatus* | Moldy malt | Malt worker's lung |
| *Penicillium casei* | Moldy cheese | Cheese worker's lung |
| *Penicillium frequentans* | Moldy cork dust | Suberosis |
| *Cryptostroma corticale* | Moldy maple bark | Maple bark stripper's lung |
| *Aureobasidium pullulans* | Moldy redwood dust | Sequoiosis |
| *Graphium* spp. | | |
| **Amoebae** | | |
| *Naegleria gruberi* | Contaminated water | Humidifier lung |
| *Acanthamoeba castellani* | | |
| **Animal proteins** | | |
| Avian proteins | Bird droppings, feathers | Bird breeder's lung |
| Rodent proteins | Urine, sera, pelts | Animal handler's lung |
| Wheat weevil | Infested flour | Wheat weevil lung |
| **Chemicals** | | |
| Toluene diisocyanate | Paints, coatings | Isocyanate lung |
| Hexamethylene diisocyanate | | |
| Diphenylmethane diisocyanate | Polyurethane foam | |
| Trimellitic anhydride | Epoxy resins, paints | TMA pulmonary hemorrhage-anemia syndrome |

lymphocytes from sensitized animals to unexposed, nonsensitized animals results in a hypersensitivity pneumonitis-like disease when the latter animals are subsequently exposed to the specific antigen by inhalation. Alveolar macrophages may also play an important role in the pathogenesis of the disease by processing and presenting inhaled antigen to T-helper lymphocytes, as well as by releasing cytokines, which may help to amplify the inflammatory response. Because only a small number of exposed persons ever develop hypersensitivity pneumonitis, the underlying mechanism of the disease may be a form of immune dysfunction in which a normal host defense response cannot be appropriately downregulated. This immune dysfunction may be, at least in part, genetically mediated. Environmental factors may also be involved since a number of studies have shown that hypersensitivity pneumonitis occurs more frequently in nonsmokers than smokers.

## Diagnosis

Inhalational exposure to antigen in a sensitized individual may result in either an acute or chronic presentation of hypersensitivity pneumonitis, depending on the exposure conditions.

The acute and more common form of presentation of hypersensitivity pneumonitis usually occurs within 4–6 hours of an intense exposure to the offending antigen. Symptoms of chills, fever, malaise, myalgia,

cough, headache, and dyspnea are commonly noted. Physical examination may reveal a relatively ill-appearing patient with bibasilar inspiratory crackles on chest auscultation. Frequently, acute hypersensitivity pneumonitis is misdiagnosed as an acute viral syndrome or pneumonia as it tends to closely mimic these conditions. Laboratory findings include peripheral blood leukocytosis with increased neutrophils and a relative decreased lymphopenia. Arterial blood gas values may show hypoxemia.

Chest radiographic findings may be completely normal even in symptomatic individuals. Typically, however, the acute phase is associated with the presence of a reticulonodular pattern. Patchy densities that tend to coalesce may also be seen. These infiltrates are usually bilaterally distributed, but a more focal presentation sometimes occurs.

Pulmonary function testing may reveal a decrease in the $FEV_1$ and FVC with an unchanged $FEV_1$/FVC ratio consistent with a restrictive impairment. A decrease in the $DL_{CO}$ reflecting impaired gas exchange is also typical of the acute presentation. The acute form generally progresses for up to 18–24 hours and then begins to resolve. Recurrence of the syndrome may subsequently occur with re-exposure to the antigen.

Recurrent low-level exposure to an appropriate antigen may result in the insidious onset of chronic interstitial lung disease with fibrosis. Progressive respiratory impairment with symptoms of dyspnea, cough, excessive fatigue, and weight loss may develop without acute episodes. Physical examination may reveal cyanosis, clubbing, and inspiratory crackles. Chest radiographic findings include diffusely increased linear markings and reduced lung size. Findings on high-resolution CT scanning of the chest include centrilobular micronodules, ground-glass opacification, patchy air-space consolidation, and linear densities. Chest CT findings can be suggestive of the diagnosis of hypersensitivity pneumonitis but are clearly not pathognomonic. Pulmonary function testing will usually show a restrictive impairment with a decreased $DL_{CO}$, although some patients may be seen with a mixed or obstructive pattern.

The diagnosis of hypersensitivity pneumonitis should be suspected in patients with episodic respiratory symptoms and evidence of fleeting infiltrates on chest radiographs or restrictive impairment on pulmonary function testing. A careful history may elicit the onset of respiratory symptoms with exposure to the offending antigen. The temporal relationship of symptom development after exposure is crucial to the diagnosis. Additional supporting evidence is provided by the remission of symptoms and signs after cessation of exposure to the antigen and their reappearance on re-exposure.

Serological studies demonstrating specific IgG precipitating antibodies by the traditional double-immuno diffusion technique will be positive in most patients with hypersensitivity pneumonitis, although such antibodies are also frequently detected in exposed individuals who are healthy. False-positive results may be obtained with the use of more sensitive assays for IgG, such as ELISA. False-negative results are frequently due to the failure to test for the correct antigen. Most commercially available hypersensitivity pneumonitis panels involve only a limited number of common antigens. Skin tests have little role in the diagnosis of hypersensitivity pneumonitis.

Inhalational challenge studies with the suspected antigen may assist in the diagnosis of hypersensitivity pneumonitis. Antigen extracts may be administered in an aerosolized form followed by serial pulmonary function testing. Specific challenge testing should only be conducted by a laboratory experienced in the technique. While such challenges provide the "gold standard" method of confirming a direct relationship between a suspected offending antigen and the disease process, workplace studies involving the actual conditions of patient exposure are safer and usually easier to conduct.

As noted above, analysis of BAL fluid obtained by fiberoptic bronchoscopy in patients with hypersensitivity pneumonitis often demonstrates an increased percentage of T lymphocytes that are primarily CD8+ suppressor cells. In sarcoidosis, another condition characterized by increased T lymphocytes in BAL, the predominant cells are of the CD4+ helper subtype.

Lung biopsy may be necessary to make the diagnosis in difficult cases such as those with the chronic form and an insidious presentation of dyspnea. Open lung biopsy is preferred as transbronchial biopsy may not provide adequate tissue for pathologic differentiation of hypersensitivity pneumonitis from other diseases such as sarcoidosis. In acute or early chronic (subacute) hypersensitivity pneumonitis, there is patchy infiltration of predominantly lymphocytes in a bronchocentric distribution, usually with accompanying epithelioid (ie, noncaseating) granulomas. The granulomas are likely what appear as centrilobular micronodules on (HRCT). In chronic hypersensitivity pneumonitis, peribronchiolar inflammation remains prominent and bronchiolitis obliterans is common. Large histiocytes with foamy cytoplasm may be seen in the alveoli and interstitium. Interstitial fibrosis with honeycombing occurs in advanced disease, by which time granulomas may no longer be evident.

## Treatment

The key to successful treatment of hypersensitivity pneumonitis is avoidance of the offending antigen. As described for occupational asthma, this may be achieved by product substitution or institution of effective engineering controls. Respiratory protective equipment may also be appropriate in situations where possible exposure is only occasional. If persistence of symptoms occurs despite engineering control measures and respiratory protective equipment, complete removal of the worker from exposure is necessary.

Corticosteroids remain the mainstay of treatment of patients with severe or progressive hypersensitivity pneumonitis, despite the lack of controlled data regarding the effect of these agents on the disease process. An empiric trial of prednisone (1 mg/kg/d), with monitoring of chest radiographic and pulmonary function changes 1 month after starting the trial is a reasonable approach. Therapy should be continued until there is significant clinical improvement. If bronchospasm is present, beta-agonists should be administered. Supplemental oxygen should be given to patients with hypoxemia, and intensive care unit support may be needed in particularly severe acute cases.

Workers with a diagnosis of hypersensitivity pneumonitis should have frequent follow-up especially if continued exposure to antigen is possible. Significant pulmonary morbidity may occur if persistent exposure is allowed.

## INHALATION FEVERS

Inhalation fever refers to several syndromes that are characterized by short-term but debilitating flu-like symptoms after exposure to organic dusts, poly-

Table 20–5. Some agents causing inhalation fever.

| Agent | Syndrome |
|---|---|
| **Metals** <br> Zinc <br> Copper <br> Magnesium | Metal fume fever |
| **Teflon pyrolysis products** <br> Polytetrafluoroethylene | Polymer fume fever |
| **Bioaerosols** <br> Contaminated water <br> Moldy silage, compost, <br> wood chips <br> Sewage sludge <br> Cotton, jute, hemp, flax dust <br> Grain dust | Humidifier fever <br> Organic dust toxic <br> syndrome <br><br> Mill fever <br> Grain fever |

mer fumes, and metal fumes (Table 20–5). In addition to fever, the symptoms include chills, myalgia, headache, malaise, cough, and chest discomfort. In contrast to occupational asthma and hypersensitivity pneumonitis, which require susceptibility and/or sensitization, the attack rate for the inhalation fevers is high, ie, most people will experience symptoms as a result of high-level exposure to the etiologic agents.

## Metal Fume Fever

Inhalation of certain freshly formed metal oxides can cause metal fume fever, an acute, self-limiting, flu-like illness. The most common cause of this syndrome is the inhalation of zinc oxide, which is generated from molten bronze or welding galvanized steel. The oxides of only two other metals, copper and magnesium, have been proven to cause metal fume fever. When zinc is heated to its melting point, zinc oxide fumes are generated. The particle size of the generated fumes ranges from 0.1–1.0 μm in diameter, although aggregation with the formation of larger particles readily occurs. The underlying pathogenesis of metal fume fever is incompletely understood. However, there is evidence from controlled human exposure studies that zinc oxide fume inhalation induces a leukocyte recruitment to the lungs with an associated release of cytokines, which causes systemic symptoms.

It is estimated that more than 700,000 workers in the United States are involved in welding operations so that the potential for inhalational exposure and metal fume fever is great. The clinical syndrome begins 3–10 hours after exposure to zinc oxide. The initial symptom may be a metallic taste associated with throat irritation and followed within several hours by the onset of fever, chills, myalgia, malaise, and a nonproductive cough. Occasionally, nausea, vomiting, and headache are noted. Physical examination during the episode may reveal a febrile patient with crackles on auscultation of the chest. Laboratory evaluation frequently reveals a leukocytosis with a

left shift and an elevated serum lactate dehydrogenase. The chest radiograph, pulmonary function tests, and arterial blood gas measurement are usually normal. Transient chest radiographic infiltrates, reduced lung volumes and $DL_{CO}$ have been reported in severe cases. Signs and symptoms generally peak at 18 hours and resolve spontaneously with complete resolution of abnormalities within 1–2 days.

Treatment of metal fume fever is entirely symptomatic. Control of elevated body temperature by antipyretics and oxygen therapy for hypoxemia may be required. There is no evidence that steroid therapy is of any benefit. Prevention relies on appropriate engineering controls and/or personal protective equipment to reduce exposure. There are no good data on the long term sequelae of repeated exposures.

## Polymer Fume Fever

A syndrome similar to metal fume fever may occur after inhalation of combustion products of polytetrafluoroethylene (Teflon) resins. The properties of Teflon—strength, thermal stability, and chemical inertness—make it a widely used product in the manufacture of cooking utensils, electric appliances, and insulating material. When Teflon is heated to temperatures greater than 300 °C, numerous degradation products are formed that appear to cause the syndrome. Exposure to such combustion products can occur during welding of metal coated with Teflon, during the operation of molding machines, and while smoking cigarettes contaminated with the polymer.

Exposure to a high concentration of polymer fumes causes a fever to develop within several hours. Often this occurs toward the end of the workshift or in the evening after work. The symptoms, signs, and laboratory findings of polymer fume fever are essentially the same as those of metal fume fever. The syndrome is self-limiting and resolves within 12–48 hours. Exposure to very high concentrations of polymer fumes may lead to the development of severe chemical pneumonitis with pulmonary edema. In such cases, the symptoms, signs, and laboratory features are similar to pulmonary edema from other causes.

## Organic Dust Toxic Syndrome

Inhalation of various bioaerosols contaminated with fungi, bacteria, and/or endotoxins can cause an acute febrile syndrome known as organic dust toxic syndrome (ODTS). Exposures to moldy silage, moldy wood chips, compost, sewage sludge, grain dust ("grain fever"), cotton dust ("mill fever"), animal confinement building environments, and contaminated humidifier mist ("humidifier fever") have been associated with the development of inhalation fever. The clinical syndrome of ODTS is essentially identical described above for metal or polymer fume fever. Severe pulmonary inflammatory reactions have been described with massive exposures but are rare.

# METAL-INDUCED LUNG DISEASE

## Hard-Metal

Hard metal is a cemented alloy of tungsten carbide with cobalt, although other metals such as titanium, tantalum, chromium, molybdenum, or nickel may also be added. These cemented carbides have found wide industrial use because of their properties of extreme hardness, strength, and heat resistance. Their major use is in the manufacture of cutting tools and drill tip surfaces.

Workers exposed to hard metal are at risk for developing interstitial lung disease, so-called "hard-metal disease," and occupational asthma. The putative cause of both these disease processes is cobalt. Some workers may present with features of both hard-metal-induced airway and parenchymal diseases. Workers at risk for these disease are those engaged in the manufacture of the alloy, grinders and sharpeners of hard metal tools, diamond polishers and others who use discs containing cobalt, and metal coaters who use powdered hard metal. Occupational asthma due to cobalt in hard-metal workers is similar to that caused by other low-molecular-weight sensitizer agents.

Workers with hard-metal disease typically complain of symptoms of dyspnea on exertion, cough, sputum production, chest tightness, and fatigue. Physical examination may reveal evidence of crackles on chest auscultation, reduced chest expansion, clubbing, and, in advanced cases, cyanosis. Chest radiographs may show bilateral rounded and/or irregular opacities with no pathognomonic features. Pulmonary function tests tend to show both a restrictive ventilatory impairment and a decreased $DL_{CO}$. The diagnosis of hard-metal disease often is made on the basis of pathologic examination of lung tissue rather than by clinical evaluation. The histologic findings are those of interstitial pneumonitis, frequently of the giant cell type (GIP), and interstitial fibrosis. Characteristic multinucleated giant histiocytes may be seen in BAL fluid as well.

The primary treatment of hard-metal disease is removal of the affected worker from further exposure. Relatively rapid progression to impairment is not infrequent and resolution after cessation of exposure may not occur. Complete removal from cobalt exposure is advisable because a case has been reported of a worker who developed rapidly fatal lung disease with continued exposure. Because hard-metal disease is often progressive, empiric therapy with corticosteroids may be required.

## Beryllium

Beryllium is a light-weight, tensile metal that has a high melting point and good alloying properties. It has a wide range of applications in modern industrial processes. Although beryllium is no longer used in the manufacture of fluorescent light tubes, it is commonly used in the ceramics, electronics, aerospace, and nuclear weapons/power industries. Workers at risk are those involved in processes that generate airborne beryllium, including melting, casting, grinding, drilling, extracting, and smelting of beryllium. Acute beryllium-induced pneumonitis can occur after high-intensity exposure but has largely disappeared due to improved workplace control of exposures. Chronic beryllium disease, which involves sensitization to the metal through a cell-mediated (type IV) mechanism, still occurs after lower-level exposures in susceptible workers. Latency from time of initial beryllium exposure to the development of clinically manifest disease ranges from months to many years.

Chronic beryllium disease is a granulomatous inflammatory disorder that is very similar to sarcoidosis. In fact, the histologic findings in chronic beryllium disease are identical to those of sarcoidosis, ie, epithelioid (noncaseating) granulomas with mononuclear cell infiltrates and varying degrees of interstitial fibrosis. Chronic beryllium disease usually affects only the lungs, but involvement of skin, liver, spleen, salivary glands, kidney, and bone may occur. Extrapulmonary involvement is more common in sarcoidosis.

Workers with chronic beryllium disease commonly present with insidious onset of dyspnea on exertion, cough, and fatigue. Anorexia, weight loss, fever, chest pain, and arthralgias may also occur. Physical examination findings are usually confined to the lungs, with crackles being the most common, but may be absent with mid disease. Palpable hepatosplenomegaly and lymphadenopathy may be present a small proportion of patients.

Chest radiographic findings are ill-defined nodular or irregular opacities and hilar adenopathy. The latter is seen somewhat less frequently (up to 40% of patients) than in sarcoidosis and rarely occurs in the absence of parenchymal changes. The small nodular opacities are sometimes more prominent in the upper lung zones and may coalesce into more conglomerate masses.

Pulmonary function testing may be normal with mild disease, but there is usually a restrictive, obstructive, or mixed pattern of impairment and a reduced $DL_{CO}$. Resting arterial hypoxemia and further desaturation with exercise are common with more severe disease.

Often a meticulously obtained occupational history is required to suggest beryllium as the causative agent. Because of the similarity between chronic beryllium disease and sarcoidosis, demonstration of beryllium sensitization is necessary to confirm the diagnosis. A relatively specific blood lymphocyte transformation test (LTT) is available in which the beryllium-specific uptake of radiolabeled DNA precursors by the patient's lymphocytes cultured in vitro is quantitated. The sensitivity of the LTT for chronic beryllium disease is approximately 90% using peripheral blood lymphocytes and can be increased if lung lymphocytes obtained from BAL are used. The blood LTT can also be used to screen for sensitization among beryllium-exposed workers.

The current criteria for the diagnosis of chronic beryllium disease are the following: (1) a history of beryllium exposure: (2) a positive peripheral blood or BAL LTT; and (3) the presence of epithelioid granulomas and mononuclear infiltrates, in the absence of infection, in lung tissue. This approach relies on the LTT to confirm sensitization to beryllium and transbronchial biopsy of lung tissue to confirm the presence of disease.

Because the disease process involves a type of hypersensitivity, a worker with chronic beryllium disease should be completely removed from further beryllium exposure. A trial of corticosteroids is warranted in symptomatic workers with documented pulmonary physiologic abnormalities as this may induce a remission in some. If steroid therapy is initiated, objective parameters of response such as chest radiographs and pulmonary function test results should be serially monitored in order to adjust appropriately the dose and duration of treatment. Chronic beryllium disease has the propensity to develop into chronic irreversible pulmonary fibrosis so careful monitoring of affected workers is necessary.

## Other Metals

Inhalation of relatively high concentrations of cadmium, chromium, or nickel fumes or mercury vapor can cause toxic pneumonitis. Occupational exposure to certain metals (eg, antimony, barium, iron, tin) can lead to deposition of sufficient radiodense dust that chest radiographs demonstrate opacities in the absence of lung parenchymal inflammation and fibrosis.

## PNEUMOCONIOSES

The pneumoconioses are a group of conditions resulting from the deposition of mineral dust in the lung and the subsequent lung tissue reaction to the dust.

## Silicosis

Silicosis is a parenchymal lung disease that results from the inhalation of silicon dioxide, or silica, in crystalline form. Silica is a major component of rock and sand. Workers with potential for exposure are miners, sandblasters, foundry workers, tunnel drillers, quarry workers, stone carvers, ceramic workers, and silica flour production workers.

Exposure to silica can lead to one of three disease patterns: (1) chronic simple silicosis, which usually follows greater than 10 years of exposure to respirable dust with less than 30% quartz; (2) subacute/accelerated silicosis, which generally follows

shorter, heavier exposures, ie, 2–5 years; and (3) acute silicosis, which is often seen following intense exposure to fine dust of high silica content over a several month period.

Chronic silicosis is characterized by the formation of silicotic nodules in the pulmonary parenchyma and the hilar lymph nodes (Figure 20–5). The lesions in the hilar lymph nodes may calcify in an "egg shell" pattern that, while only occurring in a small proportion of cases, is virtually pathognomonic for silicosis. Lung parenchymal involvement tends to have a predilection for the upper lobes. The coalescence of small silicotic nodules into larger fibrotic masses, called progressive massive fibrosis (PMF), may complicate a minority of cases. Progressive massive fibrosis tends to occur in the upper lung fields, may obliterate blood vessels and bronchioles, causes gross distortion of lung architecture, and leads to respiratory insufficiency.

Accelerated silicosis is similar to chronic silicosis except that the time span is shorter and the complication of PMF is seen more frequently.

Acute silicosis is a rare condition seen in workers who are exposed to very high concentrations of free silica dust with fine particle size. Such exposures frequently occur in the absence of adequate respiratory protection. The characteristic findings differ from chronic silicosis in that the lungs show consolidation without silicotic nodules and the alveolar spaces are filled with fluid similar to that found in pulmonary alveolar proteinosis. Acute silicosis leads to death in most cases.

Alveolar macrophages play an important role in the pathogenesis of silicosis as these cells ingest inhaled silica and then release cytokines that recruit and/or stimulate other cells. Although crystalline silica can be cytotoxic secondary to direct chemical

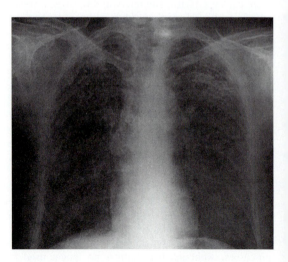

**Figure 20–5.** Radiographic changes of simple silicosis.

damage to cellular membranes, the primary effect of inhaled silica on macrophages is activation. The silica-activated macrophages recruit and activate T lymphocytes, which in turn recruit and activate a secondary population of monocyte-macrophages. The activated macrophages produce cytokines, which stimulate fibroblasts to proliferate and to produce increased amounts of collagen.

There are few symptoms and signs of chronic simple silicosis. The diagnosis is usually made by chest radiographs, which usually reveal small round opacities (< 10 mm in diameter) in both lungs, with a predilection for the upper lung zones. If an adequate occupational history is obtained from the patient along with a thorough review of the chest radiographs, the diagnosis of silicosis should not present any great difficulty. Pulmonary function testing in patients with simple silicosis is usually normal but occasionally may demonstrate evidence of a mild restrictive ventilatory defect and decreased lung compliance. In addition, a mild obstructive impairment is occasionally found in patients with simple silicosis, often due to chronic bronchitis caused by nonspecific dust effects and/or smoking. With complicated silicosis involving progressive fibrosis (nodules ≥ 10mm in diameter), increasing dyspnea is noted, initially with exertion and then progressing to dyspnea at rest. Complicated chronic silicosis is associated with greater reductions in lung volumes, decreased diffusing capacity, and hypoxemia with exercise.

There is an increased incidence of mycobacterial disease, both typical and atypical in silicosis. Fungal diseases (especially cryptococcosis, blastomycosis, and coccidioidomycosis) are also seen with greater frequency. The mechanism by which the immune-inflammatory responses to inhaled silica lead to the increased incidence of mycobacterial and fungal infections is not clearly understood.

No treatment for silicosis is currently known so that management is directed toward the prevention of progression and the development of complications. Continued exposure should be avoided and surveillance for tuberculosis should be instituted. In tuberculin skin-test positive silicotic workers, isoniazid (300 mg/d) prophylaxis for a full year is currently recommended. In acute silicosis, therapeutic whole-lung lavage has been employed to physically remove silica from the alveoli.

The prognosis for patients with chronic silicosis is good, especially if they are removed from exposure. Mortality remains high, however, in those who develop PMF.

## Asbestosis

Asbestos is the name for the fibrous forms of a group of mineral silicates. The types of asbestos that have been used commercially are chrysotile, amosite, crocidolite, anthophyllite, tremolite, and actinolite, with chrysotile being far and away the most com-

monly used. The durability, heat resistance, and ability to be woven into textiles of asbestos led to a wide variety of industrial applications. Major occupational exposures occurred with asbestos mining and milling, manufacture or installation of insulation for ships or buildings, manufacture of friction materials for brake linings and clutch facings, asbestos cement manufacture, asbestos textile manufacture, and asbestos-containing spray products for decorative, acoustical, and fireproofing purposes.

Asbestosis refers to the diffuse interstitial pulmonary fibrosis caused by inhalation of asbestos fibers. The inhaled fibers are primarily deposited at the bifurcations of conducting airways and alveoli where they are phagocytosed by macrophages. The initial injury is characterized by damage to the alveolar epithelium, incomplete phagocytosis by and activation of alveolar and interstitial macrophages, and release of proinflammatory cytokines as well as cytotoxic oxygen radicals by activated macrophages. A peribronchiolar inflammatory response ensues involving fibroblast proliferation and stimulation, which may eventually lead to fibrosis. Many factors are felt to play a role in disease initiation and progression, including the type and size of fiber, the intensity and duration of exposure, history of cigarette smoking, and individual susceptibility. A dose-response relationship exists such that asbestosis is more common in workers with a higher exposure level. Once asbestosis has begun it may progress irrespective of removal from continued exposure. Finally, there is a considerable latency period (10–20 years) between exposure and development of clinically apparent disease.

The diagnosis of asbestosis is made by a thorough exposure history, clinical examination, appropriate imaging studies, and pulmonary function testing. The symptoms of asbestosis are indistinguishable from any other gradually progressive interstitial pulmonary fibrosing disorder, with progressive dyspnea and nonproductive cough being the most prominent. Bibasilar crackles with a "Velcro" quality can be auscultated over the posterolateral chest in the mid to late phase of inspiration. The crackles of asbestosis are unaffected by coughing.

Imaging studies that are helpful in the evaluation of asbestos-exposed patients are the chest radiograph and HRCT. The chest radiograph shows characteristic small, irregular or linear opacities distributed throughout the lung fields but more prominent in the lower zones. There is loss of definition of the heart border and hemidiaphragms. The most useful radiographic finding is the presence of bilateral pleural thickening, which does not commonly occur with other diseases causing interstitial pulmonary fibrosis (Figure 20–6). Diaphragmatic or pericardial calcification is almost a pathognomonic sign of asbestos exposure. The ILO classification system is often used in the United States to rate the degree of profusion of

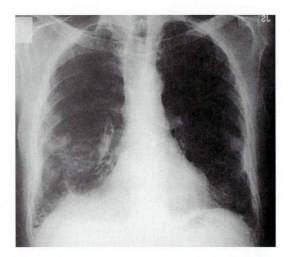

**Figure 20–6.** Radiographic changes of asbestosis.

small, irregular opacities and of pleural thickening on the chest radiograph. Conventional chest CT is more sensitive than chest radiography for the detection of pleural disease but not for parenchymal disease. High-resolution CT scanning is the most sensitive imaging method for detecting early asbestosis.

Depending on the severity of disease, pulmonary function testing will show varying degrees of restrictive impairment and decreased $DL_{CO}$. Because asbestosis begins as a peribronchiolar process, reduced flow rates at low lung volumes, indicative of small airways obstruction, may be seen.

As for silicosis, there is no known treatment for asbestosis. Fortunately, only a minority of those exposed are likely to develop radiographically evident disease, and among these, most do not develop significant respiratory impairment. Workers with asbestosis should be removed from further asbestos exposure as the risk that parenchymal scarring will progress appears to increase with cumulative asbestos exposure. Any other factors that may contribute to respiratory disease should be reduced or eliminated. This is especially true of cigarette smoking as there is some evidence that it may contribute to the initiation and progression of asbestosis.

The substitution of other fibrous materials for asbestos and the institution of strict environmental controls where it is still present have led to a dramatic reduction of occupational exposures to asbestos. Medical surveillance of all currently exposed workers in the United States is required by Occupational Safety and Health Administration (OSHA) regulation.

## Coal Workers' Pneumoconiosis

Coal workers' pneumoconiosis is the term used to describe parenchymal lung disease due to the inhala-

tion of coal dust. Miners who work at the coal face in underground mining or drillers in surface mines are at greatest risk of contracting this disease. A heavy coal dust burden is required to induce coal workers' pneumoconiosis, and the condition is rarely seen in those who have spent less than 20 years underground.

The coal macule is the primary lesion in coal workers' pneumoconiosis. It is formed when the inhaled dust burden exceeds the amount that can be removed by alveolar macrophages and mucociliary clearance. This leads to retention of coal dust in the terminal respiratory units. Prolonged retention causes lung fibroblasts to secrete a limiting layer of reticulin around the dust collection, or macule, near the respiratory bronchiole. Progressive enlargement of the macule may weaken the bronchiole wall to create a focal area of centrilobular emphysema; coalesence of small macules into larger lesions may occur. Initially there is a predilection for the upper lung lobes but with progression of the disease the lower lobes become involved. As for silicosis, coal workers' pneumoconiosis can be characterized as simple (radiographic lesions < 10 mm in diameter) or complicated (lesions ≥ 10 mm in diameter). Only a small proportion of miners (less than 5%) develop complicated or progressive fibrotic disease. Progressive massive fibrosis, identical to that described above for silicosis, may occur.

The symptoms of cough and sputum production are common among coal miners and are often the result of chronic bronchitis from dust inhalation rather than coal workers' pneumoconiosis. As with silicosis, simple coal workers' pneumoconiosis is often asymptomatic. The symptoms and signs associated with complicated disease are the same as those described above for silicosis. Progressive massive fibrosis almost invariably leads to respiratory insufficiency and death.

The chest radiograph in simple coal workers' pneumoconiosis shows the presence of small, rounded opacities in the lung parenchyma. Often seen first in the upper lung zones, these opacities may involve the lower zones in the later stage of the disease. Calcification of the hilar lymph nodes is not seen unless there is concomitant silica exposure. Complicated coal workers' pneumoncocciosis/PMF is diagnosed when large parenchymal opacities are present.

Caplan's syndrome may occur in coal miners with rheumatoid arthritis and is characterized by the appearance of rapidly evolving rounded densities on chest radiographs. These have a propensity to cavitate and histologically are composed of layers of necrotic collagen and coal dust. The pulmonary manifestations of Caplan's syndrome may precede or coincide with the onset of arthritis.

Pulmonary function findings vary with the stage of disease in a manner similar to that described for silicosis. In simple disease, there are usually no significant pulmonary function abnormalities. In complicated disease, either a restrictive or mixed restrictive and obstructive pattern may occur with a decreased diffusing capacity and abnormal arterial blood gases. It is important to remember that an obstructive ventilatory impairment in a coal miner may be due to chronic bronchitis, coal workers' pneumoconiosis or both.

Simple coal workers' pneumoconiosis usually follows a benign course. Unlike silicosis, no increase is seen in either pulmonary tuberculosis or fungal infections of the lung. In complicated disease, the affected worker may have mild to severe respiratory symptoms and significant impairment. In such cases, depending on the degree of impairment, the worker should be removed from continued dust exposure. In the United States, underground miners are able to participate in a federally run medical surveillance program that provides free periodic chest radiographs. If coal workers' pneumoconiosis is evident on the chest radiograph, the affected miner has the right to work in a low-dust job in the mine without loss of pay. In addition, personal dust exposure is monitored to confirm that exposures remain low.

Prevention of coal mine dust-related respiratory disease depends primarily on effective control of exposure to coal mine dust. In the United States, good progress has been made in reducing the incidence and prevalence of coal workers' pneumoconiosis since the passage in 1969 of the Coal Mine Health and Safety Act, which established programs to monitor dust levels in mines and to provide radiographic surveillance of miners. Despite the reduction in prevalence of coal worker's pneumoconiosis that has occurred since 1969, the number of death certificates listing the disease remains approximately 2000 per year.

## Other Pneumoconioses

Other mineral dusts capable of causing pulmonary parenchymal fibrosis include graphite (which causes disease similar to coal workers' pneumoconiosis), kaolin and diatomaceous earth (which cause silicosis-like disease), and talc and mica (which cause disease that has features of both silicosis and asbestosis). A metal dust that can cause pneumoconiosis is aluminum oxide, which can form fibers under certain conditions.

## CHRONIC BRONCHITIS

Chronic bronchitis is characterized by inflammation of the bronchial tree and is manifested by persistent cough productive of sputum on most days for at least three months of the year for at least two successive years. The inhalation of irritant dusts, fumes, and gases can cause chronic simple bronchitis, ie,

persistent sputum production without airflow obstruction (Table 20–6). Whether workers with chronic simple bronchitis are at risk for the development of chronic airflow obstruction and permanent respiratory impairment is an area of controversy that has yet to be completely resolved. The development of permanent respiratory impairment may be dependent on a variety of host factors such as preexisting nonspecific airway hyperresponsiveness, protease-antiprotease activity, and whether there is concomitant cigarette smoking.

### Diagnosis

The diagnosis of chronic bronchitis is straightforward and based entirely on whether the worker's history is consistent with the definition given above. Once chronic bronchitis has been diagnosed, establishing a causal role for an occupational exposure is also based on the history obtained from the worker. Symptoms of cough and sputum production that are temporally associated with workplace exposure should suggest the diagnosis. Smoking workers are at greater risk of developing respiratory symptoms with exposure to other irritants and a work-related contribution to their symptoms should be considered. Upper respiratory tract inflammatory symptoms, eye irritation, and an increased incidence of symptoms among other coworkers are all features that support a work-related problem. Physical examination may demonstrate no evidence of pulmonary abnormality. Spirometry and expiratory flow-volume curves may or may not show evidence of airway obstruction. A nonsmoking worker exposed to high concentrations of an irritant at the workplace who has evidence of airway obstruction and no history of asthma should be suspected of having occupationally induced chronic bronchitis.

**Table 20–6.** Some agents causing chronic bronchitis.

**Minerals**
Coal
Oil mist
Silica
Silicates
Man-made vitreous fibers
Portland cement

**Metals**
Osmium
Vanadium
Welding fumes

**Organic dusts**
Cotton
Grain
Wood

**Smoke**
Tobacco smoke
Fire smoke
Engine exhaust

## Treatment

Because chronic bronchitis often has a multi-factorial etiology, a multifocal approach to management should be taken. If the worker smokes, cessation should be encouraged. Work exposure to the suspected agent should be reduced or eliminated. Pharmacologic agents of benefit are the beta$_2$-agonists, inhaled steroids, and inhaled anticholinergic agents. Periodic follow-up with particular attention to symptoms and worsening airway obstruction on serial spirometry is warranted.

The prognosis of workers with chronic irritant-induced bronchitis has not been well described. There are data, however, which suggest that accelerated loss of ventilatory function can occur. In light of this, it may be prudent to assume that all workers with chronic work-related bronchitis are at risk of developing permanent respiratory impairment. Those with worsening symptoms or lung function abnormalities should be considered for removal from further exposure. Reduction of exposure to conditions capable of causing chronic bronchitis through engineering controls or respiratory protective equipment is necessary to prevent further cases.

## PLEURAL DISORDERS

The pleura is the serous membrane that lines the lungs, the mediastinum, the diaphragm, and the rib cage. It is divided into the *visceral pleura,* which lines the lung surface, and the *parietal pleura,* which lines the remaining structures. The primary cause of occupationally-induced pleural disease is asbestos, although talc and mica can cause benign pleural disease and zeolite can cause mesothelioma.

### Benign Pleural Effusions

Pleural effusions resulting from asbestos exposure may occur in up to 3% of exposed workers. The risk of developing an effusion is greater in those with heavy exposure. Benign asbestos effusions tend to develop within 5–20 years of the onset of exposure.

A pleural effusion can be attributed to asbestos if the following criteria are met: (1) a significant history of occupational exposure with an appropriate latent period since onset of exposure; (2) exclusion of other known causes of pleural effusion; and (3) a repeat evaluation of the effusion within a minimum of two years confirms that it is benign.

The majority of workers who have pleural effusions from asbestos exposure are asymptomatic. Physical examination in those with large effusions may show diminished rib cage expansion, dullness to percussion, and decreased breath sounds on the side of the effusion. Chest radiographs typically show small to moderately large, unilateral pleural effusions. Bilateral involvement occurs in about 10% of cases of benign asbestos effusions. Pleural thickening may be noted, although often the effusion is the first manifestation of asbestos-induced disease. Diffuse pleural thickening involving both pleural surfaces and obliteration of the costophrenic angle may develop in the wake of benign asbestos effusions. Thoracentesis will obtain pleural liquid that is a sterile exudate with no specific findings, although increased eosinophils are suggestive of an asbestos etiology.

It is essential to exclude other etiologies of pleural effusion, especially tuberculosis and malignancy. Regular follow-up with repeat thoracentesis if pleural fluid persists is essential. There is no known treatment. Recurrences occur, but in most cases, the effusion clears spontaneously within a year without any obvious residual pleural disease.

### Pleural Plaques

Pleural plaques are circumscribed areas of pleural thickening that are the most common radiographic findings due to chronic asbestos exposure. Plaques usually involve the parietal pleural surface and tend to occur over the central portions of the hemidiaphragm and along the inferior posterolateral aspect of the lower ribs.

Bilateral pleura plaques are almost invariably due to past asbestos exposure and their prevalence is related to both the intensity of exposure and the duration since onset of exposure. Workers with a greater exposure have a higher chance of developing plaques. In workers without asbestosis, plaques rarely cause signs and symptoms. The diagnosis is usually made from a routine chest radiograph. When plaques lie parallel to the beam, they appear as slightly to moderately protuberant linear or ovoid opacities along the costal or diaphragmatic margins. If calcified, they have an irregular, unevenly dense appearance. Although oblique x-ray views are recommended by some, chest CT scanning provides the most sensitive and specific technique for confirming the presence of plaques. Pathologically, the plaques are composed mainly of collagen with little accompanying inflammation. Asbestos fibers can be demonstrated in plaque tissue by electron microscopy, although this is not required for routine clinical diagnosis.

A worker with a past history of asbestos exposure and pleural plaques on chest radiograph should be evaluated for the presence of asbestosis. Even if no evidence of parenchymal disease is found, the worker should be monitored periodically for the possible development of this condition. Although workers with pleural plaques and no parenchymal disease typically do not develop respiratory impairment, there is evidence that heavily exposed workers with radiographic evidence of plaques, but no asbestosis, tend to have decreased lung function in comparison to workers with similar exposure histories whose chest radiographs are normal.

Because of the risk of development of bronchogenic carcinoma with asbestos exposure, cigarette smoking should be discouraged. The increased risk of lung cancer is not due to the plaques but to the cumulative dose of asbestos, the plaques merely acting as a marker of exposure.

Diffuse pleural thickening involving both visceral and parietal pleura can also result from past asbestos exposure. Such thickening is occasionally associated with a restrictive-type respiratory impairment even in the absence of asbestosis.

Neither circumscribed plaques nor diffuse pleural thickening is believed to undergo malignant transformation to mesothelioma.

## Mesothelioma

Malignant mesotheliomas are rare pleural tumors of which up to 80% occur in asbestos-exposed individuals. The exposure to asbestos may be relatively light, and the latent period between exposure and onset of disease is in the range of 30–40 years. Crocidolite and amosite appear to be the asbestos fiber types with the highest potential for inducing mesotheliomas. Exposure to the fibrous mineral, zeolite, and thoracic radiation are other risk factors for mesothelioma.

Mesotheliomas generally present with the symptoms of chest pain and dyspnea. The chest pain is often nonpleuritic and may be referred to the upper abdomen or the shoulder when there is diaphragmatic involvement. Other common symptoms are fatigue, decreased appetite, and weight loss. The clinical findings are influenced by the histological type of the tumor. Epithelial and mixed mesotheliomas are more commonly associated with large pleural effusions, while mesenchymal tumors rarely have an associated effusion. Patients with the epithelial type are more likely to have supraclavicular or axillary lymph node involvement and extension to the pericardium. Those with the mesenchymal type have a higher incidence of extrapulmonary metastases.

Chest radiographic findings may be suggestive of a pleural effusion but without either a meniscus or a contralateral shift of the mediastinal structures. In advanced cases, tumor is noted to encase the lung, the mediastinum is shifted toward the side of the tumor, and the involved hemithorax is contracted. Chest CT scans are especially helpful in the diagnosis of mesothelioma and often show a thickened pleura with a distinctive irregular or nodular internal margin.

Pleural fluid analysis shows a serosanguinous exudate that is often quite viscid. The cellular content is a mixture of mesothelial cells, differentiated and undifferentiated malignant mesothelial cells, and varying numbers of lymphocytes and polymorphonuclear leukocytes. While cytologic examination of the fluid may be suggestive of malignant mesothelioma, it is rarely diagnostic. An open thoracotomy or thoracoscopy with multiple biopsies is usually required to confirm the diagnosis. Even with adequate tissue for pathologic examination, distinguishing mesothelioma from metastatic adenocarcinoma may be difficult. Special stains and/or electron microscopy are usually required.

The treatment of malignant mesothelioma is palliative. Death from wasting or respiratory failure usually occurs within months after diagnosis. Radiotherapy, chemotherapy, and surgical treatments have been tried, but there are no good data to show that these prolong survival or improve quality of life.

## LUNG CANCER

Although cigarette smoking is the most important preventable cause of lung cancer, occupational exposures to respiratory tract carcinogens are also preventable. Estimates of the percentage of lung cancers attributable to occupational factors range from 3% to 17%. Agents both known and suspected to cause lung cancer are listed in Table 20–7. In addition, workers in several industries, including foundries, welding, printing, and rubber manufacturing, have been shown to be at increased risk of lung cancer without identification of specific carcinogenic agents.

The evaluation of any patient with lung cancer should include a careful occupational and environmental exposure history. The determination of whether a given exposure caused a cancer involves assessment of dose and latency, as well as consideration of the smoking history. When exposure to more than one carcinogen has occurred (eg, an occupational agent and tobacco smoke), both exposures may have contributed to the development of lung cancer. The management of a patient with work-related lung cancer is similar to that of any patient with lung cancer with the exception that an effort should be made

**Table 20–7.** Known and suspected lung carcinogens.

**Known**
  Asbestos
  Arsenic
  Chloromethyl ethers (eg, BCME)
  Chromium (hexavalent)
  Environmental tobacco smoke
  Mustard gas
  Nickel
  Polyaromatic hydrocarbons (eg, benzo(a)pyrene)
  Radon

**Suspected**
  Acrylonitrile
  Beryllium
  Cadmium
  Formaldehyde
  Silica
  Man-made vitreous fibers
  Vinyl chloride monomer

to prevent the exposure of other workers to the responsible agent at the patient's workplace.

## Specific Agents

**A. Asbestos:** Lung cancer is a more common cause of death due to asbestos exposure than mesothelioma. The effects of asbestos and cigarette smoke are believed to interact positively to increase the risk of lung cancer, but the magnitude of the interaction (additive or multiplicative) remains somewhat controversial and is probably dose-related. It is rare to see a lung cancer in an asbestos-exposed worker who does not smoke. Therefore, cessation of smoking as well as exposure to asbestos is necessary to prevent lung cancer among asbestos-exposed workers. Data from epidemiologic studies of heavily exposed workers support a linear relationship between level of asbestos exposure and lung cancer mortality. The nature of the dose-response relationship at lower levels of exposure is more controversial, with some data suggesting a threshold and other data suggesting that there is no "safe" level of exposure.

The mechanism of asbestos-related carcinogenesis is unclear, but it is likely that asbestos acts more as a promoting than an initiating agent. Both the physical and chemical characteristics of asbestos fibers appear to be factors in determining carcinogenic potential. Long, thin fibers are the most carcinogenic, but fibers that are more slowly cleared from the lungs (probably related to chemical characteristics) also appear to be more carcinogenic than those with a shorter residence time.

There are no distinctive features of asbestos-related lung cancer, although asbestos-related tumors occur somewhat more frequently in the lower lobes. Contrary to earlier reports, the distribution of histologic types of lung cancer is similar among asbestos-exposed workers to that of the general population. The risk of lung cancer is highest among workers with the greatest cumulative exposure to asbestos, and the latency since onset of exposure ranges from 15–30 years. The presence of asbestosis or asbestos-related pleural disease on the chest radiograph of a patient with lung cancer confirms a history of significant occupational or environmental exposure.

**B. Chloromethyl Ethers:** These compounds are alkylating agents capable of causing damage to DNA and are highly carcinogenic. In particular, occupational exposure to bischloromethyl ether (BCME) has been associated with an increased risk of small-cell carcinomas at a relatively young age. Smoking does not appear to further increase the risk among BCME-exposed workers. There are animal toxicologic data that support the carcinogenicity of BCME.

**C. Metals:** Occupational exposure to several metals has been associated with an increased risk of lung cancer. Workers exposed to arsenic in the smelting, pesticide manufacturing, and other industries have been shown to have a dose-related increased risk, although there is no animal model of arsenic-induced carcinogenesis. Exposure to hexavalent, but not trivalent, chromium has is another risk factor for lung cancer. Exposure to intermediate compounds in nickel refining, but not exposure to metallic nickel, has also been associated with increased relative risk for lung cancer.

**D. Radon:** Radon is an inert gas that is a decay product of uranium-235 and which itself decays with emission of alpha particles. Uranium miners as well as other underground miners exposed to radon have been shown to have a strikingly elevated risk of lung cancer. Exposure to radon and cigarette smoke appear to act synergistically to increase the risk of lung cancer. Small-cell carcinomas are increased disproportionately among uranium miners compared to the distribution of cell types in the general population. Although usually at much lower levels than in uranium mines, exposure to radon in homes has been estimated to be an important environmental risk factor for lung cancer in the United States.

**E. Environmental Tobacco Smoke:** Environmental tobacco smoke (ETS) is made up of both mainstream smoke exhaled by smokers as well as sidestream smoke released by burning cigarettes. There is now abundant data from epidemiologic studies to support an increased risk of lung cancer from ETS. The workplace environment can be an important source of exposure to ETS.

**F. Other Potential Lung Carcinogens:** Several agents for which either animal or epidemiologic data suggest an increased risk of lung cancer are shown in Table 20–7. These agents are listed as suspect lung carcinogens by the International Agency for Research against Cancer (IARC). Further research is needed to confirm the carcinogenic risk of exposure to these agents for humans.

# REFERENCES

## HISTORY & PHYSICAL EXAMINATION

Blanc P, Balmes JR: History and physical examination. In: Harber P, Schenker M, Balmes J (editors): *Occupational and Environmental Respiratory Disease.* Mosby, 1996.

## IMAGING STUDIES

Aberle DR, Balmes JR: Computed tomography of asbestos-related pulmonary parenchymal and pleural diseases. Clin Chest Med 1991;12:115.

## PULMONARY FUNCTION TESTING

Hankinson JL: Instrumentation for spirometry. Occupational Medicine: State of the Art Reviews 1993:397.

## BRONCHOPROVOCATION TESTING

Malo J-L, Cartier A: Bronchoprovocation testing. In: Harber P, Schenker M, Balmes J (editors): *Occupational and Environmental Respiratory Disease.* Mosby, 1996.

## TOXIC INHALATION INJURY

Balmes JR: Acute pulmonary injury from hazardous materials. In: Sullivan J, Krieger G (editors): *Hazardous Materials Toxicology: Clinical Principles of Environmental Health.* Williams & Wilkins, 1992.

Blanc PD et al: Symptoms, lung function and airway responsiveness following irritant inhalation. Chest 1993;103:1699.

Weiss SM, Lakshminarayan S: Acute inhalation injury. Clin Chest Med 1994;15:103.

## OCCUPATIONAL ASTHMA

American Thoracic Society: Official statement: Guidelines for the evaluation of impairment/disability in patients with asthma. Am Rev Respir Dis 1993;147:1056.

Bernstein IL et al: *Asthma in the Workplace.* Marcel Dekker, 1993.

Chan-Yeung M, Malo JL: Current concepts: Occupational asthma. N Engl J Med 1995;33:107.

Rylander R (editor): Endotoxins in the environment. Int J Occup Environ Health 1997;3(1):supplement.

## HYPERSENSITIVITY PNEUMONITIS

Richardson HB et al: Guidelines for the clinical evaluation of hypersensitivity pneumonitis, J Allergy Clin Immunol 1989;84:839.

Rose C: Hypersensitivity pneumonitis. In: Harber P, Schenker M, Balmes J (editors): *Occupational and Environmental Respiratory Disease.* Mosby, 1996.

## INHALATION FEVERS

Rose CS, Blanc PD: Inhalation fevers. In: Rom W (editor): *Environmental and Occupational Medicine,* 3rd ed. Lippincott–Raven, 1997.

## METAL-INDUCED LUNG DISEASE

Balmes JR: Beryllium and hard metal-related diseases. In: Rosenstock L, Cullen M (editors): *Clinical Occupational and Environmental Medicine.* Saunders, 1994.

## PNEUMOCONIOSES

Ahfield MD, Seixas NS: Prevalence of pneumoconiosis and its relationship to dust exposure in a cohort of U.S. bituminous coal miners and ex-miners. Am J Ind Med 1995;27:137.

American Thoracic Society: Official statement: Adverse effects of crystalline silica. Am J Respir Crit Care Med 1997;155:761.

Attfield M, Wagner G: Coal. In: Harber P, Schenker M, Balmes J (editors) *Occupational and Environmental Respiratory Disease.* Mosby, 1996.

Begin R: Asbestos. In: Harber P, Schenker M, Balmes J (editors): *Occupational and Environmental Respiratory Disease.* Mosby, 1996.

Davis G: Silica. In: Harber P, Schenker M, Balmes J (editors): *Occupational and Environmental Respiratory Disease.* Mosby, 1996.

Rom WN, Travis WD, Brody AR: Cellular and molecular basis of the asbestos-related diseases. Am Rev Respir Med 1991;143:408.

## CHRONIC BRONCHITIS

Kennedy S: Agents causing chronic airflow obstruction. In: Harber P, Schenker M, Balmes J (editors): *Occupational and Environmental Respiratory Disease.* Mosby, 1996.

## PLEURAL DISEASE

Begin R: Asbestos. In: Harber P, Schenker M, Balmes J (editors): *Occupational and Environmental Respiratory Disease.* Mosby, 1996.

Schwartz DA, et al: Restrictive lung function and asbestos-induced pleural fibrosis: a quantitative approach. J Clin Invest 1993;91:2685.

## LUNG CANCER

Steenland K et al: Occupational causes of lung cancer. In: Harber P, Schenker M, Balmes J (editors): *Occupational and Environmental Respiratory Disease.* Mosby, 1996.

# 21

# Cardiovascular Toxicology

*Neal L. Benowitz, MD*

Heart disease and stroke cause the majority of deaths in the United States. The major risk factors for coronary heart disease—family history, hypertension, diabetes, lipid abnormalities, and cigarette smoking—explain only a minority of the cases. Other factors such as stress and exposure to occupational or environmental toxic agents are believed to contribute to the development of heart disease, though the magnitude of the risk is unknown. This chapter focuses on cardiovascular disease caused by occupational toxic substances.

## CAUSATION IN TOXIC CARDIOVASCULAR DISEASE

The types and possible toxic causes of cardiovascular disease are shown in Table 21–1. Massive exposure may occur (eg, in acute carbon monoxide poisoning), but toxic cardiovascular disease is usually the result of chronic low-level exposures.

Problems in establishing the cause of cardiovascular disease include the following:

(1) Cardiovascular disease is common even in the absence of toxic exposures.

(2) There is usually nothing specific, either clinically or pathologically, to point to toxic cardiovascular disease.

(3) It is rarely possible to document high tissue levels of suspected toxic substances.

(4) It is difficult to establish occupational exposure levels over the 20 or more years it may take to develop cardiovascular disease.

(5) Cardiovascular toxic substances are likely to interact with other risk factors in causing or manifesting cardiovascular disease.

With these limitations in mind, this chapter will discuss current information concerning toxic cardiovascular disease.

## EVALUATION OF PATIENTS

Evaluation of patients with suspected toxic cardiovascular disease should include the following steps:

(1) Take a detailed occupational history (see Chapter 2), with attention to the temporal relationship between cardiovascular symptoms and exposure to toxic substances in the workplace.

(2) Attempt to document exposure to suspected toxic substances by obtaining industrial hygiene data and, if possible, directly monitoring worker exposure.

(3) Evaluate other cardiovascular risk factors.

(4) Perform a complete physical examination.

(5) Perform appropriate diagnostic studies, such as exercise stress testing and coronary angiography to establish the presence and extent of coronary artery disease; radionuclide angiography to establish myocardial disease and the presence of cardiomyopathy; and ambulatory electrocardiographic recordings taken on workdays and at other times to document work-related arrhythmias.

## CARDIOVASCULAR ABNORMALITIES CAUSED BY CARBON DISULFIDE

Chronic exposure to carbon disulfide appears to accelerate atherosclerosis and/or precipitate acute coronary ischemic events. Carbon disulfide is a widely used solvent, especially in the rubber and viscose rayon industries, in the manufacture of carbon tetrachloride and ammonium salts, and as a degreasing solvent. Epidemiologic studies have indicated that there is a 2.5- to 5-fold increase in the risk of death from coronary heart disease in workers exposed to carbon disulfide. For a complete discussion of the systemic effects of carbon disulfide, see Chapter 28.

### Pathogenesis

The mechanism of accelerated atherogenesis due to carbon disulfide has not been proved. One theory is that carbon disulfide reacts with amino- and thiol-containing compounds in the body to produce thiocarbamates, which are capable of complexing trace metals and inhibiting many enzyme systems. This

**Table 21–1.** Classification of cardiovascular diseases and possible toxic causes.

| Condition | Toxic Agent |
|---|---|
| Cardiac arrhythmia | Arsenic<br>Chlorofluorocarbon propellants<br>Hydrocarbon solvents (eg, 1,1,1-trichloroethane and trichloro-ethylene)<br>Organophosphate and carbamate insecticides |
| Coronary artery disease | Carbon disulfide<br>Carbon monoxide<br>Lead(?) |
| Hypertension | Cadmium<br>Carbon disulfide<br>Lead |
| Myocardial injury | Antimony<br>Arsenic<br>Arsine<br>Cobalt<br>Lead |
| Nonatheromatous ischemic heart disease | Organic nitrates (eg, nitroglycerin and ethylene glycol dinitrate) |
| Peripheral arterial occlusive disease | Arsenic<br>Lead |

causes metabolic abnormalities such as disturbances of lipid metabolism and thyroid function and can lead to elevations of low-density/lipoprotein cholesterol concentrations and hypothyroidism, which are risk factors for atherosclerosis. Inhibition of dopamine β-hydroxylase, an enzyme that converts dopamine to norepinephrine, may be responsible for some of the neuropsychiatric effects of carbon disulfide. Aldehyde dehydrogenase may be inhibited, resulting in a disulfiram-like reaction after alcohol ingestion. Other possible contributors to ischemic heart disease in workers exposed to carbon disulfide are depressed fibrinolytic activity, resulting in a greater tendency to thrombosis, and hypertension.

## Pathology

The findings are those of accelerated atherosclerotic vascular disease involving the coronary, cerebral, and peripheral arteries. Renovascular hypertension has also been reported.

## Clinical Findings

**A. Symptoms and Signs:** Acute intoxication may produce symptoms and signs of encephalopathy or polyneuropathy, including fatigue, headaches, dizziness, disorientation, paresthesias, psychosis, and delirium.

In cases of chronic exposure, patients may present with hypertension or manifestations of atherosclerotic vascular disease such as angina or myocardial infarction. An early sign of chronic carbon disulfide poisoning is abnormal ocular microcirculation, characterized by microaneurysms and hemorrhages resembling those of diabetic retinopathy. Presenile dementia, stroke, and sudden death have been reported in patients with chronic poisoning.

**B. Laboratory Findings:** Findings may include a decrease in serum thyroxine levels and an increase in serum cholesterol levels, particularly those of the very low density lipoproteins. There are no practical methods for measuring carbon disulfide levels in biological fluids.

**C. Cardiovascular Studies:** Delayed filling of the retinal arteries as measured by fluorescein angiography may be an early sign of vascular disease. The electrocardiogram sometimes shows evidence of ischemia or previous myocardial infarction. The presence of coronary artery disease may be confirmed by exercise stress testing and coronary angiography.

## Differential Diagnosis

The vascular findings in patients with chronic carbon disulfide poisoning are the same as those seen in any patient with atherosclerotic vascular disease. The most specific finding is abnormal ocular microcirculation in the absence of diabetes. The diagnosis is based on a clinical picture of premature vascular disease and a history of exposure to excessive levels of carbon disulfide for more than 5 or 10 years.

## Prevention

Carbon disulfide exposure is primarily by inhalation. The Occupational Safety and Health Administration (OSHA) recommends that workplace exposure be limited to 4 ppm (time-weighted average for a 40-hour workweek). Periodic examination of the ocular fundi may help detect early signs of vascular disease.

## Treatment

Treatment consists of removing the worker from sources of carbon disulfide exposure and providing medical measures for atherosclerotic vascular disease.

## Course & Prognosis

The course of the disease is similar to that of any atherosclerotic vascular disease. There is evidence of reversibility—at least of ocular changes—after exposure to carbon disulfide is discontinued.

## CARDIOVASCULAR ABNORMALITIES CAUSED BY CARBON MONOXIDE

Excessive carbon monoxide exposure can reduce maximal exercise capacity in healthy workers; aggravate angina pectoris, intermittent claudication, and chronic obstructive lung disease; and aggravate or induce cardiac arrhythmias. Acute intoxications can cause myocardial infarction or sudden death. Chronic high-level carbon monoxide exposure may result in congestive cardiomyopathy.

Carbon monoxide is the most widely distributed of all industrial toxic agents and accounts for the greatest number of intoxications and deaths. It is formed wherever combustion engines or other types of combustion are present. Workers at high risk include forklift operators, foundry workers, miners, mechanics, garage attendants, and firefighters. Carbon monoxide poisoning may also occur with the use of faulty furnaces or heaters, particularly improperly vented kerosene or charcoal heaters. Cigarette smoking is an important source of carbon monoxide, and occupational sources may be additive to exposure from cigarettes. The solvent methylene chloride is metabolized within the body to carbon monoxide.

For a complete discussion of carbon monoxide, see Chapter 33.

## Pathogenesis

The affinity of carbon monoxide for hemoglobin is more than 200 times that of oxygen. The binding of carbon monoxide and hemoglobin to form carboxyhemoglobin reduces the delivery of oxygen to body tissues because the oxygen-carrying capacity of hemoglobin is decreased and because less oxygen is released to tissues at any given oxygen tension (ie, there is a shift in the oxygen dissociation curve). Thus, a carboxyhemoglobin concentration of 20% represents a greater reduction in oxygen delivery than a 20% reduction in erythrocyte count. Other heme-containing proteins (eg, myoglobin, cytochrome oxidase, and cytochrome P-450) bind 10–15% of the total body carbon monoxide, but the medical significance of their binding at usual levels of exposure to carbon monoxide is unclear.

In healthy individuals exposed to carbon monoxide, the decrease in delivery of oxygen to tissues causes the cardiac output and coronary blood flow to increase to meet the metabolic demands of the heart. Although these compensatory responses allow healthy individuals to perform at normal work levels, their maximal exercise capacity is decreased. If, on the other hand, compensatory responses are limited, as in patients with coronary artery disease, carbon monoxide exposure may cause angina or myocardial infarction (Figure 21–1). Reduced exercise thresholds for the development of angina have been reported when carboxyhemoglobin concentrations are as low as 2.7% (Table 21–2). Carbon monoxide decreases the ventricular fibrillation threshold in experimental animals and may do the same in humans. This would explain why sudden death occurs in people who have coronary artery disease and are exposed to carbon monoxide, as has been reported to

occur on smoggy days in large cities. Severe carbon monoxide poisoning (carboxyhemoglobin concentrations > 50%) may cause severe hypoxic injury, including cardiovascular collapse.

Chronic exposure to carbon monoxide is thought to accelerate atherogenesis. Cigarette smokers demonstrate advanced coronary and peripheral atherosclerosis, and carbon monoxide is believed to be one of the primary etiologic factors. Several studies in animals have tested the effects of chronic high-level carbon monoxide exposure combined with feeding of atherogenic diets, and the results of some of these studies showed increased severity of atherosclerosis. Possible mechanisms include abnormal vascular permeability, increased vascular uptake of lipids, and increased platelet adhesiveness. Whether atherosclerosis is accelerated at levels of carbon monoxide commonly encountered in the workplace is unclear.

Chronic exposure to carbon monoxide results in increased red blood cell mass in response to chronic tissue hypoxia and in increased blood viscosity, which could contribute to acute cardiac events.

## Pathology

Cardiac necrosis is often observed in cases of fatal carbon monoxide poisoning and is presumably due to severe hypoxia. Myocardial infarction may occur in workers who have coronary artery disease and are exposed to high levels of carbon monoxide, particularly while performing strenuous work or exercise. Cardiomyopathy with cardiac enlargement and congestive heart failure has been described in workers with chronic high-level exposure to carbon monoxide (carboxyhemoglobin concentrations > 30%).

## Clinical Findings

**A. Symptoms and Signs:** Headache is typically the first symptom of carbon monoxide poisoning and may occur at carboxyhemoglobin concentrations as low as 10%. At higher concentrations, nausea, dizziness, fatigue, and dimmed vision are commonly reported.

In patients with angina pectoris or peripheral arterial occlusive disease, carbon monoxide exposure may reduce exercise capacity to the point of angina or claudication (Table 21–2). All workers experience a reduction in maximal exercise capacity.

In neuropsychiatric tests, findings such as increased reaction time and decreased manual dexterity may be seen at carboxyhemoglobin concentrations between 5 and 10%. At concentrations of 25%, there may be decreased visual acuity and impaired cognitive function; at 35%, ataxia; at 50%, vomiting, tachypnea, tachycardia, and hypertension; and at higher levels, coma, convulsions, and cardiovascular and respiratory depression. Myocardial ischemia may be evident at any carboxyhemoglobin concentration in susceptible individuals.

**B. Laboratory Findings:** The only finding

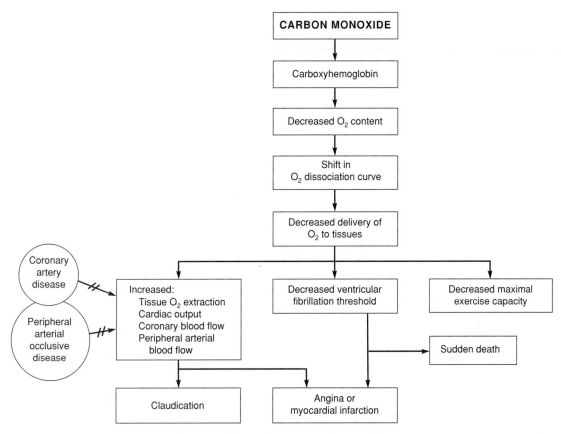

**Figure 21–1.** Cardiovascular consequences of exposure to carbon monoxide. The presence of coronary artery disease or peripheral arterial occlusive disease prevents (///) the usual compensatory increase in coronary or peripheral arterial blood flow, and this results in symptoms of arterial insufficiency.

specific for carbon monoxide intoxication is elevation of the carboxyhemoglobin concentration. Normal carboxyhemoglobin concentrations and examples of concentrations resulting from exposure to carbon monoxide in the environment and the workplace are shown in Table 21–3.

When arterial blood gases are measured, they usu-

ally show a normal or a slightly reduced arterial oxygen tension, with substantial reductions in venous $PO_2$ and oxygen content. Although respiratory alkalosis due to hyperventilation is commonly observed, there is respiratory failure in the most severe poisonings. When there is marked tissue hypoxia, lactic acidosis develops.

**Table 21–2.** Effects of carbon monoxide on exercise capacity.

| Group | Baseline Exercise Duration (sec) | Level of Exposure to Carbon Monoxide | Increase in Concentration of Carboxy-hemoglobin | Exercise Duration After Exposure (sec) | Exercise End Point |
|---|---|---|---|---|---|
| Healthy individuals | 698 | 100 ppm for 1 h | 1.7% → 4% | 662 | Exhaustion |
| Patients with angina pectoris | 224 | 50 ppm for 2 h | 1% → 2.7% | 188 | Angina |
| Patients with intermittent claudication | 174 | 50 ppm for 2 h | 1.1 → 2.8% | 144 | Claudication |
| Patients with chronic lung disease | 219 | 100 ppm for 1 h | 1.4% → 4.1% | 147 | Dyspnea |

**Table 21–3.** Normal carboxyhemoglobin concentrations and examples of concentrations resulting from exposure to carbon monoxide in the environment and the workplace.

| Source of Carbon Monoxide | Carboxyhemoglobin Concentration | |
| --- | --- | --- |
| | Average (%) | Range (%) |
| **Endogenous Metabolism** (normal level[1]) | 0.5 | . . . |
| **Environmental exposure** | | |
| Air pollution | 2 | 1.5–2.5 |
| Cigarette smoking | 6 | 3–15 |
| **Occupational exposure** (nonsmokers) | | |
| Foundry workers | 4 | 2–9 |
| Mechanics | 5 | . . . |
| Garage attendants | 7 | . . . |

[1]Carbon monoxide is normally formed as a product of metabolism of hemoglobin. Endogenous levels may be higher if there is increased hemoglobin turnover.

**C. Cardiovascular Studies:** The ECG may show ischemic changes or myocardial infarction. Various types of arrhythmias, including atrial fibrillation and premature atrial and ventricular contractions, are observed. Abnormalities seen on the ECG are usually transient, though ST–T wave abnormalities may persist for days or weeks.

### Differential Diagnosis

The most important clue to carbon monoxide poisoning is the occupational or environmental exposure history. A typical symptom, such as headache, confusion, or sudden collapse, with findings of myocardial ischemia or metabolic acidosis, should suggest the diagnosis, and carboxyhemoglobin concentrations should be measured.

### Prevention

Levels of carbon monoxide should be monitored if there are sources of combustion such as combustion engines or furnaces in the workplace. The current 8-hour threshold limit value is 25 ppm, which at the end of an 8-hour workday results in a carboxyhemoglobin concentration of 2–3% This concentration is tolerated well by healthy individuals but may impair function in people with cardiovascular or chronic lung disease. Workplace monitoring is easily done with a portable carbon monoxide meter. Biological monitoring of workers involves measuring either the carboxyhemoglobin concentration in blood or the level of expired carbon monoxide, which is directly proportionate to the carboxyhemoglobin concentra-

tion. Elevated carbon monoxide levels should be anticipated in cigarette smokers.

### Treatment

Carbon monoxide is eliminated from the body by respiration, and the rate of elimination depends on ventilation, pulmonary blood flow, and inspired oxygen concentration. The half-life of carbon monoxide in a sedentary adult breathing air is 4–5 hours. The half-life can be reduced to 80 minutes by giving 100% oxygen by face mask or to 25 minutes by giving hyperbaric oxygen (3 atmospheres) in a hyperbaric chamber.

### Course & Prognosis

Recovery is usually complete after mild to moderate carbon monoxide intoxication in the absence of a cardiac complication such as myocardial infarction. With severe carbon monoxide poisoning, particularly if coma has occurred, there may be permanent neurologic abnormalities ranging from subtle neuropsychiatric disturbances to gross motor or cognitive dysfunction to vegetative states. Abnormal findings on a CT scan of the brain (eg, lesions in the basal ganglia or the periventricular white matter) predict a poor neurologic outcome.

## CARDIOVASCULAR ABNORMALITIES CAUSED BY ORGANIC NITRATES

In the 1950s, an epidemic of sudden death in young munitions workers who hand-packed cartridges was observed. It was subsequently discovered that abrupt withdrawal from excessive exposure to organic nitrates, particularly nitroglycerin and ethylene glycol dinitrate, may result in myocardial ischemia even in the absence of coronary artery disease. Occupations in which workers may be exposed to organic nitrates include explosives manufacturing, construction work involving blasting, weapons handling in the armed forces, and pharmaceutical manufacturing of nitrates.

### Pathogenesis

Nitrates directly dilate blood vessels, including those of the coronary circulation. With prolonged exposure (usually 1–4 years), compensatory vasoconstriction develops that is believed to be mediated by sympathetic neural responses, activation of the renin-angiotensin system, or both. When exposure to nitrates is stopped, the compensatory vasoconstriction becomes unopposed (Figure 21–2). Coronary vasospasm with angina, myocardial infarction, or sudden death may result. Chest pain occurring during nitrate withdrawal has been termed "Monday morning angina" because it typically occurs 2 or 3 days after

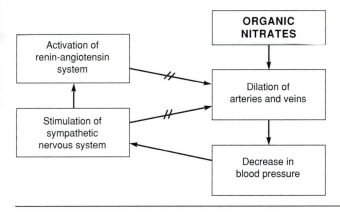

**Figure 21–2.** Mechanism of vasospasm after withdrawal from chronic exposure to nitrates. Vasoconstrictor forces antagonize (//) nitrate-induced vasodilation. Withdrawal from exposure to nitrates results in unopposed vasoconstriction and in coronary vasospasm.

the last day of nitrate exposure. Case control studies suggest a 2.5- to 4-fold increase in the risk of cardiovascular death in workers handling explosives.

## Pathology

In patients who have died following withdrawal from nitrates, there is often no or minimal coronary atherosclerosis. In one patient, coronary vasospasm was observed during angiography and the spasm was promptly reversed with sublingual nitroglycerin.

## Clinical Findings

**A. Symptoms and Signs:** Workers exposed to excessive levels of nitrates typically experience headaches and have hypotension, tachycardia, and warm, flushed skin. With continued exposure, the symptoms and signs become less prominent. After 1–2 days without exposure to nitrates—generally on weekends—there may be signs of acute coronary ischemia ranging from mild angina at rest to manifestations of myocardial infarction (eg, nausea, diaphoresis, pallor, and palpitations associated with severe chest pain), or sudden death may occur.

**B. Laboratory Findings and Cardiovascular Studies:** During episodes of pain, the ECG may show evidence of acute ischemia: ST segment elevation or depression, with or without T wave abnormalities. At other times, in the absence of pain, the ECG may be perfectly normal. Typical findings of myocardial infarction include development of a pathologic Q wave on ECG and elevation of the MB isoenzyme creatine phosphokinase (CPK) and other cardiac enzymes. Results of exercise stress testing and coronary angiography may be normal.

## Differential Diagnosis

Workers chronically exposed to nitrates may also have organic coronary artery disease, which must be identified.

## Prevention

Nitrates are extremely volatile and are readily absorbed through the lungs and skin. They can permeate the wrapping material of dynamite sticks, so workers who handle dynamite should be advised to wear cotton gloves. Natural rubber gloves should not be used, because they tend to become permeated with nitrates and may enhance absorption.

With current automated processes in explosives manufacturing, direct handling of nitrates by employees is minimized. However, levels of nitrates in the workplace environment must be controlled by adequate ventilation and by air conditioning during periods of hot weather. The current OSHA exposure limit is 0.05 ppm for nitroglycerin, but even at lower levels (0.02 ppm), personal protective gear is recommended to avoid headache. Although there are no readily available biochemical measures to detect excessive nitrate exposure, findings of progressively decreasing blood pressure and increasing heart rate during the workday are suggestive of excessive exposure. Monitoring for these signs in employees may also help prevent adverse effects of exposure to nitrates.

## Treatment

Treatment of myocardial ischemia due to nitrate withdrawal includes cardiac nitrates (eg, nitroglycerin or isosorbide dinitrate) or calcium entry blocking agents. Case reports indicate that ischemic symptoms may recur for weeks or months, indicating a persistent tendency to coronary spasm, so that long-term cardiac nitrate or calcium blocker therapy may be needed. The worker should be removed from sources of organic nitrate exposure.

## Course & Prognosis

In the absence of myocardial infarction or sudden death, anginal symptoms fully resolve after exposure to nitrate is stopped.

## CARDIOVASCULAR ABNORMALITIES CAUSED BY HYDROCARBON SOLVENTS & CHLOROFLUOROCARBONS (CFC)

Exposure to various solvents and propellants may result in cardiac arrhythmia, syncope with resultant accidents at work, or sudden death. Most serious cases of arrhythmia have been associated with abuse of or industrial exposure to halogenated hydrocarbon solvents (eg, 1,1,1-trichloroethane and trichloroethylene) or exposure to chlorofluorocarbon (Freon) propellants. Nonhalogenated solvents and even ethanol present similar risks.

Exposure to solvents is widespread in industrial settings such as dry cleaning, degreasing, painting, and chemical manufacturing. Chlorofluorocarbons are used extensively as refrigerants and as propellants in a wide variety of products and processes. For example, a pathology resident developed various arrhythmias after exposure to chlorofluorocarbon aerosols used for freezing samples and cleaning slides in a surgical pathology laboratory.

### Pathogenesis

Figure 21–3 illustrates two ways in which halogenated hydrocarbons and other solvents are thought to induce cardiac arrhythmia or sudden death. (1) At low levels of exposure, these solvents "sensitize" the heart to actions of catecholamines. For example, experimental studies have shown that the amount of epinephrine required to produce ventricular tachycardia or fibrillation is reduced after the solvents are inhaled. Catecholamine release is potentiated by euphoria and excitement due to inhalation of the solvent and also by exercise. This, in combination with

asphyxia and hypoxia, causes arrhythmia, which can result in death. (2) At higher levels of exposure, solvents may depress sinus node activity and thereby cause sinus bradycardia or arrest, or they may depress atrioventricular nodal conduction and thereby cause atrioventricular block. In some cases, they do both. Bradyarrhythmia then predisposes to escape ventricular arrhythmia or, in cases of more severe intoxication, to asystole. The arrhythmogenic action of solvents may also be enhanced by alcohol or caffeine.

### Pathology

Most cardiovascular deaths following exposure to hydrocarbons are sudden deaths. Autopsies usually reveal no specific pathologic findings. The finding of a fatty liver suggests chronic exposure to high levels of halogenated solvents or to ethanol.

### Clinical Findings

**A. Symptoms and Signs:** Symptoms of intoxication with hydrocarbon solvents or chlorofluorocarbons may include dizziness, light-headedness, headaches, nausea, drowsiness, lethargy, palpitations, or syncope. Physical examination may reveal ataxia, nystagmus, and slurred speech. The heart rate and blood pressure are usually normal, except at the time of arrhythmias, when a rapid or irregular heartbeat is sometimes accompanied by hypotension.

Convulsions, coma, or cardiac arrest may occur in severe cases of exposure to solvents. Workers who have heart disease or chronic lung disease with hypoxemia may be more susceptible to the arrhythmogenic actions of solvents.

**B. Laboratory Findings:** The concentrations

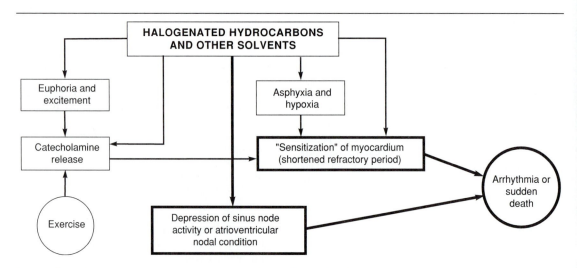

**Figure 21–3.** Mechanisms of arrhythmia or sudden death following low-level exposure (light arrows) or high-level exposure (heavy arrows) to halogenated hydrocarbons and other solvents.

of some hydrocarbons can be measured in expired air or in the blood (Chapters 29 and 38).

**C. Cardiovascular Studies:** Arrhythmias induced by solvents or chlorofluorocarbons are expected to occur only at work, while the worker is exposed to these agents. The diagnosis is based on abnormalities observed during ambulatory electrocardiographic monitoring, which consist of one or more of the following: premature atrial or ventricular contractions, recurrent supraventricular tachycardia, and recurrent ventricular tachycardia. It is essential to monitor patients on both workdays and off days and to request a log of times of exposure to solvents or chlorofluorocarbons as well as a log of symptoms of palpitations or dizzy spells. A 12-lead ECG and an exercise stress test can help determine the presence of coronary artery disease, which might increase sensitivity to hydrocarbon- or chlorofluorocarbon-induced arrhythmia.

## Differential Diagnosis

The diagnosis of solvent- or chlorofluorocarbon-induced arrhythmia is based on exclusion of other causes of arrhythmias at work (eg, the presence of a cardiac disease, metabolic disturbance, or drug abuse) and demonstration of a temporal relationship between episodes of arrhythmia and exposures to the toxic agent. The diagnosis is supported by industrial hygiene measurements documenting the level of exposure in the workplace and by objective and subjective evidence that the worker was intoxicated following exposure.

## Prevention

Preventive measures include proper handling of solvents and propellants, adequate ventilation in the workplace, and, in some cases, the use of protective respiratory equipment. Workers with heart disease—especially those with chronic arrhythmia—should be advised to avoid exposure to potentially arrhythmogenic chemicals.

## Treatment

Beta-adrenergic blocking agents may be useful in managing solvent- or chlorofluorocarbon-induced arrhythmias. In cases of episodic arrhythmia, the worker should be removed from excessive exposure or advised to use protective respiratory equipment. If a worker collapses and resuscitation is required, use of epinephrine and other sympathomimetic drugs should be avoided if possible, since they may precipitate further arrhythmia.

## Course & Prognosis

Arrhythmias are expected to fully resolve after exposure to hydrocarbons is stopped.

# CARDIOVASCULAR ABNORMALITIES CAUSED BY ORGANOPHOSPHATE & CARBAMATE INSECTICIDES

Intoxication with organophosphate and carbamate insecticides can produce diverse cardiovascular disturbances, including tachycardia and hypertension, bradycardia and hypotension, heart block, and ventricular tachycardia.

Organophosphate and carbamate insecticides are widely used in agriculture and can be applied to crops by aerial spraying or by hand. Agricultural workers may thus absorb the insecticides by inhalation of mist or via cutaneous absorption. Acute insecticide poisoning affects the circulatory system and may be fatal. Chronic poisoning may cause neuropsychiatric disturbances, as described in Chapter 32.

## Pathogenesis

Organophosphates and carbamates inhibit acetylcholinesterase, and this causes accumulation of acetylcholine at cholinergic synapses and myoneural junctions. The cardiovascular effects may vary over the time course of poisoning. Early in acute poisoning, acetylcholine stimulates nicotinic receptors at sympathetic ganglia and causes tachycardia and mild hypertension. Later, when acetylcholine acts at muscarinic receptors or blocks ganglionic transmission by hyperpolarization, it causes bradycardia and hypotension. As a consequence of autonomic imbalance and asynchronous repolarization of different parts of the heart, there may be QT interval prolongation and polymorphous ventricular tachycardia (torsades de pointes).

The excess of acetylcholine at the myoneural junctions initially causes muscle fasciculations and later causes muscle paralysis, including paralysis of the diaphragm, which results in respiratory failure or respiratory arrest. Other consequences are described below.

## Pathology

As organophosphates act on autonomic neurotransmitters, there are no specific pathologic findings.

## Clinical Findings

**A. Symptoms and Signs:** Typical symptoms of mild organophosphate or carbamate poisoning include weakness, headache, sweating, nausea, vomiting, abdominal cramps, and diarrhea. Moderate poisoning may be associated with chest discomfort, dyspnea, inability to walk, and blurred vision.

The signs are those of cholinergic excess and include small pupils, diaphoresis, salivation, lacrimation, an increase in bronchial secretions (which may resemble pulmonary edema), and muscle fasciculations. Early cardiovascular manifestations may include tachycardia and hypertension. Later, there may be bradycardia and hypotension. There is sometimes frank muscular weakness or, in severe poisoning, paralysis accompanied by respiratory failure, convulsions, or coma.

The failure of usual doses of atropine to reverse cholinergic signs is highly suggestive of the diagnosis of organophosphate or carbamate poisoning.

**B. Laboratory Findings:** The diagnosis is confirmed by the finding of markedly depressed cholinesterase activity in red blood cells. Depression to below 50% of normal is usually required for patients to have any symptoms, and depression to less than 10% of normal is usually seen in patients with severe poisoning. Plasma cholinesterase activity is usually depressed also, but this correlates less well with clinical manifestations.

Arterial blood gases may show carbon dioxide retention, hypoxia, or both.

The presence of a particular type of organophosphate may be detected in the blood or gastric fluids. Some organophosphates (eg, parathion) have metabolites that can be measured in the urine.

**C. Cardiovascular Studies:** Delayed repolarization with QT prolongation and episodes of ventricular tachycardia may be seen for up to 5–7 days after acute intoxication. The ECG also commonly shows nonspecific ST and T wave changes. A variety of arrhythmias, including premature ventricular contractions, ventricular tachycardia and fibrillation, and heart block with asystole, have been observed.

**D. Imaging:** Chest x-ray may show a pattern similar to that of pulmonary edema.

## Differential Diagnosis

The signs and symptoms of cholinergic excess are fairly specific for poisoning with cholinesterase-inhibiting insecticides. However, similar findings may be seen in people treated with cholinesterase inhibitors, such as pyridostigmine for myasthenia gravis. Small pupils may also be seen following ingestion of narcotics, clonidine, phenothiazines, and sedative drugs and in patients with pontine brain infarction or hemorrhage.

## Prevention

Most organophosphate and carbamate insecticides are rapidly absorbed following ingestion, inhalation, or contact with the skin or eyes. Continuing exposure may occur from contact with contaminated clothing or hair. Prevention requires the use of protective clothing and respirators and monitoring of red blood cell cholinesterase levels on a regular basis.

## Treatment

General measures include decontamination (removal of clothing and thorough cleaning of skin and hair), support of respiration (including mechanical ventilation in patients with respiratory failure), and support of the circulation. Specific measures include the use of pralidoxime to reverse muscular paralysis and other manifestations of excess acetylcholine and the use of atropine to reverse bronchorrhea and bradycardia.

Intensive cardiac and respiratory monitoring of patients for several days after exposure is recommended, with particular attention to the possible late development of arrhythmia or respiratory failure. Heart block and polymorphous ventricular tachycardia with a prolonged QT interval are optimally treated by cardiac pacing. The use of antiarrhythmic drugs that depress conduction (eg, quinidine, procainamide, and disopyramide) and calcium channel blockers should be avoided.

## Course & Prognosis

Recovery from acute intoxication is usually complete. Chronic intoxication may be associated with neuropsychiatric consequences (Chapters 24 and 32).

## CARDIOVASCULAR ABNORMALITIES CAUSED BY HEAVY METALS

A number of metals have been associated with disturbances in cardiovascular function, but their causative role has not been fully established.

## Antimony

Therapeutic use of antimonial compounds for treatment of parasitic infections produces electrocardiographic abnormalities—primarily T wave changes and QT interval prolongation—and has caused sudden death in some patients. Electrocardiographic changes have also been observed in workers exposed to antimony. Although these changes usually resolve after removal from exposure, a few studies have reported increased cardiovascular mortality rates in exposed workers. Studies in animals confirm that chronic exposure to antimony can produce myocardial disease.

## Arsenic

Subacute arsenic poisoning caused by ingestion of arsenic-contaminated beer has been associated with cardiomyopathy and cardiac failure. Chronic arsenic poisoning has been reported to produce "blackfoot disease," which is characterized by claudication and gangrene presumably secondary to spasms of the large blood vessels in the extremities. Arsenic exposure in drinking water is associated with an increased prevalence of hypertension. Acute arsenic poisoning can cause electrocardiographic abnormalities, and in one case it was reported to cause recurrent ventricular arrhythmia of the torsades de pointes type. A mortality study of copper smelters exposed to arsenic indicated that these workers have an increased risk of death due to ischemic heart disease.

## Arsine

Arsine gas causes red blood cell hemolysis. Massive hemolysis produces hyperkalemia, which can result in cardiac arrest. Electrocardiographic manifestations progress from high, peaked T waves to conduction disturbances and various degrees of heart block and then to asystole. Arsine may also directly affect the myocardium, causing a greater magnitude of cardiac failure than would be expected from the degree of anemia.

## Cadmium

Some epidemiologic and experimental animal studies have linked high-level cadmium exposure with hypertension, but recent epidemiologic studies have not supported the association. There is no evidence that exposure to cadmium levels found in the workplace increases the risk of cardiovascular disease.

## Cobalt

In Quebec City, Canada, in 1965 and 1966, an epidemic of cardiomyopathy occurred in heavy drinkers of beer to which cobalt sulfate had been added as a foam stabilizer. The mortality rate in affected patients was 22%, and a major pathologic finding in those who died was myocardial necrosis with thrombi in the heart and major blood vessels.

Other clinical features in affected patients included polycythemia, pericardial effusion, and thyroid hyperplasia. Cobalt is known to depress oxygen uptake by the mitochondria of the heart and to interfere with energy metabolism in a manner biochemically similar to the effects of thiamine deficiency. Since individuals receiving higher doses of cobalt for therapeutic reasons have not developed cardiomyopathy, it is possible that cobalt, excessive alcohol consumption, and nutritional deprivation acted synergistically to produce cardiomyopathy in this epidemic.

Several cases of cardiomyopathy in workers exposed to cobalt have been reported.

## Lead

Exposure to excessive levels of lead causes chronic renal diseases, and epidemiologic studies suggest that it also contributes to hypertension in the absence of renal disease. Some of the workplace studies of exposure to lead report an increased incidence of ischemic electrocardiographic changes and an increased risk of hypertensive or coronary artery disease and cerebrovascular disease in exposed workers. Nonspecific electrocardiographic changes and fatal myocarditis in the absence of hypertension have been observed in children with lead poisoning. Cardiomyopathy in moonshine drinkers has also been attributed to lead exposure. Studies in animals indicate that lead may have direct toxic effects on the myocardium.

## REFERENCES

### GENERAL

Kristensen TS: Cardiovascular diseases and the work environment: A critical review of the epidemiologic literature on chemical factors. Scand J Work Environ Health 1989;15:245.

Rosenman K: Occupational heart disease. In: Rom WN (editor). Environmental and Occupational Medicine, 3rd ed. Lippincott–Raven, 1997.

Taylor AE: Cardiovascular effects of environmental chemicals. Otolaryngol Head Neck Surg 1996; 114(2):209.

### CARBON DISULFIDE

Egeland GM et al: Effects of exposure to carbon disulphide on low density lipoprotein cholesterol concentration and diastolic blood pressure. Br J Ind Med 1992;49:287.

Peplonska B: Epidemiologic evaluation of health effects of occupational and non-occupational exposure to carbon disulfide. Med Pr 1994;45(4):359.

Vanhoorne M, De Bacquer D, De Backer G: Epidemiological study of the cardiovascular effects of carbon disulfide. Int J Epidemiol 1992;21:745.

### CARBON MONOXIDE

Allred EN et al: Short-term effects of carbon monoxide exposure of the exercise performance of subjects with coronary artery disease. N Engl J Med 1989;32:1426.

Allred EN et al: Effects of carbon monoxide on myocardial ischemia. Environ Health Perspect 1991;91:89.

American Thoracic Society: Committee of the Environmental and Occupational Health Assembly: Health effects of outdoor air pollution. Am J Respir Crit Care Med 1996;153(1):3.

Fukuhara M, et al: Circadian variations of blood pressure in patients with sequelae of carbon monoxide poisoning. Am J Hypertens 1996;9(4):300.

Hinderliter AL et al: Effects of low-level carbon monoxide exposure on resting and exercise-induced ventricular arrhythmias in patients with coronary artery disease and no baseline ectopy. Arch Environ Health 1989;44:89.

Ilano AL, Raffin TA: Management of carbon monoxide poisoning. Chest 1990;97:165.

Koskela RS: Cardiovascular diseases among foundry workers exposed to carbon monoxide. Scand J Work Environ Health 1994;20(4):286.

## ORGANIC NITRATES

Bauer JA, Nolan T, Fung HL: Vascular and hemodynamic differences between organic nitrates and nitrites. J Pharmacol Exp Ther 1997;280(1):326.

Ben-David A: Cardiac arrest in an explosives factory worker due to withdrawal from nitroglycerin exposure. Am J Ind Med 1989;15:719.

Smith RP, Wilcox DE: Toxicology of selected nitric oxide-donating xenobiotics, with particular reference to azide. Crit Rev Toxicol 1994;24(4):355.

## HYDROCARBON SOLVENTS & CHLOROFLUOROCARBONS

Eskenazi B et al: Exposure to organic solvents and hypertensive disorders of pregnancy. Am J Ind Med 1988;14:177.

Ford ES et al: Deaths from acute exposure to trichloroethylene. J Occup Environ Med 1995;37: 749.

Kaufman JD, Silverstein MA, Moure-Eraso R: Atrial fibrillation and sudden death related to occupational solvent exposure. Am J Ind Med 1994; 25:731.

Preedy VR, et al: Alcohol and the heart: Biochemical alterations. Cardiovasc Res 1996;31(1):139.

Wilcosky TC, Simonsen NR: Solvent exposure and cardiovascular disease. Am J Ind Med 1991;19:569.

## ORGANOPHOSPHATE & CARBAMATE INSECTICIDES

Adamson RH, Thorgeirsson UP: Carcinogens in foods: Heterocyclic amines and cancer and heart disease. Adv Exp Med Biol 1995;369:211.

De Bleecker J, Van Den Neucker K, Willems J: The intermediate syndrome in organophosphate poisoning: Presentation of a case and review of the literature. J Toxicol Clin Toxicol 1992;30:321.

Faroon O, Kueberuwa S, Smith L, Derosa C: ATSDR evaluation of health effects of chemicals. II. Mirex and chlordecone: health effects, toxicokinetics, human exposure. Toxicol Ind Health 1995;11(6):1.

Kass R et al: Adult respiratory distress syndrome form organophospate poisoning. Am J Emerg Med 1991; 9:32.

## HEAVY METALS

Chen CJ: Increased prevalence of hypertension and long-term arsenic exposure Hypertension 1995;25:53.

Chen CJ et al: Dose-response relationship between ischemic heart disease mortality and long-term arsenic exposure. Arterioscler Thromb Vasc Biol 1996;16(4): 504.

Christensen JM, Poulsen OM: A 1982–1992 surveillance program on Danish pottery painters: Biological levels and health effects following exposure to soluble or insoluble cobalt compounds in cobalt blue dyes. Sci Total Environ 1994;30(150):95.

Houtman JP: Trace elements and cardiovascular diseases. J Cardiovasc Risk 1996;3(1):18.

Jarvis JQ et al: Cobalt cardiomyopathy. A report of two cases from mineral assay laboratories and a review of the literature. J Occup Med 1992;34:620.

Menditto A et al: Association of blood lead to blood pressure in men aged 55 to 75 years: Effect of selected social and biochemical confounders. Environ Health Perspect 1994;102(Suppl 9):107.

Schwartz J: Lead, blood pressure, and cardiovascular disease in men. Arch Environ Health 1995;50:31.

Staessen JA, et al: Public health implications of environmental exposure to cadmium and lead: An overview of epidemiological studies in Belgium. J Cardiovasc Risk 121996;3(1):26.

Staessen J et al: Blood pressure, the prevalence of cardiovascular diseases and exposure to cadmium: A population study. Am J Epidemiol 1991;134:257.

Tomera JF, et al: Divalent cations in hypertension with implications to heart disease: Calcium, cadmium interactions. Methods Find Exp Clini Pharmacol 1994; 16(2):97.

# Liver Toxicology

**22**

*Robert J. Harrison, MD, MPH*

The liver is the target organ of many occupational and environmental chemicals and plays a central role in their detoxification and elimination. Bacterial and viral infections and certain chemical and physical agents encountered in the workplace also involve the liver. The main causes of occupational liver disease are presented in Tables 22–1, 22–4, and 22–5.

## Detection of Occupational Liver Disease

With the exception of a few chemicals that cause specific lesions (Table 22–1), hepatic injury due to industrial exposure does not differ clinically or morphologically from drug-induced damage (including damage due to ethanol). Thus, it may be difficult to differentiate occupational from nonoccupational causes on the basis of screening tests.

Occupational liver disease may be of secondary importance to damage that occurs to other organs or may occur only at high doses after accidental exposure or ingestion. While acute toxic liver injury does occur, concern is increasingly focused on chronic liver disease resulting from prolonged low-level toxic exposure. In this respect, cancer is of central concern. Because chemical studies are frequently done on animals first, the occupational health practitioner must be able to evaluate—without the assistance of adequate human studies—the results of positive carcinogenesis studies in light of actual workplace exposures (eg, methylene chloride; see Chapter 29).

In individual cases, the clinician is usually first alerted to the presence of hepatic disease by routine enzyme tests and must then make a determination about whether the cause is occupational or nonoccupational. The occupational history and results of personal or workroom air sampling are crucial to formulation of a presumptive diagnosis. It is occasionally necessary to remove the patient from exposure to the suspected workplace toxic substance to establish the workplace relationship.

## Limitations of Detection

Unfortunately, the detection of preclinical disease is made difficult by the lack of sufficiently sensitive and specific tests. It is common practice to measure liver enzymes periodically in workers exposed to a known hepatotoxin. This surveillance technique is complicated, however, by the problems of "false positives" (ie, elevated enzyme levels due to nonoccupational causes) and "false negatives" (normal values in the presence of biochemical dysfunction). In addition, little is known about the effects of multiple hepatotoxic exposures common to many occupations (eg, painters, printers, laboratory technicians). (For a detailed discussion of these limitations, see Medical Surveillance and Detection of Occupational Hepatotoxicity, below.)

## Epidemiologic Evidence of Liver Disease

Epidemiologic studies have been performed on many groups of workers exposed to hepatotoxic agents. However, relatively few workplace hepatotoxic substances have been studied in humans. Epidemiologic studies, where available, generally provide the best evidence of toxicity; however, they may be limited by inadequate study design and other factors that make conclusions difficult.

**A. Serum Aminotransferases:** Cross-sectional studies that include biochemical liver tests have been conducted among many groups of workers exposed to hepatotoxic agents—though for only a few has an adequate control group been identified. Serum aminotransferase elevations have been found in workers exposed to polychlorinated and polybrominated biphenyls (PCBs, PBBs) and in painters exposed to various solvents. Hepatocellular liver enzyme abnormalities have been found among microelectronics equipment maintenance technicians and pharmaceutical industry workers exposed to mixed solvents. Increased levels of liver enzymes have been found among chemical plant operators exposed to carbon tetrachloride but not to a mixture of chlorinated hydrocarbons. Solvent-exposed painters, printers, and degreasers did not have elevated levels of liver enzymes after adjustment for confounding due

**Table 22–1.** Chemical agents associated with occupational liver disease.

| Compound | Type of Injury | Occupation or Use |
|---|---|---|
| Arsenic | Cirrhosis, hepatocellular carcinoma, angiosarcoma | Pesticides |
| Beryllium | Granulomatous disease | Ceramics workers |
| Carbon tetrachloride | Acute hepatocellular injury, cirrhosis | Dry cleaning |
| Dimethylformamide | Acute hepatocellular injury | Solvent, chemical mfg |
| Dimethylnitrosamine | Hepatocellular carcinoma | Rocket mfg |
| Dioxin | Porphyria cutanea tarda | Pesticides |
| Halothane | Acute hepatocellular injury | Anesthesiology |
| Hydrazine | Steatosis | Rocket mfg |
| Methylene dianiline | Cholestasis | MDA production workers |
| 2-Nitropropane | Acute hepatocellular injury | Painters |
| Phosphorus | Acute hepatocellular injury | Munitions workers |
| Polychlorinated biphenyls | Subacute liver injury | Production, electrical utility |
| Tetrachloroethane | Acute or subacute hepatocellular injury | Aircraft mfg |
| Trichloroethylene | Acute hepatocellular injury | Cleaning solvent sniffing |
| Trinitrotoluene | Acute or subacute hepatocellular injury | Munitions workers |
| Vinyl chloride | Angiosarcoma | Rubber workers |

to age, alcohol consumption, medication use, or body mass index. However, house painters and carpenters were shown to have lifetime and peak solvent dose-related increases in alkaline phosphatase activity. Increased levels of liver enzymes have been reported after occupational exposure to methylene chloride, hydrazine, tetrachlordibenzo-*p*-dioxin, and polychlorinated biphenyls.

**B. Microsomal Enzyme Induction:** Using the noninvasive antipyrine clearance test, induction of the microsomal enzyme system has been demonstrated in workers exposed to various pesticides (chlordecone, phenoxy acids, DDT, lindane), halothane, PCBs, and various solvents. Functional abnormalities of liver metabolism—measured by antipyrine clearance or other noninvasive tests of liver function—are not accompanied by other clinical or laboratory signs of toxicity and so may provide a sensitive index of biologic change.

**C. Mortality Studies:** Cohort mortality studies have shown an increased mortality rate from liver cirrhosis among newspaper pressmen, spray painters, and oil refinery workers and from liver cancer among vinyl chloride, rubber, dye, and shoe factory workers. Three case-control studies have shown a statistically significant association between primary liver cancer and exposure to organic solvents, particularly among laundry workers, dry cleaners, gasoline service station attendants, asphalt workers, and bartenders.

# CHEMICAL AGENTS CAUSING LIVER TOXICITY

## Pathogenesis & Epidemiology

Occupational hepatotoxicity caused by chemicals is most frequently part of systemic toxicity involving other organ systems of primary clinical importance (eg, central nervous system depression, following exposure to hydrocarbon solvents). Occasionally, the liver toxicity is responsible for the major clinical findings (eg, carbon tetrachloride intoxication associated with renal and central nervous system damage); rarely is liver disease the sole manifestation of toxicity.

The study of hepatotoxic potential in animals is an important first step for newly-introduced chemicals. Differences among species, circumstances of exposure, and the costliness of the studies often limit extrapolation of experimental observations to the workplace. For example, while ingestion of arsenicals causes severe acute hepatic damage both in experimental animals and in humans, reports of liver disease in humans is limited to vintners exposed to arsenical pesticides.

There is no comprehensive repository of data on animal and human hepatotoxic agents. Identification of chemicals that may produce liver damage in humans has come about largely by means of clinical observation and retrospective epidemiologic studies. Some agents, such as trinitrotoluene (TNT), dimethylnitrosamine (DMA), tetrachloroethane, PCBs, and vinyl chloride, led to serious industrial hepatotoxicity before their effects on experimental animals were fully investigated. In the case of chlordecone (Kepone), human hepatotoxicity was found several years after experimental animal studies demonstrated clear evidence of liver damage following exposure.

## Routes of Exposure

Inhalation, ingestion, and percutaneous absorption are the routes by which toxic chemicals can gain entry to the body. Inhalation is probably the most important route for hepatotoxic material, particularly for the volatile solvents. Several chemicals are lipophilic and may be absorbed through the skin in sufficient quantities to contribute to hepatotoxicity (eg, TNT, 4,4-diaminodiphenylmethane, tetrachloroethylene, PCBs, dimethylformamide). In cases of liver damage by industrial agents that are not airborne, it is often difficult to distinguish between contamination of ingested material, absorption from mucous membranes, and absorption through the skin. Oral intake of hepatotoxic agents is usually of importance only in the rare case of accidental ingestion, though mouth breathing and gum and tobacco chewing can increase the amount of gaseous substances absorbed during the work day.

## Mechanisms of Toxicity

Chemical agents that cause hepatic injury may be classified into two major categories as shown in Table 22–2.

**A. Intrinsically Toxic Agents:** Agents intrinsically toxic to the liver—directly or indirectly—cause a high incidence of dose-dependent hepatic injury in exposed persons and similar lesions in experimental animals. Furthermore, the interval between exposure (under specified conditions) and onset of disease is consistent and usually short.

**1. Direct hepatotoxins–**Direct hepatotoxins—or their metabolic products—injure the hepatocyte and its organelles by a direct physicochemical effect, such as peroxidation of membrane lipids, denaturation of proteins, or other chemical changes that lead to destruction or distortion of cell membranes.

**Carbon tetrachloride** is the prototype and the best-studied example of the direct hepatotoxins, producing centrilobular necrosis and steatosis in humans and experimental animals. This agent appears to exert its hepatotoxic effects by the binding of reactive metabolites to a number of critical cellular molecules that interfere with vital cell function or cause lipid peroxidation of cell membranes.

**Chloroform** may likewise cause direct hepatic necrosis. A large number of haloalkanes (**trichloroethylene, carbon tetrabromide, tetrachloroethane**) produce hepatic injury ranging from steatosis to trivial or nondemonstrable liver damage. Their hepatotoxic potential is inversely proportionate to chain length and bond energy and directly proportionate to the number of halogen atoms in the molecule and to the atomic number of the halogen.

**2. Indirect hepatotoxins–**Indirect hepatotoxins are antimetabolites and related compounds that produce hepatic injury by interference with metabolic pathways. This may result in cytotoxic damage (degeneration or necrosis of hepatocytes) by interfering with pathways necessary for the structural integrity of the hepatocyte (morphologically seen as steatosis or necrosis) or may cause cholestasis (arrested bile flow) by interfering with the bile secretory process.

The cytotoxic indirect hepatotoxins include compounds of experimental interest (ethionine, galactosamine), drugs (tetracycline, asparaginase, metho-

**Table 22–2.** Mechanisms of toxicity of chemicals causing hepatic injury.[1]

| Category of Agent | Incidence | Experimental Reproducibility | Dose-Dependent | Example |
|---|---|---|---|---|
| **Intrinsic toxin** | | | | |
| Direct | High | Yes | Yes | Carbon tetrachloride |
| Indirect | | | | |
| Cytotoxic | High | Yes | Yes | Dimethylnitrosamine |
| Cholestatic | High | Yes | Yes | Methylene dianiline |
| **Host idiosyncrasy** | | | | |
| Hypersensitivity | Low | No | No | Phenytoin |
| Metabolic abnormality | Low | No | No | Isoniazid |

[1]Adapted from Zimmerman HJ: *Hepatotoxicity: Adverse Effects of Drugs and Other Chemicals on the Liver.* Appleton-Century-Crofts, 1978.

trexate, mercaptopurine), and botanicals (aflatoxin, cycasin, mushroom alkaloids, tannic acid). Ethanol belongs to this category by virtue of a number of selective biochemical lesions that lead to steatosis. Only one industrial chemical, 4,4'-diaminodiphenyl-methane (commonly known as methylene dianiline [MDA]), has been categorized as a cholestatic indirect hepatotoxin. Used as a plastic hardener—most commonly for epoxy resins—this agent has caused a number of epidemics (see Acute Cholestatic Jaundice, below).

**B. Agents Causing Liver Injury by Virtue of Host Idiosyncrasy:** Chemically-induced hepatic injury may be due to some special vulnerability of the individual and not the intrinsic toxicity of the agent. Liver damage in such cases occurs sporadically and unpredictably, has low experimental reproducibility, and is not dose-dependent. The injury may be due to allergy (hypersensitivity) or to production of hepatotoxic metabolites. A well-established example is halothane, which causes acute hepatitis in a small percentage of individuals with a hypersensitivity immune response.

## Hepatic Metabolism of Xenobiotics

The liver is especially vulnerable to chemical injury by virtue of its role in the metabolism of foreign compounds, or xenobiotics. The metabolism of xenobiotics is thus of central clinical interest. These chemicals, taken up by the body but not incorporated into the normal metabolic economy of the cell, are metabolized chiefly by the liver. Xenobiotic lipid-soluble compounds are well-absorbed through membrane barriers and poorly excreted by the kidney, as a result of protein binding and tubular reabsorption. Increasing polarity of nonpolar molecules by hepatic metabolism increases water solubility and urinary excretion. In this way, hepatic metabolism prevents the accumulation of drugs and other toxic chemicals in the body.

The strategic role of the liver as the primary defense against xenobiotics depends largely on cellular enzyme systems (mixed-function oxidases; MFO). The enzyme systems responsible for the metabolism of xenobiotics are attached to the membrane layers of the smooth endoplasmic reticulum. Although enzymes that catalyze the metabolism of nonpolar xenobiotics are present in the intestines, lungs, kidneys, and skin, the vast majority of metabolic conversions occur in the liver. Most xenobiotics that are toxic by the oral route are also hepatotoxic parenterally or by inhalation.

## Xenobiotic Agents Activated by the MFO System

Many hepatotoxic agents and hepatocarcinogens must be first activated by the MFO system to a toxic or carcinogenic metabolite. Examples include carbon tetrachloride, vinyl chloride, PCBs, bromobenzene, azo dyes, DMA, and allyl compounds. Electrophilic intermediates react with enzymes and regulatory or structural proteins and lead to cell death.

Many drugs, insecticides, organic solvents, carcinogens, and other environmental contaminants are known experimentally to stimulate some type of microsomal activity that is associated with the metabolism of xenobiotics. The administration of ethanol concomitantly with carbon tetrachloride enhances the toxicity of the latter, presumably via induction of the MFO system. Clinically, this may explain the well-documented synergistic effect between ethanol abuse and carbon tetrachloride toxicity in humans. Ethanol pretreatment in experimental human studies enhances the metabolic clearance of *m*-xylene and antipyrine by microsomal enzyme induction, suggesting that workers with prior alcohol consumption may be more likely to develop acute hepatotoxicity after occupational exposure.

Other mechanisms may be at work also, since a single dose of alcohol given to animals several hours prior to administration of carbon tetrachloride also potentiates toxicity. Experiments show that many other factors may affect the metabolism of xenobiotics: diet, age, sex, cigarette smoking, endocrine status, genetic factors, diurnal variations, underlying liver disease, and stress. There is considerable inter- and intraindividual variation in xenobiotic metabolism, and the relative importance of these factors in the occupational setting is not currently known. Enhanced microsomal enzyme function has been demonstrated in industrial workers exposed to hepatotoxins at levels below those shown to result in hepatic necrosis. Increasing attention has been directed to the use of noninvasive measurements of MFO in the preclinical detection of liver disease (see below).

# DISEASE PATTERNS & MORPHOLOGY OF HEPATIC INJURY

As shown in Table 22–3, occupational exposure to xenobiotics can lead to acute, subacute, or chronic liver disease.

The clinical syndromes can be associated with several types of morphologic changes, as seen by light microscopy. Hepatic injury may be clinically overt or may be discovered only as a functional or histologic abnormality. Current concern with chronic liver disease due to subtle repeated injury has generally overshadowed the problem of acute and subacute injury caused by accidental exposure.

**Table 22–3.** Morphologic patterns of liver injury.

| Type of Injury | Examples of Causes |
|---|---|
| **Acute** | |
| Cytotoxic | |
| Necrosis | |
| Zonal | Carbon tetrachloride, chloroform |
| Massive | Trinitrotoluene |
| Steatosis | Carbon tetrachloride, chloroform, phosphorus, dimethyl formamide, hydrazine |
| Cholestatic | Methylene dianiline, rapeseed oil |
| **Subacute** | Trinitrotoluene |
| **Chronic** | |
| Cirrhosis | Trinitrotoluene, polychlorinated biphenyls, tetrachloroethane |
| Sclerosis | Arsenic, vinyl chloride |
| Porphyria | Dioxin |
| Neoplasia | Arsenic, vinyl chloride |
| Steatosis | Dimethylformamide, carbon tetrachloride |
| Granuloma | Beryllium, copper |

## ACUTE HEPATIC INJURY

Acute liver disease was a cause of serious occupational liver disease in the first part of the 20th century and is still occasionally encountered. Acute hepatic injury has been reported as a result of exposure to agents listed in Table 22–4.

### Clinical Findings

Occupational exposure to xenobiotics may lead to degeneration or necrosis of hepatocytes (cytotoxic injury) or to arrested bile flow (cholestatic injury). The latent period is relatively short (24–48 hours), and clinical symptoms are often of extrahepatic origin. Anorexia, nausea, vomiting, jaundice, and hepatomegaly are often present. Severely exposed individuals who have sustained massive necrosis may have coffee-ground emesis, abdominal pain, clinically detectable reduction in liver size, rapid development of ascites, edema, and hemorrhagic diathesis.

**Table 22–4.** Agents causing acute hepatic injury (partial list).

Carbon tetrachloride
Tetrachloroethane
Trichloroethylene
Chloroform
Carbon tetrabromide
2-Nitropropane
Chlorinated naphthalenes
Elemental phosphorus
Bromobenzene
Anesthetic gases (halothane, methoxyflurane)
Dimethylformamide
Dichlorohydrin
Trichloroethane
Trinitrotoluene

This is often followed within 24–28 hours by somnolence and coma.

Morphologically, hepatic necrosis may be zonal, massive, or diffuse. Centrizonal necrosis is the characteristic lesion produced by agents listed in Table 22–4 as well as by bromobenzene, halothane, the toxin of *Amanita phalloides,* and acetaminophen. Periportal or peripheral necrosis is produced by elemental phosphorus. TNT, PCBs, and chloronaphthalenes can produce massive rather than zonal necrosis.

Various degrees of fatty change or steatosis may also be seen morphologically in association with toxicity due to carbon tetrachloride, chloroform, tetrachloroethane, dimethylformamide, trichloroethane, styrene, hydrazine, and elemental phosphorus.

### Diagnosis & Treatment

The diagnosis and treatment of acute hepatic injuries are covered under Clinical Management of Occupational Liver Disease, below.

## CARBON TETRACHLORIDE-INDUCED ACUTE HEPATIC INJURY

Carbon tetrachloride presents the classic example of an acute hepatotoxin. It was first recognized as such in the 1920s, when it was in common use as a liquid solvent, dry cleaning agent, and fire extinguisher. Since then, hundreds of poisonings and fatalities have been reported, mostly from inhalation in confined spaces.

### Clinical Findings

Clinically, immediate nervous system symptoms of dizziness, headache, visual disturbances, and confusion are observed as a result of the anesthetic properties of carbon tetrachloride. This is followed by nausea, vomiting, abdominal pain, and diarrhea during the first 24 hours. Evidence of hepatic disease usually follows after 2–4 days but may appear within 24 hours. The liver and spleen become palpable and jaundice develops, accompanied by elevated serum transaminase concentrations and prolonged prothrombin time. Renal failure (see Chapter 23) may ensue a few days after the hepatic damage becomes manifest and has in fact been the cause of death in most fatal cases. Sequelae of hepatic failure such as hypoglycemia, encephalopathy, and hemorrhage may be complications. Most instances of carbon tetrachloride toxicity have occurred with accompanying ethanol intake, which may be a potentiating factor in hepatotoxicity.

Treatment with N-acetyl cysteine (NAC) has been effective in cases of massive carbon tetrachloride ingestion. Animal studies suggest that NAC may decrease the covalent binding of carbon tetrachloride reactive metabolites, decrease the amount of carbon tetrachloride reaching the liver, or partially block lipid peroxidation.

## ACUTE HEPATIC INJURY INDUCED BY OTHER XENOBIOTICS

**Trichloroethylene** has been reported to cause acute hepatotoxicity when used as a dry cleaning agent; more recently, it has been shown to cause acute centrilobular necrosis following recreational "solvent sniffing" of cleaning fluids. This may be due to contamination with dichloroacetylene rather than to trichloroethylene itself.

**Trichloroethane** has been reported to cause acute, reversible hepatitis with fatty infiltration in several workers. A liver biopsy specimen from one trichloroethane-exposed printer showed focal bridging fibrosis and nodule formation with evidence of marked portal tract fibrosis, a pattern suggestive of macronodular or early cirrhosis.

**Carbon tetrabromide** has been reported to cause a syndrome in chemists similar to acute carbon tetrachloride hepatotoxicity.

**2-Nitropropane,** a nitroparaffin used as a solvent in epoxy resin paints and coatings, has been reported to have caused several cases of acute fulminant hepatitis following exposure in confined spaces.

The solvent **dimethylformamide** has been reported to acutely cause increased levels of liver enzymes, with liver biopsy specimens showing focal hepatocellular necrosis with microvesicular steatosis. Liver biopsy specimens from workers with longer exposures showed macrovesicular steatosis without persisting acute injury or fibrosis. Progression to cirrhosis was not demonstrated up to 22 months following exposure.

Fulminant hepatic failure has been reported in a recreational solvent abuser exposed to a mixture of **isopropyl alcohol, methyl amyl alcohol,** and **butylated hydroxytoluene** and in a worker following exposure to **dichlorohydrin** during tank cleaning.

## ACUTE CHOLESTATIC JAUNDICE

This is a rare manifestation of occupational toxicity. As mentioned above, MDA was responsible for an epidemic of cholestatic jaundice observed in Epping, England ("Epping jaundice"), in 1965. This compound, used as a hardener for epoxy resin, had spilled from a plastic container onto the floor of a van that was carrying both flour and the chemical. Acute cholestatic injury was found subsequently in 84 persons who had eaten bread made from the contaminated flour. Onset was abrupt—with abdominal pain—in 60% of the cases and was insidious in one-third. Histologic evidence of bile stasis with only slight parenchymal injury was seen in most cases,

and all victims recovered without evidence of persistent hepatic injury. Similar cases have subsequently been reported for industrial exposure during the manufacture and application of epoxy resins.

Cholestatic liver injury has been reported after accidental ingestion of denatured rapeseed oil and after ingestion of moldy grain and nuts contaminated with aflatoxin.

## SUBACUTE HEPATIC NECROSIS

This form of hepatic injury is characterized by a smoldering illness, with delayed onset of jaundice. It usually follows repeated exposure to relatively small doses of a hepatotoxin. The onset of anorexia, nausea, and vomiting accompanied by hepatomegaly and jaundice may occur after several weeks to months of exposure and may lead variably to recovery or to fulminant hepatic failure. A few patients are reported to have developed macronodular cirrhosis, though clinical data are limited.

The histologic features of subacute hepatic necrosis consist of various degrees of necrosis, fibrosis, and regeneration. In cases where the clinical course is relatively brief (2–3 weeks), necrotic features predominate. In patients with a prolonged course of several months or more, postnecrotic scarring with subacute hepatic necrosis is seen. Fortunately, subacute hepatic necrosis caused by occupational exposure is rare today.

## CHRONIC HEPATIC INJURY

Several forms of chronic liver damage can result from continuing or repeated injury caused by prolonged exposure: cirrhosis and fibrosis, hepatoportal sclerosis, hepatic porphyria, and neoplasia. Acute hepatic injury due to carbon tetrachloride exposure has been anecdotally reported to lead to chronic disease.

## CIRRHOSIS & FIBROSIS

The histologic pattern of progressive necrosis accompanied by regenerating nodules, fibrosis, and architectural distortion of the liver ("toxic cirrhosis") is well described as part of the syndrome of subacute hepatic necrosis due to **TNT tetrachloroethane,** and the **PCBs** and **chloronaphthalenes**. Additionally, some survivors of trinitrotoluene-induced injury were found to have macronodular cirrhosis.

Prolonged, repeated low-level exposure to **carbon tetrachloride** in dry cleaning plants and to **inorganic**

**arsenical insecticides** among vintners has been reported to cause cirrhosis. Micronodular cirrhosis was described in a worker with repeated exposure to a degreasing solvent containing a mixture of **trichloroethylene** and **1,1,1-trichloroethane.**

Thirteen painters with no history of drug or alcohol ingestion exposed over 6–39 years to a variety of organic solvents had persistent biopsy-verified histologic changes of steatosis, focal necrosis, and enlarged portal tracts with fibrosis. Three nurses were reported to have irreversible liver injury after years of handling cystostatic drugs, with liver biopsies showing piecemeal necrosis in one and steatosis with fibrosis in the other two.

The anesthetic agent **halothane** has been reported to cause cirrhosis and chronic active hepatitis after acute exposure.

Increased mortality due to cirrhosis has been observed among pressman, shipyard workers, metal fabrication employees, marine inspectors, and anesthesiologists. The relationship with occupational exposures among these occupations and the role of confounding factors such as ethanol or viral hepatitis remain to be determined.

## HEPATOPORTAL SCLEROSIS & HEPATIC PORPHYRIA

Portal and periportal fibrosis leading to portal hypertension ("noncirrhotic portal hypertension") has been attributed to exposure to inorganic arsenicals, thorium, and vinyl chloride. A few cases of porphyria cutanea tarda due to occupational exposure to the herbicide **2,4,5-trichlorophenoxyacetic acid** probably caused by contamination by dioxin, have been recorded. Turkish peasants developed liver disease and hepatic porphyria after ingesting wheat contaminated with the fungicide **hexachlorobenzene.**

## GRANULOMATOUS DISEASE

**Beryllium** and **copper** exposure can result in granulomatous liver disease, with hepatic granulomas located near or within the portal tracts. Clinical liver disease is usually not significant, but granulomas occasionally result in hepatomegaly, necrosis, or fibrosis.

## STEATOSIS

Steatosis is characterized morphologically by microvesicular or macrovesicular intracellular lipid formation. Steatosis may occur as a result of acute occupational exposure to elemental phosphorus, TNT, arsenical pesticides, dimethylformamide, and certain chlorinated hydrocarbons (carbon tetrachloride, methyl chloroform, and tetrachloroethane). Nonoccupational causes include diabetes, hypertriglyceridemia, and obesity. Intracellular hepatic lipid formation results from xenobiotic effects on fat metabolism. Minimal to moderate elevation in transaminase levels is seen after acute occupational exposure, with resolution in several weeks after removal.

Steatosis may also occur after chronic exposure to carbon tetrachloride or dimethyformamide. Progression from steatosis to fibrosis or cirrhosis has not been documented.

## NEOPLASIA

While many occupationally-encountered chemical agents are known to cause hepatocellular carcinoma in experimental animals, only a few are demonstrated human carcinogens.

**Vinyl chloride,** a halogenated aliphatic compound used since the 1940s in the production of polyvinyl chloride, was known to be an animal hepatotoxin in the early 1960s. Acro-osteolysis was reported in humans in 1966 (see Chapter 28). In 1974, Creech and Johnson reported 3 cases of a rare liver tumor—angiosarcoma—in employees who had been exposed to vinyl chloride for up to 20 years. Subsequent reports and surveillance activities worldwide have recorded over 75 cases of vinyl chloride-associated hepatic angiosarcoma. Pathologically, hepatic damage in association with vinyl chloride exposure appears to progress sequentially from focal hepatocyte hyperplasia, to sinusoidal dilatation, to peliosis hepatis and sarcomatous transformation of the lining of the cells of sinusoids and portal capillaries. Clinically, liver disease has usually not been recognized until the late stages of histologic damage and with the victim only a few months from death.

Medical surveillance of vinyl chloride-exposed workers has attempted to identify early histologic and structural abnormalities through the use of liver biopsy, ultrasonography, CT scans, and biochemical measures of liver function.

Hepatic angiosarcoma has also developed in vintners with long exposure to inorganic arsenic; in patients with psoriasis treated with inorganic potassium arsenite (Fowler's solution) in the 1940s and 1950s; and in patients injected with a colloidal suspension of thorium dioxide (Thorotrast), used for carotid angiography and liver-spleen scans from 1930 to 1955.

Case-control studies have shown elevated odds ratios for the development of liver cancer among workers in a variety of occupations such as clerical workers, food service workers, transport equipment operators, and workers exposed to welding fumes. Known risk factors for liver cancer have generally not been associated with these occupations, and the significance of these findings is unknown.

## INFECTIOUS AGENTS CAUSING LIVER TOXICITY (Table 22–5)

Infectious hepatotoxic agents may be of importance in the pathogenesis of both acute and chronic liver disease. Occupational exposure to infectious hepatotoxic agents may occur among hospital workers, sewer workers, emergency health care personnel; animal care, slaughterhouse, and farm workers; and laboratory workers. Additional information can be found in Chapter 16.

## HEPATITIS A

### Exposure

Hepatitis A is an occupational risk for hospital and mental institution workers as well as for teachers and other staff of day care centers and prison personnel. While contaminated food and water are common epidemic sources, hepatitis A is transmitted primarily by person-to-person contact, generally through fecal contamination. The cause of hepatitis A is the hepatitis A virus (HAV), a 27-nm ribonucleic acid (RNA) agent that is a member of the picornavirus family. Its transmission is facilitated by poor personal hygiene and intimate household or sexual contact. Transmission by blood transfusion has occurred but is rare.

Occupational transmission of hepatitis A in the hospital is uncommon, since there is little fecal excretion of the virus after the patient develops jaundice and seeks medical attention. Nevertheless, well-documented outbreaks of hepatitis A have occurred in hospitals and institutions for the mentally retarded.

### Clinical Findings & Diagnosis

The incubation period for hepatitis A is 15–50 days (average, 28–30 days). The illness caused by

**Table 22–5.** Infectious agents associated with occupational liver disease.

| Hepatitis A virus | Nursery and kindergarten staff, sewer workers |
| --- | --- |
| Hepatitis B virus | Health care workers with blood and body fluid contact |
| Cytomegalovirus | Pediatric health care workers |
| *Coxiella burnetii* | Animal care workers, farm workers, slaughterhouse workers |
| *Leptospira icterohaemorrhagiae* | Sewer workers, farm workers |

HAV characteristically has an abrupt onset, with fever, malaise, anorexia, nausea, abdominal discomfort, and jaundice. High concentrations of HAV (10 particles per gram) are found in stools of infected persons. Fecal virus excretion reaches its highest concentration during the incubation period and early in the prodromal phase; it diminishes rapidly once jaundice appears. Greatest infectivity is in the 2-week period immediately before the onset of jaundice.

A chronic carrier state with HAV in blood or feces has not been demonstrated. The fatality rate among reported cases is low (about 0.6%). The diagnosis of acute hepatitis A is confirmed by the presence of immunoglobulin M (IgM)-class anti-HAV in serum collected during the acute or early convalescent phase of the disease. IgG antibodies appear in the convalescent phase and remain positive for life, apparently conferring enduring protection against disease.

### Treatment

Treatment for hepatitis A is symptomatic, with rest, analgesics, and fluid replacement where necessary. Fulminant hepatic failure occasionally follows acute HAV infection. Orthotopic liver transplantation is well established as the appropriate treatment for severe cases.

### Prevention

Numerous studies have shown that a single intramuscular dose of 0.02 mL/kg of immune globulin (immune serum globulin; gamma globulin) given before exposure or during the incubation period of hepatitis A is protective against clinical illness. The prophylactic value is greatest (80–90%) when immune globulin is given early in the incubation period and declines thereafter. Since only 38% of acute hepatitis cases in the United States are caused by HAV, serologic confirmation of hepatitis A in the index case is recommended before treatment of contacts. Once the diagnosis of acute infection is made, close contacts should be promptly given immune globulin to prevent development of secondary cases. Such close contacts may include staff of day care facilities and institutions for custodial care—or hospital staff if an unsuspected patient has been fecally incontinent.

Routine immune globulin administration is not recommended under the usual office or factory conditions for persons exposed to a fellow worker with hepatitis A or to teachers with schoolroom contact. Food handlers should receive immune globulin when a common-source exposure is recognized. So should restaurant patrons when the infected person is directly involved in handling uncooked foods without gloves. This is especially the case when the patrons can be identified within 2 weeks after exposure and the food handler's hygienic practices are known to be deficient. Serologic screening of contacts for anti-

HAV antibodies to the hepatitis A virus before giving immune globulin is not recommended, because screening is more costly than immune globulin and would delay administration.

An inactivated hepatitis A vaccine has recently been licensed for use in the United States. Immunogenicity studies show that virtually 100% of children, adolescents, and adults develop protective levels of antibody to hepatitis A virus (anti-HAV) after completing a two-dose vaccine series (each given as intramuscular injection of 1 mL of 1440 enzyme-linked immunosorbent assay units). Protective antibodies remain for as long as 4 years, with kinetic models suggesting that protective levels of anti-HAV persisting for at least 20 years. Vaccination is recommended for persons traveling to or working in countries with intermediate or high HAV endemicity, for laboratory workers with exposure to live virus, or for animal handlers with exposure to HAV-infected primates. Consideration may be given to vaccination of food handlers in selected situations in which the risk of infection is high, although the cost-effectiveness of this approach has not been demonstrated. Consultation with local or state health authorities should precede the initiation of food handler vaccination programs. Hepatitis A vaccination is not recommended for child care workers, sewage treatment employees, or staff in institutions for the developmentally disabled.

An employee with symptoms and confirmed hepatitis A virus infection should be restricted from work until symptoms subside or for 1 week after the onset of jaundice.

## HEPATITIS B

### Exposure & Epidemiology

Hepatitis B infection (see also Chapter 16) is caused by the hepatitis B virus (HBV), a major cause of acute and chronic hepatitis, cirrhosis, and primary hepatocellular carcinoma worldwide.

High-risk health care workers with frequent blood contact include anyone having significant contact with blood, blood products, or body secretions: surgeons, oral surgeons, dental hygienists, pathologists, anesthesiologists, phlebotomists, medical technologists, respiratory therapists, emergency room personnel, and medical and surgical house staff.

The annual rate of clinically manifest hepatitis B infection in hospital workers is about 0.1%, or about 10 times that of control populations. Hospital staff with frequent blood contact have a prevalence rate of hepatitis B surface antigen (HBsAg) of 1–2% and a prevalence rate of anti-hepatitis B antibody (anti-HBs) of 15–30%, compared with healthy controls, who have rates of 0.3% and 3–5%, respectively. The risk of infection with HBV depends on the titer of virions in the infectious fluid and correlates with the presence or absence of hepatitis e antigen in the source patient. The risk of infection following percutaneous injury ranges from 2 to 40%. Infection following mucosal contact has been documented but is low. Infectious virions are not present in urine or feces, and mucosal contact with saliva poses little if any risk. Employment in a hospital without blood exposure carries no greater risk than that for the general population.

Most hospital workers experience accidental blood contact by needlestick injuries, usually during disposal and recapping of needles, administration of parenteral injections or infusion therapy, drawing blood, and handling linens and trash containing uncapped needles. Educating hospital personnel about the risks of hepatitis B and employing methods to interrupt transmission have been successful in reducing rates of infection.

Based on serologic markers of infection, HBV is also highly prevalent in certain high-risk groups, such as immigrants from areas with high HBV endemicity, clients of institutions for the mentally retarded, parenteral drug users, homosexual men, household contacts of carriers, and hemodialysis patients.

An estimated 200,000 persons in the United States, primarily young adults, become infected yearly, and one-fourth have jaundice. More than 10,000 require hospitalization, and an average 250 die of fulminant disease. A carrier state of chronic active hepatitis develops in 3–5% of infected individuals and may result in serious complications.

### Forms of Illness & Transmission

Three forms of hepatitis B are encountered in clinical practice: acute hepatitis B, inapparent sporadic episodes of unknown origin, and the chronic carrier state—detected by screening for HBsAg—in apparently healthy persons. Transmission occurs via percutaneous or permucosal routes when exposure to blood, semen, cerebrospinal fluid, saliva, or urine occurs. HBV is not transmitted via the fecal-oral route or by contamination of food or water.

### Course of Illness

The onset of acute hepatitis B is generally insidious, with anorexia, malaise, nausea, vomiting, abdominal pain, and jaundice. Skin rash, arthralgia, and arthritis can also occur. The incubation period ranges from 45 to 60 days after exposure to HBV. HBsAg can be detected in serum 30–60 days after exposure to HBV and persists for variable periods. Antibody to hepatitis B surface antigen (anti-HBs) develops after a resolved infection and indicates long-term immunity. The antibody to the core antigen (anti-HBc) develops in all HBV infections and persists indefinitely. Overall fatality rates for acute infection do not exceed 2%.

The chronic carrier state is defined as the presence

of HBsAg-positive serum on at least two occasions at least 6 months apart and is characterized by high levels of HBsAg and anti-HBc and various levels of serum transaminases, reflecting liver disease activity. The natural course of HBsAg-positive chronic active hepatitis is progressive, frequently evolving to cirrhosis, hepatocellular carcinoma, and death due to hepatic failure or bleeding esophageal varices.

Depending on the country, the estimated relative risk for developing hepatocellular carcinoma after chronic HBV infection ranges from 6- to 100-fold. Hepatocellular carcinoma usually develops after 20–30 years of persistent HBV infection accompanied by hepatocellular necrosis, inflammation, and regenerative hyperplasia. Chronic hepatitis and liver cirrhosis are important endogenous factors in the development of hepatocellular carcinoma.

### Treatment

Treatment with interferon alpha (IFN) for chronic hepatitis B infection has shown promise, with disappearance of circulating hepatitis B antigen in one-third of responders.

### Prevention

Postexposure prophylaxis should be based on the hepatitis vaccination status of the exposed person, whether the source of blood and the HBsAg status of the source is known or unknown. Guidelines for hepatitis B prophylaxis following percutaneous exposure are given in Chapter 16.

Individuals at risk for blood-borne pathogen exposure should be vaccinated with hepatitis B virus vaccine. Protective immunity is conferred in over 95% of vaccine recipients. The availability of recombinant hepatitis B vaccines has eliminated previous, albeit unwarranted concerns regarding the risk of blood-borne infections transmitted by plasma-derived vaccines. Nearly 90% of vaccine recipients have protective levels of anti-HBs 5 years after vaccination. Loss of detectable anti-HBs levels after immunization does not imply loss of protection, because studies have shown that exposure to HBV leads to an amnestic rise in anti-HBs levels after natural infection. Therefore, routine booster doses of hepatitis B vaccine are not recommended.

Measurement of prevaccination anti-HBs levels is not generally recommended, but may be performed depending on the cost of screening and the prevalence of antibody in the group to be vaccinated. Approximately 5% of immunocompetent adults fail to respond to the hepatitis B vaccine, with vaccine non-responsiveness increasing with age greater than 40, obesity, and smoking. Postvaccination anti-HBs testing may be useful in establishing immune status for postexposure treatment or for administering booster doses to vaccine nonresponders. Screening by ultrasonography and serum alpha fetoprotein measurement is indicated for patients at high risk for developing hepatocellular carcinoma.

The employee with hepatitis B virus infection and liver disease should be advised to avoid exposure to other potentially hepatotoxic agents such as ethanol or workplace solvents.

## HEPATITIS C

### Exposure & Epidemiology

Hepatitis C virus (HCV) is a single-stranded RNA virus of the family *Flaviviridae*. The virus has a striking ability to persist in the host after infection, with chronic hepatitis occurring in approximately 70% of infected individuals. Viral persistence appears to be related to rapid mutation under immune pressure, with coexistence within the host as related but immunologically distinct strains. The high rate of mutation appears to be the primary mechanism underlying the absence of effective neutralization and the development of persistent infection. In the United States alone, approximately 3.5 million people are infected with HCV, with nearly 150,000 new infections annually.

HCV is spread primarily through parenteral exposures from blood transfusions or intravenous drug abuse. Up to 40% of cases in the United States have no identified exposure source. There is minimal evidence for sexual transmission or mother-to-infant transmission of HCV. The risk of infection following occupational percutaneous exposure ranges from 3% to 10%. An infection following conjunctival mucosal exposure has been reported. HCV RNA has not been detected in the urine, feces, saliva, vaginal secretions, or semen.

### Clinical Findings & Diagnosis

Acute hepatitis C is usually a benign illness, with up to 80% of cases being anicteric and asymptomatic. The mean incubation period following transfusion-associated hepatitis C is 6–8 weeks. Mild elevations of transaminase levels occur in the acute phase; fulminant hepatic failure is rare. Persistent infection leads to liver cell destruction, possibly via direct cytopathic or immune-mediated mechanisms, with fluctuating levels of serum transaminases. Serum transaminase levels are a relatively poor indicator of the severity of disease as measured histologically.

Chronic active hepatitis or cirrhosis occurs in up to 60% of individuals with acute infection. Progression to cirrhosis appears to correlate with age at exposure, duration of infection, and degree of liver damage on biopsy. HCV is a major agent in the etiology of hepatocellular carcinoma throughout the world, with almost all cases occurring in the setting of cirrhosis. Alcohol appears to be an important cofactor in the development of complications from chronic HCV infection.

Diagnosis of HCV infection is usually based on

detection of elevated serum transaminase or anti-HCV antibody levels. Anti-HCV antibodies become detectable an average of 12 weeks following exposure but may take as long as 6 months. First-generation anti-HCV assays utilized the c100-3 antigen and were highly effective in identifying HCV-positive blood donors. The anti-c100-3 assay failed to detect HCV-infected patients for several weeks after exposure, and some HCV-infected patients never developed anti-HCV antibody. Second-generation assays added two epitopes (c22-3 and c33c) to both the enzyme-linked immunosorbent assay (ELISA) and the confirmatory recombinant immunoblot assay (RIBA-2). Antibodies to these epitopes develop much earlier after infection than do antibodies to c100-3. The second-generation assay is highly sensitive but relatively nonspecific for the detection of HCV. Nonspecificity has been associated with aged sera, hypergammaglobulinemia, rheumatoid factor–positive sera, and sera from persons recently vaccinated for influenza. Because of the nonspecificity, ELISA reactivity should be confirmed with a supplemental RIBA-2 assay. Third-generation assays incorporating an antigen in the viral NS-5 region and deleting the c100-3 antigen are awaiting licensure in the United States. The third-generation RIBA assay should resolve many RIBA-2 indeterminate patterns.

The most sensitive method to detect HCV is the measurement of HCV RNA by the polymerase chain reaction (PCR). HCV RNA is detectable by PCR in almost all patients within 1–2 weeks of exposure. In about 80% of individuals, HCV RNA persists with fluctuating serum transaminase levels.

Liver biopsy specimens from patients with chronic HCV infection may show portal inflammation, focal piecemeal necrosis, bile ductular proliferation, and characteristic lymphoid follicles within the portal tracts.

Chronic HCV infection has been associated with polyarteritis nodosa, membranous glomerulonephritis, and idiopathic Sjögren's syndrome.

### Treatment

Treatment with immune globulin or antiviral therapy for prophylaxis against HCV is not recommended. Following percutaneous or mucosal occupational exposure to HCV, baseline and follow-up HCV antibody measurements should be performed to assess the risk of seroconversion. Counseling should be provided to the exposed worker regarding the low risk of household or sexual transmission.

IFN treatment may result in a sustained clinical remission in approximately 20% of HCV-infected patients, often accompanied by loss of HCV RNA and improved histologic condition of the liver. There is a great variability in the response to IFN. Pretreatment HCV RNA levels are important predictors of response, and patients with sustained loss of HCV RNA after treatment are considered in remission and

perhaps cured of infection. Interferon is recommended for patients with compensated liver disease with sustained biochemical evidence of chronic hepatitis and showing chronic active hepatitis or active cirrhosis on liver biopsy. Patients with mild disease should be observed over time.

Hepatitis C is becoming the leading indication for orthotopic liver transplantation. Recurrence of HCV infection after transplantaion is common, although most patients usually have a benign course. Approximately 50% of viremic patients will have evidence of hepatitis on biopsy 1 year following transplantation.

### Prevention

No vaccine is currently available for HCV. Prospects for vaccine development are challenging because of the transient efficacy of neutralizing antibodies, the high frequency of mutation in critical envelope protein regions, the high rate of persistent infection, and the possibility of reinfection with both homologous and heterologous strains.

## OTHER INFECTIOUS AGENTS

**Non-A, non-B viral hepatitis** may develop after parenteral blood exposure among hospital personnel. The incidence and clinical spectrum of this disease after occupational exposure is not known. Chronic hepatitis following acute non-A, non-B hepatitis varies in frequency from 20% to 70%. The value of immune serum globulin for prophylaxis is not established.

**Cytomegalovirus** exposure is a potential risk to health care workers, particularly pediatric staff who may be pregnant and thus at risk of transmitting infection to the fetus. Cytomegalovirus may cause hepatitis, but the more serious consequence of infection for the pregnant worker may be a neonate with a congenital malformation. Convincing evidence of higher rates of seroconversion among pediatric health care workers has not been demonstrated. Nevertheless, prudent hospital policy may be to reassign seronegative employees who wish to become pregnant to jobs where there is no contact with infected patients or their biological fluids.

*Coxiella burnetii,* the agent of **Q fever,** may cause acute infection among personnel exposed to infected sheep and goats. Persons at risk include animal care technicians, laboratory research personnel, abattoir workers, and farmers. Acute hepatitis occurs in up to 50% of cases and is usually self-limited.

The clinical picture of **leptospirosis** among farm and sewer workers due to exposure to *Leptospira icterohaemorrhagiae* may also be dominated by hepatic injury.

Other causes of infectious hepatitis include **yellow fever** among forest workers (arbovirus) and **schisto-**

**somiasis** among agricultural workers (*Schistosoma mansoni, Schistosoma japonicum*).

# MEDICAL SURVEILLANCE & DETECTION OF OCCUPATIONAL HEPATOTOXICITY

## MEDICAL SURVEILLANCE FOR OCCUPATIONAL LIVER DISEASE

The choice of a surveillance test or tests to detect chemical liver disease in a working population exposed to potential hepatotoxins is determined by its specificity, sensitivity, and positive predictive value (see Diagnostic Tests for Liver Dysfunction, below). In an occupational setting, a screening test with high sensitivity (to correctly identify all those with disease) and specificity (to correctly identify all those without disease) is needed. Indocyanine green clearance and serum alkaline phosphatase have been suggested as the initial tests of choice for the surveillance of vinyl chloride workers (to reduce the number of false positives), followed by a test of high sensitivity such as serum γ-glutamyl transpeptidase (to reduce the number of false negatives). Whether this applies to other exposed groups awaits further research. In the same way, the comparative utility of other indices of liver function, such as serum bile acid measurements and noninvasive measures of microsomal enzyme activity, remains open to question.

It is currently justified to base the choice of tests on practical criteria such as noninvasiveness, simplicity of test performance, availability, and adequacy of test analysis and cost. Although serum transaminases have a relatively high sensitivity for detection of liver disease, their low specificity limits the practical utility of periodic measurement in a worker population exposed to potential hepatotoxins. Nevertheless, serum transaminases remain the test of choice for routine surveillance of such populations.

Clearance tests have been successfully used in research settings but are not recommended for daily clinical or surveillance practice until further prospective studies in well-defined groups are completed. It is not known whether reversible changes in microsomal enzyme activity in workers exposed to hepatotoxins are harmless and adaptive or potentially harmful. On the basis of current knowledge, the consequences of changes in microsomal enzyme activity cannot be accurately assessed.

So-called preemployment "baseline" measurement of serum transaminases may be helpful in establishing causality for purposes of workers' compensation where a claim is made alleging industrial liver disease. Routine medical surveillance involving measurement of serum transaminase levels should be conducted only when exposure assessment suggests a potential for hepatic injury. When the prevalence of liver disease in the population is low, the poor predictive value of an abnormal serum transaminase level after routine screening may lead to many costly diagnostic evaluations for nonoccupational liver disease.

Gray scale ultrasonography of the liver has been used in surveillance of vinyl chloride-exposed workers but has not been routinely applied in other workplace settings for surveillance of hepatic disease. Hepatic parenchymal imaging by ultrasonography has been suggested as a sensitive marker for preclinical effects among solvent-exposed dry cleaners. The use of this technique as a routine tool for medical surveillance for hepatotoxin exposure remains to be determined.

Individuals with chronic elevations of serum transaminase levels may continue to work if exposure to potential hepatotoxins is minimized through appropriate workplace controls and exposure assessment.

## DIAGNOSTIC TESTS FOR LIVER DYSFUNCTION

The ideal test for detection of liver dysfunction would be sensitive enough to detect minimal liver disease, specific enough to point to a particular derangement of liver function, and capable of reflecting the severity of the underlying pathophysiologic problem. Unfortunately, no such laboratory test is available, and "liver function tests" are used instead (Table 22–6).

**Table 22–6.** Tests for evaluation of liver disease.

**Biochemical tests**
  Serum enzyme activity
    Serum alkaline phosphatase
    Serum lactate dehydrogenase
  Serum bilirubin
  Urine bilirubin
**Tests of synthetic liver function**
  Serum albumin
  Prothrombin time
  Alpha-fetoprotein
  Serum ferritin
**Clearance tests**
  Exogenous clearance tests
    Sulfobromophthalein
    Indocyanine green
    Antipyrine test
    Aminopyrine breath test
    Caffeine breath test
  Endogenous clearance tests
    Serum bile acid
    Urinary D-glucaric acid

Broadly speaking, these tests encompass tests of biochemical evidence of cell death and hepatic synthesis as well as actual physiologic liver dysfunction. In addition, radiologic and morphologic evaluations are often used to delineate the nature of liver disease and as such may be viewed as tests of liver function. Biochemical tests and tests of synthetic function are commonly indicated for routine use; clearance tests are not widely available and not indicated for routine use.

Most epidemiologic studies in which measurement of serum enzyme levels is used to determine the hepatotoxicity of solvents have found no effect of ongoing exposure. Bile acids and other tests of metabolic function have generally been shown to be more sensitive indicators of hepatic effect from organic solvents, at levels of exposure below those expected to cause elevation of serum enzyme levels. It is not clear if these more sensitive measures of hepatic function may predict subsequent disease in workers exposed to hepatotoxins

## Biochemical Tests for Liver Disease

**A. Serum Enzyme Activity:** The tests most commonly used to detect liver disease are serum glutamic-oxaloacetic transaminase (SGOT), also called aspartate aminotransferase (AST); and serum glutamic-pyruvic transaminase (SGPT), also called alanine aminotransferase (ALT). Transaminase release is due to release of enzyme protein from liver cells as a result of cell injury. Elevations of serum aminotransferase levels may occur with minor cell injury, making such determinations useful in the early detection and monitoring of liver disease of drug or chemical origin. However, transaminase levels may be elevated in viral, alcoholic, or ischemic hepatitis as well as extrahepatic obstruction, limiting the specificity of these tests. In addition, significant elevations of transaminase levels have been noted in a few normal, healthy subjects due to diets high in sucrose, and false positives have been reported in patients receiving erythromycin and aminosalicylic acid and during diabetic ketoacidosis. Conversely, significant liver damage may be present in individuals with normal levels of transaminases. A serum AST/ALT ratio of less than 1, especially when the transaminase levels are below 300 IU/L, may be suggestive of the diagnosis of occupational liver disease.

The height of transaminase elevation in liver disease does not correlate with the extent of liver cell necrosis on biopsy and therefore has little prognostic value.

**B. Alkaline Phosphatase:** Serum alkaline phosphatase activity may originate from liver, bone, intestine, or placenta. Measurement of serum 5-nucleotidase may be used to determine the tissue origin of an elevated alkaline phosphatase; if elevated, it generally implies that the source of alkaline phosphatase is hepatobiliary, not bony. Toxic liver injury that results in disturbances in the transport function of the hepatocyte or of the biliary tree may cause elevation of serum alkaline phosphatase activity. Increased serum alkaline phosphatase levels may also be noted in the third trimester of pregnancy as well as normally in persons over age 50, in patients with osteoblastic bone disorders, and with both intrahepatic and extrahepatic cholestatic disease.

Assay of alkaline phosphatase enzymatic activity in serum in anicteric individuals is particularly useful in detecting and monitoring suspected drug- or chemical-induced cholestasis; it is not helpful in screening individuals for toxic liver injury except when there is primary involvement of the biliary network.

**C. Serum Bilirubin:** Hyperbilirubinemia may be classified as conjugated or unconjugated. Conjugated hyperbilirubinemia indicates dysfunction of the liver parenchyma or bile ducts and may be found in Dubin-Johnson syndrome and Rotor's syndrome and in viral hepatitis, drug- or toxin-induced hepatitis, shock liver, and metastatic disease of the liver. Unconjugated hyperbilirubinemia may be seen in Gilbert's disease, uncomplicated hemolytic disorders, and congestive heart failure.

Serum bilirubin is of some value in detecting toxic cholestatic liver injury but is frequently normal in the presence of more common cytotoxic damage. It is probably most useful in the presence of severe acute liver damage; although patients with fulminant hepatitis may be anicteric, the level of serum bilirubin is of prognostic importance in chemical and alcoholic hepatitis, primary biliary cirrhosis, and halothane hepatitis.

**D. Urine Bilirubin:** Bilirubin in the urine is direct bilirubin, since indirect bilirubin is tightly bound to albumin and not filtered by the normal kidney. A positive urine bilirubin test can confirm clinically suspected hyperbilirubinemia of hepatobiliary origin or may predate the appearance of overt icterus and thus serve as a useful screening test. Quantitative analysis of urine bilirubin is of no diagnostic significance.

**E. Other Biochemical Tests:**

**1. Serum $\gamma$-glutamyl transferase (SGGT)** is considered a more sensitive indicator than aminotransferases of drug-, virus-, chemical-, and alcohol-induced hepatocellular damage. Because of its lack of specificity, however, one must interpret abnormalities in conjunction with other tests.

**2. Liver-specific enzymes,** such as ornithine carbamyl dehydrogenase, phosphofructose aldolase, sorbitol dehydrogenase, and alcohol dehydrogenase, are less clinically useful than the aminotransferases, glutamyl transferases, or alkaline phosphatases.

**3. Serum lactate dehydrogenase** may originate from myocardium, liver, skeletal muscle, brain or kidney tissue, and red blood cells. Isoenzyme fractionation may determine the hepatic origin (lactate dehydrogenase 5) but is generally too nonspecific for purposes of evaluating toxic chemical liver injury.

## Tests of Synthetic Liver Function

Measurement of **serum albumin** concentrations may be a useful index of cellular dysfunction in liver disease. It is of little value in differential diagnosis.

Because all the clotting factors are synthesized by the liver, acute liver injury can result in prolongation of the **prothrombin time,** which is dependent on the activities of factors II, V, VII, and X. Measurement of prothrombin time is useful chiefly in fulminant hepatic failure, where a markedly elevated prothrombin time has prognostic significance, or in advanced chronic liver disease. It is a relatively insensitive indicator of liver damage and of little value in differential diagnosis.

High serum concentrations of alpha-fetoprotein are present in 70% of patients with primary hepatocellular carcinoma in the United States, and serial determinations may aid in monitoring the response to therapy or detecting early recurrence. **Alpha-fetoprotein** has no utility for surveillance in the occupational setting.

**Serum ferritin** levels accurately reflect hepatic and total body iron stores. Serum ferritin is useful in screening for idiopathic genetic hemochromatosis as a cause of liver disease but has no utility for surveillance in the occupational setting.

## Clearance Tests

Tests that measure the clearance of substances by the liver provide the most sensitive, specific, and reliable means of detecting the early phase of liver disease. Clearance tests may be used to determine the specificity of increased enzyme activity, to detect liver disease not reflected in abnormalities of serum enzymes, and to determine when recovery has occurred in reversible liver disease. This is especially the case when decreases in the functional state of the liver occur in patients with liver disease without active necrosis, including fatty liver, and inactive cirrhosis in the absence of clinical abnormalities or abnormal enzymes.

In the occupational setting, measures of hepatic functional capacity have been used epidemiologically to demonstrate liver dysfunction in the absence of clinical or serologic abnormalities. The clinical utility of clearance tests in screening for chemical liver injury—or in confirming occupational etiology of disease in workers with known liver dysfunction—has yet to be precisely determined.

**A. Exogenous Clearance Tests:** Exogenous clearance tests are given to detect liver function by the administration of various test substances to the individual.

**1. Sulfobromophthalein (BSP)–**Practical use of hepatic clearance as a diagnostic measure began with BSP. Its use has been discontinued because of side effects of phlebitis, severe local skin reactions, and occasionally fatal anaphylactic reactions.

**2. Indocyanine green–**Hepatic uptake of indocyanine green, a tricarbocyanine anionic dye, is an active process dependent upon sinusoidal perfusion, membrane transport, and secretory capacity. The dye is not metabolized or conjugated by the liver and is excreted directly into the bile. After a single intravenous injection of indocyanine green, clearance is calculated from serial dye levels at 3, 5, 7, 9, 12, and 14 minutes or by ear densitometry. Unlike BSP, indocyanine green causes negligible toxicity or allergic reactions.

Studies of workers exposed to vinyl chloride have shown that indocyanine green clearance after a dose of 0.5 mg/kg is the most sensitive test for subclinical liver injury and has a specificity exceeded only by serum alkaline phosphatase. A dose-response relationship has also been found between cumulative exposure to vinyl chloride and indocyanine green clearance. This has not been demonstrated in other groups of workers exposed to occupational hepatotoxins, and indocyanine green for detection of subclinical liver disease cannot yet be recommended for routine use.

**3. Antipyrine test–**This is the most widely used in vivo index of hepatic microsomal enzyme activity. Antipyrine is completely and rapidly absorbed from the gastrointestinal tract, distributed in total body water, and almost completely metabolized by the liver via three major oxidative pathways. The rate of elimination is virtually independent of hepatic blood flow, with first-order kinetics of elimination and a half-life of about 10 hours in normal subjects. At 24–48 hours after an orally administered dose of 1 g, antipyrine clearance can be calculated by serial plasma or salivary measurements. It has been shown that clearance can be calculated from a single salivary sample collected at least 18 hours after dosing, permitting a simpler, more convenient method of study. Repeat tests cannot be done less than 3 days apart, and in order to avoid the induction of antipyrine metabolism in the individual, an interval of 1 week is recommended.

The antipyrine test has undergone the most extensive study of all clearance tests in the detection of subclinical liver disease in occupational settings. It has been used to detect mean differences in hepatic enzyme activity between workers exposed to solvent mixtures and unexposed controls. Clinically, asymptomatic chlordecone-exposed workers had increased antipyrine clearance and biopsy-proved liver disease that normalized after exposure was terminated.

**4. Aminopyrine breath test–**The aminopyrine breath test has the advantage of being simple, noninvasive, safe, and relatively cheap. Clinical studies have documented the use of aminopyrine breath tests in patients with chronic advanced liver disease, but the sensitivity and specificity of the test for detection of subclinical chemical liver injury in asymptomatic populations have not been assessed.

After oral administration of about 2 $\mu$Ci of $^{14}$C-aminopyrine, the labeled methyl group will be oxidized by the microsomal enzyme system and ultimately excreted as $^{14}CO_2$. Breath samples are collected 2 hours after administration, and the specific activity of $^{14}CO_2$ is measured in a liquid scintillation counter. The test requires physical rest from dose to breath sampling.

**5. Caffeine breath test**–Inhaled $^{14}$C-labeled caffeine, labeled at one or all three methyl groups, followed by exhaled breath $^{14}CO_2$ measurement, has recently been introduced as a noninvasive means of studying hepatic microsomal enzyme function. It has not yet undergone evaluation in asymptomatic worker populations.

**B. Endogenous Clearance Tests:**

**1. Serum bile acids**–Serum bile acid measurement may be useful in further medical workup for the individual with persistent enzyme abnormalities. Bile acids are synthesized by the liver and undergo enterohepatic circulation. Serum levels of bile acids are normally low in a fasting state ($< 6$ $\mu$mol/L) and reflect only hepatic excretory function and not synthesis rate or volume distribution. Fasting bile acid levels are increased in relation to the degree of liver disease and impairment in excretion.

Depending on the population screened, the positive predictive value of an abnormal ($> 8.4$ $\mu$mol/L) serum bile acid test ranges from 10% (general population) to 94% (hospitalized population with biopsy-proved hepatobiliary disease). In a large workplace study of vinyl chloride-exposed workers, measurement of serum bile acids was found to have a sensitivity of 78%, a specificity of 93%, and a positive predictive value of 10%.

**2. Urinary D-glucaric acid**–Urinary D-glucaric acid (UDGA) has been used as an indirect measure of liver induction. D-Glucaric acid, a product of carbohydrate metabolism, is produced via the glucuronic acid pathway after initial xenobiotic metabolism. The mechanism for UDGA induction has not been elucidated, but UDGA excretion is correlated with microsomal enzyme content. Operating room personnel exposed to isoflurane and nitrous oxide have increased UDGA excretion.

Serum bile acids have been suggested as a more sensitive indicator of hepatic dysfunction than biochemical tests for liver toxicity. A dose-dependent increase in the concentration of serum bile acids has been observed in workers exposed to hexachlorobutadiene and trichloroethylene. Other standard tests of liver function were normal in these workers. The significance of these findings and their clinical correlation with disease outcome have yet to be determined.

# CLINICAL MANAGEMENT OF OCCUPATIONAL LIVER DISEASE

## Occupational & Medical History

A careful occupational history of exposure to known human hepatotoxins should be obtained in every case of suspected occupational liver disease. The past medical history of liver disease should be noted. The review of symptoms should include those of acute central nervous system toxicity, such as headache, dizziness, and lightheadedness, since the presence of these symptoms may indicate excessive solvent exposure.

Nonoccupational causes of liver disease should be carefully evaluated. Steroid use, glue-sniffing, or other recreational solvent use should be determined. Travel to areas with endemic parasitic or viral diseases may be a significant risk for infectious hepatitis. A history of hobbies involving exposure to hepatotoxins should be taken. Previous blood transfusion, percutaneous exposures (eg, tattoos, needlesticks, ear piercing, or acupuncture), or intravenous drug use may be risk factors for viral hepatitis. A relationship between obesity and elevated liver enzyme levels has been reported. Numerous medications may be hepatotoxic.

Use of protective work practices (such as respiratory protection, gloves, and work clothes) should be described, as this may indicate the extent of pulmonary and skin absorption. Material Data Safety Sheets (Chapter 2) should be obtained on the relevant products used. Airborne contaminant monitoring data (Chapter 37) should be requested and reviewed for excessive exposure. Inquiry should be made of the employer about other employees with possible liver disease.

## Physical Examination

Acute liver disease due to occupational exposure may present with right upper quadrant tenderness, hepatospenomegaly, or jaundice. Mild hepatotoxicity may cause few physical findings. Examination of the respiratory tract or skin should be performed depending on the route of exposure. Chronic liver disease may result in stigmata such as spider angiomata, palmar erythema, testicular atrophy, ascites, or gynecomastia.

## Differential Diagnosis

Other causes of occupational liver disease should be ruled out—particularly infectious and alcohol- and drug-induced hepatitis. The most common cause of elevated serum transaminase is ingestion of ethanol. If a history of excessive ethanol ingestion is elicited, the serum transaminase measurement should be repeated after 3–4 weeks of abstinence. If serum transaminase levels are normal on follow-up, ethanol should be suspected as the probable cause. Persistent serum transaminase elevation may represent chronic alcoholic hepatitis or continued occupational exposure.

The onset of liver disease after exposure to a known or suspected hepatotoxin is suggestive of occupational liver disease, particularly if normal liver function tests before exposure can be documented. Even if preexposure tests are normal, liver disease may develop coincidentally without relation to workplace exposure.

## Management of Acute Liver Disease

The most common clinical problem is the individual with elevated serum transaminase levels on routine screening who may have occupational exposure to a known hepatotoxin. Nonoccupational causes of liver disease should be carefully ruled out and the workplace inspected for the presence of hepatotoxic exposures. If an occupational cause is suspected, the individual should be immediately removed from exposure for 3–4 weeks. The serum transaminase measurement should then be repeated; with few exceptions, serum transaminase concentrations will normalize following removal from exposure. A persistently elevated serum transaminase concentration suggests a nonoccupational cause of liver disease or, rarely, chronic occupational liver disease.

Although there is little evidence that individuals with nonoccupational liver disease are more susceptible to further liver damage due to occupational exposure, it is prudent to carefully monitor them for evidence of worsening liver damage. Appropriate engineering controls and personal protective equipment should be made available to reduce potential hepatotoxic exposures. If there is evidence of worsening liver disease or if exposure cannot be satisfactorily reduced, the individual should be reassigned.

Aside from removing the individual from exposure to the offending agent, there is no specific treatment for acute occupational liver disease.

## Management of Chronic Liver Disease

Persistent abnormalities in liver function tests after removal from exposure have rarely been reported, and a thorough search for other causes should always be conducted. Occasionally, chronic liver disease may follow acute chemical hepatitis or years of low-dose exposure.

Hepatic ultrasonography or CT scanning may suggest hepatic steatosis or fibrosis. Liver biopsy is usually not helpful in differentiating occupational from nonoccupational liver disease and is rarely indicated.

Treatment of hepatocellular carcinoma due to occupational exposure does not differ from that of disease due to other causes.

## REFERENCES

Alter HJ: To C or not to C: These are the questions. Blood 1995;85:1681.

Brodkin CA et al: Hepatic ultrasound changes in workers exposed to perchloroethylene. Occup Environ Med 1995;52:679.

Driscoll TR et al: Concentrations of individual serum or plasma bile acids in workers exposed to chlorinated aliphatic hydrocarbons. Br J Ind Med 1992;49:700.

Gerberding JL: Management of occupational exposures to blood-borne viruses. N Engl J Med 1995;332:444.

Herip DS: Recommendations for the investigation of abnormal hepatic function in asymptomatic workers. Am J Ind Med 1992;21:331.

Hodgson MJ, Van Thiel DH, Goodman-Klein B: Obesity and hepatotoxins as risk factors for fatty liver disease. Br J Ind Med 1991;48:690.

Katkov WN, Dienstag JL: Hepatitis vaccines. Gastroenterol Clin North Am 1994;24:143.

Redlich CA et al: Clinical and pathological characteristics of hepatotoxicity associated with occupational exposure to dimethylformamide. Gastroenterology 1990;99:748.

Rees D et al: Solvent exposure, alcohol consumption and liver injury in workers manufacturing paint. Scand J Work Environ Health 1993;19:236.

Zimmerman HJ: Hepatotoxicity. Disease-a-month 1993;39:675.

# Renal Toxicology

**23**

*Rudolph A. Rodriguez, MD*

Although occupational and environmental exposures are known to cause both acute and chronic renal dysfunction, physicians rarely consider these exposures to be important causes of renal disease. In the United States, approximately 200,000 patients currently have end-stage renal disease (ESRD) requiring renal replacement therapy at a cost of over 6 billion dollars per year. The etiology of the renal failure in a significant percentage of these patients is never fully elucidated, and the diagnosis of renal disease of occupational origin is rarely considered. The true incidence of renal failure secondary to occupational and environmental exposures in the United States is not known. However, these exposures represent potentially preventable causes of renal failure. Even if occupational and environmental exposures account for only a small percentage of the causes of ESRD in the United States, the significant morbidity, mortality, and costs associated with renal replacement therapy could be potentially prevented.

The kidney is especially vulnerable to occupational and environmental exposures. Approximately 20% of the cardiac output goes to the kidneys, and a fraction of this is then filtered; this is represented by the glomerular filtration rate (GFR). The GFR is normally 125 mL/min or 180 L/d. Along the nephron, this filtrate is largely reabsorbed and then concentrated and acidified. Thus, occupational and environmental toxins can be highly concentrated in the kidney, and as the pH of the filtrate changes, some toxins can exist in certain ionic forms. These factors help explain the pathophysiologic mechanisms involved in certain toxins. For example, lead and cadmium cause much of their renal ultrastructural damage in the proximal tubule, where two-thirds of the filtered load is reabsorbed.

Following relatively high-dose exposure to certain organic solvents, metals, or pesticides, acute renal failure may develop within hours to days. The renal lesion is usually acute tubular necrosis. The clinical picture is usually dominated by the extrarenal manifestations of these exposures, and if the other organ systems recover, renal recovery is the rule. Chronic renal failure or ESRD may also develop after certain exposures. The renal lesion in these cases is usually chronic interstitial nephritis, and lead nephropathy is a prime example. However, glomerular lesions are also seen after selected exposures such as organic solvents or silicosis; in general, glomerular lesions after occupational or environmental exposures are very uncommon.

The renal evaluation of patients thought to have renal disease associated with an environmental or occupational exposure should be guided by the history, physical examination, and clinical presentation of the renal disease. The time course will separate acute from chronic renal disease. In acute renal failure, the urine sediment is usually diagnostic of acute tubular necrosis. Most chronic renal diseases associated with exposure to agents such as lead or cadmium present with chronic interstitial nephritis characterized by tubular proteinuria (usually less than 2 g/24 h) and a urinary sediment usually lacking any cellular elements. A nephritic sediment is suggestive of a proliferative renal lesion and has been associated only with a few exposures, such as organic solvents. The nephrotic syndrome, characterized by more than 3.5 g of protein/24 h, edema, and hypercholesterolemia, has also been associated with exposure to some heavy metals, including mercury.

Monitoring workers for the possible renal effects of occupational exposures is very difficult because of the lack of sensitive and specific tests of renal injury. Serial measurement of the traditional tests such as creatinine or blood urea nitrogen (BUN) is inadequate, because these tests do not become abnormal until significant renal damage has occurred. The newer tests of renal injury include high-molecular-weight proteinuria (albuminuria, ferritin), low-molecular-weight proteinuria ($\beta$-2-microglobulin, retinol-binding protein), enzymuria (N-acetylglucosaminidase, alanine aminopeptidase, lactate dehydrogenase [LDH], and tubular antigenuria [BB50]). Most of these tests were designed to detect early renal tubular damage. Unfortunately, their use is limited by many factors; for instance, some are unstable at certain urine pHs, others return to normal levels within a few days of the exposure despite renal damage, and others exhibit large interindividual variations. Most importantly, unlike microalbuminuria, which is able to predict future nephropathy in insulin-dependent diabetics, the predictive value of these newer tests has not been validated. More studies are needed before these newer renal tests can routinely be used to monitor renal injury in the workplace.

# ACUTE RENAL DYSFUNCTION

A large number of occupational and environmental toxins can cause acute renal failure, usually after high-dose exposure. Although the extrarenal manifestations of the particular toxic exposure usually dominate the clinical presentation and course, the characteristics and time course of the acute renal failure are very similar in all exposures. In the vast majority of cases, acute tubular necrosis is the renal lesion that develops. Hours to days after the exposure, the acute tubular necrosis is manifested by decreased urine output, usually in the oliguric range of less than 500 mL/d. The urinalysis typically is diagnostic of acute tubular necrosis, with renal tubular cells, muddy brown granular casts, and little or no protein. The presence of red blood cells, white blood cells, or casts of either cell type is not typically seen with acute tubular necrosis and suggests the presence of a glomerulonephritis. Increases in BUN and creatinine and in electrolyte abnormalities develop as expected in acute renal failure, and patients may require dialysis until the renal function recovers. After 1–2 weeks, recovery from acute tubular necrosis is usually heralded by the onset of a diuresis.

Hemodialysis and/or hemoperfusion have almost no role in accelerating the clearance of occupational and environmental toxins. For these techniques to be effective, toxins must have a low apparent volume of distribution and molecular weight, a low affinity to plasma proteins, and low tissue binding properties. For example, charcoal hemoperfusion can result in almost complete removal of circulating paraquat, but because of high tissue binding, only small amounts of total body paraquat are removed. Consequently, hemoperfusion does not affect the prognosis in paraquat poisoning. These extracorporeal techniques are effective only after a few intoxications, which include certain alcohols, salicylate, lithium, and theophylline.

## ACUTE RENAL DYSFUNCTION CAUSED BY HEAVY METALS

Significant exposure to any of the divalent metals—chromium, cadmium, mercury, and vanadium—is capable of producing acute tubular necrosis. Of these metals, the only one encountered in industrial settings in high enough concentrations to produce acute tubular necrosis with notable frequency is cadmium. Exposure to cadmium in toxic amounts is usually through inhalation, and the classic history of exposure that is of workers welding cadmium-plated metals. Welders exposed to cadmium fumes present with coughing and progressive pulmonary distress leading to adult respiratory distress syndrome. Renal failure occurs rapidly in the form of acute tubular necrosis. Severe exposure is capable of producing bilateral cortical necrosis.

## ACUTE RENAL DYSFUNCTION CAUSED BY ORGANIC SOLVENTS

In the occupational setting, the lungs are the most common route of absorption of hydrocarbons. Inhaled hydrocarbons then quickly pass into the pulmonary circulation. Transcutaneous absorption is also an important route of absorption for solvents. Organic solvents are lipophilic and are therefore distributed in highest concentration in the fat, liver, bone marrow, blood, brain, and kidneys.

### 1. HALOGENATED HYDROCARBONS

**Carbon Tetrachloride**

Carbon tetrachloride ($CCl_4$) is used as an industrial solvent and as the basis for manufacture of fluorinated hydrocarbons. It was once used as a household cleaning agent and as a component of fire extinguisher fluid under the brand name Pyrene.

After acute exposure, patients typically present with confusion, somnolence, nausea, and vomiting. Mucous membrane irritant effects, such as burning eyes, may occur, though some workers may be symptom-free for several days following exposure and then present with complaints of vomiting, abdominal pain, constipation, diarrhea, and in some cases fever. Physical findings may be compatible with the acute abdomen at this stage of illness, and many patients have been improperly subjected to laparotomy for that reason.

After 7–10 days of illness, there may be a decline in urine output even to the point of anuria. Patients with carbon tetrachloride intoxication may show signs of prerenal azotemia as demonstrated by a low urinary sodium excretion and by improvement after volume repletion. Sinicrope (1984) postulated that in some cases of carbon tetrachloride toxicity, renal failure results from volume depletion which develops after protracted vomiting and poor fluid intake. Volume repletion restored renal function in their patients. They postulated that the severe prerenal state may then lead to acute tubular necrosis. This is consistent with animal studies, which have not been able to produce significant renal lesions with carbon tetrachloride exposure. If the hepatotoxicity is severe, patients may also develop hepatorenal syndrome.

## Other Aliphatic Halogenated Hydrocarbons

Other aliphatic halogenated hydrocarbons are nephrotoxic, some to a greater and some to a lesser degree than carbon tetrachloride.

**Ethylene dichloride** ($C_2H_4Cl_2$) is used as a solvent for oils, fats, waxes, turpentine, rubber, and some resins; as an insecticide and fumigant; and in fire extinguishers and household cleaning fluids. It is slightly less potent as a renal toxicant than carbon tetrachloride but causes far greater central nervous system toxicity. Ingestion or heavy inhalation may produce acute tubular necrosis similar to that encountered with mercury poisoning.

**Chloroform** ($CCl_3H$) is more nephrotoxic than carbon tetrachloride and produces proximal tubule cell damage in animal models.

**Trichloroethylene** ($C_2HCl_3$) has a number of industrial uses and has been used as an anesthetic agent as well. Acute renal failure has followed inhalation of this agent and has occurred in persons using it as a solvent for cleaning. Although it is partially unsaturated, it has toxic effects comparable to those of carbon tetrachloride and chloroform.

**Tetrachloroethane** (1,1,2,2,-tetrachloroethane; $C_2H_2Cl_4$) is an excellent solvent for cellulose acetate and is by far the most toxic of the halogenated hydrocarbons.

**Vinylidene chloride** (1,1-dichloroethylene; $C_2H_2Cl_2$) is a monomer used in the manufacture of plastics and is not used as a solvent. Its toxicology is similar to that of carbon tetrachloride.

**Ethylene chlorohydrin** (2-chloroethyl alcohol; $C_2H_4ClOH$) is used as a solvent and as a chemical intermediate. It is far more toxic than any of the other aliphatic halogenated hydrocarbons. Unlike the others, it penetrates the skin readily and is absorbed through rubber gloves. Its mechanism of toxicity is not well understood.

## 2. NONHALOGENATED HYDROCARBONS AS A CAUSE OF ACUTE RENAL FAILURE

## Dioxane

Dioxane is a cyclic diether, colorless and with only a faint odor, freely soluble in water. The vapor pressure of dioxane is quite low, so that respiratory overexposure is rare. Although dioxane is less toxic than the halogenated hydrocarbons, toxicity can be insidious, and large amounts can be inhaled without warning. Injury may become apparent hours after exposure.

Clinically, patients present with anorexia, nausea, and vomiting. Jaundice is uncommon. In fatal cases, clinical presentation may resemble an acute abdominal emergency. Urine output decreases on about the third day of illness.

## Toluene

There have been several reports of acute renal failure occurring with toluene inhalation ("glue-sniffing"); most case reports describe reversible acute tubular necrosis, with a few documenting acute interstitial nephritis. However, metabolic acidosis associated with toluene abuse is much more common. The two mechanisms involved overproduction of hippuric acid and reduction of excretion of net acid (primarily $NH_4+$) in some abusers. Sodium and potassium depletion also commonly occurs in these patients.

## Alkyl Derivatives of Ethylene Glycol

The principal derivatives of ethylene glycol used commercially are the **monoethyl ether** (cellosolve), the **monomethyl ether** (methylcellosolve), and the **butyl ether** (butylcellosolve).

The three compounds are similar pharmacologically, with increasing toxicity in the order listed above. All can be absorbed through the skin or lungs as well as through the gastrointestinal tract. These agents are irritants of skin and mucous membranes and act as central nervous system depressants, with resultant symptoms of headache, drowsiness, weakness, slurred speech, staggering gait, and blurred vision. The renal injury caused by these ethers is not related to the oxalic aciduria caused by the parent compounds, which are dialcohols.

## Phenol

Phenol (carbolic acid) causes local burns and may be absorbed both through the lungs and transdermally.

Although phenol causes severe local burns, systemic symptoms may also occur. These include headache, vertigo, salivation, nausea and vomiting, and diarrhea. In severe intoxication, urinary albumin excretion may be increased. Red cells and casts are found in the urine. The potentially disastrous consequences of transdermal absorption should not be underestimated.

Patients may present with hypothermia, which is followed by convulsions. The urine may be dark, and oliguria may develop. Phenol is metabolized to hydroquinone, which, when excreted in the urine, may be oxidized to colored substances, causing the urine to change to green or brown (carboluria). Prolonged exposure has been reported to result in proteinuria.

## Pentachlorophenol

Pentachlorophenol is used as a preservative for timber and as an insecticide, herbicide, and defoliant. It is readily absorbed through the skin.

In addition to causing acute renal failure, pentachlorophenol causes a hypermetabolic state, with hyperpyrexia and vascular collapse. Workers exposed to pentachlorophenol in clearly subtoxic doses may present with reversible decreased proximal tubular function as manifested by reduced tubular resorption of phosphorus. When these workers are reexamined after a 21-day vacation, renal function—both glomerular filtration rate and proximal tubular function—has returned to normal.

## Dinitriphenols & Dinitro-o-Cresols

These agents have been used as pesticides and herbicides. After absorption, they uncouple oxidative phosphorylation. Fatal hyperpyrexia has been reported.

Although patients develop acute renal failure, it is not known whether this is a direct effect of the agents or secondary to the metabolic consequences, such as myoglobinuria.

## ACUTE RENAL DYSFUNCTION CAUSED BY UNIDENTIFIED PESTICIDES

### Exposure, Pathogenesis, & Clinical Findings

A reduction in glomerular filtration rate—as well as tubular reabsorption of phosphate suggestive of mild proximal tubular dysfunction—has occurred in some agricultural workers. Changes in tubular function and in glomerular filtration rate occur in conjunction with depression of serum cholinesterase, suggesting that organophosphates may be responsible for these changes in renal function.

In an ethically questionable study, prisoners in a New York State prison were fed **carbaryl**. This pesticide is similar in action to the organophosphates, and the prisoners likewise demonstrated a decrease in glomerular filtration rate and tubular resorption of phosphate. There is no evidence that structural damage occurs after exposure to any of these agents.

**Organic mercurials** are used as fungicides. Absorption of these agents in agricultural workers has been reported to lead to nephrotic syndrome in the case of methoxymethyl mercury silicate, and a dose-dependent increase in the urinary excretion of $\gamma$-glutamyl transpeptidase has been reported in the case of phenyl mercury, indicating a direct nephrotoxic effect of this class of compounds.

## ACUTE RENAL DYSFUNCTION CAUSED BY ARSINE

### Exposure

Arsine ($AsH_3$) is a heavy gas and is the most nephrotoxic form of arsenic. It is produced by the action of acids on arsenicals, usually during coal or metal processing operations. Exposure to arsine may be insidious, since even as simple an operation as spraying water on metal dross may liberate arsine. Arsine is also used in the semiconductor industry. It may be shipped over long distances, with potential for public health disaster, since arsine is an extremely toxic gas.

### Clinical Findings

Arsine is primarily hemotoxic and is a potent hemolytic agent after acute or chronic exposure. The first signs of poisoning are malaise, abdominal cramps, nausea, and vomiting. This may take place immediately or after a delay of up to 24 hours. Renal failure results from acute tubular necrosis secondary to hemoglobinuria.

### Treatment & Prognosis

Acute tubular necrosis may be delayed by treatment with mannitol and hemodialysis immediately after exposure. However, exchange transfusion is necessary to prevent further hemolysis. Recovery from acute tubular necrosis induced by arsine may not be complete, and there is evidence that residual interstitial nephritis may result.

## ACUTE RENAL DYSFUNCTION CAUSED BY PHOSPHORUS

Ingestion of only a few milligrams of elemental yellow phosphorus may produce acute hepatic and acute renal necrosis. Chronic exposure may result in proteinuria, though the kidney is not the primary organ affected by phosphorus.

# CHRONIC RENAL DYSFUNCTION

## BALKAN ENDEMIC NEPHROPATHY

The prototypic renal disease associated with an environmental exposure is Balkan endemic nephropathy (BEN). BEN highlights the difficulties involved in identifying specific toxins that may cause renal disease. In the late 1950s, BEN was first described as an interstitial nephropathy associated with urinary tract tumors. It is endemic to rural areas along the Sava,

Danube, and Morava Rivers in Serbia, Croatia, Bosnia-Herzegovina, Bulgaria, and Rumania. The prevalence of BEN may be as high as 20,000 in areas where the disease is endemic. It strikes predominantly farm workers in the fifth to sixth decade. Most victims have resided for at least 20 years in villages where the disease is endemic, and children are not affected.

Patients present with abnormalities of tubular function, including renal tubular acidosis, glycosuria, and hyperuricosuria with hypouricemia. Proteinuria is usually less than 1 g/d, and patients do not develop acute nephritis or nephrotic syndrome. Not all patients with chronic renal failure will progress to ESRD. Renal pathologic changes include interstitial fibrosis and periglomerular fibrosis; there is no inflammatory component, and glomeruli are normal. Papillary transitional cell cancer is seen in 30–40% of patients with BEN. Anemia seems to be out of proportion to the degree of renal failure in these patients.

Many etiologies have been proposed to account for BEN, but few seem likely. Both lead and cadmium have been excluded as possibilities. Aristolochic acid has been found in flour obtained from wheat contaminated with the seeds of *Aristolochia clematis* in areas of endemicity. Aristolochic acid is known to be a renal toxin, but more studies are needed before the true cause of BEN is known.

## HERBAL NEPHROPATHY/ ANALGESIC NEPHROPATHY

When evaluating patients suspected of having renal disease associated with environmental or occupational exposures, it is very important to exclude herbal and analgesic nephropathy. Both commonly present with chronic interstitial nephritis, as do most occupationally related renal disease. Chinese herb nephropathy was first described in 1991; physicians in Belgium noted an increasing number of young women presenting with ESRD following exposure to Chinese herbs at a weight reduction clinic. The renal pathologic changes and the association with papillary transitional cell cancer were very similar to those due to BEN. In fact, aristolochic acid was the common denominator found in weight reduction formulas, and it has been incriminated as the cause of Chinese herb nephropathy.

Most herbal remedies are safe, but adulteration of these herbal remedies is fairly common. The common contaminants that may cause renal disease include botanicals (eg, aristolochic acid), synthetic drugs (eg, nonsteroidal anti-inflammatory drugs [NSAIDs], and diazepam), and heavy metals (eg, lead and cadmium). Renal dysfunction due to NSAIDs may present in three different forms. The most common form is hemodynamic renal failure after the loss of prostaglandin-mediated afferent arteriolar vasodilation. This then leads to afferent arteriolar vasoconstriction in patients with preexisting volume depletion. NSAIDs can also cause acute renal failure secondary to acute interstitial nephritis, which is usually accompanied by nephrotic range proteinuria. Both forms of renal failure are reversible with discontinuation of the offending NSAID, although the renal failure due to interstitial nephritis is usually more severe and may require dialysis support. The third form of renal dysfunction is papillary necrosis, which is not reversible and which occurs after many years of high doses of NSAIDs. Papillary necrosis more commonly occurs after chronic phenacetin use. Phenacetin is no longer available in the United States. It is controversial whether chronic acetaminophen use causes papillary necrosis.

In addition to NSAIDs and aristolochic acid, herbal remedies may contain heavy metals such as lead, cadmium, or mercury; the renal disease associated with these metals is discussed in the following sections.

## CHRONIC RENAL DYSFUNCTION CAUSED BY LEAD

Although organic lead, which is used as an additive to gasoline, is not nephrotoxic, its combustion products are. Lead is released into the environment at a rate of approximately 60 million kg per year as inorganic lead through the combustion of gasoline. Its environmental fate is unknown. Lead can be absorbed from the gastrointestinal tract or the lungs. Gastrointestinal absorption is approximately 10% in adults and 50% in children. Within 1 hour of absorption by the gut, lead is concentrated in bone (90%) and kidneys. The biological half-life ranges from 7 years to several decades.

Although the link between lead exposure and small, contracted kidneys was noted by Lanceraux in 1863, the modern awareness of lead nephropathy originated with the Australian experience. Acute lead poisoning in childhood was very common in Queensland between 1870 and 1920, when lead paint was still being used. Twenty years later, a follow-up study of children hospitalized for acute lead poisoning found that more than 30% of these children had chronic nephritis, hypertension, or proteinuria. Gouty arthritis was noted in approximately 50% of patients. Epidemiologic data in the United States have also confirmed the link between lead exposure and chronic renal failure, hypertension, and gout.

Experimental models of lead nephropathy found that administration of continuous high-dose lead to rats over a 1-year period resulted in a significant reduction in GFR, and the renal pathologic tests revealed the characteristic proximal tubule intranuclear inclusions that are prominent early in human lead nephropathy. After 6 months of lead exposure, focal tubular atrophy and interstitial fibrosis appeared, and after 12 months, enlarged, dilated tubules were noted. Chelation of lead with dimercaptosuccinic acid (DMSA) resulted in an increase in GFR in rats, but the tubulointerstitial disease did not reverse. Continuous low-level lead exposure in rats did not produce significant changes in renal function and produced only mild alterations in renal morphology after 12 months.

Many studies have noted an approximate incidence of gout of 50% among subjects with lead nephropathy. The possible mechanisms of saturnine gout include decrease renal clearance of uric acid, crystallization at low urate concentrations, and lead-induced formation of guanine crystals. Human studies have found that patients with gout and renal insufficiency have significantly higher urinary lead excretion after chelation than do subjects with gout and normal renal function or subjects with no gout and renal insufficiency. These findings implicate lead as the cause of both the gout and the renal insufficiency in these patients.

Hypertension has been associated with acute lead intoxication, but the relationship between chronic lead exposure and hypertension is controversial. Many large population studies have found a direct correlation between blood lead levels and zinc protoporphyrin and blood pressure. The possible mechanisms linking lead and hypertension include increased intracellular calcium, inhibition of the Na+, K+-ATPase, direct vasoconstriction, and alterations in the renin-angiotensin-aldosterone axis. Human studies have also investigated the role that lead plays in the association of hypertension and renal failure. In patients with hypertension and renal insufficiency, the amount of mobilizable lead correlated directly with the serum creatinine concentration; however, the amount of mobilizable lead was not elevated in patients with hypertension and normal renal function or those with renal insufficiency and no hypertension. This study also implicates lead as the cause of both the renal insufficiency and hypertension.

### Presentation

The classic presentation for lead nephropathy is chronic renal insufficiency accompanied by a history of hypertension and gout. However, the diagnosis of lead nephropathy should also be considered in patients with chronic renal insufficiency and low-grade proteinuria, even without gout or significant hypertension. The urinalysis usually reveals 1+ to 2+ proteinuria but is otherwise normal, without cells or cellular casts. Twenty-four–hour urine collection usually has nonnephrotic range proteinuria in the range of 1–2 g, and renal ultrasonography typically shows small, contracted kidneys. Renal biopsy reveals nonspecific tubular atrophy, interstitial fibrosis, and minimal inflammatory infiltrates, and the arteriolar changes are indistinguishable from nephrosclerosis and appear even in patients with lead exposure and no history of hypertension. Electron microscopy

shows mitochondrial swelling and increased numbers of lysosomal dense bodies within proximal tubule cells; intranuclear inclusion bodies are usually present in the early stages of lead exposure but are often absent after chronic exposure or after lead chelation.

### Diagnosis

The diagnosis is considered after documenting significant lead exposure. Serum lead levels are not useful unless elevated, since low serum levels do not exclude chronic lead exposure. The EDTA lead mobilization test correlates well with bone lead levels. Two grams of EDTA with lidocaine are given intramuscularly in two divided doses 8–12 hours apart, and urine is then collected for 72 hours in patients with chronic renal insufficiency or for 24 hours in patients with normal renal function. Total excretion greater than 600 μg of lead chelate over 3 days is indicative of significant lead exposure. Tibial K x-ray fluorescence measurements also correlate well with bone lead levels and should eventually replace the painful EDTA mobilization test.

### Treatment

Lead nephropathy is one of the few preventable renal diseases. Whether renal function improves with treatment is controversial, but in some patients treatment has resulted in a modest improvement in GFR or, at the minimum, a slowing of the progression of the renal insufficiency. Treatment consists of continued EDTA injections thrice weekly, with the goal of normalizing the urinary lead chelate to less than 600 μg. The oral lead chelator (DMSA) is currently being studied and should replace EDTA as the treatment of choice for lead exposure. However, the safety and efficacy of chronic DMSA and EDTA in patients with moderate to severe renal insufficiency have not been well studied, and should be used with caution in these patients.

### CHRONIC RENAL DYSFUNCTION CAUSED BY CADMIUM

Cadmium, which is found primarily as cadmium sulfide in ores of zinc, lead, and copper, accumulates with age, having a biological half-life in humans in excess of 10 years. The use of cadmium has doubled in the United States every decade in the 20th century because it is commonly used in the manufacturing of nickel-cadmium batteries, pigments, glass, metal alloys, and electrical equipment.

From 40% to 80% of accumulated cadmium is stored in the liver and kidneys, with one-third in the kidneys alone. Cadmium is also a contaminant of tobacco smoke, and in the absence of occupational exposure, accumulation is substantially greater in smokers than in nonsmokers. Nonindustrial exposure is primarily via food, and only about 25% of ingested cadmium is absorbed. "Normal" daily dietary intake varies between 15 and 75 mg/d in different parts of the world, though only a small fraction of this amount (0.5–2.5 mg/d) is absorbed. The cadmium body burden of a 45-year-old nonsmoker in the United States is about 9 mg, while in Japan the total is about 21 mg. Although clinical disease has been recognized among the general population in Japan, this has not been the case in the United States, where cadmium has been generally regarded as an exclusively industrial hazard. This may represent failure to assign the correct cause to conditions commonly regarded as the result of aging.

After exposure to cadmium, the blood concentration rises sharply but falls after a matter of hours as the cadmium is taken up by the liver. In red blood cells and soft tissues, cadmium is bound to metallothionein, which is a low-molecular-weight polypeptide. This cadmium-metallothionein complex is filtered at the glomerulus, undergoes endocytosis in the proximal tubule, and is later degraded in the lysosomes. The adverse effects of cadmium on the proximal tubule are probably mediated by unbound cadmium, which can interfere with zinc-dependent enzymes.

The principal target organs for cadmium toxicity after chronic low-dose exposure are the kidneys and lungs. Once a critical concentration of 200 μg/g of renal cortex is achieved, the renal effects such as Fanconi's syndrome become evident. Hypercalciuria with normocalcemia, hyperphosphaturia, and distal renal tubular acidosis all contribute to the osteomalacia, pseudofractures, and nephrolithiasis seen in certain patients. Many of the symptoms usually originate from the increased calcium excretion that accompanies the renal tubular dysfunction. Ureteral colic from calculi is seen in up to 40% of patients subjected to industrial exposure. "Itai-Itai" disease is a painful bone disease associated with pseudofractures in Japan, and it is attributed to local cadmium contamination of food staples by polluted river water. Osteomalacia is associated with the diminished renal tubular reabsorption of calcium and phosphate, the increased amount of parathyroid hormone and the subsequent decreased hydroxylation of vitamin D.

The role of cadmium in the induction of chronic interstitial nephritis is controversial. Despite finding a direct correlation between the number of years of exposure to cadmium and both urinary excretion of β-2 microglobulin and multiple tubular abnormalities, only small increases in serum creatinine levels have been documented in cadmium workers following long-term exposure. However, workers should be monitored closely. Renal cadmium toxicity should be suspected in patients with low-molecular-weight proteinuria, urinary calculi, multiple tubular abnormalities, and a urine cadmium concentration greater than 10 μg/g of urine creatinine. There is no definitive treatment except removal from the exposure and treatment of osteomalacia if present.

## CHRONIC RENAL DYSFUNCTION CAUSED BY MERCURY

### Exposure

Occupational mercury poisoning usually results from inhalation of metal fumes or vapor—though toxicity has been reported after exposure to oxides of mercury, mercurous or mercuric chloride, phenylmercuric acetate, mercuric oxide, and mercury-containing pesticides.

Divalent mercury is quite nephrotoxic when ingested, accumulates in the proximal tubule, and can produce acute renal failure in doses as low as 1 mg/kg. Although acute tubular necrosis will result after administration of mercuric chloride ($HgCl_2$), such exposures occur either rarely or not at all as occupational hazards.

The two forms of renal disease resulting from mercury toxicity are acute tubular necrosis and nephrotic syndrome. In humans, acute tubular necrosis will develop after ingestion of 0.5 g of $HgCl_2$, and in rats, $HgCl_2$ is routinely used to produce an experimental model of acute tubular necrosis. There have also been sporadic case reports of nephrotic syndrome after mercury exposure. These may be idiosyncratic reactions, and, accordingly, occupational studies have not been able to find an association between mercury exposure and proteinuria. Membranous nephropathy, minimal change disease, and anti-glomerular basement membrane antibody deposition have all been reported following mercury exposure.

Mercuric chloride can induce membranous nephropathy in certain rat strains. Before the development of the basement membrane immune deposits seen in membranous nephropathy, an autoimmune glomerulonephritis with linear immunoglobulin G (IgG) deposits along the glomerular capillary wall is first seen, but no pulmonary findings are seen as in Goodpasture's syndrome. A T-cell–dependent polyclonal B-cell activation is responsible for the IgG deposits. As in humans, removal from mercury exposure, which can be vapor or injections, results in reversal of the proteinuria in these rat models.

### Diagnosis

The clinical presentation in patients with acute renal failure from acute tubular necrosis is usually dominated by the extrarenal manifestations of mercury toxicity. When the history of mercury exposure is available, the diagnosis of acute tubular necrosis from mercury toxicity is not difficult. On the other hand, it is more difficult to attribute glomerular disease such as membranous nephropathy to mercury exposure. Although elevated blood and urine mercury concentrations are consistent with significant exposure, these concentrations do not correlate with renal disease. Spontaneous resolution of the proteinuria following removal from the source of mercury exposure is consistent with mercury-mediated glomerular disease.

## Treatment

The mainstay of treatment is removal from the source of mercury exposure and chelation with British anti-lewisite (dimercaprol BAL). BAL is given intramuscularly. Following an initial dose of up to 5 mg/kg, 2.5 mg/kg is given twice daily for 10 days. DMSA is an oral chelating agent that can be used in the treatment of lead poisoning. Because of its convenience as an oral chelator, it is being studied in the treatment of mercury poisoning. It has been successfully used in isolated human cases; in studies in rats, it successfully decreased mercury levels in the kidneys.

## CHRONIC RENAL DYSFUNCTION CAUSED BY BERYLLIUM

### Exposure

Beryllium is encountered in the manufacture of electronic tubes, ceramics, and fluorescent light bulbs and in metal foundries. Its absorption through the gut is very poor, so that the principal route of entry into the body is by inhalation.

### Clinical Findings

The main manifestation of berylliosis is as a systemic granulomatous disease involving primarily the lungs but also the bone and bone marrow, the liver, the lymph nodes, and many other organs. Kidney damage occurs not as an isolated finding but only in conjunction with other forms of toxicity. In the kidneys, berylliosis can produce granulomas and interstitial fibrosis. Beryllium nephropathy is associated with hypercalciuria and urinary tract stones. Renal stone disease is common in berylliosis and may occur in up to 30% of patients. Parathyroid hormone levels are depressed, and the presumed mechanism of hypercalciuria is increased calcium absorption through the gut similar to that encountered in sarcoidosis. Hyperuricemia is also characteristic of beryllium nephropathy.

## CHRONIC RENAL DYSFUNCTION CAUSED BY URANIUM

It is unclear whether uranium is responsible for significant occupationally-related renal disease in humans. Uranium can cause acute renal failure in experimental models, and the pathologic changes are consistent with acute tubular necrosis. During the Manhattan Project, acute tubular necrosis occurred in men working on the atomic bomb. Whether uranium can cause chronic renal failure remains controversial. Although a previous study of workers in a uranium-

refining plant revealed an increase in urinary $\beta_2$-microglobulin excretion, the study did not document decreased renal function and the urinary $\beta_2$-microglobulin level was still in the normal range.

## CHRONIC RENAL DYSFUNCTION DUE TO SILICOSIS

Silicosis is a form of pneumoconiosis associated with pulmonary exposure to silica. Extremely heavy exposure can result in a generalized systemic disease resembling collagen vascular disease, such as systemic lupus erythematosus. Inhalation of silica may trigger an autoimmune disease in sensitive individuals, and in fact, the occurrence of positive antinuclear antibody is increased in patients with silicosis.

The possible association of silica and glomerulonephritis is suggested by animal studies, case-control studies, and multiple case reports. Animals experimentally exposed to silica actually seem to develop acute interstitial nephritis with deposition of silica in the kidney. This fact has led to speculation that silica may contribute to analgesic nephropathy as a result of the widespread use of silicates in analgesic preparations. Certain studies have found that patients with silicosis have a high prevalence of albuminuria, impaired renal function, and glomerular abnormalities at autopsy. A case-control study examined occupational histories in normal controls and ESRD patients and found an increase in the odds ratio (for ESDR) in patients with previous exposure to silica. The reported cases of possible silica-associated glomerular disease include glomerular proliferation with occasional crescents, subendothelial and membranous deposits, and tubular degeneration. The renal silica content was elevated in most of the patients in whom it was measured. Interestingly, not all patients reported to have possible silica-associated nephropathy had pulmonary disease.

## CHRONIC RENAL DYSFUNCTION CAUSED BY ORGANIC SOLVENTS

Solvent exposure may occur in many industries—including the petrochemical, aerospace, and other industries—where there is use of paints, degreasers, and fuels. There have been a number of intriguing case reports over the last 20 years of anti-glomerular basement membrane antibody-mediated glomerulonephritis occurring after solvent exposure. However, it remains unclear whether the solvent exposure is truly causal in these cases. Membranous nephropathy has also been reported after long exposure to mixed organic solvents. There have now been at least six case-control studies investigating occupational exposures and renal disease, and although most of these studies have major limitations, they are impressive in that they consistently have found an increased odds ratio between solvent exposure and a variety of renal diseases. The limitations of these studies include recall bias, lack of interviewer blinding to disease status, absence of information on the amount of solvent exposure, and the use of improper control groups, usually composed of chronically ill subjects unlikely to be part of the workforce. Cross-sectional epidemiologic studies with solvent-exposed populations have provided only weak evidence for mild tubular dysfunction.

Animal studies have shown that solvents can cause acute renal damage at high doses, and only mild chronic renal changes have been produced with chronic low-dose exposure. There are no animal models for immunologic renal disease caused by solvents.

It is clear that solvent exposure at high doses may lead to acute renal failure due to acute tubular necrosis, but whether solvent exposure is associated with glomerulonephritis remains unknown. Solvent exposure is common, and glomerulonephritis is rare, which suggests that if the association does exist, certain host factors are necessary for this idiosyncratic reaction to develop.

## CHRONIC RENAL DISORDERS CAUSED BY CARBON DISULFIDE

### Exposure History & Clinical Findings

Carbon disulfide is used in the manufacture of rayon and neoprene tires. A variety of renal disorders are reported, along with accelerated atherosclerosis. The latter may affect the renal circulation and lead to renal dysfunction, hypertension, proteinuria, and renal insufficiency. The renal effects of carbon disulfide are probably a direct result of its atherogenic effect and not related to direct nephrotoxicity.

## END-STAGE RENAL DYSFUNCTION DUE TO AGENTS THAT ALTER RENAL METABOLISM (Xenobiotic Substances)

### Exposure History

Certain individuals are more likely than others to develop renal damage from exposure to toxic materials. Thus, acute renal failure may develop in alcoholic patients after exposure to subtoxic doses of halogenated hydrocarbons or to the analgesic acetaminophen. Contact with occupational or environmental hazards may similarly reduce the threshold for the appearance of overt renal damage after exposure to a generally subtoxic dose of a second substance. Recent work has demonstrated that certain organic substances with variable biological half-lives are capable of inducing aryl hydrocarbon hydrolases in both the liver and the kidneys of the mouse.

Experiments suggest that response to a toxic agent may be predetermined by prior exposure to chemicals capable of inducing enzyme synthesis (eg, P-450, aryl hydrocarbon hydrolase), which results in increased metabolism of xenobiotics. These agents permanently—albeit imperceptibly—predispose the individual to react unfavorably when challenged by a second toxic chemical. Identification of the potential role of these substances in modulating the course of a renal disease—long after exposure—will be difficult both clinically and epidemiologically.

## REFERENCES

### GENERAL

de Broe ME, D'Haese PC, Nuyts GD, Elseviers MM: Occupational renal diseases. Curr Opin Nephrol Hypertens 1996;5(2):114.

Hook JB: Toxic responses of the kidney. Chap 11 in: *Casarett and Doull's Toxicology,* 4th ed. Macmillan, 1991.

Kosnett MJ: Medical surveillance for renal endpoints. Occup Med: State Of The Art Rev 1990;5:531.

Price RG, et al: Development and validation of new screening tests for nephrotoxic effects. Hum Exp Toxicol 1996;15:Supplement.

Wedeen RP: Renal diseases of occupational origin. Occup Med: State Of The Art Rev 1992;7:449.

### METALS: LEAD

Batuman V: Lead nephropathy, gout, and hypertension. Am J Med Sci 1993;305:241.

Bernard AM, et al: Renal effects in children living in the vicinity of a lead smelter. Environ Res 1995;68(2):91.

Khalil-Manesh F et al: Experimental model of lead nephropathy. I. Continuous high-dose lead administration. Kidney Int 1992;41:1192.

Khalil-Manesh F et al: Experimental model of lead nephropathy. II. Effect of removal from lead exposure and chelation treatment with dimercaptosuccinic acid. Environ Res 1992;58:35.

Khalil-Manesh F, Gonick JC, Cohen AH: Experimental model of lead nephropathy. III. Continuous low-level lead administration. Arch of Environ Health 1993;48: 273.

Kim R et al: A longitudinal study of low-level lead exposure and impairment of renal function. JAMA 1996;275:1177.

Nolan CV, Shaikh ZA: Lead nephrotoxicity and associated disorders: biochemical mechanisms. Toxicology 1992:73;127.

Sanchez-Fructuoso AI, et al: Occult lead intoxication as a cause of hypertension and renal failure. Nephrol Dial Transplant 1996;11:1775.

Staessen JA et al: Impairment of renal function with increasing blood lead concentrations in the general population. N Engl J Med 1992;327:151.

Verbeck MM, et al: Environmental lead and renal effects in children. Arch Environ Health 1996;51(1):83.

## METALS: CADMIUM

Jarup L, Elinder CG: Incidence of renal stones among cadmium exposed battery workers. Br J Ind Med 1993;50:598.

Lauwerys RR, et al: Cadmium: Exposure markers as predictors of nephrotoxic effects. Clin Chem 1994; 40(7):1391.

Roels HA et al: Health significance of cadmium induced renal dysfunction: A five year follow up. Br J Ind Med 1989;46:755.

Savolainen H: Cadmium-associated renal disease. Ren Fail 1995;17(5):483.

Staessen JA, et al: Public health implications of environmental exposure to cadmium and lead: An overview of epidemiological studies in Belgium. J Cardiovasc Risk 1996;3(1):26.

van Sittert NJ et al: A nine year follow up study of renal effects in workers exposed to cadmium in a zinc ore refinery. Br J Ind Med 1993;50:603.

## METALS: MERCURY

Boogaard PJ, et al: Effects of exposure to elemental mercury on the nervous system and the kidneys of workers producing natural gas. Arch Environ Health 1996;51(2):108.

Honda N, Hishida A: Pathophysiology of experimental nonoliguric acute renal failure. Kidney Int 1993;43: 513.

Hua J et al: Autoimmune glomerulonephritis induced by mercury vapour exposure in the Brown Norway rat. Toxicology 1993;79:119.

Kanluen S, Gottlieb CA: A clinical pathologic study of four cases of acute mercury inhalation toxicity. Arch of Pathol Lab Med 1991;115:56.

Nuyts GD, et al: New occupational risk factors for chronic renal failure. Lancet 1995;346(8966):7.

Ratcliffe HE, Swanson GM, Fischer LJ: Human exposure to mercury: A critical assessment of the evidence of adverse health effects. J Toxicol Environ Health 1996;49(3):221.

## METALS: BERYLLIUM

Newman L: Beryllium disease. In: Rom WN (editor): Environmental and Occupational Medicine, 3rd ed. Lippincott–Raven, 1997.

## METALS: URANIUM

Dang HS, Pullat VR, Sharma RC: Distribution of uranium in human organs of an urban Indian population and its relationship with clearance half-lives. Health Phys 1995;68(3):328.

Mao Y, et al: Inorganic components of drinking water and microalbuminuria. Environ Res 1995;71(2):135.

Morris SC, Meinhold AF: Probabilistic risk assessment of nephrotoxic effect of uranium in drinking water. Health Phys 1995;69(6):897.

Russell JJ, Kathren RL, Dietert SE: A histological kidney study of uranium and nonuranium workers. Health Phys 1996;70(4):466.

## NONMETALS

Hotz P, et al: Subclinical signs of kidney dysfunction following short exposure to silica in the absence of silicosis. Nephron 1995;70(4):438.

## HYDROCARBONS

Carlisle EJF et al: Glue-sniffing and distal renal tubular acidosis: Sticking to the facts. J Am Soc Nephrol 1991;1:1019.

Nelson NA, Robins TG, Port FK: Solvent nephrotoxicity in humans and experimental animals. Am J Nephrol 1990;10:10.

Roy AT, Brautbar N, Lee DBN: Hydrocarbons and renal failure. Nephron 1991;58:385.

Steenland NK et al: Occupational and other exposures associated with male end-stage renal disease: A case/control study. Am J Public Health 1990;80:153.

## BALKAN NEPHROPATHY

Ceovic S, Hrabar A, Saric M: Epidemiology of Balkan endemic nephropathy. Food Chem Toxicol 1992; 30:183.

Ferluga D et al: Renal function, protein excretion, and pathology of Balkan endemic nephropathy. III. Light and electron microscopic studies. Kidney Int 1991; 40(Suppl 34):S-57.

Plestina R: Some features of Balkan endemic nephropathy. Food Chem Toxicol 1992;30:177.

Stefanovic V, Polenkovic MH: Balkan Nephropathy: Kidney disease beyond the Balkans? Am J Nephrol 1991;11:1.

Wedeen RP: Environmental renal disease: Lead, cadmium and Balkan endemic nephropathy. Kidney Int 1991;40(Suppl 34):S-4.

## HERBAL NEPHROPATHY/ ANALGESIC NEPHROPATHY

Abt AB et al: Chinese herbal medicine induced acute renal failure. Arch Intern Med 1995; 155:211.

Cosyns JP et al: Chinese herbs nephropathy: A clue to Balkan endemic nephropathy. Kidney Int 1994;45: 1680.

De Smet PAG: Aristolochia species. In: *Adverse Effects of Herbal Drugs*. Springer-Verlag, 1992.

Diamond JR, Pallone TL: Acute interstitial nephritis following use of Tung Shueh pills. Am J Kidney Dis 1994;24:219.

Mohan SB, Tamilarasan A, Buhl M: Inhalational mercury poisoning masquerading as toxic shock syndrome. Anaesth Intensive Care 1994; 22:305.

Perneger TV, Whelton PK, Klag MJ: Risk of kidney failure associated with the use of acetaminophen, aspirin, and nonsteroidal antiinflammatory drugs. N Engl J Med 1994;331:1675.

Sandler DP, Burr FR, Weinberg CR: Nonsteroidal antiinflammatory drugs and the risk for chronic renal disease. Ann Intern Med 1991;115:165.

Vanherweghem JL et al: Rapidly progressive interstitial fibrosis in young women: Association with slimming regimen including Chinese herbs. Lancet 1993;341: 387.

## PESTICIDES & HERBICIDES

Ragoucy-Sengler C, Pileire B: A biological index to predict patient outcome in paraquat poisoning. Hum Exp Toxicol 1996;15(3):265.

Tsatsakis AM, Perakis K, Koumantakis E: Experience with acute paraquat poisoning in Crete. Vet Hum Toxicol 1996;38(2):113.

## ARSINE

Hendriksson J, et al: The toxicity of organoarsenic-based warfare agents: In vitro and in vivo studies. Arch Environ Contam Toxicol 1996;30(2):213.

Klimecki WT, Carter DE: Arsine toxicity: Chemical and mechanistic implications. J Toxicol Environ Health 1995;46(4):399.

## OTHER XENOBIOTICS

Monks TJ, et al: The kidney as a target for biological reactive metabolites: Linking metabolism to toxicity. Adv Exp Med Biol 1996;387:203.

# 24

# Neurotoxicology

*Yuen T. So, MD, PhD*

The nervous system is vulnerable to a wide range of insults from environmental or occupational toxins. Despite the presence of selective permeability barriers separating the systemic circulation from the brain and peripheral nerves, metals, gases, solvents, and other chemicals penetrate sufficiently to cause deleterious effects. Many descriptions of neurotoxicity exist through the history of civilization, from lead poisoning described by Greek physicians before the birth of Christ and homicidal use of arsenic by Nero to more recent accounts of the Minamata Bay epidemic (organic mercury) and glue-sniffer's neuropathy (hexacarbons).

Disorders of the nervous system manifest in a diverse manner. Each region of the neuraxis—brain, spinal cord, peripheral nerve, or muscle—responds differently to toxic injuries. Within any given region, different cell populations also react differently. This "selective vulnerability" is important because, depending on the location and type of neuronal dysfunction, toxicity may culminate in a wide spectrum of symptoms and signs. Possible syndromes may include some combination of headache, pain, cognitive and psychiatric disturbances, visual changes, seizures, ataxia, tremors, rigidity, weakness, and sensory loss.

The extent and severity of neurologic deficits are difficult to assess with precision. Despite extraordinary advances in neuroimaging techniques over the past two decades, present tools such as computed tomography (CT) and magnetic resonance imaging (MRI) for the most part provide only visualization of macroscopic structural changes. While these tests have been invaluable in detecting neoplastic, inflammatory, and infectious disorders of the nervous system, they have been far less helpful in documenting neurotoxic injuries. Imaging studies of cerebral functions, such as positron emission tomography (PET) and functional MRI, hold great promises but are still in their infancy. For the time being, the main role of imaging studies in the occupational medicine setting is to exclude neurologic diseases that mimic neurotoxic disorders. Neurologic evaluation of patients is largely dependent on bedside history and physical examination, supplemented by traditional diagnostic tests such as electroencephalography (EEG), nerve conduction study and electromyography (EMG), and neuropsychological testing.

With few exceptions, the pathophysiology of most neurotoxins is not well understood. Animal models of toxin exposure provide at best a rough guide to human disease. For ethical reasons, it is nearly impossible to study the effects of toxins under controlled conditions in humans. Much of our current knowledge is gained from clinical observations of intense exposures during accidents or chronic heavy occupational exposures that occurred prior to tightening of workplace standards. Extrapolation of these classic observations to other situations is problematic. For instance, for many compounds, there is considerable controversy concerning the exposure level and duration necessary to cause neurologic injury. It has been especially difficult to ascertain the sequelae of chronic low-level exposure, a situation particularly likely to be encountered by today physicians.

## GENERAL PRINCIPLES

Despite our incomplete understanding in many of these diseases, several generalizations have been useful in the clinical approach to these disorders.

1. A clear dose-toxicity relationship exists in the majority of neurotoxic exposures. In general, neurologic symptoms appear only after a cumulative exposure reaches a threshold level. Individual susceptibility varies over a limited range, but idiosyncratic reactions seldom occur.
2. Toxins typically cause a nonfocal or symmetrical neurologic syndrome. This is perhaps one of the most useful rules in the routine evaluation of neurotoxic disorders. Significant asymmetry, such as weakness or sensory loss of one limb or one side of the body with complete sparing of the contralateral side, should suggest an alternative cause.
3. There is usually a strong temporal relationship

between exposure and the onset of symptoms. Immediate symptoms after acute exposure are usually attributable to the physiologic effects of the chemical (eg, cholinergic effects of organophosphates). These symptoms subside quickly with elimination of the chemical from the body. Delayed or persistent neurologic deficits that occur after toxic exposures (for example, organophosphate-related delayed neuropathy) are generally due to pathologic changes in the nervous system. Recovery is still possible, but tends to be slow and incomplete.

4. Although the nervous system generally has a limited capability to regenerate, some recovery is typically possible after removal of the insulting agent. As a corollary, continuing neurologic deterioration more than a few months after cessation of exposure to a toxin generally argues a causative role of the toxin.

5. Multiple neurologic syndromes are possible from a single toxin. Different neuron populations and different areas of the nervous system react differently to the neurotoxin. Furthermore, the level and duration of exposure as well as physiologic variables such as the subject's age influence the clinical manifestations. A well-known example is lead toxicity, which may lead to an acute confusional state, chronic mental slowing, or a peripheral neuropathy.

6. Few toxins present with a pathognomonic neurologic syndrome. Symptoms and signs may be mimicked by many psychiatric, metabolic, inflammatory, neoplastic, and degenerative diseases of the nervous system. It is therefore important to exclude other neurologic diseases with appropriate clinical examination and laboratory investigations.

The principles outlined above have been invaluable in the diagnostic evaluation of patients. However, there are a few noteworthy exceptions. One is the phenomenon of "coasting." This refers to the continuing deterioration sometimes seen for up to a few weeks after discontinuation of toxic exposure. Coasting has been well documented in toxic neuropathies caused by pyridoxine (vitamin $B_6$) abuse and vincristine chemotherapy. The delay reflects the time necessary for the pathophysiologic steps to evolve to neuronal injury and death.

Another possible exception is illustrated by a hypothesis used to explain the pathogenesis of chronic degenerative diseases such as Parkinson's disease, amyotrophic lateral sclerosis, and Alzheimer's dementia. It has been postulated that an environmental or toxic exposure may reduce the functional reserve of the brain. The patient, however, remains asymptomatic until aging or other biological events further deplete the neuronal pool over many more years. Symptoms appear only when neuronal attrition reaches a threshold level. The hypothesis predicts a long latent period between toxic exposure and symptom manifestation. Although present evidence does not completely support an environmental cause, age-related neuronal attrition is an important concept in our understanding of neurodegenerative diseases. The prevalence and severity of these disorders increase with age. Attrition may explain the occasional observation of continued deterioration for many years after cessation of a toxic exposure (eg, extrapyramidal dysfunction after manganese poisoning).

## APPROACH TO PATIENTS

A confident diagnosis of a neurotoxic disorder can only be made after the documentation of all of the following: (1) a sufficiently intense or prolonged exposure to the toxicant; (2) an appropriate neurologic syndrome based on knowledge about the putative toxin; (3) evolution of symptoms and signs over a compatible temporal course; and (4) exclusion of other neurologic disorders that may account for a similar syndrome.

A detailed history of the nature, duration, and intensity of the exposure is essential in every evaluation. What are the potential toxins? What is the mode of exposure? How long and how intense are the exposures? Are there other confounding factors such as alcoholism, psychosocial issues, and possibility of secondary gains? Chronic exposures are especially difficult to assess. Not only is it essential to assess the average intensity and total duration of exposure, intermittent peak exposures are important to quantify as they may play a vital role in the pathogenesis of neurologic dysfunction.

The toxicology history should be followed by a detailed characterization of the neurologic complaints. Patients frequently use descriptors like weakness, dizziness, forgetfulness, pain, and numbness to refer to vastly different personal experience. Dizziness may mean vertigo from vestibular dysfunction, gait imbalance from sensory loss, or simply a nonspecific sense of ill feeling. Fatigue or asthenia may be referred to as weakness. Fatigue implies reduced endurance or a disinclination for physical activity rather than true weakness. Fatigue may be seen in association with depression, various systemic illnesses, and a wide range of neurologic diseases. Only weakness specifically implies motor system dysfunction. Each patient's complaints therefore should not be accepted at face value. It is especially useful to inquire about the functional consequences of the neurologic deficits. Questioning about activities of daily living is particularly useful, both to better understand the nature of the complaints and to provide a reasonably objective assessment of severity.

Documentation of the temporal course of the disease is very important. Symptoms may appear acutely (minutes or days), subacutely (weeks or months), or chronically (years). Fluctuating symptoms may suggest recurrent exposures or unrelated superimposed factors. Recovery after discontinuation of exposure helps to implicate the exposure. By contrast, continuing progression of deficits beyond the "coasting" period argues against an etiologic role of the exposure.

## Central Nervous System (CNS)

Symptoms and deficits depend on which groups of brain or spinal cord neurons are primarily affected (Table 24–1). The most common syndrome is probably an encephalopathy from diffuse dysfunction of cortical or subcortical structures. The manifestations are usually neuropsychiatric. In addition, acute encephalopathy may be associated with significant and sometimes severe alteration in the level of consciousness. Some toxicants cause relatively selective injury to the vestibular system or the cerebellum, resulting in disequilibrium, vertigo, gait or limb ataxia. Basal ganglia involvement may lead to an extrapyramidal syndrome of bradykinesia, tremors, and rigidity. This may resemble idiopathic Parkinson's disease for all practical purposes.

Evaluation of cognitive complaints should include at least a mini-mental state examination. Referral to neuropsychological testing may be needed in patients with prominent cognitive complaints to better understand the pattern and severity of the cognitive deficits. Good patient cooperation and an experienced interpreter are necessary for meaningful neuropsychological testing. Patients with gait unsteadiness, dizziness, or vertigo should be examined for cranial nerve or cerebellar deficits. The evaluation should include testing of gait, tandem walk, and Romberg sign. The examiner should also note extraocular movements, the presence or absence of nystagmus, hearing deficits, limb ataxia, and sensory deficits. Tremors, if present, should be characterized with the outstretched hands, with the hands at rest, and with the hands performing pointing maneuvers. Muscle tone should be tested for rigidity. Rapid tapping of the fingers, hands, or feet is a useful test of the motor system. Along with formal strength testing, it should be part of the routine neurologic examination.

Laboratory tests, such as brain or spinal cord imaging studies (eg, MRI), lumbar puncture, EEG, and evoked potentials, are often needed to detect unrelated neurologic diseases that mimic neurotoxic disorders.

## Peripheral Nervous System

Peripheral nervous system disorders lead to sensory disturbances and weakness, often accompanied by impairment of the deep tendon reflexes on physical examination (Table 24–1). Of the various components of the peripheral nervous system, the peripheral nerve is by far the most vulnerable to exogenous toxins. Since toxins reach the nerves systemically and affect all nerves simultaneously, the resulting syndrome is a symmetrical peripheral neuropathy. This is also often referred to as a polyneuropathy, in contrast to the mononeuropathy that is more frequently the result of local mechanical injury (see Chapter 8). With the exception of the relatively common alcoholic myopathy, toxic myopathy is uncommon.

The hallmark of most polyneuropathies is the distal distribution of the clinical symptoms and signs. The most common syndrome is subacute onset of tingling or numbness experienced in a symmetrical, stocking-and-glove distribution. Neuropathic pain is

**Table 24–1.** Neurologic symptoms and signs.

| Syndrome | Neuroanatomy | Symptoms and Signs | Examples |
|---|---|---|---|
| Acute encephalopathy | Diffuse—cerebral hemispheres | Varying combination of headache, irritability, disorientation, convulsions, amnesia, psychosis, lethargy, stupor, and coma | Acute exposure to many toxins at sufficient doses |
| Chronic encephalopathy | Diffuse—cerebral hemispheres | Cognitive and psychiatric disturbances | Chronic or low-dose exposure to many toxins |
| Parkinsonism | Basal ganglia and other extrapyramidal motor pathways | Tremor, rigidity, bradykinesia, gait instability | Manganese, carbon monoxoide, methanol |
| Motor neuron disease | Spinal cord motor neurons | Muscle atrophy, weakness | Lead, manganese |
| Myeloneuropathy (myelopathy and polyneuropathy) | Spinal cord and peripheral nerves | Paresthesias, sensory loss, hyperreflexia, Babinski's sign, gait ataxia | Nitrous oxide, organophosphates, n-hexane |
| Polyneuropathy | Peripheral sensory, motor, and autonomic nerve fibers | Paresthesias, numbness, weakness, loss of deep tendon reflexes, more rarely—autonomic failure | Many toxins at sufficient doses (see Table 24–2) |

sometimes present, and is described variously as burning, deep aching, or lancinating. Pain may be evoked by normally innocuous stimuli such as touching or stroking of the skin, a phenomenon known as hyperpathia or allodynia. Involvement of the motor nerve fibers manifests as muscle atrophy and weakness. These deficits may appear first in the distalmost muscles (ie, the intrinsic foot and hand muscles). More severe cases may involve muscles of the lower legs and forearms, leading to bilateral foot drop or wrist drop.

Physical examination of patients with peripheral nervous system disorders should include testing of muscle strength, sensation, and tendon reflexes of all four extremities. Are the sensory and motor deficits relatively symmetrical? Are the feet more affected than the hands? Since the longest axons are the most vulnerable, neurologic deficits are frequently more severe in the feet than in the hands. Prominent sensory impairment in the hands without signs of neuropathy in the feet is probably more likely to be caused by carpal tunnel syndrome than a systemic polyneuropathy. Most polyneuropathies are accompanied by diminished or absent stretch reflexes of the Achilles tendons and demonstrable sensory impairment in the toes. Testing of these functions should therefore be included in any screening examination of the peripheral nervous system.

The clinical pattern of sensory and motor nerve involvement is useful in the differential diagnosis of peripheral neuropathy (Table 24–2). The most nonspecific syndrome is a distal, symmetrical, sensorimotor polyneuropathy. This is indistinguishable from the neuropathies due to common systemic diseases such as alcoholism, uremia, diabetes mellitus, and vitamin $B_{12}$ deficiency. Some toxins such as lead cause a neuropathy with prominent weakness. The differential diagnosis of such a neuropathy is relatively narrow, and encompasses a few hereditary and immunologic neuropathies.

There are literally hundreds of possible causes of peripheral neuropathies. Nontoxic causes of neuropathy should be investigated and excluded before a diagnosis of toxic neuropathy can be considered. Moreover, approximately one-half to two-thirds of all polyneuropathies remain undiagnosed despite thorough investigation. Thus, the absence of an alternate etiology does not necessarily implicate a toxin. Aside from the presence of sufficient exposure and compatible syndrome, the diagnosis quite frequently depends on the documentation of progressive sensory or motor deficits during exposure, and recovery of function months or years after cessation of exposure.

Nerve conduction studies and EMG are the primary tools in the laboratory evaluation of neuromuscular disorders. These two tests are often performed together, and the term EMG has often been used loosely to refer to both tests. These tests are described in detail in Chapter 8. Nerve conduction and

**Table 24–2.** Toxic polyneuropathies.

**Mostly sensory or sensorimotor polyneuropathy (little or no weakness)**
Acrylamide
Metals: arsenic, mercury, thallium
Carbon disulfide
Ethylene oxide
Methyl bromide
Polychlorinated biphenyls (PCB)
Thallium

**Predominantly motor polyneuropathy or sensorimotor polyneuropathy (significant weakness)**
Metals: lead, arsenic, mercury
Hexacarbons: n-hexane, methyl n-butyl ketone
Organophosphates

**"Purely" sensory neuropathy (disabling sensory loss with no weakness)**
Pyridoxine abuse
Cis-platinum

**Cranial neuropathy**
Trichloroethylene (trigeminal neuropathy)
Thallium

**Prominent autonomic dysfunction**
Acrylamide
N-hexane (glue-sniffer)
Thallium
Vacor (PNU)

**Possible association with neuropathies (mostly anecdotal)**
Methyl methacrylate
Dioxin
Carbon monoxide
Benzene
Pyrethrins

EMG studies, occasionally supplemented by nerve biopsy, are important in the pathophysiologic characterization of peripheral neuropathies. A fundamental categorization subdivides neuropathies into those with primary degeneration of nerve axons (axonal neuropathy) and those with significant myelin breakdown (demyelinative neuropathy). Discussion of classification of polyneuropathies is beyond the scope of this chapter. Diagnostic management is best left to experienced specialists.

There has been recent interest in the use of quantitative sensory testing (QST) in the occupational health setting. The methodology makes use of special equipment to deliver precisely calibrated sensory stimuli. These tools reduce the inter-examiner variability and provide quantitative parameters for longitudinal follow-up of patients. They are therefore useful in the documentation of progression or recovery from toxic exposures (see Chapter 8).

## NEUROLOGIC DISORDERS DUE TO SPECIFIC TOXINS

It is impossible to review all the major neurotoxic disorders in this chapter. The reader is referred to the corresponding chapters on specific toxins for more detailed discussion on general toxicology and health effects. The discussions below are restricted to neurologic complications.

## Acrylamide

The population most at risk of developing neurologic toxicity are workers who handle monomeric acrylamide in the production of polyacrylamides. A second at risk group are those exposed to monomeric acrylamide used in grouting. Intoxication occurs by inhalation or skin absorption. Features of poisoning include local skin irritation, weight loss, lassitude, and neurologic symptoms of central and peripheral nervous system involvement.

Acute exposure typically causes a confusional state, manifestating as disorientation, memory loss, and gait ataxia. These symptoms are largely reversible, although irreversible dysfunction occurs rarely after very intense exposure. Chronic lower dose exposure sometimes leads to dizziness, increased irritability, emotional changes, and sleep disturbances. The primary site of action of acrylamide, however, is the peripheral nerve. A neuropathy may develop as a delayed manifestation a few weeks after acute exposure or insidiously after chronic exposure. Both sensory and motor nerves are affected, leading to sensory loss, weakness, ataxia, and loss of tendon reflexes. The loss of reflexes especially may be generalized, unlike other toxic neuropathies in which only distal reflexes are lost. Autonomic involvement such as hyperhidrosis and urinary retention are common.

Acrylamide causes abnormal accumulation of neurofilaments in axons. In this respect, its action is similar to that of organic solvents, notably the hexacarbons. Unlike hexacarbons, secondary demyelination does not occur. Nerve conduction studies typically show a neuropathy accompanied by little or no slowing of nerve conduction velocities, (ie, a neuropathy predominantly with features of axonal degeneration).

## Arsenic

Acute intoxication by arsenical compounds leads to nausea, vomiting, abdominal pain, and diarrhea. Dermatologic lesions such as hyperkeratosis, skin pigmentation, skin exfoliation, and Mees' lines occur in many patients 1–6 weeks after onset of disease. Occasionally, systemic symptoms may be accompanied by seizures and encephalopathy.

Peripheral neuropathy is the most common neurologic manifestation, and may occur after either acute or chronic exposure. After a single toxic dose, an acute polyneuropathy develops within 1–3 weeks. This neuropathy mimics Guillain-Barré syndrome in many ways. Symmetrical paresthesias and pain may occur in isolation or may be accompanied by distal weakness. With progression of neuropathy, sensory and motor deficits spread proximally. Shoulder and pelvic girdle weakness is common in severe cases,

but respiratory failure is rare. Chronic exposure leads to a more insidious sensorimotor polyneuropathy, although there is no agreement for a threshold limit.

The previously used chelating agent dimercaprol (British Anti-Lewisite, BAL) should no longer be used. Two agents, meso-dimercaptosuccinic acid (DMSA) and 2,3-dimercapto-1-propanesulfonic acid (DMPS), are less toxic and are probably more effective than BAL. Even without treatment, peripheral neuropathy improves slowly after cessation of exposure.

## Carbon Disulfide

Even relatively brief inhalation exposure to toxic levels (300 ppm or above) of carbon disulfide causes an acute organic brain syndrome. Dizziness and headache are early symptoms, followed by delirium, mania, or mental dulling. At even higher concentrations (above 400 ppm), it has a narcotizing effect, leading eventually to convulsion, coma, and death.

Data on chronic exposure primarily come from workers exposed during viscose rayon manufacturing. Reliable exposure-toxicity relationships has not been established. Long-term exposure for many years has been associated with a distal sensorimotor polyneuropathy, presenting as paresthesias and pain in the distal legs, loss of Achilles reflexes, and evidence of involvement of sensory and motor axons on nerve conduction study. A nonspecific brain syndrome of fatigue, headache, and sleep disturbances has been attributed to carbon disulfide. Association with Parkinsonism has also been suggested by case-control study. However, for any given patient, a cause-effect relationship is difficult to ascertain.

## Carbon Monoxide

Inhaling low concentrations of carbon monoxide in the range of 0.01–0.02% may cause headache and mild confusion. A higher concentration of 0.1–0.2% often results in somnolence or stupor, and inhalation of 1% for more than 30 minutes is usually fatal. Neurologic deficits are a result of cerebral hypoxia. Early symptoms include headache, dizziness, and disorientation. More severe hypoxia is accompanied by a varying combination of tremor, chorea, spasticity, dystonia, rigidity, and bradykinesia. Recovery from the hypoxia may be incomplete. Residual dementia, spasticity, cortical blindness, or Parkinsonian features are relatively common.

Occasionally, patients recover completely after acute exposure only to present again 1–4 weeks later with acute disorientation, apathy, or psychosis. Neurologic examination often reveals an encephalopathy with prominent signs of frontal lobe and extrapyramidal dysfunction. Physical findings include bradykinesia, retropulsion, frontal release signs, spasticity, and limb rigidity. The major risk factors for this delayed encephalopathy are a significant period of unconsciousness and an advanced age. CT or MRI of patients during the symptomatic stage often show lesions in bilateral subcortical white matter, basal ganglia, and thalamus. Involvement of the globus pallidus is especially common. Significant recovery is possible and may take one or more years. Some residual memory deficits and Parkinsonism are common.

The effect of long-term exposure to extremely low levels of carbon monoxide is unclear. A wide range of nonspecific symptoms—anorexia, headache, personality changes, and memory disturbances—have been attributed to carbon monoxide, but the cause-effect relationship has not been proven.

## Hexacarbons (n-hexane and methyl-n-butyl ketone)

n-Hexane and methyl n-butyl ketone represent a group of volatile organic compounds widely used in homes and industries as solvents and adhesives. Human disease is due to a toxic intermediary metabolite γ-diketone 2,5-hexanedione. The acute euphoric effect of these compounds leads to their abuse as a recreational drug. The most well-known syndrome is a distal symmetric sensorimotor polyneuropathy, the so-called "glue-sniffers' neuropathy." Early symptoms are paresthesias and sensory loss. Weakness follows and initially involves distal muscles. Proximal musculatures are affected in more severe cases. Patients complain of frequent tripping because of ankle weakness. Autonomic symptoms are uncommonly present in very severe cases. Nonspecific CNS symptoms such as insomnia and irritability may be present. On examination, sensory loss and weakness are readily demonstrable on examination. Achilles stretch reflexes are lost early in the disease. Recovery begins after a few months of abstinence and may be incomplete. In some instances, spasticity and hyperreflexia appear paradoxically during the recovery stage. In these cases, there is probably significant degeneration of central axons, and the CNS signs are initially masked by the severe neuropathy.

A less dramatic polyneuropathy was recognized in the 1960s in workers of the shoe and adhesive industries, well before the recognition of the glue-sniffer's neuropathy. The exposure to n-hexane was less intense and more chronic than the glue-sniffers. The clinical features are essentially similar, although the syndrome evolves more slowly and results in less severe deficits.

n-Hexane neuropathy has a distinctive neuropathology. Multiple foci of neurofilament accumulations form inside nerve axons. Secondary demyelination is common and is probably a result of the axonal pathology. Because of the demyelination, nerve conduction studies show severe slowing of motor nerve conduction velocities. Cerebrospinal fluid protein content is typically normal, in contrast to most other demyelinating neuropathies that are associated with elevated CSF protein. This combination

of findings provides an important clue towards an etiologic diagnosis.

## Lead

Acute high-level lead exposure, typically from accidental ingestion or industrial exposure, results in a syndrome of abdominal colic and intermittent vomiting, accompanied by neurologic symptoms such as headache, tremor, apathy, and lethargy. CNS symptoms typically appear in adults at blood levels of 40–50 μg/dL or higher. Children are more vulnerable than adults, probably because of the immaturity of the blood-brain barrier. Behavioral disturbances and neuropsychologic impairment may be present at blood levels as low as 10 μg/dL. More massive intoxication leads to convulsions, cerebral edema, stupor, or coma, and eventually transtentorial herniation. Chronic low-level exposure to lead is responsible for impaired intellectual development in children. Studies have linked chronic exposure to decreased global IQ as well as a wide range of behavioral disturbances such as poor self-confidence, impulsive behavior, and shortened attention span.

Peripheral neuropathy is a well-recognized complication of chronic lead poisoning in adults. The neuropathy has a striking predilection to motor axons with little, if any, sensory symptoms. In many ways, it mimics motor neuron diseases such as amyotrophic lateral sclerosis (Lou Gehrig's disease). The classic descriptions emphasize wrist drop and foot drop. More commonly, toxicity manifests as generalized proximal and distal weakness and loss of the tendon reflexes. Significant sensory impairment is absent. Neuropathy is often accompanied by systemic symptoms and signs such as anorexia, weight loss, constipation, abdominal pain, and anemia. Nerve conduction studies show a predominantly motor neuropathy with axonal loss and minimal or no conduction velocity slowing. EMG shows denervation and reinnervation in weak muscles. These findings are not specific to lead poisoning. Specific laboratory markers are important for diagnosis. Diagnostic markers, as well as treatment, are discussed in Chapter XX.

## Mercury

Like many other toxins, mercury poisoning causes a nonfocal encephalopathy. In its early stage, the encephalopathy is characterized by euphoria, irritability, anxiety, and emotional lability. More severe exposure leads to confusion and an altered level of consciousness. Patients may develop tremor and cerebellar ataxia. Hearing loss, visual disturbances, hyperreflexia, and Babinski's sign may be present. All the above symptoms may be encountered in intoxication from organic mercury, metallic mercury, mercury vapor, or inorganic salts. Organic mercury poisoning typically presents with prominent CNS disturbances with little or no peripheral nervous system involvement. Neuropathy is primarily associated with inorganic mercury. A subacute predominantly motor neuropathy has been reported after metallic mercury or mercury vapor exposure. The syndrome mimics Guillain-Barré syndrome, but nerve conduction study and nerve biopsy suggest axonal loss rather than demyelination.

## Methanol

The neurotoxicity of methanol is largely due to formaldehyde and formate, the end products of alcohol dehydrogenase and aldehyde dehydrogenase. Most cases are due to accidental ingestion or occupational exposure. Neurologic symptoms usually appear after a latent period of 12–24 hours after intoxication. Patients suffer from headache, nausea, vomiting, and abdominal pain. Tachypnea, if present, indicates significant metabolic acidosis. Visual symptoms ranging from blurring to complete blindness appear early. These are accompanied by an encephalopathy, ranging from mild disorientation to convulsion, stupor, or coma. In severely affected individuals, bilateral upper motor neuron signs such as hyperreflexia, weakness, and Babinski's sign are present. Brain CT or MRI often reveal infarction or hemorrhage localized characteristically in bilateral putamin. Treatment depends on reversal of the metabolic acidosis, competitive inhibition of the conversion of methanol to formaldehyde (by administration of ethanol), and swift removal of methanol by gastric lavage or hemodialysis.

## Nitrous Oxide

Excessive exposure to nitrous oxide, usually in the setting of substance abuse, causes a myeloneuropathy indistinguishable from vitamin $B_{12}$ deficiency. Patients present with paresthesias in the hands and feet. Gait ataxia, sensory loss, Romberg sign, and leg weakness may be present. Tendon reflexes may be diminished or lost (peripheral neuropathy) or may be pathologically brisk (spinal cord involvement; ie, myelopathy). Nitrous oxide inactivates vitamin $B_{12}$ and interferes with vitamin $B_{12}$-dependent conversion of homocystine to methionine. Serum vitamin $B_{12}$ and Schilling test are often normal, whereas serum homocystine level may be elevated. Repeated exposures are necessary to cause symptoms in normal individuals. Of interest is the observation that a brief exposure to nitrous oxide (eg, during anesthesia) is sufficient to precipitate symptoms in patients with presymptomatic vitamin $B_{12}$ deficiency. This is a vivid illustration of how the biological state may rarely affect individual susceptibility to a toxin.

## Organophosphates

Commonly used organophosphates (OP) are highly lipid-soluble and are rapidly absorbed through the skin or mucous membranes. All these compounds share a common property of inhibiting the enzyme acetylcholinesterase. Several distinct syndromes are possible, depending on the time lapse after acute intoxication.

The acute neurologic effects of organophosphates are those of muscarinic and nicotinic overactivity. Symptoms are usually apparent within hours of exposure. These include abdominal cramps, diarrhea, increased salivation, sweating, miosis, blurred vision, and muscle fasciculations. Convulsions, coma, muscle paralysis, and respiratory arrest occur with severe intoxication. Unless there are secondary complications due to anoxia or other insults to the brain, these symptoms improve with atropine treatment and after metabolism and excretion of the compound. Recovery is usually complete within one week, even though acetylcholinesterase activity level may be only partially restored.

An intermediate syndrome occurs within 12–96 hours of exposure and is a result of excessive cholinergic stimulation of nicotinic receptors in skeletal muscles. This leads to blockade of neuromuscular junction transmission. Weakness of proximal muscles, neck flexors, cranial muscles, and even respiratory muscles may be evident. Sensory function is spared. Electrodiagnostic testing is useful in diagnosis. The most characteristic finding is the appearance of repetitive muscle action potentials after single electrical stimulus applied to motor nerves. Another finding is a decremental motor response to repetitive nerve stimulation.

A delayed syndrome of peripheral neuropathy occurs 1–4 weeks after acute exposure. There is little or no correlation between its onset and the severity of acute or intermediate symptoms. Organophosphates inhibit another enzyme, neuropathy target esterase (NTE), forming an OP-NTE complex. This inhibition becomes irreversible when the OP-NTE complex undergoes a second step known as "aging" (loss of a R group from the OP molecule). Compounds that lead to aging are neurotoxic, resulting in the delayed polyneuropathy. Paresthesias and cramping pain in the legs are often the first symptoms. Sensory loss is usually mild on physical examination. Weakness begins distally and progresses to involve proximal muscles. Weakness dominates the clinical picture and at times may be very severe. Spasticity and other upper motor neuron signs suggesting concomitant spinal cord involvement are present in some patients. Cranial neuropathy or autonomic dysfunction are unusual. Recovery is slow and incomplete, and is dependent on the degree of motor axons loss. Those with significant spasticity tend to recover less satisfactorily.

How inhibition and aging of NTE eventually cause neuronal damage is unclear. Although NTE activity may be measured in lymphocytes, it usually normalizes by the time neuropathy appears. All the neurotoxic compounds are phosphates, phosphoramidates, or phosphonates. Important examples are tricresyl phosphates (eg, triorthocresyl phosphate or TOCP), mipafox, leptophos, trichlorphon, trichlornate, dichlorovos, and methamidophos. Of these, TOCP has probably caused the largest number of neuropathies. The so-called jake paralysis was due to drinking extracts of contaminated Jamaica ginger during the prohibition era. Other well-known outbreaks included contamination of cooking oil in Morocco and gingli oil in Sri Lanka.

Erythrocyte acetylcholinesterase levels may be depressed because of the recent exposure. Its clinical utility is limited by the wide range of normal levels. Also, low level does not predict development of delayed neuropathy. By the time neuropathy appears, nerve conduction studies show an axonal polyneuropathy affecting motor greater than sensory axons. These findings are not pathognomonic for organophosphate, but are useful to distinguish this neuropathy from other causes of acute weakness such as Guillain-Barré syndrome and neuromuscular junction disorders.

Persistent subtle neuropsychologic impairment after an episode of acute poisoning may be more prevalent than previously thought. Chronic low-level exposure to organophosphates has also been linked to an encephalopathy with forgetfulness and other cognitive dysfunctions as chief complaints.

## Miscellaneous Organic Solvents

Clinically important exposure to organic solvents occurs primarily as a result of industrial contact or volitional abuse. Most organic solvents possess acute narcotizing properties. Brief exposure at high concentrations causes a reversible encephalopathy. Coma, respiratory depression, and death occur after extremely high exposures. Chronic exposure to moderate or high levels of solvent can cause a dementing syndrome, with personality changes, memory disturbances, and other nonspecific neuropsychiatric symptoms. A sensorimotor polyneuropathy may also be present, either as the only manifestation or in combination with CNS dysfunction. The better known syndromes are either discussed under specific headings or are tabulated in Table 24–3.

Despite general agreement on the acute and chronic effects of moderate to high dose effects of organic solvents, there is considerable uncertainty about the effect of chronic low-level exposures. The sequelae of low-level exposure has been variously termed painters' syndrome, chronic toxic encephalopathy, or psycho-organic solvent syndrome. The neurologic symptoms are diverse and nonspecific. They include headache, dizziness, asthenia, mood and personality change, inattentiveness, forgetfulness, and depression. The scientific literature regarding this syndrome largely consists of epidemiologic studies of exposed workers and provides conflicting results. A large number of studies have reported higher than expected incidence of cognitive and psychiatric impairment, electrophysiologic abnormalities, and cerebral atrophy in exposed subjects. The testing methodology of these studies, however, have been criticized. A few studies using control groups matched for age, education, and socioeconomic status have not identified significant differences between exposed subjects and controls.

The controversy remains unresolved. Some physicians make the diagnosis of psycho-organic solvent syndrome in exposed individuals whenever compatible symptoms are present and another neurologic disease is not identified by laboratory evaluations. This practice is unjustified, as the syndrome is not sufficiently specific to be distinguished from depression, other affective disorders, conversion reaction, malingering, and various mild injuries of the brain. Each individual case should be examined critically. Additional useful clues may include the temporal relationship between symptoms and exposure, documentation of neurologic recovery after cessation of exposure, and careful neurologic examination for evidence of nonorganic neurologic signs. A confident diagnosis is often impossible, even after thorough evaluation.

**Table 24–3.** Neurological manifestations of toxins not discussed in text.

| Toxins | Acute Exposure | Chronic Exposure |
| --- | --- | --- |
| Carbamates | Cholinergic overactivity (similar to organophosphates) | Encephalopathy, tremor, polyneuropathy |
| Ethylene oxide | Encephalopathy | Sensorimotor polyneuropathy |
| Manganese | None (symptoms take weeks or months to develop) | Parkinsonism (tremor, rigidity, gait disturbances), encephalopathy, possible motor neuron disease |
| Organotin | Encephalopathy, visual disturbances | Encephalopathy, visual disturbances, hearing loss, vertigo |
| Thallium | Subacute polyneuropathy after massive exposure, encephalopathy | Sensorimotor polyneuropathy |
| Toluene | Euphoria or narcosis, encephalopathy | Cerebellar ataxia, tremor, encephalopathy |
| Trichloroethylene | Euphoria or narcosis, encephalopathy trigeminal neuropathy | Trigeminal neuropathy, encephalopathy |

## REFERENCES

### METALS

Carpenter DO: The public health significance of metal neurotoxicity. Cell Mol Neurobiol 1994;14:591.

Davis LE et al: Methylmercury poisoning: Long-term clinical, radiological, toxicological, and pathological studies of an affected family. Ann Neurol 1994; 35:680.

Goldstein GW: Neurologic concepts of lead poisoning in children. Pediatric Annals 1992;21:384.

Oh SJ: Electrophysiological profile in arsenic neuropathy. J Neurol Neurosurg Psychiat 1991;54:1103.

Schaffer SJ, Campbell JR: The new CDC and AAP lead poisoning prevention recommendations: Consensus versus controversy. Pediatric Annals 1994;23:592.

Wennberg A: Neurotoxic effects of selected metals. Scand J Work Environ Health 1994;20:65.

### ORGANOPHOSPHATES

De Bleecker J, Van den Neucker K, Colardyn F: Intermediate syndrome in organophosphorus poisoning: A prospective study. Crit Care Med 1993;21:1706.

Lotti M: The pathogenesis of organophosphate polyneuropathy. Crit Rev Toxicol 1991;21:465.

Rosenstock L et al: Chronic central nervous system effects of acute organophosphate pesticide intoxication. Lancet 1991;338:223.

### SOLVENTS

Baker EL: A review of recent research on health effects of human occupational exposure to organic solvents. A critical review. J Occ Med 1994;36:1079.

Chang YC: Patients with n-hexane induced polyneuropathy: A clinical follow up. Br J Industr Med 1990; 47:485.

Graham DG et al: Pathogenetic studies of hexane and carbon disulfide neurotoxicity. Crit Rev Toxicol 1995;25:91.

Juntunen J: Neurotoxic syndromes and occupational exposure to solvents. Environ Res 1993;60:98.

Triebig G et al: Neurotoxicity of solvent mixtures in spray painters. II. Neurologic, psychiatric, psychological, and neuroradiologic findings. Int Arch Occ Environ Health 1992;64:361.

Yamanouchi N et al: White matter changes caused by chronic solvent abuse. Am J Neurorad 1995;16:1643.

### MISCELLANEOUS DISORDERS

Anger WK: Human behavioral neurotoxicology. In: Rom WN (editor): Environmental and Occupational Medicine, 3rd ed. Lippincott–Raven, 1997.

Bleecker M: Toxic peripheral neuropathy. In: Rom WN (editor): Environmental and Occupational Medicine, 3rd ed. Lippincott–Raven, 1997.

Green R, Kinsella LJ: Current concepts in the diagnosis of cobalamine deficiency. Neurology 1995;45:1435.

### SUGGESTED READING

Aminoff MJ: *Electrodiagnosis in Clinical Neurology,* 3rd ed. Churchill Livingstone, 1992.

Berger AR, Schaumburg HH: Effects of occupational and environmental agents on the nervous system. In: Bradley WG et al (editors): *Neurology in Clinical Practice,* 2nd ed. Butterworth, 1996.

Windebank AJ: Metal neuropathy. In: Dyck PJ, Thomas PK (editors): *Peripheral Neuropathy,* 3rd ed. Saunders, 1993.

# Female Reproductive Toxicology  **25**

*Ana Maria Osorio, MD, MPH, & Gayle C. Windham, PhD, MSPH*

The occurrence of adverse reproductive outcomes is of great concern to the individuals and families involved. This is especially true if the individuals perceive they are living or working in areas with potential exposure to hazardous agents. Concern has been fueled by incidents such as the contamination of fish with methyl mercury in Minimata Bay, Japan, due to a release from a manufacturing plant. Consumption of the contaminated fish by pregnant women resulted in an epidemic of mental retardation, cerebral palsy and developmental delay in their offspring. Use of polychlorinated biphenyl (PCB) contaminated cooking oil in Taiwan resulted in intrauterine growth retardation and hyperpigmentation of the skin in infants of exposed women. In recent years, there have been concerns about the reproductive effects of occupational exposure to anesthetic gases, solvents, and video display terminals. In addition to mercury and PCBs, only a few substances have been shown to have strong associations with adverse reproductive outcomes in humans such as lead and ionizing radiation. However, a larger number of agents are suspected to cause reproductive harm based on the animal literature and toxicological assessment.

Relatively little research has been devoted to these outcomes until the last decade or two. Adverse reproductive effects can be very stressful for affected families. In addition to the individual concerns, the societal burden of these adverse health outcomes includes high medical costs for compromised infants, and the increasing use of advanced technology to achieve conception and monitor pregnancy. Another reason to better understand reproductive outcomes is that they may act as sentinels for detecting occupational and environmental hazards. Reproductive effects have a relatively short latency between exposure and clinical health event as compared to the long latency for cancer. If workers or community residents are protected from exposures that are harmful to reproduction or the fetus, they will usually be protected from other health effects associated with these exposures as well. Although the extent to which workplace and environmental hazards affect reproductive function is unknown, these hazards are potentially preventable.

Measures that can be taken to prevent further exposure include substitution or containment of the suspect hazard. Thus, preventing exposure should be a primary goal in the health care provider's overall assessment of the patient's situation.

## POPULATION AT RISK

In 1994, women aged 16 years or older represented 39.8% of the US population or 103.5 million individuals (Figure 25–1). During this time, there were 60.2 million women in the civilian labor force with 56.6 million (94%) of these women employed (Figure 25–2). The percentage of women in the US workforce (age 16 or older) has increased dramatically in a relatively short period: 38.1% in 1970 to 45.4% in 1990. The highest birth rates are found among women aged 15–44 years. Women within this reproductive age group merit special attention with respect to potential reproductive toxicant exposures in the workplace. The majority of female employees are found within the technical sales and administrative support, managerial and professional, and service industry categories (Table 25–1). Table 25–2 indicates the leading occupations for women, some of which have potential exposures to known reproductive toxicants (eg, chemotherapeutic agents, anesthetic gases, ionizing radiation and biological agents among health care workers). In addition, there is an increasing number of women in occupations traditionally held by men and where there is potential for exposure to reproductive hazards. In 1991, 31% of janitors and cleaners were women, 19% of laborers (except for construction), 8% of engineers, 3% of heavy truck drivers, and 1% of carpenters. When women are employed in jobs traditionally held by men, there can be difficulty in obtaining personal protective equipment that fits, accessing separate change rooms and wash areas and getting health and

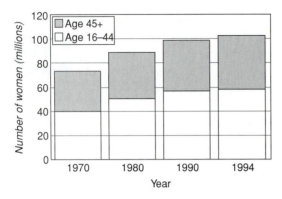

**Figure 25–1.** US female population by age group for selected years. US Dept. of Labor, Handbook of Labor Statistics, 1989.

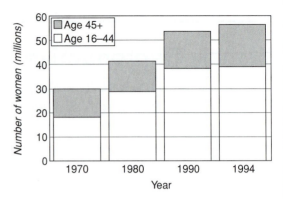

**Figure 25–2.** US female employment by age group for selected years. Us Dept. of Labor, Employment and Earnings, 1971, 1981, 1991, and 1995.

safety information that is gender specific, where appropriate. Also, women may be exposed to reproductive hazards in the environment, which can be more difficult to detect than in the workplace. Often times, these environmental hazards may be local exposures but some are of nationwide interest, such as the widespread use of pesticides that persist in the environment and food chain.

# REPRODUCTIVE OUTCOMES & RATES

A number of adverse reproductive effects may result from exposure to chemical and physical agents either pre- or post-conception. These effects range from infertility to birth defects in the infant. Several of these outcomes are quite frequent and represent a serious public health concern. Accurate data on the rates of

these outcomes are difficult to obtain because of lack of national monitoring systems and methodologic differences in individual epidemiological studies. Nevertheless, a range of prevalence rates can be estimated (Table 25–3). Approximately 10% of couples in the United States are infertile, which is defined as an inability to conceive during 12 months of unprotected intercourse. Additional couples may experience periods of subfertility or delayed conception. After conception, there may occur a continuum of reproductive loss from the time of implantation to term. Up to 50% of embryos may be lost after implantation (the earliest time at which conception can be detected), with approximately 15% of pregnancies ending in clinically detected spontaneous abortion (SAB) and 2–3% ending in stillbirth (Table 25–3). Of all liveborn infants, 5–7% are of low birthweight (LBW), 15% are born prematurely, and approximately 3% will have a congenital anomaly. The causes for most of these outcomes are unexplained. However, there are a few known risk factors, such as older maternal age associated with increased rates of SAB and black race associated with increased rates of LBW.

**Table 25–1.** Employment of women by major occupational group, age 16 or older, 1991, United States (number in millions). US Dept. of Labor, *Employment and Earnings*, January 1995.

| Occupational Group | Number of Women Employed (Millions) | % Distribution Among All Women Employed |
|---|---|---|
| Managerial and professional (eg, teachers) | 16.3 | 29 |
| Technical, sales and administrative support (eg, health techs sales personnel secretaries) | 24.0 | 42 |
| Service (eg, good, health, cleaning, personal) | 10.1 | 18 |
| Precision production, craft and repair (eg, mechanics construction) | 1.2 | 2 |
| Operators, fabricators, and laborers (eg, machine operators, assemblers, inspectors) | 4.3 | 8 |
| Farming, forestry and fishing (eg, farm operators, managers) | 0.7 | 1 |

**Table 25–2.** Ten leading occupations of employed women, age 16 or older, 1991, United States (number in millions). US Dept. of Labor, *1993 Handbook on Women Workers: Trends & Issues,* 1994.

| Occupation | Number of Women Employed (Millions) | % Women Among All Employed (Both Genders) |
|---|---|---|
| Secretaries | 3.76 | 99 |
| Managers and administrators (not elsewhere classified) | 2.66 | 34 |
| Cashiers | 2.02 | 81 |
| Bookkeepers, accounting and auditing clerks | 1.75 | 92 |
| Registered nurses | 1.62 | 95 |
| Nursing aides, orderlies, and attendants | 1.34 | 89 |
| Elementary school teachers | 1.31 | 86 |
| Sales supervisors and proprietors | 1.28 | 34 |
| Waiters and waitresses | 1.11 | 82 |
| Sales workers, other commodities | 1.03 | 71 |

# REPRODUCTIVE & DEVELOPMENTAL PHYSIOLOGY & SENSITIVE PERIODS

## GERM CELL DEVELOPMENT & MENSTRUAL CYCLE FUNCTION

The female reproductive cycle is a complex process regulated by the autonomic nervous and endocrine systems and mediated by the hypothalamic-pituitary axis (Figure 25–3). Unlike males, the female germ cells (oogonia) develop and begin the first meiotic division in utero, with no new generation after birth. The oocytes remain arrested until ovulation occurs, which may be from 20 to 30 years later. From the millions of oocytes present at birth, the number is reduced to 400,000 at puberty, with only 300–500 of these oocytes maturing during a woman's reproductive life-span.

Under hormonal stimulation at the start of each menstrual cycle, a group of primary follicles begins to develop. Release of the follicle stimulating hormone (FSH) leads to the selection and growth of a dominant follicle, which produces estrogen to support proliferation of endometrial tissue during the follicular phase of the cycle. Increasing concentration of estrogen leads to a midcycle release of the gonadotropins, FSH, and luteinizing hormone (LH) and results in the rupture of the follicle and extrusion of

**Table 25–3.** Prevalence of selected adverse reproductive outcomes in the United States.[1]

| Endpoint | Frequency per 100 | Unit |
|---|---|---|
| Infertility | 8–12 | Couples |
| Recognized spontaneous abortion | 10–20 | Women or pregnancies |
| Birthweight <2500 g | 4–7 | Livebirths |
| Preterm (≤37 wks) | 14–18 | Livebirths |
| Stillbirth | 2–4 | Stillbirths and livebirths |
| Infant death | 1 | Livebirths |
| Birth defects (through 1 year of life) | 2–5 | Livebirths |
| Chromosomal anomalies in livebirths | 0.2 | Livebirths |

[1]Compiled from multiple sources including vital records reports, California Birth Defects Monitoring Program and Guidelines for Studies of Human Populations Exposed to Mutagenic and Reproductive Hazards, Bloom, ed.

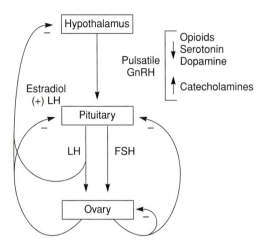

**Figure 25–3.** Feedback regulation of the hypothalamic-pituitary-ovarian axis. With permission from McGraw-Hill Companies: Scialli AR and Zinaman MJ (eds.): *Reproductive Toxicology and Infertility,* 1993.

the ovum. The remaining granulosa cells form the corpus luteum, which secretes increasing amounts of progesterone and other hormones (Figure 25–4). In the absence of fertilization, the corpus luteum degenerates. The subsequent decrease in ovarian steroids leads to sloughing of the endometrium and menstruation occurs after a 12- to 14-day luteal phase. Although this general pattern of menstrual function is known, it is important to note that there is much interwoman variation and that the exact mechanisms are not well understood. Endocrine control of the reproductive process might be disrupted by chemicals and could lead to menstrual disorders and infertility. This is especially true for those chemicals with steroid-like activity (eg, certain pesticides and dioxins).

If a sperm successfully fertilizes an ovum, the ovum completes a second meiotic division and forms a zygote. This zygote undergoes several rapid cell divisions as it is transported down the fallopian tube to the uterus. Because the germ cells are present from birth and many exposures occur during a woman's life, there is great potential for genetic or cytotoxic harm to the oocytes. It is postulated that the cumulative effects of occupational, environmental, and other exposures may explain the increased incidence of chromosomal abnormalities and spontaneous abortion that occurs as maternal age increases. But because the greatest potential for genetic damage is most likely to occur during replication and division of the genetic material, the actual sensitivity during the relatively long dormant period is unknown. Genetic damage could result in lack of fertilization or unsuccessful implantation, which can be seen clinically as infertility, or could lead to later fetal loss (since much chromosomal damage is incompatible

with life). Preconception mutagenesis might also result in a birth defect in an infant. Certain mutagenic chemicals are in use in industry, such as organic solvents, ethylene oxide, and metals (eg, arsenic and nickel). Oocyte destruction could lead to infertility or early menopause, but such a specific effect of an occupational or environmental agent has not been documented in humans.

## DEVELOPMENT OF THE FETUS

The dividing zygote reaches the uterus about 1 week after fertilization. Approximately 1 week later, implantation is complete with the establishment of placental circulation by around day 17 after ovulation. The placental villi secrete human chorionic gonadotropin (hCG), which is necessary to maintain pregnancy. In addition, the placenta takes over the secretion of estrogen and progesterone after the corpus luteum degenerates. The next 6 weeks are called the embryonic period and are the most critical for development as all the major organ systems are formed in precise sequence during this time (Figure 25–5). During the subsequent fetal period, growth and organ maturation continue until term. In particular, the central nervous, genitourinary, and immune systems continue to develop throughout pregnancy. The period of most rapid fetal growth is considered to occur during the last trimester. Full term is typically 38 weeks after conception, with a normal fetal weight of 3000–3600 g and length of 19–20 inches (360 mm).

Exposures during week 1 and 2 after conception may cause early pregnancy loss if they interfere with tubal transport, implantation, or endocrine control or if they are cytotoxic to the fetus itself. Such a loss may only appear as a late or heavy menstrual flow. With increasingly sensitive laboratory assays available, women trying to conceive or being studied for pregnancy outcome can have these very early losses detected by a short rise and subsequent fall in hCG. The embryo may be less sensitive to structural damage at this time since differentiation has not yet begun and damage is potentially correctable by the rapidly dividing cells. Thus, congenital anomalies are unlikely to result from very early embryo exposures.

The greatest susceptibility to fetotoxic or teratogenic agents occurs during the embryonic period, when major morphologic abnormalities may be induced. The timing of an effect can be very specific. The damage is most likely to occur from exposure just before or during early organogenesis. Although different agents administered at the same time may cause the same anomaly, the same agent given at two different times may induce different anomalies. Known or suspected human teratogens include antineoplastic drugs, DES, lead, and ionizing radiation (Table 25–4). As noted earlier, preconception exposure may also have an effect by inducing genetic

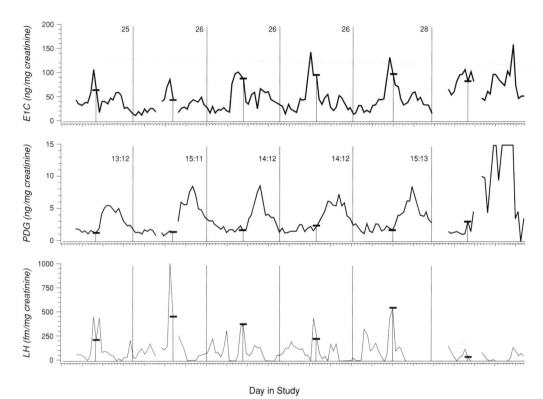

**Figure 25–4.** Examples of sex steroid (estrogen and progesterone) and luteinizing hormone metabolite profiles. E1C = estrogen metabolite, PDG = progesterone metabolite, and LH = luteinizing hormone. Long vertical lines indicate first day of bleeding during each cycle, with the number indicating cycle length. Short vertical lines topped by a horizontal bar indicate probable day of ovulation in each cycle. Data from 6 cycles of a subject in Women's Reproductive Health Study. *Courtesy of K. Waller, California Department of Health Services.*

damage or by later release during the physiologic stress of pregnancy, if the toxicant persists in the mother. Also, this period is when the highest rates of pregnancy loss occur, with approximately 60–75% of recognized losses in the first trimester. Approximately 35% of aborted conceptuses are karyotypically abnormal and another 30% have morphologic abnormalities.

Exposure after the first trimester may induce minor morphologic abnormalities or growth deficits. As the endocrine, central nervous, and other systems are still developing, their respective function might be affected by exposures during this time. Organic mercury, tobacco smoke, and lead are examples of substances that have adverse effects with exposure later in pregnancy (Table 25–4). Potentially, carcinogens could cross the placenta and exert an effect at any stage of development.

## POSTNATAL DEVELOPMENT & LACTATION

The young infant continues development after birth, with general body growth and central nervous

system maturation the most obvious changes. Adverse effects of prenatal exposures may be detected as later deficits in growth and behavior or mental function (eg, fetal alcohol syndrome). Because alcohol is a type of solvent, there may be a "fetal solvent syndrome" that needs to be evaluated. Prenatal maternal cigarette smoking has been shown to be strongly related to sudden infant death syndrome and is thought to be related to growth.

Infant development may also be affected by postnatal exposures: Environmental exposures may be present in the residence or community, and parental occupational exposures may be brought home on clothing or delivered through breast-feeding. Contamination of breast milk occurs primarily by passive diffusion. Thus, low molecular weight, lipophilic, nonpolar substances can have higher concentrations in breast milk than in maternal serum. Substances with higher milk to plasma ratios (>3) include the PCBs and DDT residues. Depending on the chemical structure, substances may have different half-lives in milk. For example, PCBs may take 5–8 months to clear, whereas alcohol is cleared in a few hours. Lactation is the main route of excretion for toxicants that bioaccumulate in maternal adipose tissue. Although

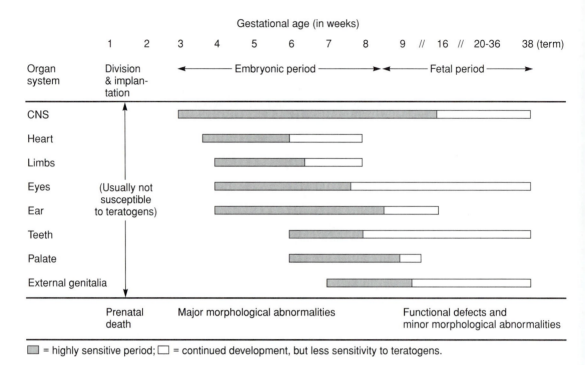

Gestational age (in weeks)

Figure 25–5. Critical periods of fetal development by organ system. Adapted from Moore HL and Persaud TVN, *The Developing Human.* Saunders, 1993.

acute toxicity in infants from contaminated breast milk has been reported (eg, PCBs), the effects of low-level chronic exposures have not been well-studied. Therefore, most pediatricians would continue to recommend the benefits of breast-feeding, except for unusual exposure circumstances. Details of postnatal effects are beyond the scope of this chapter.

## MATERNAL PHYSIOLOGIC CHANGES

A number of physiologic changes and medical complications can occur in the pregnant woman that might be affected by occupational or environmental exposures. These could be evaluated as reproductive end points, but very little research has been conducted in this area. These changes are noteworthy for the way in which they may modify fetal exposures or require accommodation in the workplace. For example, increased tidal volume and respiratory rate of the pregnant woman may increase the absorbed dose of aerosolized chemicals. An increased metabolic rate may also lead to changes in metabolism of specific compounds, leading to a different effective dose. Pregnant women can also experience fatigue and nausea. The nausea may increase sensitivity to substances with strong odors or tastes. Thus, potential changes in exposure dose and common consumption

patterns (eg, caffeinated or alcoholic beverages) could occur.

## SCIENTIFIC LITERATURE

Risk assessment of reproductive or other hazards in the workplace or environment involves the following components: hazard identification, dose-response assessment, exposure assessment, and risk characterization. The clinician may be involved in one or more of these steps when evaluating the risk for a patient or worker. This section will focus on the first two components, with discussion of the remaining topics later in this chapter.

### ANIMAL STUDIES

When evaluating a patient with potential exposure to reproductive toxicants, the clinician needs to identify chemicals and physical hazards in the workplace or environment via warning signs, product labels, material safety data sheets (MSDSs), and purchase orders. A review of both the animal and human liter-

**Table 25–4.** Human evidence for adverse female reproduction or developmental effects of selected agents. Compiled from multiple sources including original reports, Bloom, and Welch (see references).

| Agent | Human Outcomes[1] | Strength of Data[2] |
|---|---|---|
| Anesthetic gases | Sub-fertility, SAB, BDs | +/? |
| Anti-neoplastic drugs | SAB, BDs | ++ |
| Arsenic | SAB, LBW | + |
| Carbon disulfide | SAB/menstrual disorders | +/? |
| Carbon monoxide | SAB, LBW | + |
| DDT | Menstrual disorders | ? |
| Dioxins | Menstrual disorders, SAB, BDs | ? |
| Electro-magnetic fields (EMF) | SAB/childhood cancer | ?/+ |
| Ethylene glycol ethers | SAB | ++ |
| Ethylene oxide | SAB | + |
| Lead | Infertility, SAB, preterm, neurologic | ++ |
| Mercury | Menstrual disorders, SAB/LBW, CNS malformation, cerebral palsy | +/++ |
| Physical stress | Preterm, LBW/SAB | +/? |
| PCBs | LBW, hyperpigmentation/menstrual disorders | ++/? |
| Radiation, ionizing | Infertility, menstrual disorders, SAB, BDs, childhood cancer | ++ |
| Solvents, organic | Menstrual disorders, SAB/BDs | +/? |
| Tobacco smoke | Fetal loss/LBW | +/++ |
| Video display terminals (VDT) | SAB, BDs | – |

[1]All have shown at least limited positive effects in animals. SAB = spontaneous abortion, LBW = low birthweight or decreased weight, BDs = birth defects.
[2]++ = strong evidence, + = limited evidence, ? = preliminary or conflicting evidence, – = no association.

ature should be conducted. However, many chemicals and physical hazards have not been adequately studied with respect to reproductive hazards in animals, let alone in humans. Some good databases exist for those hazards that have been evaluated (see references). Because of the scarcity of human data dealing with reproductive effects, it is important to develop an understanding of the animal research process. Animal studies are meaningful for humans with respect to whether there is any harm but not necessarily predictive as to the specific type of effect. In animal studies, severe effects on the mother can occur with no teratogenic effects on the offspring. On the other hand, toxic effects on the offspring with no effect on the mother should be treated as primary effects on the embryo or fetus and not as maternal toxicity.

In the evaluation of the animal literature and its relevance to humans, the following aspects of each study need to be considered: consistency with other animal studies with respect to patterns of exposure, abnormal health outcomes, and causal association; concordance with reproductive biology; and biological plausibility of the mechanism of action. Furthermore, it is important to assess the quality of the animal study design and analysis: (1) Are mammalian species used that are predictive of human response? (2) Is the route of administration relevant to the human exposure? (3) Is the timing, duration, and magnitude of exposure appropriate? (4) Are the animal end points predictive of adverse reproductive outcomes in humans? (5) Are the abnormal reproductive effects occurring at doses that do not cause systemic toxicity and thus do not potentially interfere with mating? (6) Is there adequate study power (the probability of the study to detect a true effect)? (7) Is there observation of variability between litters rather than variation within litters (because litter mates tend to respond in a similar manner)?

From those animal studies that meet all or most of these criteria, the dose-response relationship can be assessed. When possible, it is important to ascertain the no observed adverse effect level (NOAEL), which is the highest dose level at which no biologically adverse effects occur. If sufficient data are not available to determine the NOAEL, then the lowest observed adverse effect level (LOAEL) for a given compound can be used. Whichever level is used, it is customary to apply an uncertainty factor (also called a safety factor) to the animal level when estimating the "safe" exposure level for humans. This estimated human exposure level is called the reference dose and can incorporate an uncertainty factor that usually ranges from 10 to 1000 (depending on the degree of uncertainty of the information used). On average, humans are 10 times as sensitive as the most sensitive animal species being tested. Therefore, safety factors used in dose-response extrapolations from animals to humans are not necessarily truly "safe."

## EPIDEMIOLOGIC STUDIES

Well-conducted epidemiologic studies should provide the best means of evaluating whether a specific agent, or group of agents, adversely affects human reproduction and development. Human studies can not be controlled as can animal experiments, so certain criteria or a weight-of-evidence type scheme is often used in evaluating whether a substance can be reasonably considered as having an adverse effect.

## 1. STUDY DESIGNS

The basic study designs used to examine the association of an exposure and possible outcomes include the cross-sectional, case-control, and cohort studies, which are discussed thoroughly in Appendix A. The **cross-sectional design** is the simplest and has been used often in occupational and environmental reproductive studies. In these studies, there is potential selection bias because the population existing in the workplace at the time of study may not be representative of the workforce during the time of previous exposure. For example, women with live births may leave the workforce (at least for a period of time) to care for their infants, whereas women experiencing SABs may continue to work and are at greater risk for subsequent SABs. On the other hand, women who experience adverse outcomes that they associate with a workplace exposure may change jobs. The **case-control study** is most appropriate for evaluating relatively rare diseases in large populations (eg, birth defects or childhood cancers). Because the outcome of interest is specified at the onset, the continuum of reproductive effects that may result from a given exposure cannot be evaluated. The **cohort study** is the preferred study design for most reproductive outcomes. A prospective cohort study allows

specific measures of an exposure and potential confounders to be ascertained at the etiologically relevant time periods.

The cohort and case-control studies are considered hypothesis-testing studies and are usually conducted after a possible association has been suggested by previous observations or a documented group exposure. For example, an acute clinician may recognize a series of cases that seem to have a factor in common. This situation is most likely to occur with a rare disease or new syndrome and was instrumental in identifying such associations as thalidomide and severe limb defects, and DES and vaginal clear cell carcinoma. A reported cluster of adverse outcomes occurring in a group of persons is a common way for environmental and occupational problems to be brought to attention, but such clusters often remain unexplained on further investigation.

Valuable data could be obtained from surveillance systems, but there are few established systems in place for adverse reproductive outcomes other than birth defects. Reasons for this include the fact that not all outcomes attract medical attention or require hospitalization (eg, SABs and subfertility), so they are more difficult to ascertain and are associated with less financial impact for society.

## 2. EXPOSURE ASSESSMENT

Although the methods used to measure occupational or environmental exposure are beyond the scope of this chapter, a brief overview of issues specific to evaluating exposure with respect to reproductive outcomes is presented. It should be kept in mind that the exposures of three individuals may be involved (eg, each parent and the fetus/offspring).

To cause damage to a fetus, an agent must be absorbed into the maternal blood stream and cross the placenta. Similarly, to affect fertility or the reproductive cycle, an agent must reach the appropriate organs via the blood stream. This process is affected by individual metabolism and the molecular structure of the compound. Some chemicals react with the first tissues they encounter, such as the lungs or skin, and are not absorbed into the blood stream unless they are ingested (eg, acids, chlorine, and asbestos). Once in the blood stream, agents that are of low molecular weight, are lipophilic, and are in a nonionized state are most likely to cross the placenta. Maternal metabolism may result in a metabolite that is more or less toxic to the fetus than the original substance. Unless chronic exposure results in a steady-state level in the body, the rapidity with which a substance is cleared can also affect its toxicity. Often, these issues are beyond the scope of epidemiologic studies but should be considered within the overall body of evidence about the toxicity of a substance.

In epidemiologic studies, exposures can be ascertained from interviews, existing records, or biomarkers. If exposure history is obtained by retrospective **interview,** the possibility of biased recall among cases or misclassification due to lack of records or diminished memory is of concern. Recall may be affected by the length of time since pregnancy, the outcome of the pregnancy, whether subsequent pregnancies have occurred, and changes in exposures. However, pregnancy is a well-defined period and typically a major event in a woman's life, so recall bias may not be as great a problem for pregnancy outcome studies. Ascertainment of current exposure status for cohort studies limits possible recall bias, but women may not be aware of all their exposures. In interview studies, asking one spouse about the other may not provide sufficiently accurate information.

**Existing records** often do not provide detailed information, but rather serve to group women broadly. For example, residence on the birth certificate might be used to assign likelihood of an environmental exposure. However, residence at delivery may not reflect residence in the first trimester (the critical period), nor does it account for individual behavioral differences, such as how much time is spent out of the area at work. Similarly, occupational registries may be used to group women by broad exposures, but specific work-site practices will be unknown. The most accurate occupational exposures are obtained by an industrial hygienist, but such studies are also likely to be more costly or limited in sample size to allow for more detailed study.

**Laboratory measurement** of exposure may be done in a prospective study or on stored biological samples and provides a quantification of exposure that is less likely to be biased. Techniques for measuring environmental levels have been developed for many agents, including radon, electromagnetic fields, solvents, pesticides, and dust levels. Measurements on biological samples provide an indication of internal dose, which would be more biologically relevant. A number of difficulties can arise with these types of studies, eg, small sample size or selection bias due to the higher costs and greater participation required of subjects. Sampling at one point in time may not reflect the critical exposure period, particularly if the substance is cleared rapidly.

As noted, it is important to consider the timing of exposure in an epidemiologic study. An association with an exposure at the critical time is more relevant, and such information may be useful for excluding the possibility of a particular effect if the timing is wrong. In addition to timing, a dose-response relationship is usually examined. However, this relationship may not be evident with reproductive outcomes because different doses may result in different outcomes (eg, birth defect vs fetal death).

## 3. HEALTH ENDPOINTS & STUDY DESIGN ISSUES

Numerous end points have been examined in reproductive and developmental toxicity studies (Table 25–3). The definition and ascertainment of these outcomes as well as potential confounders are summarized in Table 25–5. For a factor to be a confounder, it must be related to both the end point and exposure in the study of interest. Lack of control for one of the variables in the list does not imply the study is deficient if the investigators found this factor did not act as a confounder in their study or had reason to believe the factor would not be associated with the exposure of interest.

Many of the pregnancy outcomes in Table 25–3 are relatively frequent and lend themselves to a prospective study design. One design is to enroll women when they come in for a prenatal visit and then ascertain pregnancy outcomes by medical records, vital records, or both. However, the detection of SAB is dependent on the time at which the pregnancy is clinically recognized. Women who have had prior losses and are worried about an exposure may seek medical attention sooner than other women and thus more of their losses will be detected. This problem may be handled by using statistical methods in which pregnancies are included in risk sets only for the weeks of gestation the women were under observation. Also, a case-control design can be used to study SAB. If SABs are ascertained from medical or laboratory records, a certain percentage of early losses will be missed, which may be related to exposure status. Recently, studies have been conducted that collect periodic urine samples (daily samples or samples taken around the menstrual period) for the measurement of hCG and subclinical loss or for ovulation detection. These studies are very labor-intensive, and the types of participants may represent a selected population.

In contrast to fetal loss, congenital anomalies at birth are not common and thus a case-control study design is usually used. The primary concerns with these types of studies are ascertainment of relevant cases, selection of control subjects, and possible recall bias. Classification of defects is problematic because they may have varying etiologies and any single defect will be extremely rare. Many defects are not evident at birth; therefore, additional postnatal follow-up may be necessary to identify relevant cases.

Birthweight is recorded fairly accurately at birth and has been the subject of much perinatal research using a variety of study designs. There is a strong association between birthweight and subsequent mortality and morbidity. Mean birthweight is often categorized as low birthweight (LBW, < 2500 g). However, this category includes infants who are of

**Table 25–5.** Developmental and reproductive outcomes, definitions, and source of ascertainment.

### A. Developmental outcomes

| Outcome | Definition | Source of Ascertainment | Possible Confounders |
|---|---|---|---|
| Clinical spontaneous abortion | Fetal loss by 20 weeks | Interview, MDs or MRs Pregnancy test | Mat. age, prior SAB, smoking, alcohol, gest. age at preg. recognition |
| Early, or sub-clinical loss | Loss by 6–8 weeks Short rise and fall in hCG level | Urinary assay (days 5–20 after ovulation) | Same as clinical (unknown) |
| Congenital anomalies | Varies—structural, physiologic, genetic major & minor | Problematic—vital records incomplete. MRs, MDs, or registries | Few known-mat. age, prior hx, gender, race (defect specific) |
| Fetal growth | LBW: <2500 g IUGR: ≤10th percentile weight-for-age Preterm: <37 weeks | Vital records (accuracy of gest. age), MRs, interview | Mat. age, race, SES, parity, mat. weight & gain, prior hx, prenatal care, gest. age, gender, multiple birth, nutrition, smoking, stress |
| Fetal, neonatal, or infant death | FD: 21 wks-term ND: 1st month of life ID: 1st year | Vital records (under-report FDs), MRs | Vary by timing & cause: mat. age, race, SES, parity, infant gender, multiple birth, birthweight & gest. age |

### B. Reproductive outcomes

| Outcome | Definition | Source of Ascertainment | Possible Confounders |
|---|---|---|---|
| Infertility | No conception in 12 mos. unprotected intercourse or specific dx (eg, tubal disease, ovulatory factor, cervical factor, endometriosis) | Interview or survey Vital records crude | Mat. age, STD hx, IUD or OC use hx, smoking, weight (?), stress (?) |
| Time to conception | Continuous = mos. of unprotected intercourse, or Categorize (3, 6, 12 mos) | Interview Diary | See above, frequency of intercourse |
| Menstrual cycle dysfunction | Cycle length (<24, >34 days), bleed characteristics, pain, anovulation, long FP or short LP | Interview, BBT or cervical mucous test, hormone measurements in serum or urine | Mat. age, obesity, alcohol abuse, smoking, stress, exertion, some drugs or medical conditions (more work needed) |
| Age at menopause | Cessation of menstruation: mean about 50 years, but peri-menopausal many years prior | Interview, MDs, hormone levels | Smoking, age at menarche, preg. hx |

Definitions: MD = Medical Doctor, physician records; MR = medical (hospital) records, LBW = low birthweight, IUGR = intrauterine growth retardation, SAB = spontaneous abortion, FD = fetal death, ND = neonatal death, ID = infant death.
Abbreviations: BBT = Basal body temperature, STD = sexually transmitted disease, OC = oral contraceptives, IUD = intrauterine device, FP = follicular phase, LP = luteal phase.

low weight because they are born prematurely as well as those who are growth retarded for their age. These two groups may be etiologically different and experience different risks of mortality. To distinguish these, investigators can examine LBW among only term infants or intrauterine growth retardation (IUGR, defined as births below the 10th percentile on standard-weight-for-gestational-age curves).

Perinatal deaths include a variety of causes with a number of classification schemes developed to summarize them. For occupational or environmental factors, it is useful to distinguish between prepartum and peripartum stillbirths because a toxic effect is more likely to be related to death in utero. When infant deaths are examined, neonatal deaths are found to be most likely related to exposures or conditions of pregnancy and postnatal deaths are seen to also reflect conditions of infancy.

The reproductive end points in Table 25–5B are less well studied epidemiologically than pregnancy outcomes. This is partly due to the fact that the population at risk is harder to determine and such outcomes have only recently come under more public concern. Like some of the pregnancy outcomes, fertility problems may reflect a variety of causes, from genetic damage in gametes to tubal occlusion to a hormonal imbalance. Infertility and subfertility are often studied retrospectively as it is difficult to assemble a population of women trying to become pregnant. The definition of infertility is based on waiting time and may include some people in which no physiologic change has occurred and thus lead to misclassification of true fertility. If cases are limited to a medically diagnosed population, the study may be biased by a differential likelihood of seeking treatment among the couples. Often, control subjects are difficult to select for these studies. For example, using women giving birth as controls may include some individuals that had previously experienced some subfertility.

Because of the insensitivity of infertility to short-term effects, time to pregnancy has been the subject of more recent study on the effects of exposures. Retrospectively, women who are pregnant or have recently delivered can be questioned about past use of contraception. The choice of a reference date about when exposures are determined in controls

is critical. If the time of conception is used, women who had been trying unsuccessfully before that time may have changed their exposures and the true period at risk (when contraception is stopped) will not be included. Prospective studies may be conducted by having women keep diaries of when their menstrual periods occur, when they have intercourse, and when they use contraception to identify cycles truly "at risk" of pregnancy. These methods allow a more accurate assessment of time to pregnancy.

Menstrual cycle function has been the least well-studied of the reproductive end points. This end point is best studied prospectively with the use of diaries to record signs and symptoms. Cycle length can be used as a crude measure of function, but normal lengths may mask such problems as insufficient luteal phase and progesterone production. Studying such defects requires accurate determination of day of ovulation and measurement of hormone patterns. These types of studies are difficult to conduct in population-based groups but have become relatively easier by the recent development of cost-efficient serial sample laboratory assays. Such studies may be well-suited to an occupational

## BIRTH DEFECTS SURVEILLANCE—JOHN HARRIS, MD, MPH

Birth defects are a significant health problem and a leading cause of infant mortality in the United States. One in 33 babies is born with a serious birth defect (structural congenital anomaly). Several state, national, and international birth defects registries have been put in place in the past few decades. The best of these registries are surveillance systems based on active examination of medical records. Data from the Birth Defects Monitoring Program (BDMP) within the California Department of Health Services show that the total birth defects rate (number of defects per 1000 births) is approximately similar across all races, maternal ages, and social classes. Included in the BDMP are the following types of birth defects: structural defects (eg, missing limbs and malformed hearts), birth defect patterns (eg, fetal alcohol syndrome), and chromosomal abnormalities. The more common conditions include heart defects (1 in 200 births), pyloric stenosis (1 in 550), cleft lip/palate (1 in 550), Down's syndrome (1 in 900), spina bifida/neural tube defects (1 in 1400), and limb defects (1 in 1750).

The causes of most birth defects are unknown and for this reason many occupational and environmental factors are suspect. Population-based birth defects data are an important tool in evaluating occupational and environmental concerns. Information from birth defects registries can be used in the following ways: (1) Case-control research studies allow the evaluation of exposures such as maternal or paternal occupation, pesticides, and electromagnetic fields, as well as the traditional personal factors of diet, family history, illnesses, and medications. (2) Investigation of reports of disease clusters (birth defect outbreaks) is a type of follow-up activity associated with the routine monitoring of disease trends in a given population. (3) Targeted surveillance can be conducted around a specific site of occupational or environmental concern. Examples of specific target sites include those receiving contaminated drinking water or those in which toxic spills have occurred. The tracking of rates of birth defects among different geographic areas and over time can identify suspicious patterns that lead to more in-depth studies. However, the expected number of defects in small local populations may be too variable to reach a definitive conclusion about the association between the exposure and the birth defect.

cohort, in which a well-defined worker population is assembled and because a smaller number of participants is needed as contrasted to pregnancy studies.

## SELECTED REPRODUCTIVE HAZARDS

Few chemicals have been adequately studied in terms of their reproductive effects. Only about 5% of agents used in industry have been assessed. Most exposure standards are not based on reproductive effects. More evidence is available from animal rather than human studies, but direct extrapolation to the human cannot always be made. Although epidemiologic studies can be more difficult to interpret because of the methodologic issues described, a number of potential reproductive or developmental hazards have been identified (Table 25–4). The agents that have been shown conclusively to be reproductive toxicants in humans (other than medications) are few and include ionizing radiation, mercury, lead, and polychlorinated biphenyls (PCBs). Tobacco smoke is a complex mixture of thousands of substances and includes some agents with known animal toxicity, such as cadmium, nicotine, carbon dioxide, and polyaromatic hydrocarbons (PAHs). Active smoking during pregnancy has been strongly associated with LBW and intrauterine growth retardation. Currently, the effects of environmental tobacco smoke (ETS) are of great interest because of the large number of people exposed, especially at the workplace. ETS appears to have a small but consistent effect on lowering mean birthweight. High ETS exposures may have an effect similar to light smoking.

Questions about whether employment per se has any harmful affect on pregnancy outcome have been evaluated, with the general consensus that it does not. Physical exertion at work has been a cause of concern because of the extreme effects seen in professional athletes and dancers. The American College of Obstetricians and Gynecologists has published guidelines on exertion levels during later stages of pregnancy that indicate that moderate or light exertion levels should be safe throughout pregnancy. Heavy lifting, prolonged standing, or repetitive stooping and bending are recommended to be discontinued early during the second trimester. The most consistent effect of physical exertion (particularly prolonged standing and rotating shifts) seems to be on preterm delivery and possibly low birthweight. Less consistent results are seen for the associations with SAB and fecundability.

Most of the toxic agents in Table 25–4 have been examined in occupational settings, where exposures tend to be higher than those encountered in the environment and relatively easier to document. However,

the known hazards mentioned have been encountered environmentally from long-term use and disposal by industry as well as from acute releases. The following section will highlight three examples from the literature.

## 1. VIDEO DISPLAY TERMINALS

In 1980, a Canadian report of a cluster of severe malformations in women working with video display terminals (VDTs) led to extensive public and scientific interest. Soon after, at least 10 additional clusters were reported consisting primarily of birth defects and SABs. A review of eight subsequent analytic studies from the United States, Scandinavia, and Canada did not generally support an association of adverse reproductive outcomes with VDT work. However, one study conducted in California showed an 80% excess risk of SAB among women who used VDTs more than 20 hours/week in the first trimester. This study further fueled the debate and led to several other studies. A NIOSH study was conducted to specifically address the conflicting results of the earlier studies. This study had the advantage of measuring electromagnetic fields (EMF) at typical workstations used by women in the two cohorts of telephone operators (one group used VDTs and the other did not). However, the study design did not allow evaluation of any effects due to psychosocial or physical stress. The primary difference in exposure was that VDT users had higher abdominal exposure to very low frequency EMFs, but the extremely low frequency fields (ELFs) were similar. The investigators found no increased risk of SAB with VDT use as ascertained from company records nor any relationship with higher hours of use. A meta-analysis based on seven of the most recent studies found a pooled odds ratio of 1.0 for VDT use and SAB, but this figure is unadjusted for confounders. A Finnish report not included in the meta-analysis found no association of SAB and reported VDT use but did show an elevated risk (odds ratio, 3.4) among women who used VDTs with a high level of extremely low frequency magnetic fields. Thus, some scientists have recommended additional research on women with high exposures to ELF magnetic fields.

Fewer studies have examined birth defects and only one found an increased risk with greater hours of use of VDTs. Two studies have examined fetal growth; one showed a slight, nonsignificant trend for risk of intrauterine growth retardation with greater hours of use, and the other study found no association. In summary, the concerns raised in the lay press about VDT use from the initial cluster investigations were not readily allayed by the subsequent epidemiologic studies showing little increased risk. Although VDT use per se does not appear to be associated with increased risk, the concern now has shifted to magnetic fields that are present in *all* workplaces and homes. Furthermore, stress associated with VDT use in some settings may play a role in adverse outcomes.

## 2. ANESTHETIC GASES

The possible risk of adverse reproductive outcome with exposure to anesthetic gases first came to attention in 1967 from a small study in Russia. A number of large studies were published in the 1970s suggesting higher risks of miscarriage, infertility, and congenital malformations associated with anesthetic gas exposure among anesthetists, operating room nurses, and dental assistants. On this basis, NIOSH issued recommended standards for occupational exposure for these agents (nitrous oxide, halothane, ethane). However, some of these studies suffered from the following methodologic problems: lack of control for confounders, inclusion of multiple pregnancies that may not have occurred during exposure periods, potential recall bias, and low response rates. A mail questionnaire survey in Sweden documented a nonresponse bias and found less evidence for adverse effects of anesthetic gas exposure. In addition, two later registry-based studies in Sweden and Finland did not find any associations. In later studies of occupational groups using anesthetic gases, exposures may have been decreased by use of better protective measures, such as improved ventilation and waste gas recapture systems. Although the ideal study has not yet been conducted, the evidence to date can be considered suggestive. Hospital staff may be exposed to other hazards that could confound an association with anesthetic gases. In particular, ionizing radiation, antineoplastic drugs, and sterilizing agents (eg, ethylene oxide) have been identified as reproductive hazards in epidemiologic studies from Finland.

## 3. SOLVENTS

Solvents may well be one of the most pervasive chemical exposures of women as they include many compounds used in the workplace and the home. In the early 1980s, solvent exposure was considered a potential reproductive hazard when increased risks for adverse outcomes were identified among laboratory workers in Scandinavia. However, these studies had no evaluation of exposure to specific solvents or other hazards. In some industries (eg, dry cleaning and pharmaceutical industries), use of specific solvents such as perchlorethylene, methylene chloride, toluene, and xylene has been seen to be associated with concurrent elevation in SAB risk. Several case-control studies have shown associations of solvent exposure and cardiac and other congenital anom-

alies. Suggestive study findings have indicated a potential association between solvent use and fetal growth. Many of these epidemiologic studies suffer from crude exposure assessment. Recent interest has focused on exposures in the growing semiconductor industry, which employs a largely female workforce. A collaborative study of 14 semiconductor companies nationwide was recently completed. Risks for SAB were found to be slightly increased in two cohorts, and fecundability was reduced in a prospective cohort. The researchers have implicated exposures to photoresist and developer solvents (eg, glycol ethers and xylene) and fluoride compounds as the primary etiologic agents. However, some researchers have commented that concurrent exposure to other agents may be involved and questioned the lack of precise biological monitoring data in the study design.

# REPRODUCTIVE ASSESSMENT

The medical evaluation of the patient with a potential exposure to a reproductive hazard follows the traditional components of history taking, physical examination, and laboratory assessment, with an emphasis on both health and exposure parameters. In addition, special consideration is needed in the assessment, communication, and management of reproductive risk for the patient.

## MEDICAL EVALUATION

In the clinical setting, infertility is defined as an inability to conceive after 12 months of unprotected intercourse. Potential causes for infertility in the female include ovulatory dysfunction, tubal or pelvic factors, and uterine or cervical factors. It is estimated that the cause of infertility is due to male factors in 40% of the affected couples, female factors in 40–50%, and no known etiology in 10–20%. For the infertility work-up, the male partner needs to be assessed concurrently (see Chapter 26). Adverse pregnancy outcomes include spontaneous abortion, stillbirth, prematurity, congenital birth defects, and low birth weight (Tables 25–3 and 25–5). A full discussion of the diagnosis and treatment of various obstetric and gynecologic conditions is beyond the scope of this chapter. However, the following is a general overview of the types of evaluation techniques that can be used to assess the female reproductive system.

## 1. INTERVIEW

The patient interview should cover the following areas: demographic data, general medical history (including medications, street drugs, alcohol, and tobacco), work history, and reproductive history (including menstrual function, past pelvic surgeries or gynecological procedures, pregnancy and birth outcomes, sexually transmitted diseases, contraception, and familial illness). It is important to ask about potential exposure to any known or suspect reproductive hazards and confounders cited in Tables 25–4 and 25–5.

## 2. PHYSICAL EXAMINATION

This examination should assess the physical integrity of the genital system and rule out any extraneous mass or abnormality.

## 3. LABORATORY

A hormonal profile can be obtained in the assessment of potential fetal loss (hCG and LH), ovarian function (progesterone and estrogen metabolites), and pituitary function (LH and FSH). A wide range of tests and assays are available and need to be selected based on the medical conditions under consideration. During field biological monitoring studies, urine samples are relatively easy to collect for hormonal assays. For certain hazards, exposure burden may be estimated via exhaled breath, blood, urine, and other biological tissue measurements.

## RISK ASSESSMENT

As described earlier, the risk assessment process follows four basic steps: (1) **Hazard identification** of any hazardous agents being used by patient. This includes review of the patient history and collection of pertinent MSDS document and product labels. (2) **Hazard evaluation** to determine whether a given substance or physical agent is a reproductive hazard. This involves the utilization of technical informational sources to access the appropriate medical and scientific literature. If no reproductive information is found in the scientific literature, it is important to consider other health end points as indications of human toxicity. (3) **Exposure assessment**: This is performed by estimating the level of exposure via patient work history, potential routes of exposure, nature and pattern of symptoms, industrial hygiene data, and biological monitoring results. (4) **Risk categorization** with respect to the reproductive system. This activity is based on information gathered in the first three steps and considers: toxicity, timing and extent of exposure, potency, severity of outcome, and degree of uncertainty in animal and human studies.

Often, not all of the needed information is available and an educated guess is necessary. It is very helpful to have established contacts for additional consultation when a more difficult risk assessment is involved. Potential contacts include local or state health departments, university medical centers, poison control centers, NIOSH, EPA, ATSDR, OSHA, and the Association of Occupational and Environmental Clinics. Access to on-line literature databases is very useful (eg, REPRORISK, REPROTOX, and TERIS; see references).

## RISK COMMUNICATION

Building on the information gathered during the risk assessment process, risk communication is the logical follow-up by which the involved person or persons obtain the information needed to make informed and independent decisions about health and safety risks. In general, there is an underlying principle that needs to be acknowledged and sensitively dealt with: the threat or actual fact of reproductive dysfunction or adverse reproductive outcome has a profound impact on an individual's life. All questions must be answered truthfully and completely. A description of the limitations in knowledge may be needed. The timing of exposure and of the first contact with the involved person is very important. When possible, the risk communication is conducted prior to actual exposure in order to intervene at the primary prevention stage. The options available for the female worker should be presented in such a way that the medical impact as well as the economic consequences of decisions are understood and discussed. The medical confidentiality of the involved individual must be maintained. It is imperative that the employer, involved employee(s), and medical consultant work together in resolving a particular situation, as well as in developing a general policy on reproductive hazards in the workplace that involves both genders. Ideally, this policy is developed within a safety committee composed of representatives from management and labor and consultants in occupational medicine and industrial hygiene.

## RISK MANAGEMENT

Once the risk assessment and risk communication have occurred, risk management completes the sequence. *In order of priority,* the following actions may be considered for a given reproductive hazard situation: (1) **Exposure reduction or elimination:**

Replacement of hazards with safer agents; improved engineering controls; safer work practices; and personal protective equipment (the latter should not be the primary mode of protection—emphasis should be placed on the other actions). Exposure reduction or elimination is the most desirable option and should be attempted in all situations involving a reproductive hazard. (2) **Temporary job transfer**: Remove individual from work environment in which reproductive hazard exists. Problems may occur when there is no nonexposed job location. Transfer needs to occur before conception (which is not always planned) and this may require a written request from the personal physician (who may not be familiar with the work setting). Thus, this option should be considered when there is a high-risk situation and exposure reduction/elimination is not possible. (3) **Disability leave**: This option may need to be considered by the personal physician. Paid leave is subject to company policy, and temporary pregnancy disability leave must be treated the same as any other medical disability leave. The early embryo sensitivity period has already occurred with potential workplace exposure by the time a disability leave is granted. There is no guarantee that the medical disability will be approved, and benefits rarely are equivalent to the individual's current wage. This option should be considered when there is a high-risk situation in which the employer will not reduce exposure and a temporary transfer is not possible. (4) **Remove individual from work**: This is the least desirable action. It is illegal for an employer to terminate the affected individual due to pregnancy. A woman may choose to quit work because of personal reasons, but it is important to help her evaluate all options and to understand the possible consequences. This option is to be considered only when all other options have been explored and the woman is comfortable with the possible consequences.

## LEGAL ISSUES & WORKPLACE STANDARDS

In the lawsuit involving International Union, UAW vs Johnson Controls, Inc., the US Supreme Court held that an employer violated Title VII's ban on sex discrimination by excluding all women who could not prove their sterility from production jobs in a lead-battery factory. The Court indicated that a policy directed only at fertile women is overt discrimination on the basis of sex regardless of the scientific evidence of heightened safety concerns for mothers or potential mothers. In addition, any policies or actions taken by the employer must not violate existing laws prohibiting discrimination on the basis of pregnancy, childbirth, or related medical conditions. Employers cannot require that an individual be sterilized as a condition of employment. If an employee disabled by pregnancy, childbirth, or a related medical condition transfers to a less hazardous job, an employer must allow her to return to her original job or a similar one when the disability has resolved.

OSHA has the mandate to promulgate standards that protect workers from adverse health effects (including reproductive effects) resulting from workplace hazards. However, there are only four agents with OSHA standards based partially on reproductive effects: dibromochloropropane (DBCP), lead, ethylene oxide, and ionizing radiation. It should be recognized that many chemical and physical agents found in the workplace are not covered by an OSHA standard and those standards that do exist for the most part are not based on reproductive end points. This is why the risk assessment process should be implemented at any worksite that has potential reproductive hazards present.

## REFERENCES

### ANESTHESIA & OTHER HAZARDS AMONG HEALTH CARE WORKERS

Ahlborg G, Hemminki K: Reproductive effects of chemical exposures in the health professions. JOEM 1995; 37:956.

Evans JA et al: Infertility and pregnancy outcome among magnetic resonance imaging workers. JOM 1993;35:1191.

Guirguis SS et al: Health effects associated with exposure to anesthetic gases in Ontario hospital personnel. Br J Ind Med 1990;47:490.

Rowland A et al: Nitrous oxide and spontaneous abortion in female dental assistants. Am J Epidemiol 1995;141:531.

Rowland A et al: Reduced fertility among women employed as dental assistants exposed to high levels of nitrous oxide. N Engl J Med 1992;237:993.

Saurel-Cubizolles MJ, Job-Spira N, Estrym-Behar E: Ectopic pregnancy and occupational exposure to antineoplastic drugs. The Lancet 1993;341:1169.

### BIRTH DEFECTS

Stierman L: Birth defects in California: 1983–1990. Birth Defects Monitoring Program, California Department of Health Services, 1994.

Yielding KL: Primary and secondary risk factors for birth defects. Environ Health Perspect 1993;101 (Suppl 3):285.

## EMPLOYMENT & PREGNANCY OUTCOMES

Brandt LPA, Negro-Vilar A: Stress and other environmental factors affecting fertility in men and women. Overview. Environ Health Perspect 1993;101(Suppl 2):297.

Plowchalk D, Meadows MJ, Mattison DR: Female reproductive toxicity. In: Paul M (editor): *Occupational and Environmental Reproductive Hazards: A Guide for Clinicians.* Williams & Wilkins, 1993.

Zhang J, Wen-Wei C, David L: Occupational hazards and pregnancy outcomes. Am J Ind Med 1992;21:397.

## MEDICAL EVALUATION

Cheung AP: Clinical approach to female reproductive problems. In Gold EB, Lasley BL and Schenker MB.(editors) *Occupational Medicine: State of the Art Reviews* 9(3):415,1994.

Lasley BL, Shideler SE: Methods for evaluating reproductive health of women. In: Gold EB, Lasley BL, Schenker MB (editors): *Occupational Medicine: State of the Art Reviews* 1994;9(3):415.

## METALS

Andrews KW, Savitz DA, Hertz-Picciotto I: Prenatal lead exposure in relation to gestational age and birth weight: A review of epidemiologic studies. Am J Ind Med 1994;26:13.

Antilla A, Sallman M: Effects of parental occupational exposure to lead and other metals on spontaneous abortion. JOEM 1995;37:915.

## PESTICIDES

Garry VF et al: Pesticide appliers, biocides, and birth defects in rural Minnesota. Environ Health Perspect 1996;104:394.

Nurminen T: Maternal pesticide exposure and pregnancy. JOEM 1995;37:935.

## METHYL MERCURY

Gilbert SG, Grant-Webster KS. Neurobehavioral effects of developmental methyl mercury exposure. Environ Health Perspect 1995;103(Suppl 6):135.

Harada M: Minamata disease: methylmercury poisoning in Japan caused by environmental polution. Crit Rev Toxicol 1995;25(1):1.

Rowland A et al: The effect of occupational exposure to mercury vapour on the fertility of female dental assistants. Occup Environ Med 1994;51:28.

World Health Organization: Environmental health criteria 101, methyl mercury. WHO, Geneva, 1990.

## PHYSICAL EXERTION

American College of Obstetricians and Gynecologists (ACOG) Council on Scientific Affairs: Effects of pregnancy on work performance. JAMA 1984;251:1995.

Eskenazi B et al: Physical exertion as risk factor for spontaneous abortion. Epidemiology 1994;5:6.

Fenster L et al: A prospective study of work-related physical exertion and spontaneous abortion. Epidemiology 1997;8:66.

Florack EI, Zielhuis GA, Rolland R: The influence of occupational physical activity on the menstrual cycle and fecundability. Epidemiology 1994;5:14.

Klebanoff MA, Shiono PH, Carey JC: The effect of physical activity during pregnancy on preterm delivery and birth weight. Am J Obstet Gynecol 1990;163:1450.

Nurminen T: Female noise exposure, shift work and reproduction. JOEM 1995;37:945.

## POLYCHLORINATED BIPHENYLS (PCBS) & DIOXINS

Guo YL, Lambert GH, Hsu C-C: Growth abnormalities in the population exposed in utero and early postnatally to polychlorinated biphenyls and dibenzofurans. Environ Health Perspect 1995;103(Suppl 6):117.

Lindstrom G et al: Workshop on perinatal exposure to dioxin-like compounds: I. Summary. Environ Health Perspect 1995;103:135.

Hsieh SF et al: A cohort study of mortality and exposure to polychlorinated biphenyls. Arch Environ Health 1996;51(6):417.

## RISK ASSESSMENT & COMMUNICATION

Ahlborg G et al: Assessment of reproductive risk at work. Int J Occup Environ Health 1996;2(1):59.

Taskinen H, Viskum S: Communication concerning the risks of occupational exposures in pregnancy. Int J Occup Environ Health 1996;2(1):64.

## SOLVENTS

Lindbohm ML: Effects of parental exposure to solvents on pregnancy outcome. JOEM 1995;37:909.

Sallmen M et al: Reduced fertility among women exposed to organic solvents. Am J Ind Med 1995;27:699.

Schenker MB et al: Reproductive and other health effects of semiconductor work: the semiconductor health study. Am J Ind Med 1995;28:635.

Shaw GM, Malcoe LH, Katz E: Maternal workplace exposures to organic solvents and congenital cardiac anomalies. J Occup Med Toxicol 1992;1:371.

Taskinen H et al: Laboratory work and pregnancy outcome. J Occup Med 1994;3:311.

Windham GC et al: Exposure to organic solvents and adverse pregnancy outcome. Am J Ind Med 1991;20:241.

## TOBACCO EXPOSURE

Ahlborg G: Health effects of environmental tobacco smoke on the offspring of non-smoking women. J Smoking-Rel Dis 1994;5:107.

DiFranza JR, Lew RA: Effect of maternal cigarette smoking on pregnancy complications and Sudden Infant Death Syndrome. J Fam Pract 1995;40:385.

United States Department of Health and Human Services: The health consequences of smoking for women: A report of the Surgeon General. US Department of Health and Human Services, Public Health Service, Office of the Assistant Secretary for Health, Office of Smoking and Health, 1980.

## VIDEO DISPLAY TERMINALS (VDTS) & ELECTROMAGNETIC FIELDS (EMFS)

Delpizzo V: Epidemiological studies of work with display terminals and adverse pregnancy outcomes (1984–92). Am J Ind Med 1994;26:465–480.

Lindbohm ML et al: Magnetic fields of video display terminals and spontaneous abortion. Am J Epidemiol 1992;136:1041.

Lindbohm ML, Hietanen M: Magnetic fields of video display terminals and pregancy outcome. JOEM 1995;37:952.

Parazzini F et al: Video display terminal use during pregnancy and reproductive outcome—a meta-analysis. J Epidemiol Commun Hlth 1993;47;265.

Schnorr T et al: Video display terminals and the risk of spontaneous abortion. N Engl J Med 1992;324:727.

Shaw GM, Croen LA: Human adverse reproductive outcomes and electromagnetic field exposures: review of epidemiologic studies. Environ Health Perspect Suppl 1993;101:107.

Windham GC et al: Use of video display terminals during pregnancy and the risk of spontaneous abortion, low birthweight, or intrauterine growth retardation. Am J Indust Med 1990;18:675.

## GENERAL REFERENCES

Moore KL, Persaud TVN: *The Developing Human: Clinically Oriented Embryology*. Saunders, 1993.

Paul M: *Occupational and Environmental Reproductive Hazards: A Guide for Clinicians*. Williams & Wilkins, 1993.

Scialli AR, Zinaman MJ (editors): *Reproductive Toxicology and Infertility*. McGraw-Hill, 1993.

Terracciano GJ, Lemasters GK, Amler RW (editors): Standardized Assessment of Birth Defects and Reproductive Disorders in Environmental Health Field

Studies. ATSDR, Public Health Services, US Department of Health and Human Services, 1996.

Welch LS: Reproductive and Developmental Hazards. Case Studies in Environmental Medicine #19. Agency for Toxic Substances and Disease Registries, US Department of Health and Human Services, 1993.

## GENERAL RESOURCE LIST

Agency for Toxic Substances and Disease Registry (ATSDR), 1600 Clifton Road, Mail Stop E28, Atlanta, GA 30333, 404-639-0700.

Association of Occupational and Environmental Clinics (AOEC), 1010 Vermont Avenue NW, Washington DC 20005, 202-347-4976.

Environmental Protection Agency (EPA), 401 M Street SW, Washington DC 20460, 202-260-7751.

National Institute of Environmental Health Sciences (NIEHS), National Institutes of Health, PO Box 12233, Research Triangle Park, NC 27709, 919-541-3345.

National Institute for Occupational Safety and Health (NIOSH), 200 Independence Avenue SW, Washington DC 20201, 1-800-35-NIOSH.

Occupational Safety and Health Administration (OSHA), US Dept of Labor, 200 Constitution Avenue NW, Washington DC 20210, 202-249-8148. Establishes, enforces and provides consultation regarding national occupational health and safety standards.

Reproductive Toxicology Center (REPROTOX), Columbia Hospital for Women Medical Center, 2425 L Street, NW, Washington DC 20037, 202-293-5137. Computer data base dealing with reproductive and developmental hazards.

REPRORISK, Micromedex, Inc, 600 Grant Street, Denver, CO 80203, 303-831-1400. Computer data base dealing with reproductive and developmental hazards.

Teratogen Information System (TERIS), Dept of Pediatrics, TRIS WJ-10, University of Washington, Seattle, WA 98195, 206-543-2465. On-line access to data base and CD-ROM available.

# 26

# Male Reproductive Toxicology

*Ana Maria Osorio, MD, MPH*

In studying male reproductive toxicants, the ultimate aim is to protect the reproductive health of men and the health of their offspring, which is fundamentally important for the health of future generations. The occurrence of adverse reproductive outcomes is of great concern to the individuals and families involved. This is especially true if the individuals perceive that they are living or working in areas with potential exposure to hazardous agents. Adverse reproductive effects can be very stressful for affected families. Existing human information on this subject is very sparse and inadequate for the reproductive assessment of most suspect compounds and physical agents.

Another reason to better understand male reproductive functions is that they may act as sentinels for detecting occupational and environmental hazards. Reproductive effects have a relatively short latency between exposure and detectable health event (such as abnormal semen profile) as compared to the long latency for cancer. If workers or community residents are protected from exposures that are harmful to reproduction, they will usually be protected from other health effects associated with these exposures as well. While the extent to which workplace and environmental hazards affect reproductive function is unknown, these hazards are potentially preventable. Measures that can be taken to prevent further exposure include substitution or containment of the suspect hazard. Thus, preventing exposure should play a primary role in the health care provider's overall assessment of the patient's situation.

## REPRODUCTIVE OUTCOMES & RATES

### DEFINITIONS

A number of adverse reproductive effects may result from male exposure to chemical and physical agents. These effects range from infertility to birth defects in the infant. **Infertility** is present when a couple has not conceived after one year of unprotected sexual intercourse. **Sexual dysfunction** refers to decreased libido (decreased interest in sexual activity) and can be manifested by erectile dysfunction in men. Semen abnormalities can include **azoospermia** (complete absence of sperm), **oligospermia** (decreased sperm count), **teratospermia** (abnormally shaped sperm), and **asthenospermia** (sperm showing decreased motility). Abnormal birth outcomes include the following: **spontaneous abortion** (fetal loss prior to the 28th gestational week), **stillbirth** (fetal loss after the 28th week), **congenital defect** (abnormal appearance or function at birth), **prematurity** (birth prior to the 37th week of gestation), and **low birth weight** (weight < 2500 g at birth).

## POPULATION RATES

Accurate data on the rates of these outcomes are difficult to obtain because of lack of national monitoring systems and methodological differences in individual epidemiological studies. Nevertheless, a range of prevalence rates can be estimated (Table 26–1). Approximately 10% of couples in the United States are infertile. Additional couples may experience periods of subfertility or delayed conception. After conception, there may occur a variety of reproductive losses ranging from implantation to term. Up to 50% of embryos may be lost after implantation (the earliest time at which conception can be detected), with approximately 15% of pregnancies ending in clinically detected spontaneous abortion (SAB) and 2–3% ending in stillbirth (Table 26–1). Of all liveborn infants, 5–7% are of low birthweight (LBW), 15% are born prematurely, and approximately 3% will have a congenital anomaly. The causes for most of these outcomes are unexplained. However, there are a few known risk factors such as older maternal age (associated with increased rates of SAB) and African-American race (associated with increased rates of LBW).

**Table 26–1.** Prevalence[1] of selected adverse reproductive outcomes in the United States.

| Endpoint | Frequency per 100 | Unit |
|---|---|---|
| Azoospermia | 1 | Men |
| Infertility | 8–12 | Couples |
| Recognized spontaneous abortion | 10–20 | Pregnancies or women |
| Low birthweight | 4–7 | Livebirths |
| Prematurity | 14–18 | Livebirths |
| Stillbirth | 2–4 | Stillbirths + Livebirths |
| Birth defects (through 1 year of life) | 2–5 | Livebirths |
| Chromosomal anomalies in livebirths | 0.2 | Livebirths |
| Severe mental retardation | 0.4 | Children <age 16 |

[1]Compiled from multiple sources including vital records reports, California Birth Defects Monitoring Program and Guidelines for Studies of Human Populations Exposed to Mutagenic and Reproductive Hazards, Bloom (editor). Definition of terms in section on Reproductive Outcomes and Rates.

# REPRODUCTIVE PHYSIOLOGY

Although this section will focus on male-mediated exposure associated with reproductive and developmental abnormalities, it is important to note that maternal and fetal exposures also need to be assessed for a complete evaluation. It is recognized that more prolonged direct sources of exposure to the products of conception occur in the woman, and that maternal exposure can continue postnatally during lactation. However, changes in fertility have been reported in both sexes and genetic changes can be transmitted by either parent. An extensive discussion of fetal and postnatal development can be found in the Female Reproductive Toxicology chapter (Chapter 25).

## MALE REPRODUCTIVE SYSTEM

Appropriate hormonal balance is necessary for the adequate function of the male reproductive system (Figure 26–1). Hypothalamic, pituitary, and gonadal interactions include the following: (1) Hypothalamus produces gonadotropin-releasing hormone (GnRH); (2) Pituitary gland produces follicle-stimulating hormone (FSH) and luteinizing hormone (LH); and (3) The testis produces sperm (germ cell) from the germinal epithelium, testosterone from the Leydig cell, and Sertoli cell factor (SCF). The GnRH stimulates the pituitary gland production of FSH and LH. The FSH and LH exert a negative feedback effect on the hypothalamus and stimulate the testis. The SCF or inhibin causes a feedback inhibition of the pituitary gland hormones. The Sertoli cell in the seminiferous tubules is the site of spermatogenesis. Finally, there is testosterone feedback effect on the pituitary and hypothalamic hormones as well as the germ cell (sperm) and Sertoli cell. Testosterone causes the development and growth of sexual organs and secondary male characteristics (increased muscle mass, beard growth, axillary and pubic hair, deepening of the voice, libido and other sexual behavior).

In general, spermatogenesis involves two major sites within the testis (Figure 26–2). Starting from a germ cell, it takes 74 days for the development through the stages of spermatogonium, spermatocyte, and spermatid into a mature spermatozoon (or sperm) in the seminiferous tubules of the testis. During the next 12 days, the sperm travels along the epididymis for eventual ejaculation. Thus, approximately three months are required to complete the maturation and transport of the sperm.

## TERATOLOGY

There are important issues in teratology to be considered when evaluating male reproductive function. Preconception exposure may act directly on the germ cell (sperm). This condition could lead to either no fertilization or an aberration of the zygote and an eventual early and unrecognized abortion or birth defect. The reproductive toxicant may affect the embryo even when exposure occurs prior to conception either to the mother or father. Thus, one must consider infertility, spontaneous abortions, and birth defects in assessing men exposed to suspect reproductive toxicants.

Another important aspect to consider is that spermatogenesis involves a continuously replicating cell population (in the billions), while oogenesis occurs prenatally with a finite population at birth (only 400 oocytes ovulated during the reproductive years) and is depleted by approximately age 50. Therefore,

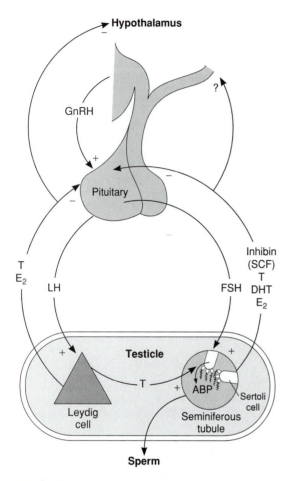

**Figure 26–1.** Hypothalamic, pituitary, and testicular interactions involved in hormonal homeostasis necessary for adequate male reproductive function. Notations: FSH (follicle-stimulating hormone), GC (germ cell), GnRH (gonadotropin releasing hormone), LC (Leydig cell), LH (luteinizing hormone), SC (Sertoli cell), and SCF (Sertoli cell factor) or Inhibin, T (testosterone), $E_2$ (estradiol), DHT (dihydrotestosterone), ADP (androgen-binding protein).

chemical or physical agents whose toxicity depends on cell division will have greater effect on the male germ cell. A complete evaluation of a male exposed to a reproductive hazard should take into account the large variability in individual susceptibility to reproductive agents, the environmental, occupational, and lifestyle factors of both parents, and the possibility that a toxic effect may lead to a clinically inapparent abnormality at the birth of the offspring.

## POTENTIAL MECHANISMS OF ACTION

Most male reproductive hazards can be characterized by having one or more of the following potential

mechanisms of action: central nervous system or endocrine abnormality (decreased libido and fertility as possible reproductive outcomes), direct testicular toxicity (decreased fertility as possible outcome), spermatogenesis or germ cell damage in the form of morphologic change, decreased cell number, abnormal motility or chromosomal abnormality (decreased fertility, fetal loss, congenital malformations, childhood developmental disabilities, and cancers as possible outcomes), and toxicants in the semen leading to abnormal sperm motility or direct action on the uterus or fetus (all of the prior possible outcomes). Although the focus of this chapter is on direct male reproductive effects, the potential for take-home exposure from the workplace needs to be concurrently assessed in the evaluation of a worker.

## SCIENTIFIC LITERATURE

Risk assessment of reproductive or other hazards in the workplace or environment involves the following components: hazard identification, dose-response assessment, exposure assessment, and risk characterization. The clinician may be involved in one or more of these steps when evaluating the risk for a patient or worker. This section will focus on the first two components with discussion of the remaining topics later in this chapter.

### ANIMAL STUDIES

When evaluating a patient with potential exposure to reproductive toxicants, the clinician needs to identify chemicals and physical hazards in the workplace or environment via warning signs, product labels, material safety data sheets (MSDSs), and purchase orders. A review of both the animal and human literature should be conducted. However, many chemicals or physical hazards have not been adequately studied with respect to reproductive hazards in animals, let alone in humans. Some good data bases exist for those hazards that have been evaluated (see references). Because of the scarcity of human data dealing with reproductive effects, it is important to develop an understanding of the animal research process. Animal studies are meaningful for humans with respect to the potential for harm, but not necessarily predictive as to the specific type of effect.

In the evaluation of the animal literature and its relevance to humans, the following aspects of each study need to be considered: consistency with other animal studies with respect to patterns of exposure,

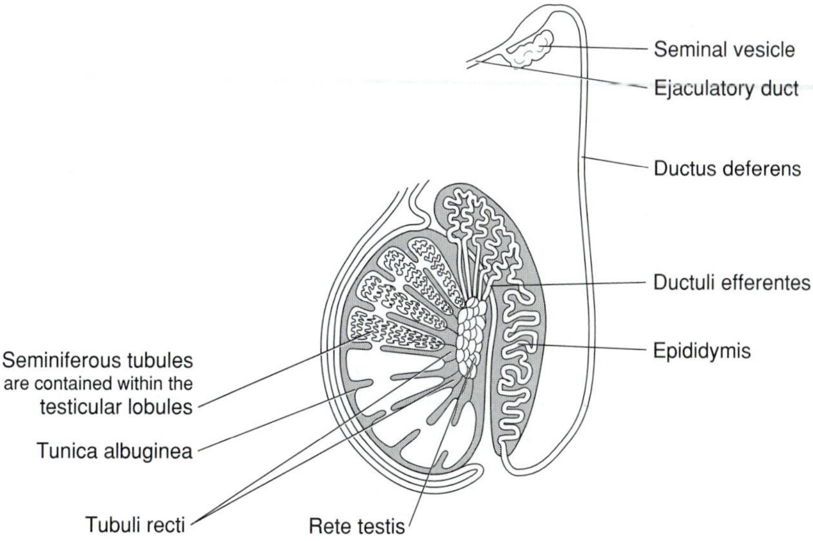

**Figure 26–2.** Cross-sectional view of the testis and adjacent structures.

abnormal health outcomes, and causal association; concordance with reproductive biology; and biological plausibility of the mechanism of action. Furthermore, it is important to assess the quality of the animal study design and analysis: (1) Are mammalian species used that are predictive of human response?; (2) Is the route of administration relevant to the human exposure?; (3) Is the timing, duration, and magnitude of exposure appropriate?; (4) Are the animal end points predictive of human adverse reproductive outcomes?; (5) Are the abnormal reproductive effects occurring at doses that do not cause systemic toxicity and thus do not potentially interfere with mating?; (6) Is there adequate study power (the probability of the study to detect a true effect)?; and (7) Is there observation of variability between litters rather than variation within litters (because litter mates tend to respond in a similar manner)?

From those animal studies that meet all or most of the criteria described, the dose-response relationship can be assessed. Whenever possible, it is important to ascertain the no observed adverse effect level (NOAEL), which is the highest dose level at which no biologically adverse effects occur. If sufficient data are not available to determine the NOAEL, then the lowest observed adverse effect level (LOAEL) for a given compound can be used. Whichever level is utilized, it is customary to apply an uncertainty factor (also called a safety factor) to the animal level when estimating the "safe" exposure level for humans. This estimated human exposure level is called the reference dose and can incorporate an uncertainty factor that usually ranges from 10 to 1000 (depending on the degree of uncertainty of the information used). On average, humans are ten times as sensitive as the most sensitive animal species being tested. Therefore, safety factors used in dose-response extrapolations from animals to humans are not necessarily truly "safe."

## EPIDEMIOLOGICAL STUDIES

Well-conducted epidemiological studies should provide the best means of evaluating whether a specific agent, or group of agents, adversely affects *human* reproduction and development. Human studies cannot be controlled as can animal experiments, so certain criteria or a weight-of-evidence type scheme are often used in evaluating whether a substance can be reasonably considered as having an adverse effect.

### Study Designs

The basic study designs used to examine the association of an exposure and possible outcomes include the cross-sectional, case-control, and cohort studies that are discussed thoroughly in Appendix A. The **cross-sectional design** is the simplest and has been used often in occupational and environmental reproductive studies. If the mechanism of action is thought to be interference with spermatogenesis, this study design is useful because there is a relatively short, three month lag period between exposure and abnormal health outcome. However, if direct germinal epithelium damage is being considered as the mechanism of action, there is potential selection bias because the population existing in the workplace at the time of study may not be representative of the work force during the time of prior exposure. The **case-control study** is most appropriate for evaluating relatively rare diseases in large populations (eg, birth defects or childhood cancers). Because the outcome of interest is specified at the onset, the continuum of reproductive effects which may result from a given exposure cannot be evaluated. The **cohort study** is the preferred study design for most reproductive outcomes. A prospective cohort study allows specific measures of an exposure and potential confounders to be ascertained at the etiologically relevant time periods. In addition, a cohort design allows repeated measurements to be conducted of tests (eg, semen analysis), which tend to have relatively high individual variability.

The cohort and case-control studies are considered hypothesis-testing studies and are usually conducted after a possible association has been suggested by previous observations or a documented group exposure. For example, an acute clinician may recognize a series of cases which seem to have a factor in common. This situation is most likely to occur with a rare disease or new syndrome and was instrumental in identifying associations such as thalidomide and severe limb defects, and DES and vaginal clear cell carcinoma. A reported cluster of adverse outcomes occurring in a group of people is a common way for environmental and occupational problems to be brought to attention, but such clusters often remain unexplained upon further investigation.

Valuable data could be obtained from surveillance systems, but there are few established systems in place for adverse reproductive outcomes other than birth defects. Reasons for this include the fact that not all outcomes attract medical attention or require hospitalization (eg, semen abnormalities, SABs, and subfertility). As a result, these outcomes are more difficult to ascertain and are associated with less financial impact for society.

### Exposure Assessment

Although the methods used to measure occupational or environmental exposure are beyond the scope of this chapter, a brief overview with issues specific to evaluating male exposure associated with reproductive outcomes will be presented. In addition, it should be kept in mind that the exposures of three individuals may be involved (eg, each parent and the embryo/fetus/offspring).

To affect fertility or spermatogenesis, an agent must reach the appropriate organs via the blood stream (eg, chemical agent) or physical change (eg, radiation or excessive heat). Some chemicals react with the first tissues they encounter, such as the lungs or skin, and are not absorbed into the blood stream unless they are ingested (eg, acids, chlorine, and asbestos). Unless a chronic exposure results in a steady-state level in the body, the rapidity with which a substance is cleared can also affect its toxicity. Often, these issues are beyond the scope of epidemiological studies but should be considered within the overall body of evidence about the toxicity of a substance.

In epidemiological studies, exposures can be ascertained from interviews, existing records, or biomarkers. If exposure history is obtained by retrospective **interview**, there is the possibility of biased recall among cases or misclassification due to lack of monitoring records or diminished memory. Recall may be affected by changes in exposures. Ascertainment of current exposure status for cohort studies limits possible recall bias, but men may not be aware of all their exposures. In interview studies, asking one spouse about the other may not provide sufficiently accurate information.

**Existing records** often do not provide detailed information, but rather serve to group men broadly. For example, the residence listed on a birth certificate might be used to assign the likelihood of an environmental exposure. However, residence at delivery may not reflect residence of the father, nor does it account for individual differences, such as how much time is spent out of the area at work. Similarly, occupational registries may be used to group men by broad exposures, but specific work-site practices will be unknown. The most accurate occupational exposures would be obtained by an industrial hygienist, but such studies are also likely to cost more or be limited in sample size to allow for more detailed study.

**Laboratory measurement** of exposure may be done in a prospective study, or on stored biological samples, and provides a quantification of exposure that is less likely to be biased. Techniques for measuring environmental levels have been developed for many agents including radon, electromagnetic fields, solvents, pesticides, and dust levels. Measurements on biological samples provide an indication of internal dose, which would be more biologically relevant. A number of difficulties can arise with these types of studies, including small sample size or selection bias due to the higher costs and greater participation required of subjects. Sampling at one point in time may not reflect the critical exposure period, particularly if the substance is cleared rapidly.

As noted earlier, it is important to consider the timing of exposure in an epidemiological study. An association with an exposure at the critical time is more relevant and such information may be useful for excluding the possibility of a particular effect if the timing is wrong. In addition to timing, a dose-response relationship is usually examined.

In summary, exposure assessment in epidemiological studies may involve problems with unknown exposure levels, unknown biological indicators, poor sources of information on exposure, imprecise exposure timing, and complication with multifactorial exposure sources.

### Biological Outcomes

There is variable quality in the detection and mea-

**Table 26–2.** List of sample sizes needed to detect a twofold increase for selected reproductive outcomes.[1] Sample size refers to the number of study units (men, pregnancies, or livebirths) evenly divided between exposed and nonexposed groups with an alpha of 0.05 and a beta of 0.20 (80% power).

| Outcome | Sample Size Needed | Unit |
|---|---|---|
| Infertility | 322 | Couples |
| Fetal loss (spontaneous abortions and stillbirths) | 322 | Pregnancies |
| Low birthweight (<2500 g) | 586 | Livebirths |
| Major congenital malformation | 631 | Livebirths |
| Severe mental retardation | 8,986 | Livebirths |

[1]Compiled from multiple sources, including vital records reports, California Birth Defects Monitoring Program and Guidelines for Studies of Human Populations Exposed to Mutagenic and Reproductive Hazards, Bloom (editor). Definition of terms in section on Reproductive Outcomes and Rates.

surement of biological end points for male reproductive toxicity studies. For specific male reproductive conditions and male-mediated reproductive outcomes, the range of conditions includes sexual dysfunction, endocrine changes, semen abnormalities, chromosomal anomalies, infertility, and abnormalities in the fetus and offspring. The spectrum of birth outcome end points are discussed in the Chapter 25. Case ascertainment methods can include the following: birth certificates, hospital records, surveillance programs (eg, birth defects registries), medical insurance forms, reproductive history questionnaires and semen analyses. The latter two methods tend to be the most useful type of case ascertainment because of relatively more precise male information as opposed to the usually inadequate paternal information found in birth outcome records.

## Statistical Issues

For selected reproductive end points, the needed number of study participants for adequate statistical power is shown in Table 26–2 and Table 26–3. One advantage of conducting studies of semen analysis is that relatively fewer participants are needed and there is a direct measurement of the abnormality being studied (eg, abnormal number, motility, and shape of sperm). It should be noted that the general population normal ranges for these semen end points are inadequate because of differences in laboratory proficiency and techniques. It is preferable to test for internal trend within a given worker group or community group or to obtain an appropriate control group. Although fewer participants are needed for semen studies, there may be a problem in selecting the most appropriate reference group.

## Confounding Factors

Potential confounders need to be considered in the evaluation of men exposed to occupational or environmental reproductive hazards. For a factor to be a confounder, it must be related to both the end point and the exposure in the study of interest. Lack of control for a known confounder in prior studies does not imply the study is deficient if the investigators found this factor did not act as a confounder in their study or had reason to believe the factor would not be associated with the exposure of interest. Potential confounding factors in male reproductive studies include the following: personal characteristics (paternal age), medical conditions (recent infection, trauma to the gonads, impaired autoimmune status, high fever, mumps orchitis, diabetes, prostatitis, varicocele, and hydrocele), drugs (marijuana, estrogen, chlorambucil, cyclophosphamide, and nitrofurantoin), and habits (tobacco, alcohol, and frequent saunas or hot tub use). In conducting occupational studies, a potential confounder may be an environmental agent such as exposure to solvents, metals, pesticides, excess heat, ionizing radiation, and neurotoxins in nonworkplace settings. Conversely, one needs to assess workplace hazards when conducting community-based reproductive studies.

**Table 26–3.** Sample size needed for semen parameter outcomes with a 5% significance test and 80% power to detect a 25% change in the mean value between exposed and nonexposed men.[1]

| Outcome | Sample Size Needed | Unit |
|---|---|---|
| Sperm count | 214 | Men |
| Sperm morphology | 26 | Men |

[1]Derived from Guidelines for Studies of Human Populations Exposed to Mutagenic and Reproductive Hazards, Bloom (editor).

## SELECTED EXAMPLES OF REPRODUCTIVE HAZARDS

Few chemicals have been adequately studied in terms of their reproductive effects. Only about 5% of agents used in industry have been assessed. Most exposure standards are not based on reproductive effects. More evidence is available from animal than human studies, but direct extrapolation to the human cannot always be made. Although epidemiological studies can be more difficult to interpret because of the methodological issues described earlier, a number of potential reproductive or developmental hazards have been identified (Table 26–4). The agents that have been shown conclusively to be reproductive toxicants in humans (other than medications) are few and include dibromochloropropane (DBCP), ionizing radiation, and lead.

Recently, much discussion has been given to reports of the general decline in semen quality over the past several decades. Several studies have noted an alleged decrease in sperm count with one report going back as far as 50 years. In addition, one study reported a concurrent decrease in motility and normally formed sperm for a 20-year period: mean sperm concentration decreased by 2.1% per year (89 million/mL in 1973 to 60 million/mL in 1992) and concurrent annual decrease of percent motile (0.6% per year) and percent normal morphology (0.5% per year). Over time, the method for evaluating sperm count (unlike the other semen quality parameters) has not changed and is thought to be less susceptible to chronological differences in laboratory technique. This decline in semen quality has coincided with reports of increased rates of testicular cancer and cryptorchidism in certain countries (eg, France and the United Kingdom, respectively). Possible explanations that have been given for this decline include: estrogen exposure in utero, diet, lifestyle factors, and environmental pollution due to the increased world-

**Table 26–4.** Human evidence[1] for adverse male reproductive effects of selected agents.

| Agent | Human Outcomes | Strength of Data[2] |
|---|---|---|
| Alcohol | Azoospermia, testicular atrophy | + |
| Boron | Oligospermia | + |
| Cadmium | Reduced fertility | + |
| Carbon disulfide | Oligospermia, asthenospermia, and teratospermia | ++ |
| Carbaryl | Teratospermia | + |
| Chlordecone[3] | Oligospermia, asthenospermia, and teratospermia | ++ |
| Chloroprene | Asthenospermia, teratospermia, and decreased libido | ++ |
| Dibromochloropropane[3] | Azoospermia, oligospermia, and hormonal changes | ++ |
| 2,4-Dichlorophenoxyacetic acid (2,4-D) | Oligospermia and teratospermia | + |
| DDT (dichlorodiphenyl-trichloroethane)[3] | Detected in semen of infertile men | + |
| Estrogens | Oligospermia | ++ |
| 2-Ethoxyethanol | Oligospermia and teratospermia | + |
| Ethylene dibromide[3] | Oligospermia, asthenospermia, and teratospermia | + |
| Ethylene glycol ethers | Oligospermia | + |
| Excessive heat | Oligospermia | ++ |
| Lead | Oligospermia, teratospermia, and asthenospermia | ++ |
| Manganese | Decreased libido and impotence | + |
| Mercury, inorganic | Decreased libido and impotence | + |
| Microwave radiation | Decreased sperm count and motility | + |
| Radiation, ionizing | Decreased sperm count | ++ |
| Radiation, microwave | Oligospermia and asthenospermia | + |
| Vinyl chloride | Decreased libido and impotence | + |

[1]Compiled from multiple sources, including Guidelines for Studies of Human Populations Exposed to Mutagenic and Reproductive Hazards, Bloom (editor); Reproductive and Developmental Hazards. Case Studies in Environmental Medicine #19, Welch LS, Paul M: Occupational and Environmental Reproductive Hazards: A Guide for Clinicians (see references).
[2]Notation: ++ = strong evidence, + = limited evidence.
[3]Use banned in the United States.
Definition of terms in section on Reproductive Outcomes and Rates.

wide use of chemicals (especially compounds with estrogen-like activity). Some researchers reject these conclusions because the patients in these studies are mostly semen donors, vasectomy candidates, or infertility clinic patients and thus not representative of the general male population. In light of the conflicting scientific opinions, it would be useful to identify a geographically defined target group of men that can be periodically sampled in the future so that the potential for selection bias is diminished.

The majority of toxic agents in Table 26–4 have been examined in occupational settings where exposures tend to be higher than those encountered in the environment and relatively easier to document. In general, most occupational crises with documented adverse reproductive effects have involved male workers (eg, dibromochloropropane, exogenous estrogens, and kepone). However, known reproductive hazards have been also encountered environmentally from long-term use and disposal by industry as well as acute releases. The following section will highlight three examples from the literature.

## Dibromochloropropane

DBCP (1,2-Dibromo-3-chloroporpane) is noteworthy as the first documented outbreak of a male reproductive hazard in the workplace. DBCP is a nematocide that is associated with reproductive and developmental abnormalities in animals. These animal effects include oligospermia, asthenospermia, and testicular and seminiferous tubule atrophy. Workers exposed to DBCP in chemical production facilities have shown exposure-dependent testicular toxicity. The following associations have been noted in DBCP exposed workers: azoospermia, oligospermia, increased plasma FSH levels, and histological abnormalities of the testicular tissue (decrease or absence of germ cells in seminiferous tubules). Decreased fertility was experienced among workers with testicular changes and the most extreme FSH elevations were found in workers who did not recover after a period of no exposure. Thus, this compound represents one of the few well-established male reproductive toxicants and provided the stimulus for subsequent increased activity in male-mediated reproductive research in the work setting.

## Lead

Lead is one of the most studied occupational and environmental agents and has a broad range of effects on multiple organ systems. Male reproductive effects have been found with both organic and inorganic lead exposures. Organic lead compounds, unlike the inorganic form, can be absorbed dermally. Sexual dysfunction (decreased libido, abnormal erectile function, and premature ejaculation) has been noted in case reports after ingestion of fuels containing organic lead. A case series of tetraethyl lead intoxicated men revealed reversible semen abnormalities: oligospermia,

azoospermia, asthenospermia, and teratospermia. Inorganic lead case reports have noted decreased libido, (including erectile problems) and abnormal ejaculations. Endocrine changes (decreased testosterone and increased LH levels) have been observed in clinic-based case series. In men not exposed to high levels of lead, detectable sperm lead concentrations have been reported that are less than that found in whole blood but greater than that of serum.

Epidemiological studies have utilized semen analyses to better quantify male reproductive outcomes. A cross-sectional survey of 150 male lead battery workers was conducted in Romania. Blood lead levels ranged from 23 to 75 µg/dL with a mean lead exposure duration of 3.5 years. Oligospermia, asthenospermia, and teratospermia were noted in a dose-response fashion. There were certain methodological problems with this study: (1) Both masturbation and coitus interruptus were allowed in semen collection. The latter method is not normally accepted because of the potential of semen mixing with the body fluids of the partner; (2) No environmental exposure data was presented; (3) The dose-response curve was constructed allowing multiple results from the same subject; and (4) The controls included 50 plant technicians and office workers who were not assessed for comparability. This study provided the basis for the consideration of reproductive effects in establishing the OSHA lead standard.

Lead exposure was evaluated among 18 battery workers and 18 cement workers in Italy. There was a statistically significant decrease in median sperm count and increase in prevalence of oligospermia for the battery workers. Participation rates were low, with 47% for the exposed and 22% for the comparison group. The exposed group had a mean BLL of 61 µg/dL and mean ZPP of 208 µg/dL. In contrast, the nonexposed group had a mean BLL of 18 and a mean ZPP of 24. Oligospermia was noted at a BLL as low as 40 µg/dL.

In summary, semen abnormalities (oligospermia, asthenospermia, and teratospermia) have been detected in the range of 40–139 µg/dL. Also, hormonal disturbances have been documented for men at BLLs as low as 44 µg/dL (testosterone), and 10 µg/dL (FSH and/or LH). Because the current OSHA Lead Standards (general industry and construction) require the removal of workers from workplace exposures when BLLs reach 50 µg/dL, there may not be adequate protection of those men trying to conceive children. Consideration needs to be given to the lowering of the medical removal BLL to a safer concentration. In 1990, the National Institute for Occupational Safety and Health (NIOSH) set a national goal to eliminate worker exposures resulting in BBLs in excess of 25 µg/dL by the year 2000. There should be adequate counseling and guidance that addresses these concerns for the male (and female) worker intending to attempt conception.

## Ionizing Radiation

Recent interest in the male reproductive hazards of ionizing radiation is the result of a study in the United Kingdom. The study found that childhood leukemia was associated with paternal employment at a nuclear power plant (relatively low ionizing radiation exposure except for periodic acute unintentional releases). One potential problem in the dose reconstruction for the study is that only cumulative external radiation was measured with no assessment of internal emitters (radiation source resulting from internally deposited radioactive material unintentionally ingested or inhaled) as part of the potential body burden among the exposed male workers. The highest risk occurred in fathers with a total dose of > 10 mSv (one milliSeivert is equivalent to one rad) during the six months prior to conception and for fathers with a total lifetime dose of > 100 mSv (10 rads) prior to conception.

Tissues with rapidly dividing cells, such as the testicular germinal epithelium, tend to be more sensitive to ionizing radiation. In rat studies, paternal exposure to high doses (360–5040 mSv) has induced malignancies, primarily lymphocytic leukemia, in the first and second generation progeny. Animal studies have demonstrated the following effects resulting from ionizing radiation exposure: paternal exposure and subsequent altered sperm in male progeny, DNA damage, testicular growth retardation and necrosis, oligospermia, and decreased breeding activity.

Various human case reports also suggest male reproductive effects from ionizing radiation: atrophy and sclerosis of testicular germinal epithelium in a radiologist working in 1923 with very high exposure levels; brief periods of sterility in men after extensive exposure to 10–15 rads; temporary azoospermia associated with levels of 100–200 rads, and permanent azoospermia at 200–600 rads. Two eastern European studies reported significantly increased reproductive effects (oligospermia and asthenospermia) in male workers exposed to ionizing radiation. A Romanian study found significant increases in the prevalence of oligospermia, asthenospermia, and teratospermia among exposed workers. The exposures ranged from 0.48–3.5 rads and lasted from 2–22 years. These latter two studies were clinical series that evaluated highly exposed workers using traditional semen analysis techniques and which lacked any description of the control group being used.

The current mean annual dose of less than 41 mSv (4.1 rads) is seen in federal radiation processing plants in the United States. Thus, an epidemiological study using more precise exposure and male reproductive outcome measurements would be needed to assess the risk to current workers who are exposed to relatively lower levels than those found in the literature.

## REPRODUCTIVE ASSESSMENT

The medical evaluation of the patient with a potential exposure to a reproductive hazard follows the traditional components of history taking, physical examination, and laboratory assessment with an emphasis on both health and exposure parameters. In addition, special consideration is needed in the assessment, communication, and management of reproductive risk for the patient.

## MEDICAL EVALUATION

In the clinical setting, infertility is defined as an inability to conceive after 12 months of unprotected intercourse. Potential causes for infertility in the female include: ovulatory dysfunction, tubal or pelvic factors, and uterine or cervical factors. It is estimated that the cause of infertility is due to male factors in 40% of the affected couples, female factors in 40–50%, and no known etiology in 10–20%. For the infertility and adverse pregnancy outcome work-up, the female partner needs to be assessed concurrently (see Female Reproductive Toxicology Chapter). A full discussion of the diagnosis and treatment of various urological and other related medical conditions is beyond the scope of this chapter. However, the following is a general overview of the types of evaluation techniques that can be utilized to assess the male reproductive system.

### Reproductive History

The patient interview should cover the following areas: demographic data (eg, both maternal and paternal age if birth outcome is being assessed), general medical history (eg, febrile illnesses, trauma, infections and structural abnormalities of the genitourinary system, and past surgeries), drug use (including medications, street drugs, alcohol, and tobacco), habits (eg, saunas and hot tubs usage), work history, and reproductive history (eg, past problems of infertility, and pregnancies and birth outcomes for each sexual partner). It is important to ask about potential occupational and environmental exposure to any known or suspect reproductive hazards cited in Table 26–4.

### Physical Examination

This examination should focus on the physical integrity of the genital system to rule out any extraneous mass or abnormality, and the presence of secondary sex traits. A physical abnormality may impede spermatogenesis, ejaculation, and erection (eg, varicocele, hydrocele, hypospadias, and cryptorchism). It is important to evaluate testicular size, prostate tenderness, and the presence of any structural anomalies. Testicular size averages 4.6 cm in length and 12–25 mL in volume, with the seminiferous tubules accounting for 95% of the testicular volume. Hypovirilization and infertility can indicate Klinefelter's syndrome (47, XYY, often associated with small testes and occurring in 0.2% of adult men) or viral orchitis.

### Hormonal Profile

A variety of hormonal tests are available and selection needs to be based on the medical conditions under consideration. A preliminary hormonal profile that can be obtained for field surveys includes the following: FSH and LH (pituitary function) and testosterone (testicular function). For field biological monitoring surveys, blood samples are relatively easy to collect for hormonal assays, but care must be taken to obtain samples at standardized times to avoid diurnal variability problems. The FSH is decreased in individuals with azoospermia, such as the DBCP episode. With a normal testosterone and an increased FSH, a decrease in spermatogenesis will occur and is usually associated with severe germinal epithelium damage. If there is a sperm abnormality with normal LH and testosterone, then an obstruction to the reproductive system can be ruled out. If both LH and testosterone are low, then a hypothalamic or pituitary abnormality is likely. When there is a high level of testosterone and a low level of LH, an autonomous or exogenous source of testosterone needs to be considered. Finally, having both LH and testosterone elevated would suggest an autonomous LH secretion or resistance to testosterone action.

### Semen Analysis

Analysis of semen parameters can be conducted by both traditional and computer-aided semen analysis (CASA) methods. The basic parameters of interest are ejaculate volume, sperm count or concentration, motility, morphology, swim velocity (direct measurement obtainable via CASA), and the presence of any suspect toxicant. The subsequent normal ranges discussed are to be used as general guidelines for the interpretation of a semen profile. There is much variability in the quality of semen analysis by laboratory and the CASA may not be available at all reproductive/infertility laboratories. Since the normal ranges for semen characteristics may vary by laboratory, it is important to review the ranges provided by the laboratory being used.

The sperm concentration refers to the number of sperm per milliliter of ejaculate, with a normal range of 20–250 mill/mL. Normal ejaculate volumes are 2–6 mL. Sperm motility is the percentage of motile sperm, with a normal sample showing greater than 40% motile sperm. When using CASA, the normal sperm velocity is approximately greater than 24 μm/sec. Morphology refers to the percentage of normal (oval) and abnormal sperm head, midpiece, and tail shapes. The 10 general categories of sperm morphology include oval/normal, microcephalic, macrocephalic, tapered head, double head, headless, no head or tail, amorphous head, immature forms, and abnormal tails. Normal morphology is greater than 50% normally shaped sperm.

When semen analyses are used for epidemiological or screening purposes, certain aspects need to be addressed. There is a need to conduct concurrent motility and count measures, because most cells are nonmotile or poorly motile. Thus, sperm count alone is not recommended. For count and motility, it is very important to note time since last ejaculation (48–72 hours maximum for accurate reading). It is important to conduct all semen analyses at the same laboratory because of the high inter-laboratory variability. Optimally, a semen sample should be analyzed within one hour of production so that the sperm remain viable for analysis. A standardized semen collection procedure needs to be established and followed by the individual being evaluated. Masturbation is recommended (preferably with no sexual partner, condom, or lubricant use), with the collection of semen in specially provided containers. It is extremely important that the entire volume of ejaculate be collected and that the specimen not be subjected to extreme temperatures in transport to the analysis site. Multiple samples from the same individual can show much variability; therefore, serial measurements are preferred. Most infertility evaluations involve three subsequent samples on separate days. Finally, there are potential barriers to cooperation from individuals being recruited for participation in a study: (1) Highly motivated subjects are needed for the study, yet the individual is usually asymptomatic and may not understand the usefulness of an evaluation; (2) Religious and cultural taboos may be encountered; and (3) There may be a lack of available sperm due to a pre-existing medical condition such as vasectomy or impotency.

### Other Tests

Other male reproductive tests are available for further evaluation but are not usually included in epidemiological field studies. These tests include, but are not limited to, the following: GnRH challenge, thyroid profile, testicular biopsy, postcoital test, sperm-oocyte interaction, and anti-sperm antibodies. In azoospermia or severe oligospermia, a testicular biopsy can assess the seminiferous tubules and Leydig cell histology for fibrosis and lack of spermatogenesis. The postcoital test involves the interaction of sperm examined in mucus following intercourse. If the index sperm penetrates a donor mucus but not the sexual partner's mucus, the mucus of the sexual partner may be a problem. The patient's sperm is considered abnormal if no penetration of either mucus occurs. The sperm-oocyte interaction test uses the zona pellucida of a hamster oocyte to evaluate if the patient's sperm is able to fuse (the capacitation and acrosomal reaction needed for eventual conception). Anti-sperm antibodies on the sperm surface are a form of immunologic infertility and are sometimes a result of prior surgical reversal of a vasectomy. Furthermore, a wide range of medical tests and assays may be indicated for the underlying medical conditions thought to be present. Lastly, the assessment of body burden for certain exposures may be estimated via exhaled breath, blood, urine, and other biological tissue measurements.

## RISK ASSESSMENT

As described earlier, the risk assessment process follows four basic steps: (1) **Hazard identification** of any hazardous agents being used by patient. This includes review of the patient history and collection of pertinent MSDS document and product labels; (2) **Hazard evaluation** to determine whether a given substance or physical agent is a reproductive hazard. This involves the utilization of technical informational sources to access the appropriate medical and scientific literature. If no reproductive information is found in the scientific literature, it is important to consider other health end points as indication of human toxicity; (3) **Exposure assessment**, performed by estimating the level of exposure via patient work history, potential routes of exposure, nature and pattern of symptoms, industrial hygiene data, and biological monitoring results; and (4) **Risk categorization** with respect to the reproductive system. This activity is based on information gathered in the first three steps and considers the following factors: toxicity, timing and extent of exposure, potency, severity of outcome, and degree of uncertainty in animal and human studies.

Oftentimes, not all of the needed information is available and an educated guess is necessary. It is very helpful to have established contacts for additional consultation when a more difficult risk assessment is involved. Potential contacts include: local or state health departments, university medical centers, poison control centers, NIOSH, EPA, ATSDR, OSHA, and the Association of Occupational and Environmental Clinics. Access to on-line literature data bases is very useful (eg, REPRORISK, REPROTOX, and TERIS; see References).

## RISK COMMUNICATION

Building on the information gathered during the risk assessment process, risk communication is the logical follow-up by which the involved person or persons obtain the information needed to make informed and independent decisions about health and safety risks. In general, there is an underlying principle that needs to be acknowledged and sensitively dealt with: the threat or actual fact of reproductive dysfunction or adverse reproductive outcome has a profound impact on an individual's life. All questions must be answered truthfully and completely. A description of the limitations in knowledge may be needed. The timing of exposure for the male and of the first contact with the involved female partner is very important. Whenever possible, the risk communication is conducted prior to actual exposure in order to intervene at the primary prevention stage. The options available for the male worker should be presented in such a way that the medical impact as well as the economic consequences of decisions are understood and discussed. The medical confidentiality of the involved individual should be maintained at all costs. It is imperative that the employer, involved employee(s), and medical consultant work together in resolving a particular situation, as well as in developing a general policy on reproductive hazards in the workplace that involves both genders. Ideally, this policy should be developed within a safety committee composed of representatives from management and labor, and consultants in occupational medicine and industrial hygiene.

## RISK MANAGEMENT

Once the risk assessment and risk communication have occurred, risk management completes the sequence. In order of priority, the following actions may be considered for a given reproductive hazard situation: (1) **Exposure reduction or elimination**: Replace hazards with safer ones; improved engineering controls, safer work practices, and personal protective equipment (this should not be the primary mode of protection—emphasis should be placed on the other actions). Exposure reduction or elimination is the most desirable option and should be attempted in all situations where a reproductive hazard exists; (2) **Temporary job transfer**: Remove individual from work environment where reproductive hazard exists. This option is very rarely performed for men considering having children. Problems may occur when there is no nonexposed job location. This option should be considered when there is a high risk situation and exposure reduction/elimination is not possible; (3) **Disability leave**: This option usually is considered by the personal physician for the pregnant woman facing reproductive hazards; and (4) **Remove individual from work**: This is the least desirable action and is usually reserved for the female worker. For female workers, it is illegal for an employer to terminate an affected woman due to pregnancy. An individual may choose to quit work because of personal reasons, but it is important to help the individual evaluate all the other options and to understand the possible consequences. This option is to be considered only if all the other options have been explored and the individual is comfortable with the possible consequences.

# LEGAL ISSUES
# & WORKPLACE STANDARDS

In the lawsuit involving International Union, UAW versus Johnson Controls, Inc., the United States Supreme Court held that an employer violated Title VII's ban on sex discrimination by excluding all women who could not prove their sterility from production jobs in a lead-battery factory. The Court indicated that a policy directed only at fertile women is overt discrimination on the basis of sex regardless of the scientific evidence of heightened safety concerns for mothers or potential mothers. In addition, any policies or actions taken by the employer must not violate existing laws prohibiting discrimination on the basis of pregnancy, childbirth, or related medical conditions. Employers cannot require that an individual be sterilized as a condition of employment. If an employee disabled by pregnancy, childbirth, or a related medical condition transfers to a less hazardous job, an employer must allow her to return to her original job or a similar one when the disability has resolved. Thus, the workplace must be made safe and reproductive hazard information must be provided for both men and women.

OSHA has the mandate to promulgate standards that protect workers from adverse health effects (including reproductive effects) resulting from workplace hazards. However, there are only four agents with OSHA standards based partially on reproductive effects: dibromochloropropane (DBCP), lead, ethylene oxide, and ionizing radiation. It should be recognized that many chemical and physical agents found in the workplace are not covered by an OSHA standard and those standards that do exist for the most part are not based on reproductive end points. This is why the risk assessment process discussed earlier should be implemented at any work site that has potential reproductive hazards present.

# REFERENCES

### DIBROMOCHLOROPROPANE

Agency for Toxic Substances and Disease Registry (ATSDR): Toxicological Profile for Dibromochloropropanes: 1,2-Dibromo-3-chloropropane. US Department of Health and Human Services, 1991.

Levy BS (editor): Dibromochloropropane. Intl J Occup Environ Health 1997;3(4):special issue.

Potashnik G, Porath A: Dibromochloropropane (DBCP): A 17-year reassessment of testicular function and reproductive performance. J Occup Environ Med 1995; 37(11):1287.

### LEAD

Alexander BH et al: Semen quality of men employed at a lead smelter. Occup Environ Med 1996;53(6): 411.

ATSDR (Agency for Toxic Substances and Disease Registry): Toxicological profile for lead. ATSDR, US Public Health Service, Publ. No. TP-92-12,1993.

Bonde JP: The risk of male subfecundity attributable to welding of metals. Int J Androl 1993;(Suppl 1):1.

Gennart JP et al: Fertility of male workers exposed to cadmium, lead, or manganese. Am J Epidemiol 1992; 135:1208.

Todd AC et al: Unraveling the chronic toxicity of lead: An essential priority for environmental health. Environ Health Perspect 1996;104(1):141.

### OTHER AGENTS

Egeland GM et al: Total serum testosterone and gonadotrophins in workers exposed to dioxin. Am J Epidemiol 1994;139(3):272.

Gardner MJ et al: Results of a case-control study of leukemia and lymphoma among young people near Sellafield nuclear plant in West Cumbria. Br Med J 1990;300:423.

Gilbert ES et al: Analyses of combined mortality data on workers at the Hanford Site, Oak Ridge National Laboratory, and Rocky Flats Nuclear Weapons Plant. Rad Res 1989;120:19.

### RISK ASSESSMENT AND COMMUNICATION

Ahlborg G et al: Assessment of reproductive risk at work. Intl J Occ Env Health 1996;2(1):59.

Taskinen H, Viskum S: Communication concerning the risks of occupational exposures in pregnancy. Intl J Occ Env Health 1996;2(1):64.

### SEMEN QUALITY IN THE GENERAL POPULATION

Auger J et al: Decline in semen quality among fertile men in Paris during the past 20 years. N Engl J Med 1995;332(5):281.

Carlsen E et al: Declining semen quality and increasing incidence of testicular cancer: Is there a common cause? Environ Health Perspect 1995;103(7):137.

Giwercman A et al: Evidence for increasing incidence of abnormalities of the human testis: A review. Environ Health Perspect 1993;101(Suppl 2):65.

Irvine DS: Falling sperm quality. Br Med J 1994;309: 476.

## GENERAL REFERENCES

Bonde JP, Giwercman A, Ernst E: Identifying environmental risk to male reproductive function by occupational sperm studies. Occup Environ Med 1996; 53(8):922.

Lahdetie J: Occupational- and exposure-related studies on human sperm. J Occup Environ Med 1995;37(8):922.

Negro-Vilar A: Stress and other environmental factors affecting fertility in men and women. Environ Health Perspect 1993;24:587.

Paul M: *Occupational and Environmental Reproductive Hazards: A Guide for Clinicians.* Williams & Wilkins, 1993.

Scialli AR, Zinaman MJ (editors): *Reproductive Toxicology and Infertility.* McGraw-Hill, 1993.

Tas S, Lauwerys R, Lison D: Occupational hazards for the male reproductive system. Crit Rev Toxicol 1996; 26(3):261.

Terracciano GJ, Lemasters GK, Amler RW (editors): Standardized Assessment of Birth Defects and Reproductive Disorders in Environmental Health Field Studies. ATSDR, Public Health Services, US Department of Health and Human Services, 1996.

Waalkes MP, Rehm S: Cadmium and prostate cancer. J Toxicol Environ Health 1994:43:251.

Welch LS: Reproductive and Developmental Hazards. Case Studies in Environmental Medicine #19. Agency for Toxic Substances and Disease Registries, US Department of Health and Human Services, 1993.

## GENERAL RESOURCE LIST

Agency for Toxic Substances and Disease Registry (ATSDR), Atlanta, Georgia, 770-639-0700. Develops and disseminates publications on health effects of toxic agents for health care providers.

Association of Occupational and Environmental Clinics (AOEC), 1010 Vermont Avenue NW, Washington DC 20005, 202-347-4976.

Environmental Protection Agency (EPA), 401 M Street SW, Washington DC 20460, 202-260-7751.

National Institute for Occupational Safety and Health (NIOSH), Information Hotline, Cincinnati, OH, 800-356-4674.

National Institute of Environmental Health Sciences (NIEHS), National Institutes of Health, PO Box 12233, Research Triangle Park, NC 27709, 919-541-3345.

Occupational Safety and Health Administration (OSHA), US Dept of Labor, 200 Constitution Avenue NW, Washington DC 20210, 202-249-8148. Establishes, enforces, and provides consultation regarding national occupational health and safety standards.

Reproductive Toxicology Center (REPROTOX), Columbia Hospital for Women Medical Center, 2425 L Street, NW, Washington DC 20037, 202-293-5137. Computer data base dealing with reproductive and developmental hazards

REPRORISK, Micromedex, Inc, 600 Grant Street, Denver, CO 80203, 303-831-1400. Computer data base dealing with reproductive and developmental hazards.

Teratogen Information System (TERIS), Dept of Pediatrics, TRIS WJ-10, University of Washington, Seattle, WA 98195, 206-543-2465. On-line access to data base and CD-ROM available.

# Section IV.
# Occupational Exposures

# Metals

27

*Richard Lewis, MD, MPH*

The diverse and valuable physical characteristics of metals have resulted in their extensive use in industry. These materials also bring a wide array of potential health hazards into the workplace and as such are of particular importance in occupational medicine. Metals are used in the construction, automotive, aerospace, electronics, and other manufacturing industries as well as in paints, pigments, plastics, and catalysts. Because of such widespread potential exposure, familiarity with the toxicity of metals is critical for the health and safety professional.

Metals exert biological effects chiefly through the formation of stable complexes with sulfhydryl groups and other ligands. These binding properties also form the basis for chelation therapy in the treatment of metal toxicity.

Metals are stable, which explains their wide use in structural materials. This stability also accounts for their pervasiveness in the workplace and in the environment generally. Biological reactivity of many metals results in accumulation in selective organs and tissues and in a potential for chronic toxicity. Meticulous attention to personal and workplace hygiene is essential for the reduction of chronic exposure and the prevention of health effects.

Metals are rarely used in their pure form, usually being present in alloys. They may also be bound to organic materials, which alters their physical characteristics and toxicity. Other forms, such as hydrides and carbonyls, are highly toxic and may be formed accidentally when the parent metal reacts with acids.

## Acute Metal Toxicity

Acute toxicity usually occurs after ingestion of metal-containing compounds or inhalation of high concentrations of metal fumes or gaseous metal compounds. In modern industrial operations, this type of exposure is unusual, often being due to unexpected chemical reactions or to burning or brazing in enclosed spaces. Awareness of the acute toxicity of metals, combined with a careful occupational history, will help in the detection of acute health effects that require specific treatment, such as chelation therapy.

Most metals can be measured in blood or urine to confirm the diagnosis of acute poisoning.

## Chronic Metal Toxicity

Research into the health effects of low-level exposure to metals continues to suggest that physiologic alterations may occur at levels that previously had been considered safe. Neurologic and neurophysiologic effects, nephrotoxicity, reproductive toxicity, teratogenicity (including behavioral alterations), and carcinogenicity remain at the forefront of current research. Medical surveillance and biological monitoring programs in industrial settings are important for determining acceptable levels of exposure. Prevention of chronic toxicity remains a challenge for workers exposed to metals, particularly lead.

## ALUMINUM

### Essentials of Diagnosis
- Respiratory/skin irritation.
- Chronic bronchitis and pulmonary fibrosis.
- ?Neurologic dysfunction.

### Exposure Limits
Metal dust/aluminum oxide
  ACGIH TLV: 10 mg/m$^3$ TWA
Welding fumes
  ACGIH TLV: 5 mg/m$^3$ TWA

### General Considerations
Aluminum is a lightweight metal with electrical conductive properties. Aluminum oxide ores are abundant in the earth's crust, with bauxite being the primary source of this raw material. Aluminum metal is produced through refining of ore and electrolytic reduction. Recycling of aluminum cans and containers is now a significant source of aluminum. This is a nonessential element in humans.

### Use
The light weight and ease of processing of aluminum have led to widespread application in auto

bodies, aircraft, tanks, and military equipment. A significant portion of aluminum is used for cans, containers, and wrapping. Aluminum siding is used in construction. Alumina (aluminum oxide) is used as a filler in ceramic materials. Aluminum chloride is used in antiperspirants. Other uses of aluminum compounds include pigments, paints, and catalysts. Medically, aluminum hydroxide is used as an antacid and has been used in the past to reduce phosphate accumulation in uremia.

## Occupational & Environmental Exposure

Exposure to aluminum occurs during welding of aluminum metal. Dust from handling of aluminum oxide powders is another important source of respiratory exposure. In the aluminum reduction industry, workers may be exposed to aluminum fume, as well as fluorides and polynuclear aromatic hydrocarbons.

## Absorption, Metabolism, & Elimination

Aluminum may be absorbed after inhalation of dust and fume. Gastrointestinal absorption is minimal, although accumulation and toxicity were observed after intake of high doses of aluminum hydroxide in persons with chronic renal failure. Urinary excretion is the primary route of elimination. The biological half-life is variable (days to months) and is dependent on the source and duration of exposure.

## Clinical Findings

**A. Symptoms and Signs:** Aluminum oxide and other aluminum dusts can cause drying and irritation of the eyes, nose, and throat. Nosebleeds may occur if exposures are excessive. Chronic inhalation of dusts and powders has been reported to cause pulmonary fibrosis. This has at times been related to the formation of granulomas. Increased respiratory symptoms, airway obstruction, and asthma may also occur in more heavily exposed workers and welders. In potroom workers, chronic obstructive lung disease and an excess risk of lung cancer may be related to exposure to polynuclear aromatic compounds, fluorides, or other irritants.

Excessive intake of aluminum compounds in uremia has been a cause of encephalopathy ("dialysis dementia") in patients with uremia. The association between aluminum accumulation in the brain and the development of Alzheimer's disease and other neurologic disorders remains controversial. While dose-dependent neurotoxicity has been demonstrated after oral intake of aluminum hydroxide, the relationships are less clear in occupational and environmental exposure settings. Medical use of aluminum compounds may also lead to osteomalacia.

**Laboratory Findings:** Laboratory testing may reveal either obstructive or restrictive deficits in pulmonary function. Chest x-rays may show nodules or granulomas or merely a diffuse increase in interstitial markings. Biological monitoring of either blood or urine levels may correlate with exposure. Results may be variable, however, and values have not been correlated with the risk of toxicity.

## Treatment

Removal from exposure is the primary treatment when potential health effects related to aluminum occur in the workplace. Deferoxamine has been used to treat dialysis dementia but is associated with side effects such as hypotension and skin rash.

## Prevention

Workers exposed to aluminum powders should use proper respiratory protection. Irritant symptoms are prevented through ventilation and dust control measures. Medical surveillance should include periodic assessment of respiratory symptoms, spirometry and chest x-rays.

# ANTIMONY

## Essentials of Diagnosis

*Acute effects:*
- Respiratory and mucous membrane irritation.
- Gastrointestinal distress.
- Dermatitis.
- Hemolysis and anuria (stibine gas).

*Chronic effects:*
- Pustular dermatitis.
- Pneumoconiosis.
- Electrocardiographic abnormalities.
- Lung cancer (antimony trioxide production).

## Exposure Limits

Antimony
   ACGIH TLV: 0.5 mg/m$^3$ TWA
   OSHA PEL: 0.5 mg/m$^3$ TWA
   NIOSH REL: 0.5 mg/m$^3$ TWA
Stibine
   ACGIH TLV: 0.1 ppm TWA
   OSHA PEL: 0.1 ppm TWA

## General Considerations

Antimony is a soft metal found as oxides and sulfides in a variety of ores. Antimony ores often contain significant quantities of arsenic and lead.

## Use

Pure antimony metal is used in the manufacture of semiconductor devices, both as a dopant compound for silicon and as a substrate material in the manufacture of intermediate crystals. Antimony alloys are used in the production of battery grids, type castings, bearings, and cable sheaths. Antimony compounds are also used in munitions, glass and pottery, fire retardants, paints and lacquers, rubber compounds, chemical catalysts, and solder. Antimonials have been used medicinally in the treatment of leishmaniasis, schistosomiasis, and filariasis.

## Occupational & Environmental Exposure

Mining and smelting operations have resulted in significant worker exposure to antimony dusts and fumes. These exposures have been complicated by concomitant exposure to lead, arsenic, and sulfur dioxide. Health effects attributed to exposure to antimony during refining and extraction include respiratory tract irritation, gastrointestinal complaints, dermatitis, and pneumoconiosis. Exposure to antimony trisulfide in the manufacture of abrasive grinding wheels has been associated with an increase in electrocardiographic abnormalities and sudden death among workers. Antimony trioxide and antimony trichloride, both used in the microelectronics industry, are strongly irritating to tissues and membranes.

Stibine gas ($SbH_3$), a hemolytic toxin similar to arsine, may be formed when antimony alloys are processed with certain reducing acids. Stibine is also used as a grain fumigant.

Parenteral administration of antimonial compounds for medicinal purposes has been associated with electrocardiographic changes, alterations in liver function, and hemolysis. Poisoning has also occurred after storage of acidic foods and beverages in containers lined with enamels containing antimony.

## Absorption, Metabolism, & Excretion

Soluble forms of antimony are readily absorbed after inhalation. Antimony is excreted largely in the urine. The trivalent form is excreted less rapidly than the pentavalent form as a result of red blood cell uptake.

Insoluble forms are excreted slowly in the urine and may be detectable years after exposure has ceased.

## Clinical Findings

### A. Symptoms and Signs:

**1. Acute exposure**–Acute exposure to antimony dusts and fumes causes intense irritation of the eyes, throat, and respiratory tract. Systemic toxicity may follow inhalation of dusts or fumes. Nausea, vomiting, abdominal pain, and bloody diarrhea may also be present. Inhalation of stibine causes headache, fatigue, abdominal pain, jaundice, and anuria due to massive hemolysis.

**2. Chronic exposure**–Chronic inhalation may result in dryness of the throat, dysosmia, and bronchitis as well as complaints of fatigue, headache, and anorexia. Complaints of dizziness may indicate a cardiac rhythm disturbance.

Chronic skin exposure to antimony compounds may cause pustular dermatitis. Other chronic effects include perforation of the nasal septum, bleeding gums, conjunctivitis, and laryngitis. Spontaneous abortions, menstrual disorders, and excretion of antimony in breast milk have been reported in exposed women.

Antimony is suspected of being a human carcinogen. Workers engaged in antimony trioxide production have been found to have an excess incidence of lung cancer. In addition, the high incidence of urinary bladder tumors in persons treated for schistosomiasis may be related to past treatment with antimonial agents.

### B. Laboratory Findings: The red cell county may be low. Hemoglobinuria and red blood cell casts are a sign of stibine-induced hemolysis and suggest acute renal and hepatic failure. Hepatitis is a rare but serious complication of antimonial drug therapy and could occur in settings where there is acute overexposure to other antimony compounds. Electrocardiographic changes after therapeutic use or industrial exposure include T wave changes and rhythm disturbances.

Acute inhalation of antimony trichloride has resulted in acute pulmonary edema with hypoxemia and diffuse pulmonary infiltrates. Rounded opacities in the mid lung fields on chest x-ray are consistent with pneumoconiosis in workers chronically exposed to antimony ores or dusts. Pulmonary function impairment may be present on spirometry related to either acute or chronic exposure.

The presence of antimony in urine is diagnostic of past exposure but does not necessarily correlate with severity of exposure or health effects. Urine concentrations in nonexposed individuals are generally less than 0.001 mg/L. In acute exposure (such as after intravenous therapy), levels may exceed 2 mg/L. Occupational exposures generally result in levels of 0.1–0.3 mg/L.

## Prevention

Personal protective devices should be worn where there is potential exposure to antimony dusts or fumes. Biological monitoring of urinary antimony levels confirms exposure and may be useful for diagnosis if markedly elevated in acute overexposure.

## Treatment

Pulmonary function and electrocardiographic monitoring are indicated when acute exposure is suspected (significant inhalation or ingestion). The occupational history will aid in the diagnosis of antimony poisoning, concentrating on acute releases of antimony fumes or vapors and work in confined spaces in patients with acute respiratory or systemic symptoms.

Irritant exposure to soluble antimony dusts or liquids is treated by removal from further exposure and cleansing of exposed skin. Chelation with dimercaprol or penicillamine is indicated when significant cardiovascular, pulmonary, or hepatic impairment occurs in patients with suspected acute exposure.

Stibine-induced hemolysis requires exchange transfusion.

## ARSENIC

### Essentials of Diagnosis

*Acute effects:*
- Nausea, vomiting, diarrhea.
- Intravascular hemolysis, jaundice, oliguria (arsine).
- Cardiovascular collapse.

*Chronic effects:*
- Hyperkeratosis and hyperpigmentation (melanosis).
- Peripheral neuropathy.
- Anemia.
- Cardiac and peripheral vascular disease.

### Exposure Limits

Arsenic
ACGIH TLV: 0.01 mg/m$^3$ TWA
OSHA PEL: 0.01 mg/m$^3$ TWA
NIOSH REL: 2 μg/m$^3$ ceiling (15 minutes)
Arsine
ACGIH TLV: 0.05 ppm TWA
OSHA PEL: 0.05 ppm TWA
NIOSH REL: 2 μg/m$^3$ ceiling (15 minutes)
ACGIH BEI: 50 μg/g creatinine

### General Considerations

Arsenic occurs in numerous ferrous and nonferrous ores. It is found in air, water, and food, and important industrial contributions are from smelting operations, pesticide use, and effluents from geothermal power plants. Arsenic is ubiquitous in living organisms, though it is not an essential trace element in humans.

The toxicity of arsenic varies greatly with the chemical state. Pure elemental arsenic and organic arsenic compounds (found in many seafoods) are virtually nontoxic, while trivalent arsenic trioxide and arsine gas are potent acute poisons.

### Use

Metallic arsenic is used as an alloy, primarily for hardening lead in battery grids, bearings, and cable sheaths. Arsenic trioxide and arsenic pentoxide are used in the manufacture of calcium, copper, and lead arsenate pesticides. Arsenic compounds are used as pigments and refining agents in glass and as preservatives in tanning and taxidermy. Copper acetoarsenite is used as a wood preservative. Arsenic compounds are also used as herbicides and desiccants for cotton harvesting. Arsanilic acid is used in veterinary pharmaceuticals and feed additives. Arsine gas and other arsenic compounds are used in the microelectronics industry, as a source of dopant arsenic atoms, and in the manufacture of gallium arsenide substrates.

### Occupational & Environmental Exposure

Exposure to arsenic compounds, primarily in the form of arsenic trioxide, occurs in the smelting of lead, copper, gold and other nonferrous metals. Readily volatilized arsenic trioxide is concentrated in flue dust and can be condensed and recovered in a cooling chamber. Furnace and flue maintenance operations carry a high risk of exposure. Arsenic may also be found in fly ash from coal boilers and present a hazard during maintenance operations. Pesticide manufacture and smelting operations have resulted in substantial contamination of the air and water in surrounding communities.

Metal workers may be exposed to airborne arsenic trioxide or to arsine. Workers engaged in the manufacture and application of arsenical pesticides, herbicides, and preservatives have the potential for significant arsenic exposure. Forestry and farm workers may be exposed to residual arsenic compounds after their use in the field. In the microelectronics industry, workers may be exposed to arsenic in handling source materials or finished product or in maintenance operations. Arsine exposure may also occur in this industry, but it is usually controlled through the use of closed systems. Arsine may be formed accidentally when nascent hydrogen is formed in the presence of arsenic or when water or acid reacts with metal arsenides. Pharmaceutical manufacturers may be exposed to arsanilic acid and other arsenic compounds.

Nonoccupational exposure has resulted from ingestion of contaminated well water, dried milk, soy sauce, and moonshine whiskey. Dietary intake is related to pesticide residues, feed additives, and bioaccumulation of arsenic in marine organisms. Organic arsenic compounds present in seafood are not metabolized and are excreted unchanged. Exposure may occur through burning of arsenic-treated wood and from smoking cigarettes made of tobacco sprayed with arsenical pesticides.

### Absorption, Metabolism, & Excretion

Arsenic compounds are absorbed after ingestion or inhalation. Skin absorption is limited. The arsenic is readily taken up by red blood cells and then deposited in the liver, kidney, muscle, bone, skin, and hair. Trivalent arsenic (+3) avidly binds to sulfhydryl groups and interferes with numerous enzyme systems, including those involved in cellular respiration, glutathione metabolism, and DNA repair. This binding also accounts for the persistence of arsenic in the hair and nails. Pentavalent arsenic (+5) and arsine are converted to trivalent arsenic in vivo. The majority of the absorbed trivalent arsenic is metabolized to dimethylarsinic acid (DMA) and monomethylarsonic acid (MMA) and excreted in the urine with a half-life of 10 hours. Organic arsenic compounds are excreted unchanged in the urine.

## Clinical Findings

### A. Symptoms and Signs:

**1. Acute exposure–**Symptoms of acute arsenic poisoning may develop minutes to hours after ingestion and consist of nausea, vomiting, abdominal pain, and copious blood-tinged diarrhea. Cold, clammy skin, muscle cramps, and facial edema may be present. Seizures, coma, and circulatory collapse precede death. A dose of 120 mg of arsenic trioxide may be fatal. Liver enlargement and oliguria may also occur.

Persons who recover may develop delayed peripheral neuropathy, presenting after several weeks as symmetric distal sensory loss. The lower extremities are usually more affected than the upper. Motor involvement extending to total paralysis may also occur.

Acute exposure to arsine results in intravascular hemolysis. Other complaints include headache, nausea, and chest tightness. Exposure to 10 ppm rapidly causes delirium, coma, and death.

The triad of abdominal pain, jaundice, and oliguria should strongly suggest arsine exposure. Physical examination may reveal bronzing of the skin and hepatosplenomegaly.

**2. Chronic exposure–**Distal paresthesias or anesthesia indicate arsenic-induced peripheral neuropathy. In more severe cases, motor involvement may be evident as well, with weakness and reflex loss. Chronic exposure to arsine gas has been reported to cause a syndrome similar to arsenic trioxide. Symptoms of sore throat, cough, and phlegm production may be due to chronic exposure to irritant arsenic dusts. Complaints of asthenia and fatigue may be due to arsenic-induced anemia. Other effects that have been reported include cardiac failure, liver disease, and renal disease. Environmental exposure in Taiwan resulted in the induction of peripheral vasospasms and gangrene, termed "blackfoot disease." This has not occurred in the occupational setting.

Dermatologic manifestations of chronic exposure to arsenic compounds are common, principally after long-term ingestion of arsenic in drinking water or for medicinal purposes. Arsenical keratoses are raised punctate or verrucous lesions occurring primarily on the palms and soles. Enlarging masses or ulcerations should suggest Bowen's disease, basal cell carcinoma, and squamous cell carcinoma, which are all increased in persons with chronic arsenic exposure. In some individuals, a diffuse bronze hyperpigmentation develops, characterized by interspersion of 10-mm macules of hypomelanosis. Alopecia may occur. Some arsenic compounds may cause an irritant dermatitis as well.

Several epidemiologic studies of smelting operations have revealed an increase in lung cancer in workers exposed to arsenic. Other cancers that have been reported in association with arsenic exposure include leukemia, lymphoma, and angiosarcoma of the liver.

Arsenic crosses the placenta and may cause fetotoxicity, decreased birth weight, or congenital malformations.

**B. Laboratory Findings:** Acute and chronic exposure to arsenic may cause anemia and leukopenia, and arsine-induced hemolysis results in anemia, hyperbilirubinemia, and hemoglobinuria. Hematuria and proteinuria indicate renal injury. Liver damage may result in elevation of serum enzymes and bilirubin. The ECG may reveal rhythm or conduction disturbances. Delayed sensory conduction velocities in a distal symmetric distribution may be seen on nerve conduction studies.

Total urine arsenic levels are useful in confirming recent exposure. The measurement of DMA and MMA eliminate confusion with dietary sources of organic arsenic compounds. Nonexposed persons will have levels less than 10 µg/g of creatinine. Workers exposed to 0.01 mg/m$^3$ will have levels of 50 µg/g of creatinine. Acute poisoning usually causes levels exceeding 1000 µg/g of creatinine. Hair and nail arsenic levels may be useful in detecting systemic absorption of arsenic, primarily due to ingestion. These are also subject to external contamination and are of little use in the industrial setting.

Tissue biopsy will confirm the diagnosis of skin or respiratory cancer. Careful medical and occupational histories are necessary to determine the relationship of these common cancers to arsenic exposure.

## Prevention

The use of engineering controls to contain sources of exposure to arsenic compounds will reduce exposure in smelting, metallurgy, and pesticide manufacturing operations. Personal protective equipment should be worn when performing maintenance work or during application of arsenic compounds. Medical surveillance should concentrate on skin and respiratory complaints as well as liver, hematologic, renal, and nervous system function. Biological monitoring of arsenic in urine will complement industrial hygiene efforts to control exposure.

## Treatment

Treatment following acute ingestion is by induced emesis followed by administration of activated charcoal and a cathartic. Shock is treated with aggressive intravenous fluid resuscitation and pressor agents as indicated. If the diagnosis is confirmed, therapy with dimercaprol, 3–4 mg/kg every 4 hours for the first 2 days is administered. This should be continued at 3 mg/kg every 12 hours until urine arsenic is below 50 μg/d. Sources of further exposure should be eliminated after treatment.

Arsine poisoning requires careful monitoring of the hematocrit and renal function. Alkaline diuresis will reduce the precipitation of hemoglobin in renal tubules and the resultant renal impairment. Elevation of plasma-free hemoglobin greater than 1.5 mg/dL or oliguria is an indication for exchange transfusion. Hemodialysis is indicated if acute renal failure develops. Dimercaprol is not effective in arsine poisoning.

## Prognosis

In acute arsenic poisoning, survival for more than 1 week is usually followed by complete recovery. Complete recovery from chronic arsenic poisoning may require 6 months to 1 year.

## BERYLLIUM

### Essentials of Diagnosis
- Tracheobronchitis, pneumonitis.
- Granulomatous pulmonary disease.
- Dermatitis (ulceration and granulomas).
- Eye, nose, and throat irritation.
- Lung cancer.

### Exposure Limits
ACGIH TLV: 0.002 ppm TWA
OSHA PEL: 0.002 ppm TWA, 0.005 ppm ceiling (30 minutes)
NIOSH REL: Do not exceed 0.5 μg Be/m$^3$

### General Considerations
Beryllium is a lightweight, gray metal with high tensile strength. It is extracted from beryl ore after grinding and heating using either a sulfate or fluoride process and electrolytic reduction. Bertrandite ($4BeO.2SiO_2.H_2O$), although lower in beryllium content (0.1–3%), provides a source of acid-soluble beryllium that is more easily extracted.

### Use
The unique properties of beryllium are ideally suited for the production of hard, corrosion-resistant alloys for use in the aerospace industry. Beryllium alloys (primarily copper) are used in nonsparking tools, bushings, bearings, and electronic components. Beryllium is used in nuclear reactors as a moderator to retard neutrons, a reflector to prevent neutron leakage, and a fuel source. Beryllium oxide combines high thermal conductivity with high electrical resis-

tance for use in ceramics, microwave tubes, and semiconductors. The use of beryllium in the manufacture of fluorescent and neon lamps was discontinued in 1949 after numerous cases of beryllium toxicity were reported in that industry.

### Occupational & Environmental Exposure
Exposure to beryllium in the past has occurred mainly in grinding, roasting, and milling of beryl ore, though recognition of the toxicity of beryllium has resulted in dramatic improvement in environmental conditions in these operations. Mining of beryl ore has not been associated with adverse health effects. Workers involved with the newer applications for beryllium in the aerospace, nuclear, and electronics industries may be less aware of its potential hazards. Workers engaged in the production and fabrication of beryllium alloys may be exposed to dusts and fumes. Persons residing in neighborhoods surrounding beryllium roasting operations have the potential for chronic low-level exposure to beryllium compounds, though there are strict emission standards for these operations.

### Absorption, Metabolism, & Excretion
Beryllium compounds are poorly absorbed after inhalation, ingestion, or skin contact. Beryllium may be retained in the lung or deposited in bone, liver, and spleen. Renal excretion is slow and variable and serves primarily to confirm exposure, since levels are usually undetectable in nonexposed individuals. The development of chronic toxicity does not appear to be dose-dependent and may involve a hypersensitivity reaction. Pathologically, beryllium toxicity is a systemic disease, evidenced by the presence of noncaseating granulomas in numerous tissues, including lung, liver, skin, and lymph nodes.

### Clinical Findings
**A. Symptoms and Signs:**
**1. Acute or subacute exposure–**Acute or subacute exposure to beryllium dusts or fumes has irritant effects on the eyes, mucous membranes, and respiratory tract. Burning eyes, sinus congestion, epistaxis, and sore throat may be presenting complaints. Affected tissues may be swollen, hyperemic, and ulcerated. Tracheobronchitis is characterized by cough, chest pain, and dyspnea. In severe cases, a chemical pneumonitis may develop, manifested by tachypnea, hemoptysis, cyanosis, and rales. Death has occurred as a result of pulmonary edema and respiratory failure.
**2. Chronic exposure–**Chronic berylliosis may develop after many years of exposure or following a single acute exposure. Exertional dyspnea is the usual presenting complaint, often accompanied by fatigue, weight loss, cough, and chest pain. On physical exam-

ination, there may be rales, hepatosplenomegaly, lymphadenopathy, and clubbing. In longstanding cases, there may be evidence of pulmonary hypertension such as jugular venous distention, a right ventricular heave, and an accentuated $P_2$ on cardiac auscultation. Exacerbations of symptoms may occur following trauma, systemic illness, or pregnancy.

After skin contact, beryllium may cause an irritant or allergic dermatitis, characterized by erythema, papules, and vesiculation. After penetration of the skin through a cut or abrasion, there may be development of a granuloma that may ulcerate through the skin surface.

Beryllium metal, beryl ore, and several beryllium alloys and compounds are proved animal carcinogens, causing both lung cancers and osteogenic sarcomas in several species. Several recent studies suggest that workers with beryllium exposure are also at an excess risk for developing lung cancer. Exposures should be reduced to the lowest feasible levels.

**B. Laboratory Findings:** In cases of acute pneumonitis, there is arterial hypoxemia with diffuse pulmonary infiltrates. In chronic beryllium disease, there may be hypergammaglobulinemia, anemia, elevated liver enzymes, hyperuricemia, and hypercalciuria. Pulmonary function studies may reveal a reduced forced expiratory volume in 1 second ($FEV_1$), a reduced $FEV_1$/forced vital capacity (FVC) ratio, or both. The carbon monoxide diffusing capacity is usually impaired. In contrast to sarcoidosis, the serum angiotensin-converting enzyme levels are usually normal and the Kveim test is negative. Biopsy of affected tissues will reveal noncaseating granulomas.

Elevated urine levels of beryllium (> 0.02 mg/L) confirm exposure. Skin testing can confirm hypersensitivity to beryllium compounds but also carries the risk of sensitization and should be avoided. Bronchoalveolar lavage (BAL) may demonstrate lymphocyte alveolitis with an increase in T-cells. Lymphocyte transformation tests (LTT) are a useful alternative and are effective in assessing individual reactivity to beryllium compounds. A positive LTT may be present without evidence of disease. X-ray findings include diffuse bilateral nodular or linear infiltrates, often with bilateral hilar adenopathy. Nodular densities suggestive of possible lung cancer need to be carefully assessed.

## Prevention

Operations that generate beryllium dusts or fumes should be enclosed and vented. Wet processes are preferred to reduce the generation of dust. Eye, skin, and respiratory protection are required during cleaning and maintenance operations. Awareness of beryllium toxicity and training and care in handling beryllium compounds will prevent inadvertent overexposure in newer industrial applications. Medical surveillance should include periodic chest x-rays and measurement of pulmonary function.

## Treatment

Treatment of acute pneumonitis should include supplemental oxygen and corticosteroids. Chronic beryllium disease may also respond to steroids, starting with prednisone, 60 mg orally daily, and tapering slowly. Skin lesions should be thoroughly cleansed and treated with topical steroids.

## Prognosis

Berylliosis is a chronic disease that may persist and progress even after cessation of exposure. Prevention and early detection are critical.

## BORON

### Essentials of Diagnosis

- Respiratory and mucous membrane irritation (boron halides, diborane, borax, boric acid).
- Central nervous system effects (boron hydrides, boric acid).
- Skin irritation (borax, borates).

### Exposure Limits

Borates (anhydrous)
ACGIH TLV: 1 mg/m$^3$ TWA
OSHA PEL: 10 mg/m$^3$ TWA
Boron oxide
ACGIH TLV: 10 mg/m$^3$ TWA
NIOSH REL: 10 mg/m$^3$ TWA
Pentaborane
ACGIH TLV: 0.005 ppm TWA
OSHA PEL: 0.005 ppm TWA, 0.015 ppm STEL
Diborane
ACGIH TLV: 0.1 ppm TWA
OSHA PEL: 0.1 ppm TWA

### General Considerations

Boron is a metalloid element that occurs in bedded deposits and lake brines. Borax ($Na_2B_4O_7.10H_2O$) and kernite ($Na_2B_4O_7.4H_2O$) are important mineral sources of boron. Boron compounds are produced by the exothermic reduction of boron trioxide with magnesium. The major deposits of boron minerals are found in the United States, Turkey, and Russia.

### Use

A major use for boron compounds is in the manufacture of glass, including insulating and textile fiberglass. Enamels, glazes, coatings, soaps, and cleansers also contain boron compounds. Boron compounds have been used as propellants in jet fuels and as gasoline additives. Boron is an important dopant element in the manufacture of semiconductor devices. Other diverse uses for boron are in herbicides, solar batteries, welding rods, nuclear reactors, flame retardants, abrasives, adhesives, and plastics. Boric acid has been used medicinally as a topical antiseptic.

## Occupational & Environmental Exposure

Workers employed in the mining and refining of boron minerals may have exposures to dusts containing boric acid. The highly toxic boron hydrides (diborane, pentaborane, and decaborane) are encountered in the production of high-energy fuels and in the rubber industry. The boron halides (boron tribromide, boron trichloride, and boron trifluoride) are used as catalysts and, along with diborane, are important sources of dopant boron atoms in the microelectronics industry. Glass workers, paint and soap manufacturers, and welders may have exposure to boron compounds.

## Absorption, Metabolism, & Excretion

Boron compounds are readily absorbed after inhalation or ingestion. Some boron compounds such as boric acid are also absorbed after skin contact. Excessive absorption may lead to accumulation in the brain. Excretion is primarily renal.

## Clinical Findings

**A. Symptoms and Signs:** The toxicity of boron is highly dependent on the source of exposure. Boron oxide, borax, and boric acid may all cause respiratory, eye, and skin irritation at high concentrations. Excessive absorption of these compounds may result in central nervous system depression, gastrointestinal distress, skin desquamation, and renal damage. Chronic exposure to boron compounds may cause alopecia. Menstrual disturbances in women have also been reported. In animal experiments, exposure to boron resulted in gonadotoxic effects, including reduction in testicular weight, sperm count, and sperm motility.

Exposure to diborane gas causes acute respiratory irritation, resulting in cough and chest tightness. Pulmonary edema may develop. Exposure to pentaborane and decaborane has been associated with severe central nervous system effects, including encephalopathy, seizures, and coma. Acute exposure may result in prolonged mental and behavioral disturbances.

Boron halides hydrolyze to the corresponding halogen acid on contact with moist surfaces. Exposure may cause eye, skin, and respiratory tract irritation as well as pulmonary edema.

**B. Laboratory Findings:** There may be evidence of renal failure, with proteinuria and hematuria. Liver enzyme levels may be elevated. The EEG may show evidence of a diffuse encephalopathy. Serum borate levels above 20 mg/L indicate excessive exposure.

## Prevention

Workers should be advised to avoid skin contact with highly concentrated or irritating boron com-

pounds through the use of gloves and protective garments. Every effort should be made to prevent worker exposure to boron halides and boron hydrides through engineering controls and process enclosure. Although borax and boric acid are upper respiratory irritants at concentrations greater than 4 mg/m$^3$, there is no evidence that they cause impairment of respiratory function. Medical surveillance of workers with exposure to boron hydrides should concentrate on the respiratory system and the nervous system.

## Treatment

Supportive measures and anticonvulsants should be used as indicated. Careful monitoring of respiratory function is indicated after acute inhalation. Hemodialysis will remove borates from the circulation.

# CADMIUM

## Essentials of Diagnosis

*Acute effects:*
- Fever, chills, dyspnea (metal fume fever).
- Chemical pneumonitis.
- Renal failure.
- Gastrointestinal disturbance.

*Chronic effects:*
- Proteinuria.
- Fanconi's syndrome.
- Osteomalacia.
- Emphysema.
- Anemia.
- Anosmia.
- Lung cancer.

## Exposure Limits

Cadmium
OSHA: 2.5 µg/m$^3$ 8-hour TWA
ACGIH TLV: 2.0 µg/m$^3$ 8-hour TWA
NIOSH REL: Reduce exposure to lowest feasible concentration.
BEI ACGIH: 5.0 µg/g creatinine

## General Considerations

Cadmium is a soft, silver-white, electropositive metal that is finding increasing industrial applications. Although greenockite (cadmium sulfide), the principal cadmium mineral, is rare, cadmium is commonly present in zinc, lead, and copper ores. Cadmium is a by-product of the smelting and refining of these ores and is recovered by electrolysis and distillation. Cadmium is a nonessential mineral for humans and is present in biological tissues as a result of environmental exposure.

## Use

The primary use of cadmium compounds is in electroplating. Cadmium imparts corrosion resistance to steel, iron, and a variety of other materials for use in automotive parts, aircraft, marine equipment, and industrial machinery. Cadmium alloys are used in high-speed bearings, solder, and jewelry. Cadmium sulfides and selenides are used as pigments in rubber, inks, resins, paints, textiles, and ceramics, particularly where heat stability and alkali resistance are desirable. Cadmium stearate is used as a stabilizer in plastics—primarily in polyvinyl chloride (PVC) film. Nickel-cadmium batteries are used in motor vehicles and rechargeable household appliances. Cadmium is also used in photoelectric cells and in semiconductors.

## Occupational & Environmental Exposure

Workers may be exposed to cadmium in the smelting and refining of zinc, lead, and copper. The recovery and refining of cadmium compounds is associated with potential exposure to high levels of dusts and fumes. Cadmium exposure may occur in the manufacture of batteries, paints, and plastics. Welders and brazers may be exposed to cadmium oxide fumes when working with cadmium-containing solders or welding rods or when working on materials that have been coated with cadmium. Exposures may also occur at electroplating operations.

Nonoccupational exposure occurs primarily through dietary intake. Air and water contamination may be significant in areas surrounding zinc smelters. Ingestion of contaminated water in Japan led to an epidemic of osteoporosis ("Itai itai") in the 1940s. Ingestion of food that has been improperly stored in containers which have been glazed with cadmium may result in acute poisoning. Cigarette smoke is another source of chronic cadmium exposure in humans.

## Absorption, Metabolism, & Excretion

Cadmium may be absorbed through inhalation or ingestion. Skin absorption is negligible under ordinary circumstances. After inhalation, 10–40% may be absorbed, depending on particle size and chemical composition. Gastrointestinal absorption is usually less than 10% but may be increased in the presence of iron, protein, calcium, or zinc deficiencies.

In the bloodstream, cadmium is bound to plasma proteins. Most is found within erythrocytes, where it is bound to hemoglobin and metallothionein, an inducible low-molecular-weight protein named for its high affinity for certain metals. Cadmium accumulates in the liver and kidneys, where binding to metallothionein protects against cellular damage.

Excretion is primarily through the kidneys, with a biological half-life of 8–30 years. Renal excretion of cadmium increases after chronic exposure due to impaired proximal tubular reabsorption, a manifestation of cadmium induced nephrotoxicity.

## Clinical Findings

### A. Symptoms and Signs:

**1. Acute exposure**–Acute inhalation of cadmium oxide fumes has accounted for several industrial fatalities. After a delay of several hours, workers complain of sore throat, headache, myalgias, nausea, and a metallic taste. Fever, cough, dyspnea, and chest tightness follow, simulating metal fume fever. In severe cases, this progresses to a fulminant chemical pneumonitis with pulmonary edema and death due to respiratory failure. Acute hepatic and renal injury may also occur. Acute exposure may result in chronic pulmonary fibrosis. Ingestion of cadmium compounds results in nausea, vomiting, headache, abdominal pain, liver injury, and acute renal failure.

**2. Chronic exposure**–The most frequent manifestation of chronic exposure to cadmium is proteinuria. Initially, there is increased excretion of low-molecular-weight proteins, such as $\beta_2$-microglobulin. With continued exposure, this progresses to Fanconi's syndrome, with aminoaciduria, glycosuria, hypercalciuria, and phosphaturia. Renal tubular dysfunction can result in nephrolithiasis and osteomalacia. Bone pain and pathologic fractures are related to renal calcium and phosphorus wasting and impaired synthesis of vitamin D. Chronic inhalation of cadmium dusts and fumes may also result in respiratory impairment and emphysema. Other effects that have been reported include anosmia and anemia.

Cadmium is a human carcinogen, reported as a cause of lung cancer in several studies of smelting and plating operations. An excess in genitourinary and prostate cancers has also been reported, but this has not been a consistent observation. Cadmium persists in tissues and has been used to induce tumors (sarcomas) in laboratory animals.

Teratogenic effects and testicular effects have been observed in laboratory animals as well, though human reproductive effects have not been reported.

### B. Laboratory Findings:

**1. Acute inhalation**–Evaluation of acute inhalations should include an arterial blood gas evaluation, a chest x-ray, spirometry, and assessment of renal and hepatic function. Hypoxemia, diffuse pulmonary infiltrates, and a reduction in $FEV_1$, FVC, and diffusing capacity for carbon monoxide indicate excessive exposure and impending respiratory failure. Later, the chest x-ray may reveal bronchopneumonia. Blood and urine cadmium levels are useful in acute exposure. Normal blood and urine cadmium levels are 1 μg/L and 1 μg/g creatinine, respectively. After acute cadmium fume inhalation, these may rise to 3 mg/L and 0.36 mg/L.

**2. Chronic exposure**–For workers exposed to air levels of cadmium in excess of 2.5 μg/m³, the Occupational Safety and Health Administration requires both biological monitoring and medical examinations. The biological monitoring includes urine and blood cadmium levels, as well as measurement of urinary $\beta_2$-microglobulin levels. Periodic medical examinations are triggered by the biological monitoring results (Tables 27–1 and 27–2). Cigarette smoking may contribute to urine cadmium levels. $\beta_2$-microglobulin levels are a sensitive indicator of cadmium renal toxicity, although exercise, febrile illness, nephrotoxic medications, and other kidney disorders may also affect this test. A complete blood count may reveal a decrease in serum hemoglobin. Evaluation of pulmonary function may reveal airway obstruction and reduction in diffusing capacity for carbon monoxide. Bone x-rays should be performed to look for abnormal mineralization and pathologic fractures in cases where Itai itai is suspected.

## Prevention

Processes that result in the production of cadmium oxide fumes should be enclosed. Local exhaust ventilation and personal protective measures should be used to minimize exposure to cadmium dusts. Strict attention to workplace and personal hygiene will lessen the potential for chronic exposures. Smoking must be prohibited where there is potential exposure to cadmium. Welding on cadmium-treated metal or brazing using cadmium-containing solders should be performed only in areas that are properly ventilated. Air-supplied respirators should be used in enclosed spaces.

Biological monitoring should focus on the early detection of proteinuria, before severe irreversible proximal renal tubular dysfunction occurs. Urine cadmium levels should be kept below 3 μg/g creatinine to prevent renal injury.

## Treatment

Persons who have suffered acute inhalation of cadmium oxide fumes should be thoroughly evaluated for evidence of acute lung injury. Admission to the hospital for observation is indicated if excessive exposure is

**Table 27–2.** Medical examination for cadmium workers.

**Medical and occupational history**
Focusing on cadmium exposure; smoking; renal, cardiovascular, musculoskeletal, and respiratory conditions; reproductive concerns; use of nephrotoxic medications, recent physical exercise, recent febrile illnesses.

**Physical examination**
Blood pressure, respiratory system, genitourinary system, prostate examination (men over 40 years), respirator medical clearance.

**Diagnostic testing**
Pulmonary function testing.
Chest x-ray.
Complete blood count.
Blood urea nitrogen, creatinine.
Urinalysis, urinary protein measurement.

suspected based on the history or clinical findings. Respiratory support may be required. In severe acute poisoning, chelation with calcium disodium edetate (EDTA) may be indicated. Renal function should be closely monitored, since chelation may increase renal toxicity. Dimercaprol should not be used.

Individuals who manifest chronic toxicity (renal impairment, emphysema, bone disease) should be removed from further exposure. Supplementation with calcium and vitamin D is indicated if calcium wasting or bone disease is present.

## CHROMIUM

### Essentials of Diagnosis
- Sinusitis, septal perforation.
- Allergic and irritant dermatitis, ulcers.
- Respiratory irritation, bronchitis, asthma.
- Lung cancer.

### Exposure Limits
Chromium metal
   ACGIH TLV: 0.5 mg/m$^3$ TWA

**Table 27–1.** Biological monitoring program for cadmium.

| Actions | Biological Monitoring Result |
|---|---|
| Annual biological monitoring<br>Medical examination every 2 years | Urine cadmium ≤3 μg/g creatinine<br>$\beta_2$-Microglobulin ≤300 μg/g creatinine<br>Cadmium in blood ≤5 μg/liter whole blood |
| Semiannual biological monitoring<br>Medical examination annually<br>Exposure assessment<br>Exposure control | Urine cadmium 3–15 (7[1]) μg/g creatinine<br>$\beta_2$-Microglobulin 300–1500 (750[1]) μg/g creatinine<br>Cadmium in blood 5–15 (10[1]) μg/liter whole blood |
| Mandatory removal<br>Medical examination<br>Exposure assessment | Urine cadmium >5 (7[1]) μg/g creatinine<br>$\beta_2$-Microglobulin >1500 (750[1]) μg/g creatinine<br>Cadmium in blood >15 (10[1]) μg/liter whole blood |

[1]New limits go into effect in 1999.

Chromium (III) compounds
    ACGIH TLV: 0.5 mg/m$^3$ TWA
Chromium (VI) compounds
    ACGIH TLV: 0.05 mg/m$^3$ TWA (soluble)
    ACGIH TLV: 0.01 mg/m$^3$ (insoluble)
    NIOSH REL: 1 $\mu$mg/m$^3$ TWA
    BEI ACGIH: 30 $\mu$g/g creatinine (end of week/
      end of shift)

## General Considerations

Chromium is a hard, brittle gray metal. Elemental chromium does not occur naturally but is widely distributed as chromite (FeOCr$_2$O$_3$) or ferrochromium. Chromite is obtained through both underground and open cast mining. Ferrochromium is produced by the reduction of chromite with carbon in an electric furnace. Chromium metal is obtained primarily through reduction of chromic oxide with aluminum powder. Chromates are produced by high temperature roasting of chromite in an oxidizing atmosphere. The valence states that are of primary industrial interest are hexavalent (Cr [VI], chromate) and, to a lesser extent, trivalent (Cr [III], chromic) chromium. The valence state is critical for the toxicity of chromium compounds.

## Use

The primary use of chromium is in plating. Numerous applications include automotive parts, household appliances, tools, and machinery, where the coating imparts corrosion resistance and a shiny, decorative finish. Chromium-iron alloys, alone or with the addition of nickel or manganese, are used to produce a variety of durable, high-strength stainless steels. Chromium alloys with nickel (nichrome) have high electrical resistance for use in electrical appliances. Chromates and dichromates are used as pigments and preservatives in paints, dyes, textiles, rubber, and inks. The radioisotope $^{56}$Cr is used in nuclear medicine to label erythrocytes.

## Occupational & Environmental Exposure

Exposure to chromium begins with mining and crushing operations, where there may be exposure to dusts of chromic oxide. The greatest occupational hazard historically has been in the processing of chromite ore to produce chromates, where workers were found to have a high incidence of lung cancer. Exposure to chromium fumes occurs in the production and fabrication of stainless steel. Arc welding of stainless steel also results in exposure to chromium compounds.

Electroplaters are exposed to chromic acid mists. Workers may be exposed to chromates through their use in the paint, textile, leather, glass, and rubber industries and in lithography, printing, and photography. Certain cements have a high chromium content.

Chromium is found in low concentrations in water, urban air, and a variety of foods.

## Absorption, Metabolism, & Excretion

Chromium compounds may be absorbed through the gastrointestinal tract, the lungs, or the skin. The soluble hexavalent forms are much more readily absorbed than the insoluble trivalent forms. Intracellularly, hexavalent chromium is converted to the trivalent form, which binds avidly to proteins and nucleic acids, resulting in chromium toxicity. Chromium is an essential trace element in humans and animals, and chromium deficiency results in impaired glucose tolerance. Chromium does not generally accumulate in tissues, though inhaled insoluble forms may remain in the lung. Excretion is primarily renal, and urine levels have been found to correlate with recent airborne exposure to soluble chromium compounds.

## Clinical Findings

**A. Symptoms and Signs:** Acute exposure to high concentrations of chromic acid or chromates will cause immediate irritation of the eye, nose, throat, and respiratory tract, resulting in burning, congestion, epistaxis, and cough. Chronic exposure may cause ulceration, bleeding, and erosion of the nasal septum. Cough, chest pain, and dyspnea may indicate exposure to irritant levels of soluble chromium compounds or the development of chromium-induced asthma. Weight loss, cough, and hemoptysis in a chromium worker should suggest the development of bronchogenic carcinoma.

Dermatologic manifestations are common in chromium workers. Penetration of the skin will cause painless erosive ulceration with delayed healing. These commonly occur on the fingers, knuckles, and forearms. Localized erythematous or vesicular lesions at points of contact or generalized eczematous dermatitis should suggest sensitization.

Ingestion of chromium compounds has caused nausea, vomiting, abdominal pain, and prostration. Death is due to uremia.

Chromium is a proven human carcinogen. Workers involved in chromate production, chrome plating, and chrome alloy work have all been found to have an increased incidence of lung cancer. The chromium compounds responsible for human cancers have not been identified, but hexavalent chromium compounds (chromates) are animal carcinogens and are mutagenic in microbial assay systems. Insoluble chromium compounds may accumulate in respiratory tissues leading to carcinogenicity. Trivalent chromium is not mutagenic in these same in vitro systems.

**B. Laboratory Findings:** With massive exposure, there will be evidence of renal and hepatic damage. Proteinuria and hematuria will precede anuria and uremia. A reduction in the $FEV_1/FVC$ ratio on spirometry may be seen after acute irritant exposure or in workers with chromium-induced asthma. Skin allergy can be confirmed by patch testing. Chest x-ray changes consistent with pneumoconiosis have rarely been reported in workers exposed to trivalent chromium compounds. Persistent cough, hemoptysis, or a mass lesion on chest x-ray in a chromium worker should prompt a thorough evaluation for possible lung cancer.

## Prevention

Reduction of exposure to airborne soluble hexavalent chromium compounds and improved worker hygiene will reduce the respiratory and nasal complications. Surveillance for nasal irritation or septal perforation will identify high-risk jobs or workers to direct exposure control efforts. Avoidance of skin contact—particularly contact with damaged or inflamed skin—will reduce the risk of developing chrome ulcers or skin sensitization. Prompt evaluation for skin sensitization will prevent the development of severe or chronic dermatitis. The value of sputum cytology to screen for lung cancer is unproved.

Exposure to hexavalent chromium compounds should be reduced to the lowest feasible levels to reduce the risk of lung cancer. Chromium workers should also be encouraged to stop smoking. Biological monitoring of urine chromium levels may be useful as an assessment of recent exposure. Workers exposed to 0.05 mg/m³ of water soluble Cr(VI) fume may show an increase in urine chromium of 10 μg/g creatinine over a work shift or a level of 30 μg/g creatinine at the end of the work week.

## Treatment

Persons who have suffered acute inhalation injury should be admitted to the hospital for observation. Supplemental oxygen and bronchodilators may be required. Careful attention to fluid and electrolyte balance is indicated in the setting of acute renal injury. Chromium-induced nasal and skin ulcerations should be treated with a 10% ointment of $CaNa_2$ EDTA (calcium disodium edetate) and an impervious dressing with frequent application to prevent formation of persistent, insoluble Cr (III). Persons who develop chromium respiratory or skin allergy should be removed from further exposure if they cannot be adequately protected.

## LEAD

### Essentials of Diagnosis

*Inorganic—acute effects:*
- Abdominal pain (colic).
- Encephalopathy.
- Hemolysis.
- Acute renal failure.

*Inorganic—chronic effects:*
- Fatigue and asthenia.
- Arthralgias and myalgias.
- Anemia.
- Peripheral neuropathy (motor).
- Neurobehavioral disturbances and chronic encephalopathy.
- Impaired fertility.
- Gout and gouty nephropathy.
- Chronic renal failure.

*Alkyl lead compounds:*
- Fatigue and lassitude.
- Headache.
- Nausea and vomiting.
- Neuropsychiatric complaints (memory loss, difficulty in concentrating).
- Delirium, seizures, coma.

### Exposure Limits

Lead, inorganic, dusts, and fumes
   ACGIH TLV: 0.05 mg/m³ TWA
   OSHA PEL: 0.05 mg/m³ TWA
   BEI ACGIH: 30 μg/dL
Tetraethyl lead
   ACGIH TLV: 0.1 mg/m³ TWA (skin)

### General Considerations

Lead is a soft, malleable, blue-gray metal characterized by high density and corrosion resistance. Lead occurs in many ores in concentrations of 1–11%. The ores of commercial interest include the sulfide (galena), the carbonate (cerussite), and the sulfate (anglesite). Lead is concentrated through wet grinding and flotation prior to smelting. Smelting is a three-step process, involving blending, sintering, and blast furnace reduction. Lead bullion and slag are further refined through pyrometallurgic or electrolytic processes to remove copper, arsenic, antimony, zinc, tin, bismuth, and other metal contaminants. In the United States, over one-third of the lead produced is recovered from secondary sources of lead scrap.

Lead serves no useful biological function in humans. The release of lead into the environment from automobile emissions, old paint, and the burning of coal—and its subsequent bioaccumulation in many organisms, including humans—has profound public health implications. Over the past 25 years, there has been growing concern over the health effects of low-level lead exposure and the "normal" body burden of lead. In the occupational setting, the "no effect" level for lead exposure is being scrutinized as more sensitive measures of the physiologic effects of lead are studied.

### Use

The primary use of lead is in the manufacture of storage batteries. In the chemical and building industries, lead alloys (chiefly with antimony and tin) are used in pipes and cable sheathing, where they impart resistance to acids and moisture. Tin-lead alloys are used in solder for electrical applications. Lead compounds are used in paints and plastics as pigments and stabilizers. Lead glazes impart brilliance and hardness to ceramics.

Lead is used in construction for attenuation of sound and vibration and for the shielding of radioactivity. Tetraethyl lead and tetramethyl lead are used primarily as antiknock agents in gasoline, though this use has declined significantly. Other uses include ammunition (lead shot), bronze and brass, cosmetics, and jewelry.

## Occupational & Environmental Exposure

Inhalation and ingestion are potential routes of lead exposure in mining, particularly the more soluble carbonate and sulfate ores. Grinding and sintering operations generate high levels of lead dust and fume. Workers engaged in the reclamation of lead from secondary sources have potential exposure to lead as well as other metal contaminants. Exposure is a constant hazard in the manufacture of lead batteries. Paint and pigment manufacturers are exposed to lead additives. Painters may also be exposed to lead, especially during fine spray-painting operations. Torch burning to remove lead-based paints generates significant quantities of lead fume. Welders and brazers may be exposed to lead alloys, fluxes, and coatings. Workers in munitions plants and rifle ranges may have exposure to lead dust, particularly indoors. Glass-makers, artists, and pottery workers may unknowingly be exposed to high levels of lead in pigments and glazes.

Environmental exposure may occur near lead smelters as a result of air, soil, and water contamination. Urban residents have exposure to lead from automobile exhausts. Children in older, low-income housing may ingest lead paint chips from decaying structures or be exposed to lead in house dust. Ingestion of moonshine whiskey is another source of acute lead poisoning. Improperly fired ceramics may release lead, especially into acidic foods and beverages.

Herbal remedies, lead-based cosmetics, gasoline sniffing, and retained bullets are less conventional sources of lead poisoning. Lead contamination of tap water from lead pipes is an important source of lead exposure in many older homes.

## Absorption, Metabolism, & Excretion

Inhalation and ingestion are the primary routes of absorption of lead compounds. Approximately 40% of inhaled lead oxide fumes is absorbed through the respiratory tract. Absorption of particulate lead dust depends on particle size and solubility. Roughly 5–10% of ingested lead compounds are absorbed from the gastrointestinal tract. Iron and calcium deficiencies and high-fat diets may increase the gastrointestinal absorption of lead. Gastrointestinal absorption is greater in infants and children than in adults.

In the bloodstream, the majority of the absorbed lead is bound to erythrocytes. The free diffusible plasma fraction is distributed to brain, kidney, liver, skin, and skeletal muscle, where it is readily exchangeable. The concentrations in these tissues are highest with acute, high-dose exposure. Lead crosses the placenta, and fetal levels correlate with maternal levels. Bone constitutes the major site of deposition of absorbed lead, where it is incorporated into the bony matrix similar to calcium. The lead in dense bone is only slowly mobilized and gradually increases with time.

Intracellularly, lead binds to sulfhydryl groups and interferes with numerous cellular enzymes, including those involved in heme synthesis. This binding accounts for the presence of lead in hair and nails. Lead also binds to mitochondrial membranes and interferes with protein and nucleic acid synthesis.

Excretion is slow over time, primarily through the kidney. Fecal excretion, sweat, and epidermal exfoliation are other routes of excretion. The half-life of lead is long, estimated to be from 5 to 10 years. This varies with the intensity and duration of exposure and the ultimate body burden accumulated. Bone diseases (osteoporosis, fractures) pregnancy, and hyperthyroidism may lead to increased release of stored lead and elevated blood lead levels.

Water-insoluble alkyl lead compounds are readily absorbed through intact skin. Respiratory and gastrointestinal absorption are significant as well. Tetraethyl and tetramethyl lead are converted to the trialkyl metabolites that are responsible for toxicity. The fat solubility of these compounds accounts for their accumulation in the central nervous system. Alkyl lead compounds are ultimately converted to inorganic lead and are excreted in the urine.

## Clinical Findings

**A. Symptoms and Signs:**

**1. Inorganic lead–**

**a. Acute exposure–**After acute or subacute exposure to lead through either ingestion or inhalation, the presenting symptoms are usually gastrointestinal. Cramping, colicky abdominal pain, and constipation are often present early. Abdominal pain may be severe, suggesting biliary colic or appendicitis. Nausea, vomiting, and black, tarry stools may also accompany the acute presentation.

Neurologic manifestations of lead encephalopathy include headache, confusion, stupor, coma, and seizures and are more common in children. Funduscopic examination may reveal papilledema or optic neuritis. In severe cases, oliguria and acute renal failure may develop rapidly.

**b. Chronic exposure–**In the occupational setting, chronic lead intoxication is a slow, insidious disease with protean manifestations. Fatigue, apathy, irritability, and vague gastrointestinal symptoms are early signs of chronic lead intoxication. Arthralgias and myalgias may involve the extremities of axial structures. As exposure continues, central nervous system symptoms progress, with insomnia, confusion, impaired concentration, and memory problems. Long-term exposure can lead to a distal motor neuropathy presenting with wrist drop. Progression to frank lead encephalopathy with seizures and coma is rare in adults but may occur.

Other presenting symptoms include loss of libido and infertility in men and menstrual disturbances and spontaneous abortion in women. Gouty arthritis and nephropathy have also been associated with chronic lead exposure.

Physical examination may reveal pallor due to anemia. Jaundice may be present in the setting of acute hemolysis. A blue-gray pigmentation ("lead line") may be present on the gums. Neurologic examination may reveal weakness, particularly of the distal extensor muscles.

In men, there is limited evidence of altered spermatogenesis. Lead crosses the placenta, and maternal exposure prior to and during pregnancy can result in fetal exposure and toxicity.

**2. Alkyl lead–**The presenting symptoms of alkyl lead intoxication are neurologic. Anorexia, insomnia, fatigue, weakness, headache, depression, and irritability are early symptoms. These progress to confusion, memory impairment, excitability, dysesthesias (eg, insects crawling on the body), mania, and toxic psychosis. In severe cases, delirium, seizures, coma, and death may occur in several days.

**B. Laboratory Findings:** Blood lead levels are an indication of recent exposure (days or weeks). Whole blood lead levels in nonexposed individuals range from 5 to 15 µg/dL. The correlation of blood lead levels with symptoms will depend on the duration and intensity of exposure. A new worker with high-level exposure may have symptoms with lead levels of 50–60 µg/dL while long-term workers may be asymptomatic with levels over 80 µg/dL. Subtle effects of lead on the central and peripheral nervous system may occur with levels between 40 and 80 µg/dL. The current OSHA standard requires that lead levels be maintained below 40 µg/dL. Anemia is a frequent manifestation of lead intoxication in children but is unusual in adults. The anemia is usually normochromic. Increased red cell turnover and frank hemolysis may be present, with basophilic stippling of the red blood cells and reticulocytosis. Altered heme synthesis, evidenced by an increase in protoporphyrin—measured as either free erythrocyte protoporphyrin (FEP) or zinc protoporphyrin (ZPP)— begins when blood lead levels exceed 40 µg/dL. Delta-aminolevulinic acid dehydratase (delta-ALAD), an enzyme inhibited by lead, may also be increased, though measurement of this enzyme is not readily available.

Proximal renal injury may result in Fanconi's syndrome, with aminoaciduria, glycosuria, and phosphaturia. Impaired uric acid excretion results in hyperuricemia. Elevations of BUN and serum creatinine indicate impaired renal function. Liver involvement may be suggested by mild elevations of serum aminotransferases. Nerve conduction studies may reveal delayed motor conduction velocities even without overt peripheral neuropathy. Neuropsychiatric evaluation may reveal evidence of intellectual impairment and behavioral alterations.

In the past, a $CaNa_2EDTA$ (calcium disodium edetate) lead mobilization test has been used to assess lead in individuals with normal blood lead levels. This is no longer in favor and probably not indicated. The test will confirm past lead exposure but is still only indirect evidence of lead toxicity. Chronic accumulation of lead in bone is best measured by x-ray fluorescence and bone densitometry.

## Prevention

Workplace hygiene is critical in the prevention of excessive lead exposure. Clean areas for eating should be provided. Showering and cleaning of work garments are mandatory and should be provided at the plant to prevent exposure of children in the home. For processes that have the potential for generation of airborne dusts and fumes, respiratory protection should be provided.

Medical surveillance is required under the OSHA Lead Standard for workers exposed in excess of the Action Level of 30 µg/m³ for over 30 days per year, regardless of the use of respiratory protection. The program should include the following medical and biological monitoring procedures:

**Whole blood lead levels:**

(1) Every 6 months if < 40 µg/dL.

(2) Every 2 months if > 40 µg/dL until two consecutive determinations are < 40 µg/dL.

(3) Monthly during medical removal from exposure.

**Medical examinations (Table 27–3):**

(1) Yearly, if any blood lead level exceeded 40 µg/dL.

(2) Prior to assignment in an area where air lead levels are at or above the Action Level.

(3) As soon as possible, if a worker develops signs or symptoms or lead intoxication.

**Removal from exposure to lead:**

(1) Workers whose lead levels exceed 60 µg/dL, unless the last lead level is < 40 µg/dL.

(2) Workers whose last three lead levels or lead

**Table 27–3.** Medical examination of lead-exposed workers.

**Medical and occupational history**
  Focusing on lead exposure history; personal and
  workplace hygiene; gastrointestinal, hematologic, renal,
  reproductive, and neurologic problems.
**Physical examination**
  Focusing on the gums and on the gastrointestinal, hema-
  tologic, renal, reproductive, and neurologic systems.
  Pulmonary status should be evaluated in workers required
  to wear respiratory protective devices.
**Blood pressure measurement**
**Blood testing**
  Blood lead level.
  Zinc protoporphyrin or free erythrocyte protoporphyrin.
  Hemoglobin, hematocrit, and peripheral smear.
  Serum creatinine.
  Urinalysis, with microscopic examination.
**Other tests**
  As clinically indicated.

levels over the past 6 months (whichever is longer) exceed 50 µg/dL unless the last lead level is < 40 µg/dL.

(3) Workers who have an increased risk of material impairment of health from exposure to lead.

Worker removal due to elevated blood lead levels is the responsibility of the employer and should be undertaken without regard to worker health. Workers may be returned to exposure if two consecutive blood lead levels are less than 40 µg/dL.

Removal due to risk of substantial health impairment is a medical decision and should not be based solely on blood lead levels. Workers removed because of risk of health impairment may be returned when the final medical determination is that the worker is no longer at risk.

The occupational physician may encounter workplaces (particularly small operations) where workers have elevated blood lead and ZPP levels but are asymptomatic. In these instances, removal of an entire workforce from exposure is clearly not feasible. A program of frequent medical and biological monitoring should be instituted while industrial hygiene, engineering, and personal protective measures are instituted to reduce exposures to acceptable levels.

**Treatment**

In all cases of suspected lead intoxication in adults, the first step in management is removal from exposure. This may mean removal from the workplace if hygienic conditions are such that secondary exposure is significant. The decision about whether chelation therapy is needed depends on the intensity and duration of exposure and the clinical signs and symptoms. The primary indication for treatment of adults is brief, high-level exposure causing acute manifestations (encephalopathy, hemolysis, renal injury). The combined measurement of blood lead and

ZPP may help in management: An elevated blood lead (> 60 µg/dL) with a normal ZPP (< 100 mg/dL) suggests a recent increase in exposure.

Much more difficult is the management of the worker with vague complaints, such as abdominal pain, fatigue, muscle aches, or irritability. In a young worker with short-term exposure and an elevated blood lead level (> 60–80 µg/dL), these could be considered indications for treatment both to ameliorate symptoms and reduce the body burden. In long-term lead workers, removal from exposure remains the treatment of choice, chelation being reserved for those with severe manifestations (ie, frank encephalopathy).

While vague symptoms of ill health can occur as a result of exposure to lead, these nonspecific findings may be related to other health problems. Generally, symptoms related to lead will gradually improve after removal from exposure and reduction in blood lead levels. Symptoms that persist or worsen following removal from exposure should not be assumed to be due to lead and should prompt appropriate diagnostic evaluations.

**A. Acute Poisoning:** After poisoning by ingestion, emesis and then catharsis should be induced. Hydration is essential to reduce acute renal injury. In adults, the use of chelation therapy should be reserved for patients with significant symptoms or signs of toxicity. The patient should be hospitalized and treatment overseen by a physician who has experience with chelation therapy. The protocol recommended by Rempel (1989) is for adult patients, not for children. If the BUN and urinalysis are normal, 2 g of $CaNa_2EDTA$ in 1000 mL of 5% dextrose in water is infused intravenously over 24 hours. This is repeated daily for 5 days until a total of 10 g of $CaNa_2EDTA$ has been administered. Urinalysis, BUN, and serum creatinine should be monitored daily; if proteinuria, hematuria, or renal dysfunction is observed, $CaNa_2EDTA$ treatment should be discontinued.

An oral medication, 2,3 dimercaptosuccinic acid (succimer, Chemet), is approved in the United States for treatment of children with lead levels in excess of 45 µg/dL. The dose is 10 mg/kg every 8 hours for 5 days. Higher doses (up to 30 mg/kg) have been used in adults. This has been demonstrated to markedly increase lead excretion. Treatment must be carefully supervised to monitor for side effects (neutropenia, GI complaints, skin rashes). Rebound elevation of lead levels may also occur after treatment.

**B. Chronic Poisoning:** Results of the lead mobilization test together with the presence of significant symptoms or signs of toxicity should support the decision to treat with the same hospital protocol set forth above. If acute renal failure ensues, discontinue $CaNa_2EDTA$ treatment and institute hemodialysis.

**C. Lead Encephalopathy:** Lead encephalopathy is extremely rare in the occupational setting. When it occurs, it is a medical emergency. Treatment with chelation therapy should be instituted as described above. Cerebral edema should be treated and seizures controlled by a physician experienced in the care of such patients. Owing to the rarity of this problem in the occupational setting, it is wise to establish a consultative relationship with a physician whose background includes medical management of lead encephalopathy cases.

**D. Chronic Overexposure:** For workers with mild symptoms, removal from exposure is the treatment of choice. Chelation may not be effective for workers with long-term exposure (and an excessive body burden of lead), and treatment with $CaNa_2$ EDTA may cause acute tubular necrosis. Prophylactic chelation should not be used and is prohibited by the OSHA Lead Standard.

**E. Organic Level:** In acute alkyl lead intoxication, chelation therapy is of no benefit. Treatment should be directed at the presenting symptoms as indicated.

## Prognosis

Early diagnosis and treatment of lead toxicity will generally result in complete recovery. Once renal or neurologic impairment has occurred, only partial recovery may be expected.

## MANGANESE

### Essentials of Diagnosis

- Parkinsonlike syndrome.
- Behavioral changes, psychosis.
- Pneumonia.

### Exposure Limits

Manganese elemental and inorganic compounds
    ACGIH TLV: .02 mg/m³ TWA
Manganese cyclopentadienyl tricarbonyl
    ACGIH TLV: 0.1 mg/m³ TWA

### General Considerations

Manganese is a brittle gray metal that is abundant in the earth's crust, soils, and sediments and in biological materials. The most important source of manganese for commercial use is manganese dioxide, occurring as pyrolusite. Manganese is an essential trace element in humans and other living organisms. Manganese is present in highest concentrations in cells with high levels of metabolic activity, and several manganese-dependent enzyme systems have been identified.

### Use

Ferromanganese, an iron alloy containing over 80% manganese metal, is essential in the large-scale production of steel. Manganese is also used as a depolarizer in dry cell batteries and as an oxidizing agent in the chemical industry. Manganese is used in the manufacture of matches, paints, and pesticides. The manganese carbonyls, particularly methylcyclopentadienyl manganese tricarbonyl (MMT), is used as an antiknock agent in unleaded gasoline and in jet fuel. The manganese carbonyls are also used as a source of pure manganese metal in the electronics industry.

### Occupational & Environmental Exposure

Exposure to manganese dioxide occurs in the mining, smelting, and refining of manganese ores. Manganese exposure also occurs near crushing operations and reduction furnaces engaged in the production of ferrous and nonferrous alloys and in steel production. The use of manganese-containing welding rods is another source of potential worker exposure.

Exposure may also occur in the chemical industry and in the electronics industry. Workers engaged in the manufacture of fuels containing MMT may have respiratory or skin contact with this highly toxic liquid. Combustion of manganese containing fuels evolves primarily manganese oxides.

### Absorption, Metabolism, & Excretion

Manganese fumes may reach the alveoli and be absorbed after inhalation. Larger particles are ingested after mucociliary clearance from the lungs. Gastrointestinal absorption is generally low (10%) but may be increased in persons who are iron deficient. MMT may be absorbed after ingestion, inhalation, or skin contact.

Manganese is primarily excreted in the bile and may undergo enterohepatic recirculation. The biological half-life of manganese is approximately 30 hours, though in chronically exposed workers this may be shortened to 15 hours. Blood and urine levels are elevated in exposed workers but do not correlate with toxicity. Variations in manganese homeostasis may account for individual susceptibility to the development of toxic effects.

### Clinical Findings

**A. Symptoms and Signs:**

**1. Acute exposure**–Dermal and respiratory exposure to MMT results in slight burning of the skin followed by the development of headache, a metallic taste, nausea, diarrhea, dyspnea, and chest pain. On the basis of animal studies, acute overexposure to MMT could cause chemical pneumonitis, hepatic toxicity, and renal toxicity.

**2. Chronic exposure**–Industrial exposure to manganese has more frequently resulted in chronic effects on the nervous system, usually after several years. The earliest manifestations are vague symptoms of fatigue, headache, apathy, and behavioral disturbances. Episodes of excitability, garrulousness, and sexual arousal have been termed "manganese psychosis." With continued exposure, there is development of a syndrome that closely resembles Parkinson's disease. Speech becomes slow and monotonous, and the worker develops a masked facies. Tremor, bradykinesia, gait disturbance, and micrographia may all be present, resulting in a syndrome identical to idiopathic parkinsonism. Excessive salivation and sweating and vasomotor disturbances may also occur. Exposure to MMT has not been associated with nervous system toxicity, though experience with this compound is limited.

Worker exposure to manganese dust has also been associated with increased susceptibility to pneumonia and respiratory infections, often refractory to treatment. An inhibitory effect of manganese dioxide on pulmonary macrophage function may be responsible for this effect.

**B. Laboratory Findings:** Laboratory findings are usually normal. Minor decreases in leukocyte and red blood cell counts may be seen. Liver enzyme elevations have also been reported. Elevation of the protein level in cerebrospinal fluid often accompanies central nervous system toxicity.

Measurement of elevated urine manganese levels or finding an increase in urine manganese levels after a dose of calcium disodium edetate, a manganese chelator, serve to confirm exposure. Levels do not correlate with the degree of toxicity. Blood levels are of no value.

## Prevention

Manganese exposure should be reduced by the use of closed systems, local exhaust ventilation, and respiratory protection. Dermal and respiratory exposure to MMT should be prevented through use of proper personal protective equipment. Medical surveillance should focus on nervous system symptoms and changes in behavior to identify affected workers while the condition is still reversible. Careful neurologic examinations should be performed routinely on all exposed workers. Workers with exposure to MMT should also have periodic assessment of respiratory, liver, and kidney function.

## Treatment

Pneumonia should be treated with appropriate antibiotics as well as removal from exposure until the disease has cleared.

After skin contact with MMT, the affected areas should be cleansed immediately to reduce skin absorption. Workers who develop respiratory symptoms after inhalation of MMT should be admitted to the hospital for observation. Liver and kidney function should be monitored.

In workers with chronic exposure to manganese, the nervous system effects are reversible if they are detected early. Subjective symptoms may be the only manifestations at this stage. Once signs of parkinsonism have developed, the condition may be permanent, though progression will cease after exposure is terminated. Treatment with levodopa as for idiopathic parkinsonism is effective. Calcium disodium edetate chelation will increase urinary excretion of manganese but is ineffective in reversing the nervous system effects.

# MERCURY

## Essentials of Diagnosis

*Inorganic mercury:*
- Acute respiratory distress.
- Gingivitis.
- Tremor.
- Erethism (shyness, emotional lability).
- Proteinuria, renal failure.

*Organic mercury (alkyl mercury compounds):*
- Mental disturbances.
- Ataxia, spasticity.
- Paresthesias.
- Visual and auditory disturbances.

## Exposure Limits

Alkyl compounds
ACGIH TLV: 0.01 mg/m$^3$ TWA, 0.03 mg/m$^3$ STEL
Vapor (all forms except alkyl)
ACGIH TLV: 0.025 mg/m$^3$ TWA
Aryl and inorganic compounds
ACGIH TLV: 0.1 mg/m$^3$
BEI ACGIH: urine: 35 µg/g creatinine; blood: 15 µg/L (end of week/end of shift)

## General Considerations

Mercury is a heavy, silvery-white metal that is a liquid at room temperature. Its high vapor pressure presents the constant inhalation hazard in settings where elemental mercury is handled. Mercury is present in numerous classes of rocks and is recovered primarily from cinnabar ore (HgS). Ore is mined using both surface and underground methods. Mercury is recovered through heating in furnaces and retorts. While mercury is ubiquitous in nature, environmental contamination and subsequent bioaccumulation—particularly in seafood—has led to strict emission controls. Mercury is not considered to be an essential element in humans.

## Use

A major use of mercury is in the manufacture of control instruments, tubes, rectifiers, thermometers, barometers, batteries, and electrical devices. Mercury is used in brine cells for the electrolytic production of chlorine and caustic soda and as a catalyst in polyurethane foams. Use of alkyl mercury compounds (methyl mercury and ethyl mercury) as grain fumigants and antimildew agents has been banned in the United States—replaced by less toxic mercury compounds. Mercury is used in plating, jewelry, tanning, and taxidermy. Use in the felt industry in the 19th century led to extensive poisoning ("mad as a hatter"), and such use has been discontinued also. Mercury amalgams are used in dentistry. Mercury has been used in medicinal preparations (eg, mercurial diuretics) in the past, but these have been largely replaced by less toxic agents.

### Occupational & Environmental Exposure

All workers involved in the extraction and recovery of mercury are at high risk for exposure to mercury vapor. Maintenance work on furnaces, flues, and retorts is an important potential source of exposure. Workers in chlorine plants are also at risk, though most operate using closed systems.

Workers engaged in the manufacture of electrical equipment requiring mercury may be exposed through spillage or careless handling. Metal-reclaiming workers may be exposed to mercury as well as other heavy metals. In production areas where mercury is used as a catalyst, workers may be exposed through improper storing and handling or during maintenance operations. Dentists, dental technicians, and other laboratory workers may be exposed if mercury is not handled carefully. Short-term peak exposures may occur during certain dental procedures. Workers may be exposed to alkyl mercury compounds during the production and application of organic mercury fungicides.

Several epidemics of organic mercury poisoning have occurred as a result of environmental contamination from industrial effluents and improper use of grain fumigants. Release of organic mercury into Minimata Bay in Japan resulted in accumulation of methyl mercury in seafood, poisoning thousands of individuals ("Minimata disease"). Similar mass poisonings have occurred after consumption of grain treated with alkyl mercury compounds. Air and water contamination with inorganic mercury from the burning of coal and from chlorine plants has had less dramatic consequences but has been a significant source of background exposure.

### Absorption, Metabolism, & Excretion

Elemental mercury is absorbed after the inhalation of mercury vapor. Ingested elemental mercury forms globules that are poorly absorbed from the gastrointestinal tract. Soluble mercurial salts ($Hg^{2+}$) and aryl mercury compounds are also absorbed after inhalation and to a limited extent after ingestion. Alkyl mercury compounds are readily absorbed through all routes—inhalation, ingestion, or skin contact.

Inorganic and aryl mercury compounds are distributed to many tissues, primarily the brain and kidney. There they bind to sulfhydryl groups and may interfere with numerous cellular enzyme systems. Metallothionein (a low-molecular-weight protein rich in sulfhydryl groups) production is increased after mercury exposure and may exert a protective effect in the kidney. Alkyl mercury compounds have a tight carbon-mercury bond and accumulate in the central nervous system. In the bloodstream, the majority of the absorbed alkyl mercury is found in the red blood cells.

Both organic and elemental mercury compounds readily cross the blood-brain barrier and the placenta and are secreted in breast milk. After inhalation, elemental mercury is rapidly oxidized by red blood cells, protecting the nervous system. Peak exposures may be more hazardous, since the rate of exodation may be inadequate to protect the target tissue. All mercury compounds are eliminated slowly in the urine, feces, saliva, and sweat. The average half-life in humans is 60 days for inorganic mercury and 70 days for alkyl mercury compounds. Mercury also binds to thiol groups and may be measured in the hair and nails.

### Clinical Findings

#### A. Symptoms and Signs:

**1. Inorganic mercury**–Inhalation of high concentrations of mercury vapor or soluble mercury salts usually is a result of work in enclosed spaces. Cough, dyspnea, inflammation of the oral cavity, and gastrointestinal complaints occur shortly after exposure. These may be followed by the development of a chemical pneumonitis with cyanosis, tachypnea, and pulmonary edema. Renal injury is a particular concern after exposure to mercuric chloride and presents as an initial diuresis followed by proteinuria and oliguric renal failure. After recovery from the acute illness, neurologic symptoms similar to those seen with chronic overexposure may develop. Ingestion of soluble mercury compounds results in gastrointestinal complaints of nausea, vomiting, diarrhea, and abdominal pain, which may be followed by renal and neurologic sequelae.

Chronic exposure to inorganic mercury compounds results primarily in effects on the nervous system. Neuropsychiatric manifestations include changes in personality, shyness, anxiety, memory loss, and emotional lability. Tremor is an early sign of neurotoxicity. Initially, the tremor is fine and occurs at rest, progressing with further exposure to an intention tremor interrupted by coarse jerking movements. A comparison with prior handwriting may demonstrate the tremor. Head tremor and skeletal ataxia may also occur. A sensory peripheral neuropathy is usually present with distal paresthesias. Hallucinations and dementia are late manifestations.

Other findings after excessive chronic exposure include inflammation of the oral cavity, manifested by salivation, gingivitis, and dental erosions. A bluish linear pigmentation may be present on the teeth or gums. Reddish-brown pigmentation of the lens may be apparent on slit lamp examination. Renal injury usually results in proteinuria without frank renal failure. Excessive sweating and an eczematous skin eruption may also be present.

**2. Organic mercury–**Exposure to alkyl mercury compounds results in the insidious onset of progressive nervous system effects. The earliest symptoms are of numbness and tingling of the extremities and lips. Loss of motor coordination follows, with gait ataxia, tremor, and loss of fine movement. Constriction of the visual fields, central hearing loss, muscular rigidity, and spasticity occur with exaggerated deep tendon reflexes. Behavioral changes, fits of laughter, and intellectual impairment may be prominent. Erythroderma, desquamation, and other skin rashes may be present. Renal disease is rare. Neurotoxicity in infants exposed in utero in the Minimata Bay epidemic resembled cerebral palsy.

**B. Laboratory Findings:** After acute inhalation, there may be hypoxemia (as shown by arterial blood gas measurements) and diffuse infiltrates on chest x-ray. Proteinuria indicates renal injury. The earliest manifestations of renal effects are increased excretion of low-molecular-weight proteins, including N-acetyl-$\beta$-glucosaminidase, $\beta_2$-microglobulin, and retinol-binding protein.

Measurement of mercury in blood and urine will confirm the diagnosis. Gross renal or neurologic manifestations are unusual unless urine mercury levels exceed 500 $\mu$g/g creatinine. Subtle nervous system effects have been detected in workers with levels of 50–150 $\mu$g/g creatinine, and early renal effects (low-molecular-weight proteinuria with normal renal function) have been detected when urine mercury levels chronically exceed 50 $\mu$g/g creatinine. Normal concentrations in nonexposed individuals are less than 0.01 mg/L in whole blood and less than 10 $\mu$g/g creatinine in urine. Substantial seafood consumption may result in higher levels. A high ratio of whole blood mercury to plasma mercury suggests alkyl mercury intoxication. Hair and nail levels may be elevated in intoxication but are subject to external contamination.

## Prevention

Awareness of the constant hazard of mercury vapor exposure along with proper handling of materials and meticulous attention to workplace hygiene will reduce potential exposures. Use of proper ventilation and respiratory protection is required in all operations that use mercury compounds. Special attention should focus on maintenance workers. Care in the handling and disposal of mercury compounds will prevent inadvertent contamination of the workplace. Control of industrial emissions will prevent contamination of waterways and seafood. Grain fumigation with mercury compounds should be restricted.

Medical surveillance of mercury-exposed workers should include a careful history and neurologic examination as well as periodic urinalyses. A sample biological monitoring program is shown in Table 27–4. Urine levels fluctuate, and periodic monitoring or group monitoring will be more representative of ongoing exposure. Greater accuracy may be obtained by adjusting to urine creatinine.

## Treatment

After acute exposure to mercury, prompt treatment with dimercaprol (5 mg/kg intramuscularly) should be instituted. Respiratory distress and renal failure should be treated appropriately. Penicillamine is also effective for acute poisoning.

Individuals manifesting symptoms of chronic mercury toxicity should be removed from further exposure. The decision to give treatment in such cases depends on the severity of the symptoms and whether evidence of neurologic or renal toxicity is present. There is limited evidence that chronic mercury poisoning may respond to treatment with the investigational drug 2,3-dimercaptopropane-1-sulfonate (100 mg orally 3 times daily, increasing to 4 times daily, for several weeks). The neurologic sequelae of alkyl mercury poisoning are irreversible, emphasizing the need for prevention.

## NICKEL

### Essentials of Diagnosis

*Nickel compounds (except nickel carbonyl):*
- Allergic contact dermatitis, eczema.
- Sinusitis, anosmia.
- Asthma.
- Nasal and lung cancer.

*Nickel carbonyl:*
- Headache, fatigue, gastrointestinal symptoms.
- Cough, dyspnea.
- Interstitial pneumonitis.
- Delirium, coma.

### Exposure Limits

Nickel, insoluble and soluble
    ACGIH TLV: 0.05 mg/m$^3$
    OSHA PEL: 1 mg/m$^3$ TWA (metal)
    OSHA PEL: 0.1 mg/m$^3$ (soluble)

### General Considerations

Nickel is a hard, silver-white, malleable, magnetic

**Table 27–4.** Biological monitoring program for mercury.[1]

| Air Exposure | Urine Hg Level | Action |
|---|---|---|
| >50 µg/m³ | >100 µg/g creatinine | Remove from exposure until <50<br>Medical examination if over 150 or if two consecutive levels exceed 100<br>Repeat measurement weekly |
| 50 µg/m³ | 75–100 µg/g creatinine | Monitor weekly<br>Perform hygiene assessment to limit exposure |
| 25–50 µg/m³ | 50–75 µg/g creatinine | Monitor monthly |
| 25 µg/m³ | 35–50 µg/g creatinine | Monitor quarterly |
| <25 µg/m³ | <35 µg/g creatinine | Monitor semiannually |

[1] Approximate equivalents if adjusted to a specific gravity of 1.024: 100 µg/g creatinine = 150 µg/L; 75 µg/g creatinine = 100 µg/L; 50 µg/g creatinine = 75 µg/L; 35 µg/g creatinine = 50 µg/L.

metal that has wide industrial application. Pentlandite—$(FeNi)_9S_8$—the primary commercial ore, is often deposited with other iron and copper sulfides. Nickel sulfide is concentrated by flotation and magnetic separation prior to roasting. Nickel is refined by electrolysis or the Mond process, in which treatment with carbon monoxide leads to the formation of nickel carbonyl—$Ni(CO)_4$. Nickel occurs naturally in a variety of vegetables and grains.

## Use

The major use of nickel is in the production of stainless steel, where it may be present in concentrations of 5–10%. Nickel alloys with other metals, such as copper (Monel metal), supply durability and fabricating properties for applications in food and dairy processing equipment, chemical synthesis, and the petroleum industry. Coins, tableware and utensils, springs, magnets, batteries (nickel-cadmium), and spark plugs also utilize nickel alloys. Soluble nickel salts are used in electroplating to impart lustrous, polishable, corrosion-resistant surfaces to parts and equipment. Nickel compounds are also used as catalysts and pigments.

## Occupational & Environmental Exposure

Exposure to nickel compounds may occur during mining, milling, roasting, sintering, and refining operations. In the Mond process, workers may also be exposed to highly toxic nickel carbonyl gas. Workers engaged in the production of nickel alloys—as well as those involved in the fabrication and welding of these materials—may also be exposed to nickel dusts and fumes. In electroplating shops, workers may have respiratory and skin exposure to soluble nickel salts. Workers using nickel as a catalyst may be exposed to nickel powders. Air levels may be elevated in communities surrounding roasting and sintering plants. Nickel and (presumably) nickel carbonyl are contaminants in cigarette smoke.

## Absorption, Metabolism, & Excretion

Nickel is poorly absorbed from the gastrointestinal tract. Soluble nickel compounds and nickel carbonyl are readily absorbed after inhalation.

In plasma, nickel is bound to albumin and "nickelplasmin," a metalloprotein. Absorbed nickel does not accumulate in tissues and is excreted in the urine with a half-life of approximately 1 week.

Nickel is excreted to a lesser extent in sweat and bile. Insoluble nickel compounds may accumulate in the respiratory tract—a factor that may contribute to carcinogenicity. Nickel readily crosses the placental barrier and can be measured in fetal tissue.

## Clinical Findings

**A. Symptoms and Signs:** The most common manifestations of exposure to soluble nickel compounds are dermatologic. Nickel is a common cause of allergic contact dermatitis (usually nonoccupational) and may cause erythema and vesiculation at points of contact in sensitized individuals. Chronic eczematous dermatitis involving the hands and arms may also develop in nickel workers, particularly in electroplating shops where there is exposure to liquids and aerosols. Exposure to high levels of soluble nickel aerosols may also cause rhinitis, sinusitis, anosmia, and septal perforation. Cough and wheezing should suggest the possibility of nickel-induced asthma, though this is uncommon. Nickel fumes may cause an illness resembling metal fume fever.

Exposure to nickel carbonyl causes headache, fatigue, nausea, and vomiting. These symptoms usually resolve when the affected individual is removed to fresh air. In severe cases, there is a delay of 12–36 hours before development of a diffuse interstitial pneumonitis, with fever, chills, cough, chest pain, and dyspnea. Delirium, seizures, and coma may occur prior to death.

Exposure to nickel compounds in refining and nickel subsulfide roasting operations has caused an increase in nasal and respiratory cancers in humans. Smaller studies of workers exposed to pure nickel dust, nickel oxides, and nickel alloys have not shown an excess in respiratory cancers. Nickel, nickel subsulfide, nickel carbonyl, and other nickel compounds are carcinogenic in laboratory animals. Nickel should be considered a human respiratory carcinogen, and worker exposure should be reduced to the lowest feasible levels, particularly in refining and roasting operations.

**B. Laboratory Findings:** The diagnosis of nickel skin allergy can be confirmed by patch testing or lymphocyte transformation testing. Nickel-induced asthma may result in an elevated eosinophil count. After exposure to nickel carbonyl, there is a moderate leukocytosis, hypoxemia, and a reduction in lung volumes and carbon monoxide diffusing capacity consistent with acute pneumonitis. Liver enzyme levels may be elevated. In evaluating persons who have been exposed to nickel carbonyl, urine nickel levels greater than 100 µg/L indicate moderate exposure while levels in excess of 500 µg/L indicate severe exposure.

## Prevention

Skin and respiratory protection should be used where there is potential exposure to nickel dusts, fumes, or soluble nickel aerosols and liquids. Extreme caution should be used in handling gaseous nickel carbonyl. Medical surveillance should concentrate on the skin and respiratory system, with prompt removal of those who develop dermal or respiratory allergy. A biological threshold level of 10 µg/L in plasma is recommended for workers exposed to nickel compounds. A maximum level of 10 µg/L in the urine is recommended for workers exposed to nickel carbonyl.

## Treatment

Nickel dermatitis should be treated with topical steroids and removal from further exposure. Extremely sensitive individuals may not be able to work where there is any further exposure to nickel, even with proper personal protection. Nickel sensitivity is permanent. Respiratory tract irritation will resolve after removal from exposure.

Individuals who have been exposed to nickel carbonyl should be admitted to a hospital to be monitored for the development of pulmonary complications and systemic toxicity. An 8-hour urine collection should be sent for nickel measurement. If exposure is found to be excessive (urine nickel 100 µg/L), treatment should be instituted with sodium diethyldithiocarbamate (Dithiocarb). This may be given orally in a dosage of 50 mg/kg in divided doses as follows:

50% of total dose at time 0
25% of total dose at 4 hours
15% of total dose at 8 hours

10% of total dose at 16 hours and then an additional dose equivalent to 10% of the total dose every 8 hours until symptoms have resolved or urine nickel is below 50 µg/L.

In comatose or acutely ill persons, the drug may be given in a dose of 25 mg/kg intramuscularly every 4 hours, increasing to 100 mg/kg depending on the clinical condition.

## PHOSPHORUS

### Essentials of Diagnosis
- Necrosis of the jaw.
- Dermal burns.
- Respiratory irritation.
- Hepatic and renal injury.

### Exposure Limits

Phosphorus (yellow)
  ACGIH TLV: 0.1 mg/m$^3$ TWA
  OSHA PEL: 0.1 mg/m$^3$ TWA
Phosphine
  ACGIH TLV: 0.4 mg/m$^3$ TWA, 1 mg/m$^3$ STEL
  OSHA PEL: 0.4 mg/m$^3$ TWA, 1 mg/m$^3$ STEL
Phosphorus oxychloride
  ACGIH TLV: 0.6 mg/m$^3$ TWA, 3 mg/m$^3$ STEL
  OSHA PEL: 0.6 mg/m$^3$ TWA
Phosphoric acid
  ACGIH TLV: 1 mg/m$^3$ TWA, 3 mg/m$^3$ STEL

### General Considerations

Phosphorus is an essential element for energy metabolism in many biological systems. In nature, phosphorus does not occur free but is found in rock in the mineral apatite (tricalcium phosphate). Phosphorus rock is crushed and heated, liberating elemental phosphorus, which is then condensed and submerged in water to prevent spontaneous combustion in air. Two allotropes—the highly toxic white (yellow) form and red phosphorus—are of industrial importance. Elemental phosphorus is converted to phosphoric acid, phosphine, and phosphorus chlorides and sulfides for specific industrial applications.

### Use

The use of white phosphorus in matches was banned after the turn of the century after numerous workers developed severe, disabling jaw necrosis ("phossy jaw"). This has been replaced by the less toxic red phosphorus and phosphorus sesquisulfide. White phosphorus is still used in explosives, fireworks, smoke bombs, and rodenticides. Phosphoric acid is used in the production of superphosphate fertilizers. In the microelectronics industry, phosphorus is used as a dopant for silicon and for substrate material in mixed crystals. Phosphorus compounds are used in the manufacture of a variety of chemicals, including organophosphate pesticides (refer to Chapter 32).

## Occupational & Environmental Exposure

Workers may be exposed to white phosphorus during production of explosives, pesticides, or other phosphorus compounds. Production workers engaged in the manufacture of matches and fertilizers may handle large quantities of phosphorus compounds. Semiconductor manufacturers may use elemental phosphorus, phosphorus chlorides, and phosphine as sources of phosphorus atoms. Phosphine may escape during the storage of ferrosilicon. Phosphine may also be liberated through the accidental wetting of zinc phosphide rodenticides or aluminum phosphide grain fumigants or during the manufacture of acetylene from calcium carbide. Accidental or suicidal ingestion of phosphorus-containing fireworks or rodenticides has been a cause of nonoccupational poisoning.

## Absorption, Metabolism, & Excretion

Phosphorus may be absorbed after inhalation, ingestion, or skin contact. Spontaneous combustion in air leads to extensive tissue destruction of the skin, eyes, and mucous membranes. In the liver, phosphorus interferes with protein and carbohydrate metabolism and inhibits glycogen storage. Fat deposition in the liver is increased. Chronic exposure to phosphorus causes subepiphyseal bone formation with impaired vascularity, leading to bone necrosis. Excretion of inorganic phosphate is primarily through the kidney.

## Clinical Findings

### A. Symptoms and Signs:

**1. Acute exposure**–Ingestion of yellow phosphorus is followed in 1–2 hours by development of nausea, vomiting, and abdominal pain owing to local tissue injury. Phosphorescent vomitus and smoking stools may be clues to the diagnosis. Systemic manifestations, including uremia, jaundice, and liver enlargement, develop after several days. Hypocalcemic tetany with carpal and pedal muscle spasms may also develop. In severe cases, cardiac arrhythmias and coma may precede death.

Phosphorus burns may result following spontaneous combustion, when contaminated skin surfaces dry. Second- and third-degree phosphorus burns with blistering are characterized by slow healing. Absorption of phosphorus in severe cases may result in systemic phosphorus toxicity.

Inhalation of phosphorus compounds may cause bronchospasm with cough, chest tightness, and wheezing. Local tissue necrosis may cause hemoptysis. In severe cases, chemical pneumonitis may develop, with respiratory failure due to pulmonary edema followed by arrhythmias and signs of systemic phosphorus poisoning.

Inhalation of phosphine gas causes headache, fatigue, nausea, vomiting, and excessive thirst as well as cough, chest tightness, and shortness of breath. Neurologic symptoms include ataxia, paresthesias, tremor, and diplopia. Death may occur in 1–2 days from respiratory failure, cardiovascular collapse, or convulsions.

**2. Chronic exposure**–The main hazard from chronic exposure to yellow phosphorus was the development of jaw necrosis. This usually presents as a dental affliction followed by chronic suppuration. Persistent bacterial infection imparts a fetid odor to the breath. Other forms of phosphorus have not been associated with this condition. Workers exposed to irritant phosphorus compounds may develop obstructive lung disease and chronic bronchitis.

### B. Laboratory Findings:
Findings in acute intoxication with phosphorus compounds include elevated liver enzymes, hyperbilirubinemia, hematuria, proteinuria, and leukopenia. Profound hypocalcemia may occur. After acute inhalation injury, arterial hypoxemia may be present. Pulmonary function tests may show obstruction or a mixed obstructive and restrictive pattern with an impaired diffusing capacity for carbon monoxide.

Perihilar infiltrates on chest x-ray suggest a chemical pneumonitis or pulmonary edema. X-ray changes in phosphorus-induced jaw necrosis include degeneration, sequestration, and necrosis.

## Prevention

Phosphorus must be handled with extreme care, using wet processes to avoid accidental exposure and spontaneous combustion. Skin, eye, and respiratory protection should be worn when handling phosphorus compounds. Awareness of the potential sources of exposure to phosphine gas will prevent accidental injury. Medical surveillance should concentrate on dental hygiene and respiratory, liver, and kidney function. There is currently no method for biological monitoring of workers exposed to phosphorus compounds.

## Treatment

After ingestion, gastric lavage should be performed with 5–10 L of tap water and vomiting should be induced. Mineral oil should then be administered. Hypocalcemia should be treated with calcium gluconate 10%, 10 mL intravenously, with close monitoring of serum calcium. Cardiac rhythm should be closely monitored during calcium repletion. Skin and eye burns should be treated with copious irrigation. A topical solution of 3% copper sulfate will neutralize phosphorus on the skin; however, extensive use may result in excessive absorption of copper. Phosphorus-induced bone necrosis may respond to drainage and appropriate antibiotic therapy. Surgical excision and bone grafting may be necessary in patients with extensive necrosis.

## SELENIUM

### Essentials of Diagnosis

*Acute effects:*
- Respiratory, mucous membrane, and skin irritation.
- Skin burns.

*Chronic effects:*
- Fatigue, lassitude.
- Gastrointestinal complaints.
- Garlic odor of breath and sweat.
- Dermatitis, paronychia, alopecia.
- Conjunctivitis.

### Exposure Limits

ACGIH TLV: 0.2 mg/m$^3$ TWA
OSHA PEL: 0.2 mg/m$^3$ TWA

### General Considerations

Selenium is a metalloid element that is distributed widely in igneous rock, sedimentary rock, and mineral ores, particularly in sulfur and copper deposits. Selenium for commercial use is obtained primarily through extraction from slimes produced in the electrolytic refining of copper. Selenium exists in three forms: a red amorphous powder, a gray hexagonal semiconducting crystal, and a red crystal. Selenium is an essential trace element in humans, serving as a cofactor for glutathione peroxidase in the prevention of oxidative damage in erythrocytes.

Selenium has also been found to be teratogenic in animals. An isolated report found four spontaneous abortions and one congenital malformation among 10 women exposed to sodium selenite in a laboratory.

### Use

Selenium is used in the manufacture of glass and plastics to impart a red tint or to neutralize green discoloration. The photoconducting properties of selenium are useful in rectifiers and photoelectric cells. Selenium is used to alter the machinability of steel and to increase the rate of vulcanization of rubber. Selenium is also used medicinally in dandruff shampoos and topical antifungal lotions. Selenium is used in paint pigments, animal feeds, and veterinary medicines. Selenium hexafluoride is used as a gaseous insulator in transformers.

### Occupational & Environmental Exposure

Workers engaged in the smelting and refining of copper may be exposed to airborne selenium fumes and selenium oxide dust. Refinery and metal workers may also be exposed to hydrogen selenide through the reaction of acid with metal selenides. Elemental selenium is encountered in the electronics, glass, ceramics, plastics, and rubber industries. Formulators may be exposed to selenium in the production of pharmaceuticals and animal feed. Selenium is available commercially in dandruff shampoos and mineral supplements. Agricultural use of sodium selenite as a pesticide and selenium contamination of phosphate fertilizers has led to soil and groundwater contamination.

### Absorption, Metabolism, & Excretion

Selenium compounds may be absorbed through the lungs, gastrointestinal tract, or damaged skin. Selenium is metabolized to organic forms in the liver. Dimethylselenium is excreted through the lungs and imparts a garlic odor to the breath. Trimethylselenium is excreted in the urine. Elevated levels may be seen for several weeks following exposure.

### Clinical Findings

**A. Symptoms and Signs:**

**1. Acute exposure**–Acute inhalation of selenium fumes, selenium oxide dust, selenium oxychloride vapor, hydrogen selenium, or selenium hexafluoride may cause severe respiratory irritation, resulting in cough, chest pain, and dyspnea. In severe cases, a chemical pneumonitis with pulmonary edema may develop. Neurologic, hepatic, and renal damage may occur. Selenium oxide may cause severe skin burns.

**2. Chronic exposure**–Chronic exposure to selenium compounds may result in nonspecific complaints of fatigue and lassitude. Gastrointestinal complaints of nausea and indigestion may be present. There is a strong garlic odor to the breath and sweat. Chronic airborne exposure may cause conjunctivitis, termed "rose eye." Dermatologic manifestations include irritant or allergic dermatitis, painful paronychia, and loss of hair and nails. Reddish skin and hair discoloration may also be present.

The role of selenium in the development of cancer in humans is uncertain. A protective effect has been proposed but not confirmed. Selenium has caused liver tumors in laboratory animals.

**B. Laboratory Findings:** Laboratory evaluation is usually nondiagnostic. Liver enzyme elevations and anemia may be seen. Measurement of selenium in the urine will confirm overexposure, normal concentrations being less than 150 µg/L.

### Prevention

Respiratory and skin protection should be used where exposure to high levels of airborne selenium compounds cannot be controlled through other means. Medical surveillance should focus on gastrointestinal and dermatologic complaints. The detection of a garlic odor in an exposed individual should suggest excessive absorption. Urine selenium should remain below 100 μg/L in individuals exposed to air levels of 0.1 mg/m$^3$.

## Treatment

Prompt evacuation and resuscitation should be undertaken in cases of acute inhalation. Burns of the skin should be irrigated with a solution of 10% aqueous sodium thiosulfate followed by use of a 10% sodium thiosulfate cream. Administration of ascorbic acid may lessen the offensive garlic odor of exposed individuals. Chelation is contraindicated and may cause renal damage.

## TELLURIUM

### Essentials of Diagnosis

- Respiratory irritation.
- Garlic odor.
- Fatigue, somnolence.
- Dryness of mouth and skin.
- Anhidrosis.
- Blue-black skin discoloration.

### Exposure Limits

ACGIH TLV: 0.1 mg/m$^3$ TWA
OSHA PEL: 0.1 mg/m$^3$ TWA

### General Considerations

Tellurium is a bright silvery metalloid element that shares many characteristics with selenium. Its distribution in rock and ore deposits is similar to that of selenium, though tellurium is much rarer. Tellurium—like selenium—is obtained primarily by extraction from anodic slimes formed as a by-product in copper refining. Tellurium compounds are generally less toxic than the corresponding selenium compounds. Although present in various concentrations in human tissues, tellurium is not considered an essential trace element for humans.

### Use

Tellurium is used in the vulcanization of rubber to increase durability. Like selenium, tellurium is finding increasing use in electronics, primarily in the manufacture of rectifiers and semiconductors. Tellurium imparts corrosive resistance in steel and is used as a carbide stabilizer for iron. Tellurium is used in numerous alloys, catalysts, pigments, and photographic chemicals.

### Occupational Exposure

Workers in the rubber industry may be exposed to tellurium compounds. Tellurium exposure may also occur in the refining of copper, silver, gold, lead, and bismuth and in foundries. Workers in the glass, ceramic, and electronics industries may also be exposed to tellurium.

### Absorption, Metabolism, & Excretion

Soluble tellurium compounds are absorbed after inhalation or ingestion. Metabolism to dimethyl telluride results in the characteristic garlicky odor. Excretion is primarily through the urine and bile. Tellurium accumulates in liver and bone, and excretion may be prolonged after exposure.

### Clinical Findings

**A. Symptoms and Signs:**

**1. Acute exposure–**Acute inhalation of tellurium fumes, tellurium oxide, hydrogen telluride, or tellurium hexafluoride may result in acute respiratory irritation. Acute exposure is followed by development of the characteristic garlicky odor of the breath and sweat. A blue-black discoloration of the skin may also develop. Fatigue, nausea, and other systemic complaints may be present.

**2. Chronic exposure–**Chronic exposure produces garlic breath, a metallic taste, fatigue, somnolence, dryness of the mouth, and anhidrosis. Tellurium has been found to have adverse neurologic and reproductive effects in experimental animals. Demyelination, congenital hydrocephalus, and aspermatogenesis have been reported. There have been no reports of similar effects in humans.

**B. Laboratory Findings:** Laboratory tests are nonspecific. Hemolysis may occur after exposure to hydrogen telluride.

### Prevention

Exhaust ventilation and personal protective equipment should be used where there is potential exposure to tellurium fumes. Periodic air monitoring and careful attention to workplace hygiene will reduce the chance for chronic exposure. Medical surveillance should focus on complaints of unusual odors, metallic taste, or dry or discolored skin. Urinary tellurium levels should be kept below 0.05 mg/L. Pregnant women should not work directly with tellurium compounds.

### Treatment

Supportive therapy should be instituted as indicated. Pulmonary status should be monitored after acute inhalation. Severe hemolysis should be treated with exchange transfusion. Chelation is contraindicated because of its renal toxicity. Ascorbic acid reduces the garlicky odor but may also result in renal toxicity.

# THALLIUM

## Essentials of Diagnosis

*Acute effects:*
- Alopecia.
- Gastrointestinal distress.
- Ascending paralysis, coma.

*Chronic effects:*
- Alopecia.
- Weakness, fatigue.
- Peripheral neuropathy.

## Exposure Limits

ACGIH TLV: 0.1 mg/m$^3$ TWA
OSHA PEL: 0.1 mg/m$^3$ TWA

## General Considerations

Thallium is a heavy metal that occurs in the earth's crust as a minor constituent in iron, copper, sulfide, and selenide ores. Thallium can be recovered from flue dusts, either from pyrite ($FeS_2$) roasting or from lead and zinc smelting. Thallium can be prepared as both water-soluble (sulfate, acetate) and water insoluble (halide) salts.

## Use

Thallium sulfate was used as a medicinal in the treatment of syphilis, gonorrhea, gout, and tuberculosis in the 19th century. Abandoned because of its toxicity, it enjoyed a brief resurgence as a depilatory in the 1920s. $^{201}$TlCl is currently used in myocardial imaging for the diagnosis of cardiac ischemia.

Thallium salts have been used extensively as rodenticides in the form of impregnated grain (Thalgrain) and pastes (Zelio). Numerous accidental and suicidal poisonings led to the banning of these compounds in the United States in 1972. Currently, thallium is finding increasing uses in the manufacture of electronic components, optical lenses, imitation jewelry, dyes, and pigments.

## Occupational & Environmental Exposure

At highest risk for exposure are those engaged in the production of thallium salt derivatives. In addition, workers in the electronics and optical industries have potential exposure to thallium compounds. Thallium exposure can occur at smelters, particularly in the maintenance and cleaning of ducts and flues. Thallium-containing pyrite is also used in cement production.

Environmental exposure can occur in the vicinity of smelting operations through air and water contamination. Thallium exposure in a community surrounding a cement plant in Germany was attributed to ingestion of vegetables grown in thallium-contaminated soil. Water pollution from smelters may contaminate seafood. Thallium chloride has been found in potassium chloride salt substitutes.

## Metabolism & Mechanism of Action

Thallium—and especially its soluble salts—is readily absorbed through the gastrointestinal tract, skin, and respiratory system. Ingestion of 0.5–1 g may be lethal. Thallium is rapidly distributed intracellularly throughout all body tissues. Elimination is slow and occurs through intestinal and renal secretion in a ratio of 2:1. Thallium behaves much like potassium and binds avidly to several enzyme systems, including Na$^+$-K$^+$ ATPase. Thallium binds to sulfhydryl groups and interferes with cellular respiration and protein synthesis. Binding to riboflavin may contribute to its neurotoxicity.

## Clinical Findings

### A. Symptoms and Signs:

**1. Acute exposure**–Gastrointestinal symptoms predominate early and include pain, nausea, vomiting, hemorrhage, and diarrhea. Cardiac abnormalities include tachycardia and hypertension. Neurologic manifestations usually begin with pain, hyperesthesia, and hyperreflexia in the lower extremities. This may rapidly progress to areflexia, hypesthesia, and paralysis depending on the amount ingested. Ataxia, agitation, hallucinations, and coma may occur in severe cases. Alopecia, primarily of scalp and body hair, occurs at the end of the first week; however, black pigmentation of the hair root may be seen earlier. Mees' lines of nails and gingival pigmentation occur. Anhidrosis occurs early owing to destruction of sweat glands.

**2. Chronic exposure**–In chronic intoxication, the onset of symptoms is insidious. Alopecia and dry skin may be the only complaint. Fatigue and asthenia are frequent. Insomnia and behavioral dysfunction, cranial nerve involvement, and dementia may be presenting symptoms. Endocrine dysfunction includes impotence and amenorrhea.

**B. Laboratory Findings:** Findings are generally nonspecific. Hypokalemia and alkalosis may be present. Elevated liver enzyme levels in severe cases reflect centrilobular necrosis. Proteinuria and renal tubular necrosis can occur. The ECG may show signs of hypokalemia. The EEG reveals nonspecific slow wave activity in severe cases. Nerve conduction studies are consistent with axonal degeneration, though demyelination has been seen pathologically.

The diagnosis is confirmed by demonstrating elevated thallium levels in the urine. Normal levels range from 0 to 10 μg/L. Hair and nail levels may be elevated in chronic exposure. Levels in workers should be maintained below 50 μg/L.

## Differential Diagnosis

Thallium intoxication should be considered in every case of peripheral neuropathy of unknown cause. The acute presentation may suggest lead poisoning; however, basophilic stippling of red blood cells is absent. The absence of urobilinogen in the urine distinguishes thallium poisoning from acute intermittent porphyria. In chronic intoxication from industrial exposure, the presentation may suggest depression, hypothyroidism, or organic brain syndrome.

## Prevention

Proper skin and respiratory protection are essential. Eating and smoking should not be permitted in areas where thallium compounds are handled. Thallium is a cumulative toxin, and biological monitoring of urine levels should be considered where there is chronic exposure to thallium compounds.

The banning of thallium-containing pesticides has reduced the frequency of thallium poisoning in the United States, but these compounds may still be encountered and are still available in other countries.

## Treatment

In acute cases, emesis should be induced. Treatment with Prussian blue (potassium ferric cyanoferrate II) in a dose of 1 g three times daily will bind secreted thallium in the gut. This should be administered with a cathartic to avoid constipation. Activated charcoal should be used as an alternative. Potassium chloride will exchange with thallium in cells and increase renal excretion. This should be administered cautiously, since the rise in serum thallium levels may transiently worsen symptoms. Chelating agents have not been shown to be effective. In chronic intoxication, removal from exposure is the treatment of choice. Recovery is generally complete, though permanent blindness and hair loss have been reported.

## TIN

### Essentials of Diagnosis

*Inorganic:*
- Respiratory and mucous membrane irritation.
- Benign pneumoconiosis (stannosis).

*Organic:*
- Mild to severe skin irritation.
- Headache, visual disturbances.
- Seizures, coma.

### Exposure Limits

Tin, inorganic compounds
  ACGIH TLV: 2 mg/m$^3$ TWA
  OSHA PEL: 2 mg/m$^3$ TWA

Tin, organic compounds
  ACGIH TLV: 0.1 mg/m$^3$ TWA
  OSHA PEL: 0.1 mg/m$^3$ TWA

### General Considerations

Tin is a soft, pliable, silvery metal used extensively for its corrosion resistance properties. Cassiterite ($SnO_2$), or tinstone, is the primary commercial ore, with sulfide ores, such as stanniote ($Cu_2FeSn_2$) and tealite ($PbZnSnS_2$), being of lesser importance. Ores extracted by dredging are subjected to high temperature reduction in smelting operations to obtain tin for commercial use. An increasing proportion of tin production, particularly in the United States, is through recycling of tin-plated scrap metal and tin alloys.

### Use

The primary use of tin is for plating, where it imparts resistance to acids and the atmosphere. Tin-plated iron and steel are used for canning, in household utensils, and for decorative purposes. A tin-lead alloy is used for soldering electronic components. Tin alloys include bronze, babbitt metal, and pewter and are used in printing, bearings, and jewelry. Stannous fluoride is used in toothpastes. Organotin compounds are used as stabilizers in plastics and oils; as catalysts in curing silicone rubber; as preservatives in textiles and leather; and as pesticides in marine paints.

### Occupational & Environmental Exposure

At smelting operations, workers may be exposed to tin oxide fumes when pouring molten tin and tin oxide dust during bagging and filter maintenance. Exposure to sulfur dioxide is a hazard in the roasting of sulfide ores of tin. Plating operations, utilizing molten tin drip tanks, may expose workers to tin oxide dust and fumes. Workers engaged in the manufacture of tin solder and other alloys are also exposed. Exposure to the highly toxic organotin compounds may occur in paint formulation and the manufacture of plastics. The use of organotin paints to protect boat hulls may result in contamination and poisoning of marine organisms in harbors. Divalent organotin compounds are used in the production of PVC film, urethanes, and silicone rubber. Trivalent organotin compounds are used as biocides and may be encountered as preservatives in textiles, leathers, glass, and paper products.

### Absorption, Metabolism, & Excretion

Inorganic tin is poorly absorbed from the gastrointestinal tract. Most of the ingested dose is excreted in the feces. Absorbed tin is found in many tissues, including the reticuloendothelial system in the liver and spleen. Renal excretion is minor. Inhaled compounds remain in the lung. Organic compounds may be absorbed by inhalation, ingestion, or through the skin. Excretion is dependent on chemical composition and is through both the biliary tract and the kidney.

## Clinical Findings

### A. Symptoms and Signs:

**1. Inorganic**–Workers exposed to tin dusts in high concentrations may complain of eye, throat, and respiratory irritation. Long-term exposure may result in significant chest x-ray findings, since tin is radiopaque. Changes in pulmonary function have not been associated with exposure to tin compounds. Exposure to tin fumes may cause metal fume fever (see Zinc).

**2. Organic**–Acute exposure to trimethyl and triethyl tin may cause severe skin irritation followed by central nervous system effects. Headache, lassitude, and visual disturbances may occur. In severe cases, nervous system toxicity may result in seizures and coma. Recovery in nonfatal cases may be delayed. Chronic exposure to organotin compounds may cause an erythematous skin rash and folliculitis, particularly over the lower abdomen and thighs.

### B. Laboratory Findings:
After chronic exposure to inorganic tin, the chest x-ray may reveal nodular densities throughout the lung fields. Abnormal spirometry should suggest concomitant exposure to silica or other fibrogenic agents. Acute toxicity due to organotin compounds may be manifested by evidence of abnormal renal and hepatic function as well as abnormal findings on the EEG. Elevated urinary levels or organotin compounds will confirm the diagnosis but are not readily available.

## Prevention

Enclosure and ventilation of dipping and bagging operations will reduce exposure to tin oxide dusts and fumes. Respiratory protection should be used during maintenance. Organotin compounds should be handled with extreme care to avoid inhalation and skin contact. Medical surveillance should focus on the respiratory system of inorganic tin workers and the skin and nervous system in workers exposed to organic tin compounds.

## Treatment

Irritant and dermatologic effects will resolve after removal from exposure. After dermal exposure to organotin compounds, the skin should be extensively cleansed with a strong detergent and water to prevent delayed absorption. Neurologic, hepatic, and renal toxicity should be treated as indicated clinically.

# VANADIUM

## Essentials of Diagnosis
- Respiratory irritation.
- Asthma.
- Green discoloration of the tongue.

## Exposure Limits
Vanadium pentoxide
ACGIH TLV: 0.05 mg/m$^3$ TWA

## General Considerations

Vanadium is a soft, gray metal that is nonoxidizing in acids and seawater. The principal commercial ores are vanadium sulfide and lead-zinc vanadate. Vanadium is also found in uranium-bearing sandstones in sufficient quantities for commercial extraction. Various levels of vanadium are found in fossil fuels and contribute to environmental contamination.

## Use

The primary use of vanadium is in production of ferrovanadium, in which as little as 0.05–5% vanadium imparts greater strength and elasticity. Vanadium alloys supply hardness and durability for high speed cutting and drilling tools. Vanadium is also used as a catalyst for high-temperature polymerization, as a mordant in dyeing, and as a colorant in ceramics and glass. Organic vanadium compounds are used as catalysts and coatings.

## Occupational & Environmental Exposure

Exposure to vanadium pentoxide dusts and fumes may occur during milling and roasting. Workers using vanadium compounds for alloys or additives will have contact with pure source materials. A particular inhalation hazard exists in cleaning fuel dusts from oil and coal furnaces where high levels of vanadium pentoxide may accumulate. Fossil fuel burning power stations may emit vanadium compounds, resulting in environmental contamination and air pollution.

## Absorption, Metabolism, & Excretion

Vanadium compounds may be absorbed after inhalation or ingestion. The lung content has been shown to be increased in miners and in persons living in proximity to effluents from the burning of fossil fuels. Excretion is primarily renal, with little accumulation in bone.

## Clinical Findings

**A. Acute Exposure:** Acute exposure to high levels of vanadium pentoxide dusts or fumes results in profuse lacrimation, eye irritation, epistaxis, cough, and bronchitis. Pneumonia may follow acute exposures. Sensitivity to vanadium, resulting in cough and bronchospasm at lower levels of exposure, is consistent with allergic asthma. Skin irritation or allergy may also occur.

**B. Chronic Exposure:** With chronic exposure, green discoloration of the tongue may occur. Plasma cholesterol has been found to be lowered in workers exposed to vanadium. Pulmonary function tests may reveal an obstructive pattern. Patch testing may be used to confirm dermal sensitization to vanadium compounds.

## Prevention

Proper respiratory protection should be worn when handling vanadium compounds and when cleaning oil and coal furnace flues. Medical surveillance should screen for respiratory and dermatologic complaints, which suggest chronic overexposure or development of respiratory or skin allergy.

## Treatment

Ascorbic acid and calcium disodium edetate are protective in experimental animals, though there is no human experience with these compounds. Persons who develop respiratory or dermatologic allergy should be permanently removed from exposure.

## ZINC

### Essentials of Diagnosis

*Zinc oxide:*
- Headache, metallic taste.
- Fever, chills, myalgias.
- Cough, chest pain.

*Zinc chloride:*
- Severe skin and eye burns.
- Respiratory irritation.
- Pulmonary edema.

### Exposure Limits

Zinc oxide fume
  ACGIH TLV: 5 mg/m$^3$ TWA, 10 mg/m$^3$ STEL
  OSHA PEL: 5 mg/m$^3$ TWA, 10 mg/m$^3$ STEL
Zinc oxide dust
  ACGIH TLV: 10 mg/m$^3$ TWA
  OSHA PEL: 10 mg/m$^3$ TWA
Zinc chloride fume
  ACGIH TLV: 1 mg/m$^3$ TWA, 2 mg/m$^3$ STEL
  OSHA PEL: 1 mg/m$^3$ TWA, 2 mg/m$^3$ STEL

### General Considerations

Zinc is a silver-white metal with a blue tinge that is widely distributed in nature. Zinc deposits frequently contain cadmium, iron, lead, and arsenic. Zinc is recovered through flotation and separation followed by either smelting or electrolytic refining.

Zinc is an essential element for humans and is found in all tissues. Many different enzyme systems require zinc for normal functioning. Daily intake of zinc in the diet is between 10 and 15 mg.

### Use

A major application of zinc is in the galvanizing of steel and other metals, where a coating is applied through dipping or electroplating. Purified zinc metal is die cast for use in automotive parts, electrical equipment, tools, machinery, and toys. Zinc oxide is used as a pigment and in the vulcanizing of rubber. Zinc chloride is used in welding and soldering fluxes, wood preservatives, dry cell batteries, oil refining, smoke bombs, dental cement, and deodorants. Zinc forms alloys with many metals, including copper to form brass.

### Occupational & Environmental Exposure

Exposure to zinc sulfide in mining and ore extraction is less significant than exposure to other heavy metal contaminants. In zinc ore roasting operations, there is potential exposure to zinc oxide dusts and fumes. Workers engaged in fabricating or welding of galvanized metal may have exposure to zinc oxide fumes. Zinc chloride exposure occurs in welding and soldering as well as with its use in manufacturing. Zinc alloy production and brass work involve exposure to zinc compounds. Ingestion of acidic foods and beverages from galvanized food containers has resulted in zinc poisoning.

### Absorption, Metabolism, & Excretion

Only 20–30% of ingested zinc is absorbed from the gastrointestinal tract. Zinc may also be absorbed after inhalation of fumes. Circulating zinc is bound to plasma proteins (metallothionein and albumin) and is found in erythrocytes. Zinc is distributed widely in tissues, most of it in striated muscle. Absorbed zinc is excreted in pancreatic fluid, bile, and sweat, with only 20% excreted in the urine.

### Clinical Findings

**A. Symptoms and Signs:** The most characteristic manifestation of occupational zinc toxicity is the development of metal fume fever after exposure to zinc oxide fumes. Several hours after exposure, the worker develops headache and a sweet metallic taste, followed by muscle and joint pains and fatigue. Fever, chills, profuse sweating, cough, and chest pain occur 8–12 hours after exposure, usually when the worker is at home. The symptoms resolve spontaneously after 24–48 hours, resembling an acute viral syndrome. The condition occurs more frequently early in the week, suggesting that tolerance may develop. Chronic sequelae do not occur.

Contact with zinc chloride may cause serious skin and eye burns even after brief contact. Chronic skin exposure may cause an eczematous dermatitis or skin sensitization.

Inhalation of zinc chloride fumes causes sinus and throat irritation, cough, hemoptysis, and dyspnea. Pulmonary edema and pneumonia may develop following excessive exposure. Ingestion of soluble zinc compounds causes nausea, vomiting, and diarrhea due to irritation of the gastrointestinal tract.

**B. Laboratory Findings:** The onset of symptoms of metal fume fever is accompanied by leukocytosis of 15,000–20,000/$\mu$L and a transient fall in $FEV_1$, FVC, and carbon monoxide diffusing capacity on pulmonary function testing. The chest x-ray is usually normal but may reveal hazy infiltrates in the mid lung fields. A significant drop in lung function or diffuse pneumonitis should suggest possible exposure to nitrogen dioxide or cadmium oxide. Nonspecific elevation of LDH and other serum enzyme levels may occur. Urine and plasma zinc levels may also be elevated.

After zinc chloride inhalation, findings of arterial hypoxemia and pulmonary infiltrates are consistent with acute chemical pneumonitis. Zinc chloride skin allergy can be confirmed by patch testing.

## Prevention

Proper ventilation of high-temperature processes involving zinc will reduce exposure to zinc oxide dusts and fumes. Proper local exhaust ventilation should be provided when welding on galvanized metal and brazing on brass. Proper eye and skin protection should be used when handling zinc chloride. Home remedies purported to prevent metal fume fever, including milk and vitamin C, have no scientific basis. Medical monitoring for zinc exposed workers should concentrate on dermatologic and respiratory effects. Urine zinc levels have been found to range up to 0.7 mg/L in persons exposed to zinc below the current ACGIH limit.

## Treatment

No specific treatment is indicated for metal fume fever, though bacterial infections of the lungs should be ruled out through careful clinical evaluation. Zinc chloride skin and eye burns should be irrigated immediately with copious amounts of water. Eye irrigation with 1.7% $CaNa_2EDTA$ for 15 minutes should be instituted as soon as possible to prevent the development of corneal opacities. Persons with suspected zinc chloride inhalation should be observed closely. Persons who develop chronic dermatitis and zinc skin allergy should be removed from further exposure.

# WELDING

Welding is a joining process with wide application in manufacturing and the building trades. Through the application of heat or pressure, welding joins metals with a lightweight bond, with strength and resistance approaching that of the parent metal.

Welding is a labor-intensive activity. Even though automated welding methods are finding increasing applications, manual arc welding remains the principal welding process.

## Health Hazards of Welding

Welders work with a wide variety of materials under varied conditions and are exposed to many health hazards, including air contaminants (metal fumes, particulates, gases); physical agents such as radiation (infrared, ultraviolet), noise, and electricity; and ergonomic stress.

The common air contaminants of different welding processes are listed in Tables 27–5 and 27–6. **Shielded metal arc (SMA)** welding of mild steel, or "stick welding," is the most common use of welding. The main exposure is to iron oxide, and pulmonary deposition of this nonfibrogenic particulate has resulted in the development of a benign pneumoconiosis. Exposure to manganese and fluoride fumes may be considerable when certain welding rods are used.

The corrosion-resistant properties of stainless steel are due to a high concentration of chromium (18–30%). Nickel and manganese may also be present in different stainless steel alloys. Exposure to chromium [including Cr (VI)], nickel, and manganese may be considerable, particularly with **gas metal arc (GMA)** processes. The stainless steel sur-

**Table 27–5.** Air contaminants of selected welding processes.

| Process | Base Metal | Contaminants |
|---------|-----------|--------------|
| Shielded metal arc (stick welding) | Mild steel | Dust, iron oxide, manganese |
| Shielded metal arc (stick welding) | Stainless steel | Chromium, nickel, manganese, fluorides |
| Gas metal arc (MIG) | Stainless steel | Chromium, nickel, manganese, nitrogen oxides, ozone |
| Tungsten inert gas (TIG) | Aluminum | Ozone, aluminum oxide |
| Gas, brazing, cutting | Variable | Nitrogen oxides, cadmium oxide, metal fume |

**Table 27–6.** Potential hazards of welding processes.

| Air contaminants | |
|---|---|
| Metals | |
| Iron oxide | Benign pneumoconiosis |
| Manganese | Neurotoxicity, pneumonia |
| Cadmium oxide | Acute lung injury |
| Zinc oxide | Metal fume fever |
| Chromium | Lung cancer, allergy |
| Nickel | Lung cancer, allergy |
| Fluoride | Skin or respiratory irritation |
| Gases | |
| Ozone | Respiratory irritation, asthma |
| Nitrogen oxides | Acute lung injury |
| Carbon monoxide | Systemic poisoning |
| **Physical hazards** | |
| Radiation | |
| Ultraviolet | Photokeratitis, skin erythema, |
| Infra-red | Burns, cataracts(?) |
| Electricity | Electric shock, electrocution |
| Noise | Hearing loss |
| Ergonomic stress | Muscle strain |

**Table 27–7.** Coatings and contaminants encountered in welding.

| | |
|---|---|
| Galvanized metal | Zinc oxide |
| Paints | Lead, cadmium, isocyanates, aldehydes, epoxies |
| Biocides | Organic mercury, organic tin |
| Chlorinated solvents | Phosgene |
| Rustproofing | Phosphorus, phosphine |
| Alloys, sheet metal | Cadmium, nickel, manganese, beryllium |
| Solders | Rosin, colophony |

face reflects ultraviolet radiation, with formation of oxides of nitrogen and ozone. Low hydrogen welding of stainless steel generates high concentrations of fluoride fumes.

Most aluminum welding uses the **tungsten inert gas (TIG)** method. As with stainless steel, the gas-shielded process results in formation of ozone due to the action of ultraviolet radiation on the nascent oxygen in the atmosphere. Total dust and aluminum oxide generation are also considerable.

Brazing and **gas welding** both generate metal fume. An acetylene torch is used to generate an intense flame. Exposure to cadmium oxide from cadmium-containing silver solder has caused acute lung injury and death after brazing in enclosed spaces. Similar consequences have occurred from generation of the oxides of nitrogen during gas welding. In all cases, improper ventilation was the critical factor in creating the hazard.

Radiation and heat result in the most common injuries to welders: photokeratitis (welder's flash) and thermal burns. These are often related to improper use of protective goggles, gloves, and screens. Flying sparks or debris may cause burns or eye injury as well. Noise exposure may exceed 80 dB in welding processes, particularly cutting or gouging operations; in plasma welding (where intense heat is generated), levels may approach 120 dB. Environmental conditions will also influence noise generation. Electrical shock is a constant hazard and requires careful grounding and shielding of cables and equipment. Most manual processes place isometric stress on the welder, particularly involving the shoulders and the upper extremities.

Coatings or contaminants may present additional hazards (Table 27–7), particularly when their presence and potential hazard are unknown or unsus-

pected. The formation of toxic gases, fumes, or vapors is usually due to the heating of a coated or treated metal, although phosgene exposure is related to the action of ultraviolet radiation or heat on chlorinated hydrocarbon vapors (similar to the formation of ozone from oxygen and oxides of nitrogen from nitrogen).

Soldering is not associated with significant exposure to metal fumes because the temperatures are low. Potential contamination of the workplace with lead dust requires careful attention to hygiene. Some fluxes, such as rosin, are skin sensitizers and may cause allergic dermatitis or asthma.

## Clinical Findings

### A. Acute Exposure:

**1. Photokeratitis**–Photokeratitis is the result of exposure of the cornea to ultraviolet radiation in the 280- to 315-nm range (UVB). The duration of exposure necessary to induce this effect varies with the distance from the arc and the light intensity. Following exposure of the unprotected eye to the welding arc for several seconds, the worker develops pain, burning, or a feeling of "sand or grit" in the eye. Physical examination shows conjunctival injection, and slit lamp examination may reveal punctate depressions over the cornea. The condition is self-limited, resolving in several hours. Careful examination for foreign bodies or evidence of thermal ocular injury is mandatory.

**2. Metal fume fever**–(See Zinc, above.) Metal fume fever is a benign, self-limited condition characterized by the delayed onset (8–12 hours) of fever, chills, cough, myalgias, and a metallic taste. A history of welding on galvanized metal suggests the diagnosis.

**3. Upper respiratory irritation**–Upper respiratory tract irritation may result from exposure to a variety of welding contaminants, including dusts, ozone, aluminum oxide, nitrogen oxides, cadmium oxide, and fluorides. Asthma may also be triggered as a result of nonspecific irritation or allergy (chromium, nickel).

**4. Lung injury**–While unusual, exposure to oxides of nitrogen and cadmium oxide may cause acute lung injury and delayed pulmonary edema. A history of gas welding or brazing in enclosed or poorly ventilated spaces or sheet metal work should raise this concern and serve as an indication for careful medical evaluation and observation.

**5. Musculoskeletal trauma**–Injuries resulting from isometric stress on the upper extremity during welding may present as symptomatic shoulder and neck pain following prolonged activity. Asymptomatic muscle damage may result in slight increases in creatine phosphokinase levels in serum.

**6. Thermal burns and electrical injuries**–See Chapter 12.

**B. Chronic Exposure:**

**1. Siderosis**–Siderosis (see Chapter 20) results from accumulation of nonfibrogenic iron oxide particles in the lung. While the radiographic appearance may be dramatic, with evidence of diffuse reticulonodular densities, reports of deficits of pulmonary function have been inconsistent, suggesting a mild or minimal effect. In welders who have also been exposed to crystalline silica or asbestos, radiographic differentiation of hemosiderosis from pulmonary fibrosis is difficult. Pleural thickening or calcification has not been related to welding in the absence of asbestos exposure.

**2. Other chronic effects**–Welders report an excess of respiratory symptoms and have increased work absences from respiratory diseases. Demonstration of clear deficits in pulmonary function attributable to welding have been inconsistent. At present, there is limited evidence that welding results in chronic respiratory impairment. In the evaluation of a welder with chronic lung disease, a careful medical and occupational history is essential, focusing on both welding exposures and other confounding factors.

Studies of lung cancer in welders have also been inconsistent, sharing the limitations of many of the respiratory studies. Some researchers attribute the small excess in lung cancer cases seen in several studies to exposure to chromium and nickel in welding of stainless steel, a small proportion of all welding exposures. Studies involving welders who worked in shipyards during the first half of this century will be confounded by significant secondary exposure to asbestos.

Other studies have indicated that welders may have decreased sperm counts and be at risk for adverse reproductive outcomes. Subtle neuropsychological effects have also been reported.

## Prevention

Most acute injuries or poisonings related to welding processes are preventable. Strict adherence to appropriate safety procedures will prevent burns, eye injuries, and electric shock. Awareness of the potential hazards, with attention to the provision of adequate ventilation, is the best safeguard against accidental overexposure to air contaminants. In enclosed spaces, air-supplied respirators are essential, particularly with processes that result in generation of nitrogen oxides.

Carefully designed and controlled studies in the future will better assess the potential impact of welding on respiratory function and on the development of lung cancer. These effects, if present, will certainly be minimized by measures to reduce welding exposures through engineering, ventilation, and proper use of personal protection.

## Treatment

Photokeratitis and metal fume fever require no specific treatment, though other diagnoses should be excluded. Welders suspected of having acute overexposure to nitrogen oxides, phosgene, or cadmium oxide should be observed for possible development of pulmonary edema. Treatment of pulmonary edema and respiratory insufficiency related to these agents is supportive. Asthmatics bothered by nonspecific irritant effects related to welding may benefit from improved ventilation and respiratory protection, though cartridge respirators will not prevent exposure to irritant gases. Frank allergic asthma to specific agents may require removal from further exposure.

Burns and radiation injuries are discussed in Chapter 12.

## REFERENCES

### ALUMINUM

Armstrong B et al: Lung cancer mortality and polynuclear aromatic hydrocarbons: A case-cohort study of aluminum production workers in Arvida, Quebec, Canada. Am J Epidemiol 1994;139:250.

Bast-Pettersen R et al: Neuropsychological deficit among elderly workers in aluminum production. Am J Ind Med 1994;25:649.

Flodin U et al: Bronchial asthma and air pollution at workplaces. Scand J Work Environ Health 1996; 22(6):451.

Gitelman HJ et al: Serum and urinary aluminum levels of workers in the aluminum industry. Ann Occup Hyg 1995;39:181.

Hanninen H et al: Internal load of aluminum and the central nervous system function of aluminum welders. Scand J Work Environ Health 1994;20:(4)279.

Jederlinic PJ et al: Pulmonary fibrosis in aluminum oxide workers. Investigation of nine workers, with pathologic examination and microanalysis in three of them. Am Rev Respir Dis 1990;142:1179.

Kilburn KH, Warshaw RH: Irregular opacities in the lung, occupational asthma, and airways dysfunction in aluminum workers. Am J Ind Med 1992;21:845.

Kongerud J, Samuelsen SO: A longitudinal study of respiratory symptoms in aluminum potroom workers. Am Rev Respir Dis 1991;144:10.

Ljunggren KG, Lidums V, Sjögren B: Blood and urine concentrations of aluminum among workers exposed to aluminum flake powders. Br J Ind Med 1991;48:106.

## ANTIMONY

Bailly R et al:Experimental and human studies on antimony metabolism: Their relevance for the biological monitoring of workers exposed to inorganic antimony. Br J Ind Med 1991;48:93.

De Wolff FA: Antimony and health. Br Med J 1995;310:1216.

Jones RD: Survey of antimony workers: Mortality 1961–1992. Occup Environ Med 1994;51:772.

Leonard A, Gerber GB: Mutagenicity, carcinogenicity and teratogenicity of antimony compounds. Mutat Res 1996;366(1):1.

## ARSENIC

Arbouine MW, Wilson HK: The effect of seafood consumption on the assessment of occupational exposure to arsenic by urinary arsenic speciation measurements. J Trace Elem Electrolytes Health Dis 1992;6: 153.

Conner EA et al: Biological indicators for monitoring exposure/toxicity from III-V semiconductors. J Exp Anal Environ Epidemiol 1993;3:431.

Enterline PE, Day R, Marsh GM: Cancers related to exposure to arsenic at a copper smelter. Occup Environ Med 1995;52:28.

Farmer JG, Johnson LR: Assessment of occupational exposure to inorganic arsenic based on urinary concentrations and speciation of arsenic. Br J Ind Med 1990;47:342.

Hertz-Picciotto I, Smith AH: Observations on the dose-response curve for arsenic exposure and lung cancer. Scand J Work Environ Health 1993;19:217.

Klimecki WT, Carter DE: Arsine toxicity: Chemical and mechanistic implications. J Toxicol Environ Health 1995;46(4):399.

Risk M, Fuortes L: Chronic arsenicalism suspected from arsine exposure: A case report and literature review. Vet Hum Toxicol 1991;33:590.

Sheehy JW, Jones JH: Assessment of arsenic exposures and controls in gallium arsenide production. Am Ind Hyg Assoc J 1993;54:61.

## BERYLLIUM

Kreiss K et al: Epidemiology of beryllium sensitization and disease in nuclear workers. Am Rev Respir Dis 1993;148:985.

Meyer KC: Beryllium and lung disease. Chest 1994;106:942.

Mroz MM et al: Reexamination of the blood lymphocyte transformation test in the diagnosis of chronic beryllium disease. J Allergy Clin Immunol 1991;88:54.

Newman LS, Orton R, Kreiss K: Serum angiotensin converting enzyme activity in chronic beryllium disease. Am Rev Respir Dis 1992;146:39.

Steenland K, Ward E: Lung cancer incidence among patients with beryllium disease: A cohort mortality study. J Natl Cancer Inst 1991;83:1380.

Ward E et al: A mortality study of workers at seven beryllium processing plants. Am J Ind Med 1992;22:885.

## BORON

Culver BD et al: The relationship of blood- and urine-boron to boron exposure in borax workers and usefulness of urine-boron as an exposure marker. Environ Health Perspect 1994;102:133.

Hu X et al: Dose related acute irritant symptom responses to occupational exposure to sodium borate dusts. Br J Ind Med 1992:49:706.

Penland JG: Dietary boron, brain function, and cognitive performance. Environ Health Perspect 1994;103 (Suppl 7):65.

Woods WG: An introduction to boron: History, sources, uses, and chemistry. Environ Health Perspect 1994; 102(Suppl 7):5.

## CADMIUM

Anonymous: Cadmium and cadmium compounds. IARC Monogr Eval Carcinog Risks Hum 1993; 58:119.

Armstrong R et al: Longitudinal studies of exposure to cadmium. Br J Ind Med 1992;49:556.

Bernard A et al: Association between NAG-B and cadmium in urine with no evidence of a threshold. Occup Environ Med 1995;52:177.

Houtman JP: Trace elements and cardiovascular diseases. J Cardiovasc Risk 1996;3(1):18.

Jarup L, Elinder CG: Dose-response relations between urinary cadmium and tubular proteinuria in cadmium-exposed workers. Am J Ind Med 1994;26:759.

Kahan E et al: Adverse health effects in workers exposed to cadmium. Am J Ind Med 1992;21:527.

Roels H et al: Markers of early renal changes induced by industrial pollutants. III. Application to workers exposed to cadmium. Br J Ind Med 1993;50:37.

Staessen JA: Public health implications of environmental exposure to cadmium and lead: An overview of epidemiological studies in Belgium. J Cardiovasc Risk 1996;3(1):26.

Thun MJ, Elinder CG, Friberg L: Scientific basis for an occupational standard for cadmium. Am J Ind Med 1991;20:629.

Trevisan A et al: Biological monitoring of cadmium exposure: reliability of spot urine samples. Int Arch Occup Environ Health 1994;65:373.

van Sittert NJ et al: A nine year follow up study of renal effects in workers exposed to cadmium in a zinc ore refinery. Br J Ind Med 1993;50:603.

## CHROMIUM

Huvinen M et al: Respiratory health of workers exposed to low levels of chromium in stainless steel production. Occup Environ Med 1996;53(11):741.

Johansen M, Overgaard E, Toft A: Severe chronic inflammation of the mucous membranes in the eyes and upper respiratory tract due to work-related exposure to hexavalent chromium. J Laryngol Otol 1994;108:591.

Lees PS: Chromium and disease: Review of epidemiologic studies with particular reference to etiologic information provided by measures of exposure. Environ Health Perspect 1991;92:93.

Lin SC et al: Nasal septum lesions caused by chromium exposure among chromium electroplating workers. Am J Ind Med 1994;26:221.

Park HS, Yu HJ, Jung KS: Occupational asthma caused by chromium. Clin Exp Allergy 1994;24:676.

Pastides H et al: A retrospective-cohort study of occupational exposure to hexavalent chromium. Am J Ind Med 1994;25:663.

Satoh N et al: Chromium-induced carcinoma in the nasal region. A report of four cases. Rhinology 1994;32:47.

## LEAD

Balbus-Kornfeld JM et al: Cumulative exposure to inorganic lead and neurobehavioural test performance in adults: An epidemiological review. Occup Environ Med 1995;52:2.

Cardenas A et al: Markers of early renal changes induced by industrial pollutants. II. Application to workers exposed to lead. Br J Ind Med 1993;50:28

dos Santos AC et al: Occupational exposure to lead, kidney function tests, and blood pressure. Am J Ind Med 1994;26:635.

Fayerweather WE, Karns ME, Nuwayhid IA, Nelson TJ: Case-control of cancer risk in tetraethyl lead manufacturing. Am J Ind Med 1997;31(1):28.

Gennart JP et al: Fertility of male workers exposed to cadmium, lead, or manganese. Am J Epidemiol 1992;135:1208.

Goyer RA: Results of lead research: Prenatal exposure and neurological consequences. Environ Health Perspect 1996;104(10):1050.

Grandjean P, Jacobsen IA, Jorgensen PJ: Chronic lead poisoning treated with dimercaptosuccinic acid. Pharmacol Toxicol 1991;68:266.

Hu H, Aro A, Rotnitzky A: Bone lead measured by X-ray fluorescence: Epidemiologic methods. Environ Health Perspect 1995;103 (Suppl 1):105.

Lee BK et al: Provocative chelation with DMSA and EDTA: Evidence for differential access to lead storage sites. Occup Environ Med 1995;52:13.

Porru S et al: The utility of health education among lead workers: The experience of one program. Am J Ind Med 1993;23:473.

Rempel D: The lead-exposed worker. JAMA 1989;262:532.

Schwartz BS et al: Decrements in neurobehavioral performance associated with mixed exposure to organic and inorganic lead. Am J Epidemiol 1993;137:1006.

Skerfving S et al: Biological monitoring of inorganic lead. Scand J Work Environ Health 1993;19(Suppl 1):59.

Staessen JA et al: Impairment of renal function with increasing blood lead concentrations in the general population. N Engl J Med 1992;327:151.

Winder C, Bonin T: The genotoxicity of lead. Mutat Res 1993;285:117.

Zhang J: Investigation and evaluation of zinc protoporphyrin as a diagnostic indicator in lead intoxication. Am J Ind Med 1993;24:707.

Zhang W et al: Early health effects and biological monitoring in persons occupationally exposed to tetraethyl lead. Int Arch Occup Environ Health 1994;65:395.

## MANGANESE

Huang CC et al: Progression after chronic manganese exposure. Neurology 1993;43:1479.

Kishi R et al: Subjective symptoms and neurobehavioral performances of ex-mercury miners at an average of 18 years after the cessation of chronic exposure to mercury vapor. Mercury Workers Study Group. Environ Res 1993;62:289.

Loranger S, Zayed J: Environmental and occupational exposure to manganese: A multimedia assessment. Int Arch Occup Environ Health 1995;67:101.

Lucchini R et al: Neurobehavioral effects of manganese in workers from a ferroalloy plant after temporary cessation of exposure. Scand J Work Environ Health 1995;21:143.

Nelson K et al: Manganese encephalopathy: Utility of early magnetic resonance imaging. Br J Ind Med 1993;50:510.

Sierra P et al: Occupational and environmental exposure of automobile mechanics and nonautomotive workers to airborne manganese arising from the combustion of methylcyclopentadienyl manganese tricarbonyl (MMT). Am Ind Hyg Assoc J 1995;56:713.

Sjögren B et al: Effects on the nervous system among welders exposed to aluminum and manganese. Occup Environ Med 1996;53(1):32.

## MERCURY

Andersen A et al: A neurological and neurophysiological study of chloralkali workers previously exposed to mercury vapour. Acta Neurol Scand 1993;88:427.

Cardenas A et al: Markers of early renal changes induced by industrial pollutants. I. Application to workers exposed to mercury vapour. Br J Ind Med 1993;50:17.

Chang YC, Yeh CY, Wang JD: Subclinical neurotoxicity of mercury vapor revealed by a multimodality evoked potential study of chloralkali workers. Am J Ind Med 1995;27:271.

Ellingsen DG et al: Assessment of renal dysfunction in workers previously exposed to mercury vapour at a chloralkali plant. Br J Ind Med 1993;50:881.

Ellingsen DG et al: Incidence of cancer and mortality among workers exposed to mercury vapour in the Norwegian chloralkali industry. Br J Ind Med 1993;50:875.

Ellingsen DG et al: Relation between exposure related indices and neurological and neurophysiological effects in workers previously exposed to mercury vapour. Br J Ind Med 1993;50:736.

Kishi R et al: Subjective symptoms and neurobehavioral performances of ex-mercury miners at an average of 18 years after the cessation of chronic exposure to mercury vapor. Mercury Workers Study Group. Environ Res 1993;62:289.

O'Carroll RE et al: The neuropsychiatric sequelae of mercury poisoning. The Mad Hatter's disease revisited. Br J Psychiatry (July)1995;167(1):95.

Sallsten G, Barregard L, Schutz A: Decrease in mercury concentration in blood after long term exposure: A kinetic study of chloralkali workers. Br J Ind Med 1993;50:814.

## NICKEL

Angerer J, Lehnert G: Occupational chronic exposure to metals. II. Nickel exposure of stainless steel welders—biological monitoring. Int Arch Occup Environ Health 1990;62:7.

Kurta DL, Dean BS, Krenzelok EP: Acute nickel carbonyl poisoning. Am J Emerg Med 1993;11:64.

Muir DC et al: Cancer of the respiratory tract in nickel sinter plant workers: Effect of removal from sinter plant exposure. Occup Environ Med 1994;51:19.

Rendall RE, Phillips JI, Renton KA: Death following exposure to fine particulate nickel from a metal arc process. Ann Occup Hyg 1994;38:921.

Shen HM, Zhang QF: Risk assessment of nickel carcinogenicity and occupational lung cancer. Environ Health Perspect 1994;102(Suppl 1):275.

## PHOSPHORUS

Dutton CB et al: Lung function in workers refining phosphorus rock to obtain elementary phosphorus. J Occup Med 1993;35:1028.

## SELENIUM

Fan AM: The carcinogenic potential of cadmium, arsenic, and selenium and the associated public health and regulatory implications. J Toxicol Sci 1990; 15(Suppl 4):162.

Larner AJ: Alzheimers's disease, Kuf's disease, tellurium and selenium. Med Hypotheses 1996;47(2):73.

## TELLURIUM

Hryhorczuk DO, Aks SE, Turk JW: Unusual occupational toxins. Occup Med 1992;7:567.

Morgan DL et al: Acute pulmonary toxicity of copper gallium diselenide, copper indium diselenide, and cadmium telluride intratracheally instilled into rats. Environ Res 1995;7(1):16.

## THALLIUM

Shabalina LP et al: Methods of diagnosis of thallium intoxication and its antidote therapy. Med Tr Prom Ekol 1996;10:25.

## TIN

Hryhorczuk DO, Aks SE, Turk JW: Unusual occupational toxins. Occup Med 1992;7:567.

Nuyts GD et al: New occupational risk factors for chronic renal failure. Lancet 1995;346(8966):7.

## VANADIUM

Hryhorczuk DO, Aks SE, Turk JW: Unusual occupational toxins. Occup Med 1992;7:567.

Kucera J, Lener J, Mnukova J: Vanadium levels in urine and cystine levels in fingernails and hair of exposed and normal persons. Biol Trace Elem Res 1994;43:327.

Leonard A, Gerber GB: Mutagenicity, carcinogenicity and teratogenicity of vanadium compounds. Mutat Res 1994;317(1):81.

## ZINC

Ameille J et al: Occupational hypersensitivity pneumonitis in a smelter exposed to zinc fumes. Chest 1992;101:862.

Blanc P et al: An experimental human model of metal fume fever. Ann Intern Med 1991;114:930.

Gordon T et al: Pulmonary effects of inhaled zinc oxide in human subjects, guinea pigs, rats, and rabbits. Am Ind Hyg Assoc J 1992;53:503.

Malo JL, Cartier A, Dolovich J: Occupational asthma due to zinc. Eur Respir J 1993;6:447.

## WELDING

Billings CG, Howard P: Occupational siderosis and welders' lung: A review. Monaldi Arch Chest Dis 1993; 48:304.

Beach JR et al: An epidemiologic investigation of asthma in welders. Am J Respir Crit Care Med 1996;154(5):1394.

Blanc PD et al: Cytokines in metal fume fever. Am Rev Respir Dis 1993;147:134.

Chinn DJ et al: Respiratory health of young shipyard welders and other tradesmen studied cross sectionally and longitudinally. Occup Environ Med 1995;52:33.

Danielsen TE et al: Incidence of cancer among welders of mild steel and other shipyard workers. Br J Ind Med 1993;50:1097.

Flodin U et al: Bronchial asthma and air pollution at workplaces. Scand J Work Environ Health 1996; 6:451.

Knudsen LE et al: Biomonitoring of genotoxic exposure among stainless steel welders. Mutat Res 1992;279:129.

Moulin JJ et al:A mortality study among mild steel and stainless steel welders. Br J Ind Med 1993;50:234.

Nielsen J et al: Small airways function in aluminium and stainless steel welders. Int Arch Occup Environ Health 1993;65:101.

Ozdemir O et al: Chronic effects of welding exposure on pulmonary function tests and respiratory symptoms. Occup Environ Med 1995;52(12):800.

Sjögren et al: Exposure to stainless steel welding fumes

and lung cancer: a meta-analysis: Occup Environ Med 1994;51:335.

Stridsklev IC et al: Biologic monitoring of chromium and nickel among stainless steel welders using the manual mental arc method.Int Arch Occup Environ Health 1993;65:209.

Vandenplas O et al: Occupational asthma due to gas metal arc welding on mild steel. Thorax 1995;50: 587.

Wang ZP et al: Asthma, lung function, and bronchial responsiveness in welders. Am J Ind Med 1994;26: 741.

# 28

# Chemicals

*Robert J. Harrison, MD, MPH*

This chapter covers selected chemicals of particular importance to the occupational health practitioner. Solvents, plastics, pesticides, and gases are covered in subsequent chapters.

## ACIDS & ALKALIS

Acids and alkalis are of great importance as industrial chemicals. When ranked by volume of production, the inorganic acids and alkalis (including chlorine and ammonia) comprise 8 of the major 50 chemicals produced yearly in the United States.

## 1. ACIDS

### Essentials of Diagnosis

*Acute effects:*
- Irritative dermatitis, skin burn.
- Respiratory irritation, pulmonary edema.

*Chronic effects:*
- Hydrofluoric acid: osteosclerosis.
- Nitric acid (oxides of nitrogen): bronchiolitis fibrosa obliterans.
- Chromic acid: nasal ulceration, perforation, skin ulceration.
- Sulfuric acid: laryngeal cancer.

### Exposure Limits
Sulfuric acid
   ACGIH TLV: 1 mg/m$^3$, 3 mg/m$^3$ STEL
   OSHA PEL: 1 mg/m$^3$ TWA
   NIOSH REL: 1 mg/m$^3$ TWA
Phosphoric acid
   ACGIH TLV: 1 mg/m$^3$ TWA, 3 mg/m$^3$ STEL
   OSHA PEL: 1 mg/m$^3$ TWA, 3 mg/m$^3$ STEL
   NIOSH REL: 1 mg/m$^3$, 3 mg/m$^3$ STEL
Hydrochloric acid
   ACGIH TLV: 5 ppm ceiling
   OSHA PEL: 5 ppm ceiling
   NIOSH REL: 5 ppm ceiling

Chromic acid (Cr VI)
   ACGIH TLV: 0.05 mg/m$^3$ TWA
   OSHA PEL: 0.01 mg/m$^3$ ceiling
   NIOSH REL: .001 mg/m$^3$
Hydrofluoric acid
   ACGIH TLV: 3 ppm TWA
   OSHA PEL: 3 ppm TWA
   NIOSH REL: 3 ppm TWA, 6 ppm ceiling
Nitric acid
   ACGIH TLV: 2 ppm TWA, 4 ppm STEL
   OSHA PEL: 2 ppm TWA
   NIOSH REL: 2 ppm TWA, 4 ppm STEL

### General Considerations
An inorganic acid is a compound of hydrogen and one or more other elements (with the exception of carbon) that dissociates to produce hydrogen ions when dissolved in water or other solvents. The resultant solution has the ability to neutralize bases and turn litmus paper red. Inorganic acids of greatest industrial use are chromic, hydrochloric, hydrofluoric, nitric, phosphoric, and sulfuric acids. Inorganic acids share certain fire, explosive, and health hazards.

Organic acids and their derivatives include a broad range of substances used in nearly every type of chemical manufacture. All have primary irritant effects depending on the degree of acid dissociation and water solubility.

### Use, Production, & Occupational Exposure
  A. **Inorganic Acids:**
  **1. Sulfuric acid**–Sulfuric acid is the leading chemical in production volume, with annual US production exceeding 89 billion lb. It is less costly than any other acid, can be easily handled, reacts with many organic compounds to produce useful products, and forms a slightly soluble salt with calcium oxide or calcium hydroxide. The majority of sulfuric acid is used in the manufacture of phosphate and other fertilizers, petroleum refining, production of ammonium sulfate, iron and steel pickling, explosives and other nitrates and synthetic fiber manufacture, and as a

chemical intermediate. Workers with potential exposure to sulfuric acid include electroplaters, jewelers, metal cleaners, picklers, and storage battery makers. Occupational exposure can occur both by skin contact and by inhalation of sulfuric acid mist. A NIOSH study of lead acid battery plants found exposure to average 0.18 mg/m$^3$ and in some cases to be as high as 1.7 mg/m$^3$. NIOSH estimates that over 775,000 workers are potentially exposed to sulfuric acid.

**2. Phosphoric acid**–Phosphoric acid is used predominantly in the manufacture of fertilizers and agricultural feeds, in water treatment, and as a component of detergents and cleansers. US yearly production is over 25 billion lb. Other uses include the acid treatment (pickling) of sheet metal, chemical polishing of metals, as a tart flavoring agent for carbonated beverages, as a refractory bonding agent, and for boiler cleaning, textile dying, lithographic engraving, and rubber latex coagulation. Occupational exposure occurs primarily to the liquid acid by skin contact. NIOSH estimates that over 1.2 million workers are potentially exposed to phosphoric acid.

**3. Chromic acid**–Chromic acid is produced by roasting chromite ore with soda ash and treatment with sulfuric acid to form chromic acid anhydride, chromic acid (chromium trioxide), and dichromic acid. Chromic acid is used in chromium plating, process engraving, cement manufacturing, anodizing, metal cleaning, tanning, and in the manufacture of ceramic glazes, colored glass, metal cleaning, inks, and paints. Without local exhaust ventilation, occupational exposure to chromic acid mist during metal-plating operations can range up to several milligrams per cubic meter, but with a local exhaust system this can be markedly reduced to near undetectable limits. NIOSH estimates that over 126,000 workers are exposed to chromic acid.

**4. Nitric acid**–Nitric acid is produced from the oxidation of ammonia in the presence of a catalyst to yield nitric oxide, which is then further oxidized and absorbed in water to form an aqueous solution of nitric acid. Nitric acid is used to produce ammonium and potassium nitrate, explosives, adopic acid, isocyanates, fertilizers, nitroparaffins, and nitrobenzenes. Over 17 billion lb are produced annually in the United States. Occupational exposure can occur by topical contact with the liquid acid as well as by inhalation of nitrogen oxides evolved when nitric acid reacts with reducing agents (metals, organic matter) or during the combustion of nitrogen-containing materials (welding, glass blowing, underground blasting, and decomposition of agricultural silage). Reports of occupational exposure to nitric acid are limited to measurements of nitrogen oxides that evolved by these reactions. NIOSH estimates that over 297,000 workers are exposed to nitric acid.

**5. Hydrochloric acid**–Hydrochloric acid is an aqueous solution of hydrogen chloride and is used in steel pickling, chemical manufacturing, oil and gas well acidizing, and food processing. Annual US production exceeds 6 billion lb. Hydrochloric acid gas may also evolve from thermal degradation of polyvinyl chloride, a hazard to firefighters. NIOSH estimates that over 1.2 million workers are potentially exposed to hydrochloric acid.

**6. Hydrofluoric acid**–Hydrofluoric acid (hydrogen fluoride) is a colorless liquid manufactured by reaction of sulfuric acid with calcium fluoride in heated kilns. It evolves as a gas and is then condensed as liquid anhydrous hydrogen fluoride. Hydrofluoric acid is used as an intermediate in the production of fluorocarbons, aluminum fluoride, and cryolite; as a gasoline alkylation catalyst; and as an intermediate in the production of uranium hexafluoride. It is used in metal cleaning, glass etching, and polishing applications. Occupational exposure can occur both by direct skin contact and by inhalation of fumes. NIOSH estimates that over 189,000 workers are potentially exposed to hydrofluoric acid.

**7. Organic acids**–Among the saturated monocarboxylic acids, **formic acid** is used mainly in the textile industry as a dye-exhausting agent, in the leather industry as a deliming agent and neutralizer, as a coagulant for rubber latex, and as a component of nickel plating baths.

**Propionic acid** is used in organic synthesis, as a mold inhibitor, and as a food additive.

The unsaturated monocarboxylic acid **acrylic acid** is widely used in the manufacture of resins, plasticizers, and drugs.

The aliphatic dicarboxylics **maleic**, **fumaric**, and **adipic acids** find use in the manufacture of synthetic resins, dyes, surface coatings, inks, and plasticizers.

The halogenated **acetic acids** are highly reactive chemical intermediates used in glycine, drug, dye, and herbicide manufacture.

**Glycolic acid** and **lactic acid** are widely used in the leather, textile, adhesive, and plastics industries, and lactic acid is also used as a food acidulant.

## Metabolism & Mechanism of Action

Both inorganic and organic acids, by virtue of their water solubility and acid dissociation, will cause direct destruction of body tissue, including mucous membranes and skin. The extent of direct skin damage depends on the concentration of acid and length of exposure, while the damage to the respiratory tract by inhalation of acid mists will depend in addition on particle size. **Hydrofluoric acid**, one of the most corrosive of the inorganic acids, readily penetrates the skin and travels to deep tissue layers, causing liquefaction necrosis of soft tissues and decalcification and corrosion of bone. The intense pain that may accompany hydrogen fluoride burns is attributed to the calcium-precipitating property of the fluoride ion, which produces immobilization of tissue calcium and an excess of potassium that stimulates nerve endings. The fluoride ion may also bind body calcium, causing life-threatening systemic hypocalcemia after acute skin exposure or osteosclerotic bone changes after chronic exposure to hydrogen fluoride mist.

## Clinical Findings

### A. Symptoms & Signs:

**1. Acute exposure**–All acids act as primary irritants of the skin and mucous membranes.

**a. Skin**–All acids on contact with the skin cause dehydration and heat release to produce first-, second-, or third-degree burns with pain. Sensitization is rare. Hydrofluoric acid solutions of less than 50% may cause burns that may not become apparent for 1–24 hours; stronger solutions cause immediate pain and rapid tissue destruction, appearing reddened, pasty-white, blistered, macerated, or charred.

**b. Respiratory effects**–Inhalation of vapors or mists causes immediate rhinorrhea, throat burning, cough, burning eyes, and conjunctival irritation. High concentrations may cause shortness of breath, chest tightness, pulmonary edema, and death from respiratory failure. Inhalation of acid vapors or mists generally causes immediate symptoms due to high water solubility in mucous membranes, but respiratory effects may be delayed for several hours. Noncardiogenic pulmonary edema has been reported following acute inhalation exposure to sulfuric acid fumes, with almost complete recovery except for slightly decreased diffusion capacity on pulmonary function testing. For **nitric acid** exposure with oxides of nitrogen, overexposure tends to produce delayed symptoms 1–24 hours after inhalation, beginning with dyspnea followed by pulmonary edema and cyanosis. Three workers died of rapidly progressive pulmonary edema of delayed onset following inhalation of fumes from an accidental nitric acid explosion. Postmortem electron microscopy of lung tissue suggested increased permeability as a result of microvascular injury.

Chlorine species are highly reactive, resulting in a variety of dose-related lung effects ranging from respiratory mucous membrane irritation to pulmonary edema. Obstructive or restrictive pulmonary defects can result immediately following exposure, with complete resolution over a few days to weeks in most individuals. A few patients have long-term, persistent obstructive or restrictive pulmonary deficits or increased nonspecific airway reactivity after high-level exposure to chlorine gas. Tobacco smoking may increase the risk of adverse effects following chlorine inhalation.

To evaluate the effects of sulfuric acid contained in acid aerosols and ozone, normal and asthmatic subjects have been experimentally exposed to both sulfuric acid and ozone. No significant symptomatic or physiological effects of exposure to either sulfuric acid or ozone were found in healthy subjects; asthmatic subjects had significant changes in lung function and bronchial reactivity when exposed to ozone but not to sulfuric acid alone.

**c. Systemic effects**–One death has been reported as a result of persistent hypocalcemia following exposure to hydrofluoric acid involving 2.5% of total body surface area. Systemic toxicity involving gastrointestinal hemorrhage, acute renal failure, and hepatic injury has been reported following chromic acid ingestion.

**2. Chronic exposure**–

**a. Skin**–Chromate compounds can be allergens and can cause pulmonary as well as skin sensitization, but **chromic acid** results only in direct irritant dermatitis. Ulceration of the skin and ulceration and perforation of the nasal septum have been reported following chronic exposure to 0.1 mg/m$^3$ of chromic acid.

**b. Dental erosion**–Exposure to inorganic and organic acid fumes is reported to cause tooth surface loss. An increase in periodontal pockets but not oral mucous membrane lesions was found among acid-exposed workers.

**c. Respiratory effects**–Bronchiolitis fibrosa obliterans—a chronic interstitial lung disease—has been described after acute pneumonitis from nitric acid and oxides of nitrogen. No significant change in lung function was found among workers exposed to **phosphoric acid** while refining phosphorus.

**d. Systemic effects**–Osteosclerosis has been found in workers exposed to **hydrofluoric acid** and fluoride-containing compounds. Farmers with **formic acid** exposure have increased renal ammoniagenesis and urinary calcium excretion, possibly as a result of interaction with the oxidative metabolism of renal tubular cells.

**e. Cancer**–Studies of workers exposed to **sulfuric acid** mists show an excess risk of laryngeal cancer. The International Agency for Research on Cancer (IARC) concludes that there is sufficient evidence that occupational exposure to strong inorganic acid mists containing sulfuric acid is carcinogenic (Group I).

For **chromic acid**, IARC concludes that there is sufficient evidence of carcinogenicity in humans and animals (Group I). NIOSH recommends that chromic acid be regulated as a carcinogen.

An increase in the number of sister-chromatid exchanges has been found in lymphocytes of workers exposed to acid aerosols at a **phosphate** fertilizer factory.

IARC finds that **hydrochloric acid** is not classifiable in terms of carcinogenicity to humans (Group 3). The lung cancer risk was not increased among a cohort of chemical manufacturing workers exposed to hydrogen chloride.

**B. Laboratory Findings:** In cases where inhalation exposure may cause more extensive mucosal irritation, the chest x-ray may show interstitial or alveolar edema, and hypoxemia may be evident by arterial blood gas analysis. Nonspecific abnormalities in liver and kidney function have been reported following massive inhalation exposures to **sulfuric acid** and **hydrofluoric acid**.

Urine fluoride levels can be used as biological indices of exposure in hydrofluoric acid intoxication, with a normal mean value in urine of 0.5 mg/L (recommended occupational postshift urinary biological standard of 7 mg/L).

### Differential Diagnosis

There are many respiratory irritants (see Chapter 20), including gases such as ammonia, phosgene, halogens (chlorine, bromine), sulfur dioxide, and ozone; solvents such as glycol ethers; and dusts such as fibrous glass. The symptoms and clinical course of lung disorders due to these substances and to the acids discussed in this chapter do not differ; thus, the history is essential. Likewise, hundreds of industrial chemicals may cause direct irritant dermatitis.

### Prevention

**A. Work Practices:** When possible, highly corrosive acids should be replaced by acids that present less hazard, and if use of corrosives is essential, only the minimum concentration should be used. Proper storage practices should include fire-resistant buildings with acid-resistant floors, retaining sills, and adequate drainage; containers should be adequately protected against impact, kept off the floor, and clearly labeled. Wherever possible, handling should be done through sealed systems or the substances transported in safety bottle carriers. Decanting should be done with special siphons or pumps. The potential for violent or dangerous reactions (eg, when water is poured into nitric acid) can be avoided by appropriate training.

Where processes produce acid mists (as in electroplating), local exhaust ventilation should be installed. Workers potentially exposed to splashes or spills must wear acid-resistant hand, arm, eye, and face protection, and respiratory protection should be available for emergency use.

Emergency showers and eyewash stations should be strategically located.

**B. Medical Surveillance:** Preplacement and periodic examinations should include a medical history of skin and respiratory disease and examination of the skin, teeth, and lungs. For potential hydrofluoric acid exposure near or above the permissible exposure limit, periodic postshift urinary fluoride in excess of 7 mg/L (adjusted for urine specific gravity of 1.024) may indicate poor work practices. Elemental analysis of hair for fluoride has been correlated with fluoride levels in serum and urine.

### Treatment

Immediate on-site first aid treatment of acid burns to the eye or skin is copious flushing with running water with removal of all contaminated clothing. First-degree burns or second-degree burns involving a small area can generally be treated at the on-site medical facility with debridement and application of suitable burn dressings. All other acid burns should be treated at a hospital emergency facility.

For hydrofluoric acid burns, the definitive treatment is aimed at deactivation of the fluoride ion in tissue with calcium, magnesium, or quaternary ammonium solution. If the hydrogen fluoride concentration is 20% or more or if the patient has been exposed to a long delay of a lower concentration—or if a large tissue area has been affected by a lower concentration—then calcium gluconate solution should be used. The latter, prepared by mixing 10% calcium gluconate with an equal amount of saline to form a 5% solution, is infiltrated with a small needle in multiple injections (0.5 mL/cm$^2$ of tissue) into and 5 mm beyond the affected area. Dramatic pain relief should occur. Vesicles and bullae should be carefully debrided, with removal of necrotic tissue; if periungual or ungual tissues are involved, the nail should be split to the base. A burn dressing is then applied along with calcium gluconate 2.5% gel or magnesium sulfate paste. Hydrofluoric acid burns of the hand have been successfully treated with repeated application of an occlusive glove over topical calcium carbonate gel. Repeated intra-arterial infusion over 4 hours with 10 mL of 10% calcium chloride diluted with 40 mL of normal saline has also been recommended for the treatment of hydrofluoric acid extremity burns. Careful monitoring of serum magnesium and calcium levels is required. If the hydrogen fluoride concentration is 20% or less and only a small surface area is involved, the burn can be flushed with water and then treated with 10% magnesium sulfate solution under a soft dressing.

The eye burned with hydrogen fluoride should be copiously irrigated and then evaluated by an ophthalmologist. One percent calcium gluconate in normal saline can be used as an irrigant.

Systemic effects from absorption should be anticipated from skin burns from hydrogen fluoride of greater than 50% concentration or from extensive burns at any concentration. Hypocalcemia can be life-threatening and should be monitored by repeated measurement of serum calcium and electrocardiography for QT interval prolongation. Ten percent calcium gluconate intravenously with adequate hydration should be used for calcium depletion.

For inhalation of acid vapors or mists, the victim should be immediately removed from the source of exposure and treated on-site with 100% oxygen. If there are symptoms of shortness of breath, chest tightness, or persistent cough, the patient should be evaluated at the hospital. Upper body or facial burns are a clue that inhalation may have occurred with possible lower airway damage. Evaluation should include a chest x-ray and arterial blood gas analysis for oxygen. Hypoxemia should be treated with 100% oxygen by mask, or by intubation in the event of severe hypoxemia, acidosis or respiratory distress. Fluid balance should be carefully monitored and intracardiac pressure measured directly if necessary. Bronchospasm may be treated with inhaled bronchodilators or intravenous aminophylline, and steroids if necessary. The benefits of steroids in the management of noncardiogenic pulmonary edema due to acid inhalation are unknown, but the drugs may be used empirically to speed recovery and prevent the subsequent development of interstitial lung disease. Nebulized calcium gluconate has been reported for treatment of inhalational exposure to hydrofluoric acid.

## 2. ALKALIS

### Essentials of Diagnosis

*Acute effects:*
- Skin and eye burns.
- Respiratory irritation.

*Chronic effects:*
- Corneal opacities of the eye (untreated).
- Obstructive lung disease.

### Exposure Limits

Sodium hydroxide
    ACGIH TLV: 2 mg/m$^3$ TWA
    OSHA PEL: 2 mg/m$^3$ TWA
    NIOSH REL: 2 mg/m$^3$ ceiling (15 minutes)
Potassium hydroxide
    ACGIH TLV: 2 mg/m$^3$ ceiling
    OSHA PEL: 2 mg/m$^3$ ceiling
Calcium oxide
    ACGIH TLV: 2 mg/m$^3$ TWA
    NIOSH REL: 2 mg/m$^3$ TWA

### General Considerations

Alkalis are caustic substances that dissolve in water to form a solution with a pH higher than 7.0. These include ammonia, ammonium hydroxide, calcium hydroxide, calcium oxide, potassium hydroxide, potassium carbonate, sodium hydroxide, sodium carbonate, and trisodium phosphate. The alkalis, whether in solid form or concentrated liquid form, are more destructive to tissue than most acids. They tend to liquefy tissues and allow for deeper penetration, depending on concentration, duration of contact, and area of the body involved.

### Use, Production, & Occupational Exposure

In the United States, all **sodium hydroxide** (caustic soda) is produced by the electrolysis of sodium or potassium chloride in mercury cells. In this process,

pure saturated brine is decomposed by electric current to liberate chlorine gas at the anode and sodium metal at the cathode. The latter reacts with water to form sodium hydroxide. Most caustic soda is produced as a 50% aqueous solution. Sodium hydroxide is used in pulp and paper production, water treatment, and manufacture of a wide variety of organic and inorganic chemicals, soaps and detergents, textiles, and alumina. Annual US production is over 25 billion lb. NIOSH estimates that over 2.8 million workers are potentially exposed to sodium hydroxide.

**Sodium carbonate** (soda ash) is produced by the ammonium chloride process, by the reaction of sodium chloride and sulfuric acid, or by leaching out rock deposits. Sodium carbonate is used in glass manufacturing, as a component of cleaning-product formulations, in pulp and paper processing and water treatment, and as a chemical intermediate. Annual US production exceeds 20 billion lb. NIOSH estimates that over 200,000 workers are potentially exposed to sodium carbonate.

**Potassium carbonate** (potash) is produced by carbonating potassium hydroxide solutions obtained by electrolysis. Potassium carbonate is used in the manufacture of soap, glass, pottery, and shampoo; in tanning and finishing leather; in photographic chemicals, fire-extinguishing compounds, and rubber antioxidant preparations; and as an alkalizer and drainpipe cleaner. Annual US production exceeds 3.3 billion lb. NIOSH estimates that over 475,000 workers are potentially exposed to potassium carbonate.

**Potassium hydroxide** (caustic potash) is produced by electrolysis of potassium chloride solution and is used a chemical intermediate for potassium carbonate, potassium phosphate, soaps, tetrapotassium pyrophosphate, liquid fertilizers, dyestuffs, and herbicides. Annual US production exceeds 3.1 billion lb. NIOSH estimates that about 6700 workers are potentially exposed to potassium hydroxide.

**Calcium oxide** (quicklime) is made by calcining limestone. Calcium oxide is used in metallurgy as a flux in steel production, for ammonia recovery in the Solvay process for sodium carbonate, in construction applications and water purification and softening, in beet and sugar cane refining, in Kraft paper pulp production, and in sewage treatment. Annual US production exceeds 38 billion lb. NIOSH estimates that over 725,000 workers are potentially exposed to calcium oxide.

### Metabolism & Mechanism of Action

Occupational exposure to the alkalis is primarily by direct contact with the eyes, skin, and mucous membranes. Inhalation of caustic mists is generally limited by the irritant properties of the compound. Contact of the eyes with alkalis will cause disintegration and sloughing of corneal epithelium, corneal opacification, marked edema, and ulceration. Alkaline compounds will combine with skin tissue to form albuminates and with natural fats to form soaps. They gelatinize tissue and result in deep and painful destruction. Accidental or intentional ingestion of alkalis may cause severe esophageal necrosis with subsequent stenosis.

## Clinical Findings

### A. Symptoms & Signs:

**1. Acute exposure–**In contrast to acids, skin contact with the alkalis may not elicit immediate pain but may start to cause immediate damage with erythema and tissue necrosis within minutes to hours. Splashes of alkali to the eyes, if not rapidly treated within minutes, may result in corneal necrosis, edema, and opacification.

Irreversible obstructive lung injury has developed after acute inhalation of sodium hydroxide in a poorly ventilated space. Three patients suffered severe skin and inhalational injuries following exposure to "black liquor" used in the pulp and paper industry. Fatal injury has occurred after a relatively brief inhalation and dermal contact with a hot concentrated caustic solution. Acute tracheobronchitis and respiratory failure as a result of high-dose ammonia inhalation may result in permanent, severe, and fixed airways obstruction. Bronchiolitis obliterans has been reported due to occupational exposure to incinerator fly ash.

**2. Chronic exposure–**Chronic exposure to caustic dusts for years does not significantly increase the mortality rate. Long-term sodium hydroxide inhalation has been reported to cause severe obstructive airway disease with significant air-trapping. Chronic exposure to ammonia over 7.5 ppm is significantly associated with pulmonary function decrements among swine production facility workers. An increased prevalence of coughing, wheezing, and ocular and nasal irritation was reported among community residents exposed to alkali dust. Corneal opacities have resulted from untreated corneal alkali burns.

### B. Laboratory Findings: No laboratory tests are of value in the diagnosis and management of problems resulting from alkali exposure.

## Differential Diagnosis

Many other industrial chemicals, including acids, may cause eye and skin burns.

## Prevention

### A. Work Practices: Insofar as possible, solutions of caustics should be handled in closed systems that will prevent contact with or inhalation of the chemical. All persons with potential exposure to caustics should wear the proper protective clothing

and equipment, such as a full-face shield, safety goggles, apron or suit, rubber gloves, and boots.

Emergency showers and eyewashes must be located where eye or skin contact may occur.

### B. Medical Surveillance: Medical examination of the eyes, skin, and respiratory tract are recommended for all workers with caustic exposure.

## Treatment

Sodium and potassium hydroxide may cause more extended and deeper damage as a result of rapid penetration through ocular tissues. Alkali burns of the eye and skin should be treated within minutes by copious irrigation with water and removal of all contaminated clothing. First aid treatment with prompt and continuous eye irrigation is essential to prevent permanent corneal damage and visual loss. Topical use of a synthetic metalloproteinase inhibitor has been shown to reverse or stop the progression of corneal ulceration following an experimental alkali burn. A physician or health practitioner should be consulted for eye burns and careful examination of the eye performed. If damage is suspected, follow-up with an ophthalmologist is recommended.

## ACRYLAMIDE & ACRYLONITRILE

## 1. ACRYLAMIDE

## Essentials of Diagnosis

*Acute effects:*
- Dermatitis.

*Chronic effects:*
- Peripheral neuropathy.

## Exposure Limits

ACGIH TLV: 0.03 mg/m$^3$ TWA
OSHA PEL: 0.03 mg/m$^3$ TWA
NIOSH REL: 0.03 mg/m$^3$ TWA, skin

## General Considerations

Pure acrylamide is a white crystalline solid at room temperature and is highly soluble in water. It is a vinyl monomer with high reactivity with thiols and with hydroxy and amino groups. Commercial acrylamide is shipped in 50% aqueous form in stainless steel drums, tank trucks, and cars. Acrylamide manufacture is from the catalytic hydration of acrylonitrile.

## Use

The major use of acrylamide monomer is in the production of polymers, which are useful as flocculators. Polyacrylamides are used for waste and water treatment flocculants, in products for sewage dewatering, and in a variety of products for the water treatment industry. Other uses include strengtheners for papermaking and retention aids, drilling-mud additives, textile treatment, and surface coatings. One of the more important uses is as a grouting agent, particularly in mining and tunnel construction. NIOSH estimates that over 10,000 workers are potentially exposed to acrylamide.

### Occupational & Environmental Exposure

Monomer manufacturing workers are potentially exposed to acrylamide, as are papermaking workers, soil stabilization workers, textile workers, and well drillers. Intoxication has been reported in the manufacture of acrylamide monomer, in the handling of a 10% aqueous solution in a mine, in the production of flocculators, in the use of a resin mixture containing residual monomer, and in the production of polymers while manufacturing papercoating materials. One nonoccupational incident occurred in Japan, where a family ingested well water containing 400 ppm acrylamide.

### Metabolism & Mechanism of Action

Acrylamide is easily absorbed in animals following all routes of administration. Quantitative data on absorption or excretion in humans are not available. Following intravenous administration in rats, acrylamide is distributed throughout total body water within minutes and then excreted largely in the urine with a half-life of less than 2 hours. Protein-bound acrylamide or acrylamide metabolites have a half-life in blood and possibly in the central nervous system of about 10 days. The primary metabolite of acrylamide is N-acetyl-S-(3-amino-3-oxypropyl) cysteine and is excreted predominantly in the urine.

### Clinical Findings

**A. Symptoms & Signs:** Acrylamide polymer may cause dermatitis but does not cause neurotoxicity. The monomer can produce numbness and tingling of hands, and weakness of the hands and legs. Acrylamide is neurotoxic in many experimental animals.

Over 60 cases of acrylamide-associated neurotoxicity have been reported in humans. Similar to the neuropathy associated with the hexacarbons *n*-hexane and methyl-*n*-butyl ketone, acrylamide neuropathy is considered a typical example of a dying-back disorder, where degeneration begins at the distal ends of the longest and largest fibers and spreads proximally. In most cases toxicity results from skin contact and dermal absorption, though it may be absorbed by inhalation as well. The neurologic features of acrylamide intoxication vary depending on the speed of intoxication. In the Japanese family who ingested contaminated well water, encephalopathy with confusion, disorientation, memory disturbances, hallucinations, ataxia, and peripheral

neuropathy developed in approximately 1 month. Reported time to onset of symptoms in occupational cases has varied from 4 weeks to about 24 months. Clinically, acrylamide peripheral neuropathy affects both motor and sensory nerve fibers predominantly in the distal limbs. Difficulty in walking and clumsiness of the hands are usually the first symptoms, followed by numbness of the feet and fingers. Distal weakness is found on examination, with loss of tendon reflexes and vibration sensation. Evidence of excessive sweating affecting predominantly the extremities has been commonly reported, along with redness and exfoliation of the skin. In acute cases, central nervous system involvement may result in truncal ataxia, lethargy, and dysarthria. Major histologic findings are swelling of axons and/or decrease in large diameter axons. The axonopathy is reversible slowly over time, but complete recovery depends on the severity of intoxication. Only the acrylamide monomer is neurotoxic.

Acrylamide has been found to increase the tumor yield in mice. Two cohort mortality studies have shown no significant excess of cancer among acrylamide-exposed workers. IARC has concluded that there is sufficient evidence in experimental animals for acrylamide to be classified as a carcinogen (Group 2A).

**B. Laboratory Findings:** Electrophysiologic studies of workers with signs and symptoms of neurotoxicity have shown only a slight effect on maximal conduction velocity of either motor or sensory fibers. Sensory nerve action potentials are usually reduced and are the most sensitive electrophysiologic test.

Sural nerve biopsies performed on two patients during recovery from acrylamide neuropathy showed axonal degeneration affecting mainly large-diameter fibers.

### Differential Diagnosis

The combination of truncal ataxia with peripheral neuropathy—predominantly motor—accompanied by excessive sweating and redness and peeling of the skin makes the diagnosis of acrylamide-associated neurotoxicity likely. Other occupational toxic agents associated with peripheral neuropathy must be considered (see Chapter 24), along with the presence of other underlying metabolic diseases, drug use, and endocrine disorders.

### Prevention

**A. Work Practices:** Mechanized bag loading of polymerization reactors, closed-line transfer of liquid acrylamide, and other closed-system processes are important to minimize exposure. Where necessary, personal protective equipment designed to prevent dermal and inhalation exposure to acrylamide should be available.

**B. Medical Surveillance:** Preplacement and

periodic examinations should exclude symptomatic peripheral neuropathies. Hemoglobin adducts have been used to monitor occupational exposure to both acrylamide and acrylonitrile. A neurotoxicity index involving electrophysiological measures was correlated with urinary 24-hour mercapturic acid levels, hemoglobin adducts of acrylamide, employment duration, and vibration sensitivity. Vibration threshold may be a sensitive indicator of early neurotoxicity due to acrylamide exposure.

## Treatment

Skin contaminated with acrylamide should be washed immediately with soap and water and contaminated clothing removed. There is no known treatment for acrylamide intoxication. Removal from exposure is the only effective measure that can be taken. Full recovery has been observed in most cases after 2 weeks to 2 years, though in severe cases some residual abnormalities have been noted.

## 2. ACRYLONITRILE

### Essentials of Diagnosis

*Acute effects:*
- Respiratory irritation, nausea, and dizziness, irritability, followed by
- Convulsions, coma, and death.

*Chronic effects:*
- Nausea, dizziness, headache, apprehension, fatigue.

### Exposure Limits

ACGIH TLV: 2 ppm TWA
OSHA PEL: 2 ppm TWA, 10 ppm ceiling (15 minutes)
NIOSH REL: 1 ppm TWA, 10 ppm ceiling (15 minutes)

### General Considerations

Acrylonitrile is a volatile colorless liquid with a characteristic odor resembling that of peach seeds, discernible at 20 ppm or less. It is a highly reactive compound. Pure acrylonitrile polymerizes readily in light, and storage requires the addition of polymerization inhibitors. Its vapors are explosive and flammable in the range of 3–17% and may release hydrogen cyanide on burning.

### Use

Acrylonitrile was not an important product until World War II, when it was used in the production of oil-resistant rubbers. Nearly all world production of acrylonitrile is now based on a process where propylene, ammonia, and air are reacted in the vapor phase in the presence of a catalyst. Hydrogen cyanide and acrylonitrile are the chief by-products formed; the latter undergoes a series of distillations to produce acrylonitrile.

Much of acrylonitrile monomer is used for the manufacture of acrylic fibers for the apparel, carpeting, and home furnishings industries. Acrylonitrile-containing plastics, particularly the resins acrylonitrile-butadiene-styrene (ABS) and styrene- acrylonitrile (SAN), are used in pipe and pipe fittings, automotive parts, appliances, and building components. Nitrile elastomers are used for their oil and hydrocarbon-resistant properties in the petrochemical and automobile industries. Acrylonitrile is also used to make acrylamide.

### Occupational & Environmental Exposure

Potential exposure to acrylonitrile may occur in monomer-, fiber-, resin- and rubber-producing plants. Potential exposure to acrylonitrile in acrylic fiber production is greatest when the solvent is removed from newly formed fibers and during decontamination of acrylonitrile processing equipment, loading, surveillance of the processing unit, and product sampling. Annual US production exceeds 3 billion lb. NIOSH estimates that over 81,000 workers are potentially exposed to acrylonitrile.

### Metabolism & Mechanism of Action

Acrylonitrile is readily absorbed in animals following ingestion or inhalation. There is a biphasic half-life of 3.5 hours and 50–77 hours, with elimination predominantly in the urine. Acrylonitrile is metabolized to cyanide, and its metabolites are eliminated in the urine. In humans, absorption can occur both through inhalation and skin contact. The acute toxicity of acrylonitrile in humans is thought to be due to the action of cyanide, and thiocyanate is detected in blood and urine of workers. Acrylonitrile is an electrophilic compound and binds covalently to nucleophilic sites in macromolecules. Hemoglobin adducts have been used for exposure assessment in experimental animal studies. It has been postulated that the mutagenic effect of acrylonitrile is due to glycidonitrile, a reactive intermediate able to alkylate macromolecules.

### Clinical Findings

**A. Symptoms & Signs:** A few deaths have been reported from acrylonitrile exposure, with respiratory distress, lethargy, convulsions, and coma at 7500 mg/m$^3$. Acrylonitrile was implicated in four cases of toxic epidermal necrosis, which developed 11–21 days after the victims returned to houses fumigated with a 2:1 mixture of carbon tetrachloride and acrylonitrile. One patient had measurable blood cyanide levels at autopsy. Symptoms of acute poisoning are described as irritability, respiratory irritation, limb weakness, respiratory distress, dizziness, nausea, cyanosis, collapse, convulsions, and cardiac arrest; these resemble cyanide poisoning.

Chronic human toxicity has been reported in rubber workers exposed to 16–100 ppm of acrylonitrile for periods of 20–45 minutes, with complaints of nasal irritation, headache, nausea, apprehension, and fatigue.

Acrylonitrile is carcinogenic in rats after 1 year of feeding and inhalation, inducing brain tumors and stomach papillomas. An excess risk of colon and lung cancers occurred among acrylonitrile polymerization workers from a textile fibers plant. Epidemiologic studies have suggested that acrylonitrile is associated with an increased lung cancer risk with a latency period of 20 years and that it should be regarded as probably carcinogenic in humans. However, a meta-analysis of mortality studies among acrylonitrile-exposed cohorts did not reveal evidence for carcinogenicity. IARC has concluded that there is sufficient evidence in experimental animals for acrylonitrile to be classified as a carcinogen (Group 2A).

**B. Laboratory Findings:** Chromosomal analysis of workers exposed to acrylonitrile has not shown an increase in aberrations. Elevated serum cyanide or urine thiocyanate levels may be found in cases of acute intoxication.

## Differential Diagnosis

Acute poisoning with acrylonitrile may mimic cyanide intoxication.

## Prevention

**A. Work Practices:** Controls have proved effective in reducing employee exposure to acrylonitrile. NIOSH has recommended that acrylonitrile be handled in the workplace as a potential human carcinogen and has published detailed recommendations for adequate work practices.

**B. Medical Surveillance:** Preplacement and annual medical examinations should include special attention to the skin, respiratory tract, and gastrointestinal tract and to the nonspecific symptoms of headache, nausea, dizziness, and weakness that may be associated with chronic exposure.

Treatment kits for acute cyanide intoxication (see Chapter 33) should be immediately available to trained medical personnel at each area where there is a potential for release of or contact with acrylonitrile.

Biological monitoring may be useful to reflect exposure to acrylonitrile. The relationship between the degree of exposure to acrylonitrile and the urinary excretion of thiocyanate and acrylonitrile was determined in Japanese workers from acrylic fiber factories. A mean postshift urine thiocyanate concentration of 11.4 mg/L (specific gravity, 1.024) was found to correlate with an 8-hour average acrylonitrile exposure of 4.2 ppm. Normal urinary thiocyanate levels in nonsmokers does not exceed 2.5 mg/g of creatinine. Mean urinary acrylonitrile levels of 30 μg/L in Dutch plastics workers were found to correlate with a mean 8-hour TWA exposure level of 0.13 ppm and were used to monitor adequate work practices.

## Treatment

Treatment of acute intoxication with acrylonitrile is similar to that of cyanide poisoning (see Chapter 33).

# AROMATIC AMINES

## Essentials of Diagnosis

*Acute effects:*
- Dermatitis.
- Asthma.
- Cholestatic jaundice.
- Methemoglobinemia.

*Chronic effects:*
- Bladder cancer.

## Exposure Limits

Aniline
   ACGIH TLV: 2 ppm TWA
   OSHA PEL: 5 ppm TWA
   NIOSH REL: Reduce exposure to lowest feasible concentrations
p,p′-Methylene dianiline
   ACGIH TLV: 0.1 ppm TWA
   NIOSH REL: Reduce exposure to lowest feasible concentration
Naphthylamines
   OSHA PEL: Stringent workplace controls. Occupational carcinogen
   ACGIH TLV: Confirmed human carcinogen
   NIOSH REL: Reduce exposure to lowest feasible concentrations
Benzidine-based dyes
   NIOSH REL: Reduce exposure to lowest feasible concentration.
   ACGIH TLV: 0.01 ppm TWA
   NIOSH REL: 3 μg/m$^3$ (lowest detectable concentration)
o-Toluidine
   ACGIH TLV: 2 ppm TWA
   OSHA PEL: 5 ppm TWA
   NIOSH REL: Reduce exposure to lowest feasible concentrations

## General Considerations

The aromatic amines are a class of chemicals derived from aromatic hydrocarbons such as benzene, toluene, naphthalene, anthracene and diphenyl, etc, by the replacement of at least one hydrogen atom by an amino group. Some examples are shown below.

Aniline

o-Toluidine

Benzidine

MBOCA

## Use

Aromatic amines are used mainly in the synthesis of other chemicals.

The principal commercial use of benzidine is as a chemical intermediate in dye manufacture and security printing and as a laboratory reagent. At present, benzidine dihydrochloride is the only form commercially produced in the United States. At least 16 benzidine-based dyes are produced in the United States, with a total production of 1–2 million lb. Two-thirds are used by the textile industry, 17% for the paper and pulp industry, 10% for the leather tanning industry, and about 7% for the aqueous ink and plastics industries. NIOSH estimates that approximately 1,500 workers are potentially exposed to benzidine.

Aniline is used as a chemical intermediate in the production of methylenediisocyanate, rubber products, dyes, pesticides, pigments, and hydroquinones. Annual US production exceeds 1.2 billion lb. NIOSH estimates that almost 42,000 workers are potentially exposed to aniline. p,p′-Methylenedianiline is used as a chemical intermediate in the production of polyurethanes, dyes, and polyamide and polyimide resins and fibers and as a laboratory analytic reagent. NIOSH estimates that over 15,000 workers are potentially exposed to p,p′-methylenedianiline. o-Toluidine is used as a component of printing textiles, in the preparation of ion exchange resin, as an antioxidant in rubber manufacture, and in the synthesis of dyestuffs. NIOSH estimates that over 30,000 workers are potentially exposed to o-toluidine. MBOCA has been used as a curing agent in urethane and epoxy resins. It is no longer commercially manufactured in the United States. NIOSH estimates that approxi-

mately 125 employees are potentially exposed to MBOCA.

Because of the demonstrated carcinogenicity of b-naphthylamine, its manufacture and use has been banned in many countries. Production of b-naphthylamine ceased in the United States in 1972.

## Metabolism & Mechanism of Action

The aromatic amines are nearly all lipid-soluble and are absorbed through the skin. Metabolism is largely via the formation of hydroxylamine intermediates. These metabolites are transported to the bladder as N-glucuronide conjugates and hydrolyzed by the acid pH of urine to form reactive electrophiles that bind to bladder transitional epithelial DNA. Animal studies have demonstrated that bladder epithelial prostaglandin H synthetase can activate aromatic amines that then bind to nucleic acids.

## Clinical Findings
### A. Symptoms & Signs:
**1. Acute exposure–**

**a. Dermatitis–**Because of their alkaline nature, certain amines constitute a direct risk of dermatitis. Many aromatic amines can cause allergic dermatitis, notably p-aminophenol and p-phenylenediamine. The latter was known for "fur dermatitis" and caused asthma among fur dyers.

**b. Respiratory effects–**Asthma due to p-phenylenediamine has been reported.

**c. Hemorrhagic cystitis–**Hemorrhagic cystitis can result from exposure to o- and p-toluidine and 5-chloro-o-toluidine. The hematuria is self-limited, and no increase in bladder tumors has been subsequently noted.

**d. Hepatic injury–**Cholestatic jaundice has resulted from industrial exposure to diaminodiphenylmethane, which also caused toxic jaundice due to contaminated baking flour ("Epping jaundice") (see Chapter 22). The hepatitis has been reversible after cessation of exposure.

**e. Methemoglobinemia–**Acute poisoning by aniline and its derivatives results in the formation of methemoglobin. A significant elevation of methemoglobin levels has been demonstrated in adult volunteers after ingestion of 25 mg of aniline. The mean lethal dose has been estimated to be between 15 and 30 g, although death has followed ingestion of as little as 1 g of aniline. It has been postulated that a toxic metabolite, phenylhydroxylamine, is responsible for the methemoglobin. Peak levels of methemoglobin are observed within 1–2 hours after ingestion. Cyanosis becomes apparent at levels of methemoglobin of 10–15%, and headache, weakness, dyspnea, dizziness, and malaise occur at levels of 25–30%. Concentrations above 60–70% may cause coma and death.

**f. Bladder cancer–**An excess of bladder tumors was recognized in 1895 among German workers who used aromatic amines in the production of synthetic dyes. British dyestuffs workers had a high risk for the development of bladder cancer. In the United States, bladder cancer occurred in workers exposed to β-naphthylamine or benzidine in the manufacture of dyes, with a mean latency period of 20 years from onset of exposure.

Workers involved in the production of auramine and magenta from aniline and those working with 4-aminobiphenyl have an increased risk of bladder tumors. Workers exposed to 4-chloro-*o*-toluidine have been observed to have a 73-fold excess of bladder cancer. Animal studies have shown an increased risk of bladder tumors after exposure to benzidine, *o*-toluidine, *o*-dianisidine-based dyes and MBOCA and other aromatic amines.

IARC considers benzidine carcinogenic to humans (Group 1A) and MBOCA probably carcinogenic to humans (Group 2A). IARC has concluded that there is sufficient evidence in experimental animals for the carcinogenicity of *o*-toluidine and p,p′-methylenedianiline (Group 2B) and finds limited evidence for the carcinogenicity of aniline in animals (Group 3).

Results from cohort and case-control studies strongly support the association between occupational aromatic amine exposure (benzidine, naphthylamines, MBOCA, *o*-toluidine) and bladder cancer.

**B. Laboratory Findings:** Methemoglobin levels can help in the detection of excess absorption of the single-ring aromatic compounds. Normal individuals have methemoglobin concentrations of 1–2%. A biological threshold limit value of 5% has been proposed.

Determination of the metabolites *p*-aminophenol and *p*-nitrophenol can be useful to monitor exposure to aniline and nitrobenzene. After 6 hours of exposure to 1 ppm of nitrobenzene, the urinary concentration of *p*-aminophenol should not exceed 50 mg/L, and the recommended biological threshold value is 10 mg/L.

Levels of free MBOCA in the urine can be used to monitor exposure to this compound. Levels of free MBOCA in urine should be minimized to the limit of detection and used as an index of the adequacy of existing work practices and engineering controls.

For workers exposed to the known or suspected carcinogenic aromatic amines, periodic screening of urine for red blood cells and evidence of dysplastic epithelium may detect early bladder cancer.

### Differential Diagnosis

Aliphatic nitrates (eg, ethylene glycol dinitrate), aliphatic nitrites, inorganic nitrites, and chlorates may also cause methemoglobinemia.

Occupation-associated bladder cancer may account for 10–15% of all cases of bladder cancer.

Cigarette smoking, with inhalation of carcinogenic arylamines (eg, 2-aminonaphthalene), is also a significant risk factor.

### Prevention

**A. Work Practices:** Every effort should be made to eliminate use of the carcinogenic aromatic amines by substitution of safer alternatives. Appropriate engineering controls for manufacturers of polyurethane products who use MBOCA—particularly the use of automated systems and local exhaust ventilation—can successfully reduce the potential for exposures. Since most cases of aniline exposure occur through skin and clothing contamination, emphasis should be given to provision of appropriate gloves and protective clothing.

For the benzidine-based dyes, worker exposure should be reduced to the lowest feasible levels through appropriate engineering controls, including the use of closed-process systems, liquid metering systems, walk-in hoods, and specific local exhaust ventilation. Dust levels can be minimized by the use of dyes in pellet, paste, or liquid form. Restricted access to areas with potential exposure and provision of suitable protective clothing and respirators should be instituted.

**B. Medical Surveillance:** Preemployment and periodic measurement of postshift urinary *p*-aminophenol is useful for biological monitoring of aniline exposure. Similarly, periodic postshift urine samples for free MBOCA can be an important adjunct to industrial hygiene measures of exposure.

The ACGIH-recommended biological exposure limit (BEI) for *o*-toluidine, MBOCA, and aniline is methemoglobin in blood in excess of 1.5% during or at the end of the workshift. Biological monitoring by high-pressure liquid chromatography (HPLC) methods for analysis of urinary *o*-toluidine, aniline, and MBOCA may be useful. Measurement of MDA using sensitive gas chromatography-mass spectrometry (GC-MS) assay in urine has been correlated with hemoglobin adducts of MDA in polyurethane production workers and may serve as a sensitive index of exposure (particularly for dermal exposure) at levels below air monitoring detection limits. Hemoglobin adducts have also been used for biological monitoring of workers exposed to 3-chloro-4-fluoroaniline.

High-risk populations with past or current exposure to carcinogenic aromatic amines should be screened on a periodic basis with exfoliative bladder cytology. Positive findings are followed up with direct urologic examination.

### Treatment

The definitive treatment of methemoglobinemia caused by aniline poisoning is administration of the reducing agent methylene blue. However, an excessive amount of methylene blue may itself provoke the formation of methemoglobin. Additionally, the ability of methylene blue to reduce methemoglobin can be impaired by hereditary G6PD deficiency and can precipitate frank hemolysis. The recommended dose of methylene blue for the initial management of methemoglobinemia is 1–2 mg/kg of body weight intravenously, equivalent to 0.1–0.2 mL of a 1% solution. Maximal response to methylene blue usually occurs within 30–60 minutes. Repeated doses should be spaced about 1 hour apart and based on methemoglobin levels; most patients, unless they are anemic, can tolerate a level of 30% or less. Methylene blue administration should be discontinued if either a negligible response or an increase in methemoglobin levels results after two consecutive doses or if the total dose exceeds 7 mg/kg. It is advisable to continue to monitor methemoglobin levels even after an initial response to methylene blue, since there is a potential for continued production of methemoglobin by aniline.

Treatment of bladder cancer associated with aromatic amine exposure is identical to that of nonoccupationally associated bladder tumors.

Early detection through screening programs may improve prognosis.

## CARBON DISULFIDE

### Essentials of Diagnosis

*Acute effects:*
- Irritability, manic delirium, hallucinations, paranoia.
- Respiratory irritation.

*Chronic effects:*
- Coronary artery disease.
- Neurobehavioral abnormalities.
- Retinal microaneurysms.
- Peripheral neuropathy with ascending symmetric paresthesias and weakness.

### Exposure Limits

ACGIH TLV: 10 ppm TWA
OSHA PEL: 4 ppm TWA, 12 ppm STEL
NIOSH REL: 1 ppm TWA, 10 ppm ceiling

### General Considerations

Carbon disulfide is a colorless volatile solvent with a strong, sweetish aroma. The average odor threshold of 1 ppm is below the permissible exposure limit; therefore, carbon disulfide is a material with good warning properties. It evaporates at room temperature, and its vapor is 2.6 times heavier than air; it may form explosive mixtures in a range of 1–50% by volume in air.

### Use

Carbon disulfide is used in the manufacture of rayon, cellophane, carbon tetrachloride, and rubber chemicals and as a grain fumigant. Annual US production exceeds 300 million lb. NIOSH estimates that over 45,000 workers are potentially exposed to carbon disulfide.

### Occupational & Environmental Exposure

In the production of viscose rayon, carbon disulfide is added to alkali cellulose to yield sodium cellulose xanthate. The latter is dissolved in caustic soda to yield viscose syrup, which can be spun to form textile yarn, tire yarn, or staple fiber or cast to form cellophane. Exposure to high concentrations of carbon disulfide can occur during the opening of sealed spinning machines and during cutting and drying.

### Metabolism & Mechanism of Action

Inhalation is the major route of absorption in occupational exposure, and 40–50% of carbon disulfide in inhaled air is retained in the body. Excretion of carbon disulfide by the lung accounts for 10–30% of absorbed dose, and less than 1% is excreted unchanged by the kidney. The remainder is excreted in the form of various metabolites in the urine.

Carbon disulfide is metabolized by formation of dithiocarbamates and reduced glutathione conjugates as well as by oxidative transformation. Thiourea, mercapturic acids, and the glutathione conjugate 2-thiothiazolidine-4-carboxylic acid (TTCA) can be detected in urine of exposed workers. Formation of dithiocarbamate may account in part for the nervous system toxicity of carbon disulfide, while oxidation yields carbonyl sulfide, a hepatotoxic metabolite. Carbon disulfide reacts with protein amino functions to form adducts of dithiocarbamate, which then undergo oxidation or decomposition to an electrophile, which reacts with protein nucleophiles to result in protein cross-linking. Cross-linked neurofilaments may then accumulate within axonal swellings.

### Clinical Findings
#### A. Symptoms & Signs:
**1. Acute exposure–**Acute carbon disulfide intoxication was described in the 1920s from the viscose rayon industry, involving exposure to concentrations of hundreds or thousands parts per million. Signs and symptoms included extreme irritability, uncontrolled anger, rapid mood changes (including manic delirium and hallucinations) paranoid ideas, and suicidal tendencies.

Exposure to 4800 ppm of carbon disulfide for 30 minutes may cause rapid coma and death. High concentrations of vapor may cause irritation of the eyes, nose, and throat; liquid carbon disulfide may cause second- or third-degree burns.

**2. Chronic exposure–**Chronic effects of lower-level exposure to carbon disulfide include the following:

**a. Eye**–Viscose rayon workers have been reported to have a high incidence of eye irritation. A high incidence of retinal microaneurysms and delayed fundal peripapillary filling by fluorescein angiography has been reported in Japanese and Yugoslavian workers exposed to carbon disulfide. Finnish studies have not confirmed these findings, and whether eye damage occurs below 20 ppm (8-hour TWA) is still unknown.

**b. Ear**–High-frequency hearing loss and vestibular symptoms of vertigo and nystagmus may occur.

**c. Heart**–Epidemiologic studies indicate that workers exposed to carbon disulfide are at increased risk for cardiovascular disease mortality. A correlation has been found between blood pressure or lipoprotein levels and exposure to carbon disulfide.

**d. Nervous system**–Studies have shown neurobehavioral changes in psychomotor speed, motor coordination, and personality in workers exposed to low concentrations (5–30 ppm) of carbon disulfide. There is a reduction in peripheral nerve conduction upon exposure to less than 10 ppm, although clinical symptoms of polyneuropathy are not present. Distal latency, motor nerve conduction velocity, and sensory amplitude were found to be sensitive indicators of polyneuropathy in viscose rayon workers exposed to carbon disulfide. Lower levels of exposure have been correlated with decreased slow fiber conduction velocity with prolongation of the refractory period of the peroneal nerve. Impaired motor and sensory nerve conduction has been demonstrated in prospective studies of workers exposed to carbon disulfide near the TLV. Extrapyramidal symptoms with atypical parkinsonism and cerebellar signs have been reported.

**e. Reproductive effects**–Carbon disulfide exposure was associated with a significant effect on libido and potency but not on fertility or semen quality. Women exposed to concentrations of less than 10 ppm may have an increased rate of menstrual abnormalities, spontaneous abortions, and premature births.

**B. Laboratory Findings:** Nonspecific elevations of liver enzymes and creatinine have been reported in acute intoxication. With chronic exposure, peripheral nerve conduction velocity can be decreased and neurobehavioral testing may show abnormalities in psychomotor skills and measures of personality function.

Urinary metabolites that catalyze the reaction of iodine with sodium azide can be used to detect exposure above 16 ppm (iodine-azide reaction). The concentration of end-of-shift urinary TTCA is related to exposure and can detect uptake as low as 10 ppm over the whole working shift. The ACGIH BEI is 5 mg of 2-TTCA per g of creatinine in urine at the end

of a shift. Heavy physical work and greater skin contact are correlated with higher TTCA levels.

## Differential Diagnosis

Cardiac disease from carbon disulfide intoxication must be differentiated from atherosclerotic heart disease due to other causes. Peripheral polyneuropathy should be distinguished from that due to alcohol, drugs, diabetes, and other toxic agents. Neuropsychiatric symptoms may be due to depression, posttraumatic stress syndrome, or other toxic exposures such as organic solvents.

## Prevention

**A. Work Practices:** Control of exposure must rely largely on engineering controls, with enclosure of processes and machines and proper use of ventilation systems. Operator rotation and respiratory protection during peak exposures should be implemented. Potential sources of ignition are prohibited in areas where carbon disulfide is stored or handled, and the substance must not be allowed to accumulate to concentrations higher than 0.1%. Impervious clothing, gloves, and face shields should be worn to prevent skin contact.

**B. Medical Surveillance:** Initial medical examination should include the central and peripheral nervous system, eyes, and cardiovascular system. Visual acuity should be measured and a baseline electrocardiogram obtained. Periodic medical surveillance to detect early signs or symptoms of toxicity should include questions regarding cardiac, nervous system, and reproductive function, with evaluation of blood pressure, peripheral nerve function, and mental status. Neurobehavioral testing, exercise electrocardiography, and nerve conduction velocity testing may be indicated. Measurement of finger tremor frequencies may provide an early indication of chronic carbon disulfide intoxication. Single photon emission computed tomography (SPECT) scans have not been of diagnostic value in workers with neurobehavioral effects from carbon disulfide exposure.

Measurement of TTCA in urine collected at the end of the workshift following the first workday is the test of choice for biological monitoring. Five milligrams per gram of creatinine corresponds to an 8-hour exposure (TWA) to the current TLV. The widely used iodine-azide test is insensitive at carbon disulfide levels of less than 16.7 ppm.

The presence of preexisting neurologic, psychiatric, or cardiac disease should be considered relative contraindications for individual exposure.

## Treatment

Skin and eye contact with carbon disulfide should be treated immediately by washing with large amounts of water, and all contaminated clothing should be removed. No specific treatment is available for chronic carbon disulfide toxicity.

## CHLOROMETHYL ETHERS

### Essentials of Diagnosis

*Acute effects:*
- Respiratory irritation.
- Skin rash.

*Chronic effects:*
- Lung cancer.

### Exposure Limits

ACGIH TLV: 0.001 ppm TWA
OSHA PEL: Stringent workplace controls
NIOSH REL: Reduce exposure to lowest feasible
    concentration

### General Considerations

The haloethers bis(chloromethyl) ether (BCME) and chloromethyl methyl ether (CMME) are highly volatile colorless liquids at room temperature, miscible with many organic solvents. The haloethers are alkylating agents, which are highly reactive in vivo. Technical grade CMME contains 1–8% BCME as an impurity.

### Use

BCME is formed when formaldehyde reacts with chloride ions in an acidic medium. It has been used in the past primarily for chloromethylations (eg, in the preparation of ion exchange resins), where a polystyrene resin is chloromethylated and then treated with an amine.

### Occupational & Environmental Exposure

Occupational exposure to the chloromethyl ethers occurs in anion exchange resin production. Since 1948, approximately 2000 workers have been exposed to BCME in ion exchange resin manufacture where exposure levels ranged from 10 to 100 ppb. Currently, exposure to BCME in the manufacture of ion exchange resins is limited to one plant in the United States. NIOSH estimates that only a few US workers are potentially exposed to BCME.

BCME may also be a potential hazard in the textile industry, where formaldehyde-containing reactants and resins are used in fabric finishing and as adhesives in laminating and flocking fabrics. Thermosetting emulsion polymers containing methylacrylamide as binders may liberate formaldehyde on drying and curing and then form BCME in the presence of available chloride. A NIOSH study of textile finishing plants found from 0.4 ppb to 8 ppb BCME

in the workroom air. This led to the use of low-formaldehyde resins and chloride-free catalysts.

### Clinical Findings

**A. Symptoms & Signs:**

**1. Acute exposure**–The chloromethyl ethers are potent skin and respiratory irritants. There are no reported cases of acute overexposure to either BCME or CMME.

**2. Chronic exposure**–Both BCME and CMME are carcinogenic and mutagenic in animal and cellular test systems. When rats are exposed to 0.1 ppm of BCME by inhalation for 6 hours a day, 5 days a week, for a total of 101 exposures, a high incidence of esthesioneuroblastomas and squamous cell carcinoma of the respiratory tract is observed. Both BCME and CMME produce skin papillomas and squamous tumors on direct application or subcutaneous injection. In humans, an excess of lung cancer has been suspected since 1962. An industry-wide survey of plants using chloromethyl ethers has documented a strikingly increased risk of lung cancer in exposed workers. Over 60 cases of BCME-associated lung cancer have been identified, with oat cell the principal histologic type. The historical average timeweighted exposure in these cases has been estimated to be between 10 and 100 ppm, and the latency period between exposure and lung cancer ranges from 5 to 25 years. An increasing incidence is observed with intensity and length of exposure. In addition, the risk of lung cancer is increased in smokers versus nonsmokers. The mortality rate from respiratory tract cancer is significantly (almost 3 times) higher among chlormethyl ether-exposed workers, with a latency of 10–19 years. The risk of cancer among exposed workers declines after 20 years from first exposure.

NIOSH recommends that BCME be regulated as a potential human carcinogen. IARC considers BCME carcinogenic to humans (Group 1A).

**B. Laboratory Findings:** The lung carcinoma associated with BCME and CMME presents in similar fashion to nonoccupationally associated carcinoma. Chest radiography may show a mass that should lead to appropriate diagnostic testing. Alternatively, sputum cytology may be abnormal in the presence of a normal chest x-ray and thus may be useful as a screening technique in individual cases. Sputum cytology may be of some value in the follow-up of workers exposed to known carcinogens who remain at risk for many years following exposure.

### Differential Diagnosis

Known occupational lung carcinogens include asbestos, arsenic, chromium, and uranium, and so a careful occupational history should be obtained from an individual who presents with lung carcinoma.

## Prevention

**A. Work Practices:** Enclosed chemical processes are essential to reduce exposure below 1 ppb, and continuous monitoring has been utilized successfully to warn of excessive exposures to BCME and CMME. As the number of potentially exposed workers has markedly declined since the 1970s, medical follow-up of past exposed workers has assumed a greater role.

**B. Medical Surveillance:** Preplacement and annual lung examination should be included in medical surveillance of exposed workers. Periodic sputum cytology may be of value in detecting early lung cancer.

## Treatment

The treatment of lung carcinoma associated with BCME/CMME exposure does not differ from that of nonoccupational cases.

## DIBROMOCHLOROPROPANE

### Essentials of Diagnosis

*Acute effects:*

- Oligospermia, azoospermia.

### Exposure Limits

OSHA PEL: 1 ppb TWA
NIOSH REL: Reduce exposure to lowest feasible concentration

### General Considerations

Dibromochloropropane is a brominated organochlorine nematocide which was used extensively since the 1950s on citrus fruits, grapes, peaches, pineapples, soybeans, and tomatoes. Millions of pounds were produced in the United States. In 1977, employees at a California pesticide formulation plant were found to be infertile, and further investigation documented azoospermia and oligospermia among workers exposed to dibromochloropropane. In DBCP-exposed men with both azoospermia and elevation in FSH level, follow-up evaluation has generally shown permanent destruction of germinal epithelium. In the United States, its use is restricted to a soil fumigant against plant-parasitic nematodes in pineapples. NIOSH estimates that approximately 175 workers are potentially exposed to DBCP.

A 17-year follow-up of DBCP-exposed workers found sperm count recovery at 36–45 months in three of nine azoospermic and three of six oligozoospermic men, with no improvement thereafter. A significant increase in plasma levels of follicle-stimulating hormone and luteinizing hormone was found in the most severely affected workers, with incomplete recovery of sperm count and motility.

No correlation has been found between DBCP contamination in drinking water and mortality rates from leukemia or gastric cancer. NIOSH recommends that DBCP be regulated as a potential human carcinogen. IARC finds that there is sufficient evidence of carcinogenicity in animals (Group 2B). Birth outcomes (low birth weight and birth defects) did not differ among DBCP-exposed workers or community residents exposed to DBCP-contaminated drinking water.

## DIMETHYLAMINOPROPIONITRILE

Dimethylaminopropionitrile was a component of catalysts used in manufacture of flexible polyurethane foams. In 1978, NIOSH reported urinary dysfunction and neurologic symptoms among workers at facilities which used dimethylaminopropionitrile. Workers at polyurethane manufacturing plants developed neurogenic bladder dysfunction after the introduction of a catalyst containing dimethylaminopropionitrile. Workers had urinary retention, hesitancy, and dribbling. Examination showed a pattern of decreased sensation confined to the lower sacral dermatomes, abnormal retention of contrast material on intravenous pyelogram, or abnormal cystometrograms. Nerve conduction velocity studies were normal. Symptoms of persistent sexual dysfunction were found 2 years after the original epidemic, and one worker had residual sensorimotor neuropathy. Following these findings, production of catalysts containing dimethylaminopropionitrile was voluntarily discontinued.

Dimethylaminopropionitrile appears to be a unique example of a neurotoxin that produces localized autonomic dysfunction without peripheral nervous system damage. Urotoxic effects may be related to metabolism via a cytochrome P-450-dependent mixed-function oxidase system, with formation of reactive-intermediate metabolites that interfere with axoplasmic transport. The discovery of this toxicity by an alert clinician underscores the role of the community practitioner in the discovery of new occupational diseases.

## ETHYLENE OXIDE

### Essentials of Diagnosis

*Acute effects:*

- Respiratory tract irritation.
- Skin rash.
- Headache, drowsiness, weakness.

*Chronic effects:*

- Increased sister chromatid exchanges in lymphocytes.
- Possible increased risk of cancer.

## Exposure Limits

ACGIH TLV: 1 ppm TWA

OSHA PEL: 1 ppm TWA, 5 ppm excursion limit (15 minutes)

NIOSH REL: Less than 0.1 ppm TWA, 5 ppm ceiling (10 min/d)

## General Considerations

Ethylene oxide is a colorless flammable gas with a characteristic etherlike odor. At elevated pressures, it may be a volatile liquid. It is completely miscible with water and many organic solvents. The threshold of detection in humans is about 700 ppm but is quite variable, and smell cannot be relied on to warn of overexposure. To reduce the explosive hazard of ethylene oxide used as a fumigant or sterilant, it is often mixed with carbon dioxide or halocarbons (15% ethylene oxide and 85% dichlorofluoromethane).

## Use

Ethylene oxide is used in the manufacture of ethylene glycol (used for antifreeze and as an intermediate for polyester fibers, films, and bottles), nonionic surface-active agents (used for home laundry detergents and dishwashing formulations), glycol ethers (used for surface coatings), and ethanolamines (for soaps, detergents, and textile chemicals). It is used as a pesticide fumigant and as a sterilant in hospitals, medical products manufacture, libraries, museums, beekeeping, spice and seasoning fumigation, animal and plant quarantine, transportation vehicle fumigation, and dairy packaging. Annual US production exceeds 6.7 billion lb. NIOSH estimates that over 270,000 workers are potentially exposed to ethylene oxide.

## Occupational & Environmental Exposure

Most ethylene oxide is used as a chemical intermediate in plants where closed and automated processes generally maintain exposure levels below 1 ppm. The greatest potential for worker exposure occurs during loading or unloading of transport tanks, product sampling, and equipment maintenance and repair.

Although only about 0.02% of production is used for sterilization in hospitals, NIOSH estimates that 75,000 health care workers have potential exposure to ethylene oxide. Approximately 10,000 ethylene oxide sterilization units are in use in 8100 hospitals in the United States. Field surveys of hospital gas sterilizers have generally found that 8-hour time-weighted average exposures to ethylene oxide are below 1 ppm. However, occupational exposure may be several hundred parts per million for brief periods during the opening of the sterilizer door, in the transfer of freshly sterilized items to the aeration cabinet or central supply area, during tank changes, and at the gas discharge point.

## Metabolism & Mechanism of Action

Ethylene oxide is absorbed through the skin and respiratory tract. It is an alkylating agent that binds to DNA and may cause cellular mutation.

## Clinical Findings

### A. Symptoms & Signs:

**1. Acute exposure**–Ethylene oxide is irritating to the eyes, respiratory tract, and skin, and at high concentrations it can cause respiratory depression. Symptoms of upper respiratory tract irritation occur at between 200 and 400 ppm, and above 1000 ppm ethylene oxide may cause headache, nausea, dyspnea, vomiting, drowsiness, weakness, and incoordination. Direct contact of the skin or eyes with liquid ethylene oxide can result in severe irritation, burns, or contact dermatitis.

**2. Chronic exposure–**

**a. Reproductive effects**–Ethylene oxide is toxic to reproductive function in both male and female experimental animals. In humans, a retrospective study of reproductive function in Finnish hospital sterilizing staff has shown a higher rate of spontaneous abortions in women exposed to ethylene oxide.

**b. Carcinogenic effects**–Chronic inhalation bioassays in rats have shown that ethylene oxide results in a dose-related increase in mononuclear cell leukemia, peritoneal mesothelioma, and cerebral glioma. Intragastric administration of ethylene oxide in rats produces a dose-dependent increase of squamous cell carcinomas of the forestomach. IARC considers ethylene oxide to be carcinogenic to humans (Group 1). Studies have shown a dose-related increase in chromosonal aberrations and sister chromatid exchange in lymphocytes and micronuclei in bone marrow cells of exposed workers; cancers of the lymphatic and hematopoietic systems in humans and experimental animals; a dose-related increase in the level of hemoglobin adducts; and gene mutations and heritable translocations in germ cells of animals. NIOSH recommends that ethylene oxide be treated as a potential human carcinogen.

Retrospective cohort mortality studies have suggested an excess of lymphatic hematopoietic cancers in ethylene oxide-exposed workers.

Based on the animal and human data regarding carcinogenicity, NIOSH lowered the 8-hour TWA to below 0.1 ppm. As exposure of hospital personnel are generally short-term peak exposures, NIOSH recommends a short-term exposure limit of 5 ppm as well.

**c. Neurologic toxicity**–Impairment of sensory and motor function has been observed in animals exposed to 357 ppm ethylene oxide over 48–85 days, and four cases of peripheral neuropathy were described among workers exposed to a leaking sterilizing chamber for 2–8 weeks. Neurotoxicity has been reported following chronic ethylene oxide exposure, including neuropsychological abnormalities, lower P300 amplitude, and peripheral neuropathy.

**d. Other**–Occupational asthma has also been reported following acute exposure.

**B. Laboratory Findings:** No specific finding is characteristic of ethylene oxide exposure. Lymphocytosis has been noted after acute exposure. Where inhalation results in respiratory symptoms, the chest radiograph may show interstitial or frank alveolar edema. Where suspect, a complete blood count may be helpful in the diagnosis of leukemia. Cytogenetic analysis (ie, sister chromatid exchange) of peripheral lymphocytes cannot be used in individual cases to quantitate exposure or estimate cancer risk.

### Differential Diagnosis

The mixture of chlorofluorocarbons found in sterilant cylinders may also produce upper respiratory symptoms on inhalation exposure. Many other genotoxicants, including cigarette smoke and other alkylating agents, may cause an increase in sister chromatid exchanges and chromosomal aberrations, so these findings cannot be specifically linked to ethylene oxide unless these causes are excluded.

### Prevention

**A. Work Practices:** Proper engineering controls are essential that reduce short-term exposures to hospital sterilizer staff during procedures where ethylene oxide levels have been found to be greatest. An NIOSH survey has found that engineering controls are extremely effective in hospitals in reducing ethylene oxide exposure during sterilization. These include effective sterilization chamber ethylene oxide purging, local exhaust ventilation at the sterilizer door, adequate ventilation of floor drains, efficient handling of product carts from sterilizer to aerator, and installation of ethylene oxide tanks in ventilated cabinets. Self-contained breathing apparatus or airline respirators are the only respirators acceptable for ethylene oxide and must be worn when concentrations of ethylene oxide are unknown, as when entering walk-in chambers or for emergency response.

**B. Medical Surveillance:** Preplacement and periodic examinations should include attention to the pulmonary, hematologic, neurologic, and reproductive systems. A white blood cell count should be obtained at least initially and at periodic intervals if exposure to ethylene oxide is over 0.5 ppm 8-hour TWA or if intermittent exposures exceed 5 ppm. Cytogenetic monitoring has been used by industries willing to maintain exposures below those causing any observable increase above preexposure baseline levels.

A significant decrease in hematocrit and hemoglobin level, an increase in lymphocyte percentages, and a relative decrease in neutrophil percentages have been seen in ethylene oxide-exposed female hospital workers in the United States. Other studies have not demonstrated the utility of the complete blood count as a screening test for medical surveillance of ethylene-oxide exposed hospital workers. Biological monitoring studies of ethylene oxide-exposed workers show an increase in chromosomal aberrations, sister chromatid exchanges, micronuclei, and hemoglobin adducts. Personnel trained in emergency response for use of self-contained breathing apparatus should be evaluated for cardiorespiratory fitness with pulmonary function or exercise testing.

### Treatment

Removal from the work environment after inhalation of the gas should be immediate. If respiratory symptoms are evident, oxygen should be administered and the victim brought to the emergency ward. Any contaminated clothing should be immediately removed and, where appropriate, the skin thoroughly washed with soap and water. A chest radiograph should be obtained if warranted by respiratory symptoms, and the patient should be observed for several hours for the onset of pulmonary edema. No other specific treatment is indicated.

## FORMALDEHYDE

### Essentials of Diagnosis

*Acute effects:*
- Eye irritation causing lacrimation, redness, and pain.
- Cough, chest tightness, shortness of breath.
- Skin irritation, contact dermatitis.

*Chronic effects:*
- Bronchitis, exacerbation of asthma.

### Exposure Limits

ACGIH TLV: 1 ppm TWA, 2 ppm STEL
OSHA PEL: 1 ppm TWA, 2 ppm STEL
NIOSH REL: 0.016 ppm TWA, 0.1 ppm ceiling
(15 minutes)

### General Considerations

Formaldehyde is a colorless, flammable gas with a pungent, irritating odor. Known to physicians as a tissue preservative and disinfectant, formaldehyde is a basic feedstock of the modern chemical industry. It may also be encountered as formalin (37–50% formaldehyde), methyl aldehyde, methanal (methanol-formaldehyde mixture), methylene glycol, paraform, or paraformaldehyde (a linear copolymer of formaldehyde).

### Use

The largest use for formaldehyde is the manufacture of urea-formaldehyde and amino and phenolic resins and as an intermediate in the manufacture of ethylene-diaminetetraacetic acid, methylene dianiline, hexamethylenetetramine, and nitriloacetic acid. Other important uses include wood industry products, molding compounds, foundry resins, adhesives for insulation, slow-release fertilizers, manufacture of permanent-press finishes of cellulose fabrics, and formaldehyde-based textile finishes. Total annual US production exceeds 7.9 billion lb. It is a byproduct of the incomplete combustion of hydrocarbons and is found in small amounts in automobile exhaust and cigarette smoke. NIOSH estimates that over 1.3 million workers are potentially exposed to formaldehyde.

## Occupational & Environmental Exposure

Occupational exposure to formaldehyde above 1 ppm occurs in the production of formaldehyde resin and plastics and in the manufacture of apparel, plywood particle board and wood furniture, paper, and paperboard; workers at risk include ureaformaldehyde foam insulation dealers and installers, mushroom farmers, embalmers, and laboratory workers. NIOSH industrial hygiene surveys have found formaldehyde levels up to 8 ppm in hospital autopsy rooms and up to 2.7 ppm in gross anatomy laboratories. Embalmers report more frequent symptoms of respiratory irritation with exposures during embalming exceeding permissible limits. Formaldehyde exposures in gross anatomy dissection may exceed exposure limits, causing significantly increased upper respiratory symptoms and decrements in airflow during exposure. Several studies have shown respiratory irritation from exposure to formaldehyde and wood dust. Wildland firefighters may be exposed to formaldehyde as a result of vegetation combustion.

Residential exposure to formaldehyde up to several parts per million occurs from urea-formaldehyde foam insulation (UFFI) and particle board in mobile homes. Levels of formaldehyde are highest in new residences and decline with a half-life of 4–5 years for mobile homes and less than 1 year for UFFI homes. Mean levels for mobile homes are about 0.5 ppm and for UFFI homes about 0.1 ppm. Diurnal and seasonal variations in exposure levels may occur. Respiratory irritant effects are significantly associated with formaldehyde exposure in mobile homes. Residents of homes insulated with urea-formaldehyde foam had a higher prevalence of respiratory symptoms than did residents of control homes but had no demonstrated changes in various hematologic or immunologic parameters.

## Metabolism & Mechanism of Action

Formaldehyde is formed intracellularly as $N^5,N^{10}$-methylenetetrahydrofolic acid, an important metabolic intermediate. Exogenous formaldehyde can be absorbed by inhalation, ingestion, or dermal absorption. Over 95% of an inhaled dose is absorbed and rapidly metabolized to formic acid by formaldehyde

dehydrogenase. Formaldehyde disappears from plasma with a half-life of 1–1.5 minutes, so that an increase cannot be detected immediately following inhalation exposure to high concentrations. Most formaldehyde is converted to $CO_2$ via formate, and a small fraction is excreted in the urine as formate and other metabolites.

Formaldehyde interacts with macromolecules such as DNA, RNA, and protein. This probably accounts for its carcinogenic effect.

## Clinical Findings

### A. Symptoms & Signs:

**1. Acute exposure**–Formaldehyde vapor exposure causes direct irritation of the skin and respiratory tract. Both direct irritation (eczematous reaction) and allergic contact dermatitis (type IV delayed hypersensitivity) occur. After a few days of exposure to formaldehyde solutions or formaldehyde-containing resins, the individual may develop a sudden urticarial eczematous reaction of the skin of the eyelids, face, neck, and flexor surfaces of the arms. Allergic contact dermatitis may occur from exposure to cosmetics and personal-care products, dishwashing liquids, water-based paints, or photographic products. There appears to be no relationship between cutaneous disease from formaldehyde and personal or family history of atopy.

Direct irritation of the eyes, nose, and throat occurs among most people exposed to 0.1–3 ppm of formaldehyde vapor. The odor threshold is 0.05–1 ppm, and some individuals may therefore note irritation of the upper respiratory tract at or just above the odor threshold. Shortness of breath, cough, and chest tightness occur at 10–20 ppm. Exposure to 50–100 ppm and above can cause pulmonary edema, pneumonitis, or death. Irritant symptoms due to formaldehyde exposure do not elicit a significant immunologic response with elevated levels of IgE or IgG antibody to formaldehyde-human serum albumin.

### 2. Chronic exposure–

**a. Cancer**–Squamous cell carcinomas of the nasal epithelium were induced in rats and mice exposed for prolonged periods (up to 2 years). Biochemical and physiologic studies in rats have shown that inhaled formaldehyde can depress respiration, inhibit mucociliary clearance, stimulate cell proliferation, and cross-link DNA and protein in the nasal mucosa.

Some epidemiologic studies have suggested that occupational exposure to formaldehyde may increase the risk for lung cancer (particularly among hourly workers with higher levels of cumulative exposure), whereas other studies have found no association between formaldehyde exposure and deaths from malignant respiratory disease. Inconsistent results have been observed in studies of nasopharyngeal cancer and exposure to formaldehyde, but a recent meta-analysis suggests an increased risk for nasopharyngeal cancer with high levels of exposure. Three cases of malignant melanoma of the nasal mucosa have been reported in persons occupationally exposed to formaldehyde. IARC has found sufficient evidence in animals, but not humans, for the carcinogenicity of formaldehyde (Group 2A). NIOSH recommends that formaldehyde be regulated as a potential human carcinogen.

**b. Occupational asthma** has been reported as a result of formaldehyde resin dust, with studies reporting workers with asthma and positive specific bronchial challenge to formaldehyde. One patient with formaldehyde-induced asthma had positive IgE and IgG titers to formaldehyde-human serum albumin and positive cutaneous reactivity but negative methacholine and specific challenge test. A study of medical students exposed to formaldehyde (including those with asthma) reported no changes in symptoms or lung function over a 7-month period. No significant changes in lung function or bronchial reactivity have been seen in normal subjects or asthmatics exposed to test concentrations of formaldehyde. Workers exposed to formaldehyde have significantly greater cross-shift reduction in forced expiratory volume in 1 second and significantly more lower respiratory symptoms than do unexposed controls. However, the rate of decline of lung function in formaldehyde-exposed workers is not greater than expected.

Chronic formaldehyde exposure has been linked anecdotally to a variety of neuropsychologic problems, but there is no evidence to substantiate these reports.

Spontaneous abortions in cosmetologists and laboratory workers have been significantly associated with the use of formaldehyde-based disinfectants and formalin, respectively.

**B. Laboratory Findings:**

**1. Liver and kidney–**Routine tests of hepatic and renal function are generally unremarkable. Measurement of formic acid in the urine is generally not helpful due to the short half-life of formaldehyde.

**2. Skin–**If contact dermatitis is suspected, patch testing should be performed with appropriate concentrations of formaldehyde.

**3. Respiratory system–**Cough, shortness of breath, or wheezing may be associated with decreased forced expiratory volume in 1 second ($FEV_1$) by pulmonary function testing. Peak flow recordings while at work may show a decrease in maximal airflow during or after exposure to formaldehyde. After exposure to over 20–30 ppm of formaldehyde, chest x-rays may show interstitial or alveolar edema, with resultant reduction in arterial oxygen content on blood gas analysis.

### Differential Diagnosis

Numerous workplace gases and vapors may produce symptoms of upper respiratory tract irritation. Symptoms of eye and throat irritation among office workers may be due to inadequate ventilation, cigarette smoke, or glues and solvents emitted from newly installed synthetic materials. Correlation of symptoms with measured levels of formaldehyde in indoor environments may be difficult.

### Prevention

**A. Work Practices:** Safety goggles or a full-length plastic face mask should be worn where splashing is possible. At air concentrations above the permissible exposure limit, a full facepiece respirator with organic vapor cartridge is required. Protective neoprene clothing and boots and gloves impervious to formaldehyde should be worn to prevent skin contact.

**B. Medical Surveillance:** Biologic monitoring using urinary formate concentration is not useful with the possible exception of populations where ambient formaldehyde concentrations are greater than 1 ppm. A preplacement history of asthma or allergy should be obtained, along with a baseline $FEV_1$ and forced vital capacity (FVC).

Low-level exposure to formaldehyde during embalming is associated with cytogenetic changes in epithelial cells of the mouth and in blood lymphocytes. These cytogenetic effects may be useful markers in biological monitoring of formaldehyde-exposed workers. Various pathologic changes have been observed in the nasal mucosa of formaldehyde-exposed workers, including ciliary loss, goblet cell hyperplasia, squamous metaplasia, and mild dysplasia.

### Treatment

In case of eye and skin contact, immediately flush the contaminated area with water for 15 minutes and remove any contaminated clothing. Immediate removal to fresh air is required for inhalation exposure, with administration of oxygen for shortness of breath or hypoxemia. For formaldehyde exposure exceeding 20–30 ppm, emergency department observation with periodic evaluation of respiratory status is necessary for 6–8 hours.

## NITRATES: NITROGLYCERIN & ETHYLENE GLYCOL DINITRATE

### Essentials of Diagnosis

*Acute effects:*
- Headache.
- Angina.
- Fall in blood pressure.

*Chronic effects:*
- Sudden death.
- Increased incidence of ischemic heart disease.

### Exposure Limits

Nitroglycerin
ACGIH TLV: 0.05 ppm TWA

OSHA PEL: 0.2 ppm ceiling
NIOSH REL: 0.1 mg/m$^3$ ceiling (20 minutes)
Ethylene glycol dinitrate
ACGIH TLV: 0.05 ppm TWA
OSHA PEL: 1 mg/m$^3$ ceiling
NIOSH REL: 0.1 mg/m$^3$ ceiling (20 minutes)

## General Considerations

Nitroglycerin (glyceryl trinitrate, trinitropropanetriol) and ethylene glycol dinitrate (dinitroethanediol) are liquid nitric acid esters of monohydric and polyhydric aliphatic alcohols. Those of the tetrahydric alcohols (erythritol tetranitrate, pentaerythritol tetranitrate) and the hexahydric alcohol (mannitol hexanitrate) are solids. They are less stable than aromatic nitro compounds.

Nitroglycerin is readily soluble in many organic solvents and acts as a solvent for many explosive ingredients, including ethylene glycol dinitrate. It is an oily liquid at room temperature with a slightly sweet odor. The sensitivity of nitroglycerin decreases with decreasing temperature, so ethylene glycol dinitrate may be added to nitroglycerin-bearing dynamites to depress the freezing point. Explosions of nitroglycerin may occur when the liquid is heated or when frozen nitroglycerin is thawed.

Ethylene glycol dinitrate is an oily colorless liquid that is more stable and less likely than nitroglycerin to explode when it burns.

## Use, Production, & Occupational Exposure

Alfred Nobel first used a mixture of nitroglycerin with diatomaceous earth and later a more stable mixture of nitroglycerin, sodium nitrate, and wood pulp to form dynamite. The major application of nitroglycerin is in explosives and blasting gels, as in low-freezing dynamite in mixture with ethylene glycol dinitrate. Other explosive uses are in cordite in mixture with nitrocellulose and petroleum and in blasting gelatin with 7% nitrocellulose. Nitroglycerin also has medical therapeutic applications for the treatment of angina.

Nitroglycerin may be manufactured by a process in which glycerin is added to a mixture of nitric and sulfuric acids. Dynamite is formed by adding "dope," or mixtures of sodium nitrate, sulfur, antacids, and nitrocellulose. Ethylene glycol dinitrate is made by nitration of ethylene glycol with mixed acid.

Occupational exposures to nitroglycerin and ethylene glycol dinitrate can occur during their manufacture and during the manufacture and handling of explosives, munitions, and pharmaceuticals. Skin absorption for both nitroglycerin and ethylene glycol dinitrate has not been quantitated but is generally greater than respiratory absorption. Air sampling in dynamite plants where both nitroglycerin and ethylene glycol dinitrate are manufactured and used to produce explosives have shown that short-term

higher exposures (in the range of 2 mg/m$^3$ of ethylene glycol dinitrate) occur among mixers, cartridge fillers, and cleanup or maintenance workers. NIOSH estimates that over 38,000 workers are potentially exposed to nitroglycerin.

## Metabolism & Mechanism of Action

Both nitroglycerin and ethylene glycol dinitrate pass readily through the skin. Although there is an excellent correlation of blood nitrate ester levels with airborne exposures, skin absorption is more significant. Both nitroglycerin and ethylene glycol dinitrate are hydrolyzed to inorganic nitrates. The biological half-life of both nitroglycerin and ethylene glycol dinitrate is about 30 minutes. Both act directly on arteriolar and venous smooth muscle, causing vasodilation within minutes with a consequent drop in blood pressure and an increase in regional myocardial blood flow. The headache associated with nitrate esters is secondary to cerebral vessel distention.

The tolerance that develops after 2–4 days of continuous exposure appears to be due to an increased sympathetic compensatory mechanism.

The pathogenesis of sudden death due to nitroglycerin and ethylene glycol dinitrate has been postulated to be a rebound vasoconstriction resulting in acute hypertension or myocardial ischemia. NIOSH has recommended that workplace exposure to nitroglycerin and ethylene glycol dinitrate be controlled so that workers are not exposed at concentrations that will cause vasodilation, as indicated by the development of throbbing headaches or decreases in blood pressure. At this exposure level, workers should be protected against work-related angina pectoris, other signs or symptoms of ischemia or cardiac damage, and sudden death.

## General Considerations
### A. Symptoms & Signs:
**1. Acute exposure**–Symptoms of acute illness include loss of consciousness, severe headache, difficulty in breathing, weak pulse, and pallor. Tolerance to these effects develops in dynamite production workers after 1 week of exposure, but symptoms recur upon return to work after an absence of 2 days or more. The headache associated with nitroglycerin ("powder headache") frequently begins in the forehead and moves to the occipital region, where it can remain for hours or days. Associated symptoms include depression, restlessness, and sleeplessness. Alcohol ingestion may worsen the headache.

An acute drop in mean blood pressure of 10 mg Hg systolic and 6 mg Hg diastolic occurs on return to work after 2–3 days off. Mean blood pressure measurements increase over the week as compensatory mechanisms develop.

Blood pressure reduction has been noted after exposure to 0.5 mg/m$^3$ for 25 minutes, and some workers develop headaches after inhalation exposure of more than 0.1 mg/m$^3$. Both irritant and allergic contact dermatitis due to nitroglycerin have been reported.

**2. Chronic exposure**–Angina pectoris and sudden death have been described among dynamite workers handling nitroglycerin and ethylene glycol dinitrate. In affected workers, the angina usually occurs on the weekend or early in the work shift following periods away from work. The angina is relieved by reexposure to nitroglycerin or ethylene glycol dinitrate in contaminated clothes or by taking nitroglycerin sublingually. Sudden deaths without premonitory angina have also been recorded in dynamite workers. There is an excess risk of cardiac disease among nitroglycerin and ethylene glycol dinitrate workers.

Other reported chronic effects include symptoms of Raynaud's phenomenon and peripheral neuropathy. At high concentrations, the aliphatic nitrates may give rise to methemoglobinemia. A retrospective cohort mortality study of munitions workers exposed to niroglycerin and dinitrotoluene did not show a chronic effect on cardiovascular disease risk. Similarly, nitrate fertilizer workers have not shown an increased risk of cancer.

**B. Laboratory Findings:** Coronary angiography has shown normal coronary arteries in workers with angina, and atheromatous coronary vessels have not generally been found on autopsy of workers who died suddenly. The incidence of ectopy is not increased in dynamite workers, and electrocardiograms may be normal. Abnormalities in digital plethysmography show changes in the digital wave pulse with inhalation exposures of 0.12–0.41 mg/m$^3$.

### Differential Diagnosis

An increased incidence of cardiovascular disease has been found in carbon disulfide-exposed workers. Sudden cardiac death may occur after exposure to carbon monoxide or to hydrocarbon solvents.

### Prevention

**A. Work Practices:** Avoidance of headaches, blood pressure reduction, angina, or sudden death is best achieved by reduction of exposure through proper work practices. Control of exposure is best accomplished by closed systems, local ventilation, and the use of proper seals, joints, and access ports. The danger of detonation can be minimized by the use of nonsparking equipment, prevention of smoking and open flames, and other safety measures. Natural and synthetic rubber gloves will accelerate absorption of nitrate esters, so only cotton or cotton-lined gloves should be worn. Dermal contact with nitrates should be minimized, because this may be an important route of absorption.

**B. Medical Surveillance:** Preplacement and periodic examination should stress a history of cardiovascular disease and physical examination of cardiac abnormalities. A small experimental study in humans has shown that urinary N-methylnicotinamide may have potential as a biomarker for nitrate exposure, but further studies are necessary to determine its importance in the occupational setting. Methemoglobin is not sensitive for routine monitoring of exposure.

### Treatment

Treatment of cardiac symptoms due to nitrate ester exposure does not differ from that of symptoms of coronary insufficiency due to underlying coronary artery disease. Sublingual nitroglycerin should be used immediately for anginal symptoms. New onset angina or a change in anginal patterns should be evaluated by noninvasive cardiac imaging or angiography if indicated.

## NITROSAMINES

### Essentials of Diagnosis

*Acute effects:*
• Liver damage.

*Chronic effects:*
• Probable human carcinogen (selected).

### Exposure Limits

OSHA PEL: Stringent workplace controls
ACGIH TLV: Suspected human carcinogen
NIOSH REL: Reduce exposure to lowest feasible concentration

### General Considerations

N-Nitrosamines have the general structure shown below:

$$
\begin{array}{c}
R' \\
| \\
N - N = O \quad \text{Nitrosyl group} \\
| \\
R
\end{array}
$$

where R and R′ can be alkyl or aryl or aryl, eg, N-nitrosodimethylamine (NDMA), N-nitrosodiethylamine (NDEA), N-nitrosodiethanolamine (NDELA), and N-nitrosodiphenylamine (NDPhA). Derivatives of cyclic amines also occur, eg, N-nitrosomorpholine (NMOR) and N-nitrosopyrrolidine (NPyR). N-Nitrosamines are volatile solids or oils and are yellow because of their absorption of visible light by the N–N = O group.

Reactions of nitrosamines involve mainly the nitroso group and the C = H bonds adjacent to the amine nitrogen. Enzymatic reactions leading to the formation of carcinogenic metabolites is thought to occur at the alpha carbon.

NDMA        NDEA        NDELA

NDPhA        NMOR        NPyR

## Use, Production, & Exposure

Nitrosamines are formed by the reaction of a secondary or tertiary amine with nitrite ion in an acidic medium, according to the general equation shown below:

$$NH + NO_2^- \xrightarrow{H^+} N-N{=}O$$

Appreciation of the carcinogenicity of the nitrosamines has led to their characterization in many occupational and environmental circumstances. Humans may be exposed to nitrosamines in several ways: formation in the environment and subsequent absorption from food, water, air, or industrial and consumer products; formation in the body from precursors ingested separately in food, water, or air; from the consumption or smoking of tobacco; and from naturally occurring compounds.

The greatest exposure to the population as a whole occurs from cigarette smoking and the ingestion of nitrite-preserved meats.

## Occupational Exposure

NDMA was used in the United States until 1975 in the production of dimethylhydrazine, a rocket propellant. Exposures ranged up to 36 μg/m³. In surveys, a fish meal factory was found to contain NDMA at 0.06 μg/m³, a plant that manufactured surface-active agents contained NDMA at 0.8 μg/m³, a chrome tannery had NDMA at 47 μg/m³, and the rubber industry contained levels of NMOR as high as 248 μg/m³. NDMA and

NEMA have been found in foundries and leather tanneries. NDMA and NDEA have been detected in the workroom air of a rubber footwear plant.

NDMA has been used as an industrial solvent, antioxidant, and rubber accelerator. NIOSH estimates that approximately 750 workers are potentially exposed to NDMA. NDEA has been used as a gasoline and lubricant additive, antioxidant, and stabilizer. The major uses of NDPhA have been in the rubber industry as an antiscorching agent or vulcanization retarder. NDPhA reacts with other amines in the rubber to form N-nitrosamines. NIOSH estimates that over 1000 workers are potentially exposed to NDPhA. There is no commercial production of NMOR, NDELA, or NPyR.

Synthetic cutting fluids may contain up to 3% NDELA. Direct contact with cutting fluids and the presence of airborne mists provide the opportunity for ingestion or skin absorption.

Certain classes of pesticides have been found to contain identifiable N-nitroso contaminants formed during synthesis or as a result of interaction with nitrate fertilizers applied simultaneously to crops. EPA requires testing for nitrosamines of suspect formulation.

**A. Tobacco & Tobacco Smoke:** The largest nonoccupational exposure to preformed nitrosamines is derived from tobacco products and tobacco smoke, which may contain NDMA, NDEA, NPyR, and others. Nitrosamine content is greater in sidestream smoke and from cigars.

**B. Foods:** Low levels of nitrosamines occur in several types of food, including cheese, processed meats, beer, and cooked bacon.

**C. Cosmetics:** Many cosmetics, soaps and shampoos are contaminated with NDELA as a result of the nitrosation of triethanolamine by bactericides.

**D. In Vivo Nitrosation:** Nitrate can be reduced to nitrite in vitro and in human saliva in vivo. The reaction of ingested nitrites with amines will yield in vivo nitrosamines in the acidic medium of the stomach. Main contributors to gastric nitrite load are vegetables, cured meats, baked goods, cereals, fruits, and fruit juices.

## Metabolism & Mechanism of Action

The nitrosamines are rapidly metabolized after skin or gastrointestinal absorption, with a biological half-life for NDMA of several hours. NDMA is enzymatically demethylated to form monomethylnitrosamine, which then yields an unstable diazohydroxide. The carcinogenic action of the nitrosamines is attributed to this electrophilic species, which can covalently react with DNA.

## Clinical Findings
**A. Symptoms & Signs:**
**1. Acute exposure**–Two cases of industrial

poisoning due to NDMA were reported in 1937 in chemists producing an anticorrosion agent. They developed headaches, backache, abdominal cramps, nausea, anorexia, weakness, drowsiness, and dizziness; both workers developed ascites and jaundice, and one died with diffuse hepatic necrosis. Five family members who ingested lemonade accidentally contaminated with NDMA developed nausea, vomiting, and abdominal pain within a few hours, and two died 4 and 5 days later with generalized bleeding. Postmortem examination showed hepatic necrosis.

**2. Chronic exposure**–Liver cirrhosis has been reported following chronic exposure to NDMA.

About 85% of over 200 nitrosamines tested in animals have been found to be carcinogenic, inducing tumors of the respiratory tract, esophagus, kidney, stomach, liver, and brain. N-Nitrosodimethylamine, NDMA, NDEA, NDphA, NDELA, NPyR, and NMOR have been shown to be carcinogenic in many animal species and are transplacental carcinogens.

The tools of molecular epidemiology have been increasingly used to estimate cancer risks from occupational exposure. In one study, analyses of lung tissue have found higher levels of 7-methyl-dGMP (a metabolic product of N-nitrosamines) in association with specific genotypes. Genetic polymorphisms may be predictive of carcinogen adduct levels and may therefore predict the risk of cancer following carcinogen exposure. Studies of workers exposed to metalworking fluids (MWFs) indicate an association between MWF and stomach, pancreatic, laryngeal, and rectal cancer. Although it remains to be determined which specific constituents of MWFs are responsible for the increased risk of various cancers, N-nitrosamines are one of the suspect chemicals. IARC considers that NDEA and NDMA are probably carcinogenic to humans (Group 2A) and that NDELA, NMOR, and NPyR are possibly carcinogenic to humans (Group 2B). NIOSH recommends that NDMA be regulated as a potential human carcinogen.

Nitrates may be found in drinking water and have been associated in epidemiologic studies with a greater risk of gastric cancer. Case-control studies of gastric cancer and occupational exposures have suggested a slight increase in risk associated with exposure to nitrosamine.

**B. Laboratory Findings:** In the few fatalities reported, elevated liver enzymes consistent with hepatic necrosis were noted.

### Prevention

**A. Work Practices:** Nitrosamines should be handled in well-ventilated fume hoods. To minimize the potential for formation of nitrosamines, nitrate-containing materials should not be added to MWFs containing ethanolamines. Reduction of nitrosamine exposure in the rubber industry includes the avoidance of compounds that give rise to nitrosamines. Adequate engineering controls should be instituted

for working with raw polymers, elastomers, and rubber parts containing dialkylamine compounds that may emit nitrosamine when heated.

**B. Medical Surveillance:** Increased single-strand DNA breaks in peripheral mononuclear cells have been found in metalworkers exposed to NDELA in cutting fluids. Screening for mutagenicity of cutting fluids containing nitrite and NDELA has been suggested as a means to assess risk of hazardous exposure. Use of biological samples for nitrosamine exposure has not been adequately evaluated. No specific medical surveillance for nitrosamines is recommended.

### Treatment

There is no treatment for nitrosamine exposure.

## PENTACHLOROPHENOL

### Essentials of Diagnosis

*Acute effects:*
- Skin and respiratory tract irritation.
- Systemic collapse.

*Chronic effects:*
- Skin rash (chloracne secondary to chlorodibenzodioxin).

### Exposure Limits

ACGIH TLV: 0.5 mg/m$^3$ TWA
OSHA PEL: 0.5 mg/m$^3$ TWA
NIOSH REL: 0.5 mg/m$^3$ TWA

### General Considerations

Pentachlorophenol (PCP) is a crystalline solid with low water solubility and a characteristic pungent phenolic odor. Its commercial production proceeds readily by the direct chlorination of phenol in the presence of chlorine and a catalyst or by the alkaline hydrolysis of hexachlorobenzene; both processes result in 4–12% tetrachlorophenol and less than 0.1% of trichlorophenol in the final product. In addition, the required elevated temperatures to produce PCP result in the formation of condensation products, including the toxic dimers dibenzo-*p*-dioxin and dibenzofuran. Analyses of commercial PCP have reported ranges of chlorinated dioxins and furans from 0.03 to 2510 parts per million. Tetrachlorodibenzodioxin has been found in a commercial sample of PCP, but it was not the most toxic 2,3,7,8-isomer. Thus, evaluation of the health effects of PCP must be considered separately from those of its impurities.

### Use

PCP is used as a wood preservative, herbicide, defoliant, fungicide, and chemical intermediate in the production of pentachlorophenate. A 0.1% solution in mineral spirits, fuel oil, or kerosene is commonly applied as a wood preservative. PCP is used in pressure treatment of lumber at a 5% concentration. About 80% is used by the wood preserving industry to treat wood products such as railway ties, poles, pilings, and fence posts. Treated wood products have a useful product life 5 times that of untreated wood, resulting in significant economic savings and conservation of timber resources. PCP is usually applied to wood products as a 5% solution in mineral spirits, fuel oil, or kerosene. In the United States, commercial and industrial use of PCP as a preservative is concentrated in the south, southeast, and northwest. The remaining 20% is used in production of sodium PCP, in plywood and fiberboard waterproofing, in termite control, and as a herbicide for use in rights-of-way and industrial sites. PCP is registered by the EPA as a termiticide, fungicide, herbicide, algicide, and disinfectant and as an ingredient in antifouling paint. It can be applied as a microbial deterrent in the preservation of wood pulp, leather, seeds, rope, glue, starch and cooling tower water. NIOSH estimates that over 26,000 workers are potentially exposed to PCP.

Because of the risk of teratogenicity and fetotoxicity, the EPA since 1984 has required that PCP products in concentrations of 5% or less be used only by certified applicators and has restricted the use of PCP on products that may contact bare skin, food, water, or animals.

## Occupational & Environmental Exposure

Occupational exposure to PCP occurs primarily in the gas, electric service, and wood preservative industries. Air sampling at 25 wood treatment plants using PCP showed an average exposure of 0.013 mg/m$^3$, and newer automated processes and closed systems at larger facilities are further reducing exposure. Acute exposure may occur with the opening of pressure vessel doors or in tank cleaning, solution preparation, and the handling of wood after treatment. Hand application of PCP may also pose a risk of overexposure. Dermal exposure is the principal route, either through direct contact with PCP or through contact with treated wood. Skin contamination with PCP may be an important route of exposure, including glove contamination after direct contact with PCP-treated wood.

Nonoccupational exposure to PCP can occur after the wood has been treated and shipped, where handling may result in dermal exposure. Six months after treatment, PCP will be present on the wood surface at a concentration of about 0.5 mg/ft$^2$. Elevated levels of PCP have been found in the blood and urine of residents of log homes where the logs have been dipped in PCP prior to construction; air samples showed an indoor air concentration of up to 0.38 μg/m$^3$ 5 years after construction.

## Metabolism & Mechanism of Action

Absorption of PCP in the occupational setting is largely through inhalation and skin absorption. The latter is increased when PCP is dissolved in organic solvents. PCP is mainly excreted in urine as free PCP and as a conjugate with glucuronic acid. Pharmacokinetics were characterized in a single-dose oral administration study by first-order absorption, enterohepatic circulation, and first-order elimination, with 74% of the oral dose of PCP excreted unchanged within 8 days. The half-life for elimination was approximately 30 hours. However, in chronically exposed workers during 2- to 4-week vacations, the terminal half-life of elimination ranges from 30–60 days.

Acute intoxication with PCP is due to interference with cellular electron transport and the uncoupling of oxidative phosphorylation in mitochondria and endoplasmic reticulum. Interaction with energy-rich phosphate compounds results in hydrolysis and free energy release, leading to a hypermetabolic state with peripheral tissue hyperthermia.

## Clinical Findings
### A. Symptoms & Signs:
**1. Acute exposure–**

**a. Skin–**Commercial PCP can cause skin irritation after single exposures to more than a 10% concentration of the material or after prolonged or repeated contact with a 1% solution. Skin sensitization has not been demonstrated. Chloracne may occur after exposure to PCP contaminated with dioxins and dibenzofurans, particularly associated with direct skin contact.

**b. Eye, nose, and throat–**Irritation can occur at levels above 0.3 mg/m$^3$, but higher concentrations can be tolerated by those accustomed to the compound.

**c. Systemic intoxication–**Systemic intoxication due to PCP became evident in the 1950s after 2 workers died following cutaneous exposure in a wood-dipping operation. Since that time, fatalities from PCP have occurred among chemical production workers, herbicide sprayers, and wood manufacturers. A unique poisoning tragedy occurred in 20 babies wearing diapers inappropriately laundered in 23% sodium pentachlorophenate; two babies died.

Acute intoxication is characterized by the rapid onset of profuse diaphoresis, hyperpyrexia, tachycardia, tachypnea, weakness, nausea, vomiting, abdominal pain, intense thirst, and pain in the extremities. An intense form of muscle contraction is observed before death. Postmortem examination of one acutely intoxicated worker showed cerebral edema with fatty degeneration of the viscera. The minimum lethal dose of PCP in humans is estimated to be 29 mg/kg.

**d. Other–**Occupational exposure to PCP does not cause adverse effects on the peripheral nervous system. Consistent immunologic effects have not been demonstrated following prolonged exposure to PCP. Community residents in China exposed to sodium PCP used for the eradication of schistosomiases were found to have higher than normal blood lipid levels of dibenzodioxin and dibenzofuran congeners.

**2. Chronic exposure–**Chronic exposure to PCP is associated with conjunctivitis, chronic sinusitis, and bronchitis. Chloracne among PCP wood treatment workers is probably due to dioxin contaminants. In animal studies, pure PCP does not elicit acne.

Bone marrow aplasia has been reported after exposure to PCP. Cytogenetic studies of PCP-exposed workers have not demonstrated increased sister chromatid exchanges or chromosomal breakage. An increased risk for non-Hodgkin's lymphoma has been observed following exposure to PCP and phenoxyacetic acids. IARC finds that pentachlorophenol is possibly carcinogenic to humans (Group 2B). The EPA has concluded that the use of PCP poses a risk of oncogenicity because of the contaminants hexachlorodibenzodioxin and hexachlorobenzene.

PCP and its contaminants cause teratogenic and fetotoxic effects in test animals, but little is known concerning adverse reproductive outcomes in humans.

**B. Laboratory Findings:** Acute intoxication with PCP can result in elevation of blood urea and creatinine, with metabolic acidosis and increased anion gap. Increased serum LDH activity and reduced creatinine clearance have been measured in chronically PCP-exposed workers.

Blood levels of PCP in fatal cases have ranged from 40–170 mg/L. Urine levels have ranged from 29–500 mg/L in fatal cases, and from 3–20 mg/L in nonfatal cases of intoxication. In PCP-exposed workers, mean urine PCP levels were 0.95–1.31 mg/L. In nonoccupationally exposed individuals in the United States, urine values of PCP average 6.3 μg/L, with a range from 1–193 μg/L, and an average of 15μg/L in hemodialysis patients.

### Differential Diagnosis

Acute intoxication can be confused with hyperthermia from other causes, including heat stroke or sepsis. Symptoms of respiratory irritation may be due to the solvent carrier or other occupational irritants. Chloracne is associated with polychlorinated biphenyls, polychlorinated dibenzodioxins, or polychlorinated dibenzofurans.

### Prevention

**A. Work Practices:** Appropriate respiratory protection must be worn where exposure to PCP may exceed permissible limits, particularly in higher-risk operations such as formulating plants and pressure vessel and tank maintenance. Gloves of nitrile and polyvinyl chloride provide the best protection against both aqueous sodium pentachlorophenate and PCP in diesel oil. Clothing contaminated with PCP must be removed, left at the workplace, and laundered before reuse. Washing and showering facilities should be available to prevent contamination of food, drink, and family. Coating PCP-treated logs of home interiors with a sealant will reduce PCP levels in the residents.

**B. Medical Surveillance:** Preemployment urine analysis for PCP should be performed and repeated at intervals. Samples should be collected prior to the last shift of the work week and PCP measured by methods that incorporate hydrolysis. The recommended ACGIH Biological Exposure Index is 2 mg of total PCP per milligram of creatinine in urine or 5 mg of free PCP per milligram of creatinine in plasma before the last shift of work. Discontinuation of PCP exposure will not result in persistent excretion of total PCPs in urine.

Routine medical surveillance should include attention to skin and mucous membrane irritation and skin rash. Hot weather appears to be a predisposing factor for PCP intoxication, so exposure to PCP should be minimized during those times. Significant skin absorption of PCPs may occur and can be documented by urinary PCP monitoring.

### Treatment

Solutions of PCP spilled on the skin are treated with prompt and thorough washing with soap and water. Eyes should be flushed for 15 minutes in water. All contaminated shoes and clothing should be immediately removed.

In the event of acute PCP intoxication, adequate intravenous hydration and efforts to maintain normal body temperature are essential to prevent cardiovascular collapse. Rapid onset of muscular spasms may prevent intubation and resuscitation, so careful monitoring of respiratory status is critical. Metabolic acidosis should be treated with sodium bicarbonate. Atropine sulfate is contraindicated.

## POLYCHLORINATED BIPHENYLS

### Essentials of Diagnosis

*Acute effects:*
- Skin rash (chloracne).
- Eye irritation.
- Nausea, vomiting.

*Chronic effects:*
- Weakness, weight loss, anorexia.
- Skin rash (chloracne).
- Numbness and tingling of extremities.
- Elevated serum triglycerides.
- Elevated liver enzymes.

## Exposure Limits

ACGIH TLV: 0.5 mg/m$^3$ TWA (54% chlorine)
OSHA PEL: 1 mg/m$^3$ TWA (42% chlorine)
NIOSH REL: 1 μg/m$^3$

## General Considerations

Polychlorinated biphenyls (PCBs) are a large family of chlorinated aromatic hydrocarbons prepared by the chlorination of biphenyl. Commercial products are a mixture of PCBs with variable chlorine content and are named according to the percentage of chlorine. In addition, all PCBs are contaminated with small but highly toxic concentrations of polychlorinated dibenzofurans. Outbreaks of PCB-associated disease were probably due to these contaminants.

## Use

Between 1930 and 1975, about 1.4 billion lb of PCBs were produced in the United States. The fire-resistant nature of PCBs, combined with their outstanding thermal stability, made them excellent choices as hydraulic and heat transfer fluids. They were also used to improve the waterproofing characteristics of surface coatings and have been used in the manufacture of carbonless copy paper, printing inks, plasticizers, special adhesives, lubricating additives, and vacuum pump fluids. In the United States, commercial PCBs were marketed under the name Aroclor. In 1977, the manufacture, processing, distribution, and use of PCBs were banned by Congress. However, as of 1980, an estimated 750 million tons was still in use (about half of all PCBs purchased by US industries), primarily in electrical transformers, capacitors, and voltage regulators in electric light fixtures.

## Occupational & Environmental Exposure

NIOSH estimates that approximately 450 employees are potentially exposed to PCBs Much larger numbers are at risk of exposure due to accidental contamination. Leakage of PCBs from capacitors and transformers while in storage, shipment, or maintenance results in transient exposure risks for utility repair crews, railroad maintenance workers, building engineers, and custodians. Improper storage of used PCB electrical equipment may result in environmental contamination and community exposure. Electrical fires occurring in transformers containing PCBs may release polychlorinated dibenzofurans and polychlorinated dibenzodioxins formed through incomplete combustion of PCBs and chlorinated benzenes. Incidents of widespread building contamination due to PCB transformer fires have occurred in Binghamton, San Francisco, Chicago, and Miami. The EPA estimated that in 1984 approximately 107,000 transformers were in use or in storage for reuse, posing a significant risk to the general public if leakage or fire should occur.

## Metabolism & Mechanism of Action

Chlorinated biphenyl compounds are readily absorbed through the respiratory tract, gastrointestinal tract and skin. Distribution is primarily into fat. Biphenyls are metabolized in the liver as the primary site of biotransformation. PCB mixtures cause induction of the hepatic microsomal monooxygenase systems. Induction is related to chlorination, and PCB mixtures containing higher percentages of chlorine are more potent than mixtures with lower levels of chlorination. More highly chlorinated isomers are also more resistant to metabolism and therefore are more persistent. Hydroxy metabolites can be detected in bile, feces, and breast milk, but urinary excretion is quite low. This leads to bioaccumulation in fat at low exposure levels and the persistence of PCBs in fatty tissue years after exposure. The formation of electrophilic arene oxide metabolites may cause DNA damage and the initiation of tumor growth.

## Clinical Findings of Toxicity

### A. Symptoms & Signs:

**1. Acute**–Acute exposure to PCBs results in mucous membrane irritation and nausea and vomiting. Transient skin irritation may result from direct handling of PCBs containing mixtures of solvents.

In the mass food poisoning incident due to rice oil contamination in western Japan in 1968 (Yusho, or rice oil disease), ingestion of PCBs resulted in chloracne. Chloracne probably results from interference with vitamin A metabolism in the skin, with disturbances of the epitheilial tissues of the pilosebaceous duct. Typical chloracne presents with cystic or comedonal lesions over the face, ear lobes, retroauricular region, axillae, trunk, and external genitalia and may occur at any age. Yusho patients also showed dark pigmentation of the gingivae, oral mucosa, and nails, with conjunctival swelling. It is not clear whether all or some of these findings were due to trace contamination of the PCBs with dibenzofurans; the latter compound may have increased during cooking.

**2. Chronic**–In addition to the acute symptoms of upper respiratory tract irritation, chronic workplace exposure to PCBs has also resulted in chloracne. The relationship between dose of exposure and the appearance of chloracne is inconsistent, though chloracne persists for years after exposure has ceased.

Adverse reproductive effects of PCBs have been reported in many animal species; these include failure of implantation, increased number of spontaneous abortions, and low birth weight of litters. Adverse reproductive effects in humans have not been conclusively demonstrated. In Yu-cheng ("oil-disease"), mothers were exposed to PCBs and their heat degradation products from the ingestion of contaminated rice oil in 1979. Children of these mothers were born growth retarded, with dysmorphic physical findings, delayed cognitive development, and increased activity levels. Rare cases of chloracne and, more commonly, nail abnormalities have been found in Yu-cheng children. Prenatal exposure to PCBs predicted poorer short-term memory function in offspring of women who consumed PCB-contaminated fish. PCBs fed to test animals produce hepatocellular carcinomas. Some cohort studies and case reports of workers exposed to PCBs have suggested an increased risk of pancreatic cancer, cancer of the brain, and malignant melanoma. Other studies have found no evidence of excess cancer risk associated with PCB exposure.

Congeners of PCB elicit weak estrogenic and other endocrine responses in animals, probably based on physicochemical properties mimicking natural hormones. Epidemiologic studies have not show an increased risk of breast or endometrial cancers in association with occupational or environmental PCB exposure. Despite the presence of PCBs in breast milk, no association between breast milk exposure and any measured outcome has been observed.

PCBs alter immune function by decreasing the cell-mediated immune response. Cytogenetic analysis of peripheral blood lymphocytes has shown increased chromosome aberrations and sister chromatid exchanges among PCB-exposed workers.

**B. Laboratory Findings:** Mild elevations of serum triglyceride concentrations have been found in Yusho patients and occupationally exposed individuals. PCB-exposed workers have been reported to have significant correlations between the serum PCB level and the $\gamma$-glutamyl transpeptidase level. Nerve conduction velocity was decreased and serum transaminase concentrations increased. These tests have limited diagnostic value.

Owing to widespread environmental contamination and bioconcentration, PCB residues are detectable in blood and fat tissue of nonoccupationally exposed individuals. Serum and plasma levels have ranged to 42 parts per billion (ppb), with means from 2.1 to 24.2 ppb. Fat levels have ranged to 6600 ppb (wet weight basis), with mean values from 800 to 1700 ppb. Levels vary with location, diet, and laboratory.

If exposure to PCB is suspected, serum or fat levels of PCBs may be measured to document absorption. In a steady state, serum is as good a reflection of body burden as is fat. Results must be interpreted in light of established normals for geographic area and laboratory technique. PCBs can be measured in human tissue by a variety of analytic methods and have been variously reported as total PCB content related to a commercial mixture, as quantification of chromatographic peaks, or by characterization of specific congeners. Analysis of coplanar, mono-or-tho-substituted and di-ortho-substituted PCB levels in human blood may be useful following acute or chronic exposure. These more toxic congeners contribute significantly to dioxin toxic equivalents in blood from US adults. Unfortunately, the relationship between symptoms or signs and PCB levels in serum or fat is variable.

## Differential Diagnosis

Occupational exposure to PCBs may be accompanied by exposure to chlorinated dibenzodioxin and dibenzofuran contaminants and may be responsible for chronic toxicity. Concurrent exposure to solvents is important, because these substances may cause chronic fatigue and elevated liver enzymes. Mild chloracne should not be confused with other papular rashes. A biopsy may be necessary to establish the diagnosis.

## Prevention

**A. Work Practices:** Work practices to avoid exposure to PCBs include the use of special PCB-resistant gloves and protective clothing. Adequate ventilation should be maintained during spill cleanup or maintenance of vessels containing PCBs; if this is not possible, approved respirators should be provided. Provision should be made for proper decontamination or disposal of contaminated clothing or equipment. Locations where PCBs are stored should be clearly posted as required by law. Environmental sampling may be necessary to ensure adequate worker protection or safety for public reentry to contaminated areas. Reentry or cleanup levels have been established for dioxins and PCBs to protect workers who reoccupy buildings following a PCB fire. Persistent health effects after PCB transformer fires include self-reported unexplained weight loss, muscle pain, frequent coughing, and sleep problems. These symptoms may be due to stress or recall bias and may not be specifically linked to the toxic effects of PCBs.

**B. Medical Surveillance:** Workers intermittently exposed to PCBs should have a baseline skin examination and liver function tests. Follow-up examination can be limited to symptomatic individuals and those exposed as a consequence of accidental contamination. Routine serum and fat PCB measurements are not recommended.

## Treatment

Acute exposure should be treated by immediate decontamination of the skin with soap and water to prevent skin absorption. No specific measures are available for respiratory tract or skin absorption.

No treatment is available for chronic PCB toxicity. Chloracne is treated with topical therapy for symptomatic relief.

# POLYCYCLIC AROMATIC HYDROCARBONS

## Essentials of Diagnosis

*Acute effects:*
- Dermatitis, conjunctivitis (coal tar pitch volatiles).

*Chronic effects:*
- Excess cancer rates in selected occupations.

## Exposure Limits

Coal tar products (volatiles)
    ACGIH TLV: Confirmed human carcinogen
    OSHA PEL: 0.2 mg/m$^3$ TWA (benzene-soluble fraction)
    NIOSH REL: 0.1 mg/m$^3$ TWA
Naphthalene
    ACGIH TLV: 10 ppm TWA, 15 ppm STEL
    OSHA PEL: 10 ppm TWA, 15 ppm STEL
    NIOSH REL: 10 ppm TWA, 15 ppm STEL
Bitumens
    NIOSH REL: 5 mg/m$^3$ ceiling (15 minutes)
Carbon black
    ACGIH TLV: 3.5 mg/m$^3$ TWA
    OSHA PEL: 3.5 mg/m$^3$ TWA
    NIOSH REL: 3.5 mg/m$^3$ TWA; in presence of polycyclic aromatic hydrocarbons, 0.1 mg/m$^3$ TWA
Anthracene
    ACGIH TLV: 0.2 mg/m$^3$ TWA
    OSHA PEL: 0.2 mg/m$^3$ TWA
    NIOSH REL: 0.01 mg/m$^3$ TWA (cyclohexane extractable fraction)
Benzo(*a*)pyrene
    ACGIH TLV: suspected human carcinogen, no TWA
    OSHA PEL: 0.2 mg/m$^3$ TWA
    NIOSH REL: 0.1 mg/m$^3$ (cyclohexane extractable fraction)

## General Considerations

Polycyclic aromatic hydrocarbons are organic compounds consisting of three or more aromatic rings that contain only carbon and hydrogen and share a pair of carbon atoms. They are formed by pyrolysis or incomplete combustion of such organic matter as coke, coal tar and pitch, asphalt, and oil. The composition of the products of pyrolysis is dependent on the fuel, the temperature, and the time in the hot area. Polycyclic aromatic hydrocarbons are emitted as vapors from the zone of burning and condense immediately on soot particles or form very small particles themselves. Such processes always lead to a mixture of hundreds of polycyclic aromatic hydrocarbons. Compounds with three or four aromatic rings predominate. Carcinogenic polycyclic aromatic hydrocarbons are found among those with five or six rings. The simplest fused ring is naphthalene. Some important polycyclic aromatic hydrocarbons in the occupational environment are shown below.

Naphthalene

Anthracene

Benzo(*a*)pyrene

## Use, Production, & Exposure

Pure polycyclic aromatic hydrocarbons have no direct use except for naphthalene and anthracene.

**Anthracene** is used in the manufacture of dyes, synthetic fibers, plastics, and monocrystals; as a component of smoke screens; in scintillation counter crystals, and in semiconductor research. NIOSH estimates that over 2300 workers are potentially exposed to anthracene.

**Benzo(*a*)pyrene** is used as a research chemical and is not produced commercially in the United States. NIOSH estimates that almost 900 workers are potentially exposed to benzo(*a*)pyrene.

**Bitumens** are contained in road-paving, roofing, and asphalt products. NIOSH estimates that over 471,000 workers are potentially exposed to asphalt.

The majority of **carbon black** is used as a pigment for rubber tires, with the remainder used in a variety of products such as paint, plastics, printing inks, pigment in eye cosmetics, carbon paper, and typewriter ribbons. Annual US production exceeds 3 billion lb. NIOSH estimates that about 125 employees are potentially exposed to carbon black.

**Creosote** is used extensively as a wood preservative, usually by high-pressure impregnation of lumber, and as a constituent of fuel oil, lubricant for die molds, and pitch for roofing. Creosote contains over 300 different compounds, the major components of which are polycyclic aromatic hydrocarbons, phenols, cresols, xylenols, and pyridines. NIOSH estimates that about 240 workers are potentially exposed to cresosote during production.

**Coal tar pitch** is used as a raw material for plastics, solvents, dyes, and drugs; crude or refined coal tar products are used for waterproofing, paints, pipe coatings, roads, roofing, and insulation; as a sealant, binder, and filler in surface coatings; and a modifier in epoxy resin coatings. NIOSH estimates that over 19,000 workers are potentially exposed to coal tar pitch.

**Naphthalene** is used as a chemical intermediate in the production of phthalic anhydride, carbamate insecticides, β-naphthol, sulfonic acids, and surfactants and as a moth repellent and tanning agent. NIOSH estimates that over 112,000 workers are potentially exposed to naphthalene. Polycyclic aromatic hydrocarbons as contaminants can be found in air, water, food, and cigarette smoke as well as in the industrial environment.

## Occupational Exposure

**A. Coal Tars & Products:** Exposures to PAHs may occur among carbon black production workers, wildland firefighters, petroleum tanker deck crews, meat smokehouse workers, and printing press room operators. The most important source of polycyclic aromatic hydrocarbons in the air of the workplace is coal tar. Tars and pitches are black or brown, liquid or semisolid products derived from coal, petroleum, wood, shale oil, or other organic materials. Coal tars are by-products of the carbonization of coal to produce coke or natural gas. The coke-oven plant is the principal source of coal tar. Coal tar pitch and creosote are derived from the distillation of coal tar. Numerous polycyclic aromatic hydrocarbons have been identified in coal tar, coal tar pitch, and creosote. Coal tar pitch volatiles are the volatile matter emitted into the air when coal tar, coal tar pitch, or their products are heated, and they may contain several polycyclic aromatic hydrocarbons.

The major use for coal tar pitch is as the binder for aluminum smelting electrodes; other uses include roofing material, surface coatings, pipe-coating enamels, and as a binder for briquettes and foundry cores. Creosote is used almost exclusively as a wood preservative.

Occupational exposure to polycyclic aromatic hydrocarbons in coal tar and pitches may occur in gas and coke works, aluminum reduction plants, iron and steel foundries, coal gasification facilities, and during roof and pavement tarring and the application of coal-tar paints.

**B. Carbon Black:** Carbon black is derived from the partial combustion (pyrolysis) of natural gas or petroleum. It is primarily used in pigmenting and reinforcing rubber products and in inks, paints, and paper.

**C. Bitumens:** Bitumens are viscous solids or liquids derived from refining processes of petroleum. They are principally used for road construction when mixed with asphalt, in roofing felt manufacture, in pipe coatings, and as binders in briquettes. Occupational exposure may occur in these operations.

**D. Soots:** Soots are mixtures of particulate carbon, organic tars, resins, and inorganic material produced during incomplete combustion of carbon-containing material. Occupational exposure is primarily to chimney soot; potential exposure occurs to chim-ney sweeps, brick masons, and heating unit service personnel.

## Environmental Exposure

Polycyclic aromatic hydrocarbons occur in the air primarily as a result of coal burning and settle on soil, where they may leach into water. They are found in smoked fish and meats and form during the broiling and grilling of foods. They are inhaled in cigarette smoke from the burning of tobacco.

## Metabolism & Mechanism of Action

Polycyclic aromatic hydrocarbons are readily absorbed by the skin, lungs, and gastrointestinal tract of experimental animals and are rapidly metabolized and excreted in the feces. In humans, they are largely absorbed from carrier particles via the respiratory route. They are activated by aryl hydrocarbon hydroxylase to a reactive epoxide intermediate, then conjugated for excretion in urine or bile. The reactive epoxide may covalently bind with DNA and probably accounts for the carcinogenic activity.

## Clinical Findings

**A. Symptoms & Signs:**

**1. Acute exposure**–Acute inhalation exposure to naphthalene may cause headache, nausea, diaphoresis, and vomiting. Accidental ingestion has caused hemolytic anemia. Naphthalene may also cause erythema and dermatitis on repeated skin contact.

Exposure to coal tar products may cause phototoxicity, with skin erythema, burning, and itching (see Chapter 18), and eye burning and lacrimation.

**2. Chronic exposure**–Many polycyclic aromatic hydrocarbons are carcinogenic in animals. Often, benzo(a)pyrene (BaP) is measured to indicate the presence of polycyclic aromatic hydrocarbons where exposure to carcinogens is suspect.

Evidence for human carcinogenicity was initially described by Percivall Pott in 1775 when he associated scrotal cancer in chimney sweeps with their prolonged exposure to tar and soot. Subsequently, scrotal cancer in mulespinners exposed to shale oil and workers exposed to pitch have been reported.

IARC considers coal tar pitch volatiles to be carcinogenic to humans (Group 1), benzo(a)pyrene and creosote possibly carcinogenic to humans (Group 2A), and carbon black possibly carcinogenic to humans (Group 2B). NIOSH considers that coal tar products, carbon black, and anthracene are carcinogenic and recommends that exposures be limited to the lowest feasible level. There is evidence that extracts of refined bitumens are carcinogenic in animals. There are insufficient data to assess cancer risk among workers exposed to bitumens (such as highway maintenance workers and road pavers).

Excess respiratory and prostate cancer mortality has been found among coke oven workers, respiratory cancer mortality among foundry workers, bladder and lung cancer mortality among aluminum smelter workers, and lung and stomach cancer mortality among roofers. One cohort mortality study of workers exposed to chlorinated naphthalenes did not find excess cancer risk.

Exposure-related respiratory effects in carbon black-exposed workers have included reduction in airflows, symptoms of chronic bronchitis, and small opacities on chest x-ray.

Occupational creosote exposure is a risk for squamous papilloma and carcinoma of the skin.

**B. Laboratory Findings:** Photopatch testing may demonstrate photodermatitis in workers with occupational exposure to coal tar pitch and fumes.

### Differential Diagnosis

Exposure to other known or potential carcinogenic exposure in the work environment should be investigated.

### Prevention

**A. Work Practices:** Reduction of emissions from coke ovens, aluminum works, foundries, and steel works is essential. Where gaseous emissions occur during loading or transferring of heated coal tar products, fume and vapor control systems will reduce personal exposure. Skin exposure to tars, pitches, and oils containing polycyclic aromatic hydrocarbons is avoided by wearing gloves and changing contaminated work clothes.

**B. Medical Surveillance:** Periodic examination of workers exposed to coal tar pitch volatiles should include a history of skin or eye irritation and physical examination with attention to the skin, upper respiratory tract, and lungs. Urinary 1-hydroxy-pyrene (1-OHP) has been used for biological monitoring of coal liquefaction workers, coke oven workers, foundry workers, aluminum smelter pot-room workers, electrode paste plant workers, graphite electrode production workers, automotive repair workers, carbon black production workers, and road pavers. Good correlation has been found between airborne polycyclic aromatic hydrocarbon exposure and urinary 1-OHP, with significant contribution from dermal exposure. Urinary 1-napthol has been used as a biomarker of polycyclic aromatic hydrocarbon exposure among naphthelene oil distillation workers, foundry workers, and creosote-impregnated wood assemblers. Enzyme radioimmunoassay techniques to measure polycyclic aromatic hydrocarbon-DNA adducts in white blood cells have also been used as a biomarker of polycyclic aromatic hydrocarbon exposure among several types of polycyclic aromatic hydrocarbon-exposed workers, including foundry workers, coke oven workers, aluminum smelter pot-room workers, roofers, and

wildland firefighters. Dietary sources of polycyclic aromatic hydrocarbons (eg, charbroiled food) and cigarette smoking contribute to polycyclic aromatic hydrocarbon-DNA adduct or urinary 1-OHP levels and should be evaluated as confounding factors. Tetrahydrotetrol metabolites of benzo(*a*)pyrene in urine may also prove to be useful for biomonitoring of polycyclic aromatic hydrocarbon exposures.

### Treatment

Photodermatitis should be treated with cortisone-containing preparations, barrier creams, or removal from exposure.

## STYRENE

### Essentials of Diagnosis

*Acute effects:*
- Eye, respiratory tract, and skin irritation.

*Chronic effects:*
- Weakness, headache, fatigue, dizziness.
- Neuropsychological deficits, color vision loss, sensory nerve conduction slowing.

### Exposure Limits

ACGIH TLV: 50 ppm TWA, 100 ppm STEL
OSHA PEL: 100 ppm TWA, 200 ppm maximum period of 5 minutes in 3 hours
NIOSH REL: 50 ppm TWA, 100 ppm ceiling (15 minutes)

### General Considerations

Styrene, also known as vinyl benzene and phenylethylene, has the chemical formula $C_6H_5CH:CH_2$. It is a colorless volatile liquid at room temperature with a sweet odor at low concentrations. The odor threshold of 1 ppm is below the permissible exposure limit, and the material has adequate warning properties. Styrene monomer must be stabilized by an inhibitor to prevent exothermic polymerization, a process that may cause explosion of its container.

### Use

Commercial styrene was first produced in the 1920s and 1930s. During World War II, styrene was important in the manufacture of synthetic rubber. Over 90% of styrene is produced by the dehydrogenation of ethylbenzene. Styrene is used as a monomer or copolymer for polystyrenes, for acrylonitrile-butadiene-styrene (ABS) resins, styrene-butadiene rubber (SBR), styrene-butadiene copolymer latexes, and styrene-acrylonitrile (SAN) resins. Styrene is also used in glass-reinforced, unsaturated polyester resins used in construction materials and boats and in the manufacture of protective coatings. Annual US production exceeds 11 billion lb, with production of styrene polymers exceeding 9 billion lb. NIOSH estimates that over 330,000 workers are potentially exposed to styrene.

## Occupational & Environmental Exposure

In closed polymerization processes, worker exposure to styrene is generally low, but exposure peaks may occur during cleaning, filling, or maintenance of reaction vessels or during transport of liquid styrene. Styrene exposure during manual application of resins (hand lamination) or spraying in open molds may exceed exposure limits. Exposures should be reduced through general and local ventilation systems or through the use of automated processes and closed molds.

The most significant exposure to styrene occurs when it is used as a solvent-reactant for unsaturated polyester products that have been reinforced with fibrous glass. Reinforced plastics/composites are used in the manufacture of boats, storage tanks, wall panels, tub and shower units, and truck camper tops. In this process, alternating layers of chopped fibers or woven mats of fibrous glass are hand-applied with catalyzed resin; up to 10% of the styrene may evaporate into the workplace air as the resin cures. Average styrene exposures in plants where the reinforced products are manufactured can range from 40–100 ppm, with short-term individual exposures up to 150–300 ppm. In a NIOSH study of the reinforced plastics industry, directly exposed workers engaged in the manufacture of truck parts and boats had the highest exposure to styrene, with a mean 8-hour TWA of 61 and 82 ppm, respectively.

## Metabolism & Mechanism of Action

Occupational exposure occurs mainly via inhalation, with about 60% of inhaled styrene retained by the lungs. Percutaneous absorption is not significant. In closed polymerization processes, worker exposure to styrene is generally low, but exposure peaks may occur during cleaning, filling, or maintenance of reaction vessels, or during transport of liquid styrene. Styrene exposure during manual application of resins (hand lamination) or spraying in open molds may exceed exposure limits. Exposures should be reduced through general and local ventilation systems or through the use of automated processes and closed molds. After short-term exposure, the venous half-life of styrene is approximately 40 minutes. The half-lives of mandelic acid and phenylglyoxylic acid are about 4 and 8 hours, respectively. In the chronically exposed worker, the half-life for mandelic acid excretion may range from 6–9 hours.

## Clinical Findings

### A. Symptoms & Signs:

**1. Acute exposure**–Concentrations of styrene from 100–200 ppm may cause eye and upper respiratory tract irritation. Styrene is a defatting agent and a primary skin irritant, resulting in dermatitis. Experimental human exposure to several hundred parts per million causes typical alcohol-organic solvent anesthetic symptoms, with listlessness, drowsiness, impaired balance, difficulty in concentrating, and decrease in reaction time. There have been no reports of fatalities due to styrene exposure.

**2. Chronic exposure**–Weakness, headache, fatigue, poor memory, and dizziness can occur in workers chronically exposed to styrene in concentrations of less than 100 ppm. Mean reaction time and visuomotor performance may be decreased in exposed workers. The incidence of abnormal EEGs was significantly greater as well.

Studies of styrene-exposed workers have shown detectable blood levels of styrene-7,8-oxide, with dose-related increases in lymphocyte DNA adduct levels, styrene-7,8-oxide hemoglobin adduct levels, single-strand DNA breaks, chromosomal aberrations, lymphocyte micronuclei, and sister chromatid exchanges. Reduction of styrene exposure can prevent adverse cytogenetic effects. Several studies of styrene-exposed workers have demonstrated an association between styrene exposure and degenerative disorders of the nervous system, pancreatic cancer, and lymphohematopoietic cancer. Significant associations have been observed in large European studies between the risk of leukemia and the time elapsed since first exposure to styrene. Other authors suggest that these findings may be confounded by concomitant exposures to other solvents or have not been replicated consistently across studies. IARC considers styrene possibly carcinogenic to humans (Group 2B).

A variety of neurotoxic effects have been observed after styrene exposure, including electroencephalographic abnormalities, sensory nerve conduction slowing, prolonged somatosensory evoked potentials, and neuropsychological deficits. Styrene exposure among glass-reinforced-plastic workers and plastic-boat manufacturing workers has been associated with early color and contrast vision dysfunction. No effect on hearing acuity has been observed. Moderate exposure to styrene has been associated with an altered distribution of lymphocyte subsets.

Styrene may be embryotoxic or fetotoxic in animals. Human reproductive studies (spontaneous abortions, congenital malformations, low birth weight, or reduced fertility) have been inconsistent or limited by methodologic shortcomings.

### B. Laboratory Findings: In one study, styrene-exposed workers had elevated $\gamma$-glutamyl transferase values. No other blood test is specific for styrene toxicity.

The most reliable indicator of styrene exposure is mandelic acid in the urine. Postshift mandelic acid levels in urine show a good correlation with average TWA styrene exposure over the range of 5–150 ppm.

Levels of 500 mg of mandelic acid per liter of urine may indicate recent exposure to at least 10 ppm of styrene. A concentration of 1000 mg of mandelic acid per liter of urine corresponds to an average 8-hour TWA styrene exposure of 50 ppm.

### Differential Diagnosis

Exposure to other solvents during the production of styrene and in the manufacture of reinforced plastic products may cause similar symptoms of central nervous system toxicity such as headache, fatigue, and memory loss.

### Prevention

**A. Work Practices:** Styrene poses a significant fire hazard, and proper handling and storage are essential to prevent ignition of the liquid and vapor and a potential explosive reaction. Closed-process systems are recommended. Intensive local exhaust ventilation is the best way to reduce styrene vapor concentrations during construction of large reinforced plastic objects, though dilution ventilation is widely used to reduce styrene vapor exposure in the boat industry.

When worker exposure cannot be adequately controlled by engineering controls, protective clothing and respirators may be needed. Where workers may come into contact with liquid styrene, appropriate gloves, boots, overshoes, aprons, and face shields with goggles are recommended. Polyvinyl alcohol and polyethylene gloves and protective clothing give good protection against styrene. To prevent eye irritation at moderately low concentrations, full-face-piece respirators are recommended.

**B. Medical Surveillance:** Initial medical evaluation should include a history of nervous system disorders and an examination with particular attention to the nervous system, respiratory tract, and skin. Annual medical examinations should be performed on all workers with significant air exposure above the action level or with potential for significant skin exposure. The ACGIH recommended Biological Exposure Index is 240 mg of phenylglyoxylic acid per gram of creatinine or 300 mg of mandelic acid per gram of creatinine in urine or 0.55 mg/L in venous blood, at the end of the work shift. Styrene in exhaled air has also been used as an indicator of low-level styrene exposure. Measurement of monoamine oxidase type B activity in platelets and the glycophorin A assay have also been suggested as biomarkers of styrene exposure.

### Treatment

Hands should be washed after skin exposure, and clothing saturated with styrene should be immediately removed. In the case of eye contact, flush the eye immediately with copious amounts of water for 15 minutes. No specific treatment is recommended for acute or chronic styrene exposure.

## 2,3,7,8-TETRACHLORODIBENZO-P-DIOXIN

### Essentials of Diagnosis

*Acute effects:*
- Eye and respiratory tract irritation.
- Skin rash, chloracne.
- Fatigue, nervousness, irritability.

*Chronic effects:*
- Chloracne.
- Soft tissue sarcoma, non-Hodgkin's lymphoma, Hodgkin's disease.

### Exposure Limits

NIOSH REL: Lowest feasible concentration

### General Considerations

Polychlorinated dibenzo-*p*-dioxins (PCDDs) and polychlorinated dibenzofurans (PCDFs) are two large series of tricyclic aromatic compounds that exhibit similar physical, chemical, and biological properties.

PCDFs

PCDDs

However, there is a pronounced difference in potency among the different PCDD and PCDF isomers. The most extensively studied is the 2,3,7,8-tetrachlorodibenzo-*p*-dioxin isomer (2,3,7,8-TCDD). "Dioxin" is the name used for at least 75 chlorinated aromatic isomers, including 22 isomers of the tetrachlorinated dioxin. 2,3,7,8-TCDD is the specific dioxin identified as a contaminant in the production of 2,4,5-trichlorophenol (TCP), 2-(2,4,5-trichlorophenoxy)propionic acid (Silvex), and 2,4,5-trichlorophenoxyacetic acid (2,4,5-T). In its pure form, 2,3,7,8-TCDD is a colorless crystalline solid at room temperature, sparingly soluble in organic solvents and insoluble in water. The degree of toxicity of the dioxin compounds is highly dependent on the number and position of the chlorine atoms; isomers with chlorination in the four lateral positions (2,3,7,8) have the highest acute toxicity in animals. Under laboratory conditions, 2,3,7,8-TCDD is one of the most toxic synthetic chemicals known.

The chlorinated dibenzofurans are contaminants found in some polychlorinated biphenyl compounds

(PCBs) used in transformers and capacitors, including the most toxic 2,3,7,8-tetrachlorinated dibenzofuran.

## Use

2,3,7,8-TCDD is formed as a stable by-product during the production of TCP. Normally, 2,3,7,8-TCDD persists as a contaminant in TCP in amounts ranging from 0.07 to 6.2 mg/kg. Production of 2,4,5-T and Silvex ceased in the United States in 1979, although stockpiles are still being distributed and used. Agent Orange, used in Vietnam as a defoliant during the 1960s, was a 50:50 mixture of esters of the herbicides 2, 4-D and 2,4,5-T. Ten to twelve million gallons was sprayed over 3–4 million acres in Vietnam; the 2,3,7,8-TCDD concentration was about 2 ppm in Agent Orange available after usage was stopped.

The combustion of 2,4,5-T can result in its conversion to small amounts of 2,3,7,8-TCDD. Polychlorinated biphenyls can be converted to PCDFs. Soot from PCB transformer fires may be contaminated with more than 2000 μg/g of PCDFs, including the most toxic 2,3,7,8- isomers. A complex mixture of PCDDs and PCDFs may occur in fly ash from municipal incinerators. 2,3,7,8-TCDD is not used commercially in the United States, and NIOSH estimates that only 14 employees are potentially exposed to dioxin.

## Occupational & Environmental Exposure

Occupational exposure to 2,3,7,8-TCDD can occur during the production and use of 2,4,5-T and its derivatives. Since 1949, there have been 24 accidents in chemical plants manufacturing chlorinated phenols in which workers were exposed to PCDDs. The explosion of a TCP chemical plant in 1976 in Seveso, Italy, exposed some 37,000 residents of surrounding communities to 2,3,7,8-TCDD.

Workers may be exposed to PCDDs during the production of TCP, 2,4,5-T, and pentachlorophenol. Herbicide sprayers using 2,4,5-T or Silvex have been exposed to 2,3,7,8-TCDD during application. Environmental contamination occurred from spraying waste oil that contained 2,3,7,8-TCDD for dust control on the ground in Missouri. Workers exposed to slag and fly ash from older municipal waste incinerators may have increased blood concentrations of PCDDs and PCDFs. The EPA banned most uses of 2,4,5-T and Silvex in 1979, though their use was allowed on sugarcane and in orchards, and miscellaneous noncrop uses were permitted. In October 1983, EPA published its intent to cancel the registration of all pesticide products containing 2,4,5-T or Silvex. It is not possible to accurately estimate the number of US workers currently exposed to 2,3,7,8-TCDD during decontamination of worksites, from waste materials contaminated with 2,3,7,8-TCDD, or from cleanup after fires in transformers containing polychlorinated biphenyls.

## Metabolism & Mechanism of Action

2,3,7,8-TCDD is an extremely lipophilic substance and is readily absorbed following an oral dose in the rat. It accumulates mainly in the liver and after a single dose is largely eliminated unmetabolized in the feces with a whole-body half-life of about 3 weeks. After repeated dosing in small laboratory animals, it is stored in adipose tissue. The retention in humans is not known. Dermal absorption may be important in workers exposed to phenoxy acids and chlorophenols. Exposure to 2,3,7,8-TCDD as a vapor will normally be negligible because of its low vapor pressure.

Dioxin-like compounds are characterized by high-affinity binding to the Ah receptor, and most biological effects are thought to be mediated by the ligand-Ah receptor complex. A second protein is required for DNA-binding capability and transcriptional activation of target genes. Growth factors, free radicals, the interaction of 2,3,7,8-TCDD with the estrogen transduction pathway, or protein kinases may also play a role in signal transduction mechanisms. Relative potency factors have been assigned to the dioxin-like compounds on the basis of a comparison of potency with that of 2,3,7,8-TCDD. Each chemical is assigned a toxic equivalency factor (TEF), some fraction of 2,3,7,8-TCDD, and the total toxic equivalency of the mixture (TEQ) is the sum of the weighted potencies. TEF values have been calculated for PCDDs, PCDFs, and dioxin-like PCBs.

## Clinical Findings

### A. Signs & Symptoms:

**1. Acute exposure–**In some animals, 2,3,7,8-TCDD is lethal in doses of less than 1 μg/kg. Acute toxicity results in profound wasting, thymic atrophy, bone marrow suppression, hepatotoxicity, and microsomal enzyme induction.

In humans, the acute toxicity of 2,3,7,8-TCDD is known from accidental release due to runaway reactions or explosions. A process accident in Nitro, West Virginia, in 1949 was followed by acute skin, eye, and respiratory tract irritation, headache, dizziness, and nausea. These symptoms subsided within 1–2 weeks and were followed by an acneiform eruption; severe muscle pain in the extremities, thorax, and shoulders; fatigue, nervousness, and irritability; dyspnea, complaints of decreased libido, and intolerance to cold. Workers exhibited severe chloracne, hepatic enlargement, peripheral neuritis, delayed prothrombin time, and increased total serum lipid levels. A follow-up study 30 years later found persistence of chloracne in 55% but no evidence of increased risk for cardiovascular disease or for hepatic, renal, or nervous system damage.

**2. Chronic exposure–**In animals, 2,3,7,8-TCDD is a teratogen and is toxic to the fetus. Two-year feeding studies in rats and mice have demonstrated an excess of liver tumors; the feeding level at which no observable effects in rats occurred was 0.001 μg/kg/d.

Chloracne can result within several weeks after exposure to 2,3,7,8-TCDD and can persist for decades. Among production workers, the severity of chloracne is related to the degree of exposure. In some workplaces, exposed persons had chloracne but no systemic illnesses; in others, workers experienced fatigue, weight loss, myalgias, insomnia, irritability, and decreased libido. The liver has become tender and enlarged, and sensory changes, particularly in the lower extremities, have been reported. In exposed production workers, systemic symptoms—except for chloracne—have not persisted after exposures ceased.

Immunotoxic and reproductive effects appear to be among the most sensitive indicators of dioxin toxicity. Laboratory studies in animals suggest that dioxin-like compounds cause altered development (low birth weight, spontaneous abortions, congenital malformations) and adverse changes in reproductive health (fertility, sex organ development, reproductive behavior). 2,3,7,8-TCDD may be transferred transplacentally and via breast milk, and elevated levels of 2,3,7,8-TCDD have been detected in adult children of female chemical production workers exposed to dioxins. Three epidemiologic studies have suggested an association between paternal herbicide exposure and an increased risk of spina bifida in offspring.

A variety of immunologic effects have also been seen in animal studies. Human studies have shown alteration in delayed-type hypersensivity after exposure to dioxins. No consistent cytogenetic effects have been seen from 2,3,7,8-TCDD exposure.

2,3,7,8-TCDD may inhibit uroporphyrinogen decarboxylation, and cases of porphyria cutanea tarda among exposed workers have been reported. However, recent studies have failed to find an association between 2,3,7,8-TCDD and porphyrin levels. No association has been observed among former chlorophenol production workers between 2,3,7,8-TCDD exposure and serum transaminases levels, induction of cytochrome P-450 activity, peripheral neuropathy, chronic bronchitis or chronic obstructive pulmonary disease, and porphyria cutanea tarda. Serum dioxin levels have been positively associated with levels of luteinizing and follicle-stimulating hormone and inversely related to total testosterone levels. This finding is consistent with dioxin-related effects on the hypothalamic-pituitary-Leydig-cell axis in animals. No 2,3,7,8-TCDD-associated liver abnormalities have been seen among Vietnam veterans reporting exposure to Agent Orange.

Excess risk of soft tissue sarcoma has been associated with exposure to 2,3,7,8-TCDD and phenoxy herbicides. The National Academy of Sciences (NAS) has found sufficient evidence to indicate an association between exposure to herbicides (eg, 2-4-dichlorophenoxyacetic acid, 2,4,5-trichlorophenoxyacetic acid, and 2,3,7,8-TCDD) among Vietnam veterans and soft tissue sarcoma, non-Hodgkin's lymphoma, Hodgkin's disease, and chloracne. IARC finds that 2,3,7,8-TCDD is possibly carcinogenic to humans (Group 2B). NIOSH recommends that 2,3,7,8-TCDD be treated as a potential human carcinogen and that exposure be reduced to the lowest feasible concentration.

Increased episodes of a variety of illnesses have been observed in a long-term follow-up study of a cohort exposed to 2,3,7,8-TCDD after a chemical reactor incident.

**B. Laboratory Findings:** Abnormalities reported most consistently are elevated liver enzymes, prolonged prothrombin time, and elevated cholesterol and triglyceride levels. Urinary porphyrins may be elevated. Following the Seveso accident, the incidence of abnormal nerve conduction tests was significantly elevated in subjects with chloracne.

Very low levels of 2,3,7,8-TCDD (4–130 parts per trillion) can be detected in adipose tissue of nonexposed populations. Concentration of polychlorinated compounds in plasma may be 1000-fold less than in adipose tissue. There is a high correlation between adipose and serum 2,3,7,8-TCDD levels; serum levels are a valid measure of body burden. The correlation between plasma and adipose tissue concentrations of 2,3,7,8-TCDD with signs and symptoms is uncertain.

## Differential Diagnosis

Known causes of an acneiform eruption in the workplace include petroleum cutting oils, coal tar, and the chlorinated aromatic compounds. With systemic complaints, such as weight loss, headache, myalgias, and irritability, other underlying medical illnesses should be ruled out before attributing the disorder to 2,3,7,8-TCDD.

## Prevention

**A. Work Practices:** NIOSH recommends that 2,3,7,8-TCDD be considered a potential occupational carcinogen and that exposure in all occupational settings be controlled to the fullest extent possible. Specific guidelines for safe work practices must begin with environmental sampling to determine the presence of 2,3,7,8-TCDD contamination, including sampling of air, soil, and settled dust and wipe sampling of surfaces. For site cleanup, specific decontamination procedures should be adhered to for adequate worker protection. Protective clothing and equipment should consist of both outer and inner garments, with outer coveralls, gloves, and boots made of nonwoven polyethylene fabric. Appropriate respiratory protection must be worn, ranging from an air purifying respirator to a self-contained breathing apparatus. Follow-up sampling should be conducted after decontamination of a site to ensure adequate cleanup.

**B. Medical Surveillance:** Production workers exposed to compounds contaminated with 2,3,7,8-TCDD as well as site decontamination personnel should undergo baseline and periodic medical examination with special attention to the skin and nervous system. Baseline laboratory testing should include liver enzymes, cholesterol, and triglycerides, with follow-up as required. Effective safety measures for dioxin clean-up workers will prevent clinical or biochemical disease (chloracne, liver disease, peripheral neuropathy, porphyria cutanea tarda). There has been considerable progress in the use of serum 2,3,7,8-TCDD levels, with the characterization of 2,3,7,8-TCDD body burdens in the Ranch Hand cohort, Seveso residents, herbicide production employees, and Vietnamese civilians. Serum or adipose dioxin levels may be useful for research purposes or to assess health outcome risks for exposure reconstruction, but they are not recommended for routine medical monitoring.

## Treatment

Skin contaminated with 2,3,7,8-TCDD should be immediately washed and any contaminated clothing removed and placed in marked containers and disposed of appropriately.

Except for symptomatic treatment of chloracne, there is no treatment for acute or chronic health effects resulting from 2,3,7,8-TCDD exposure.

# VINYL CHLORIDE MONOMER & POLYVINYL CHLORIDE

## Essentials of Diagnosis

*Acute effects:*
- Respiratory tract irritation.
- Lethargy, headache.

*Chronic effects:*
- Acro-osteolysis, Raynaud's phenomenon, skin thickening.
- Hepatosplenomegaly.
- Hepatic angiosarcoma.

## Exposure Limits

OSHA PEL: 1 ppm TWA (15 minutes) 5 ppm
ACGIH TLV: 5 ppm TWA
NIOSH REL: Reduce exposure to lowest feasible concentration

## General Considerations

Vinyl chloride monomer (chloroethene) is a colorless, highly flammable gas at room temperature. It is usually handled as a liquid under pressure containing a polymerization inhibitor (phenol). It is soluble in ethanol and ether. The odor threshold is variable, so that odor cannot be used to prevent excess exposure.

## Use

The bulk of vinyl chloride monomer is used for the production of polyvinyl chloride resins. Polyvinyl chloride is used primarily in the production of plastic piping and conduit, floor coverings, home furnishings, electrical applications, recreational products (records, toys), packaging (film, sheet, and bottles), and transportation materials (automobile tops, upholstery, and mats). Vinyl chloride is used primarily as a monomer for polyvinyl chlorode resins and for the synthesis of methyl chloroform. Annual US production exceeds 14 billion lb. NIOSH estimates that over 81,000 workers are potentially exposed to vinyl chloride.

## Occupational & Environmental Exposure

A 1977 NIOSH survey of three vinyl chloride monomer plants found that the 8-hour TWA ranged from 0.07–27 ppm. Following promulgation of the OSHA standard in 1974, exposures were reduced to less than 5 ppm. The highest exposures occur in polymerization plants, particularly during reactor vessel cleaning.

Retained unreacted monomer in polyvinyl chloride products is so low that there is little risk now to polyvinyl chloride fabrication workers.

## Metabolism & Mechanism of Action

The chief route of exposure to VCM is through inhalation of the gas, though dermal absorption may be significant during manual reactor vessel cleaning. Vinyl chloride is readily absorbed through the respiratory tract. Its primary metabolite is chloroethylene oxide, which forms the reactive intermediate epoxide that can bind to RNA and DNA in vivo and may be responsible for the carcinogenicity observed in animal and human studies. The half-life of vinyl chloride monomer in expired air is 20–30 minutes. Thiodiglycolic acid is the major urinary metabolite, but it is of limited value in biomonitoring because of metabolic saturation of vinyl chloride, variable metabolism rates, and nonspecificity.

## Clinical Findings

### A. Symptoms & Signs:

**1. Acute exposure**–Vinyl chloride monomer has relatively low acute toxicity, causing respiratory irritation and central nervous system depression at high concentrations (10,000–20,000 ppm).

**2. Chronic exposure**–Chronic toxicity from vinyl chloride monomer exposure can result in hepatomegaly, osteolysis, Raynaud's phenomenon, vasalitic purpua, mixed connective tissue disease, and sclerodermalike skin lesions.

**a. Acro-osteolysis**–Symptoms of Raynaud's phenomenon, osteolysis in the terminal phalanges of some of the fingers, and thickening or raised nodules on the hands and forearms occurred rarely in workers employed in production and polymerization, especially associated with the cleaning of reactors. "Vinyl chloride disease" is a syndrome consisting of Raynaud's phenomenon, acroosteolysis, joint and muscle pain, enhanced collagen deposition, stiffness of the hands, and scleroderma-like skin changes. An increase in circulating immune complex levels, cryoglobulinemia, B-cell proliferation, hyperimmunoglobulinemia, and complement activation have been found in these patients. Susceptibility to this disease has been associated with the HLA-DR5 allele.

Vascular changes in the digital arteries of the hand associated with acro-osteolysis have been demonstrated by arteriography, and circulating immune complexes have been identified.

**b. Liver disease–**Hepatic fibrosis, splenomegaly, and thrombocytopenia with portal hypertension have occurred. The characteristic pattern of changes consists of hypertrophy and hyperplasia of hepatocytes and sinusoidal cells; sinusoidal dilation associated with damage to the cells lining the sinusoids; focal areas of hepatocellular degeneration; and fibrosis of portal tracts, septa, and intralobular perisinusoidal regions.

In 1974, three cases of hepatic angiosarcoma among polyvinyl chloride polymerization workers were reported at a plant in Louisville, Kentucky. Since then, many cohort mortality studies have documented an increased risk of hepatic angiosarcoma and cancers of the liver and biliary tract. The risk of hepatic angiosarcoma is related to the time since the first exposure, duration of employment, and the extent of exposure. IARC finds that vinyl chloride is carcinogenic to humans (Group 1), and NIOSH recommends that vinyl chloride be regulated as a potential human carcinogen. Vinyl chloride is genotoxic, causing increased chromosomal aberrations, sister chromatid exchanges, and lymphocyte micronuclei among exposed workers. An estimated 200–350 deaths from vinyl chloride-related angiosarcoma can be expected over the next 30 years.

Only two cases of hepatic angiosarcoma have been documented in the polyvinyl chloride processing-industry, suggesting a significantly lower vinyl chloride-related neoplastic risk among fabrication workers. Hemangioendothelioma has also been reported after both vinyl chloride and polyvinyl chloride exposure.

**c. Mortality studies–**Cohort mortality studies of vinyl chloride monomer-exposed workers have documented significant mortality rates for liver cancer, particularly hepatic angiosarcoma. After cessation of exposure, the increased risk of hepatic angiosarcoma continues for at least 6 years. Other than liver cancer, no excess cancer deaths have been observed.

**d. Pulmonary effects–**Cases of pneumoconiosis have been reported in workers exposed to polyvinyl chloride dust. Some polyvinyl chloride production and fabrication workers with high (>10 mg/m$^3$) exposure to polyvinyl chloride dust have reduced pulmonary function and an increased incidence of chest x-ray abnormalities. Cumulative polyvinyl chloride dust exposure has been associated with mild obstructive airway disease and a higher prevalence of small opacities on chest x-ray. One case of pneumoconiosis and systemic sclerosis following a 10-year exposure to polyvinyl chloride dust has been reported.

**e. Reproductive effects–**Decreased androgen levels and complaints of impotence, decreased libido, and sexual function have been found among male vinyl chloride-exposed workers. Few studies have evaluated the effects of vinyl chloride exposure on the reproductive function of female workers. A significant increase in congenital abnormalities has been found in communities located near a vinyl chloride-processing plant, although other studies have failed to report significant development toxicity in association with parental exposure to vinyl chloride or proximity to vinyl chloride facilities.

**B. Laboratory Findings:** There may be an increased frequency of elevated levels of liver enzymes and alkaline phosphatase in workers with vinyl chloride exposure. Fasting levels of serum bile acids and urinary coproporphyrins have been suggested as clinically useful indicators of early chemical injury in vinyl chloride monomer-exposed worker populations with asymptomatic liver dysfunction. Gray-scale ultrasonography of the liver has been helpful in identifying early hepatic injury in asymptomatic workers.

## Differential Diagnosis

Hepatic angiosarcoma has been associated with a history of arsenic exposure and thorium dioxide (Thorotrast) ingestion. Thoratrast and arsenic exposure may also cause hepatic angiosarcomas. Specific gene mutations at the p53 locus and mutant p21 proteins have been linked to vinyl chloride angiosarcoma. These findings suggest an effect of chloroethylene oxide, a carcinogenic metabolite of vinyl chloride. Serum anti-p53 antibodies or detection of serum mutant proteins may hold promise as a marker for high cancer risk among workers exposed to vinyl chloride. The vinyl chloride monomerassociated sclerotic changes in skin, with skin nodules, Raynaud's phenomenon, and osteolysis, are clinically very similar to idiopathic scleroderma; however, sclerodactyly, calcinosis, and digital pitting scars are unusual in vinyl chloride monomer disease.

## Prevention

The risk of hepatic angiosarcoma should be minimal if the 8-hour TWA is less than 1 ppm. If processing of vinyl chloride monomer production is controlled, general environmental risk is negligible.

**A. Work Practices:** Worker isolation is achieved in most polyvinyl chloride plants through the use of isolated process control rooms. For operators, cleaners, and utility employees, extensive engineering controls in polyvinyl chloride polymerization plants are required to reduce 8-hour TWA worker exposures to less than 1 ppm. Preventing worker exposure during routine maintenance and cleanup operation by adequate degassing of autoclaves and reaction vessels is essential. On-line gas chromatographic vinyl chloride monomer-specific detectors can identify leaks before large emissions develop.

Employees should be required to wear half-face supplied-air respirators when the concentration of vinyl chloride monomer exceeds 1 ppm. A full-face supplied-air respirator is required for reactor cleaning or other maintenance. Where skin contact is possible, protective uniforms, gloves, and head coverings and impervious boots are necessary.

Based on findings of pulmonary function changes and x-ray abnormalities, engineering controls to minimize polyvinyl chloride dust exposure should be taken.

**B. Medical Surveillance:** Preplacement medical examination should evaluate the presence of pre-existing liver disease. Preplacement and periodic measurement of liver enzymes is recommended by NIOSH, though the specificity and sensitivity of these tests are poor. Fasting levels of serum bile acids or plasma clearance of technetium-labeled iminodiacetate have been suggested as a sensitive measure of liver dysfunction among vinyl chloride-exposed workers. One study has suggested that an increased γ-glutamyl transpeptidase level is associated with vinyl chloride exposure, and this test may offer greater specificity for medical surveillance. Serum transaminase levels generally return to normal after removal from vinyl chloride exposure.

## Treatment

The mean survival after diagnosis of hepatic angiosarcoma is several months. Computed tomography with intravenous contrast dynamic scanning shows a characteristic isodense appearance on delayed postcontrast scans. Chemotherapy may slightly improve the duration and quality of survival. Acroosteolysis appears to be irreversible after cessation of exposure.

# REFERENCES

### ACIDS

Dayal HH et al: A community-based epidemiologic study of health sequelae of exposure to hydrofluoric acid. Ann Epidem 1992;2:213.

Hajela R et al: Fatal pulmonary edema due to nitric acid fume inhalation in three pulp-mill workers. Chest 1990;97:487.

IARC Working Group: Occupational exposures to mists and vapours from strong inorganic acids and other industrial chemicals. Working Group views and expert opinion, Lyon 15–22 October 1991. IARC Monogr Eval Carcinog Risks Hum 1992;54:1

Kirkpatrick JJ, Burd DA: An algorithmic approach to the treatment of hydrofluoric acid burns. Burns 1995;21:495.

Kirkpatrick JJ, Enion, DS, Burd DA: Hydrofluoric acid burns: A review. Burns 1995;21:483.

Sheridan RL et al: Emergency management of major hydrofluoric acid exposures. Burns 1995;21:62.

Terrill PJ, Gowar JP: Chronic acid burns: Beware, be aggressive, be watchful. Br J Plastic Surg 1990;43:699.

Tuominen M: occurrence of periodontal pockets and oral soft tissue lesions in relation to sulfuric acid fumes in the working environment. Acta Odontol Scand 1991;49:261.

### ALKALIS

Hansen KS, Isager H: Obstructive lung injury after treating wood with sodium hydroxide. J Soc Occup Med 1991;41:45.

Kuckelkorn R et al: Retrospective study of severe alkali burns of the eyes. Klin Monatsb Augenhelk 1993;203:397.

Leduc D et al: Acute and long term respiratory damage following inhalation of ammonia. Thorax 1992;47:755.

Lee Ka, Opeskin K: Fatal alkali burns. Forensic Sci Int 1995;72:219.

Rubin AE, Bentur L, Bentur Y: Obstructive airway disease associated with occupational sodium hydroxide inhalation. Br J Ind Med 1992;49:213.

Weiss SM, Lakshminarayan S: Acute inhalation injury. Clin Chest Med 1994;15:103.

Winewaker M, Douglas L, Peters W: Combination alkali/thermal burns caused by "black liquor" in the pulp and paper industry. Burns 1992;18:68.

### ACRYLAMIDE AND ACRYLONITRILE

Bachmann M, Myers JE, Bezuidenhout BN: Acrylamide monomer and peripheral neuropathy in chemical workers. Am J Ind Med 1992;21:217.

Calleman CJ: Relationships between biomarkers of exposure and neurological effects in a group of workers exposed to acrylamide. Toxico Appl Pharmacol 1994;126:361.

Deng H et al: Quantitative measures of vibration threshold in healthy adults and acrylamide workers. Int Arch Occup Environ Health 1993;65:53.

IARC: Acrylamide. IARC Monogr Eval Carcinog Risk Chem Hum 1994;60:389.

Ivanov V et al: Biological monitoring of acrylonitrile exposure through a new analytical approach to hemoglobin and plasma protein adducts and urinary metabolites in rats and humans. Int Arch Occup Environ Health 1993;65(Suppl):S103.

Myers JE, Macun I: Acrylamide neuropathy in a South African factory: An epidemiologic investigation. Am J Ind Med 1991;19:487.

Rothman KJ: Cancer occurrence among workers exposed to acrylonitrile. Scand Work Environ Health 1994;20:313.

Smith EA, Oehme FW: Acrylamide and polyacrylamide: A review of production, use, environmental fate and neurotoxicity. Rev Environ Health 1991;9:215.

US Department of Health and Human Services: Toxicological Profile for Acrylonitrile. Publication TP-90/02. US Department of Health and Human Services Agency for Toxic Substances and Disease Registry, 1990.

## AROMATIC AMINES

Choudhary G: Human health perspectives on environmental exposure to benzidine: A review. Chemosphere 1996;32:267.

Clavel et al: Occupational exposure to polycyclic aromatic hydrocarbons and the risk of bladder cancer: A French case-control study. Int J Epidemiol 1994;23:1145.

Cocker J, Nutley BP, Wilson HK: A biological monitoring assessment of exposure to methylene dianiline in manufacturers and users. Occup Environ Med 1994;51:519.

IARC: 4,4′-Methylenebis(2-chloroaniline) (MOCA): IARC Monogr Eval Carcinog Risks Hum 1993;57:271.

MMWR: NIOSH Alert: Request for assistance in preventing bladder cancer from exposure to o-toluidine and aniline. Morbid Mortal Weekly Rep 1991;40:353.

Schutze D et al: Biomonitoring of workers exposed to 4,4′-methylenedianiline or 4,4′-methylenediphenyl diisocyanate. Carcinogenesis 1995;16:573.

Sellers C, Markowitz S: Reevaluating the carcinogenicity of ortho-thouidine: A new conclusion and its implications. Regul Toxico Pharmaco 1992;16:301.

Shinka T et al: Factors affecting the occurrence of urothelial tumors in dye workers exposed to aromatic amines. Int J Uro 1995;2:243.

Shirai T: Etiology of bladder cancer. Semin Uro 1993;11:113.

Taylor JA et al: p 53 mutations in bladder tumors from arylamine-exposed workers. Cancer Res 1996;56:294.

Teass AW et al: Biological monitoring for occupational exposures to o-toluidine and aniline. Int Arch Occup Environ Health 1993;83:501.

US Department of Health and Human Services: Toxicological Profile for Benzidene. US Department of Health and Human Services Agency for Toxic Substances and Disease Registry, 1995.

US Department of Health and Human Services: Toxicological Profile for 4,4′-Methylenebis-(2-Chloroaniline). US Department of Health and Human Services Agency for Toxic Substances and Disease Registry, Atlanta, Publication TP-93/12, 1994.

Ward E et al: Excess number of bladder cancers in workers exposed to ortho-toluidine and aniline. JNCI 1991;83:501.

## CARBON DISULFIDE

Aaserud O et al: Carbon disulfide exposure and neurotoxic sequelae among viscose rayon workers. Am J Ind Med 1990;18:25.

Aaserud O et al: Region cerebral blood flow after long-term exposure to carbon disulfide. Acta Neurolo Scand 1992;85:266.

Cassitto MG et al: Carbon disulfide and the central nervous system: A 15-year neurobehavioral surveillance of an exposed population. Environ Res 1993;63:252.

Chu CC et al: Polyneuropathy induced by carbon disulphide in viscose rayon workers. Occup Environ Med 1995;52:404.

Drexler H et al: Carbon disulphide. III. Risk factors for coronary heart diseases in workers in the viscose industry. Int Arch Occup Environ Health 1995;67:5.

Ruijten MW et al: Special nerve functions and colour discrimination in workers with long term low level exposure to carbon disulphide. Br J Ind Med 1990;47:589.

US Department of Health and Human Services: Toxicological Profile for Carbon Disulfide. US Department of Health and Human Services Agency for Toxic Substances and Disease Registry, 1995.

Vanhoorne M, De Bacquer D, De Backer G: Epidemiological study of the cardiovascular effects of carbon disulphide. Int J Epidemiol 1992;21:745.

Vanhoorne M, Comhaire F, De Bacquer D: Epidemiological study of the effects of carbon disulfide on male sexuality and reproduction. Arch Environ Health 1994;49:273.

## CHLOREMETHYL ETHERS

Collingwood KW, Pasternack BS, Shore RE: An industry-wide study of respiratory cancer in chemical workers exposed to chloromethyl ethers. JNCI 1987;78:1127.

Coultas DB, Samet JM: Occupational lung cancer. Clin Chest Med 1992;13:341.

Gowers DS et al: Incidence of respiratory cancer among workers exposed to chloromethyl-ethers. Am J Epidemiol 1993;137:31.

US Department of Health and Human Services: Toxicological Profile for Bis(chloromethyl) Ether. US Department of Health and Human Services Agency for Toxic Substances and Disease Registry, 1989.

## DIBROMOCHLOROPROPANE

Potashnik G, Phillip M: Lack of birth defects among offspring conceived during or after parental exposure to dibromochloropropane (DBCP). Andrologia 1988;20:90.

Potashnik G, Porath A: Dibromochloropropane (DBCP): A 17-year reassessment of testicular function and reproductive performance. J Occup Environ Med 1995;37:1287.

Whorton MD et al: An epidemiologic investigation of birth outcomes in relation to dibromochloropropane contamination in drinking water in Fresno County,

California, USA. Int Arch Occup Environ Health 1989;61:403.

Wong O et al: Ecological analyses and case-control studies of gastric cancer and leukaemia in relation to DBCP in drinking water from Fresno County, California. Br J Ind Med 1989;46:521.

## DIMETHYLAMINOPROPIONITRILE

Baker EL et al: Follow-up studies of workers with bladder neuropathy caused by exposure to dimethylaminopropionitrile. Scand J Work Environ Health 1981;7(Suppl 4):54.

Keogh HP: Classical syndromes in occupational medicine: Dimethylaminopropionitrile. Am J Ind Med 1983;4:479.

Keogh JP et al: An epidemic of urinary retention caused by dimethylaminopropionitrile. JAMA 1980;243:746.

Kreiss K et al: Neurological dysfunction of the bladder in workers exposed to dimethylaminopropionitrile. JAMA 1980;243:741.

Mumtaz MM et al: Studies on the mechanism of urotoxic effects of N,N'-dimethylaminopropionitrile in rats and mice. 1. Biochemical and morphologic characterization of the injury and its relationship to metabolism. J Toxicol Environ Health 1991;33:1.

Mumtaz MM et al: The urotoxic effects of N,N'-dimethylaminopropionitrile 2. In vivo and in vitro metabolism. Toxicol Appl Pharmacol 1991;110:61.

## ETHYLENE OXIDE

Bisanti et al: Cancer mortality in ethylene oxide workers. Br J Ind Med 1993;50:317.

Deschamps D et al: Persistent asthma after accidental exposure to ethylene oxide. Br J Ind Med 1992;49:523.

Dretchen KL et al: Cognitive dysfunction in a patient with long-term occupational exposure to ethylene oxide. Role of ethylene oxide as a causal factor. J Occup Med 1992;34:1106.

Estrin WJ et al: Neutoxicological evaluation of hospital sterilizer workers exposed to ethylene oxide. J Toxicol Clin Toxicol 1990;28:1.

Hagmar L, Mikoczy Z, Welinder H: Cancer incidence in Swedish sterilant workers exposed to ethylene oxide. Occup Environ Med 1995;52:154.

IARC: Ethylene oxide. IARC Monogr Eval Carcinog Risk Chem Hum 1994;60:73.

Klees JE et al: Neuropsychologic "impairment" in a cohort study of hospital workers chronically exposed to ethylene oxide. J Toxicol Clin Toxicol 1990;28:21.

LaMontagne AD, Christiani DC, Kelsey KT: Utility of the complete blood count in routine medical surveillance for ethylene oxide exposure. Am J Ind Med 1993;24:191.

Norman SA et al: Cancer incidence in a group of workers potentially exposed to ethylene oxide. Int J Epidemiol 1995;24:276.

Ohnishi A, Murai Y: Polyneuropathy due to ethylene oxide, propylene oxide, and butylene oxide. Environ Res 1993;60:242.

Popp W et al: DNA-protein cross-links and sister chromatid exchange frequencies in lymphocytes and hydroxyethyl mercapturic acid in urine of ethylene oxide-exposed hospital workers. Int Arch Occup Environ Health 1994;313:81.

Schulte PA et al: Molecular, cytogenic, and hematological effects of ethylene oxide on female hospital workers. J Occup Environ Med 1995;37:313.

Shore RE, Gardner MJ, Pannett B: Ethylene oxide: An assessment of the epidemiological evidence on carcinogenicity. Br J Ind Med 1993;50:971.

Steenland K et al: Mortality among workers exposed to ethylene oxide. N Engl J Med 1991;324:1402.

Tates AD et al: Biological effect monitoring in industrial workers following incidental exposure to high concentrations of ethylene oxide. Mutat Res 1995;329:63.

US Department of Health and Human Services: Toxicological Profile for Ethylene Oxide. Publication TP-90/16, US Department of Health and Human Services Agency for Toxic Substances and Disease Registry, 1990.

van Sittert NJ et al: Monitoring occupational exposure to ethylene oxide by the determination of hemoglobin adducts. Environ Health Perspect 1993;99:217.

Verraes S, Michel O: Occupational asthma induced by ethylene oxide (Letter.) Lancet 1995;346:1434.

## FORMALDEHYDE

Akbar-Khanzadeh F et al: Formaldehyde exposure, acute pulmonary response, and exposure control options in a gross anatomy laboratory. Am J Ind Med 1994;26:61.

Alexandersson R, Hedenstierna G: Pulmonary function in wood workers exposed to formaldehyde: A prospective study. Arch Environ Health 1989;44:5.

Andjelkovich DA et al: Mortality of iron foundry workers. III. Lung cancer case control study. J Occup Med 1994;36:1301.

Blair A, Stewart PA, Hoover, RN: Mortality from lung cancer among workers employed in formaldehyde industries. Am J Ind Med 1990;17:683.

Blair A et al: Epidemiologic evidence on the relationship between formaldehyde exposure and cancer. Scand J Work Eviron Health 1990;16:381.

Gannon PF et al: Occupational asthma due to glutaraldehyde and formaldehyde endoscopy and x-ray departments. Thorax 1995;50:156.

Gardner MJ et al: A cohort study of workers exposed to formaldehyde in the British chemical industry: An update. Br J Ind Med 1993;50:827.

Gerin M et al: Cancer risks due to occupational exposure to formaldehyde: Results of a multi-site case-control study in Montreal. Int J Cancer 1989;44:53.

Grammer LC et al: Clinical and immunological evaluation of 37 workers exposed to gaseous formaldehyde. J Allergy Clin Immunol 1990;86:177.

Hansen J, Olsen JH: Formaldehyde and cancer morbidity among male employees in Denmark. Cancer Causes Control 1995;6:354.

Herbert FA et al: Respiratory consequences of exposure to wood dust and formaldehyde of workers manufacturing-oriented strand board. Arch Environ Health 1994;49:465.

Holmstrom M, Lund VJ: Malignant melanomas of the nasal cavity after occupational exposure to formaldehyde. Br J Ind Med 1991;48:9.

IARC: Formaldehyde. IARC Monogr Eval Carcinog Risks Hum 1995;62:217.

John EM, Savitz DA, Shy CM: Spontaneous abortions among cosmetologists. Epidemiology 1994;5:147.

Kilburn KH: Neurobehavioral impairment and seizures from formaldehyde. Arch Environ Health 1994;49:37.

Lemiere C et al: Occupational asthma due to formaldehyde resin dust with and without reaction to formaldehyde gas. Eur Respir J 1995;8:861.

Luce D et al: Sinonasal cancer and occupational exposure to formaldehyde and other substances. Int J Cancer 1993;53:224.

McLaughlin JK: Formaldehyde and cancer: A critical review. Int Arch Occup Environ Health 1994;66:295.

Sterling TD, Weinkam JJ: Mortality from respiratory cancers (including lung cancer) among workers employed in formaldehyde industries. Am J Ind Med 1994;25:593.

Taskinen H et al: Laboratory work and pregnancy outcome. J Occup Med 1994;36:311.

## NITRATES

Fandrem SI et al: Incidence of cancer among workers in a Norwegian nitrate fertiliser plant. Br J Ind Med 1993;50:647.

Jansen EH et al: A new physiological biomarker for nitrate exposure in humans. Toxicol Lett 1995;77:265.

Kanerva L et al: Occupational allergic contact dermatitis caused by nitroglycerin. Contact Dermatitis 1991;24:356.

Kristensen TS: Cardiovascular diseases and the work environment. A critical review of the epidemiologic literature on chemical factors. Scand J Work Environ Health 1989;15:245.

Stayner LT et al: Cardiovascular mortality among munitions workers exposed to nitroglycerin and dinitrotoluene. Scand J Work Environ Health 1992;18:34.

US Department of Health and Human Services: Case Studies in Environmental Medicine. Nitrate/Nitrite Toxicity. US Department of Health and Human Services Agency for Toxic Substances and Disease Registry, 1991.

## NITROSAMINES

Bartsch H: N-nitroso compounds and human cancer: Where do we stand? IARC Sci Publ 1991;105:1.

Cocco P et al: Occupational exposures as risk factors for gastric cancer in Italy. Cancer Causes Control 1994;5:241.

Eisen EA et al: Mortality studies of machining fluid exposure in the automobile industry. I. A standardized mortality ratio analysis. Am J Ind Med 1992;22:809.

Kato S et al: Human lung carcinogen-DNA adduct levels mediated by genetic polymorphisms in vivo. JNCI 1995;87:902.

Mirvish SS: Role of N-nitroso compounds (NOC) and N-nitrosation in etiology of gastric, esophageal, nasopharyngeal and bladder cancer and contribution to cancer of known exposures to NOC. Cancer Lett 1995;93:17.

Monarca S et al: Monitoring nitrite, N-nitrosodiethanolamine, and mutagenicity in cutting fluids used in the

metal industry. Environ Health Perspect 1993;101:126.

US Department of Health and Human Services: Toxicologic Profile for N-Nitrosodimethylamine. US Department of Health and Human Services Agency for Toxic Substances and Disease Registry, 1989.

US Department of Health and Human Services: Toxicological Profile for N-Nitrosodiphenylamine. US Department of Health and Human Services Agency for Toxic Substances and Disease Registry, 1993.

US Department of Health and Human Services: Toxicologic Profile for N-Nitrosodi-n-propylamine. US Department of Health and Human Services Agency for Toxic Substances and Disease Registry, 1989.

## PENTACHLOROPHENOL

Coenraads PJ et al: Chloracne. Some recent issues. Dermatol Clin 1994;12:569.

Colosio C et al: Toxicological ad immune findings in workers exposed to pentachlorophenol (PCP). Arch Environ Health 1993;48:81.

Hardell L, Eriksson M, Degerman A: Exposure to phenoxyacetic acids, chlorophenols, or organic solvents in relation to histopathology, stage, and anatomical localization of non-Hodgkin's lymphoma. Cancer Res 1994;54:2386.

IARC: Pentachlorophenol. IARC Monogr Eval Carcinog Risks Hum 1991;53:371.

Jorens PG, Schepens PJ: Human pentachlorophenol poisoning. Hum Exp Toxicol 1993;12:479.

Leet TL, Collins JJ: Chloracne and pentachlorophenol operations. Am J Ind Med 1991;20:815.

McConnachie PR, Zahalsky AC: Immunological consequences of exposure to pentachlorophenol. Arch Environ Health 1991;46:249.

Thind KS, Karmali S, House RA: Occupational exposure of electrical utility linemen to pentachlorophenol. Am Ind Hyg Assoc J 1991;52:547.

US Department of Health and Human Services: Case Studies in Environmental Medicine. Pentachlorophenol Toxicity. US Department of Health and Human Services Agency for Toxic Substances and Disease Registry, 1993.

US Department of Health and Human Services: Toxicological Profile for Pentachlorophenol. US Department of Health and Human Services Agency for Toxic Substances and Disease Registry, Publication TP-93/13, 1994.

## POLYCHLORINATED BIPHENYLS

Adami HO et al: Organochlorine compounds and estrogen-related cancers in women. Cancer Causes Control 1995;6:551.

Birnbaum LS: Endocrine effects of prenatal exposure to PCBs, dioxins, and other xenobiotics: Implications for policy and future research. Environ Health Perspect 1994;102:676.

Chase KH, Shields PG: Medical surveillance of hazardous waste site workers exposed to polychlorinated biphenyls (PCBs). Occup Med 1990;5:33.

Chen YC et al: A 6-year follow-up of behavior and activity disorders in the Taiwan Yu-Cheng children. Am J Public Health 1994;84:415.

Coenraads PJ et al: Chloracne. Some recent issues. Dermatol Clin 1994;12:569.

Hsu MM, Mak CP, Hsu CC: Follow-up of skin manifestations in Yu-Cheng children. Br J Dermatol 1995; 132:427.

Kimbrough RD: Polychlorinated biphenyls (PCBs) and human health: An update. Crit Rev Toxicol 1995;25: 133.

McKinney JD, Waller CL: Polychlorinated biphenyls as hormonally active structural analogues. Environ Health Perspect 1994;102:290.

Rogan WJ, Gladen BC: Neurotoxicology of PCBs and related compounds. Neurotoxicology 1992;13:27.

Sauer PJ et al: Effects of polychlorinated biphenyls (PCBs) and dioxins on growth and development. Hum Exp Toxicol 1994;13:900.

Silberhorn EM, Glauert HP, Robertson LW: Carcinogenicity of polyhalogenated biphenyls. Am J Epidemiol 1992;136:389.

Swanson GM, Ratcliffe HE, Fischer LJ: Human exposure to polychlorinated biphenyls (PCBs): A critical assessment of the evidence for adverse health effects. Regul Toxicol Pharmacol 1995;21:136.

US Department of Health and Human Services: Case Studies in Environmental Medicine. Polychlorinated biphenyl (PCB) toxicity. US Department of Health and Human Services Agency for Toxic Substances and Disease Registry, 1990.

Yassi A, Tate R, Fish D: Cancer mortality in workers employed at a transformer manufacturing plant. Am J Ind Med 1994;25:425.

## POLYCYCLIC AROMATIC HYDROCARBONS

Armstrong B et al: Lung cancer mortality and polynuclear aromatic hydrocarbons: A case-cohort study of aluminum production workers in Arvida, Quebec, Canada. Am J Epidemiol 1994;139:250.

Burgaz S, Borm PJ, Jongeneelen FJ: Evaluation of urinary excretion of 1-hydroxypyrenes and thioethers in workers exposed to bitumen fumes. Int Arch Occup Environ Health 1992;63:397.

Chiazze L Jr, Watkins DK, Amsel J: Asphalt and risk cancer in man. Br J Ind Med 1991;48:538.

Costantino JP, Redmond CK, Bearden A: Occupationally related cancer risk among coke oven workers: 30 years of follow-up. J Occup Environ Med 1995;37: 597.

Elovaara E et al: Significance of dermal and respiratory uptake in creosote workers: Exposure to polycyclic aromatic hydrocarbons and urinary excretion of 1-hydroxypyrene. Occup Environ Med 1995;52:196.

Gardiner K: Effects on respiratory morbidity of occupational exposure to carbon black: A review. Arch Environ Health 1995;50:44.

Hansen AM et al: Correlation between work-process-related exposure to polycyclic aromatic hydrocarbons and urinary levels of alpha-naphthol, beta-naphthylamine and 1-hydroxypyrene in iron foundry workers. Int Arch Occup Environ Health 1994;65:385.

Heikkila P et al: Urinary 1-naphthol and 1-pyrenol as indicators of exposure to coal tar products. Int Arch Occup Environ Health 1995;67:211.

Levin JO, Rhen M, Sikstrom E: Occupational PAH exposure: Urinary 1-hydroxypyrene levels of coke oven workers, aluminum smelter pot-room workers, road pavers, and occupationally non-exposed persons in Sweden. Sci Total Environ 1995;163:169.

Ovrebo S et al: Biological monitoring of exposure to polycyclic aromatic hydrocarbon in an electrode paste plant. J Occup Med 1994;36:303.

Partanen T, Boffetta P: Cancer risk in asphalt workers and roofers: Review and meta-analysis of epidemiologic studies. Am J Ind Med 1994;26:721.

Quinlan R et al: Urinary 1-hydroxypyrene: A biomarker for polycyclic aromatic hydrocarbon exposure in coal liquefaction workers. Occup Med 1995;45:63.

Ronneberg A, Andersen A: Mortality and cancer morbidity in workers from aluminum smelter with prebaked carbon anodes. Part II. Cancer morbidity. Occup Environ Med 1995;52:250.

Spinelli et al: Mortality and cancer incidence in aluminum reduction plant workers. J Occup Med 1991; 33:1150.

Tremblay C et al: Estimation of risk of developing bladder cancer among workers exposed to coal tar pitch volatiles in the primary aluminum industry. Am J Ind Med 1995;27:335.

US Department of Health and Human Services: Toxicological Profile for Benzo(a)pyrene. US Department of Health and Human Services Agency for Toxic Substances and Disease Registry, 1990.

US Department of Health and Human Services: Case Studies in Environmental Medicine. Polyaromatic Hydrocarbon (PAH) Toxicity. US Department of Health and Human Services Agency for Toxic Substances and Disease Registry, 1990.

US Department of Health and Human Services: Toxicological Profile for Creosote. US Department of Health and Human Services Agency for Toxic Substances and Disease Registry, 1995.

## STYRENE

Artuso M et al: Cytogenetic biomonitoring of styrene-exposed plastic boat builders. Arch Environ Contam Toxicol 1995;29:270.

Bergamaschi E et al: Immunological changes among workers exposed to styrene. Int Arch Occup Environ Health 1995;67:165.

Bond GG et al: Mortality among workers engaged in the development or manufacture of styrene-based products—An update. Scand J Work Environ Health 1992;18:145.

Campagna D et al: Visual dysfunction among styrene-exposed workers. Scand J Work Environ Health 1995;21:382.

Checkoway H et al: Platelet monoamine oxidase B activity in workers exposed to styrene. Int Arch Occup Environ Health 1994;66:359.

Coggon D: Epidemiological studies of styrene-exposed populations. Crit Rev Toxicol 1994;24(Suppl):S107.

Compton-Quintana PJ et al: Use of the glycophorin A human mutation assay to study workers exposed to styrene. Environ Health Perspect 1993;99:297.

Edling C et al: Increase in neuropsychiatric symptoms

after occupational exposure to low levels of styrene. Br J Ind Med 1993;50:843.

Hallier E et al: Intervention study on the influence of reduction of occupational exposure to styrene on sister chromatid exchanges in lymphocytes. Int Arch Occup Environ Health 1994;66:167.

Heseltine E et al: Assessment of the health hazards of 1,3-butadiene and styrene. Meeting report. J Occup Med 1993;35;1089.

Holz O et al: Determination of low level exposure to volatile aromatic hydrocarbons and genotoxic effects in workers at a styrene plant. Occup Environ Med 1995;52:420.

IARC: Styrene. IARC Monogr Eval Carcinog Risk Chem Hum 1994;60:233.

Kogevinas M et al: Cancer mortality in a historical cohort study of workers exposed to styrene. Scand J Work Environ Health 1994;20:251.

Kolstad HA et al: Exposure to styrene and chronic health effects: Mortality and incidence of solid cancers in the Danish reinforced plastics industry. Occup Environ Med 1995;52:320.

Kolstad HA et al: Incidence of lymphohematopoietic malignancies among styrene-exposed workers of the reinforced plastics industry. Scand J Work Environ Health 1994;20:272.

Landrigan PJ: Critical assessment of epidemiological studies on the carcinogenicity of 1,3-butadiene and styrene. IARC Sc Publ 1993;127:375.

Lindbohm ML: Effects of styrene on the reproductive health of women: A review. IARC Sci Publ 1993; 127:163.

Murata K, Araki S, Yokoyama K: Assessment of the peripheral, central, and autonomic nervous system function in styrene workers. Am J Ind Med 1991;20:775.

Norppa H, Sorsa M: Genetic toxicity of 1,3-butadiene and styrene. IARC Sc Publ 1993;127:185.

Pfaffli P,Saamanen A: The occupational scene of styrene. IARC Sci Publ 1993;127:15.

Santos-Burgoa C et al: Lymphohematopoietic cancer in styrene-butadiene polymerization workers. Am J Epidemiol 1992;136:843.

US Department of Health and Human Services: Toxicological Profile for Styrene. Publication TP-91/25. US Department of Health and Human Services Agency for Toxic Substances and Disease Registry, 1992.

## 2,3,7,8-TETRACHLORODIBENZO-p-DIOXIN

Bertazzi A et al: Cancer incidence in a population accidentally exposed to 2,3,7,8-Tetrachlorodibenzo-paradioxin. Epidemiology 1993;4:398.

Birnbaum LS: Developmental effects of dioxins. Environ Health Perspect 1995;103(Suppl 7):89.

Birnbaum LS: Workshop on perinatal exposure to dioxin-like compounds. V. Immunologic effects. Environ Health Perspect 1995;103(Suppl 2):157.

Calvert GM et al: Evaluation of chronic bronchitis, chronic obstructive pulmonary disease, and ventilatory function among workers exposed to 2,3,7,8-Tetrachlorodibenzo-p-dioxin. Am Rev Respir Dis 1991;144:1302.

Calvert GM et al: Evaluation of porphyria cutanea tarda in US workers exposed to 2,3,7,8-Tetrachlorodibenzo-p-dioxin. Am J Ind Med 1994;25:559.

Calvert GM et al: Hepatic and gastrointestinal effects in an occupational cohort exposed to 2,3,7,8-Tetrachlorodibenzo-p-dioxin. JAMA 1992;267:2209.

Collins JJ et al: The mortality experience of workers exposed to 2,3,7,8-tetrachlorodibenzo-p-dioxin in a trichlorophenol process accident. Epidemiology 1993; 4:7.

Egeland GM et al: Total serum testosterone and gonadotropins in workers exposed to dioxin. Am J Epidemiol 1994;139:272.

Eriksson M, Hardell L, Adami HO: Exposure to dioxins as a risk factor for soft tissue sarcoma: A population-based case-control study. JNCI 1990;82:486.

Eskenazi B, Kimmel G: Workshop on perinatal exposure to dioxin-like compounds. II. Reproductive effects. Environ Health Perspect 1995;103(Suppl 2): 143.

Fingerhut MA et al: Cancer mortality in workers exposed to 2,3,7,8-tetrachlorodibenzo-p-dioxin. N Engl J Med 1991;324:212.

Flesch-Janys D et al: Exposure to polychlorinated dioxins and furans (PCDD/F) and mortality in a cohort of workers from a herbicide-producing plant in Hamburg, Federal Republic of Germany. Am J Epidemiol 1995;142:1165.

Halperin W et al: Induction of P-450 in workers exposed to dioxin. Occup Environ Med 1995;52:86.

Hooper K, Clark GC: Workshop on perinatal exposure to dioxin-like compounds. VI. Role of biomarkers. Environ Health Perspect 1995;103(Suppl 2):161.

Kogevinas M et al: Cancer incidence and mortality in women occupationally exposed to chlorophenoxy herbicides, chlorophenols, and dioxins. Cancer Causes Control 1993;4:547.

Kogevinas M et al: Soft tissue sarcoma and non-Hodgkin's lymphoma in workers exposed to to phenoxy herbicides, chlorophenols, and dioxins: Two nested case-control studies. Epidemiology 1995;6:396.

Lindstrom G et al: Workshop on perinatal exposure to dioxin-like compounds. I. Summary. Environ Health Perspect 1995;103(Suppl 2):135.

National Academy of Sciences, Institute of Medicine. Veterans and Agent Orange Update 1996. National Academy Press, 1996.

Orban JE et al: Dioxins and dibenzofurans in adipose tissue of the general US population ad selected subpopulations. Am J Public Health 1994;84:439.

Schecter A et al: Dioxin concentrations in blood of workers at municipal waste incinerators. Occup Environ Med 1995;52:385.

Sweeney MH et al: Peripheral neuropathy after occupational exposure to 2,3,7,8-tetrachlorodibenzo-p-dioxin (TCDD). Am J Ind Med 1993;23:845.

Tamburro CH: Chronic liver injury in phenoxy herbicide-exposed Vietnam veterans. Environ Res 1992; 59:175.

US Department of Health and Human Services: Case Studies in Environmental Medicine. US Department of Health and Human Services Agency for Toxic Substances and Disease Registry, 1990.

US Department of Health and Human Services: Toxicological Profile for Chlorodibenzofurans. Publication

TP-93/04. US Department of Health and Human Services Agency for Toxic Substances and Disease Registry, 1994.

## VINYL CHLORIDE

Giri, AK: Genetic toxicology of vinyl chloride—A review. Muta Res 1995;339:1.

Laplanche A et al: Exposure to vinyl chloride monomer: Results of a cohort study after a seven year follow up. The French VCM Group. Br J Ind Med 1992;39:134.

Lundberg I et al: Mortality and cancer incidence among PVC-processing workers in Sweden. Am J Ind Med 1993;23:313.

Newshiwat LF et al: Hepatic angiosarcoma. Am J Med 1992;93:219.

Ng TP et al: Pulmonary effects of polyvinyl chloride dust exposure on compounding workers. Scand J Work Environ Health 1991;17:53.

Ostlere LS et al: Atypical systemic sclerosis following exposure to vinyl chloride monomer. A case report and review of the cutaneous aspects of vinyl chloride release. Clin Exp Dermatol 1992;17:208.

Pirastu R et al: Mortality from liver disease among Italian vinyl chloride monomer/polyvinyl chloride manufacturers. Am J Ind Med 1990;17:155.

Riordan SM et al: Vinyl chloride related hepatic angiosarcoma in a polyvinyl chloride autoclave cleaner in Australia. Med J Aust 1991;155:125.

Simonato L et al: A collaborative study of cancer incidence and mortality among vinyl chloride workers. Scand J Work Environ Health 1991;17:159.

Sinues B et al: Sister chromatid exchanges, proliferating rate index, and micronuclei in biomonitoring of internal exposure to vinyl chloride monomer in plastic industry workers. Toxicol App Pharmacol 1991;108:37.

Studnicka MJ et al: Pneumoconiosis and systemic sclerosis following 10 years of exposure to polyvinyl chloride dust. Thorax 1995;50:583.

Trivers GE et al: Anti-p53 antibodies in sera of workers occupationally exposed to vinyl chloride. JNCI 1995; 87:1400.

US Department of Health and Human Services: Case Studies in Environmental Medicine. Vinyl Chloride Toxicity. US Department of Health and Human Services Agency for Toxic Substances and Disease Registry, 1990.

US Department of Health and Human Services: Toxicological Profile for Vinyl Chloride. Publication TP-92/20. US Department of Health and Human Services Agency for Toxic Substances and Disease Registry, 1993.

Wong O et al: An industry-wide epidemiologic study of vinyl chloride workers, 1942–1982. Am J Ind Med 1991;20:317.

# Solvents　29

*Jon Rosenberg, MD, James E. Cone, MD, MPH,*
*& Elizabeth A. Katz, MPH, CIH*

## GENERAL PROPERTIES & HEALTH EFFECTS OF SOLVENTS

A solvent is any substance—usually a liquid at room temperature—that dissolves another substance, resulting in a solution (uniformly dispersed mixture). Solvents may be classified as aqueous (water-based) or organic (hydrocarbon-based). Since most of the substances that solvents are used to dissolve in industry are organic, most industrial solvents are organic chemicals. They are commonly used for cleaning, degreasing, thinning, and extraction.

Many solvent chemicals are also used as chemical intermediates in the manufacture and formulation of chemical products. However, more workers are exposed to high levels of solvents during use of the substances as cleaners, thinners, and in pesticide formulations.

Hundreds of individual chemicals are used to make over 30,000 industrial solvents. There are physical, chemical, and toxicologic properties that help to classify this large group of chemicals into families with shared or distinguishing features. These features will be discussed first, followed by a brief summary of the commonly used industrial solvents according to their chemical families.

## PHYSICAL & CHEMICAL PROPERTIES OF SOLVENTS

### Solubility

Lipid solubility is an important determinant of the efficiency of a substance as an industrial solvent and a major determinant of a number of health effects. The potency of solvents as general anesthetics and as defatting agents is directly proportionate to their lipid solubility.

Dermal absorption is related to both lipid solubility and water solubility (since the skin behaves like a lipid-water sandwich), so that solvents such as dimethyl sulfoxide, dimethylformamide, and glycol ethers, which are highly soluble in both (amphi-pathic), are well absorbed through the skin. All organic solvents are lipid-soluble, but this solubility may differ to a significant degree.

### Flammability & Explosiveness

Flammability and explosiveness are the properties of a substance that allow it to burn or ignite, respectively. Some organic solvents are flammable enough to be used as fuels, whereas others (eg, halogenated hydrocarbons) are so nonflammable that they are used as fire-extinguishing agents. Flash point, ignition temperature, and flammable and explosive limits are measures of flammability and explosiveness. The National Fire Prevention Association (NFPA) rates flammability hazards by a numerical code from 0 (no hazard) to 4 (severe hazard). Flash points and NFPA codes are listed in Table 29–1. These properties are important to consider when selecting a solvent or substituting one solvent for another on the basis of undesirable health effects or efficacy.

### Volatility

Volatility is the tendency of a liquid to evaporate (form a gas or vapor). Other conditions being equal, the greater the volatility of a substance, the greater the concentration of its vapors in air. Since the most common route of exposure to solvents is inhalation, exposure to a solvent is highly dependent on its volatility. Solvents as a class are all relatively volatile over a wide range. Vapor pressure and evaporation rate are two measures of volatility listed in Table 29–1.

### Chemical Structure

Solvents can be divided into families according to chemical structure and the attached functional groups. Toxicologic properties tend to be similar within a group, such as liver toxicity from chlorinated hydrocarbons and irritation from aldehydes. The basic structures are aliphatic, alicyclic, and aromatic. The functional groups include halogens, alcohols, ketones, glycols, esters, ethers, carboxylic acids, amines, and amides.

| | Flash Point (°F) | NFPA Flamma-bility Code[1] | Vapor Pressure (mm Hg 25 °C) | Evapora-tion Rate[2] | TLV[3] (ppm) | Odor Thresh-old[4] (ppm) | Biologic Monitor[5] | General Hazards of Chemical Family and Unique Hazards of Specific Compounds |
|---|---|---|---|---|---|---|---|---|
| **Aliphatic** | | | | | | | | Anesthetic > irritant. |
| Pentane | −40 | 4 | 500 | 1 | 600 | 400 | | |
| n-Hexane | −10 | 3 | 150 | 1.9 | 50 | 130 | + | Peripheral neuropathy. |
| Hexane (other) | −10 | 3 | 150 | 1.9 | 500 | 130 | | Hazard relative to concen-tration of n-hexane. |
| Heptane | 25 | 3 | 50 | 2.7 | 400 | 150 | | |
| Octane | 55 | 3 | 15 | 5.9 | 300 | 50 | | |
| Nonane | 90 | 0 | 5 | 2.9 | 200 | 50 | | |
| **Alicyclic** | | | | | | | | Anesthetic > irritant. |
| Cyclohexane | 10 | 3 | 95 | 2.6 | 300 | 25 | | |
| **Aromatic** | | | | | | | | Anesthetic > irritant. |
| Benzene | 10 | 3 | 75 | 2.8 | 10(0.3) | 10 | + | Leukemia and aplastic anemia. |
| Toluene | 40 | 3 | 30 | 4.5 | 100 | 5 | + | Renal tubular acidosis, cerebellar dysfunction. |
| Xylenes (all) | 85 | 3 | 10 | 9.5 | 100 | 1 | + | |
| Ethyl benzene | 60 | 3 | 5 | 9.4 | 100 | 1 | + | |
| Cumene | 95 | 2 | 10 | 14 | 50-S | 0.1 | + | |
| Styrene | 90 | 3 | 5 | 12.4 | 50-S(20) | 0.5 | + | |
| **Petroleum distillates** | | | | | | | | Hazard relative to aliphatic and aromatic components: |
| Petroleum ether | ~ −50 | 3 | ~ 40 | ~ 1.1 | . . . | . . . | | 100% aliphatic, extremely volatile, flammable. |
| Rubber solvent | ~ −20 | 3 | . . . | ~ 2.3 | 400 | . . . | | Mostly aliphatic, extremely volatile, flammable. |
| V M & P naphtha[6] | ~ 30 | 3 | ~ 20 | ~ 7.1 | 300 | . . . | | Mostly aliphatic. |
| Mineral spirits I | ~ 100 | 3 | ~ 5 | ~ 4.4 | 100 | . . . | | |
| Aromatic petroleum naphtha | ~ 110 | 3 | ~ 5 | . . . | . . . | . . . | | Mostly aromatic. |
| Kerosene | ~ 115 | 3 | ~ 5 | . . . | . . . | . . . | | |
| **Alcohols** | | | | | | | | Irritant > anesthetic. |
| Methyl alcohol | 50 | 3 | 90 | 5.2 | 200-S | 100 | + | Acidosis, optic neuropathy. |
| Ethyl alcohol | 55 | 3 | 45 | ~ 7 | 1000 | 85 | | "Fetal alcohol syndrome" (ingestion). |
| 1-Propyl alcohol | 75 | 3 | 20 | 7.8 | 200-S | 2 | | |
| Isopropyl alcohol | 55 | 3 | 35 | 7.7 | 400 | 20 | | |
| n-Butyl alcohol | 85 | 3 | 10 | 19.6 | 50-S | 1 | | Auditory, vestibular nerve injury reported. |
| sec-Butyl alcohol | 75 | 3 | 15 | 12.3 | 100 | 2 | | |
| tert-Butyl alcohol | 50 | 3 | 15 | . . . | 100 | 50 | | |
| Iso-octyl alcohol | 185 | 2 | 0.05 | 300 | 50-S | . . . | | |
| Cyclohexanol | 155 | 2 | 1 | 150 | 50-S | 0.1 | | |
| **Glycols** | | | | | | | | Extremely low volatility. |
| Ethylene glycol aerosol | 230 | 1 | 0.05 | . . . | 39.4 | . . . | | Acidosis, seizures, renal failure (ingestion). |
| **Phenols** | | | | | | | | Irritant > anesthetic; cytotoxic, corrosive. |
| Phenol | 175 | 2 | 0.5 | . . . | 5-S | 0.05 | + | Dermal absorption of |
| Cresol | 180 | 2 | 0.2 | >400 | 5-S | . . . | | vapors. |
| **Ketones** | | | | | | | | Irritant, strong odor > anes-thetic. |
| Acetone | −5 | 3 | 20 | 1.9 | 750 | 15 | + | |
| Methyl ethyl ketone | 15 | 3 | 70 | 2.7 | 200 | 5 | + | |
| Methyl isobutyl ketone | 70 | 3 | 5 | 5.6 | 50 | 1 | | |
| Diacetone alcohol | 140 | 2 | 1 | ~ 60 | 50 | 0.1 | | |
| Mesityl oxide | 90 | 3 | 10 | 8.4 | 15 | 0.5 | | |
| Cyclohexanone | 110 | 2 | 3 | 22.2 | 25-S | 1 | | |

(continued)

| | Flash Point (°F) | NFPA Flamma-bility Code[1] | Vapor Pressure (mm Hg 25 °C) | Evapora-tion Rate[2] | TLV[3] (ppm) | Odor Thresh-old[4] (ppm) | Biologic Monitor[5] | General Hazards of Chemical Family and Unique Hazards of Specific Compounds |
|---|---|---|---|---|---|---|---|---|
| **Esters** | | | | | | | | Irritant, strong odor > anes-thetic. |
| Methyl formate | −2 | 3 | 475 | 1.6 | 100 | 600 | | Optic neuropathy from metabolism to formic acid. |
| Ethyl formate | −5 | 3 | 200 | 1.8 | 100 | 30 | | |
| Methyl acetate | 15 | 3 | 175 | 2.2 | 200 | 5 | | Optic neuropathy from metabolism to methanol. |
| Ethyl acetate | 25 | 3 | 75 | 2.7 | 400 | 5 | | |
| n-Propyl acetate | 55 | 3 | 35 | 4.8 | 200 | 0.5 | | |
| n-Butyl acetate | 75 | 3 | 10 | 5.2 | 150(20) | 0.5 | | |
| n-Amyl acetate | 85 | 3 | 5 | 11.6 | 100 | 0.05 | | Odorant ("banana oil"). |
| **Ethers** | | | | | | | | |
| Ethyl ether | −50 | 4 | 450 | 1 | 400 | 10 | | Extremely volatile, flamma-ble, explosive. |
| Dioxane | 54 | 3 | 27 | 14 | 25-S | 24 | | Carcinogenic in animals. |
| **Glycol ethers** | | | | | | | | Skin absorption without irri-tation. |
| 2-Methoxyethanol | 100 | 2 | 10 | 21.1 | 5-S | 2 | + | Reproductive toxicity in male and female animals. |
| 2-Ethoxyethanol | 110 | 2 | 5 | 28.1 | 5-S | 3 | + | Reproductive toxicity in male and female animals. |
| 2-Butoxyethanol | 340 | 2 | 1 | ~ 85 | 25-S | 0.1 | | Anemia. |
| Propylene glycol monomethyl ether | 100 | 3 | 10 | . . . | 100 | 10 | | |
| Dipropylene glycol monomethyl ether | 185 | 2 | 0.5 | . . . | 100-S | . . . | | |
| **Glycidyl ethers** | | | | | | | | Sensitizers, genetic and reproductive toxins. |
| Phenyl glycidyl ether | . . . | . . . | 0.01 | . . . | 0.1 | . . . | | Carcinogenic in animals |
| Diglycidyl ether | . . . | . . . | 0.1 | . . . | 0.1 | . . . | | |
| **Acids** | | | | | | | | Irritant > anesthetic. |
| Formic | . . . | . . . | . . . | 45 | 5 | 0.1 | | |
| Acetic | 105 | 2 | 15 | 11 | 10 | 0.5 | | |
| Propionic | . . . | . . . | . . . | 5 | 10 | 0.2 | | |
| **Amines** | | | | | | | | Irritant > anesthetic; corneal edema, visual halos. |
| Methylamine | . . . | . . . | gas | gas | 5 | 3 | | |
| Dimethylamine | . . . | . . . | gas | gas | 5 | 0.5 | | |
| Trimethylamine | . . . | . . . | gas | gas | 5 | 0.0005 | | |
| Ethylamine | <0 | 4 | gas | gas | 5–5 | 1 | | |
| Diethylamine | −9 | 3 | 240 | 2.2 | 5–5 | 0.2 | | |
| Triehylamine | 20 | 3 | 70 | 2.7 | 1–5 | 0.5 | | |
| Butylamine | 10 | 3 | 70 | 5.1 | 5-S | 2 | | |
| Cyclohexylamine | 90 | 3 | 10 | 82.9 | 10 | 2.5 | | |
| Ethylenediamine | 95 | 2 | 10 | >5000 | 10-S | 1 | | Allergic contact dermatitis, asthma. |
| Diethylene triamine | 215 | 1 | 0.5 | >400 | 1-S | . . . | | |
| Ethanolamine | 185 | 2 | 0.5 | >5000 | 3 | 2.5 | | |
| Diethanolamine | 280 | 1 | 0.05 | >5000 | 0.46-S | 0.5 | | |
| **Chlorinated hydrocarbons** | | | | | | | | Cancer in animals; liver, kid-ney, cardiac effects. |
| Methyl chloroform (1,1,1,-trichloro-ethane) | NF | 0 | 120 | 2.7 | 350 | 120 | + | |
| Trichloroethylene | . . . | 1 | 75 | 3.1 | 50 | 30 | + | Alcohol intolerance, degreaser's flush. |
| Perchloroethylene (tetrachloroethyl-ene) | NF | 0 | 20 | 6.6 | 25 | 25 | + | Carcinogenic in animals. |

*(continued)*

**Table 29–1.** Industrial solvents: Properties, odor thresholds, and exposure limits. (continued)

| | Flash Point (°F) | NFPA Flamma-bility Code[1] | Vapor Pressure (mm Hg 25 °C) | Evapora-tion Rate[2] | TLV[3] (ppm) | Odor Thresh-old[4] (ppm) | Biologic Monitor[5] | General Hazards of Chemical Family and Unique Hazards of Specific Compounds |
|---|---|---|---|---|---|---|---|---|
| Methylene chloride | NF | 0 | 420 | 1.8 | 50 | 250 | + | Metabolized to carbon mon-oxide, suspect human carcinogen. |
| Carbon tetrachloride | NF | 0 | 110 | 2.6 | 5-S | 100 | | Cirrhosis, liver cancer. |
| Chloroform | NF | 0 | 190 | 2.2 | 10 | 85 | | Suspect human carcinogen. |
| 1,1,2-Trichloro-ethane | NF | 0 | 20 | 12.6 | 10-S | . . . | | |
| 1,1,2,2-Tetra-chloroethane | NF | 0 | 10 | 19.1 | 1-S | 1.5 | | |
| **Chlorofluorocar-bons** | | | | | | | | Weak anesthetic, irritant; cardiac effects. |
| Trichlorofluoro-methane (F-11) | NF | 0 | 330 | 1.6 | 1000 | 5 | | |
| Dichlorodifluoro-methane (F-12) | NF | 0 | . . . | . . . | 1000 | . . . | | |
| Chlorodifluoro-methane (F-22) | NF | 0 | . . . | . . . | 1000 | . . . | | |
| 1,1,2,2-Tetra-chloro-2,2-difluoroethane (F-112) | NF | 0 | . . . | . . . | 500 | . . . | | |
| 1,1,2-Trichloro-1,2,2-trifluoro-ethane (F-113) | NF | 0 | 325 | 2 | 1000 | 45 | | |
| 1,2-Dichlorotetra-fluoroethane (F-114) | . . . | . . . | . . . | . . . | 1000 | . . . | | |
| Chloropentafluoro-ethane (F-115) | . . . | . . . | . . . | . . . | 1000 | . . . | | |
| **Miscellaneous** | | | | | | | | |
| Turpentine | 100 | 3 | . . . | ~ 375 | 100 | . . . | | Irritant > anesthetic; allergic contact dermatitis. |
| Dimethylsulfoxide | 200 | 1 | . . . | >300 | . . . | . . . | | Hepatotoxic > anesthetic; skin absorption. |
| Dimethylformamide | 140 | 2 | 5 | 45 | 10-S | 2 | | Smell in breath after expo-sure; skin absorption. |
| Tetrahydrofuran | 5 | 3 | 175 | 2 | 200 | 2 | | Anesthetic, irritant. |

[1]See text for explanation.
[2]Ether = 1, see text for explanation.
[3]American Conference of Governmental Industrial Hygienists (ACGIH) threshold limit value, 8-hour time-weighted average, 1994–95 adopted (1955–96 proposed change). S = "skin" designation.
[4]Population odor threshold determined by testing.
[5]Information available on biological monitoring; see Chapter 38.
[6]Varnish makers' and painters' naphtha.

# PHARMACOKINETICS OF SOLVENTS

## Absorption (Route of Exposure)

**A. Pulmonary:** Since organic solvents are gen-erally volatile liquids and since the vapors are lipid-soluble and therefore well absorbed across the alveo-lar-capillary membrane, inhalation is the primary route for occupational exposure. The pulmonary re-tention or uptake (percentage of inhaled dose that is retained and absorbed) for most organic solvents ranges from 40% to 80% at rest. Because physical la-bor increases pulmonary ventilation and blood flow, the amount of solvent delivered to the alveoli and the amount absorbed are likewise increased. Levels of physical exercise commonly encountered in the workplace will increase the pulmonary uptake of many solvents by a factor of 2–3 times that at rest.

**B. Percutaneous:** The lipid solubility of or-ganic solvents results in most being absorbed through the skin to some degree following direct contact. However, percutaneous absorption is also determined by water solubility and volatility. Solvents that are soluble in both lipid and water are most readily absorbed through the skin. Highly volatile substances are less well absorbed since they tend to evaporate from the skin unless evaporation is prevented by occlusion.

For a number of solvents, dermal absorption contributes to overall exposure sufficiently to result in a "skin" designation for the American Conference of Governmental Industrial Hygienists (ACGIH) threshold limit values (TLVs), as set forth in Table 29–1. For a few solvents, significant absorption of vapors through the skin can also occur. This is most likely to occur when solvents with a "skin" designation and low TLV are used in a situation that results in very high airborne concentrations, such as in an enclosed space with respiratory protection.

### Distribution

Since organic solvents are lipophilic, they tend to be distributed to lipid-rich tissue. In addition to adipose tissue, this includes the nervous system and liver. Since distribution occurs via the blood and since the blood-tissue membrane barriers are usually rich in lipids, solvents are also distributed to organs with large blood flows, such as cardiac and skeletal muscle. Persons with greater amounts of adipose tissue will accumulate greater amounts of a solvent over time and consequently will excrete larger amounts at a slower rate after cessation of exposure. Most solvents will cross the placenta and also enter breast milk.

### Metabolism

Some solvents are extensively metabolized and some not at all metabolized. The metabolism of a number of solvents plays a key role in their toxicity and in some cases the treatment of intoxication. The role of toxic metabolites is discussed in their respective sections for n-hexane, methyl n-butyl ketone, methyl alcohol, ethylene glycol, diethylene glycol, methyl acetate, methyl formate, and glycol ethers. A number of solvents, including trichloroethylene, are metabolized in common with ethyl alcohol (ethanol) by alcohol and aldehyde dehydrogenase. Competition for these limited enzymes accounts for synergistic effects ("alcohol intolerance" and "degreaser's flush") and may result in reactions in workers exposed to these solvents while taking disulfiram (Antabuse) for alcoholism. Chronic ethanol ingestion may induce solvent-metabolizing enzymes and lower blood solvent concentrations. Other solvents may have acute and chronic interactions similar to those of ethanol.

### Excretion

Excretion of solvents occurs primarily through exhalation of unchanged compound, elimination of metabolites in urine, or a combination of each. Solvents such as perchloroethylene that are poorly metabolized are excreted primarily through exhalation. The biological half-life of parent compounds varies from a few minutes to several days, so that some solvents accumulate to some degree over the course of the work week while others do not. However, bioaccumulation beyond a few days is not an important determinant of adverse health effects for most solvents.

### BIOLOGICAL MONITORING

Biologic monitoring can provide a more accurate measure of exposure than environmental monitoring for some solvents (see Table 29–1 and Chapter 38). This is particularly true for substances whose pulmonary absorption is affected to a large degree by physical work and those with significant dermal exposure and absorption (ie, those with ACGIH "skin" designations [Table 29–1]). Unfortunately, solvents have properties that tend to make biologic monitoring less useful or practical: (1) They tend to be rapidly absorbed and excreted, so that biological levels change rapidly over time; and (2) exposure over very short intervals is often a more important determinant of adverse health effects than 8-hour or longer exposures. However, biological monitoring has been investigated for a number of solvents. The ACGIH has recommended biological exposure indices (BEIs) for the following solvents: n-hexane, benzene, toluene, xylenes, ethyl benzene, styrene, phenol, methyl ethyl ketone, perchloroethylene, trichloroethane (methyl chloroform), trichloroethylene, dimethylformamide, and carbon disulfide. For many solvents, significant levels may be present only in exhaled air, which is currently cumbersome to sample. A number of laboratories offer whole-blood or plasma analysis of solvents. For solvents with relatively slow excretion, such as perchloroethylene and methyl chloroform, analysis of blood is a reasonable alternative to analysis of exhaled air. However, for those with relatively fast excretion (most of the rest), the timing of the sample is critical—even within minutes—and the results are therefore difficult to interpret. Most solvents distribute into several compartments in the body, so that the decline in blood levels exhibits several consecutive half-times, with the first being very short, on the order of 2–10 minutes. A blood sample taken immediately after an exposure will reflect primarily peak exposure at that time. A sample taken 15–30 minutes after termination of exposure will reflect exposure over the preceding few hours, while a sample taken 16–20 hours after exposure (prior to the next shift) will reflect mean exposure over the preceding day. The distribution of exposure over an 8-hour shift will also affect the validity of the biological sample.

# HEALTH EFFECTS OF SOLVENTS

## SKIN DISORDERS

Up to 20% of cases of occupational dermatitis are caused by solvents (see Chapter 18). Almost all organic solvents are primary skin irritants as a result of defatting, or the dissolution of lipids from the skin. The potency of solvents for defatting the skin is related directly to lipid solubility and inversely to percutaneous absorptivity and volatility. In addition to concentration and duration of exposure, a critical factor in the development of solvent dermatitis is occlusion of the exposed area of skin, such as by clothes and leaking protective clothing. A few industrial solvents can also cause allergic contact dermatitis. Scleroderma was found to be significantly associated with exposure to organic solvents in a recent case-reference study.

The most common work practice leading to solvent dermatitis is washing the hands with solvents. The occupations most commonly associated with solvent dermatitis are painting, printing, mechanics, and dry cleaning, though workers are at risk wherever solvents are used.

### Clinical Findings
**A. Symptoms & Signs:** Diagnosis is based on the typical appearance of the skin and a history of direct contact with solvents. The typical appearance ranges from an acute irritant dermatitis manifested by erythema and edema to a chronic dry, cracked eczema. Areas of skin affected by solvent dermatitis are more permeable to chemicals than unaffected skin and are susceptible to secondary bacterial infection.

**B. Laboratory Findings:** Patch testing is rarely indicated since few solvents (principally turpentine and formaldehyde) cause allergic contact dermatitis. Patch testing with actual material used in the workplace may be necessary on occasion.

### Differential Diagnosis
Consideration must sometimes be given to the possibility of other sources of irritant or allergic contact dermatitis. Use of waterless hand cleansers that contain alcohols and emollients that contain sensitizers may exacerbate or cause irritant or allergic dermatitis.

### Treatment & Prevention
Treatment of dermatitis due to solvents is the same as for contact dermatitis from other causes: topical corticosteroids, emollients, and skin care. Prevention depends upon education of workers about proper handling of solvents, use of engineering controls to minimize direct contact with solvents, provisions for alternatives to washing with solvents, and the use of solvent-resistant barrier creams or protective clothing where appropriate.

### Prognosis
The resolution of solvent dermatitis depends on elimination of direct solvent contact with involved areas of skin.

## CENTRAL NERVOUS SYSTEM EFFECTS

### 1. ACUTE CENTRAL NERVOUS SYSTEM EFFECTS

Almost all volatile lipid-soluble organic chemicals cause general, nonspecific depression of the central nervous system, or general anesthesia. Beginning with ethyl ether, a number of industrial solvents were used historically as surgical anesthetics. There is good correlation between lipid solubility, as measured by the air-olive oil partition coefficient, and anesthetic potency. However, the mechanism of action of general anesthesia by any agent is not known. Excitable tissue is depressed at all levels of the central nervous system, both brain and spinal cord. Lipid solubility—and therefore anesthetic potency—increases with length of carbon chain, substitution with halogen or alcohol, and the presence of unsaturated (double) carbon bonds.

### Clinical Findings
**A. Symptoms & Signs:** The symptoms of central nervous system depression from acute intoxication by organic solvents are the same as those from drinking alcoholic beverages. Indeed, there is currently no evidence that ethyl alcohol has any acute effects on the central nervous system other than general anesthesia. Symptoms range from headache, nausea and vomiting, dizziness, light-headedness, vertigo, disequilibrium, slurred speech, euphoria, fatigue, sleepiness, weakness, irritability, nervousness, depression, disorientation, and confusion to loss of consciousness and death from respiratory depression. A secondary hazard from these effects is increased risk of accidents. Excitatory manifestations of early intoxication are the result of depression of inhibitory functions and correspond to stage I anesthesia.

The acute effects are related to the concentration of the chemical in the nervous system, so resolution of symptoms correlates with the biological half-life, which ranges from a few minutes to less than 24 hours for most industrial solvents. However, it must be kept in mind that many solvent exposures are to mixtures of solvents and that the effects of each solvent are at least additive and may be synergistic.

Tolerance to the acute effects can occur, particularly for those compounds with longer half-lives, and is generally not metabolic in nature (ie, not due to increased rates of metabolism and excretion). The development of tolerance may be accompanied by morning "hangovers" and even frank withdrawal symptoms on weekends and vacations, alleviated by ingestion of alcohol. Additive and synergistic effects have both been described for interactions between organic solvents and with drinking alcohol.

**B. Laboratory Findings:** Biologic monitoring may provide an accurate assessment of exposure to some solvents, but there is little information on the correlation of biological levels with degrees of intoxication.

### Differential Diagnosis

Acute solvent intoxication must be distinguished from that resulting from the use of alcohol or psychoactive drugs on the basis of exposure.

### Treatment

The sole treatment for acute solvent intoxication is removal from exposure to solvents or any other anesthetic or central nervous system depressant until the signs and symptoms have completely resolved. The use of alcohol or other central nervous system depressant medication should be avoided. Analgesics for headache may be necessary, but nonnarcotic medication is usually adequate.

### Prognosis

Most symptoms resolve in a time course parallel to the elimination of the solvent and any active metabolites, though headaches may persist for up to a week or more following acute exposure. Persistence of central nervous system dysfunction following severe overexposure with coma suggests hypoxic brain damage. The occurrence of persistent neurobehavioral dysfunction following acute overexposure has been reported anecdotally and in a few case series, particularly impairment of memory.

### 2. CHRONIC CENTRAL NERVOUS SYSTEM EFFECTS

Alcohol is now well recognized as causing neurobehavioral dysfunction in chronic alcoholics. It is reasonable to assume that sufficient chronic exposure to organic solvents could also cause chronic adverse neurobehavioral effects. A variety of terms have been applied to these effects when associated with solvent exposure: chronic toxic encephalopathy, presenile dementia, chronic solvent intoxication, painter's syndrome, psychoaffective disorder, and neurasthenic syndrome.

A number of epidemiologic studies of workers chronically exposed to organic solvents have demonstrated an increased incidence of adverse neurobehavioral effects. These effects have been best demonstrated in groups of workers with relatively high exposures, such as boat builders and spray painters, and with specific types of exposure, such as to carbon disulfide (see Chapter 28). Such effects include subjective symptoms, changes in personality or mood, and impaired intellectual function as assessed by batteries of neurobehavioral tests. Decrements in short-term memory and psychomotor function are consistent findings. The nature of these tests and uncertainty about the significance of the results are discussed in Chapter 24. Dose-response data and correlation of chronic with acute effects are becoming more available. Correlation of symptoms with test results is often lacking, so that the interpretation of neurobehavioral test results in an individual must be made by experienced observers. Solvent-exposed workers are at increased risk of requiring disability pension for neuropsychiatric disorders in a number of industrialized countries.

Chronic brain damage from chronic alcoholism or drug abuse is not well understood, but similar mechanisms may be present with chronic solvent exposure. Cortical atrophy may represent the underlying pathologic changes. A recent study suggests a possible association between Alzheimer's disease and history of solvent exposure.

In addition to neuropsychological dysfunction, there are other potential chronic central neurotoxic effects of solvents that can be considered briefly here. Acute and perhaps chronic intoxication with solvents can result in vestibulo-oculomotor disturbances, presumably due to effects on the cerebellum. A syndrome called acquired intolerance to organic solvents in which dizziness, nausea, and weakness after exposure to minimal solvent vapor concentrations with normal vestibular test results has been reported.

### Clinical Findings

Symptoms commonly reported are headache, mood disturbance (depression, anxiety), fatigue, memory loss (primarily short-term), and difficulty in concentrating. Clinical examination may reveal signs of impairment in recent memory, attention span, and motor or sensory function. The Swedish Q16 questionnaire (Table 29–2) may be useful in the evaluation of workers with long-term solvent exposure.

### Diagnosis

Test results that have been associated with solvent exposure in group studies include alteration of a variety of neurobehavioral tests; pneumoencephalography, CT scan, and cerebral blood flow studies showing evidence of diffuse cerebral cortical atrophy; and electroencephalographic abnormalities, particularly diffuse low wave patterns. These tests should not be

**Table 29–2.** Swedish Q16 questionnaire for long-term solvent-exposed workers.

This questionnaire is used to help determine whether long-term *overexposure* to solvents has affected the central nervous system (brain)—answer "yes" or "no" to each question.[1]
   1. Do you have a short memory?
   2. Have your relatives told you that you have a short memory?
   3. Do you often have to make notes about what you must remember?
   4. Do you often have to go back and check things you have done (turned off the stove, locked the door, etc)?
   5. Do you generally find it hard to get the meaning from reading newspapers and books?
   6. Do you have problems with concentrating?
   7. Do you often feel irritated without any particular reason?
   8. Do you often feel depressed without any particular reason?
   9. Are you abnormally tired?
   10. Are you less interested in sex than what you think is normal?
   11. Do you have heart palpitations even when you don't exert yourself?
   12. Do you sometimes have a feeling of pressure in your chest?
   13. Do you perspire without any particular reason?
   14. Do you have a headache at least once a week?
   15. Do you often have a painful tingling in some part of your body?

[1]If a solvent-exposed worker answers "yes" to six or more of these questions, referral for more in-depth evaluation may be indicated.

used in the evaluation of individual patients without incorporating information from other sources.

Juntunen (1993) has proposed the following diagnostic criteria for chronic neurobehavioral toxicity from solvents:

A. Verified quantitative and qualitative exposure to organic chemicals which are known to be neurotoxic.
B. Clinical picture of organic central nervous system damage:
   1. Typical subjective symptoms.
   2. Pathologic findings in some of the following:
      a. Clinical neurologic status.
      b. Electroencephalography.
      c. Psychological tests.
C. Other organic diseases reasonably well excluded.
D. Primary psychiatric diseases reasonably well excluded.

## Differential Diagnosis

Primary psychiatric disease may be excluded by the presence of signs of organic brain dysfunction, but these signs are not always entirely objective or clear-cut. Drug or alcohol abuse may result in a clinical state identical to chronic solvent toxicity, distin-

guished only by history and other evidence of exposure. Diffuse organic brain disease—particularly Alzheimer's disease or, less commonly, Creutzfeld-Jacob disease—must also be considered.

## Treatment

Removal from exposure is recommended in all suspected cases. Alcohol and other central nervous system depressants should be avoided.

Depression may respond to antidepressants or other measures. Other neuropsychological symptoms may respond to psychological counseling. Treatment of chronic solvent-induced headaches involves empiric trials of medications, psychological counseling, and biofeedback therapy. Cognitive retraining is useful in some individuals with persistent memory loss documented on neuropsychological testing.

## Prognosis

A number of follow-up studies workers diagnosed as having solvent-associated neurobehavioural changes have been conducted. In general, those having symtoms but no impairment of psychometric test performance improved after removal from or reduction of solvent exposure. Severe impairment of initial test performance was often associated with persistent and sometimes worsening follow-up test performance, even if exposure was eliminated. Persistent impairment was often associated with persistent disabilities and considerable adverse social consequences.

## EFFECTS ON PERIPHERAL NERVOUS SYSTEM & CRANIAL NERVES

All organic solvents may be capable of causing or contributing to peripheral neuropathies (see also Chapter 24). However, only a few are specifically toxic to the peripheral nervous system, including carbon disulfide and the hexacarbons n-hexane and methyl n-butyl ketone. These three cause a symmetric, ascending, mixed sensorimotor neuropathy of the distal axonopathy type that can be replicated in animals. This may be referred to as a centralperipheral distal axonopathy, since the nerves in the spinal canal are also affected. Of the three substances, only n-hexane is currently in general use as an industrial solvent. Most industrial hexane is a mixture of isomers, and reports of neuropathy from hexane use are rare in the United States and more common in Italy and Japan, where cottage industries result in higher exposures. Methyl ethyl ketone, a common solvent, potentiates the neurotoxicity of the hexacarbons (n-hexane, methyl n-butyl ketone).

Trichloroethylene has been associated with isolated trigeminal nerve anesthesia. Other organic solvents such as methyl chloroform (1,1,1-trichloroethane) have been associated with peripheral neurotoxicity in case reports of occupational exposure, following exposure to mixtures of solvents, or in persons exposed to extremely high levels from deliberate "sniffing" of solvents. Limited epidemiologic evidence and case reports of solvent abusers have associated solvent exposure with sensorineural hearing loss. Toluene caused high-frequency hearing loss in rats at levels above 1000 ppm. The effects of solvents on auditory nerve function merit additional study in the future. Toluene causes vestibular dysfunction in abusers, but whether this is specific for toluene is unclear.

An increased incidence of color vision disturbances has been reported in solvent-exposed workers, with evidence to suggest a central rather than peripheral site of damage. Disturbances of olfactory function (hyposmia, parosmia) have been reported in cases of solvent-exposed individuals and anecdotally in a high percentage of long-term painters. Effects on olfaction could be due to local destruction of olfactory nerve endings in the nasal mucosa or to action at a central site.

Studies of general solvent exposure have paid little attention to the peripheral nervous system. The few that have been performed suggest that at exposures more likely to result in central nervous system effects, symptoms of peripheral neurotoxicity are uncommon but neurophysiologic function may be altered. Analogous to the effects of chronic alcoholism, solvents may be only weakly toxic to the peripheral nervous system but capable of acting additively or synergistically with dietary deficiencies or other neurotoxic agents.

### Clinical Findings

Typical symptoms of solvent-induced neuropathy are slowly ascending numbness, paresthesias, and weakness. Pain and muscle cramps are occasionally present. Physical findings include diminished sensation and strength in a symmetric pattern and, in most cases, depressed distal reflexes. Trigeminal neuropathy from trichloroethylene is restricted to loss of sensory function in the distribution of the trigeminal nerve.

### Diagnosis

The diagnosis of solvent-induced neuropathy is based on a history of illness and exposure, clinical examination, and neurophysiologic testing, as described in Chapter 24. Nerve conduction velocities may be normal or slightly depressed. Sensory conduction velocities and sensory action potential amplitude are the most sensitive. Electromyography may indicate denervation (fibrillations and positive sharp waves). The use of evoked potentials (visual and somatosensory) shows promise. Symptoms and other clinical findings are often found with absent or slight neurophysiologic abnormalities. A sural nerve biopsy

may be helpful, and in the case of hexacarbons show accumulation of neurofilaments in the terminal axon.

Neurophysiologic testing may be helpful in screening large numbers of workers, but has not been shown to be more sensitive in early detection of clinical neuropathy than clinical examinations—though periodic monitoring of n-hexane-exposed workers with nerve conduction velocity testing has been recommended.

Odor threshold testing and other tests of olfactory function should be performed in individuals with complaints of disturbances in either smell or taste.

### Differential Diagnosis

The primary differential for peripheral neuropathy is diabetes, alcoholism, drugs, familial neuropathies, and renal failure. About 25–50% of cases of peripheral neuropathy remain without etiologic diagnoses after initial evaluation excludes these causes. A chemical-related cause should be considered in all such cases.

### Treatment

Treatment consists of removal of exposure to all substances toxic to the peripheral nervous system, including alcoholic beverages. Physical therapy should be encouraged for patients with weakness; this increases muscular strength to counteract loss of neuromuscular function, improves psychological outlook, and may even improve the ability of nerves to regenerate effectively.

Careful clinical monitoring of workers exposed to substances toxic to the peripheral nervous system is important for early detection and prevention of permanent disability.

### Prognosis

Symptoms may worsen initially and then improve for up to 1 year or more. The rate of recovery is related to the rate of axonal regeneration, which is approximately 1 mm/d. An axon from the tip of the toe that has died back to the cell body in the spinal cord may take 1 year to recover. The degree of residual disability, if any, is usually proportionate to the degree of injury at the time of diagnosis and cessation of exposure. However, permanent disability should not be judged until at least 1 year after diagnosis.

## RESPIRATORY SYSTEM

All organic solvents irritate the respiratory tract to some degree. Irritation is a consequence of the defatting action of solvents, and so the same structure-activity relationships hold true for the respiratory tract as for the skin. Addition of functional groups to the hydrocarbon molecule may also increase the potency of the solvent as an irritant, as in the case of organic amine bases and organic acids, which are corrosives;

and alcohols, ketones, and aldehydes, which denature proteins at high concentrations.

Respiratory tract irritation from solvents is usually confined to the upper airways, including the nose and sinuses. Solvents that are both highly soluble and potent irritants, such as formaldehyde, cannot reach the lower respiratory tract without intolerable irritation of the upper tract. However, it is possible for less potent irritants to reach the alveoli in sufficient concentrations following extremely high overexposures, such as in spills and in confined spaces, to cause acute pulmonary edema. Severe central nervous system depression is usually also a result of such exposure. Pulmonary edema without effects on the nervous system can result from exposure to phosgene gas produced by the extreme heating (as in welding) of chlorinated hydrocarbon solvents. Exacerbation of asthma or, less commonly, induction of reactive airway dysfunction syndrome after acute exposure can occur, as with any other airway irritant.

There are few studies of chronic pulmonary effects from exposure to organic solvents. Chronic bronchitis may occur as a result of long-term exposure to the more potent irritant compounds, such as the aldehydes.

### Clinical Findings

**A. Symptoms & Signs:** Irritation of the upper respiratory tract is marked by sore nose and throat, cough, and possibly chest pain. If the eyes are not protected by vapor goggles, irritation of the eyes possibly accompanied by tearing may also occur. A few solvents are specific lacrimators, and induce pronounced tearing such that exposure may be sufficient to preclude inhalation and irritation of the respiratory tract. A productive cough indicates chemical bronchitis or the imposition of an infectious bronchitis. Manifestations of pulmonary edema include a productive cough, dyspnea, cyanosis, and rales.

**B. Laboratory Findings:** Upper airway irritation should not be associated with any laboratory abnormalities. Pulmonary edema is marked by infiltrates on chest x-ray, hypoxia and perhaps hypocapnia on arterial blood gas analysis, and impaired diffusion as shown by pulmonary function tests.

### Differential Diagnosis

Infectious bronchitis may be distinguished from chemical bronchitis by sputum analysis and possibly sputum culture, although chemical bronchitis may be followed by a superimposed infection. Solvent-induced pulmonary edema must be distinguished from infectious or aspiration pneumonitis.

### Treatment

Management of the acute pulmonary effects of solvents is the same as for any acute pulmonary irritant: administration of oxygen, bronchodilators, and other respiratory support as indicated.

### Prognosis

Upper respiratory tract irritation should resolve quickly without sequelae in the absence of infection. Once treated appropriately, patients with acute pulmonary edema from solvent overexposure should recover completely if protected from the effects of hypoxic tissue damage. Rarely, induction of reactive airway dysfunction syndrome occurs (see Chapter 20).

## EFFECTS ON THE HEART

The principal effect of organic solvents on the heart is "cardiac sensitization"—a state of increased myocardial sensitivity to the arrhythmogenic effects of epinephrine (see also Chapter 21). It can be demonstrated in animals—typically unanesthetized beagle dogs—by administration of epinephrine, either in fixed or multiple doses, before and after administration of a solvent and observation of the frequency of epinephrine-induced ventricular arrhythmias. Cases of sudden, otherwise unexplained death during abuse of solvents such as toluene in glue and trichloroethane in spot remover, usually associated with physical activity ("sudden sniffing deaths"), and occasional reports of sudden death in otherwise healthy workers overexposed to industrial solvents are probably due to cardiac sensitization.

From animal studies it appears that high—near-anesthetic or anesthetic—levels are required for this effect on an otherwise healthy heart and that all organic solvents may be capable of causing it, though potencies vary. Halogenated hydrocarbons, particularly 1,1,1-trichloroethane, trichloroethylene, and trichlorotrifluoroethane, were of higher potency in the dog, with thresholds to a particular dose of epinephrine at 0.5% (5000 ppm) of solvent vapors for 5 minutes, compared with approximately 5% (50,000 ppm) for heptane, hexane, toluene, and xylene; 10% (100,000 ppm) for propane; and 20% (20,000 ppm) for ethyl ether. Thresholds for these effects in humans, particularly with any condition predisposing to arrhythmias, are unknown.

A few solvents appear to have specific cardiovascular effects. Carbon disulfide exposure has been associated with increased risk of coronary artery disease in a number of epidemiological studies. Methylene chloride can affect cardiac function acutely, possibly on a long-term basis, through its metabolism to carbon monoxide.

### Clinical Findings

**A. Symptoms & Signs:** Cardiac sensitization should be considered when a worker exposed to high concentrations of a solvent reports dizziness, palpitations, faintness, or loss of consciousness in conjunction with or in the absence of symptoms of central nervous system depression (see above). If the victim is examined promptly, an irregular pulse or low blood pressure may be detected.

**B. Laboratory Findings:** A resting ECG may be normal or abnormal and is rarely diagnostic. For workers with symptoms suggestive of cardiac sensitization, ambulatory cardiac monitoring during exposure may be helpful.

### Differential Diagnosis

In the presence of high levels of exposure, the distinction between central nervous system depression alone and depression plus cardiac sensitization is difficult—and may not be important if all symptoms resolve with correction of overexposure. The need for evaluation for primary cardiac disease must be made on a case-by-case basis. The presence of cardiac disease does not preclude the possibility of solvent-related arrhythmias, which may occur at levels of solvent exposure lower than those usually associated with cardiac sensitization.

### Treatment

Given the high levels of exposure usually associated with cardiac sensitization, evaluation and appropriate correction of exposure are essential. If arrhythmias appear to be related to exposure and the exposure is not excessive or cannot be controlled adequately, removal from exposure is preferable to treatment with antiarrhythmic medication and continued exposure.

### Prognosis

Cases due solely to excessive exposure should resolve with correction of the workplace situation.

## EFFECT ON THE LIVER

Although it is possible that any organic solvent may cause hepatocellular damage in sufficient doses for a sufficient duration, some solvents, particularly those substituted with halogen or nitro groups, are particularly hepatotoxic. Others, such as the aliphatic hydrocarbons (cycloparaffins, ethers, esters, aldehydes, and ketones), are only weakly if at all hepatotoxic. The aromatic hydrocarbons (benzene, toluene, and xylene) appear to be weakly hepatotoxic, with only a few reports of possible liver toxicity in exposed workers. A few solvents such as acetone, with little direct hepatotoxicity themselves have been reported to potentiate the effects of alcohol on the liver.

Acute hepatic injury was frequently reported in the past from acute overexposure to carbon tetrachloride. More recently, acute hepatic necrosis and death from liver failure have been reported from exposure to 2-nitropropane used as a solvent in specialty paint products.

Dimethylformamide, present in glues and fabric coatings, has been reported to cause toxic hepatitis occasionally with persistent elevations of liver enzyme levels. Subacute liver disease has been rarely reported in modern times, while chronic liver disease, including cirrhosis, has been occasionally reported in workers exposed to carbon tetrachloride.

### Clinical Findings

**A. Symptoms & Signs:** Liver injury may be symptomless or associated with right upper quadrant pain, nausea, and vomiting. Hepatic tenderness, jaundice, dark urine, and light stool may be present.

**B. Laboratory Findings:** Diagnosis of acute hepatic injury is based on the presence of abnormal liver function tests in a pattern consistent with hepatocellular dysfunction and a history consistent with exposure to a hepatotoxic solvent in the absence of exposure to any other known hepatotoxin. A pattern of liver enzyme abnormality different from alcohol hepatitis has been reported anecdotally for a few solvents. Serum bilirubin may be elevated. Evaluation of liver injury due to occupational exposure to solvents has been hampered by the lack of sensitivity and specificity of liver function tests and their often high incidence of abnormalities in working populations. The use of serum bile acid measurements and antipyrine metabolism rates has been proposed as a sensitive screening method for solvent-related liver dysfunction. Occasionally, liver biopsy is necessary to distinguish solventinduced hepatitis from chronic active hepatitis.

Routine monitoring of liver function tests is not recommended unless there is potential exposure to a hepatotoxic dose of a solvent. Monitoring a patient after abstinence from alcohol may be necessary to evaluate the possible role of drinking. Removal of exposure with monitoring of liver function tests may be helpful in making a diagnosis.

### Differential Diagnosis

The major entity that must be differentiated is alcohol-induced liver injury; if excessive use of alcohol cannot be ruled out, a diagnosis of solvent-induced liver injury often cannot be made with confidence. Viral and other infectious forms of hepatitis must also be considered.

### Treatment

Treatment consists of removal from exposure and correction of any workplace situation that can be identified as having caused or contributed to the condition.

## EFFECT ON THE KIDNEYS

Although many organic solvents, particularly halogenated aliphatic hydrocarbons, show evidence of nephrotoxicity to animals in relatively high doses, there are few reports of renal effects in exposed workers—perhaps in part due to the lack of sensitivity and specificity of renal function tests. Acute renal failure from acute tubular necrosis has been observed in workers with acute intoxication from halogenated hydrocarbons such as carbon tetrachloride.

Animal studies indicate that halogenated aliphatic hydrocarbons damage primarily the proximal renal tubular cells. Renal tubular dysfunction—particularly renal tubular acidosis of the distal type—has been reported in solvent abusers using mainly toluene but has not been associated with occupational exposure. Acute renal failure from intrarenal deposition of oxalic acid can result from ingestion of ethylene glycol but has not been reported from other routes of exposure.

There are few studies of chronic renal effects in solvent-exposed workers. Cross-sectional studies have suggested that chronic exposure to a number of solvents or solvent mixtures may result in mild tubular dysfunction evidenced by enzymuria (increased excretion of muramidase, β-glucuronidase, and N-acetyl-β-glucosaminidase) and either normal urinalyses or proteinuria. Case control studies have suggested an association between solvent exposure and primary glomerulonephritis, particularly rapidly progressive glomerulonephritis associated with anti-glomerular basement membrane antibodies (the renal component of Goodpasture's syndrome).

### Clinical Findings

**A. Symptoms & Signs:** Solvent abusers with renal tubular acidosis have presented with weakness and fatigue, probably as a result of electrolyte abnormalities. Signs of acute intoxication (central nervous system depression) have often been present. If it occurs, chronic renal tubular dysfunction as a result of chronic solvent exposure would usually be subclinical.

**B. Laboratory Findings:** Renal tubular dysfunction from solvents may be manifested by polyuria, glycosuria, proteinuria, acidosis, and electrolyte disorders. Hypokalemia, hypophosphatemia, hyperchloremia, and hypocarbonatemia have been seen as manifestations of renal tubular acidosis in toluene abusers. Acute renal failure from halogenated solvents is similar to that from any other cause. Routine monitoring of renal function is not generally recommended for workers exposed to solvents. However, the measurement of urinary excretion of low-molecular-weight enzymes such as N-acetyl-β-glucosaminidase, β-glucuronidase, and muramidase appears to offer promise as a monitor for evidence of early tubular dysfunction.

### Differential Diagnosis

Renal tubular dysfunction, including acidosis, can be a primary disease that first manifests itself in early adulthood or may occur secondary to a variety of metabolic and hyperglobulinemic states and exposure to toxic agents, including antibiotics and heavy metals.

### Treatment

If renal tubular dysfunction is found in a worker with a high level of exposure to a solvent, observation of renal tubular function during cessation and then reinstitution of exposure may be helpful in both establishing a diagnosis and in determining the effectiveness of removal from exposure.

## EFFECTS ON BLOOD

Hematologic effects from solvents are not common. Benzene causes a dose-related aplastic anemia after months to years of exposure that may be a precursor to leukemia. Chlorinated hydrocarbons have been associated with a number of reported cases of aplastic anemia, which may be idiosyncratic or simply a spurious association. Some glycol ethers can cause either a hemolytic anemia due to increased osmotic fragility or hypoplastic anemia due to bone marrow depression.

### Clinical Findings

**A. Symptoms & Signs:** Workers with anemia from solvents have generally presented with weakness and fatigue. Aplastic anemia can present with bleeding from thrombocytopenia or infections due to neutropenia.

**B. Laboratory Findings:** Aplastic anemia from benzene may be manifested by reductions in any or all of the three cell lines, which may occur suddenly without preceding changes. The bone marrow may be hyperplastic or hypoplastic and does not always correlate with abnormalities in the peripheral blood. Hemolytic anemia from glycol ethers or other hemolytic agents is indicated by low red blood cell concentration and reticulocytosis. Monitoring of blood counts is recommended only for exposure to benzene and perhaps for the hematotoxic glycol ethers, but the results may not be predictive of anemia even for these agents.

### Differential Diagnosis

The usual causes of anemia, particularly hypoplastic anemia, must be considered.

### Treatment

The treatment of solvent-induced anemia is removal from exposure, transfusion if needed, and correction of the workplace situation if appropriate. Workers with aplastic anemia from benzene should not be reexposed to benzene.

### Prognosis

A significant percentage of workers with aplastic anemia from benzene will subsequently develop leukemia, which is frequently fatal. Other solvent-induced hematologic effects should resolve with cessation of exposure.

## CANCER POTENTIAL

Benzene is the only commonly used solvent for which there is sufficient evidence of carcinogenicity in humans. It has been associated with all types of acute and chronic leukemia. Investigation of many of the halogenated hydrocarbons has produced limited to sufficient evidence of carcinogenicity in animals, particularly hepatocellular carcinomas in mice. Most have not been adequately studied in humans. Mixed solvent exposures have been associated with increases in lymphatic and hematopoietic malignancies in some studies.

## EFFECTS ON
## REPRODUCTIVE SYSTEM

Most organic solvents easily cross the lipid barrier of the placenta and, to a lesser degree, the testes. There is concern for their potential to cause reproductive toxicity. Few studies have been conducted in humans. Case-control studies have suggested an association between maternal exposure to organic solvents and central nervous system, cardiovascular, and urinarty tract birth defects. A few studies have found an increased risk of spontaneous abortion associated with mixed solvent exposure.

With the exception of the glycol ethers, chlorinated hydrocarbons (carbon tetrachloride, trichloroethylene, and perchloroethylene), and ethyl alcohol, available animal studies have generally not revealed evidence of significant teratogenicity. Ethyl alcohol causes both structural and behavioral teratogenic effects (fetal alcohol syndrome) in both animals and women drinking more than three or four glasses of alcoholic beverages per day. Controversy exists over whether pregnant women should be advised not to drink alcoholic beverages at all during pregnancy. Since all organic solvents readily cross the placenta and reach the fetal nervous system and affect the nervous system in similar ways to alcohol, the possibility of a "fetal solvent syndrome" has been discussed. Standard teratogenicity studies would not necessarily reveal such effects, and behavioral teratogenicity studies in animals have been performed only to a limited extent. If a "fetal solvent syndrome" exists, important questions about dose-response relationships need to be addressed. For instance, what would the relationship be between effects on the mother and on the offspring? Would effects occur in offspring only at levels that produced acute intoxication in the mother, or at lower levels? And are short, high exposures worse than lower, longer exposures?

Decisions regarding exposure of pregnant workers to solvents must currently be made in the absence of definitive toxicologic data (see Chapter 25). Many solvents show evidence of fetotoxicity in animals at or near maternally toxic levels. Exposure that produces acute reversible effects on the mature maternal nervous system may produce irreversible effects on the developing fetal nervous system. Therefore, it is prudent to ensure that women who may be pregnant not be overexposed to any organic solvent. In addition, because of distribution to a possibly vulnerable fetal nervous system and the possibility of behavioral teratogenicity, exposure to organic solvents should be kept as low as possible throughout pregnancy.

There is potential for solvent exposure to males to affect reproduction directly by affecting male reproductive capacity or indirectly via damaged sperm. This is best studied in male workers chronically exposed to glycol ethers (2-methoxyethanol or 2-ethoxyethanol) who had an increased prevalence of oligospermia and azospermia and an increased likelihood of low sperm counts compared with unexposed workers (see Chapter 26).

# PREVENTION OF SOLVENT TOXICITY

## SELECTION & SUBSTITUTION
## OF SOLVENT

Selection of an initial solvent—or substitution of a less hazardous for a more hazardous solvent—must take into account both the desirable and undesirable properties of the solvents. This involves comparing not only health hazard (toxicity, dermal absorptivity, and volatility), but also flammability, explosiveness, reactivity, compatibility, stability, odor properties, and environmental fates. For example, carbon tetrachloride, perchloroethylene, trichlorotrifluoroethane, and mineral spirits are all used to some extent at the present time as dry-cleaning agents, though to different degrees than in the past. Carbon tetrachloride is by far the most toxic and for that reason is used chiefly as a spot removal agent. Perchloroethylene is less toxic than carbon tetrachloride and has replaced it for that reason. Perchloroethylene replaced mineral spirits because of the flammability of the latter; perchloroethylene and carbon tetrachloride are virtually nonflammable.

However, perchloroethylene is moderately toxic and was recently found to be carcinogenic and teratogenic in laboratory animals. Trichlorotrifluoroethane is the least toxic, but it is expensive and may contribute to depletion of the ozone layer. It is used in closed systems to decrease cost and environmental pollution by recycling, but this requires an initial capital outlay for equipment.

Obviously, the choice of solvent is complicated when advantages and disadvantages exist in different categories.

## ENGINEERING CONTROLS

The volatility of organic solvents makes engineering ingenuity to control vapors of paramount importance in many situations. Process enclosure, such as the closed system use of trichlorotrifluoroethane for dry cleaning, is common in chemical manufacturing but not in other circumstances. Spray painting and other spray operations create large quantities of aerosols and vapors, so that engineering controls such as paint spray booths are particularly critical. Effective functioning of ventilation systems is dependent upon proper design and regular mechanical maintenance, but these are commonly lacking. The substitution of water-based for solvent-based paints has been the most effective means of reducing solvent exposure from painting. Auto body repair represents the last major use of solvent-based paints that has not been partially replaced with water-based paints.

## PERSONAL PROTECTION

Respiratory protection should be used only when engineering controls are not feasible, such as in construction, confined space, and emergency response situations. The employer must conduct a comprehensive respiratory protection program. Frequently, there is improper fitting, selection, and maintenance of respirators for solvent work, resulting in poor or inconsistent protection. Knowledge of the odor threshold of a substance (Table 29–1) is necessary before using a respirator for levels above the TLV for that substance. If the average odor threshold is well below the TLV (eg, at least 10-fold) the odor will serve as an adequate warning to signal breakthrough or other failure of the respirator to provide adequate protection. A decrease in the ability to detect odors (hyposmia) has been reported from chronic exposure to solvents, and a history of hyposmia should be sought as part of the initial medical evaluation for ability to use a respirator. Some solvents such as methanol, methyl chloride, and formaldehyde are not removed by standard organic vapor filters.

Protective clothing made of the proper material should be selected on the basis of studies that show the rate of penetration of materials by the solvent used. *Guidelines for the Selection of Chemical Protective Clothing*, published by ACGIH, is a good source of this information. Protective (barrier) creams can correct or prevent loss of oils from the skin and may provide some protection against percutaneous absorption of solvents.

Some workers, such as mechanics, may be unable to use gloves and adequately perform their work. Barrier creams are not recommended as substitutes for gloves.

# SPECIFIC SOLVENTS & THEIR EFFECTS

## ALIPHATIC HYDROCARBONS

### Essentials of Diagnosis

*Acute effects:*
- Anesthesia: dizziness, headache, nausea, vomiting, sleepiness, fatigue, "drunkenness," slurred speech, disequilibrium, disorientation, depression, and loss of consciousness.
- Respiratory tract irritation: cough and sore nose and throat.

*Chronic effects:*
- Dermatitis: dry, cracked, and erythematous skin.
- Neurobehavioral dysfunction: headache, mood lability, fatigue, short-term memory loss, difficulty concentrating, decreased attention span, neurobehavioral test abnormalities, CT scan (cerebral atrophy), EEG (diffuse slow waves).
- Peripheral neuropathy (n-hexane): slowly ascending numbness, paresthesias, and weakness; normal or slightly depressed nerve conduction velocity and electromyography (denervation).

### General Considerations

Aliphatic hydrocarbons consist of carbon and hydrogen molecules in straight or branched chains. They are further divided into alkanes, alkenes, and alkynes.

### 1. ALKANES (PARAFFINS)

Alkanes are aliphatic hydrocarbons with single-bonded (saturated) carbons:

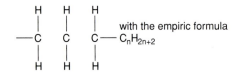

with the empiric formula $C_nH_{2n+2}$

The physical state of an alkane depends on its number of carbons:

| Carbons | State | Name |
| --- | --- | --- |
| 1–4 | Gas | Methane, ethane, propane, butane |
| 5–16 | Liquid | Pentane, hexane, heptane, octane, nonane |
| >16 | Solid | Paraffin wax |

The gases are essentially odorless, while the vapors of the liquids have a slight "hydrocarbon" odor.

## Use

A number of liquid alkanes are used in relatively pure form as solvents and also are the major constituents of a number of petroleum distillate solvents (see below). The liquid alkanes are important ingredients in gasoline, which accounts for most of the pentane and hexane used in the United States. Hexane (generally a mixture of isomers including n-hexane) is an inexpensive general use solvent in solvent glues, quick-drying rubber cements, varnishes, inks, and extraction of oils from seeds. The alkane gases are used as fuels, while paraffin wax is used for candles and other wax products.

## Occupational & Environmental Exposure

NIOSH estimates that approximately 10,000 US workers are potentially exposed to pentane and heptane, 300,000 to octane, and 2.5 million to hexane annually. Many more individuals may be exposed to these and other alkanes in gasoline, naphthas, and other petroleum products. They are common contaminants of ambient air, with levels of methane reported to be 1.2–1.5 ppm in rural areas and 2–3 ppm in urban air, while other alkanes are generally detected at more than 10-fold lower concentrations.

## Pharmacokinetics

The alkanes are well absorbed by inhalation and, to a lesser but still significant extent, through the skin. None have skin TLV designations. Approximately 75% of most inhaled alkanes will be absorbed at rest, decreasing to 50% with moderate physical labor. Unbranched hydrocarbons such as n-hexane and n-heptane are metabolized by microsomal cytochrome P-450 enzymes to alcohols, diols, ketones, and diketones, which are further metabolized to carbon monoxide or conjugated with glucuronic acid and excreted in urine.

## Health Effects

The alkanes are generally of low toxicity. The first three gases (methane, ethane, and propane) are simple inert asphyxiants whose toxicity is related only to the amount of available oxygen remaining in the environment and to their flammability and explosiveness. The vapors of the lighter, more volatile liquids, pentane through nonane, are irritants and anesthetics, while the heavier liquids, known as liquid paraffins, are primarily defatting agents. Hexane and heptane are most commonly used as general purpose solvents. They cause anesthesia, respiratory tract irritation, and dermatitis and are associated with neurobehavioral dysfunction; and the associated clinical findings, differential diagnosis, treatment, and prognosis are not different from those of other solvents (see above).

One isomer of hexane, n-hexane, causes peripheral neuropathy. A number of outbreaks of peripheral neuropathy have been described, particularly in cottage industries such as shoe and sandal making, where glues have been used containing n-hexane as a solvent. The proximate neurotoxin is the metabolite 2,5-hexanedione. Other diketones with the same spacing between ketone (carbonyl) groups, such as 3,6-hexanedione, can also cause peripheral neuropathy. A metabolite of n-heptane, 2,5-heptanedione, causes peripheral neuropathy in laboratory animal studies, but n-heptane has not been implicated in human peripheral neuropathy in the absence of concomitant exposure to n-hexane. The clinical and neurophysiologic findings of n-hexane-induced peripheral neuropathy is typical of distal axonopathies (see above and Chapter 24). Nerve biopsies are notable for swollen axons that contain increased numbers of neurofilaments. Methyl ethyl ketone and possibly methyl isobutyl ketone potentiate the neurotoxicity of n-hexane.

Exposure to n-hexane can be assessed by measuring 2,5-hexanedione in the urine or n-hexane in end-exhaled air. A concentration of 2,5-hexanedione in urine of 5 mg/L measured at the end of a work shift corresponds to exposure to a TWA of 50 ppm. However, false-positive results may be obtained as a result of confounding by α-acetylfuran if the sample pH and choice of gas-chromatographic column are not appropriate.

## 2. ALKENES (OLEFINS) & ALKYNES

Alkenes are aliphatic hydrocarbons with double (unsaturated) carbon bonds:

$$
\begin{array}{ccc}
H & H & H \\
| & | & | \\
-C=C-C- & & C_nH_{2n} \\
 & & | \\
 & & H
\end{array}
\quad \text{with the empiric formula}
$$

Dienes are alkenes with two double bonds. Alkynes are aliphatic hydrocarbons with triple carbon bonds. The physical state of alkenes and alkynes is determined by the number of carbons, as for alkanes.

## Use

The liquid alkenes are not widely used as solvents but are common chemical intermediates. The alkenes are more reactive than alkanes, a property that leads to their use as monomers in the production of polymers, such as polyethylenes from ethylene, polypropylene from propylene, and synthetic rubber and resin copolymers from 1,3-butadiene.

## Occupational & Environmental Exposure

Occupational exposure estimates are not available for most alkenes and alkynes. Occupational exposure to ethylene, propylene, and 1,3-butadiene occurs primarily through inhalation during monomer and polymer production. NIOSH estimates that 62,000 US workers are potentially exposed to 1,3-butadiene. NIOSH found mean exposure levels of 5.9 ppm in the 1,3-butadiene monomer industry. Propylene is a common air pollutant as a result of engine exhaust emissions and industrial activity, with urban atmospheric concentrations ranging from 2.6–23.3 ppb in the United States and Europe. Butadiene has been detected in urban atmospheres in the United States at concentrations ranging from 1–5 ppb, while other alkenes and alkynes have been detected at comparable concentrations.

## Pharmacokinetics

There is little information on absorption or metabolism of alkenes and alkynes. Absorption of these compounds should be similar to their corresponding alkanes. None have skin TLV designations.

## Health Effects

The alkenes are similar in toxicity to the alkanes. The unsaturated carbon bonds increase lipid solubility to some extent and therefore irritant and anesthetic potencies, compared to corresponding alkanes. n-Hexene does not cause peripheral neuropathy, unlike n-hexane.

The presence of double bonds makes the alkenes more reactive than alkanes and dienes more reactive than alkenes. This reactivity is utilized in the production of polymers but may in some cases result also in additional health hazards. 1,3-Butadiene was recently found to be carcinogenic in animals, while propylene and ethylene were not.

1,3-Butadiene is a human and animal carcinogen; elevated rates of leukemia and lymphosarcoma have been associated with occupational exposure. Both in utero embryo toxicity and male-mediated reproductive toxicity have been shown in animals. Biological monitoring can be accomplished by urinary sampling for the product of epoxybutene hydrolysis followed by gluthathione conjugation.

## ALICYCLIC HYDROCARBONS (Cyclic Hydrocarbons, Cycloparaffins, Naphthenes)

## Essentials of Diagnosis

*Acute effects:*
- Anesthesia: dizziness, headache, nausea, vomit-

ing, sleepiness, fatigue, "drunkenness," slurred speech, disequilibrium, disorientation, depression, and loss of consciousness.
- Respiratory tract irritation: sore nose and throat and cough.

*Chronic effects:*
- Dermatitis: dry, cracked, and erythematous skin.
- Neurobehavioral dysfunction: headache, mood lability, fatigue, short-term memory loss, difficulty concentrating, decreased attention span, neurobehavioral test abnormalities, CT scan (cerebral atrophy), EEG (diffuse slow waves).

## General Considerations

Alicyclic hydrocarbons consist of alkanes or alkenes arranged into cyclic or ring structures:

They have a slight "hydrocarbon" odor.

## Use

Cyclohexane is the only alicyclic hydrocarbon that is widely used as an industrial solvent. Most of the US production is used in the synthesis of nylon. Cyclopropane is used as a general anesthetic, but this is limited by its flammability and explosiveness.

## Occupational & Environmental Exposure

The use of cyclohexane in nylon production results in only limited occupational exposure. The alicyclic hydrocarbons are not reported as common environmental contaminants.

## Pharmacokinetics

Similar to their corresponding alkanes and alkenes, the alicyclic hydrocarbons are well absorbed by inhalation, while percutaneous absorption is less important. Approximately 70% of cyclohexane that is inhaled is absorbed and excreted unchanged in urine and exhaled air and as cyclohexanol in urine.

## Health Effects

The alicyclic hydrocarbons are similar in toxicity to their alkane or alkene counterparts in causing irritation and central nervous system depression. They cause anesthesia, respiratory tract irritation, and dermatitis and are associated with neurobehavioral dysfunction. The associated clinical findings, differential diagnosis, treatment, and prognosis are not different from those of other solvents (see above). Cyclohexane does not cause peripheral neuropathy.

## AROMATIC HYDROCARBONS

### Essentials of Diagnosis

*Acute effects:*
- Anesthesia: dizziness, headache, nausea, vomiting, sleepiness, fatigue, "drunkenness," slurred speech, disequilibrium, disorientation, depression, and loss of consciousness.
- Respiratory tract irritation: cough and sore nose and throat.

*Chronic effects:*
- Dermatitis: dry, cracked, and erythematous skin.
- Neurobehavioral dysfunction: headache, mood lability, fatigue, short-term memory loss, difficulty concentrating, decreased attention span, neurobehavioral test abnormalities, CT scan (cerebral atrophy), EEG (diffuse slow waves).

### General Considerations

Aromatic hydrocarbons are compounds that contain one or more benzene rings:

They are produced—directly or indirectly—chiefly from crude petroleum and to a lesser extent from coal tar. Aromatics used as solvents include benzene and the alkylbenzenes: toluene (methyl benzene), xylenes (*o*-, *m*-, and *p*-isomers of dimethyl benzenes), ethyl benzene, cumene (isopropyl benzene), and styrene (vinyl benzene). They have a characteristic "aromatic" sweet odor.

### Use

Although benzene currently has only limited use as a general industrial solvent, it is still widely used in manufacturing, for extraction in chemical analyses, and as a specialty solvent. Approximately half the benzene produced is used to synthesize ethyl benzene for the production of styrene. In the United States, gasoline contains approximately 2–3% benzene and 30–50% other aromatics. Aromatics constitute a significant percentage of a number of petroleum distillate solvents (see below). Toluene and xylenes are two of the most widely used industrial solvents—principally in paints, adhesives, and the formulation of pesticides—though about a third of the toluene used goes to produce benzene and only about one-sixth is used as a solvent. The solvent uses

of toluene and xylenes have been decreasing owing to environmental regulations because of their photochemical reactivity. Ethyl benzene is used chiefly as an intermediate in the manufacture of styrene and to a lesser extent as a solvent. Styrene is used chiefly as a monomer in the manufacture of plastics and rubber (see Chapters 30 and 31). Most of the cumene produced is used to manufacture phenol and acetone. Other aromatic compounds have a wide variety of uses but are not commonly used as solvents and so will not be discussed here.

### Occupational & Environmental Exposure

NIOSH estimates that 4.8 million workers are potentially exposed to toluene, the fourth largest number for an individual chemical. The NIOSH estimate for xylene exposure is 140,000 workers. Aromatic hydrocarbons are common environmental contaminants from engine exhaust and other industrial sources. Levels in urban air have been reported to be as high as 130 ppb toluene, 100 ppb xylenes, 60 ppm benzene, 20 ppb ethyl benzene, < 1 ppb styrene, and 330 ppb total aromatics.

### Pharmacokinetics

The pulmonary absorption values for aromatic hydrocarbons do not vary significantly as a group, ranging from approximately 50–70% at rest and decreasing to 40–60% with light to moderate work and 30–50% with moderate to heavy work. Percutaneous absorption of aromatic hydrocarbons can be significant, but only styrene and cumene currently have TLVs with skin designations.

All the aromatic hydrocarbons are extensively metabolized, their metabolic profiles varying with the substituents on the benzene ring. Benzene is metabolized mainly to phenol and excreted in urine as conjugated phenol and dihydroxyphenols, with a slow elimination phase half-time of about 28 hours. About 10% of benzene is excreted unchanged in exhaled air. Toluene is primarily metabolized to benzoic acid and excreted in urine as the glycine conjugate hippuric acid, with a half-time of about 1–2 hours. Approximately 15–20% of toluene is excreted unchanged in expired air. Xylene is almost entirely metabolized to the *o*-, *m*-, and *p*-methylbenzoic acids and excreted in urine as the glycine conjugates, *o*-, *m*-, and *p*-methylhippuric acids, with a slow elimination phase half-time of about 30 hours. About 64% of absorbed ethyl benzene is excreted in urine as mandelic acid and about 25% as phenylglyoxylic acid. The principal metabolites of the aromatic hydrocarbons are used for biologic monitoring as indicated below.

### Health Effects

The aromatic hydrocarbons are generally stronger irritants and anesthetics than the aliphatics. Substitution on benzene (toluene, xylene, ethyl benzene, and styrene) increases lipid solubility and these toxicities slightly. Aromatic hydrocarbons cause acute anesthetic effects, respiratory tract irritation, and dermatitis and are associated with neurobehavioral dysfunction. The associated clinical findings, differential diagnosis, treatment, and prognosis are not different from those of other solvents (see above).

Benzene is notable for its effects on the bone marrow: reversible pancytopenia, aplastic anemia that may itself be fatal or progress to leukemia, and all types of leukemia, but predominantly acute nonlymphocytic leukemia. There is no evidence that the substituted benzenes have any of these myelotoxic effects. Earlier reports of effects of these substances on the bone marrow were probably due to their contamination with benzene.

There have been a few anecdotal reports of liver function abnormalities in workers exposed to aromatic hydrocarbons. Renal tubular acidosis of the distal type, with serious but reversible electrolyte abnormalities, has been reported in solvent abusers exposed primarily to toluene. A syndrome of persistent cerebellar ataxia has been reported after exposure to toluene, chiefly in solvent abusers but also occasionally in workers. Toluene and xylenes have been reported to raise auditory thresholds in laboratory animals at relatively low levels of exposure.

Exposure to benzene, ethyl benzene, toluene, xylene, and styrene can be assessed by a variety of biological monitoring techniques. These are summarized in Chapter 38. Although extensive research has been conducted on the use of these techniques, given the short half-lives and acute effects of these compounds, the utility of biological monitoring for the routine assessment of exposure is limited. Little information is available on the use of biological levels in the diagnosis of acute intoxication from aromatic hydrocarbons.

## PETROLEUM DISTILLATES
### (Refined Petroleum Solvents)

### Essentials of Diagnosis

*Acute effects:*
- Anesthesia: dizziness, headache, nausea, vomiting, sleepiness, fatigue, "drunkenness," slurred speech, disequilibrium, disorientation, depression, and loss of consciousness.
- Respiratory tract irritation: cough and sore nose and throat.

*Chronic effects:*
- Dermatitis: dry, cracked, and erythematous skin.
- Neurobehavioral dysfunction: headache, mood lability, fatigue, short-term memory loss, difficulty concentrating, decreased attention span, neurobe-

havioral test abnormalities, CT scan (cerebral atrophy), EEG (diffuse slow waves).

### General Considerations

Petroleum distillate solvents are mixtures of petroleum derivatives distilled from crude petroleum at a particular range of boiling points. Each is a mixture of aliphatic (primarily alkane), alicyclic, and aromatic hydrocarbons, the relative concentration of each depending on the particular petroleum distillate fraction. They have a "hydrocarbon" or "aromatic" odor depending on the relative concentrations of aliphatic or aromatic hydrocarbons.

The major petroleum distillate solvents are shown in Table 29–3, with the number of carbon atoms, typical percentages of components, and range of boiling points of each.

### Use

Petroleum distillates are among the most common general use solvents, since they are available at low cost in large quantities. Petroleum ether (petroleum naphtha) represents an estimated 60% of the total industrial solvent usage. Approximately 1.4 billion gallons of petroleum solvents (Table 29–3) were produced in the United States. Kerosene is used as a fuel as well as a cleaning and thinning agent; about 2.3 billion gallons are produced in the United States every year.

### Occupational & Environmental Exposure

NIOSH estimates that 600,000 workers are potentially exposed to the petroleum solvents (Table 29–3) (naphtha solvents), 136,000 to the mineral spirits, and 310,000 to kerosene.

### Pharmacokinetics

The pharmacokinetics of petroleum distillate solvents are those of the individual aliphatic, alicyclic, and aromatic constituents.

### Health Effects

The hazard of a particular petroleum distillate fraction is related to concentrations of the various classes of hydrocarbons it contains (Table 29–3). Petroleum distillate solvents cause anesthetic effects, respiratory tract irritation, and dermatitis, and have been associated with neurobehavioral dysfunction; the clinical findings, differential diagnosis, treatment, and prognosis are not different from those of other solvents (above).

Most of the aliphatic fractions are alkanes, including n-hexane. Therefore, the risk of peripheral neuropathy must be considered, particularly with exposure to petroleum ether, which may contain a significant percentage of n-hexane. The benzene content of petroleum distillates should be below 1%.

**Table 29–3.** Petroleum distillate solvents.

| | Synonyms | Carbon Number | Class Components | Percentage (%) | Boiling Point (°C) |
|---|---|---|---|---|---|
| Petroleum ether | Petroleum, naphtha, ligroin, benzene | $C_{5-6}$ | Alkanes (pentanes, hexanes) | 100 | 30–60 |
| Rubber solvent | Naphtha | $C_{5-7}$ | Aliphatic Alicyclic Aromatic | 60 35 5 | 45–125 |
| Petroleum ether, high-boiling point | Light aliphatic solvent naphtha | $C_{7-8}$ | ... | ... | 80–130 |
| V M & P naphtha[1] | ... | $C_{5-11}$ | Aliphatic Aromatic | >80 <20 | 95–100 |
| Mineral spirits I | Stoddard solvent I, white spirits, petroleum distillate | $C_{7-12}$ | Aliphatic Alicyclic Aromatic | 30–50 30–40 10–20 | 150–200 |
| Mineral spirits II | Stoddard solvent II, high-flash naphtha, 140-flash naphtha | $C_{5-13}$ | Aliphatic Alicyclic Aromatic | 40–60 30–40 5–15 | 175–200 |
| Aromatic petroleum naphtha | Coal tar naphtha | $C_{8-13}$ | Aliphatic Aromatic | <10 >90 | 95–315 |
| Kerosene | Kerosine, stove oil | $C_{10-16}$ | Aliphatic Alicyclic Aromatic | ... | 163–288 |

[1]Varnish makers' and painters' naphtha.

## ALCOHOLS

### Essentials of Diagnosis

*Acute effects:*
- Respiratory tract irritation: cough and sore nose and throat.
- Anesthesia: dizziness, headache, nausea, vomiting, sleepiness, fatigue, "drunkenness," slurred speech, disequilibrium, disorientation, depression, and loss of consciousness.

*Chronic effects:*
- Dermatitis: dry, cracked, and erythematous skin.
- Optic neuropathy (methyl alcohol): blurred vision, blindness, hyperemic optic disk, and dilated pupil.

### General Considerations

Alcohols are hydrocarbons substituted with a single hydroxyl group:

$$—C—C—OH$$

They have a characteristic pungent odor. Examples of alcohols used as solvents are ethyl alcohol, methyl alcohol, and isopropyl alcohol (Table 29–1).

### Use

Alcohols are widely used as cleaning agents, thinners, and diluents; as vehicles for paints, pesticides, and pharmaceuticals; as extracting agents; and as chemical intermediates. Methyl alcohol is widely used as an industrial solvent—one-fourth of its production—and as an adulterant to denature ethanol to prevent its abuse when used as an industrial solvent. Approximately one-third of methyl alcohol used is in the production of formaldehyde. Over half of isopropyl alcohol produced is used to manufacture acetone, and the rest in a variety of solvent and chemical formulation uses. About 90% of cyclohexanol is used to produce adipic acid for nylon, the rest for esters for plasticizers. Alkyl alcohol is used solely as a chemical intermediate. The higher alcohols (> 5 carbons) are divided into the plasticizer range (6–11 carbons) and the detergent range (≥ 12 carbons). About 500 kilotons of plasticizer-range alcohols are produced annually in the United States to make esters for plasticizers and lubricants, and about 260 kilotons of detergent-range alcohols are produced to make sulfate deionizers for detergents.

### Occupational & Environmental Exposure

NIOSH estimates that approximately 175,000 workers are potentially exposed to methyl alcohol and 141,000 workers to isopropyl alcohol in the United States. Exposure to isopropyl alcohol in the home is common in the form of cleaners, cosmetics, and rubbing alcohol.

## Pharmacokinetics

The pharmacokinetics of the simple (primary) alcohols are similar. About 50% of inhaled alcohol is absorbed at rest, decreasing to 40% with light to moderate work loads. Methyl alcohol, n-butyl alcohol, isopropyl alcohol, and isooctyl alcohol are sufficiently absorbed percutaneously to be given skin TLV designations.

The primary alcohols are metabolized by hepatic alcohol dehydrogenase to aldehydes and by aldehyde dehydrogenase to carboxylic acids. The metabolic acidosis and optic neuropathy caused by methyl alcohol have been attributed to its metabolism to formic acid. Metabolic interactions of ethanol with other organic solvents, such as "degreasers' flush" in workers exposed to trichloroethylene and other chlorinated hydrocarbons, are frequently due to competition for alcohol and aldehyde dehydrogenases, with subsequent accumulation of the alcohol and aldehyde and resulting reaction. Secondary alcohols are primarily metabolized to ketones.

## Health Effects

The alcohols are more potent central nervous system depressants and irritants than the corresponding aliphatic hydrocarbons, but they are weaker skin and respiratory tract irritants than aldehydes or ketones. Respiratory tract and eye irritation usually occurs at lower concentrations than central nervous system depression and thus serves as a useful warning property. This may explain why occupational exposure to alcohols has not been implicated as causing chronic neurobehavioral effects. The TLVs for most alcohols are based on prevention of irritation.

Methyl alcohol is toxicologically distinct owing to its toxicity to the optic nerve, which can result in blindness. An extensive literature is available on this effect, which occurs primarily as a result of ingestion of methanol as an ethanol substitute or adulterant. A few poorly documented cases of blindness have been reported as a result of occupational inhalation exposure in confined spaces. The minimum oral dose causing blindness to an adult male has been estimated to be about 8–10 g; the minimum lethal dose is estimated to be 75–100 g. These amounts correspond to 8-hour exposure concentrations in air of approximately 1600–2000 ppm and 15,000–20,000 ppm, respectively. Blurred vision and other visual disturbances have been reported occasionally as a result of exposures to levels slightly above the TLV of 200 ppm. Methanol in urine can be used for biological monitoring, with 15 mg/L at the end of a work shift corresponding to an 8-hour exposure to the TLV of 200 ppm.

Inhalation exposure to ethanol and propanols result in simple irritation and central nervous system depression, though propanols may be significantly absorbed through the skin. There are a few reports of auditory and vestibular nerve injury in workers exposed to n-butyl alcohol. Isooctyl alcohol is the most industrially important of the higher alcohols, but little toxicologic information about it is available.

## GLYCOLS (DIOLS)

### Essentials of Diagnosis

*Acute effects:*
- Anesthesia (unusual due to low vapor pressure): dizziness, headache, nausea, vomiting, sleepiness, fatigue, "drunkenness," slurred speech, disequilibrium, disorientation, depression, and loss of consciousness.

*Chronic effects:*
- Dermatitis: dry, cracked, and erythematous skin.

### General Considerations

Glycols are hydrocarbons with two hydroxyl (alcohol) groups attached to separate carbon atoms in an aliphatic chain:

Examples include ethylene glycol, diethylene glycol, triethylene glycol, and propylene glycol (Table 29–1). They have a slightly sweet odor.

### Use

Glycols are used as antifreezing agents and as solvent carriers and vehicles in a variety of chemical formulations. Only ethylene glycol is in common general industrial use as a solvent, but large volumes of the others are used as vehicles and chemical intermediates. Approximately 40% of ethylene glycol is used as antifreeze, 35% to make polyesters, and 25% as solvent carriers.

### Occupational & Environmental Exposure

NIOSH estimates that nearly 2 million workers are potentially exposed to ethylene glycol, 660,000 to diethylene glycol, and 226,000 to triethylene glycol, primarily as a result of their being directly handled, heated, or sprayed.

### Pharmacokinetics

The glycols have such low vapor pressures that inhalation is only of moderate concern unless heated or aerosolized. Ethylene glycol does not have a skin TLV designation. Ethylene glycol and diethylene glycol are metabolized to glycol aldehyde, glycolic acid, glyoxylic acid, oxalic acid, formic acid, glycine, and carbon dioxide. Oxalic acid is the cause of the acute renal failure and metabolic acidosis that occur following ingestion of ethylene glycol. The first two steps in this metabolism use alcohol and aldehyde dehydrogenase and may be competitively blocked by administration of ethyl alcohol.

## Health Effects

The low vapor pressures of the glycols result in little hazard in their customary industrial use. They are not significantly irritating to the skin or respiratory tract but can produce a chronic dermatitis from defatting of the skin. The systemic toxicity of ethylene glycol commonly seen after ingestion of commercial antifreeze compounds as an alcohol substitute—seizures, central nervous system depression, metabolic acidosis, and acute renal failure—have not been reported as a result of occupational exposure.

## PHENOLS

### Essentials of Diagnosis

*Acute effects:*
- Respiratory tract irritation: cough and sore nose and throat.
- Tissue destruction (eg, hepatic necrosis with abdominal pain, jaundice, abnormal liver function tests), kidney necrosis with acute renal failure, skin necrosis with blisters and burns.
- Anesthesia: dizziness, headache, nausea, vomiting, sleepiness, fatigue, "drunkenness," slurred speech, disequilibrium, disorientation, depression, and loss of consciousness.

*Chronic effects:*
- Dermatitis: dry, cracked, and erythematous skin.

### General Considerations

Phenols are aromatic alcohols:

Examples include phenol, cresol (methyl phenol), catechol (1,2,-benzenediol, 1,2-dihydroxybenzene), resorcinol (1,3-benzenediol, 1,3-dihydroxybenzene), and hydroquinone (1,4-benzenediol, 1,4-hydroxybenzene).

### Use

The industrial use of phenols as solvents is limited by their acute toxicity. Phenol is used as a cleaning agent, paint stripper, and disinfectant, but its chief use is as a chemical intermediate for phenolic resins, bisphenol A for epoxy resins, and other chemicals

and drugs. Cresol is used as a disinfectant and chemical intermediate. Catechol is used in photography, fur dyeing, and leather tanning and as a chemical intermediate. Resorcinol is used as a chemical intermediate for adhesives, dyes, and pharmaceuticals. Hydroquinone is used in photography, as a polymerization inhibitor, and as an antioxidant.

### Occupational & Environmental Exposure

NIOSH estimates that more than 10,000 workers are potentially exposed to phenol.

### Pharmacokinetics

Phenol is well absorbed both by inhalation of vapors and by dermal penetration of vapors and liquids. Phenol and cresols have skin TLV designations. Phenol is rapidly eliminated within 16 hours, almost entirely as conjugated phenol in urine.

### Health Effects

Phenol and related compounds are potent irritants that can be corrosive at high concentrations. As a result of their ability to complex with, denature, and precipitate proteins, they can be cytotoxic to all cells at sufficient concentrations. Direct contact with concentrated phenol can result in burns, local tissue necrosis, systemic absorption, and tissue necrosis in the liver, kidneys, urinary tract, and heart. Central nervous system depression occurs, as it does with all volatile organic solvents. A concentration of total phenol in urine of 250 mg/g of creatinine at the end of a work shift corresponds to an 8-hour exposure to the TLV of 5 ppm.

## KETONES

### Essentials of Diagnosis

*Acute effects:*
- Respiratory tract irritation: cough and sore nose and throat.
- Anesthesia: dizziness, headache, nausea, vomiting, sleepiness, fatigue, "drunkenness," slurred speech, disequilibrium, disorientation, depression, and loss of consciousness.

*Chronic effects:*
- Dermatitis: dry, cracked, and erythematous skin.

### General Considerations

Ketones are hydrocarbons with a carbonyl group that is attached to two hydrocarbon groups (the carbonyl is nonterminal):

They are produced by the dehydroxylation or oxidation of alcohols. A great many ketones are in use—some used as industrial solvents are listed in Table 29–1. Acetone and methyl ethyl ketone (2-butanone) are in most common use. The ketones have a characteristic minty odor that some people find pleasant and others offensive.

## Use

Ketones are widely used as solvents for surface coatings with natural and synthetic resins; in the formulation of inks, adhesives, and dyes; in chemical extraction and manufacture; and, to a lesser extent, as cleaning agents. About one-fourth of the acetone produced is used in the manufacture of methacrylates and one-third as solvent. Almost all cyclohexanone is used to make caprolactam for nylon, but small amounts are used as solvents.

## Occupational & Environmental Exposure

The wide use of ketones is reflected in the large numbers of potentially exposed workers estimated by NIOSH: acetone, 2,816,000; methyl ethyl ketone, 3,031,000; methyl isobutyl ketone, 1,853,000; cyclohexanone, 1,190,000; isophorone, 1,507,000; and diacetone alcohol, 1,350,000. The use of many ketones has decreased owing to their regulation as photochemical reactants. Consumer exposure to acetone is common in the form of nail polish remover and general use solvent.

## Pharmacokinetics

Ketones are well absorbed by inhalation of vapors and to a lesser extent after skin contact with liquid. Only cyclohexanone has a skin TLV designation. The pulmonary retention of acetone at rest has been estimated to be about 45%. Most ketones are rapidly eliminated unchanged in urine and exhaled air and by reduction to their respective alcohols, which are conjugated and excreted or further metabolized to a variety of compounds, including carbon monoxide. Acetone is excreted in the expired air of normal, healthy individuals at about 120 ng/L.

## Health Effects

Ketones have good warning properties in that irritation or a strong odor usually occurs at levels below those that cause central nervous system depression. Headaches and nausea as a result of the odor have been mistaken for central nervous system depression. The TLVs for most ketones are set to prevent irritation. A concentration of acetone in urine of 100 mg/L at the end of a work shift corresponds to an 8-hour exposure to the TLV of 750 ppm.

Methyl n-butyl ketone causes the same type of peripheral neuropathy as n-hexane. It is metabolized to the neurotoxic diketone 2,5-hexanedione to an even greater extent than n-hexane and therefore poses an even greater hazard. The neurotoxic potential of methyl n-butyl ketone was discovered following the occurrence of a large number of cases of peripheral neuropathy in a plastics manufacturing plant in Ohio in 1974. A large volume of research has been published since, from animal neurotoxicity and metabolism studies to cell culture and mechanistic studies. However, human exposure to this substance no longer occurs, since the sole manufacturer ceased production a number of years ago. Other ketones used as solvents have not been shown to cause peripheral neuropathy, but methyl ethyl ketone (MEK) potentiates the neurotoxicity of n-hexane and methyl n-butyl ketone, probably through a metabolic interaction. Concentrations of MEK and methyl isobutyl ketone (MIBK) of 2 mg/L at the end of a work shift correspond to 8-hour exposures to the TVLs of 200 and 50 ppm, respectively.

## ESTERS

### Essentials of Diagnosis

*Acute effects:*

- Anesthesia: dizziness, headache, nausea, vomiting, sleepiness, fatigue, "drunkenness," slurred speech, disequilibrium, disorientation, depression, and loss of consciousness.
- Respiratory tract irritation: cough and sore nose and throat.

*Chronic effects:*

- Dermatitis: dry, cracked, and erythematous skin.

### General Considerations

Esters are hydrocarbons that are derivatives of an organic acid and an alcohol:

$$-\mathrm{C}=\mathrm{O}$$
$$\backslash\mathrm{O}-\mathrm{C}-$$

They are named after their parent alcohols and acids, respectively (eg, methyl acetate for the ester of methyl alcohol and acetic acid). Examples of some of the many esters used as solvents are listed in Table 29–1. They have characteristic odors that range from sweet to pungent.

### Use

Esters—particularly the lower esters—are commonly used as solvents for surface coatings. Vinyl acetate is used primarily in the production of polyvinyl acetate and polyvinyl alcohol. Other lower esters are used to make polymeric acrylates and methacrylates. Higher esters are used as plasticizers.

## Occupational & Environmental Exposure

NIOSH estimates that 70,000 workers are potentially exposed to vinyl acetate in polymer production in the United States. Large numbers of workers are potentially exposed to other esters used as industrial solvents, particularly in surface coatings.

## Pharmacokinetics

Esters are very rapidly metabolized by plasma esterases to their parent organic acids and alcohols.

## Health Effects

Many esters have extremely low odor thresholds, their distinctive sweet smells serving as good warning properties. Because of this property, n-amyl acetate (banana oil) is used as an odorant for qualitative fit testing of respirators. Esters are more potent anesthetics than corresponding alcohols, aldehydes, or ketones but are also strong irritants. Odor and irritation usually occur at levels below central nervous system depression. Their systemic toxicity is determined to a large extent by the toxicity of the corresponding alcohol. There is one report of optic nerve damage from exposure to methyl acetate as a result of metabolism to methanol and hence to formic acid (see Alcohols, above). Similarly, methyl formate may cause optic neuropathy following metabolism directly to formic acid.

# ETHERS

## Essentials of Diagnosis

*Acute effects:*
- Anesthesia: dizziness, headache, nausea, vomiting, sleepiness, fatigue, "drunkenness," slurred speech, disequilibrium, disorientation, depression, and loss of consciousness.
- Respiratory tract irritation: cough and sore nose and throat.

*Chronic effects:*
- Dermatitis: dry, cracked, and erythematous skin.

## General Considerations

Ethers consist of two hydrocarbon groups joined by an oxygen linkage:

$$—C—O—C—$$

Examples include ethyl ether and dioxane (Table 29–1). They have a characteristic sweet odor often described as "ethereal."

## Use

Ethyl ether was used extensively in the past as an anesthetic but has been replaced by agents less flammable and explosive. It is too volatile for most solvent uses except analytic extraction. It is used as a solvent for waxes, fats, oils, and gums. Dioxane (1,4-diethylene dioxide) is used as a solvent for a wide range of organic products, including cellulose esters, rubber, and coatings; in the preparation of histologic slides; and as a stabilizer in chlorinated solvents. Methoxy ter-butyl ether (MTBE) has been widely used as an oxygenated fuel additive to reduce carbon monoxide emissions.

## Occupational & Environmental Exposure

Occupational exposure to ethyl ether is largely confined to analytic laboratories. NIOSH estimates that 2500 workers are exposed to dioxane in its use as a solvent, and many more may be exposed through its use as a stabilizer in chlorinated solvents. Inhalation exposure to MTBE is widespread because of its use in gasoline.

## Pharmacokinetics

Ethyl ether is well absorbed by inhalation of vapors; its volatility limits percutaneous absorption. Over 90% of absorbed ethyl ether is excreted unchanged in exhaled air; the rest may be metabolized by enzymatic cleavage of the ether link to acetaldehyde and acetic acid. Dioxane is well absorbed by inhalation of vapors and through skin contact with liquid and has a skin TLV designation. It is metabolized almost entirely to β-hydroxyethoxyacetic acid and excreted in urine with a half-life of about 1 hour.

## Health Effects

Ethyl ether is a potent anesthetic and a less potent irritant. Higher ethers are relatively more potent irritants. Dioxane is also an anesthetic and irritant but has also caused acute kidney and liver necrosis in workers exposed to uncertain amounts. Animal cancer studies have indicated an increased incidence of tumors at about 10,000 ppm in the diet but not at about 100 ppm by inhalation. Studies in exposed workers have been inadequate. The issue of carcinogenic risk from exposure to dioxane is controversial. Exposure to gasoline containing MTBE has been associated with headache, nausea, eye irritation, dizziness, vomiting, sedation, and nosebleeds. MTBE causes liver tumors in mice and other hematologic malignancies in rats. This has raised concern about possible synergistic effects with benzene, which is also present in gasoline.

# GLYCOL ETHERS

## Essentials of Diagnosis

*Acute effects:*
- Anesthesia: dizziness, headache, nausea, vomiting, sleepiness, fatigue, "drunkenness," slurred

speech, disequilibrium, disorientation, depression, and loss of consciousness.

*Chronic effects:*

- Dermatitis: dry, cracked, and erythematous skin.
- Anemia: low erythrocyte count or pancytopenia and evidence of hemolysis or bone marrow suppression
- Encephalopathy: confusion and disorientation.
- Reproductive toxicity (laboratory animals): major malformations with maternal exposure, low sperm count, testicular atrophy, and infertility with male exposure.

## General Considerations

The glycol ethers are alkyl ether derivatives of ethylene, diethylene, triethylene, and propylene glycol (an alkyl group linked to the glycol by an oxygen). The acetate derivatives of glycol ethers are included and are considered toxicologically identical to their precursors. They are known by formal chemical names (eg, ethylene glycol monomethyl ether [EGME]); common chemical names (2-methoxyethanol, 2-ME), used here; and trade names (Methyl Cellosolve).

## Use

The glycol ethers are widely used solvents because of their solubility or miscibility in water and most organic liquids. They are used as diluents in paints, lacquers, enamels, inks, and dyes; as cleaning agents in liquid soaps, dry cleaning fluids, and glass cleaners; as surfactants, fixatives, desiccants, antifreeze compounds, and deicers; and in extraction and chemical synthesis. They are used extensively in the semiconductor industry. Since the first two members of this family, 2-methoxyethanol and 2-ethoxyethanol, were found to be potent reproductive toxins in laboratory animals and their TLVs lowered on this basis, there has been a shift in use to 2-butoxyethanol and other longer-chained ethylene glycol ethers and to diethylene and propylene glycol ethers.

## Occupational & Environmental Exposure

Over 1 million workers are potentially exposed to each of the most commonly used glycol ethers and their acetates. Accurate estimates are not available owing to the recent shifts in their use patterns. Because of their low volatility, the most important exposures occur as a result of direct contact with liquids, inhalation of vapors in enclosed spaces, and spraying or heating of the liquids to generate aerosols or vapors. These exposures can easily exceed the doses of 2-methoxyethanol and 2-ethoxyethanol that cause reproductive toxicity in laboratory animals.

Environmental exposure occurs because of the presence of some glycol ethers in consumer products, such as glass cleaners. Glass-cleaning workers have been shown to have elevated levels of butoxyacetic acid in urine despite TWA air exposure levels below 3 ppm, suggesting that the skin is the predominant route of exposure.

## Pharmacokinetics

The glycol ethers are well absorbed by all routes of exposure owing to their universal solubility. They have relatively low vapor pressures, so that dermal exposure is often of primary importance. The acetate derivatives are rapidly hydrolyzed by plasma esterases to their corresponding monoalkyl ethers. The ethylene glycol monoalkyl ethers maintain their ether linkages and are metabolized by hepatic alcohol and aldehyde dehydrogenases to their respective aldehyde and acid metabolites. The acid metabolites 2-methoxyacetic acid and 2-ethoxyacetic acid are responsible for the reproductive toxicities of 2-methoxyethanol and 2-ethoxyethanol. These metabolites are excreted in urine unchanged or conjugated to glycine and may be used as biologic indicators of exposure.

## Health Effects

Acute central nervous system depression has not been reported as an effect of occupational exposure. However, a number of cases of encephalopathy have been reported in workers exposed to 2-methoxyethanol over periods of weeks to months. Manifestations have included personality changes, memory loss, difficulty in concentrating, lethargy, fatigue, loss of appetite, weight loss, tremor, gait disturbances, and slurred speech.

Bone marrow toxicity usually manifested as pancytopenia has been reported in workers and laboratory animals exposed to 2-methoxyethanol and 2-ethoxyethanol. The longer-chain ethylene glycol monoalkyl ethers cause hemolysis by increasing osmotic fragility in laboratory animals, an effect that has not been reported to date in humans.

Male reproductive toxicity was recently demonstrated in experimental animals for 2-methoxyethanol, 2-ethoxyethanol, and their acetate derivatives. Acute or chronic exposure of mice, rats, and rabbits to low levels of these compounds by inhalation, dermal, or oral routes resulted in reductions in sperm count, impaired sperm motility, increased numbers of abnormal forms, and infertility. These effects began about 4 weeks after the onset of exposure and—in the absence of testicular atrophy—were reversible following cessation of exposure.

The testicular toxicity of the glycol ethers decreases sharply with lengthening of the alkyl group, such that beginning with and proceeding through butyl n-propyl and isopropyl they are nearly or completely inactive. The acetic acid derivatives (alkoxy acids) appear to be the active testicular toxins. In limited testing, the dimethyl ethers of ethylene glycol and diethylene glycol—but not the monomethyl ether of diethylene glycol—show some evidence of causing testicular toxicity, though the latter has not been tested at the high doses that have been shown to be teratogenic. Ethylene glycol hexyl ether, ethylene glycol phenyl ether, and the propylene glycol ethers do not appear to be toxic to either the male or female reproductive systems.

The same glycol ethers that are testicular toxins have been shown to be teratogenic in the same and additional species of laboratory animals at comparable doses. The structure-activity relationships also appear to be similar; the alkoxy acid metabolites are apparently the proximate teratogens. Major defects of the skeleton, kidneys, and cardiovascular system have been observed, with some variation in their nature and severity with species, dose, and route of administration. The ethylene glycol monoalkyl ethers with longer alkyl chains and other glycol (propylene and dipropylene) ethers have not been shown to be teratogenic with the exception of the diethylene glycol ethers, which produced typical malformations.

There have been only limited studies of reproductive effects of the glycol ethers in humans to date. However, three studies of occupationally exposed men and women have provided evidence that the effects in humans are the same as those in animals. Two recent epidemiologic studies of semiconductor workers showed that women exposed to 2-ethoxyethanol had increased risk of spontaneous abortion.

One study of male workers exposed to 2-methoxyethanol or 2-ethoxyethanol found evidence of spermatotoxicity. Since reproductive effects have been consistently produced in all species tested and their metabolism and other health effects appear to be similar in humans and laboratory animals, those compounds with reproductive effects in animals should be assumed to be potential testicular toxins and teratogens in humans. Biological monitoring may be necessary to ensure that exposure is minimized. When possible, the risk of reproductive toxicity from these compounds should be reduced by substitution of other glycol ethers or other solvents.

# GLYCIDYL ETHERS

## Essentials of Diagnosis

*Acute effects:*
• Dermatitis (primary irritant): irritation, erythema, and first and second degree burns of skin.

*Chronic effects:*
• Dermatitis (allergic contact): itching, erythema, and vesicles.

## General Considerations

The glycidyl ethers consist of a 2,3-epoxypropyl group with an ether linkage to another hydrocarbon group:

They are synthesized from epichlorohydrin and an alcohol. Only the monoglycidyl ethers are in common use and will be discussed here.

## Use

The epoxide or oxirane ring of glycidyl ethers makes these compounds very reactive, so their use is confined to processes that utilize this property, such as reactive diluents in epoxy resin systems. Epoxy resins have a wide range of applications in industry and consumer use (see Chapter 30).

## Occupational & Environmental Exposure

The primary exposure of workers and consumers is in the application of uncured epoxy resins. The epoxide groups of the ethers react to form crosslinkages within epoxy resins, so that glycidyl ethers no longer exist in a completely cured resin. However, workers may be exposed to the ethers in their manufacture and in the formulation and application of the resin system. NIOSH estimates that 118,000 workers in the United States are potentially exposed to glycidyl ethers and an additional 1 million to epoxy resins.

## Pharmacokinetics

The glycidyl ethers have low vapor pressures, so that inhalation at normal air temperatures is not usually a concern. However, the curing of epoxy resins often generates heat, which may vaporize some glycidyl ether. A number of uses such as epoxy paint require spraying and the generation of an aerosol. Although quantitative data are lacking, the glycidyl ethers should be well absorbed by all routes. They have a short biological half-life owing to their reactivity. Three metabolic reactions have been proposed: reduction to diols by epoxide hydrase, conjugation with glutathione, and covalent bonding with proteins, RNA, and DNA.

## Health Effects

Reported effects of glycidyl ethers from occupational exposure have been confined to dermatitis of both the primary irritant and allergic contact type. Dermatitis can be severe and may result in second degree burns. Asthma in workers exposed to epoxy resins may be due to exposure to glycidyl ethers.

Glycidyl ethers are positive in a number of short-term tests of genotoxicity, including mutagenicity, but none have been adequately tested for carcinogenicity. They are testicular toxins in laboratory animals, but few have been tested for teratogenicity.

## ORGANIC ACIDS

### Essentials of Diagnosis

*Acute effects:*
- Respiratory tract irritation: sore nose and throat and cough.

*Chronic effects:*
- Dermatitis: dry, cracked, and erythematous skin.

### General Considerations

Organic acids are derivatives of carboxylic acid:

$$-C \overset{\displaystyle =O}{\underset{\displaystyle OH}{\phantom{|}}}$$

Acetic acid (vinegar) is used in a variety of industrial settings, including photographic development. Other organic acids are used to a lesser extent. Most organic acids are such strong irritants that they can be considered as primary irritants and not anesthetics.

## ALIPHATIC AMINES

### Essentials of Diagnosis

*Acute effects:*
- Eye irritation, corneal edema, and visual halos.
- Respiratory tract irritation: sore nose and throat and cough.
- Dermatitis (irritant): erythema and irritation of skin.

*Chronic effects:*
- Dermatitis (allergic contact): erythema, vesicles, and itching of skin.
- Asthma (ethyleneamines): cough, wheezing, shortness of breath, dyspnea on exertion, and decreased FVC on pulmonary function testing with response to bronchodilators.

### General Considerations

Aliphatic amines are derivatives of ammonia in which one or more hydrogen atoms are replaced by an alkyl or alkanol group:

$$C - C - NH_2 \qquad\qquad -C - \overset{\displaystyle OH}{\underset{\displaystyle}{C}} - NH_2$$

(primary amine)          (alkanolamine)

They can be classified as primary, secondary, and tertiary monoamines according to the number of substitutions on the nitrogen atom; as polyamines if more than one amine group is present; and as alkanolamines if a hydroxyl group is present on the alkyl group (an alcohol). They have a characteristic odor like that of fish and are strongly alkaline.

### Use

There are a large number of aliphatic amines that have a number of uses. They are used to some extent as solvents but to a greater degree as chemical intermediates. They are also used as catalysts for polymerization reactions, preservatives (bactericides), corrosion inhibitors, drugs, and herbicides.

### Occupational & Environmental Exposure

Given the diversity of their uses, accurate estimates of the number of workers exposed to aliphatic amines are not possible. They are not common environmental pollutants.

### Pharmacokinetics

Little is known of the pharmacokinetics of the aliphatic amines in industrial use. They are well absorbed by inhalation, and some have skin designations as a result of their percutaneous absorption (Table 29–1). Metabolism is probably primarily deamination to ammonia by monoamine oxidase and diamine oxidase.

### Health Effects

The vapors of the volatile amines cause eye irritation and a characteristic corneal edema, with visual changes of halos around lights, that is reversible. Irritation will occur wherever contact with the vapors occurs, including the respiratory tract and skin. Direct contact with the liquid can produce serious eye or skin burns. Allergic contact dermatitis has been reported primarily from ethyleneamines, as has asthma.

## CHLORINATED HYDROCARBONS

### Essentials of Diagnosis

*Acute effects:*
- Anesthesia: Dizziness, headache, nausea, vomiting, sleepiness, fatigue, "drunkenness," slurred speech, disequilibrium, disorientation, depression, and loss of consciousness.
- Respiratory tract irritation: cough and sore nose and throat.

*Chronic effects:*
- Dermatitis: dry, cracked, and erythematous skin.
- Neurobehavioral dysfunction: headache, mood lability, fatigue, short-term memory loss, difficulty in concentrating, decreased attention span, neurobehavioral test abnormalities, CT scan (cerebral atrophy), EEG (diffuse slow waves).
- Hepatocellular injury: abdominal pain, nausea, jaundice, and abnormal liver function tests.
- Renal tubular dysfunction: weakness, fatigue,

polyuria, glycosuria, electrolyte abnormalities (acidosis, hypokalemia, hypophosphatemia, hypochloremia, and hypocarbonatemia), glycosuria, and proteinuria.

## General Considerations

The addition of chlorine to carbon and hydrogen

increases the stability and decreases the flammability of the resulting compounds. They have characteristic slightly pungent odors. Six chlorinated aliphatic hydrocarbons are commonly used as solvents: trichloroethylene, perchloroethylene (tetrachloroethylene), 1,1,1-trichloroethane (methyl chloroform), methylene chloride (dichloromethane), carbon tetrachloride, and chloroform. Other chlorinated aliphatic hydrocarbons such as ethylene dichloride and chlorinated aromatics such as chlorobenzenes are rarely used as general industrial solvents and will not be discussed here. Abbreviations such as TCE and TCA will not be used since they are not standardized and can lead to errors in identification.

## Use

The chlorinated hydrocarbons are used extensively as cleaning, degreasing, and thinning agents and less so as chemical intermediates. Historically, trichloroethylene was the principal solvent used in vapor degreasers, and while 80% of trichloroethylene is still used for this purpose, it is being replaced by 1,1,1-trichloroethane and chlorofluorocarbons (CFCs), which are somewhat safer, although many CFCs are being phased out because of their ozone-depleting properties. Perchloroethylene has replaced mineral spirits and carbon tetrachloride as the primary dry-cleaning solvent in two-thirds of facilities because of the flammability of the former and the toxicity of the latter.

Methylene chloride is used as a paint stripper and extraction agent. Chloroform is used for extraction and spot cleaning. Carbon tetrachloride is used primarily as a chemical intermediate and in small quantities as a spot cleaning agent. 1,1,1-Trichloroethane is used in vapor degreasers and increasingly as a general cleaning and thinning agent.

## Occupational & Environmental Exposure

Table 29–4 shows the estimated number of workers exposed and typical air and contaminated drinking water level for the common chlorinated hydrocarbon solvents. Chloroform is present in drinking water as one of the trihalogenated methanes produced as a

**Table 29–4.** Chlorinated hydrocarbon solvents: Occupational and environmental exposure data.

| Solvent | Number of Workers Exposed[1] | Ambient Air[2] | Drinking Water[3] |
|---|---|---|---|
| Trichloroethylene | 100,000 full-time 3.5 million part-time | 1 ppb | 1–30 ppb |
| Perchloroethylene | 27,000 full-time 550,000 part-time | 1–10 ppb | 1–2 ppb |
| 1,1,1-Trichloroethane | 100,000 | 1 ppb | 1–10 ppb |
| Methylene chloride | 70,000 | 0.5–5 ppb | < 1 ppb |
| Carbon tetrachloride | 160,000 | 0.1 ppb | < 1 ppb |
| Chloroform | 80,000 | < 1 ppb | < 100 ppb |

[1]NIOSH estimates.
[2]EPA-reported average urban concentrations.
[3]EPA-reported range in contaminated drinking water.

result of chlorination. EPA recently proposed a 100-ppb limit for total trihalogenated methanes, including chloroform, in drinking water.

## Pharmacokinetics

The chlorinated hydrocarbon solvents are all relatively volatile and moderately well absorbed by inhalation. Pulmonary uptake ranges from 60% to 80% at rest and decreases to 40–50% during activity. Percutaneous absorption of vapors is usually insignificant, but dermal absorption following prolonged or extensive contact of the skin with liquid can be significant.

Biological monitoring of the chlorinated hydrocarbons is based on their pattern of metabolism and excretion, which varies with their structure. 1,1,1-Trichloroethane and perchloroethylene are excreted mainly unchanged in exhaled air and metabolized and excreted only slightly as trichloroethanol and trichloroacetic acid. Therefore, biological monitoring has been conducted chiefly with exhaled air and to a lesser extent with the parent compound in blood and metabolites in urine. Accumulation of both compounds occurs to some degree with daily exposure.

In contrast, less than 10% of trichloroethylene is excreted unchanged in exhaled air. The remainder is rapidly metabolized by alcohol and aldehyde dehydrogenases via chloral hydrate to trichloroethanol and trichloroacetic acid, or to unidentified metabolites. Although the biological half-life of the parent compound is very short, trichloroethanol is an active anesthetic, and with a half-life of 10–15 hours accumulates to some extent over the course of a work week. Trichloroacetic acid, though inactive, has a much longer half-life of 50–100 hours and has been recommended for use in biological monitoring. A value of 100 mg/L in urine voided at the end of the work week corresponds to exposure to a TWA of 50 ppm trichloroethylene. However, because of large individual variability, this value can be used only to assess groups of workers and not individuals.

Methylene chloride is both excreted unchanged in exhaled air and metabolized to carbon monoxide in a dose-dependent fashion. An 8-hour exposure to methylene chloride at its prior TLV of 100 ppm results in a carboxyhemoglobin level of about 3–5% in a nonsmoker, while exposure at its current (proposed) TLV carboxyhemoglobin levels are indistinguishable from background (1–2%). Methylene chloride in blood and exhaled air can also be used as biologic indicators of exposure.

Chloroform and carbon tetrachloride are each approximately 50% excreted unchanged in exhaled air and 50% metabolized. Both can be measured in blood and exhaled air, but little information is available on biologic monitoring for either.

## Health Effects

As a class, the chlorinated hydrocarbons are more potent anesthetics, hepatotoxins, and nephrotoxins than other organic solvents. Most have been found to cause hepatocarcinomas in laboratory mice following oral administration. Evidence for carcinogenicity following inhalation has been recently demonstrated for methylene chloride and perchloroethylene, while adequate inhalation bioassays of the remainder have not been completed. Because of their common industrial use, the issue of carcinogenic risk to humans from exposure to these compounds is one of the most controversial topics in regulatory toxicology. There are surprisingly few animal studies examining their potential for reproductive toxicity, and almost none in male animals. Pertinent aspects of the toxicity of each compound will be briefly discussed.

## 1. TRICHLOROETHYLENE

The TLV of 50 ppm is based on prevention of central nervous system depression, which occurs at levels below those causing evidence of hepatic dysfunction. A National Toxicology Program (NTP) cancer bioassay in multiple rat strains conducted in an attempt to address the uncertainty over results in mice was unfortunately inadequate owing to insufficient survival in dosed animals, so that the carcinogenicity of trichloroethylene remains unresolved. Reproductive effects have been little studied. One study showed that trichloroethylene causes developmental effects and full-litter resorption in the presence of maternal toxicity (altered weight gain). It was associated with malformation suggestive of teratogenicity (microphthalmia).

## 2. PERCHLOROETHYLENE

Perchloroethylene is approximately equipotent to trichloroethylene as an anesthetic and more potent an irritant. Its TLV of 50 ppm is set to prevent both effects. An NTP inhalation bioassay provided clear evidence of carcinogenicity in mice and male rats and some evidence in female rats. Limited studies of the effects of perchloroethylene on reproduction in animals suggest that perchloroethylene may be spermatotoxic. Perchloroethylene caused full-litter resorption and delayed partutition and reduced prenatal and postnatal viability in one recent study. One case has been reported of obstructive jaundice in a newborn who was nursed in a drycleaning shop where perchloroethylene was used and was found in the mother's breast milk. Subclinical behavioral effects of perchloroethylene, including decrements in visual reproduction, pattern memory, and pattern recognition were measured in workers exposed to an estimated average concentration of 41 ppm for more than 3 years.

## 3. TRICHLOROETHANE

1,1,1-Trichloroethane is only weakly hepatotoxic, with minor injury reported following massive overexposure. It is the weakest anesthetic of this group; its TLV of 350 ppm is established to prevent this effect. Sudden deaths in situations indicative of acute overexposure have been attributed to cardiac arrhythmias as a result of cardiac sensitization. The compound is weakly positive for mutagenicity in Salmonella, but it has not been adequately tested for carcinogenicity or reproductive toxicity. Several case reports suggest the possibility of peripheral neuropathy associated with 1,1,1-trichloroethane.

## 4. CARBON TETRACHLORIDE

Carbon tetrachloride is a potent anesthetic. Both acute and chronic effects on the liver and kidneys have been reported at levels not much higher than those causing central nervous system depression. The TLV of 5 ppm (skin) was established to prevent fatty infiltration of the liver demonstrated in animals at 10 ppm and potentiated by alcohol ingestion. Deaths have occurred from both hepatic and renal necrosis, and liver cancer has been reported in workers following acute liver damage from acute overexposure. The TLV has an A2 (suspected human carcinogen) designation. There is evidence that carbon tetrachloride is fetotoxic but not teratogenic, and it causes testicular and ovarian damage in animals at toxic doses—but there is no evidence about effects at nontoxic doses.

## 5.  CHLOROFORM

Chloroform is only slightly less potent than carbon tetrachloride as an anesthetic and liver toxin. Its TLV was lowered to 10 ppm (A2) by ACGIH because of its carcinogenicity to rats (epithelial tumors of the kidney) and mice (hepatocarcinoma) and embryotoxicity to the rat at 30–300 ppm by inhalation.

## 6.  METHYLENE CHLORIDE

Methylene chloride is similar to perchloroethylene and trichloroethylene in potency as an anesthetic and liver toxin. It is unique in that it is metabolized to carbon monoxide, with formation of carboxyhemoglobin. At exposure levels above 100 ppm, carboxyhemoglobin levels can exceed 10%, so that the presence of anoxia in addition to anesthesia must be considered. The TLV was recently lowered from 100 ppm to 50 ppm to provide a wider margin of safety in preventing liver injury and lowering carboxyhemoglobin to near background levels—and in recognition of evidence for carcinogenicity in animals. Methylene chloride was fetotoxic but not teratogenic to rats and mice exposed to 1225 ppm, although it was associated with delayed ossification of the sternum in prenatally exposed rats.

## CHLOROFLUOROCARBONS (CFCS)

### Essentials of Diagnosis

*Acute effects:*
- Respiratory tract irritation: cough and sore nose and throat.
- Anesthesia: dizziness, headache, nausea, vomiting, sleepiness, fatigue, "drunkenness," slurred speech, disequilibrium, disorientation, depression, and loss of consciousness.
- Cardiac sensitization: dizziness, palpitations, faintness, loss of consciousness, and arrhythmia on ambulatory cardiac monitoring.

*Chronic effects:*
- Dermatitis: dry, cracked, and erythematous skin.

### General Considerations

CFC solvents are aliphatic hydrocarbons (methane or ethane) that contain one or more atoms each of chlorine and fluorine. Table 29–1 lists the commonly used CFC solvents.[1]

---

[1]The numbering system for chlorofluorocarbons offers a convenient method of determining their chemical formulas. The "units" digit is the number of fluorine atoms (with CFC-113, this would be 3); the "tens" digit is the number of hydrogen atoms plus 1; and the "hundreds" digit is the number of carbon atoms minus 1. (Thus, CFC-113 would contain 3 fluorine atoms, no hydrogen atoms, and 2 carbon atoms, thereby requiring 3 chlorine atoms to make trichlorotrifluoroethane.)

CFCs are often referred to as Freons, which is the trade name of CFCs manufactured by Dupont. A CFC may be formulated with another organic solvent, such as methanol or methylene chloride, in a proprietary solvent mixture.

### Use

The main solvent uses of CFCs are as cleaning and degreasing agents. CFC-113 has been used increasingly in dry cleaning in closed systems ("dry-to-dry") as a replacement for open systems ("wet-to-dry") using perchloroethylene. Other uses include refrigeration and air-conditioning fluids, propellants, foam blowing agents, vehicles for pesticides, paints, and other materials, and intermediates in the manufacture of plastics and resins. Restrictions have been placed on CFC use in general, with a phase-out scheduled for many CFCs because of their role in depletion of stratospheric ozone. The completely halogenated CFCs are those implicated in this effect. Bromine-containing compounds are widely used as fire extinguishing agents (see Chapter 30).

Five CFCs account for almost 99% of all US CFC production. The most common uses for these compounds are shown in Table 29–5.

### Occupational & Environmental Exposures

The widespread use of CFCs in industry and in consumer products has resulted in exposure of large numbers of workers and consumers and in global contamination of the environment. In homes where aerosols are used, ambient air concentrations of CFCs can be significantly higher than that outside.

### Pharmacokinetics

Very little information is available on the pharmacokinetics of CFCs. Most are probably resistant to metabolism and are excreted rapidly unchanged in exhaled air. Correlations undoubtedly exist between exposure and concentrations in exhaled air, but information is too limited to recommend biologic monitoring.

### Health Effects

The CFCs are of relatively low toxicity. All are

**Table 29–5.** Uses of chlorofluorocarbons.

| Use | Chlorofluorocarbon |
| --- | --- |
| Cleaning and degreasing | CFC-113, CFC-11 |
| Refrigeration and air conditioning | CFC-22, CFC-12, CFC-11 |
| Foam blowing | CFC-11 |
| Aerosol propellant | CFC-12, CFC-11, CFC-114 |
| Plastics manufacturing | CFC-12, CFC-22 |

anesthetics but require exposure to concentrations above 500–1000 ppm before this effect is manifested. Such levels most commonly are encountered in enclosed spaces (eg, cleaning out a degreasing tank) or when the CFC is heated (eg, using a heated vapor degreaser) or sprayed (eg, when used as propellant). They have not been associated with chronic neurobehavioral effects. They are not strong irritants.

Prolonged or frequent skin contact can cause a typical solvent dermatitis. Cardiac sensitization was first demonstrated for CFCs after a number of cases of sudden death of persons abusing CFC-11 and CFC-12 beginning in the late 1960s. An NCI bioassay of CFC-11 was negative for mice and inconclusive for rats, while CFC-22 may have caused a slight increase in salivary gland tumors in male rats. Two rarely used chlorofluorocarbons, CFC-31 and CFC-133a, were carcinogenic in a limited gavage assay in rats. CFC-22, CFC-31, CFC-142b, CFC-143, and CFC-143a are positive in one or more short-term genotoxicity tests. CFC-22, the only one of the genotoxic CFCs in common use, is a weak bacterial mutagen. A number of CFCs have been tested for teratogenicity, including CFC-11, CFC-12, CFC-21, CFC-22, CFC-31, CFC-114, CFC-123b, and CFC-142b, but because of either inadequate design or inadequate reporting no conclusions about effects can be reached. Unpublished studies have reported that CFC-22 is teratogenic in rats but not rabbits, producing microphthalmia and anophthalmia at inhalation levels of 50,000 ppm.

## ALDEHYDES

### Essentials of Diagnosis

*Acute effects:*
• Respiratory tract irritation: cough and sore nose and throat.

*Chronic effects:*
• Dermatitis: dry, cracked, and erythematous skin.
• Asthma: cough, wheezing, shortness of breath, dyspnea on exertion, and decreased FVC on pulmonary function testing reversible with bronchodilators.

### General Considerations

The aldehydes are used primarily as preservatives, disinfectants, and chemical intermediates rather than as solvents. Glutaraldehyde is commonly used in hospitals as a disinfectant. The prototype aldehyde, formaldehyde, is discussed in Chapter 28. Most aldehydes are such strong irritants that at levels that would produce anesthetic effects irritation would be intolerable. Asthma has been associated with exposure to formaldehyde and glutaraldehyde.

## MISCELLANEOUS SOLVENTS

### Turpentine

Turpentine is a mixture of substances called terpenes, primarily pinene. Gum turpentine is extracted from pine pitch, wood turpentine from wood chips. It has had greater home than industrial use as a solvent. It is irritating and anesthetic and is one of the few solvents that causes allergic contact dermatitis. The incidence of sensitization varies with the type of pine, being generally higher with European than American pines. Owing to the frequency of allergic dermatitis, the availability of turpentine is now extremely limited. Limonene is a terpene used as a solvent for printing and art paints that also causes allergic contact dermatitis.

### Dimethylformamide

Dimethylformamide is a useful solvent because of its solubility in both aqueous and lipid media. However, these properties also result in its being well absorbed by all routes of exposure. It is a potent hepatotoxin and has been associated with both hepatitis and pancreatitis following occupational exposure. This hazard precludes most general industrial solvent uses. Two recent case series have associated dimethylformamide exposure with testicular cancer. Exposure can be monitored biologically by measuring monomethylformamide and related metabolites in urine.

### Dimethyl Sulfoxide

Like dimethylformamide, dimethyl sulfoxide is soluble in a variety of media and is well absorbed by all routes of exposure. It appears to potentiate the absorption of other substances through the skin. Its use has not been associated with significant toxicity, but it has been subjected to little scientific study. It has a characteristic garlic-like or oyster-like odor that is present in exhaled air of exposed persons. Its use as a dermally applied anti-inflammatory agent is not approved by the Federal Drug Administration, though it is used in that way in veterinary medicine.

# REFERENCES

Arlien-Søborg P: *Solvent Neurotoxicity.* CRC Press, 1992.

Axelson O, Hogstedt C: The health effects of solvents. In: Zenz C, Dickerson OB, Horvath EP (editors): *Occupational Medicine,* 3rd ed. Mosby, 1994.

Baker EL: A review of recent research on health effects of human occupational exposure to organic solvents. A critical review. J Occup Med 1994;36:1079.

Borak J: Glycol ethers: A quick review. OEM Rep 1993;7: 43.

Gerr F: Health effects of occupational and environmental exposure to solvents. In: Rom WN (editor): *Environmental and Occupational Medicine,* 3rd ed. Lippincott-Raven, 1997.

Juntunen J: Neurotoxic syndromes and occupational exposure to solvents. Environ Res 1993;60:98.

Lundberg I et al: Organic solvents and related compounds. In: Rosenstock L, Cullen MR (editors): *Textbook of Clinical Occupational and Environmental Medicine.* Saunders, 1994.

Lundberg I, Lidén C: Industrial Solvents. In: Corn M (editor): *Handbook of Hazardous Materials.* Academic Press, 1993.

# 30

# Plastics

*Richard Lewis, MD, MPH*

The emergence of the plastics industry during the past 40 years has had a major impact on many other industries, including manufacturing, construction, consumer products, medical supplies, and transportation. Articles made from plastics are ubiquitous in industrialized societies, being found in appliances, automobiles, toys, home furnishings, clothing, insulation, food and beverage containers, and countless other applications. Advances in plastics technology have resulted in the development of materials with properties that match or surpass in quality and utility those of traditional materials such as metal, wood, and glass. Plastic materials are versatile and can be readily shaped to meet changing design and engineering specification.

Plastics are divided into two main classes (Table 30–1).

**Thermoplastics** are linear or branched polymers that can be repeatedly softened and reshaped with the application of heat or pressure. These materials are recyclable, though variations in formulations and additives limit the recycling of products after they have reached the consumer.

**Thermoset** plastics undergo a chemical reaction during processing that results in permanent cross-linking. The finished materials are resistant to heat and cannot be re-formed. Table 30–1 lists the major thermoplastic and thermoset polymers in current use.

## HEALTH HAZARDS IN THE MANUFACTURE OF PLASTICS

As the plastics industry has grown over the last several decades, potential health hazards in manufacturing and processing have remained important concerns for the occupational health practitioner. The hazards related to the production and use of plastics fall into three areas: resin manufacture, plastic processing, and combustion.

### Resin Manufacture

Resin manufacture involves the linking of individual chemical units, or monomers, into long chains, termed polymers. Monomer chemicals are derived chiefly from the petrochemical industry. The chemical processes involved in the formation of plastics include crude oil distillation followed by catalytic cracking and re-formation. Other chemical reactions, such as the addition of halogen, may take place prior to polymerization.

Most of the polymerization processes take place in closed systems, and the health hazards of resin manufacture are similar to those of the petrochemical industry. Workers may be exposed to vapors and dusts containing chemical intermediates, polymers, and additives during loading, mixing, pelletizing, and maintenance operations. Proper storage and handling of chemicals and additives is mandatory. Reactions must be carefully controlled to avoid chemical release or explosion. Dry mixing and pelletizing operations may generate high concentrations of airborne dusts of combustible plastic materials, presenting an explosion hazard. The use of heavy machinery requires proper safety measures to avoid worker injury.

### Plastic Processing

There are currently nearly 60,000 companies involved in plastic processing; they employ more than 1.5 million workers internationally. The plastic processing industry converts the resins into finished products. Granules and powders may be compounded with additives prior to processing, and workers in these operations may have exposures similar to those of the resin manufacturers. Thermoset and partially polymerized materials may be supplied in solid or liquid form, and workers handling these materials may be exposed to unreacted intermediates and catalysts.

Plastic processing equipment uses high temperatures and pressures and must be equipped with guards and safety rails to avoid serious burns, amputations, and crush injuries. Plastic grinding may generate polymer dust, resulting in inhalation and possible combustion hazard. The overheating of plastic

Table 30–1. Principal plastic materials.

**Thermoplastics**
  Polyethylene
  Polyvinyl chloride
  Polypropylene
  Polystyrene
  Polyester
  ABS (acrylonitrile-butadiene-styrene)
  SAN (styrene-acrylonitrile)
  Acrylics
  Nylon
  Fluoropolymers
**Thermosets**
  Phenolics
  Polyurethane
  Urea and melamine
  Epoxies
  Cellulosics

Table 30–2. Thermal degradation products of some plastics.

| Polymer | Degradation Products | Hazards |
|---------|---------------------|---------|
| Polyethylene | Carbon monoxide | S |
| Polyvinyl chloride | Hydrochloric acid, phosgene | I, R |
| Polystyrene | Styrene | S |
|  | Benzene | S, C |
| Fluoropolymers | Carbonyl fluoride | I, R |
|  | Perfluoroisobutylene | I, R |
|  | Hydrogen fluoride | I, R |
| Polyurethane | Aldehydes, ammonia | I, R |
|  | Cyanide | S |
|  | Isocyanates | I, R |
|  | Nitrogen dioxide | R |
| Phenolics | Formaldehyde | I, R, S |
|  | Aldehydes, ammonia | I, R |
|  | Cyanide | S |
|  | Nitrogen dioxide | R |

A = asphyxiant; C = carcinogen; I = mucous membrane irritant; R = respiratory irritant; S = systemic poison.

materials during processing, cleaning, and maintenance may expose workers to the thermal decomposition products of the polymer materials. Finishing operations may expose workers to a variety of other chemical compounds, such as solvents and adhesives. In addition, cutting of plastics may result in repetitive motion injuries, such as tendinitis, sprains, and carpal tunnel syndrome.

## COMBUSTION PRODUCT HAZARDS

Thermoplastic materials must be heated during processing. The temperatures required to achieve proper fluidity vary with the composition of the polymer and the additives. Overheating of plastics results in thermal decomposition and the release of oligomers, monomers, and other combustion products. The composition of the mixture of gases and vapors that are evolved is extremely complex and depends not only on the chemical constituents of the polymer but also on the temperature. Workers may be exposed to the thermal decomposition products of plastics through accidental overheating during processing or during clean-out and maintenance operations. In addition, the burning of plastic materials during fires may present a health hazard to firefighters and the public.

The main combustion hazards that have been identified for the major classes of plastic materials are listed in Table 30–2. This list is far from complete, and new degradation products will be identified as research progresses. It is important to note that while combustion hazards are primarily respiratory irritants (hydrochloric acid, aldehydes), significant pulmonary injury (oxides of nitrogen) and systemic poisoning (carbon monoxide, cyanides) may occur. The long-term health effects of exposure to combustion products are unknown.

## THERMOPLASTICS

### POLYETHYLENE

#### Essentials of Diagnosis
- Asphyxia (ethylene).
- Respiratory irritation (thermal decomposition products).

#### Exposure Limits
  Ethylene
    ACGIH TLV: Asphyxiant

#### General Considerations & Production
Polyethylene is a semicrystalline, lightweight thermoplastic, first produced in 1942. High- and low-density polyethylene resins are the two leading plastics produced internationally, totaling nearly 20 billion lb (9 billion kg) per year. Over 100 different brands of polyethylene are available.

Polyethylene is produced by the polymerization of ethylene in either continuous-flow or tubular reactors. Catalysts include chromic oxide, aluminum alkyls, titanium chloride, and t-butyl esters. Density can be altered by addition of other olefins, such as butene, hexene, octene, and vinyl acetate. Liquid polymer is then cooled and pelletized.

#### Use
A primary use of high-density polyethylene is in

the production of containers (milk bottles, drums, fuel tanks), using blow molding. Other uses include the production of trash bags, pipe and wire covering by extrusion, and the production of containers, toys, and housewares by injection molding. Low-density polyethylene has higher clarity and is used for films, coating, shrink-wrapping, and food packaging and is formed primarily by extrusion.

## Exposure

The principal hazard of exposure to ethylene is asphyxia. Catalysts used are potent irritants of the eyes, skin, and respiratory system.

When burned at 230 °C (450 °F), polyethylene gives off primarily carbon monoxide, though the respiratory irritants acrolein and formaldehyde may also be formed. Occupational asthma has been attributed to exposure to acrolein or other irritants when overheating polyethylene.

The induction of tumors (primarily sarcomas) in laboratory animals by implants of polyethylene has been attributed to solid-state carcinogenesis rather than an effect of the polymer or monomer. Intrauterine devices made of polyethylene have been associated with endometrial metaplasia, perhaps by a similar process, in humans.

## Prevention

The use of enclosed processes will prevent exposure to ethylene gas. Proper respiratory protection should be worn by persons cleaning machinery or reaction vessels. Avoiding overheating or burning polyethylene will prevent exposure to irritant aldehydes and other decomposition products. Medical surveillance of workers should focus on the respiratory system.

## Treatment

Workers overcome by ethylene in an oxygen-deficient atmosphere should be rescued by persons equipped with air-supplied respirators. Once the victim has been removed to a fresh air environment, treatment consists of cardiopulmonary resuscitation and 100% oxygen. Exposure to respiratory irritants usually results in self-limited symptoms that resolve after removal from exposure. Asthma should be treated with inhaled bronchodilators.

## POLYPROPYLENE

### Essentials of Diagnosis
- Asphyxia (propylene).
- Respiratory irritation (thermal combustion products).

### Exposure Limits
Propylene
ACGIH TLV: Asphyxiant

## General Considerations & Production

Polypropylene was first brought into production in 1957. It is characterized by high heat resistance, strength, and resistance to corrosion by chemicals such as detergents and alcohols. Production of polypropylene generally occurs in a slurry with a hydrocarbon diluent and the addition of an organometallic catalyst. High-activity catalysts improve the quality of the finished polymer. Solvent vapors are generated during drying and grinding.

## Use

Through extrusion, a major application of polypropylene is in the production of fibers for carpeting and clothing. Blow and injection molding are used to produce medical containers, syringes, battery casings, dashboards, packing materials, and components for appliances.

## Exposure

Polypropylene is an asphyxiant. As in the case of polyethylene, the main hazards are respiratory irritation due to exposure to thermal decomposition products. This may occur during the welding of pipe made from polypropylene, particularly in poorly ventilated spaces. A single study suggested that workers exposed to polypropylene fibers may be at an increased risk for developing colorectal polyps and colon cancers. Subsequent studies have not confirmed this finding. Since this is an important condition in the general population, workplace screening should be considered.

## Prevention

Awareness of the hazards from release of propylene into enclosed spaces will prevent asphyxia during maintenance and cleaning operations. Polypropylene should not be burned or heated without proper ventilation or respiratory protection.

## Treatment

Treatment is the same as that for polyethylene, above.

## POLYVINYL CHLORIDE

### Essentials of Diagnosis
- Asthma and respiratory effects: wheezing, dyspnea, cough, and chest tightness.
- Angiosarcoma: nausea, abdominal pain, weight loss, jaundice, and hepatomegaly.
- Acro-osteolysis (vinyl chloride monomer): pain, loss of bone structure at ends of phalanges.

### Exposure Limits
Vinyl chloride monomer
ACGIH TLV: 5 ppm TWA

OSHA PEL: 1 ppm TWA, 5 ppm ceiling (15 minutes)

NIOSH REL: Lowest reliable detectable concentration

## General Considerations & Production

Although polyvinyl production began in 1927, it was not until the 1970s that the toxicity and carcinogenicity of vinyl chloride monomer became widely recognized. Vinyl chloride is a gas at room temperature, and polymerization reactions take place in pressure vessels. Whereas in recent years worker exposure to vinyl chloride has been reduced significantly, many current workers in the industry may have had heavy exposure to this substance in the past. A full discussion of the occupational health hazards of vinyl chloride is found in Chapter 28.

## Use

The commercial value of polyvinyl chloride (PVC) is related to its processing versatility, strength, corrosion resistance, and cost. Rigid and flexible resins have diverse applications and are processed by a variety of molding methods. Sheet, pipe, wire and cable coating, and conduits formed by extrusion have major applications in the building and construction industries. Flexible PVC is used to form garden hoses; automobile upholstery, floor mats, and trim; baby pants; medical tubing; and intravenous solution bags. PVC can be blow-molded into bottles and is also used to coat flooring, furnishings, and clothing.

## Exposure

The potential exposure to unreacted vinyl chloride monomer was great in PVC production facilities prior to 1960, a time when exposures have been estimated to routinely exceed 1000 ppm. Workers often were lowered into reaction vessels during cleaning, resulting in significant exposure. Loading, drying, and bagging operations also resulted in significant exposure. Between 1970 and 1974, exposures were estimated to range between 100 and 200 ppm.

There were further reductions following the promulgation of the Occupational Safety and Health Administration (OSHA) standard of 1 ppm in 1974. Industrial hygiene surveys by the National Institute for Occupational Safety and Health (NIOSH) revealed a continued reduction in exposure in the production of PVC resins between 1974 and 1977, with most exposures being less than 5 ppm. The workers with greatest potential exposure included reactor operators, baggers, and maintenance workers, while exposures in PVC fabrication were generally less than 1 ppm. Since 1977, routine worker exposures in the PVC manufacturing industry are assumed not to have exceeded the current standard, but intermittent peak exposures may still occur if proper work practices are not observed.

## Clinical Findings

The main hazards in the production and processing of PVC are exposure to vinyl chloride monomer, PVC dust, and thermal decomposition products.

**A. Acute Effects:** The effects of acute massive exposure to vinyl chloride (10,000 ppm) include narcosis and chemical hepatitis.

**B. Chronic Effects:** Chronic exposure to vinyl chloride in PVC production in the 1950s and 1960s resulted in a significant excess risk of angiosarcoma of the liver. The average latency from time of first exposure to disease has been 20–25 years. For unknown reasons, the risk appears to be higher at some plants than others. While a few cases have been reported, the risk does not appear to be excessive in the PVC processing industry. Except for angiosarcoma, cancer risks for other organs have not been consistently demonstrated in the industry.

Another health effect reported in PVC production workers was acro-osteolysis. This was a combination of clubbing of the fingers and erosion of the distal tufts of the phalanges. Symptoms similar to those of Raynaud's phenomenon (pain, vasospasm) were also reported. This occurred in the early 1960s and was associated with hand cleaning of reactors. Changes in work practices and the use of proper protection have apparently eliminated this condition.

PVC dust has generally been treated as nuisance dust. There were early reports of lung effects in the 1970s. There have also been isolated case reports associating scleroderma and pulmonary fibrosis with PVC exposure. A more clearly documented condition known as meat-wrappers' asthma was observed in workers cutting PVC food wrap with a hot wire. The thermal decomposition products of PVC include hydrochloric acid, phosgene, and other irritants. With the extensive use of PVC in the construction industry, these substances present a potential hazard to firefighters.

## Prevention

Protection of workers in the PVC industry from exposure to vinyl chloride monomer will result in the reduction or elimination of the corresponding health effects, both acute and chronic. Workers should also avoid exposure to PVC dust generated during grinding, drying, or cleaning operations. Medical surveillance should be directed toward the detection of abnormal liver function in workers with potential exposure to high levels of vinyl chloride. While routine liver enzyme studies have been of limited value, current research has suggested that measurements of bile acids, von Willebrand's factor, and genetic markers may be used to detect risk or disease. Bile acid levels are elevated in the presence of chronic liver injury, and the other markers may be present in individuals at risk for angiosarcoma.

For workers exposed to PVC, periodic assessment of respiratory function is indicated.

## Treatment

Workers who have evidence of liver injury after exposure to vinyl chloride should be removed from further exposure. Angiosarcoma may be diagnosed by ultrasonography, computed tomography, magnetic resonance imaging, or angiography. Resection has been curative in a few cases. Chemotherapy has been of limited value. Acro-osteolysis is usually reversible. Respiratory irritation resulting in asthma should be treated with inhaled bronchodilators.

## POLYSTYRENE, ABS, & SAN

### Essentials of Diagnosis

- Lightheadedness and incoordination (styrene monomer).
- Altered liver function (styrene monomer): nausea and vomiting, jaundice, and hepatomegaly.
- Mucous membrane and respiratory irritation: wheezing and cough.
- Acrylonitrile and butadiene: ?cancer.

### Exposure Limits

Styrene
    ACGIH TLV: 50 ppm TWA
    OSHA PEL: 50 ppm TWA, 100 ppm STEL
Acrylonitrile
    ACGIH TLV: 2 ppm TWA
    OSHA PEL: 2 ppm TWA, 10 ppm ceiling
    NIOSH REL: 1 ppm TWA, 10 ppm ceiling (15 minutes)
1,3-Butadiene
    ACGIH TLV: 2 ppm TWA (carcinogen)
    NIOSH REL: Reduce exposure to lowest feasible concentration

### General Considerations

Styrene-based polymers were widely used in the 1940s because of the demand for synthetic rubber. This group of polymers now ranks third in total production, after polyethylene and polyvinyl chloride. The major classes of styrene-based polymers are polystyrene, acrylonitrile-butadiene-styrene (ABS), and styrene-acrylonitrile (SAN).

### Production

Styrene is produced by the catalytic dehydrogenation of ethylbenzene. More than 90% of styrene produced is used for polymers, primarily polystyrene and to a lesser extent ABS, SAN, and synthetic rubbers. Polystyrene resins are produced by the bulk polymerization process at low temperatures 48.8–93 °C (120–200 °F). The rate of polymerization increases at higher temperatures, and careful temperature monitoring is required to prevent uncontrolled reactions. A bead polymerization process in suspension is used to produce polystyrene foams. SAN resins are random, amorphous copolymers produced by suspension or emulsion. ABS resins are manufactured by a graft polymerization process in which SAN copolymers are added to polybutadiene rubber.

### Use

The major applications of polystyrene are in packaging, disposables, toys, and building materials. Foam polystyrene is used to form egg cartons, plates, cups, and food containers through extrusion. ABS copolymers combine the chemical resistance of acrylonitrile, the impact resistance of butadiene, and the rigidity and gloss of styrene for diverse applications in business machinery housings, telecommunications equipment, automobile grilles, pipe fittings, and appliances. SAN copolymers are used for appliances, battery casings, and packaging.

### Exposure

Workers engaged in the production of polystyrene resins may have exposure to unreacted styrene monomer during loading and maintenance operations. The potential for runaway reactions may result in intermittent releases of high concentrations of styrene into the workroom air if conditions are not carefully controlled. The residual monomer content of polystyrene resins is low—usually less than 0.5%—but residual monomer may be released during the heating of polystyrene. Exposure to acrylonitrile and butadiene may also occur during the production of copolymers. Inhalation is the main route of exposure, but both styrene and acrylonitrile are absorbed through the skin.

### Health Hazards

Polystyrene is biologically inert, and the main hazard is exposure to styrene monomer. High concentrations (> 100 ppm) of styrene cause irritation of the eyes and mucous membranes. Prolonged skin contact may cause dermatitis and defatting of the skin and may lead to skin absorption. Exposure to the styrene in the production of polymer resins may cause lightheadedness, dizziness, and incoordination. Workers with chronic exposure to styrene have been found to manifest changes in electroencephalograms, slowed nerve conduction velocities, and impaired performance on neuropsychological tests, suggesting both central and peripheral nervous system effects. Most of these findings were subclinical. Changes in hepatic function, including increases in serum enzymes and serum bile acids, have suggested possible hepatotoxicity. Styrene is mutagenic and has been associated with the induction of chromosomal aberrations in humans.

Acrylonitrile is a potent eye, mucous membrane, and skin irritant. Excessive exposure may result in vague symptoms of headache, fatigue, and nausea. Acrylonitrile is a chemical asphyxiant similar to cyanide, and acute exposure may be fatal. Acrylonitrile is an animal carcinogen and has been regulated in the United States as a probable human carcinogen. Human studies have not shown a cancer excess in workers exposed to acrylonitrile.

Butadiene is a gas at room temperature and an irritant of the eyes and mucous membranes and a central nervous system depressant at high concentrations. 1,3-Butadiene has been found to be an animal carcinogen. An excess risk of lymphosarcoma has been seen in workers involved in butadiene monomer production, and an excess risk of leukemia in workers making synthetic rubber.

The main combustion products of thermal decomposition of polystyrene are styrene, benzene, and carbon monoxide. With acrylonitrile copolymers, the major hazard is the production of hydrogen cyanide, ammonia, and the oxides of nitrogen.

### Prevention

Awareness of the potential neurotoxicity of styrene and concern over possible carcinogenicity of acrylonitrile and butadiene has resulted in stricter control of worker exposures to these compounds. Both respiratory and skin protection are required during loading and maintenance operations, which carry a high risk of exposure to unreacted monomers. Styrene polymers should not be welded or burned—particularly those containing acrylonitrile. Medical surveillance of styrene-exposed workers in resin manufacture should include assessment of nervous system symptoms and careful neurologic and mental status examinations. Blood testing should include liver enzyme determinations.

Biological monitoring of workers exposed to styrene can include urine metabolites (phenylglyoxylic acid and mandelic acid) or the measurement of styrene in blood or exhaled air.

Workers exposed to butadiene should have periodic complete blood counts. Hemoglobin adducts are currently being evaluated for the biological monitoring of workers exposed to acrylonitrile and butadiene.

### Treatment

Workers who develop acute or chronic nervous system symptoms related to exposure to styrene should be removed from further exposure. Skin irritation should be treated with local care and topical steroids.

Overexposure to acrylonitrile is a medical emergency. After resuscitation of the worker, contaminated clothing should be removed and the skin cleansed to eliminate further absorption. Treatment with amyl nitrite should be given as for cyanide poisoning. Alternatively, sodium nitrite and sodium thiosulfate may be given. Persons with suspected serious poisoning should be hospitalized for observation for 24–48 hours.

Skin, eye, and mucous membrane irritation due to exposure to butadiene should be treated by cleansing the affected area followed by local care.

## ACRYLICS

### Essentials of Diagnosis

- Respiratory and mucous membrane irritation: cough and wheezing.
- Allergic contact dermatitis: swelling, redness, and pruritus.
- Headache, fatigue, and irritability (methyl methacrylate monomer).

### Exposure Limits

Methylmethacrylate
    ACGIH TLV: 100 ppm TWA
    OSHA PEL: 100 ppm TWA
Methyl acrylate
    ACGIH TLV: 10 ppm TWA
    OSHA PEL: 10 ppm TWA
Ethyl acrylate
    ACGIH TLV: 5 ppm TWA, 25 ppm STEL
    OSHA PEL: 5 ppm TWA, 25 ppm STEL

### General Considerations

The acrylics are a broad group of plastics of which the main classes of monomers are the acrylate or methacrylate esters. Polyacrylonitrile and other copolymers are also included in this class.

### Production

Methyl methacrylate, the major monomer used in acrylic production, is formed through the reaction of acetone and hydrogen cyanide. This is then heated with methanol in the presence of sulfuric acid to liberate the monomer. Bulk polymerization is initiated by peroxide catalysts and liberates heat, which must be dissipated. Resins are supplied as clear sheets, pellets, or syrups.

### Use

Acrylics combine the properties of crystal clarity, environmental and chemical resistance, and pigment compatibility for use as lightweight substitutes for glass. Extruded sheet is used in lighting fixtures, signs, displays, windows, and face shields. Acrylics are also used as coatings and laminates for other plastics, metal, and wood.

### Health Hazards

Acrylic monomers are upper respiratory and mucous membrane irritants. Skin sensitization may occur, resulting in contact dermatitis after exposure to unreacted acrylic monomers. Methyl methacrylate exposure has caused symptoms of headache. Fatigue and irritability in exposed workers and central nervous system effects have been demonstrated in experimental animals. Hypotension and cardiac arrest were reported in several elderly persons in whom methyl methacrylate was used as an adhesive for hip prosthesis.

Cardiac toxicity has not been observed in industrial populations.

### Prevention

Skin contact with acrylic monomers should be avoided. In persons who develop dermatitis, patch testing should be performed to differentiate allergic from irritant effects. Once allergy has been demonstrated, workers should be removed from further exposure. Medical surveillance should include examination of the skin and respiratory system and assessment of nervous system symptoms.

### Treatment

Central nervous system effects related to exposure to acrylic monomers resolve with removal from exposure. Allergic dermatitis should be treated with topical steroids.

## FLUOROPOLYMERS

### Essentials of Diagnosis

- Polymer fume fever (fever, chills, and respiratory impairment).
- Chronic lung disease: wheezing, cough, and dyspnea.

### Exposure Limits

ACGIH TLV: There is no TLV for polytetrafluoroethylene decomposition products. Exposure should be minimized.

### General Considerations

Fluoropolymers are a class of plastics that combine properties of high resistance with low friction for application in electronics, coatings, and cable sheaths. These compounds were introduced in the 1960s and make up a small but growing class of materials.

### Production

The fluorinated monomers are produced through the fluorination of aliphatic and chlorinated hydrocarbons using hydrogen fluoride. Polytetrafluoroethylene—the main fluoropolymer resin—is polymerized in the presence of water with a peroxide catalyst. The fluoropolymers have high melt viscosity, which requires special processing and extrusion equipment capable of generating high pressures.

### Use

The fluoropolymers are resistant to solvents and used in linings and components of chemical processing equipment. The low-friction and resistance properties are used in coatings and sheathing for wire and cables. Fluoropolymers are also used for nonstick coating applications on home cookware, food processing equipment, and production line conveyer parts.

### Health Hazards

A variety of fluorinated and chlorinated hydrocarbons may be used in the production of fluoropolymer resins. Although these are usually reacted in closed systems, worker exposure during loading or maintenance operations may result in symptoms of solvent narcosis (lightheadedness, headache, and incoordination).

Exposure to the thermal decomposition of polytetrafluoroethylene has resulted in a syndrome known as "polymer fume fever" characterized by fever, chills, malaise, cough, and dyspnea several hours after exposure, with spontaneous resolution after 12–24 hours. The cause of this syndrome has not been identified, but several respiratory irritants may be evolved during the thermal decomposition of fluoropolymers, including carbonyl fluoride, perfluoroisobutylene, and hydrogen fluoride. The syndrome has been associated with the accidental or intentional overheating of fluoropolymers during processing or maintenance operations. This has also been associated with smoking cigarettes that may have been contaminated with fluoropolymer resins. In some cases, chronic respiratory impairment has occurred in workers who have experienced episodes of polymer fume fever, indicating that the condition may not necessarily be benign and self-limited.

### Prevention

Solvent compounds should be properly stored and handled to avoid excess worker exposure. Care should be taken to avoid overheating of fluoropolymers. Workers should not smoke in areas where fluoropolymers are being handled and processed. Medical surveillance should include careful questioning regarding symptoms of polymer fume fever as well as periodic assessment of pulmonary function. Industrial hygiene and engineering measures should be instituted to prevent worker exposures that result in symptoms of polymer fume fever.

### Treatment

Polymer fume fever is a self-limited condition that does not require specific treatment. If bronchospasm is evident after exposure to thermal decomposition products, bronchodilators by inhalation should be provided.

# THERMOSETS

## PHENOLICS

### Essentials of Diagnosis
- Respiratory irritation and bronchospasm: wheezing, cough, and dyspnea.
- Irritant or allergic dermatitis: swelling, redness, and pruritus.
- Possible pneumoconiosis: wheezing, cough, dyspnea, and chest tightness.

### Exposure Limits
Formaldehyde
   ACGIH TLV: .03 ppm (ceiling)
   OSHA PEL: 1 ppm TWA, 2 ppm STEL
   NIOSH REL: 0.016 ppm TWA, 0.1 ppm ceiling
      (15 minutes)
Phenol
   ACGIH TLV: 5 ppm TWA
   OSHA PEL: 5 ppm TWA
   NIOSH REL: 5.2 ppm TWA, 15.6 ppm ceiling
      (15 minutes)
Cresol
   ACGIH TLV: 5 ppm TWA
   OSHA PEL: 5 ppm TWA
   NIOSH REL: 2.3 ppm TWA

### General Considerations
The phenolics are hard crystalline resins formed by the reaction of a phenol and an aldehyde—most frequently formaldehyde. These were the first synthetic resins produced.

### Production
Phenolic resins are of two main types. Single-stage resins, or resoles, contain phenol, formaldehyde, and an alkaline catalyst. The condensation process in a charged reaction vessel is interrupted while the material is still thermoplastic, and the resin is supplied as a flake, powder, or liquid that requires heating for final curing.

The two-stage resins, or novalacs, contain excess phenol and an acid catalyst. Hexamethylene tetramine is added to the resin molding powder prior to processing to complete the cure.

### Use
Most phenolic resins produced in the United States are used for the production of plywood and other building materials, adhesives, and bonding agents and insulation. Molded products are used in the automotive industry to replace metals in transmissions, brake components, and electric motors. The electrical resistance properties of resoles are used in electrical components and for laminating surfaces. Phenolics are also used to crease resistant fabrics.

### Health Hazards
The main hazards in the production and handling of phenolic resins are skin irritation or allergic sensitization due to phenol or formaldehyde. Contact dermatitis may result from handling raw materials, resins, or finished products due to exposure to uncured resin. Phenol, formaldehyde, and hexamethylene tetramine are respiratory and mucous membrane irritants and may induce symptoms of eye irritation, cough, and congestion in sensitive individuals at concentrations near the current exposure limits. Phenol is absorbed through the skin, and chronic exposure has resulted in symptoms of fatigue, weight loss, and hepatic dysfunction. Hexamethylene tetramine is metabolized to formaldehyde, and both compounds can also cause systemic symptoms of headache, malaise, and fatigue. Exposure to powdered resins has been associated with chronic respiratory impairment and possible pneumoconiosis. Thermal decomposition products include phenol, formaldehyde, acrolein, and carbon monoxide. Formaldehyde is a suspect human carcinogen and is capable of inducing nasal cancers in experimental animals.

### Prevention
Skin protection is mandatory in the production and processing of phenolics. Respiratory protection should be used during loading and maintenance operations and when handling resin powders. Workers who develop skin problems should be patch-tested for sensitivity to both resin materials and finished polymers. Those who develop true allergy may have to be removed from further exposure. Medical surveillance should include a careful history to elicit irritant and systemic symptoms and periodic assessment of respiratory function. Urinary phenol levels may be of value in following workers with the greatest potential exposure to this compound.

### Treatment
Allergic or irritant dermatitis should be treated by application of topical steroids. Respiratory irritation resulting in bronchospasm should be treated with inhaled bronchodilators. Persons suspected of overexposure to phenol should be removed from exposure until symptoms have resolved.

## POLYURETHANE

### Essentials of Diagnosis
- Corneal burns.
- Allergic or irritant dermatitis: swelling, redness, and pruritus.
- Asthma.

## Exposure Limits

Toluene
ACGIH TLV: 0.005 ppm TWA, 0.02 ppm STEL
OSHA PEL: 0.005 TWA, 0.02 ppm STEL
NIOSH REL: 0.005 ppm TWA, 0.02 ppm ceiling (10 minutes)
Methylene bisphenyl isocyanate (MDI)
ACGIH TLV: 0.005 ppm TWA
OSHA PEL: 0.02 ppm ceiling
Methylene bis(4-cyclohexylisocyanate)
ACGIH TLV: 0.005 ppm TWA
OSHA PEL: 0.01 ppm (ceiling)

## General Considerations

Polyurethanes were first developed in the 1940s as synthetic fibers, but the main current use is in the form of flexible and rigid foams. The main health hazards are related to the use of isocyanates.

## Production

Polyurethanes are complex cellular polymers based on the reaction of isocyanates with alcohol groups (polyols) from either polyesters or polyethers. The reactions take place in the presence of a catalyst (usually an organotin compound), a blowing agent (fluorocarbon), and water. TDI is used for the production of flexible foams, while MDI is used for rigid foam. For some applications, tertiary amines such as triethylenediamine are used as cross-linking agents.

## Use

Flexible foams are used in furniture, mattresses, automobile seats, and carpet pads. Rigid foams are used for building insulation and packaging. Urethanes are also used for surface coatings to impart resistance to abrasion and chemical corrosion.

## Health Hazards

The main health hazard in the production of polyurethanes is exposure to isocyanates. These compounds can cause severe eye and skin burns. Isocyanates are potent skin sensitizers, as are tertiary amine compounds. Dermal allergy can be confirmed by patch testing. Respiratory sensitization may also occur, resulting in symptoms of chest tightness and cough. Workers who develop either dermal or respiratory sensitization may have symptoms at very low exposure levels. Thermal decomposition products include isocyanates, hydrogen cyanide, oxides of nitrogen, and carbon monoxide.

## Prevention

Eye, skin, and respiratory protection is mandatory when working with isocyanates. Exposure to uncured isocyanates may occur during loading, processing, or maintenance operations. Residual isocyanates may also be released from finished foam products. Med-ical surveillance should concentrate on respiratory symptoms and skin problems and should include periodic assessment of pulmonary function.

## Treatment

Eye contact with isocyanates should be treated by copious irrigation with water and referral to an eye specialist. Allergic dermatitis should be treated with topical steroids. Bronchospasm should be treated with inhaled bronchodilators.

## AMINO RESINS

## Essentials of Diagnosis

- Eye irritation.
- Respiratory irritation: wheezing, cough, and dyspnea.
- Allergic sensitization.

## Exposure Limits

Formaldehyde
ACGIH TLV: 1 ppm TWA, 2 ppm STEL
OSHA PEL: 1 ppm TWA, 2 ppm STEL
NIOSH REL: 0.016 ppm TWA, 0.1 ppm ceiling (15 minutes)

## General Considerations

The amino resins were first developed in the 1920s for use as resins and adhesives in glues, wood, paper, and textiles. Approximately 40% of commercial formaldehyde production is used in the production of amino resins.

## Production

The amino resins are thermoset materials, formed by the reaction of formaldehyde with an amino group, usually urea or melamine. The controlled polymerization reaction occurs in the presence of an acid catalyst and heat, with the evolution of water and formaldehyde. Amino resins are supplied as liquids, air-dried solids, or powders.

## Use

Liquid resins are used as adhesives and bonding agents in plywood and particle board or are impregnated into textiles to impart crease resistance. Molding applications include electrical devices, dinnerware, knobs, handles, and industrial laminates, where they display hardness and surface resistance properties. Urea-formaldehyde foam was used extensively in home insulation during the energy crisis of the 1970s until this use was banned in 1982.

## Health Hazards

The main health hazard in the production and use of amino resins is exposure to formaldehyde. Formaldehyde is a respiratory and mucous membrane irritant to which there appears to be great variability in individual susceptibility. Dermal sensitization may occur.

Dermal sensitization to the amino resins may also occur without evidence of sensitivity to formaldehyde. Systemic symptoms such as headache, fatigue, and nausea and irritant symptoms have been associated with the use of urea-formaldehyde insulation.

Formaldehyde is an animal carcinogen and a suspected human carcinogen. Thermal decomposition products include carbon monoxide, formaldehyde, ammonia, and cyanide.

### Prevention

Workers should avoid extensive skin contact with amino resins to prevent skin irritation or cutaneous sensitization. Materials should be kept in well ventilated areas after production to avoid accumulation of unreacted formaldehyde vapor. Medical surveillance should focus on the skin and respiratory system. Individuals who demonstrate intolerance to exposure to formaldehyde or amino resins—manifested by respiratory, skin, or systemic symptoms—should be removed from exposure if adequate ventilation or personal protection cannot be provided.

### Treatment

Respiratory irritation related to formaldehyde is usually self-limited. If bronchospasm is present, administer inhaled bronchodilators. Treat dermatitis with topical steroids.

## OTHER POLYMERS

## POLYESTERS

Polyesters are formed through a polycondensation reaction of an acid (phthalic or maleic anhydride) and an alcohol (ethylene or propylene glycol). Thermoplastic polyesters are used primarily to form soft drink containers and films.

Reinforced unsaturated polyesters are used to make boat hulls, paneling, shower stalls, and automotive bodies. The unsaturated polyester is mixed with styrene and an inhibitor (hydroquinone). A catalyst is added at the time of application to promote cross-linking and curing. The material is reinforced with a filler, usually fibrous glass, and shaped by spraying, molding, or hand application.

Exposure to polyesters does not generally result in dermatologic or respiratory irritation or sensitization. A major hazard in the reinforced plastics industry is exposure to styrene vapor during the application and curing process (see Styrene, Polystyrene).

## EPOXY RESINS

Epoxy resins are formed by the reaction of epichlorohydrin and a diglycidyl ether of the bisphenol A type. Epoxies are used primarily for protective coatings and laminates for metals, woods, and other plastics. Other uses include adhesives and bonding agents, flooring, and reinforced plastics for electrical and tooling applications. The main health hazard of exposure to epoxies is allergic dermal or respiratory sensitization, usually to low-molecular-weight oligomers of the cured resin (MW 340). Hardeners include aliphatic and cycloaliphatic amines, which are strong irritants as well as sensitizers. Epichlorohydrin reacts with nucleic acids and has been shown to induce chromosomal aberrations in lymphocytes of exposed workers.

Bisphenol A is currently under investigation as a potential endocrine toxin.

## NYLON

Nylon polymers are polyamides formed either by the polymerization of a lactam ($\varepsilon$-caprolactam) or by the reaction of an amine and a dibasic acid. A major use of nylon is in the production of fibers and filaments for textiles and furnishings. Molded compounds are used in automotive products, housewares, and appliances. The raw materials are respiratory and skin irritants. Most reactions take place in closed systems. Nylon compounds are a rare cause of allergic sensitization.

## CELLULOSICS

Cellulosics are formed by the chemical modification of naturally occurring polymers from wood and cotton. They are used for films, sheeting, tools, and personal items (brushes, pens). Exposure to organic raw wood and cotton fibers may cause allergic respiratory problems. A major hazard with the use of cellulose nitrate films was the formation of high levels of nitrogen oxides with thermal decomposition.

## ADDITIVES

A large number of organic and inorganic compounds are added to plastic materials to alter their physical and chemical properties. During the evaluation of workers for potential health effects in the plastics industry, the health professional needs to consider the toxicities of the additives in addition to the hazards of monomers or polymers. The occurrence of new health effects in a long-standing polymer operation should suggest a change in additives. The following is a brief discussion of a few of the major plastic additives.

## PLASTICIZERS

Plasticizers are added to polymers to increase flexibility, softness, and processability. Polyvinyl chloride polymers are particularly well suited to modification by the addition of plasticizers.

The major class of plasticizers is the phthalate esters. Di(2-ethylhexyl)phthalate is used extensively. This compound has been shown to have hepatotoxic effects and may be released in potentially toxic quantities from treated materials. It has recently been shown to be a carcinogen and to cause testicular toxicity in animal studies.

## COLORANTS

Inorganic and organic pigments and dyes are used to color plastics. Titanium dioxide and iron oxides are most common, but lead, cadmium, and chrome pigments are also used. Exposure to pigment dusts may occur during compounding and maintenance operations.

## FILLERS

Fillers include silica, silicates, fibrous glass, metal oxides and powders, and polymer fibers. The main hazards are respiratory exposure to fibrogenic dusts or metal dusts or skin contact with irritant fibers.

## FOAMING AGENTS

Foaming or blowing agents are used to introduce a gas or vapor into a polymer to impart a cellular structure of low density. Azodicarbonamide is most commonly used. Occupational asthma has been related to exposure to this compound in several reports. Organic solvents may also be used.

## FLAME RETARDANTS

Flame retardants include polychlorinated and polybrominated compounds, phosphate esters, and inorganic compounds. These are added to materials with construction and electrical applications. Triorthocresyl phosphate, a flame retardant, causes peripheral neuropathy after ingestion, though this effect has not been seen after industrial exposure.

## STABILIZERS

Heat stabilizers to prevent thermal decomposition are used extensively in polyvinyl chloride. These include organotin compounds, metal salts (lead, barium, cadmium, zinc), and epoxies.

## REFERENCES

Cherry N, Gautrin D: Neurotoxic effects of styrene: Further evidence. Br J Ind Med 1990;47:29.

Estlander T et al: Occupational dermatitis from exposure to polyurethane chemicals. Contact Dermatitis 1992;27:161.

Froment O et al: Immunoquantitation of von Willebrand factor (factor VIII-related antigen) in vinyl chloride to exposed workers. Cancer Lett 1992;61:201.

Fuortes LJ et al: An outbreak of naphthalene di-isocyanate-induced asthma in a plastics factory. Arch Environ Health 1995;50:337.

Gannon PF, Burge PS, Benfield GF: Occupational asthma due to polyethylene shrink wrapping (paper wrapper's asthma). Thorax 1992;47:759.

Hagmar L et al: Incidence of cancer and exposure to toluene diisocyanate and methylene dephenyldiisocyanate: A cohort based case-referent study in the polyurethane foam manufacturing industry. Br J Ind Med 1993;50:1003.

Jolanki R et al: Occupational dematoses from exposure to epoxy resin compounds in a ski factory. Contact Dermatitis 1996;34:390.

Kiec-Swierczynska MK: Occupational allergic contact dermatitis due to acrylates in Lodz. Contact Dermatitis 1996;34:419.

Lagast H, Tomenson J, Stringer DA: Polypropylene production and colorectal cancer: A review of the epidemiological evidence. Occup Med (Oxf) 1995;4 5:69.

Malo JL et al: Occupational asthma due to heated polypropylene. Eur Respir J 1994;7:415.

Marex T et al: Bronchial symptoms and respiratory function in workers exposed to methylmethancrylate. Br J Ind Med 1993;50:894.

Ostlere LS et al: Atypical systemic sclerosis following exposure to vinyl chloride monomer. A case report and review of the cutaneous aspects of vinyl chloride disease. Clin Exp Dermatol 1992;17:208.

Shusterman DJ: Polymer fume fever and other fluorcarbon pyrolysis-related syndromes. Occup Med State of the Art Rev 1993;8:519.

Simpson C et al: Hypersensitivity pneumonitis-like reaction and occupational asthma associated with 1,3-bis(isocyanatomethyl) cyclohexane pre-polymer. Am J Ind Med 1996;30:48.

Skarping G et al: 4,4'-Methylenedianiline in hydrolysed serum and urine from a worker exposed to thermal degradation products of methylene diphenyl diisocyanate elastomers. Int Arch Occup Environ Health 1995;67:73.

Swaen GM et al: Mortality of workers exposed to acrylonitrile. J Occup Med 1992;34:801.

Tarvainen K et al: Exposure, skin protection and occupational skin diseases in the glass-fibre-reinforced plastics industry. Contact Dermatitis 1993;29:119.

Tikuisis T, Phibbs MR, Sonnenberg KL: Quantitation of employee exposure to emission products generated by commercial-scale processing of polyethylene. Am Ind Hyg Assoc J 1995;56:809.

Wong O, Trent LS, Whorton MD: An updated cohort mortality study of workers exposed to styrene in the reinforced plastics and composites industry. Occup Environ Med 1994;51:386.

# 31

# The Rubber Industry

*Richard Lewis, MD, MPH*

As early as the sixth century AD, objects made from rubber were considered magical by the Aztecs and Mayas and used in religious ceremonies. In the Amazon, natives fashioned footwear from natural rubber using wood smoke (which killed bacteria) to increase strength and durability. But it was not until the early part of the 19th century that the development of waterproof footwear and garments—and tremendous public demand—resulted in the birth of the rubber industry in Great Britain and the United States.

Several historic developments served to shape the modern rubber industry. Invention of the vulcanization process by Charles Goodyear in 1839—using sulfur and heat to cross-link natural rubber molecules—as well as the use of additives to improve processing led to a demand for rubber products that exceeded the natural supplies at the time. By the end of the 19th century, rubber plants had been exported from Brazil to plantations in Southeast Asia, Sri Lanka, Indonesia, Liberia, and Zaire, which remain the primary producers of natural rubber today.

Development of the pneumatic tire and its application in the automobile industry after the turn of the century led to vast increases in rubber production along with continuing improvements in rubber processing. The growth of the petrochemical industry and advances in polymer technology, coupled with significant shortages in the supply of natural rubber during the Second World War, led to the rapid expansion of the synthetic rubber industry in the 1940s. Today, over two-thirds of all rubber produced is synthetic, primarily styrene-butadiene (SBR) rubber.

Tire manufacturing remains the leading sector of the rubber industry, consuming nearly half of all natural and synthetic rubber produced annually. This industry employs over one-half million workers in nearly 400 plants around the world. Other uses of rubber include automotive components, gaskets, wiring and cable, hoses, clothing and footwear, medical supplies, building materials, and sports and leisure equipment. The fastest-growing use of rubber products has been in the health care industry, with a high demand for rubber gloves to prevent exposure to infectious agents.

Potential exposures in the rubber industry are diverse. A single tire may require the use of 275 raw materials. Workers' exposures will vary not only with different jobs within the industry but also with changes in production techniques and material use over time. This chapter will review the basic processes involved in rubber production, focusing on the tire industry, and will highlight the occupational health issues of the industry as a whole. Specific exposures relevant to the rubber industry are discussed elsewhere in this book.

## PRODUCTION OF NATURAL RUBBER

Natural rubber is obtained primarily from a variety of trees and plants, especially the tree Hevea brasiliensis. Latex is harvested manually from trees by field workers. Preliminary processing involves filtering to remove dirt and debris and coagulation with acids (formic acid and acetic acid). The rubber is then rolled into sheets, cut, and cured with either smoke or sodium bisulfite bleach. It is then formed into bales for shipping.

The production of natural rubber shares many of the occupational health hazards of other agricultural industries. These include use of sharp cutting implements, exposure to pesticides (including sodium arsenite), and risk of tropical diseases in endemic areas. The acids and caustics used in processing are potential respiratory and skin irritants. Increasing use of processing equipment requires careful attention to safety practices to prevent worker injuries.

## PRODUCTION OF SYNTHETIC RUBBER

Synthetic rubbers are elastomers—polymeric materials similar to plastic resins. The distinction is based on the elastomer's ability to be stretched (extensibility) at room temperature and return to its original shape. Synthetic rubber in its crude state is thermoplastic but lacks strength and resiliency. Cross-linking using sulfur or other atoms during vulcanization creates a durable thermoset material of variable strength and pliability.

As in resin production for plastics, the manufacturing of synthetic rubber involves use of large volumes of raw materials. Polymerization reactions take place in enclosed vessels, limiting worker exposure to unreacted chemical intermediates. Workers may be exposed to chemical feedstocks during receiving and loading or with leaks and spills. Maintenance operations, such as the cleaning of reaction vessels, have been major sources of exposure in the past, prior to the implementation of proper venting and respiratory protection measures.

The most widely used synthetic rubber is a copolymer of **styrene and butadiene (SBR)** used extensively in tire manufacturing. This substance is produced through an emulsion polymerization reaction of aqueous styrene and butadiene. Unreacted monomers are captured and recycled. The latex polymer is coagulated with sulfuric acid and dried prior to shipping. Other chemicals such as carbon black, antioxidants, and curing agents may be added, depending on the intended use of the product.

Overexposure to unreacted styrene monomer can result in effects on the nervous system (giddiness, loss of coordination) and the liver. Worker exposure to 1,3-butadiene results primarily in mucous membrane and respiratory tract irritation at high concentrations. Both styrene and butadiene are potential mutagens. Recent studies of chemical workers involved in the production of 1,3-butadiene have found excess mortality from lymphosarcoma. Studies of synthetic-rubber workers have noted an excess of leukemia. These findings have led to much stricter control of worker exposures in the industry.

**Neoprene (polychloroprene)** combines the mechanical properties of natural rubber with increased resistance to aging, oils, and chemicals. This is used in belts, hoses, footwear, and low voltage insulation.

**Chloroprene (2-chloro-1,3-butadiene)** is flammable, and exposure to high concentrations of unreacted monomer and other chemical intermediates has caused narcosis, respiratory tract and skin irritation, alopecia, and liver and kidney damage. Studies of workers exposed to low concentrations of chloroprene in a manufacturing and polymerization plant showed no evidence of biochemical or hematologic abnormalities.

Other synthetics include **butyl rubber** (isobutylene-isoprene polymers), **nitriles** (NBR [nitrile butadiene rubber], copolymers of acrylonitrile and butadiene), and **polyurethane** elastomers (see Chapter 30). Acrylonitrile is a respiratory and mucous membrane irritant, and overexposure may mimic cyanide poisoning. Acrylonitrile is also a suspect human carcinogen.

## MANUFACTURING OF TIRES & OTHER RUBBER PRODUCTS

The manufacturing of rubber products varies from relatively simple operations, such as the production of gloves and balloons by dipping into liquid latex concentrates, to the complex 40-step process involved in tire manufacturing. The basic processes and potential environmental exposures described below in tire manufacturing are relevant to many other rubber manufacturing operations.

### Compounding & Mixing

Thousands of different chemicals may be used as rubber additives. The major **reinforcement and filler materials** are carbon black and amorphous silica, though asbestos-containing materials have been used in the past. **Vulcanizing agents** include sulfur, zinc oxide, stearic acid, and other sulfide compounds. Thiurams, thiocarbamates, and various amine- aldehyde compounds are used as **accelerators** to increase the rate of curing. Additional additives include **activators** (soaps and fatty acids), **extenders** (mineral oils), **plasticizers** (phthalates), **antioxidants** (amines, quinones), and **pigments**.

The initial step in fabrication involves the weighing and mixing of various additives with natural and synthetic rubbers—also known as master-batching. Manual weighing and filling of hoppers results in generation of large amounts of dust that can be reduced through the use of local exhaust ventilation. The materials are combined and loaded into banburies for mixing. In certain applications, the uncured rubber may be heated prior to mixing.

Other activities include the mixing of rubber with solvents to form cements for use in the manufacturing process. Up to the 1940s, solvents such as benzene, carbon disulfide, and carbon tetrachloride were used routinely. Currently, a wide variety of solvents are used in rubber cements and adhesives, including chlorinated, aliphatic, and aromatic hydrocarbons, ketones, and other petroleum derivatives. As a preventive measure, the industry has continued to substitute less toxic solvents for these applications. Mixers should be well sealed and provided with local exhaust ventilation to limit the release of solvent vapors into the workplace.

### Milling, Extrusion, & Calendering

Rubber stock is heated and milled to confer softness and plasticity for further processing. The time and the temperature of the mills govern the chemical reactions within the batch, determining the properties of the finished material. During the formation of rubber sheets, the uncured rubber is coated with an anti-tack agent to reduce sticking. Talc was used extensively for this purpose in the past but has now largely been replaced by amorphous silica (kaolin) and liquid soaps. The rubber stock is cooled in dip tanks, generating steam.

In tire manufacturing, the milled rubber sheet is extruded through a die corresponding to the tread dimensions and weight. This is cut into specified lengths, and the ends are joined manually or automatically, using cement. Rubber sheet is also formed into ply stock by calendering onto steel cord and fabrics (nylon, rayon, polyesters, and fiberglass). Fabric may be pretreated using a phenol-formaldehyde solution to improve adhesion.

All of these operations result in potential exposure to the reaction products from the unvulcanized feedstock. In addition, there is potential exposure to dust (talc, kaolin) from the antitack agents and solvent vapors from the cements.

## Product Fabrication

Many rubber products combine different materials. Tires are assembled on a drum combining ply stock, beads, sidewalls, and other components. The surface of the components may be treated with solvent (primarily naphtha) during the tire building process. Many rubber products, such as hoses, are already formed into their final shape prior to curing. Tires are sprayed with a mold release agent and placed in steel molds to impart the final shape and surface characteristics during the curing process.

## Vulcanization

The application of heat and pressure initiates the cross-linking reactions that will define the shape and characteristics of the final product. Vulcanization may take place in heated molds, ovens, autoclaves, curing pans, or curing presses employing various heat sources. The main exposure is to curing fume, a complex mixture produced by the volatilization of rubber compounds, additives, and impurities. Curing operations also result in exposure to nitrosamines.

## Finishing Operations

After vulcanization, the final products may undergo further processing, such as grinding, trimming, painting, and assembly. Potential occupational health hazards in the finishing operations involve exposure to dusts and solvent vapors, repetitive trauma, and the use of sharp instruments and machinery.

# HEALTH HAZARDS IN RUBBER MANUFACTURING

As in many other manufacturing industries, noise remains a major concern in the rubber industry. The extensive use of milling and mixing equipment, extruders, calenders, conveyers, and hydraulic tools in the tire industry results in noise levels exceeding 85 db throughout many operations. Other physical hazards include risk of thermal burns and heat stress. Ergonomic concerns include lifting (rubber bales, truck tires) and upper extremity disorders. The physical and chemical risks of the industry are summarized in Table 31–1.

## DERMATITIS

A number of accelerators and other compounds used in the rubber industry—including thiurams, amines, and mercaptobenzothiazole—are skin sensitizers causing allergic contact dermatitis in both rubber workers and users of rubber products. Many of the common rubber sensitizers are included in patch test batteries employed by dermatologists and allergists. Cross-reactivity to similar substances may oc-

**Table 31–1.** Potential hazards in tire and rubber manufacturing.

| Process | Task | Physical Hazards | Chemical Hazards |
|---------|------|------------------|------------------|
| Mixing/milling | Weighing<br>Loading<br>Mill operation | Lifting<br>Crush injury<br>Burns<br>Noise | Fillers<br>Stabilizers<br>Antioxidants<br>Vulcanizing agents<br>Uncured rubber fume |
| Tire building | Material handling<br>Cutting/splicing | Lifting<br>Upper extremity injuries<br>Lacerations | Solvents<br>Rubber cement<br>Uncured rubber |
| Curing | Material handling | Lifting<br>Heat stress | Rubber fume<br>Nitrosamines |
| Finishing | Grinding<br>Trimming<br>Painting<br>Packaging | Noise<br>Lacerations<br>Lifting | Dust<br>Paint solvents |

cur, and sensitized individuals generally need to be removed from further exposure. Latex sensitivity in health care professionals has become a leading cause of occupational skin disease.

Irritant dermatitis may be precipitated by contact with solvents, caustics, and acids. Phenols and hydroquinones can cause focal hypopigmentation (leukoderma).

Dermatitis can be prevented by avoidance of skin contact with these substances. Treatment with topical steroids and emollients is usually effective.

## RESPIRATORY DISEASE

Several studies have demonstrated a high incidence of respiratory symptoms and pulmonary function abnormalities in rubber workers. Findings consistent with mucous hypersecretion and mild airway obstruction have been reported in workers exposed to carbon black and other additives, talc, and curing fumes. Symptoms reported by these workers have included cough and phlegm production, chest colds, and episodes of bronchitis. Spirometry has shown decrements in flow rates with preservation of lung volumes. In general, the effects of smoking and workplace exposures appear to be additive.

Occupational asthma remains a concern because of the sensitization potential of several agents used in production. Asthma due to latex sensitivity has also been reported in health care workers.

The long-term impact of exposures in the rubber industry on respiratory status is uncertain. Radiographic evidence of pulmonary fibrosis (talcosis, asbestosis) has been reported only rarely in rubber workers and has been related to specific materials and work practices. Mortality studies have not shown excess mortality rates from respiratory diseases.

If the primary pulmonary insult is the inhalation of particulates and mild irritants, then improved ventilation, material substitution, and better work practices should lessen these effects. There have been few studies in recent years on respiratory effects in the industry, however, so this has yet to be demonstrated.

## CANCER

Excess deaths from various cancers have been reported in rubber workers, and the International Agency for Research on Cancer (IARC) has classified exposures in the rubber industry as carcinogenic in humans. As might be expected from the changes in materials, operations, and work conditions over the past 60 years, epidemiologic investigations have identified excesses of several different cancers in rubber workers depending on the time of the study and the population of interest. While in some instances specific causes have been identified, the fac-

tors contributing to cancer excess in rubber workers remain uncertain.

The first cancer identified in rubber workers was an excess in **bladder cancer** in Great Britain. The excess in the initial workers studied was ultimately attributed to the use of aromatic amines, primarily β-naphthylamine, as accelerators. This was discontinued in 1950, and excess bladder cancers have not been identified in other studies.

Several studies have identified an excess incidence of **gastrointestinal cancers** in rubber workers. The most consistent finding has been an increased risk of stomach cancer, with over half of the studies reporting excesses from 25% to over 100%. Excess mortality rates from cancer of the colon and esophagus have also been reported, although less consistently. Etiologic factors considered include carbon black and other particulates, nitrosamines, and curing fume, though none have been clearly implicated.

Some studies have also shown certain rubber workers to be at increased risk of developing leukemia. Solvents have been considered as the primary etiologic agents, particularly where an excess of myelogenous leukemia has been found related to use of benzene (a pliofilm process being the most publicized). Excess risks found in other studies include a risk of lymphocytic leukemia from exposure to solvents other than benzene. Studies of workers producing synthetic rubber (SBR) have also suggested an excess leukemia risk.

While rubber workers in general have not been found to be at an increased risk for developing **lung cancer**, excesses have been found in a variety of worker subpopulations. This has been associated with exposure to compounding, mixing and milling, and curing fume exposure, but the studies are inconsistent. Smoking, interactions of smoking with other exposures in the rubber industry, and chance clustering (given the extensive investigation of this industry) all remain possible explanations for the findings related to lung cancer to date.

## MEDICAL SURVEILLANCE

Health surveillance programs for rubber workers should include periodic audiometry and spirometry. If possible, the information should be standardized to allow assessment of the effectiveness of controls in high-risk areas. Physical examinations should focus on the respiratory system as well as the skin. Synthetic-rubber workers should undergo periodic assessment of hematologic status, with careful assessment of abnormalities or trends suggestive of leukemia. Despite many uncertainties regarding the true cancer risks in the rubber industry, screening for gastrointestinal cancer should be considered. These diseases are relatively common in the general population, and early detection can markedly improve the outcome, particularly for cancer of the colon.

## PREVENTION

Reduction in the release of air contaminants into the work environment through the use of proper ventilation and material substitution presents a continuing challenge for the rubber industry. Comprehensive hearing conservation programs must be in place and enforced. Given the potential risks of respiratory disease and cancer, workplace smoking restriction policies and smoking cessation programs may be extremely beneficial for rubber workers. Continuing exposure control in production of synthetic rubber should reduce the potential risk of leukemia.

## REFERENCES

Altman LC: Occupational exposure to latex. West J Med 1995;163:369.

Carlo Gl et al: Reduced mortality among workers at a rubber plant. J Occup Med 1993;35:611.

Delzell E et al: A follow-up study of synthetic rubber workers. Toxicology 1996;113:182.

Greenberg GN: Occupational risks in the rubber industry. NC Med J 1995;56:215.

Reh BD, Fajen JM: Worker exposures to nitrosamines in a rubber vehicle sealing plant. Am Ind Hyg Assoc J 1996;57:918.

Rogaczewska T, Ligocka D: Occupational exposure to coal tar pitch volatiles, benzo/a/pyrene and dust in tyre production. Int J Occup Med Environ Health 1994;7:379.

Swuste P, Kromhout H, Drown D: Prevention and control of chemical exposures in the rubber manufacturing industry in The Netherlands. Ann Occup Hyg 1993;37:117.

Vandenplas O et al: Prevalence of occupational asthma due to latex among hospital personnel. Am J Respir Crit Care Med 1995;151:54.

Weiland SK et al: Cancer mortality among workers in the German rubber industry: 1981–91. Occup Environ Med 1996;53:289.

Zuskin E et al: Longitudinal study of respiratory findings in rubber workers. Am J Ind Med 1996;30:171.

# Pesticides

# 32

*Jon Rosenberg, MD, & Michael O'Malley, MD*

As defined by the United States Federal Insecticide, Fungicide, and Rodenticide Act (FIFRA), the federal law that regulates the manufacture, sale, and use of pesticides in the United States, a pesticide is "any substance or mixture of substances intended for preventing, destroying, repelling, or mitigating any insects, rodents, nematodes, fungi, weeds, or any other forms of life declared to be pests—any substance or mixture of substances intended for use as a plant regulator, defoliant, or desiccant."

There are over 1200 chemical compounds used and marketed as pesticides in over 30,000 formulations and under different brand names. The United States uses 35–45% of the total world supply of pesticides, or about 900 million pounds annually. The greatest recent increase has been in the use of herbicides, which now account for approximately 60% of pesticide sales. Prior to World War II, most pesticides were inorganic chemicals. Currently, most pesticides are synthetic organic chemicals. Most of these can be divided into categories or families according to structure or use, with certain properties in common—including health effects on workers and others exposed to toxic quantities by various routes. The specific clinical discussions that begin on page 547 are organized in this way.

Information on identity, exposure, toxicity, and clinical management of specific pesticides is often difficult to obtain. It is therefore important to become familiar with the sources of such information that are available in any particular area of practice. This can include the county agricultural commissioner, county health officer, regional poison control center, state departments of health and agriculture, union officials, and local growers. The annual editions of the Farm Chemicals Handbook is a useful source for identifying a pesticide by common name, chemical name, trade name, and manufacturer or marketer. The United States Environmental Protection Agency (EPA) booklet entitled Recognition and Management of Pesticide Poisonings is a concise guide to diagnosis and treatment. The misnamed three volume Handbook of Pesticide Toxicology is a more definitive source of health-related information.

Although there have been regulatory requirements for toxicity testing of pesticides in the United States for a number of years, the testing for most many pesticides has been completed only recently; the regulatory and public health assessment of these data is still ongoing.

## USES OF PESTICIDES

Approximately 80–90% of all pesticides produced are used for commercial agriculture and the remainder are used for for structural pest control, horticulture, and home and garden purposes. The principal goal of pesticide application in commercial agriculture and horticulture is to reduce crop loss or decrease growing or cultivation costs in order to enhance economic returns. Structural pesticides are applied to prevent or reduce structural damage from pests (termites) or reduce the impact of pest infestations (cockroaches) that may be a threat to public health. Certain pesticides may be used specifically for protection of public health, such as drinking and swimming water treatment, disinfectants for medical facilities, and control of carriers of disease such as mosquitoes and rodents. The public health benefits of pesticides are particularly noteworthy in developing countries.

## OCCUPATIONAL & ENVIRONMENTAL PESTICIDE EXPOSURES

Typical occupational and nonoccupational pesticide exposure situations are listed in Table 32–1. The nature, extent, and route of exposure may vary among these different circumstances and the physical properties—particularly the vapor pressure—of individual pesticides (Table 32–2).

The nature of exposure depends on whether exposure is to the commercial formulation of a pesticide, as applied in a field or structure, or to the active ingredient, as occurs in a manufacturing facility. A

**Table 32–1.** Occupational and environmental pesticide exposure situations.

**Occupational exposures**
Research and development
Manufacturing: technical grade material produced in enclosed and semi-enclosed operations; exposures during leaks/spill and process repairs—packaging operations vary in degree of enclosure
Formulation: technical grade material mixed with "inert" ingredients such as solvents, and adjuvants
Transportation
Pest control
Mixing: commercial material diluted with water or other material
Loading: into tanks in planes, ground rigs, backpacks, or hand-held sprayers. Closed vs open mix/loading systems
Application: variable requirements in protective clothing
Flagging: standing at the end of fields to mark the rows to be sprayed by crop-dusting aircraft. Flagging currently being replaced by GPS flagging systems in some operations
Farm work: field workers, pickers, sorters, packers, and others who come into contact with pesticide residues on leaves and fruit. High contact work tasks include hand labor in grapes; picking row crops, such as lettuce or strawberries, results in markedly less contact—as described in results of residue transfer studies
Emergency and medical work: personnel exposed to contaminated persons and equipment in the process of responding to spills, accidents, and poisonings
**Environmental and consumer exposures**
Accidents and spills: especially ingestion by children (floor level materials—ant traps, etc)
Suicide and homicide
Home use: house and garden
Structural use: residents and occupants of buildings
Bystanders
Contamination: food, water, air
Ag-Urban interface

**Table 32–2.** Vapor pressures of common pesticides.

| Pesticide | Vapor Material Pressure (mm Hg) |
|---|---|
| **Fumigants/nematocides** | |
| Phosphine | 23,369 |
| Sulfuryl fluoride | >760 |
| Methyl bromide | 1,725 |
| Chloropicrin | 17 |
| Metam-sodium | not measurable |
| **Metam-sodium byproducts** | |
| Methyl-isothiocyanate | 16.0 |
| Carbon disulfide | 334.3 |
| Hydrogen sulfide | 15,981 |
| Methylamine | 2,324.3 |
| **Common solvents** | |
| Water | 24 |
| Toluene | 30 |
| 1,1 Dichloroethane | 234 |
| **Organophosphate contaminants** | |
| Methyl mercaptan | 1,261 |
| Ethyl mercaptan | 467 |
| N-butyl mercaptan | 83 |
| **Organophosphates** | |
| Dichlorvos (DDVP) | $1 \times 10 - 2$ |
| Mevinphos | $2 \times 10 - 3$ |
| Malathion | $1.2 \times 10 - 4$ |
| Chlorpyrifos | $2.02 \times 10 - 5$ |
| Dimethoate | $8 \times 10 - 6$ |
| Phosalone | $<10 - 9$ |
| **Carbamates** | |
| Methomyl | $5.0 \times 10 - 5$ |
| **Organochlorines** | |
| Chlordane | $1 \times 10 - 5$ |
| **Herbicides** | |
| 2,4-D | $1.4 \times 10 - 7$ |
| Cyanazine | $1.6 \times 10 - 9$ |
| Alachlor | $2.2 \times 10 - 5$ |
| Glyphosate | $<7.5 \times 10 - 8$ |
| **Fungicides** | |
| Hexachlorobenzene | $1.09 \times 10 - 5$ |
| Zinc bisdithiocarbamate (ziram) | $<7.5 \times 10 - 8$ |
| Benomyl | $<3.75 \times 10 - 10$ |
| Chlorothalonil | $5.72 \times 10 - 7$ |
| Triadimefon | $1.5 \times 10 - 7$ |

pesticide, as applied, consists of the technical grade chemical ("active" ingredient), diluents (often organic solvents), additives ("adjuvants"), and other "inert" ingredients. The pesticide is then applied mixed or unmixed as sprays, dusts, aerosols, granular, impregnated preparations, fumigants, baits, or systemics. "Inert" ingredients are not necessarily nontoxic; many are organic solvents. Most typical solvents used are petroleum distillates, but other organic solvents such as methylene chloride and propylene glycol have been used. Systemic pesticides are water-soluble chemicals that are taken up by a plant and translocated to a part of the plant where a pest, usually an insect, feeds on plant juices and ingests the pesticide. This term is also used for animal systemics, or feed-through pesticides, which are fed to an animal so that pests that feed on feces also ingest the pesticide. The use of systemic, granular, bait, and impregnated pesticide formulations can result in significantly reduced exposure during application.

Pesticides used by consumers for home and garden are often nearly identical in formulation to those used by commercial applicators or differ only in reduced concentration of active ingredient. The most serious exposures occur from accidental or deliberate ingestions. Although pesticides account for a relatively small percentage of the total childhood ingestions, a large proportion of childhood ingestions of organophosphates, carbamates, and bipiridyl herbicides (diquat and paraquat) result in serious illness or death. Children also frequently attempt to ingest pesticides used at floor or ground level, such as anticoagulant rodenticides, snail baits, and ant-traps, but these less frequently cause serious poisonings.

## PHARMACOKINETICS OF PESTICIDE TOXICITY HIGH RISK GROUPS

The highest exposures and incidences of poisonings occur in individuals involved in agricultural pest control operations: mixing, loading, applying, and flagging. Mixers and loaders are exposed to concentrated pesticides and large volumes, respectively. The use of closed systems for mixing and loading, which is required in California, but not in other states or countries, has reduced these exposures and poisonings considerably. The exposure of applicators varies with the type of application, from backpack sprayers to enclosed-cab vehicles with filtered cooled air. Leaking or poorly maintained equipment may fail and produce large overexposures with any type of application device, including closed mixing/loading systems. Exposures in most manufacturing facilities are low, due to the use of automated closed systems, but exposures that require unscheduled maintenance occur during process breakdowns or leaks. Exposures in formulating facilities may be much higher, particularly if dusty formulations (dusts, powders, granules) are produced in open systems.

## PHARMACOKINETICS OF PESTICIDE TOXICITY: ROUTES OF EXPOSURE

With fumigants and some insecticidal compounds, exposures to vapors is a significant issue (Table 32–2), as most pesticide inhalation exposures derive from aerosols generated at the time of application or from pesticide adsorbed to household or environmental dust. In manufacturing operations, inhalation exposures to aerosols or vapors may be equally significant. The most important route for most occupational exposures is dermal.

A high percentage of pesticides are absorbed across intact human skin to a significant degree, since they must be absorbed through the coverings of insects or plants to be effective. The low molecular weight and high lipid solubility of many pesticides confer this absorptivity. The ratio of dermal LD50 to oral LD50 values that are available for most pesticide provides a rough indication of degree of dermal absorption. A low ratio of dermal LD50 to oral LD50 indicates a probable high degree of dermal absorption (eg, the organophosphate insecticide mevinphos has reported oral LD50s ranging from 3.7 to 6.8 mg/kg and reported dermal LD50s ranging from 4.2 to 7.0 mg/kg).

Other pharmacokinetic considerations vary considerably among pesticide families and so are discussed below, according to family.

## EFFECTS, PREVENTION, & TREATMENT OF PESTICIDE TOXICITY

Some toxic effects of pesticides, such as cancer, require consideration as a class, since the populations shown to be at increased risk are exposed to many different types. For some effects, such as acute poisoning, there are general principles of diagnosis, treatment, and prevention. After these general remarks, the individual pesticides will be considered.

### Clinical Findings

**A. Symptoms and Signs:**

**1. Acute Exposure–**The manifestations of acute toxicity vary among pesticide families. The vast majority of acute pesticide poisonings are due to organophosphates and carbamates. However, the diagnosis of acute pesticide poisoning in general relies upon the following features: (1) Signs and symptoms consistent with exposure to one or more chemical families of pesticides (in which a relatively specific clinical constellation [toxidrome] is present); (2) A temporal relationship to known exposure to pesticides, or field work, even in the absence of known recent pesticide application. Temporal relationships will vary depending on the type of pesticide, the route and duration of exposure, and the nature of the toxic effect; and (3) Evidence of poisoning in other workers or family members.

Severe acute poisoning usually does not present a diagnostic challenge, since a history of high-level acute exposure is usually available and a full spectrum of clinical manifestations is normally present. Mild acute or subacute poisoning, however, may not be readily apparent, since the signs and symptoms are likely to be nonspecific and similar to a common illness, such as influenza, and a history of exposure may not be particularly remarkable or even known to the patient.

**2. Chronic Exposure–**Specific organ-related chronic effects are discussed in later sections. Some general considerations regarding dermatologic effects, carcinogenicity, and the reproductive toxicity of pesticides are discussed here.

**a. Dermatologic effects–**Approximately one-third of all reported pesticide-related diseases are dermatologic—about the same percentage estimated for other chemicals. Pesticides may be primary skin irritants or skin sensitizers and result in irritant or allergic contact dermatitis. A few have have been reported to cause other reactions such as contact urticaria, erythema multiforme, chloracne, and porphyria cutanea tarda. Sulfur (a fungicide) and propargite (Omite, a miticide) are common causes of irritant dermatitis when used on grapes, while the dithiocarbamates, phthalimides, and benomyl (Benlate)—all fungicides—are common causes of both irritant and allergic contact dermatitis. Paraquat is corrosive and can cause irritant dermatitis. However, because of the lack of reporting and research in pesticide-related skin disease, any pesticide must be considered for its possible role in causation of rash in an exposed worker.

The diagnosis and management of dermatitis in a worker exposed to pesticides differs little from that for dermatitis in other workers, except in the case of field workers. Diagnosis depends upon careful evaluation of the pattern of exposure and its relation to the distribution and character of subsequent skin lesions. This task may be especially difficult in cases of dermatitis in field workers who may not know what pesticide residues are present on the plants they are in contact with. They may also be exposed to plants known to cause primary irritant or allergic contact dermatitis. (For a discussion of plant-related dermatitis, see Chapter 18.) Definitive diagnosis of irritant dermatitis depends upon noting the above described correspondence between pattern of exposure and the pattern of skin reaction, in addition to recognizing the irritant properties of the suspected material(s). Allergic dermatitis can only be confirmed by diagnostic patch testing (type IV allergy) or open patch applications or prick testing (type I allergy). Patch tests are available for a number of pesticides and plants known to be sensitizers and may be made for others, provided preliminary testing of control subjects is conducted to identify the maximum nonirritating concentration of the new test material. The distinction between pesticide and plant allergy and allergic dermatitis is important from an exposure/management standpoint because irritant dermatitis can often be prevented by reducing exposure through use of personal protective equipment or administrative measures such as reentry intervals. Prevention of allergic contact dermatitis requires complete removal from exposure. Individual pesticides or weeds are generally simple to avoid, given a cooperative employer, but allergy to crop plants presents a greater problem. This is an infrequent problem with most food crops, but may be relatively frequent among nursery workers handling alstromeria, carnations, primrose, chrysanthemums, and other allergenic ornamental crops. The distinction is particularly important for field workers, since a pesticide-related cause may mean transfer from the field for several days at one time during a season, while a plant-related cause may mean permanent avoidance of a particular crop for at least part of its growing cycle.

Medical treatment consists of alleviation of symptoms with corticosteroids and moisturizers. Prevention of further exposure sufficient to cause recurrence is usually possible with protective clothing.

**b. Cancer**–No pesticides currently in use are recognized human carcinogens, with the exception of inorganic arsenic. Arguable cases may be made for the wood preservatives creosote and chromic acid and the fumigant ethylene oxide. Most occupational carcinogens have been identified in worker populations employed in chemical manufacturing. Because the current chemical industry is not labor-intensive, the number of workers required to produce chemical pesticides is relatively small and the epidemiologic studies of these workers with unique exposures to individual pesticides are necessarily limited by small numbers. For pesticides, these types of classic occupational cohort studies are therefore only capable of identifying very potent human carcinogens. Most recently, 4-chloro-ortho-toluidine (4-COT), the principle metabolite of the insecticide chlordimeform, was found to be a carcinogen in a study of 120 manufacturing workers in Germany, provoking an incidence of bladder cancer 72 times higher than background. Chlordimeform was taken off the market in 1986 when this information became known. Animal studies identified chlordimeform and 4-COT as carcinogens in the late 1970s.

Epidemiologic studies of cancer in farmers have shown a relatively consistent increase in certain cancers, notably leukemia, lymphoma, and multiple myeloma. Although these findings are suggestive of an increase in cancer due to pesticides, specific pesticides could not be incriminated and other causes related to farm work (eg, viral exposures associated with animal handling) could not be ruled out.

A few studies have examined cancer incidence in pesticide applicators. Two of these studies have indicated elevated risks for lung cancer and one for bladder cancer, without being able to attribute carcinogenicity to specific pesticides. A number of studies conducted in Sweden between the late 1970s and early 1980s have suggested (without proof) an association between phenoxy herbicides and soft tissue sarcoma, but have not been consistently replicated in other populations.

Another important issue in recent years has been the findings of the New York University (NYU) Women's Health Study (1993) that identified serum levels of the DDT metabolite DDE as a risk factor for breast cancer. The study showed a four-fold increase in relative risk of breast cancer for an elevation of serum DDE concentrations from 2.0 ng/mL (10th percentile) to 19.1 ng/mL (90th percentile). The findings of this study prompted widespread concern about organochlorines and breast cancer (Pesticide residues and breast cancer: the harvest of a silent spring?) and attempts were made to correlate secular trends in organochlorine exposures with trends in breast cancer incidence. In 1994, a study of women in the San Francisco Bay region conducted by some of the same investigators who participated in the NYU study found no relationship between serum DDE levels and breast cancer.

**B. Laboratory Findings:** For acute pesticide poisoning, laboratory findings are usually specific and timely only for cholinesterase inhibition by organophosphate and possibly carbamate pesticides. Measurement of the pesticide or its metabolites in body fluids is usually helpful only in later confirmation of diagnosis, since the information is rarely available in time to aid in management. The use of biological levels is not helpful in the diagnosis of chronic toxicity because adequate dose-response data are unavailable for most pesticides and biological levels at the time of diagnosis, if present at all, may not reflect those present during exposure.

## PESTICIDES RECOGNIZED AS ANIMAL CARCINOGENS

For a number of pesticides, most notably the halogenated hydrocarbons insecticides and fumigants and the chloroalkylthiodicarboximide and ethylene-bis-dithiocarbamate fungicides, there is evidence of carcinogenicity in animals. Table 32–3 lists pesticides known or preliminarily identified by the EPA to be associated with evidence for carcinogenicity in animals—recognizing that such evidence is often uncertain, controversial, and subject for reevaluation. It is important to realize that these and other toxicologic data were generated primarily by pesticide manufacturers in response to regulatory requirements (see below) and are generally unpublished and unavailable to persons outside the companies and regulatory agencies. The pesticides are categorized according to the ranking system by the EPA's scientific advisory panel. Compounds are usually recognized as animal carcinogens (category B2) based upon occurrence of

**Table 32–3.** Pesticide carcinogenicity data.

| Chemical | Comments | Potency | Group |
|---|---|---|---|
| Accent (nicosulfuron) | New chemical 1990 | | E |
| Acephate (OP insecticide) | Mouse liver | | C |
| Acetamide (metabol of Methomyl and Thidiocarb) | Male and female rat liver | 3.07E-3 | C |
| Acetochlor (herbicide) | Rat nasal; mouse multiple sites | 1.69E-2 | B2 |
| Acifluorfen Tackle/Blazer (herbicide) | Mouse liver; male and female | 1.1 E-1 | B2 |
| Acrylonitrile | | 5.4E-1 | B2 |
| Alachlor | Rat nasal | 8.0E-2 | B2 |
| Alar (see Daminozide) | | | |
| Aliette/Fosethy-Al | Male rat bladder | | C |
| Amdro (hydramethylnon) | Female mouse lung | | C |
| Amitraz | | 4.97E-2 | C |
| Amitrole | Rat thyroid Mouse liver | 1.1 | B2 |
| Apollo/Clofentezine | Rat thyroid | | C |
| Arsenic compounds | Human carcinogens Skin/lung | | |
| Assert (imazamethabenz-methyl)-herbicide | | | D |
| Assure (Quizalofopethyl) | Mouse liver equivocal | | C |
| Asulam; plant | Male rat/adr. pheo Metab. hydroquinone | | C |
| Atrazine | Female rat mammary | 2.22E-1 | C |
| Baygon/Propoxur | Male and female rat bladder | 3.7E-3 | B2 |
| Bayleton (triadimefon) | Male and female mouse liver | | C |
| Baytan (triadimenol) | Male and female mouse liver | | C |
| Beacon (primisulfuronmethyl) herbicide | | | D |

*(continued)*

**Table 32–3.** Pesticide carcinogenicity data. (continued)

| Chemical | Comments | Potency | Group |
|---|---|---|---|
| Benomyl | | 4.2E-3 | C |
| Bentazon (herbicide) | | | E |
| Bifenthrin | Male mouse bladder | | C |
| Boric Acid (Borax) | | | E |
| Bromacil | Male mouse liver | | C |
| Bromoxynil | Male mouse liver | | C |
| Butylate | | | E |
| Cacodylic acid | Female and male rat bladder | | |
| Cadmium (fungicide)—inactive or cancelled registrations | | 6.1 | B1 |
| Calcium Cyanamide + Hydrogen Cyanamide (growth regulator) | Mouse ovary | 6.74 E-2 | C |
| Captafol (cancelled) | Mouse lymphosarcoma | 5.1 E-2 | B2 |
| Captan | | 3.6 E-3 | B2 |
| Carbaryl | | 2.27 E-2 | |
| Carbon tetrachloride | Mouse/rat—multiple positive studies dose 47–2000 mg/kg/d | | |
| Chloramben | | 1.6E-4 | |
| Chlordane | Mouse liver | 1.3 | B2 |
| Chlordimeform (cancelled) | Mouse liver Hemangiosarcoma | 1.3 diet | B2 |
| Chlorobenzilate (cancelled) | Published studies show hepatocellular carcinomas in two strains of mice | | |
| Chlorothalonil | Female rat renal | 1.IE-2 | B2 |
| Chlorpyriphos | | | E |
| Cinch (cinmethylin) | | | D |
| Coal tar, coal tar creosote, creosote oil | Human/animal skin Carcinogen | | |
| Cyanazine | Female rat mammary | 8.4E-1 | C |
| Cyhalothrin/Karate | Eval dose select mouse | | D |
| Cypermethrin | Mouse lung | 1.9E-2 | C |
| Cyproconazole | Male mouse liver | 3.02E-1 | C |
| Cyromazine/Larvadex metabolite = melamine | Female mouse mammary | 2.4E-3 | C |
| DBCP | Liver, kidney, stomach nasal rat | 1.4 oral; 8.3 inhal | B2 |
| 2,4-D | Astrocytomas male rats at high dose only; several completely negative studies | | C |
| DDT, DDE, DDD | | 3.4E-1 2.4E-1 | B2 |
| DDVP; Dichlorvos | Female mouse stomach; male rat leukemia | 2.0E-1 | C |
| Dacthal | | | |

*(continued)*

**Table 32–3.** Pesticide carcinogenicity data. (continued)

| Chemical | Comments | Potency | Group |
|---|---|---|---|
| Daminozide | Male mouse lung | 8.7E-3 | B2 |
| Dazomet | | | D |
| DBCP | Liver, kidney, stomach, nasal, rat | 1.4 oral 8.3 inhal | B2 |
| Desmedipham | | | E |
| Diallate (cancelled) | | | |
| Dicamba | | | D |
| Dichlobenil | Male and female rat liver | | C |
| p-Dichlorobenzene | | | C |
| Dichloropropene (Telone II) | Forestomach/liver tumors in male rats; forestomach tumors in female rats; forestomach, lung, urinary bladder in female mice | Oral 1.8 E-1; Inhalation 9.66 E-2 | B2 |
| Diclofop-methyl (Hoelon) herbicide | Female and male mouse liver | 4.4E-1 | C |
| Dicofol/Kelthane | | | C |
| Dieldrin | | 16 | B2 |
| Dimethoate | Male rat Hemangiosarcoma | | C |
| Dinoseb | EPA evaluation incomplete; 1971 published mouse study negative at maximum tolerated dose | | C |
| Diquat | | | E |
| Dithyopyr | | | E |
| DPX-E9636 | | | E |
| Ebufos | | | E |
| EDB | Stomach mouse; nasal rat | 67 oral; 1.4 inhal | B2 |
| Endosulfan | | | E |
| Ethalfluralin | | | |
| Ethephon | | | E |
| Ethion | | | E |
| Ethofenprox | Female rat thyroid | 5.1E-3 | C |
| Ethofumesate | | | D |
| Ethylene oxide | Leukemia in rats and monkeys; mice show lung cancers and lymphomas; human cancer in case reports; NIOSH study showed increased risk of leukemia in US cohort; SMR = 1.55 | | |
| ETU | Rat thyroid; mouse liver | 1.1 E-1 | B2 |
| Express (tribenuron methyl) herbicide | Female rat mammary | | C |
| Fenamiphos (Nemacur) | | | E |
| Fenarimol | | | D |
| Fenbuconazole | Female mouse liver male rat thyroid | 1.65 E-2 | C |

(*continued*)

**Table 32–3.** Pesticide carcinogenicity data. (continued)

| Chemical | Comments | Potency | Group |
|---|---|---|---|
| Fenitrothion (Sumithion) | | | E |
| Fenpropathrin (Danitol) | | | E |
| Fluridone | | | E |
| Folpet | Mouse GI tract | 3. 49E-3 | B2 |
| Fomesafen (herbicide) | | 1.9E-1 | C |
| Fonofos | | | E |
| Furmecyclox | Female rat liver | 2.98 E-2 | B2 |
| Glyphosate | | | C |
| Guthion | | | E |
| Haloxyfop-Methyl Verdict (herbicide) | Male and female mouse liver | 7.39 | C |
| Harvade/Dimethipin (defoliant, growth regulator) | | | C |
| Hexachlorobenzene | Thyroid adenomas, hepatomas (hamsters); mice hepatomas | 1.7 | B2 |
| Heptachlor | | 4.5 | B2 |
| Hexaconazole (fungicide) | Rat testes | 2.3 E-2 | C |
| Hexazinone | Male and female mouse liver | | C |
| Imidacloprid | | | E |
| Imidan/Phosmet | | | C |
| Iprodione | Male and female mouse liver; rat testes | | |
| Isoxaben (herbicide) | | | C |
| Lactofen (herbicide) | Mouse liver | 1.7E-1 | B2 |
| Lindane | | 1.3 | B2/C |
| Linuron | Rat testes | | C |
| Malathion | | | D |
| Maleic hydrazide (growth retardant) | | | D |
| Mancozeb; Maneb | | use ETU potency | B2 |
| MBC (Benomyl, thiophanate methyl breakdown product) | | 4.2E-3 | C |
| Melamine; cyromazine metabolite | Male rat bladder associated with urolithiasis at high doses | | D |
| Mercapotobenzothiazole (MBT) | Male and female rat Pheochromocytomas in NTP studies | | C |
| Metalaxyl | | | E |
| Methanearsonic acid | | | |
| Methidathion | Male mouse liver | | C |
| Methiocarb (Mesurol) | | | D |
| Methoxychlor | Published studies show testicular tumors in some mouse strains 100 ppm in diet; carcinomas both sexes of rats 2000 ppm in diet | | D |

(*continued*)

**Table 32–3.** Pesticide carcinogenicity data. (continued)

| Chemical | Comments | Potency | Group |
|---|---|---|---|
| Methyl bromide | 1974 published rat study showed squamous cell cancer in stomach—reinterpreted as only inflammatory hyperplasia; gliomas noted at 1/3 MTD in male rats in study submitted to Cal-EPA; effect not seen at MTD dose | | |
| Metolachlor (herbicide) | Female rat liver | 9.6E-3 | C |
| MGK Repellent 326 (dipropyl isochihomeronate) | Male and female rat liver | 2.4E-3 M; 1.22E-3 F | B2 |
| Mirex | Hepatomas in mouse and rat at maximum tolerated dose and MTD | 1.8 | B2 |
| Molinate (Ordram) | Male rat kidney | 1.1E-1 | C |
| MON 12000 (Halosulfuron Methyl) | | | E |
| Nitrapyrin (nitrification inhibitor) | Male rat kidney; mouse inadequate | | D |
| Nitrofen/TOK | Liver cancer male and female mice; pancreatic cancer female rats | | B2 |
| Norflurazon (herbicide) | | | C |
| Oryzalin | Female rat mammary | 1.3E-1 | C |
| Oxadiazon | Male and female mouse liver | 1.4E-1 | B2 vs.C |
| Oxadixyl | Male and female rat liver | 5.3E-2 | C |
| Oxyfluorfen (Goal) herbicide | Mouse liver | 1.28E-1 | C |
| Paclobutrazol | | | D |
| Paraquat | | | E |
| Parathion | | | C |
| PCNB Pentachloronitrobenzene | Male rat thyroid | | D |
| Pendimethalin | Male and female rat thyroid | | C |
| Pentachlorophenol | | 1.29E-1 | B2 |
| Permethrin | Mouse lung and liver | 1.84E-2 | C |
| o-Phenyl-phenol and Na salt | Male rat bladder | 2.2E-3 | B2 |
| Phenipedipham (herbicide) | | | D |
| Phorate | | | D |
| Phosphamidon | | | C |
| Phostebupirim (corn insecticide) | | | E |
| Picloram (herbicide) | | | D |
| Prochloraz (fungicide) | Male and female mouse liver | 1.5E-1 | C |
| Procymidone (fungicide)— not currently registered | | m. rat 1. 92E-2 f. mouse 2.35E-2 | B2 |
| Prodiamine | Rat thyroid | | C |
| Prometon | | | |
| Pronamide (Kerb) | Mouse liver; rat thyroid and testes | 1.54E-2 | C |
| Propargite | Male and female rat jejunum | 3.1 E-2 | B2 |

(*continued*)

**Table 32–3.** Pesticide carcinogenicity data. (continued)

| Chemical | Comments | Potency | Group |
|---|---|---|---|
| Propazine | Rat mammary | | C |
| Propiconazole | Male mouse liver | | C |
| Propiolactone (antimicrobial) | | | B2 |
| Pyridaben | | | E |
| Quinclorac (herbicide) | Male rat pancreas | | C |
| Rotenone | | | D |
| Savey (hexythiazox)—mite ovicide, larvicide | Mouse liver | 3.9E-2 | C |
| Simazine | Female rat mammary | 1.2E-1 | C |
| Sulfallate (Vegadex) herbicide | Positive in NCI mouse and rat bioassays | | |
| Sulfosate (herbicide) | | | E |
| Tebuconazole | Male and female mouse liver | | C |
| Tebuthiuron (herbicide) | | | D |
| Terbutryn (herbicide)—cancelled | | 8.9 E-3 | C |
| Terrazole (etridazole—fungicide) | Male and female rats; several tumor sites. | 7.2 E-2 male 5.4 E-3 female rare tumor | B2 |
| Tetrachlorovinphos | Female mouse liver | 3.13 E-3 | C |
| Tetramethrin | | | C |
| Thiazopyr | Rat thyroid | | C |
| Toxaphene | Rat liver/thyroid | 1.1 | B2 |
| TPTH (fentin hydroxide) | Female rat pituitary | 2.8 | B2 |
| Treflan/Trifluralin | Male rat thyroid | 7.7 E-3 | C |
| Triallate (thiocarbamate herbicide) | Mouse liver | | C |
| Triasulfuron (Arber) | | | C |
| Tribufos (DEF)—cotton defoliant | | | C |
| Tridiphane (Tandem) | | 3.0E-1 | C |
| Triflumizole | | | E |
| Troysan Polyphase IPBC 55406-53-6 | | | C |
| Tycor (Ethiozin) | Male and female rat thyroid | | C |
| UDMH (daminozide B2 contaminant) | Mouse hemangiosarcoma | 8.9; 8.8 E-1; 4.6 E-1 | B2 |
| Uniconazole (fungicide) | Male mouse liver | | C |
| Vendex (Hexakis) | | | E |
| Vinclozolin (Ronilan) | | | E |
| XRD-498 (Flumtsulam) | | | E |
| Zineb | EBDC | | |

tumors in more than one strain of animals at multiple doses. For example, separate studies of the fungicide captan indicated that the compound causes adrenal and pituitary neoplasms at both low and high doses in male and female rats. The female rats showed neoplasms in the breast and ovaries, also.

Studies of the chloroalkylthiodicarboximide fungicides (including captafol and folpet as well as captan) as a whole indicated increased incidence of malignant tumors and benign tumors in experiments involving different strains of mice and rats. The primary tumor sites included the gastrointestinal tract, lymphatic system, vascular system, and endocrine system. All three compounds are classified as B2 carcinogens by the EPA.

Compounds producing tumors only at the maximum tolerated dose in a single species are classified as class C or class D, depending upon the quality of the study demonstrating the effect. For example, the fungicide fosetyl-al (Aliette or aluminum tris [-O-ethyl-phsophonate]), was classified as group C because of benign and malignant urinary bladder tumors in a study involving male Charles River rats at doses between 30,000 and 40,000 ppm. No tumors were seen in female rats in this study, nor in mice tested in another study. Because fosetyl-al is a relatively simple compound, structurally unrelated to known classes of bladder carcinogens (aniline dyes or polynuclear aromatic hydrocarbons), the observed tumors probably represent no significance for human health.

No pesticides are recognized human teratogens or female reproductive toxins. However, case reports and a few epidemiologic studies have described either teratogenicity or fetotoxicity at doses that also cause maternal toxicity. For example, in the mid 1980s, 35 workers developed acute organophosphate poisoning after entering a cauliflower field contaminated with residues of oxydemeton-methyl, mevinphos, and methomyl. A crew member who was four weeks pregnant at the time of the poisoning subsequently gave birth to a child with multiple cardiac defects, bilateral optic nerve colobomas, microphthalmia of the left eye, cerebral and cerebellar atrophy, and facial anomalies. Similarly, the massive amounts of methyl isocyanate (MIC) released from the pesticide plant at Bhopal, India was associated with an four-fold increased incidence of spontaneous abortion in women who survived the acute pulmonary syndrome that it also provoked.

A variety of descriptive studies have demonstrated ecologic associations between agricultural chemicals and various types of congenital anomalies (neural tube defects, facial cleft, renal agenesis). A 1988 study from New Brunswick, for example, found evidence of an association between the potential exposure to agricultural chemicals and three major anomalies combined, as well as spina bifida. The same study showed an association between stillbirths and exposure to agricultural chemicals during the second trimester of pregnancy. The study also described cyclic patterns of stillbirth in the agricultural Saint John River basin, correlated with agricultural activities. A variety of associations have also been reported for neural tube defects for agricultural employment and residence in areas with heavy use of agricultural chemicals. Associations have also been reported in some studies for craniofacial anomalies and exposures to herbicides. Employment in the Colombian floricultural industry has been associated with numerous adverse reproductive outcomes including abortion, prematurity, and congenital malformations.

## ANIMAL TERATOGENS, REPRODUCTIVE TOXINS, & RELATED EPIDEMIOLOGIC STUDIES

Table 32–4 is a list of pesticides with some current evidence for female reproductive toxicity in animals. Important teratogens listed include the fungicide benomyl, which produces anomalies including encephalocele, hydrocephalus, microphthalmia, and anophthalmia in various animal model systems over doses ranging from 15.6 to 125 mg/kg. Clusters of anophthalmia have been subsequently reported in Britain and Wales, speculatively associated with benomyl exposure (by means of residence in a high-use area). Fungicides in the ethylenebidithiocarbamate (EBDC) class containing the contaminant ethylene thiourea (ETU) are less consistently teratogenic in animal studies than benomyl. ETU produces malformations in rats, but not in mice, hamsters, guinea pigs, and cats, except at very high dose levels. Reported effects of bromoxynil are limited to skeletal abnormalities (a high incidence of supernumerary ribs compared to controls) at doses that also produced some maternal toxicity.

The structural similarity between the potent teratogen thalidomide and the phthalimide fungicide captan has prompted concern about limb reduction defects in agricultural workers. Descriptive studies have associated these defects with living in California agricultural areas and with employment as a farm worker (5.05 per 1000 total births versus 2.19 per 1000 total births, rate ratio = 2.3). Animal studies of teratogenic effects of captan have been largely negative, including numerous studies that included thalidomide as a positive control. One positive study was reported in rabbits, with malformations reported at the low and intermediate doses, but not at the highest dose tested.

Fungicides containing organic mercury are well-characterized perinatal poisons. Pregnant mice administered single doses of methyl mercury have anatomically normal offspring that demonstrate func-

**Table 32–4.** Animal and human teratogens and reproductive toxins.

| Teratogen | Toxicity |
|---|---|
| Arsenic acid, Arsenic pentoxide, sodium arsenate, sodium pyroarsenate | High doses of inorganic arsenic increase fetal resorptions and genitourinary defects |
| Benomyl | Encephalocele, hydrocephalus, microphthalmia, and anophthalmia in various animal model systems over doses ranging from 15.6 mg/kg to 125 mg/kg |
| Bromoxynil | Reported effects of bromoxynil are limited to skeletal abnormalities (a high incidence of supernumerary ribs compared with controls) at doses that also produced some maternal toxicity |
| Captan | Inconsistently dose-related effects in single rabbit study; others negative despite positive controls demonstrating thalidomide effects—most rodent species except hamster |
| Carbon disulfide | Fetotoxicity—at doses 25, 75, 250 mg/kg/d; malformations in a multigeneration study—hydrocephalus, microcephalus, clubfoot, tail deformations |
| Chlordecone (Kepone) | Fetotoxicity and malformations ranging from reduced ossification, edema, undescended testes, enlarged renal pelvis, and enlarged cerebral ventricles |
| Chromic acid, sodium dichromate, other chromates: defoliant for cotton and other plants; principal use as wood preservative | EPA lists as teratogen and fetotoxin |
| Cyanazine | Teratogenicity, fetotoxicity—head anomalies 25 mg/kg 6–15 days; NOEL 10 mg/kg/d—no effect in Sprague Dawley rat; fetotoxicity—NZ rabbits but no teratogenicity |
| Cyhexatin | This compound was removed from the market in 1988 secondary to adverse reproductive effects observed in animal tests |
| Dinocap | Torticollis and fetotoxicity in offspring at doses below those producing maternal toxicity |
| Dinoseb | Abdominal distension, cleft palate, torticollis at MTD; torticollis at doses below MTD; fetotoxicity |
| Ethylene oxide | Aberrations in cervical vertebrae in mice treated intravenously with 75–150 mg/kg |
| Ethylene thiourea and EBDC fungicides—maneb, zineb | ETU produces malformations in rats, but not in the mouse, hamster, guinea pig, and cat, except at very high dose levels |
| Methyldithiocarbamate (metam-sodium) | Fetotoxicity—in feeding studies reported to Cal-EPA; principal byproduct methyl-isothiocyanate negative in similar studies; other byproducts include carbon disulfide and hydrogen sulfide. The former is noted to produce malformations in feeding studies as described above |
| Methyl mercury, mercury and mercury compounds (inactive or cancelled registrations as seed treatment and paint preservative) | Pregnant mice treated with a single dose of 4–8 mg/kg methyl mercury had offspring with no structural birth defects, but the offspring showed cerebellar deficits in behavioral tests and pathologic changes in cerebellar Purkinje cells |
| Methyl bromide | Omphalocele, arterial malformations, gallbladder agenesis in studies reported to Cal-EPA |
| Nicotine | Spontaneous abortions reported in patients using transdermal nicotine to stop smoking; skeletal abnormalities at doses 25/mg/kg/d in animal studies—PDR; low birth weight associated with smoking mediated by nicotine? or by carbon monoxide? |
| Pentachlorophenol | Decreased survival and growth of their young at 30 mg/kg/d; 50 mg/kg/d on 6–15, 8–11, 12–15 toxicity in the young in the form of resorptions, subcutaneous edema, dilated ureters, and skeletal anomalies—?Only at maternally toxic doses |
| 2,3,7,8-Tetrachlorodibenzo-para-dioxin (TCDD) | Cleft palate, kidney anomalies mice/rats; fetotoxic to variety of experimental animals; mouse NOEL = 0.1 g/kg/d; male toxin at doses above those producing above effects |

(continued)

**Table 32–4.** Animal and human teratogens and reproductive toxins. (continued)

| Pesticide | Reproductive Toxicity |
|---|---|
| | **Pesticide with evidence for reproductive toxicity in male animals.** |
| Benomyl | Fungicide: dose-dependent decreases in mean testis weight and mean seminiferous tubular diameter and occlusions in efferent ductules in mice dosed with 100 mg/kg of benomyl metabolite carbendazim |
| Carbaryl | Insecticide: spermatotoxin in rodents; study in manufacturing and formulating workers indicating no effect at relatively low levels of exposure |
| Carbon disulfide | Fumigant: interferes with sperm transport in rats exposed to 600 ppm. Testes grossly and histologically normal |
| Chlordecone (Kepone) | Insecticide: testicular toxin in a number of species; infertility in manufacturing and formulating workers; no longer manufactured |
| Chlorobenzilate | Insecticide: testicular toxin in rodents; inadequate human studies (no longer registered) |
| Dibromochloropropane (DBCP) | Nematocide: testicular toxin in a number of species; alkylating agent, mutagen, carcinogen; number of reports and studies indicating infertility in formulating workers and applicators; almost all uses suspended |
| Dinoseb | Diffuse tubular atrophy/reproductive failure in rats fed up to 200 ppm; decreased sperm motility at doses down to 125 ppm |
| Ethylene dibromide | Fumigant, nematocide, testicular toxin in a number of species; alkylating agent, mutagen, carcinogen; epidemiological study indicating decreased sperm count; almost all uses suspended |
| Ethylene oxide | Dominant lethal mutations produced when male mice injected with single 150 mg/kg dose of ethylene oxide. Similar effect produced by inhalation of 1000 ppm. Decreased sperm count and motility in monkeys inhaling 50–100 ppm |
| Fenchlorphos | Spermatotoxin in cattle |
| Molinate (Ordram) | Rice herbicide; spermatotoxin in rats, not other species; epidemiologic study of manufacturing and formulating workers indicating no effect at relatively low levels of exposure |
| Triphenyltin | Fungicide; testicular toxin in rats; no human studies |

tional and histological cerebellar abnormalities. Clinical cases of in utero mercury poisoning have resulted from episodes of grain contaminated with mercury in Iraq and fish contaminated with mercury in Minimata, Japan. Currently, there are no mercury-containing seed treatment fungicides with active US registrations. Organic mercuries used as preservatives in latex paint were phased out following reported cases of acrodynia associated with their use in 1990.

## MALE REPRODUCTIVE TOXICITY

In 1977, a number of male workers were discovered to have reduced or absent sperm, infertility or sterility, and testicular atrophy as a result of exposure to dibromochloropropane (DBCP) (see Chapter 26). Similar effects were observed in animals. A short time later, workers exposed to chlordecone (Kepone) in a manufacturing facility were found to have similar testicular changes, followed by confirmatory animal tests. These episodes prompted an increase in the screening of pesticides for male reproductive toxicity. Table 32–4 also lists pesticides determined in animals to be male reproductive toxins.

## Prevention

**A. Work Practices:** Manufacturing and formulation workers, mixers, loaders, applicators, and flaggers are all directly exposed to the concentrated or dilute product and so can only be protected by engineering controls and personal protective clothing and devices. Field workers are exposed primarily to residues on plants and in soil. They are protected primarily by reentry intervals—the minimum time allowed between application of a pesticide on a field and entry into that field. The rate of degradation and the toxicity of the degradation products are important determinants of the extent and effect of exposure in this group. Pesticide degradation rates often vary among geographic regions, so that reentry intervals may need to be specific to an area or climate. One of the most common causes of acute pesticide intoxication in agriculture is the early entry of a group of field workers into a field where an acutely toxic pesticide has recently been applied.

Since skin contamination is the most important route of most occupational exposures, the focus of prevention is to reduce dermal exposure though the use of respirators by manufacturing or formulation workers or pesticide applicators. Contamination of clothing, irritated skin, heat, and sweat are all factors common in agricultural work that promote absorption through the skin. The use of protective clothing in agriculture is usually impeded by the fact that most agricultural work takes place in hot and frequently humid environments. Therefore, the need for skin protection, which is difficult to quantify, must be balanced against the risk of heat-related disorders. The use of personal protective equipment for structural pest control is sometimes hampered by the need to work in tight areas, such as crawl spaces, but the confined nature of these spaces often makes their use necessary.

**B. Medical Surveillance:** Specific medical and biological monitoring is available for cholinesterase-inhibiting organophosphate pesticides, as discussed below. For most other pesticides, surveillance is limited to general and occupational histories and physical examinations, with available tests discussed under laboratory findings for each family.

### Treatment

Treatment of pesticide poisoning in general proceeds in three steps, as described below.

**A. Decontamination:** Decontamination is the first priority, unless life-saving measures are required. In the case of acute dermal overexposure, the skin and clothing are reservoirs for continued exposure, as is the gastrointestinal tract in the case of ingestion. All clothing should be removed and placed in double plastic bags for later analysis, decontamination, or disposal. The skin and, if necessary, the hair should be washed with soap. Contamination should be checked for under the fingernails. If the eyes have been contaminated, they should be irrigated. The need for gastrointestinal lavage or activated charcoal instillation should be determined on a case-by-case basis (ie, depending on the pesticide, whether vomiting or diarrhea have occurred, and the level of consciousness). All procedures should be done in such a way as to minimize the contamination of medical personnel and equipment without compromising patient care.

**B. Specific Antidotes:** Specific antidotes are available only in the form of atropine and pralidoxime for cholinesterase-inhibiting pesticides, as discussed in detail below, and chelating agents for heavy metal pesticides such as arsenic and mercury, which rarely result in the need for treatment, except in cases of ingestion.

**C. Supportive Care:** Supportive care may be the only treatment indicated and may be lifesaving. Assessment of respiratory status and provision of appropriate ventilatory support are critical, since most fatal or serious acute pesticide poisonings are indicated, at least in part, through respiratory embarrassment or arrest. Certain medications that might otherwise be given based on clinical diagnosis may be contraindicated once the diagnosis of a specific pesti-

cide intoxication is known. An example is the use of morphine, which can precipitate cardiac arrhythmia, for pulmonary edema in the presence of organophosphate poisoning.

## REGULATION OF USE OF PESTICIDES

Pesticides are regulated differently from other chemicals in the United States and in most other countries that have chemical regulatory systems. Prior to enactment of the Federal Insecticide Fungicide and Rodenticide Act (FIFRA) in 1970, there was little regulation and testing of pesticides in the United States. Since that time, the United States Environmental Protection Agency (EPA) has applied an increasingly strict testing scheme to registration for sale and use of pesticides in the United States.

Since the discovery of irregularities and even fraud by certain commercial laboratories performing these tests under contract to manufacturers, greater attention has been paid to good laboratory practice and laboratory audits. The data required by the EPA for registration of a pesticide are set forth in Table 32–5. Until recently, access to these data was completely restricted in accordance with trade secrecy laws.

In spite of these requirements for testing, data gaps for both old and new pesticides remain serious. In 1984, the National Academy of Sciences (NAS)-National Research Council (NRC) published the results of a survey on toxicity testing for chemicals. Although testing was more complete for pesticides than for industrial chemicals (and less complete than for cosmetics and food additives), the toxicity data available for most pesticides can only be described as incomplete or inadequate.

The NAS-NRC survey identified 3350 pesticides and inert ingredients and selected 50 for evaluation. For 19 of those (38%), no toxicity information was available; for 13 (26%), there was less than minimal toxicity information (acute and subchronic only); and for only 5 (10%) was there sufficient information to allow a complete health hazard assessment. By category of testing, 59% were studied for acute effects, 51% for subchronic effects, 23% for chronic effects, 34% for reproductive effects, and 28% underwent mutagenicity studies.

Because of the data call-in program initiated by EPA in 1981 and legislation passed in California during the mid-1980s (California Senate Bill 950) that mandated filling of data gaps for all registered pesticides, a large number of new chronic studies were submitted for review by both the California and Federal EPAs. California officials reviewing the data submitted estimate that 90% of the required data has been submitted. Because of the complexities of the

**Table 32–5.** US Environmental Protection Agency (EPA) requirements for pesticide registration.

**Product chemistry**
  Production composition
  Physical and chemical characteristics
  Residue chemistry
  Environmental fate
**Hazards to humans and domestic animals**
  Acute studies
    Oral LD50: rat
    Dermal DL50: usually rabbit; inhalation LCSO: rat
    Primary eye irritation: rabbit
    Primary dermal irritation: rabbit
    Dermal sensitization
    Acute delayed neurotoxicity: organophosphates
    Subchronic studies: Required depending on nature of
      exposure
    90-day feeding: rodent, nonrodent 21-day dermal 90-day
      dermal
    90-day inhalation: rat
    90-day neurotoxicity: if acute studies positive
  Chronic studies: required for pesticides with allowable food
    residues (tolerances), or "significant" worker exposure
    Chronic feeding: 2 species, rodent and nonrodent
    Carcinogenicity: 2 species, rat and mouse preferred
    Teratogenicity: two species
    Reproduction: two generations
    Mutagenicity studies: a battery to include:
      Gene mutations
      Structural chromosomal aberrations
    Other genotoxic effects as appropriate
    Metabolism studies (pharmacokinetics)
**Hazard to nontarget organisms**
  Short-term studies
  Long-term and field studies
    Avian and mammalian testing
    Aquatic organism testing
    Plant protection
  Nontarget insect

Source: US Environmental Protection Agency, 1983.

hazard and risk assessment process, regulatory review of these data are still ongoing.

In the United States, the EPA regulates the registration, sale, and conditions of use of all pesticides and is responsible for the protection of agricultural workers exposed to pesticides. When a specific pesticide is approved for use, its use is specified as either general or restricted (to be applied only through permit to a licensed pest control operator) and it is registered and assigned an EPA registration number. The label information and use instruction, including hazard information and first-aid recommendations, are specified by the EPA. Labels contain useful information, and use of a pesticide in any way other than as specified by the label is illegal. Each pesticide is assigned a toxicity category according to its acute toxicity. Table 32–6 shows the EPA labeling categories with their hazard signal words and precautionary statements.

The Occupational Safety and Health Administration (OSHA) is responsible for the protection of manufacturing and formulation workers. A criteria document for these exposures was published by the National Institute for Occupational Safety and Health (NIOSH) in 1978. State agriculture and health departments, along with county agriculture and health departments and other state and local agencies, along with OSHA, may have a variety of regulatory or advisory functions in regard to the use of pesticides. Structural pest control—the application of pesticides to commercial and residential buildings—may fall under one or another of these jurisdictions or often through cracks in the regulatory system.

## PESTICIDES & ADDITIVES IN FOOD

There are over 300 pesticides (active ingredients) used on food in the United States. The EPA (in conjunction with the FDA) regulates the residues of pesticides and their breakdown products in foods by establishing tolerance levels, or the legal limits for residues in foods. The regulation of pesticide residues in food is a complicated and controversial process.

Tolerances for raw agricultural commodities and processed foods are established through field trials to determine the highest residues likely to occur in the course of normal agricultural procedures and practices.

Tolerances for processed foods are established by determining the degree to which the residues might become concentrated during processing, such as milling or juicing. The risks to health of pesticide residues in food are considered only after the development of proposed tolerances, through a separate process. There are inconsistencies in the way in which health effects are considered. Tolerances for raw commodities may be arrived at by considering both health risks and economic benefits of pesticides, whereas tolerances for processed food—which include all food additives such as artificial sweeteners, preservatives, chemical processing aids, animal drug residues, and packaging materials—are derived by considering only health risks. The Delaney Clause (see below) prohibiting tolerance for any additive found to cause cancer in humans or animals applies to processed foods, but not to raw foods. New tolerances are usually denied for pesticides known to be carcinogenic, but many older pesticides have been found to be carcinogenic only after food tolerances have been established. This is the case with daminozide (Alar), the growth regulator used in apples (see below). In these cases, pesticide use often continues while the EPA proceeds through a regulatory process that often takes years, generating considerable controversy.

With the exception of the occurrence of high concentrations of acutely toxic pesticides in food, such as aldicarb in watermelon (see Organophosphates

**Table 32–6.** Environmental Protection Agency (EPA) toxicity labeling categories.

| Hazard Indicator | Toxicity Category | | | |
|---|---|---|---|---|
| | I | II | III | IV |
| Oral LD50 | <50 mg/kg | 50–500 mg/kg | 500–5000 mg/kg | >5000 |
| Inhalation LD50 | <0.2 mg/L | 0.2–2 mg/L | 2–20 mg/L | >20 mg/L |
| Dermal LD50 | <200 mg/kg | 200–2000 mg/kg | 2000–20,000 mg/kg | >20,000 mg/kg |
| Eye effects | Corrosive; corneal opacity not reversible within 7 days | Corneal opacity reversible within 7 days; irritation for 7 days | No corneal opacity; irritation reversible within 7 days | No irritation |
| Skin effects | Corrosive | Severe irritation at 72 hours | Moderate irritation at 72 hours | Mild or slight irritation at 72 hours |
| Signal word | "Danger" | "Warning" | "Caution" | "Caution" |
| Precautionary statements | Fatal (poisonous) if swallowed, inhaled, or absorbed through skin. Do not breathe vapor, dust, or spray mist. Do not get in eyes or on skin or clothing | May be fatal if swallowed, inhaled, or absorbed through skin. Do not breathe vapor, dust, or spray mist. Do not get in eyes or on skin or clothing | Harmful if swallowed, inhaled, or absorbed through skin. Avoid breathing vapor, dust, or spray mist. Avoid contact with skin, eyes, or clothing | No precautionary statements required |

Source: US Environmental Protection Agency, 1983.

and Carbamates, below), the principal health concern regarding pesticide residues in food—given their usual low concentrations—is carcinogenic risk. Of approximately 8350 tolerances for raw commodities, about 2500 are for carcinogenic pesticides, as are 31 of 150 tolerances for processed foods. A committee of the National Research Council recently published Regulating Pesticides in Food: The Delaney Paradox, a report examining the issue of regulating carcinogenic pesticides in food. A small number of carcinogenic pesticides (mostly fungicides) present in a small number of foods were found to contribute most of the estimated carcinogenic effects from eating food containing residues of carcinogenic pesticides. The committee recommended a consistent standard for regulating pesticide residues in food rather than the current inconsistencies, according to whether food was raw or in processed form and old versus new tolerances. They recommended a negligible risk standard rather than the zero risk of the Delaney Clause and a focus on those pesticides that contribute to a majority of the risk. These recommendations will probably be implemented in some form by the EPA and the FDA in the future.

Monitoring for pesticide residues in food is performed by the United States Department of Agriculture (USDA) in meat and poultry and by the FDA in domestic and imported raw and processed food. A number of states and private groups also analyze samples for pesticides. The amount of sampling performed and the analytical methods used have been subjects of further controversy. Most of the methods used detect only about 50% of food-use pesticides and are designed to detect levels at or near the tolerance level, but not below that level. Thus, it is difficult on the basis of available sampling data to accurately judge the risk to consumers of current pesticide residues in food. There is increasing pressure to improve monitoring programs and to calculate risks based on a range of diets and for sensitive populations, particularly children. In California, the state EPA collects 6000–7000 samples per year in its marketplace surveillance program of more than 100 commodities. The residue screens detect approximately 200 pesticides with minimum detection limits ranging from 20 to 200 parts per billion (ppb).

The USDA program samples 12 commodities for 55 pesticides, with minimum detection limits ranging from 1 to 150 ppb. For the 1993 California program, 64% of the samples tested showed no detectable residues. An additional 22.9% had detectable residues that were less than 10% of the legal tolerances. Approximately 1.6% of the samples showed violative residues, with three-quarters representing pesticides detected on crops for which they had no legal tolerance, and one quarter representing pesticides present over the legal tolerance levels.

# MANAGEMENT OF TOXICITY DUE TO PESTICIDES

## ORGANOPHOSPHATE & CARBAMATE CHOLINESTERASE-INHIBITING INSECTICIDES

### Essentials of Diagnosis

*Acute effects:*
- Acetylcholinesterase inhibition-acetylcholine excess.
- Parasympathetic nervous system hyperactivity, neuromuscular paralysis, central nervous system dysfunction, and depression of red cell and plasma cholinesterase activity.

*Chronic effects:*
- Persistent CNS dysfunction (organophosphates): irritability, anxiety, mood lability, fatigue, impaired short-term memory, and impaired concentration for weeks or months after acute pesticide exposure.
- Organophosphate-induced delayed neuropathy: rapid onset of distal symmetric sensorimotor neuropathy.
- Dermatitis.

## General Considerations

Organophosphates are esters of phosphoric acid that exist in two forms: -thion and -oxon. The latter is shown in Figure 32–1B. Carbamates are esters of carbamic acid. The organophosphates and carbamates are considered here as a single class because they share a common mechanism of acute toxicity cholinesterase inhibition, with similar signs and symptoms of acute poisoning. The thiocarbamates and dithiocarbamates do not inhibit cholinesterase and are considered separately under fungicides and herbicides. The carbamates differ from organophosphates primarily in the transient and reversible nature of their cholinesterase inhibition, which results in a shorter duration of acute toxicity without persistent sequelae.

Together, these substances represent one of the largest and most important classes of insecticides. Commonly used compounds are listed according to acute toxicity in Table 32–7. They vary widely in their potency, and in inhibiting cholinesterase, as reflected in their LD50 values.

As a result of their widespread use and acute toxicity, the organophosphates and carbamates are the most common cause of acute insecticide intoxication. Cholinesterase inhibitors produce a relatively stereotypical clinical presentation that in conjunction with determination of cholinesterase levels makes diagnosis more accurate than with other pesticides. Specific

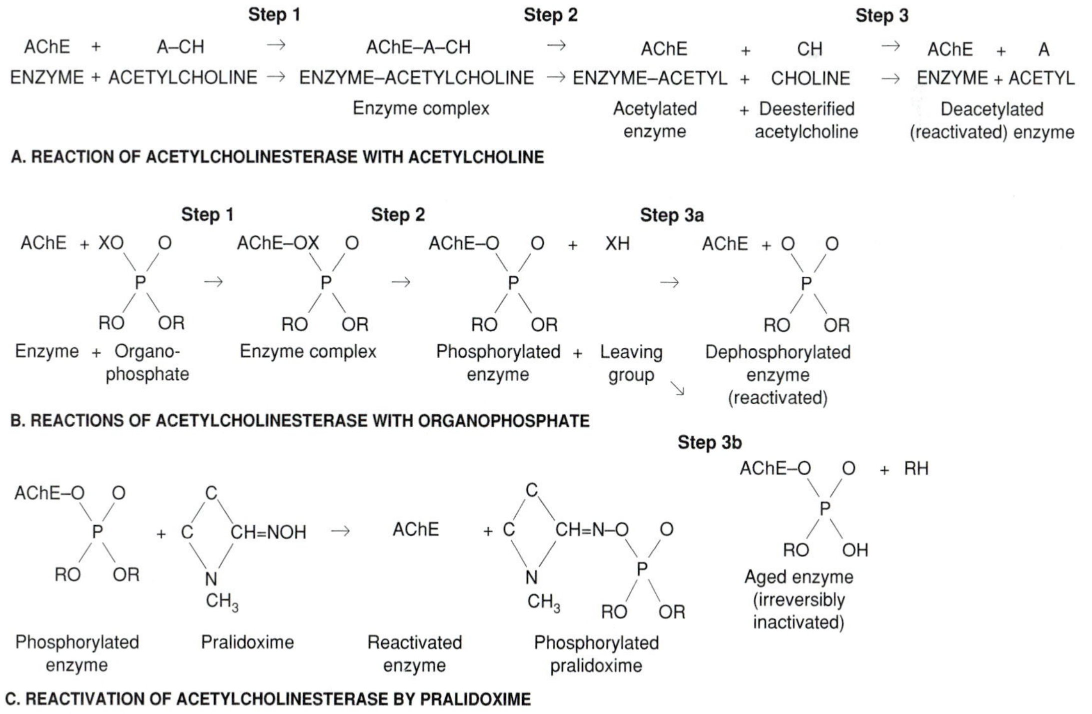

**Figure 32–1.** *A:* Reaction of acetylcholinesterase with acetylcholine. *B:* Reactions of acetylcholinesterase with organophosphate. *C:* Reactivation of acetylcholinesterase by pralidoxime.

**Table 32–7.** Organophosphate and carbamate pesticides in common use in the United States.

| Common Name | Trade Name | Oral LD50 (mg/kg) | Dermal LD50 (mg/kg) |
|---|---|---|---|
| Organophosphates: Category I Parathion | | 1–5 | 1–10 |
| Mevinphos | Phosdrin | 1–5 | 1–10 |
| Methyl parathion | | 5–10 | 50–100 |
| Carbophenothion | Trithion | 5–10 | 20 |
| EPN | | 5–10 | 20 |
| Methamidophos | Monitor | 10–20 | 100 |
| Azinphos-methyl | Guthion | 10–20 | 200 |
| Methidathion | Supracide | 20–30 | 400 |
| Dichlorvos (DDVP) | Vapona | 20–30 | 50–100 |
| Organophosphates: Category II Chlorpyrifos | Dursban, Lorsban | 50–150 | 2000 |
| Diazinon | Spectracide | 50–150 | 400 |
| Phosmet | Imidan | 50–150 | 3000 |
| Dimethoate | Cygon | 150–500 | 150 |
| Fenthion | Baytex | 150–500 | |
| Naled | Dibrom | 150–500 | 1000 |
| Trichlorion | Diptarex | 150–500 | 2000 |
| Organophosphates: Categories III and IV Acephate | Orthene | 500–1000 | 2000 |
| Malathion | | 500–1000 | 4000 |
| Stirofos (tetrachlorvinphos) | Gardona Rabon | 1000–5000 | 5000 |
| Carbamates Aldicarb | Temik | 1–5 | 1–10 |
| Carbofuran | Furadan | 5–10 | 10,000 |
| Methomyl | Lannate | 15–25 | 1000 |
| Propoxur | Baygon | 100 | 1000 |
| Bendiocarb | Ficam | 100–200 | |
| Carbaryl | Sevin | 300–600 | 2000 |

**Table 32–8.** Commonly used organophosphate pesticides with evidence for delayed neuropathy in humans and animals.

| Pesticide | In Humans | In Animals |
|---|---|---|
| Trichlorphon | + | + |
| Merphos (Folex) | + | + |
| O-Ethyl-0-p-nitrophenyl-benzene-thioophos-phonate (EPN) | ? | + |
| Methamidophos | ? | + |
| Fenthion | ? | ? |
| Trichloronate | NR | + |
| S,S,S-Tributyl phosphorotrithioate (DEF) | NR | + |
| Diisopropylfluorophosphate (DFP) | NR | + |
| Dichlorvos    NR | ? | |

? = uncertain; NR = not reported; + = reliably reported.

the only recognized human health effect of these compounds that is unrelated to cholinesterase inhibition.

## Use

**A. Organophosphates:** Organophosphate pesticides were developed following World War II as a consequence of the synthesis of the organophosphate nerve gases sarin, soman, and tabun. Since then, they have largely replaced inorganic pesticides and organochlorines as the principal insecticides used in agriculture. A number are water-soluble, which enables them to be used as systemic insecticides (demeton, dimethoate, disulfoton, phosphamidon, and trichlorphon). Many are highly toxic and therefore restricted, but are still used extensively in agriculture (eg, parathion). Others, such as malathion and diazinon, are of relatively low toxicity and are used commonly in home and garden. Dichlorvos has a very high vapor pressure and so is impregnated into pet collars and pest strips for slow release. Chlorpyrifos is perhaps the insecticide most frequently used by structural pest control operators against cockroaches and other structural pests.

**B. Carbamates:** The cholinesterase-inhibiting carbamates are all insecticides. Carbaryl has by far the largest use, owing to its low mammalian toxicity and relatively wide spectrum of activity. The others have more narrower spectrums. Aldicarb, carbofuran, and methomyl are highly water-soluble, which results in their being taken up into plants for use as systemic pesticides. Propoxur is used by structural pest control operators and in the home against cockroaches.

and nonspecific antidotes are available for treatment. A presumably small, but uncertain, percentage of patients acutely poisoned by organophosphates displays persistent central nervous system dysfunction for weeks or months after acute poisoning. A small number of organophosphate pesticides also cause a delayed neuropathy that is correlated with inhibition of the enzyme neurotoxic esterase (Table 32–8). This is

## Occupational & Environmental Exposure

Organophosphates and carbamates are applied by a variety of techniques, from aerial spraying to application. Granular and bait formulations significantly reduce exposure. These pesticides are generally rapidly degraded in the environment, though in hot, dry climates they persist to a greater degree, and longer reentry intervals (1–2 weeks) have been necessary to prevent acute poisoning of field workers. Water contamination from organophosphates has not been a major problem to date.

Carbamates as a class were generally thought to rapidly degrade in the environment and not migrate into groundwater. However, aldicarb (Temik), the most acutely toxic carbamate, has been found in groundwater and drinking water. Since aldicarb is water-soluble, it concentrates in the watery parts of fruits and vegetables. An outbreak of acute aldicarb intoxication in hundreds of consumers of watermelons in the western United States occurred in 1985 as a result of the illegal use of aldicarb on some fields of the fruit. Similar but smaller episodes had taken place earlier, following the instillation of aldicarb into the water of hydroponically grown tomatoes and cucumbers.

## Pharmacokinetics & Mechanism of Action

Organophosphates and carbamates are easily absorbed by inhalation, skin contact, and ingestion; the primary route of occupational exposure is dermal. They differ from one another in lipid solubility and therefore distribution in the body, particularly to the central nervous system.

Many commercial organophosphates are applied in the -thion (sulfur-containing) form, but readily undergo conversion to the -oxon (oxygen-containing) form (Figure 32–1B). Most of the -oxon forms have much greater toxicity than their corresponding -thion analogues. The conversion occurs in the environment, so that residues crops field workers are exposed to may be more toxic than the pesticide that was applied. Some of the sulfur is released in the form of mercaptans, which produce the typical odor of the -thion form of organophosphates. The mercaptans have very low odor thresholds, and the reactions to their noxious odor, including headache, nausea, and vomiting, are often mistaken for acute organophosphate poisoning.

The conversion from -thion to -oxon also occurs in vivo as a result of hepatic microsomal metabolism, so that the -oxon becomes the active form of the pesticide in both animal pests and humans. Hepatic esterases rapidly hydrolyze organophosphate esters, yielding alkyl phosphates and phenols, which have little, if any, toxicologic activity and are rapidly excreted. Carbamates are also metabolized by the liver and excreted as metabolites in urine without evidence of significant accumulation.

Organophosphates and carbamates exert effects on insects and mammals, including humans, by inhibiting acetylcholinesterase at nerve endings. The normal function of acetylcholinesterase is the hydrolysis, and thereby inactivation, of acetylcholine (Figure 32–1A). The reactions of organophosphates and acetylcholinesterase are shown in Figure 32–1B. The inhibition of acetylcholinesterase occurs through the formation of a pesticide-enzyme complex (step 1), a hydrolysis of the -X (leaving-group), resulting in phosphorylation of the enzyme (step 2). The enzyme can then be spontaneously dephosphorylated and reactivated (step 3a) or aged through the hydrolysis of an alkyl (-R) group, resulting in irreversible inactivation. After irreversible inactivation, normal enzyme activity can only be restored by the synthesis of new acetylcholinesterase, a process that can take up to 60 days to complete.

Carbamates initially react with acetylcholinesterase in the same fashion as organophosphates, resulting in accumulation of acetylcholine in the same distribution as organophosphates. The carbamyl enzyme product does not progress to an aging reaction but instead dissociates relatively rapidly. As a family, the carbamates have no known health effects other than those resulting from this acute, reversible inhibition of cholinesterase and resulting overactivity of acetylcholine.

The clinical manifestations of acute organophosphate or carbamate poisoning depend upon the organs where acetylcholine is the transmitter of nerve impulses, as shown in Table 32–9.

The character, degree, and duration of acute illness produced by cholinesterase-inhibiting organophosphate and carbamate pesticides are all directly related to the degree and rate of acetylcholinesterase inhibition and subsequent accumulation of acetylcholine. Rapid rates of inhibition are associated with clinical illness at levels of inhibition that may not be associated with symptoms following slower rates of inhibition. Chronic inhibition of acetylcholinesterase appears to result in tolerance to some of the acute effects. Even if tolerance occurs, chronic inhibition of acetylcholinesterase results in a state in which exposure to a dose of an organophosphate that previously would have had no effect may now lower acetylcholinesterase levels below a critical threshold and result in clinical illness. Cumulative inhibition of acetylcholinesterase is unlikely to occur from carbamates, owing to the rapidly reversible nature of the enzyme inhibition.

Organophosphate pesticides possess structural differences that result in differences in cholinesterase inhibition potency, in lipid solubility (and therefore distribution, particularly to the central nervous system) in rates of reversibility and aging, and in physical properties such as volatility. However, for both

**Table 32–9.** Signs and symptoms of acute organophosphate poisoning by site of acetylcholine neurotransmitter activity.

| System | Receptor Type | Organ | Action | Sign or Symptom |
|---|---|---|---|---|
| Parasympathetic | Muscarinic | Eye, iris muscle, ciliary muscle | Contraction | Miosis |
| Sympathetic | | | Contraction | Blurred vision |
| | | Glands: Lacrimal, salivary, respiratory gastrointestinal, urinary, sweat | Secretion | Tearing, salivation, bronchorrhea, pulmonary edema, nausea, vomiting, diarrhea, urination, perspiration |
| | | Heart: sinus node, atrioventricular node | Slowing; refractory period increased | Bradycardia, arrhythmias, Heart block |
| | | Smooth muscle: bronchial, gastrointestinal | Contraction | Bronchoconstriction |
| | | Wall, sphincter | Contraction Relaxation | Vomiting, cramps, diarrhea |
| | | Bladder, fundus, sphincter | Contraction, relaxation | Urination, incontinence |
| Neuromuscular | Nicotinic | Skeletal | Excitation | Fasciculations, cramps, followed by weakness, loss of reflexes, paralysis |
| Central nervous | | Brain | Excitation (early) | Headache, dizziness, malaise, apprehension, confusion, hallucinations, manic or bizarre behavior, convulsions |
| | | | Depression (late) | Depression of, then loss of, consciousness; respiratory depression |

organophosphates and carbamates, cholinesterase-inhibiting potency is the only characteristic of practical clinical significance. For a large proportion of patients with acute intoxication, the clinician will not know the identity of the particular pesticide or pesticides at the time of initial presentation, and decisions regarding diagnosis and management will need to be made on the basis of clinical signs, symptoms, and laboratory data.

The only known systemic health effect of organophosphate pesticides that is entirely unrelated to cholinesterase inhibition is organophosphate-induced delayed neuropathy. The pathologic lesion consists of symmetric distal axonal degeneration in the distribution of the ascending and descending nerve fiber tracts in the central and peripheral nervous systems.

The mechanism of action is unknown. Inhibition of an enzyme known as neurotoxic esterase (NTE), found in the central and peripheral nervous systems of various species, is an indicator of neurotoxic potential and a potential biological monitor for exposure to neurotoxic organophosphates. Compounds that are neurotoxic not only must inhibit NTE but must do so irreversibly through an aging process similar to that responsible for cholinesterase inhibition. Animal studies indicate that irreversible inhibi-

tion of NTE to 75% of initial activity will be followed 10–14 days later by a rapidly progressive ascending peripheral neuropathy. However, NTE does not appear to play a direct role in the pathogenesis of the neuropathy. There is no relationship between cholinesterase and NTE inhibition. The commonly used organophosphate pesticides, with evidence of neurotoxicity, are shown in Table 32–8. Carbamates do not cause delayed neuropathy.

A number of organophosphates and carbamates are known to cause primarily irritant dermatitis. Only a few, including malathion and methyl-parathion, dichlorvos, and naled are known to cause allergic contact dermatitis.

Organophosphate and carbamate compounds are alkylating agents, though generally not strong ones. A few are mutagenic, but most, if tested, have not been found to be carcinogenic in animals and none have been found, on the basis of animal studies, to pose a significant carcinogenic risk to humans. Many have not been adequately tested for reproductive toxicity. Although some are fetotoxic at doses near or at cholinesterase-inhibiting levels in maternal animals—and this is of some concern for women directly handling pesticides—none have been found (by animal studies) to pose a significant teratogenic risk to humans. Carbaryl is teratogenic to beagle dogs, but not to a number of other animal species. It is spermatotoxic in animals, but showed no evidence of that effect in one study of manufacturing workers (exposed to relatively low levels).

## Clinical Findings

**A. Symptoms and Signs:** In spite of the popularity of mnemonics such as MUDDLES or MUD-DDLES (miosis, urination, diarrhea, defecation diaphoresis, lacrimation, excitation, and salivation), the signs and symptoms of acute intoxication with organophosphates and carbamates are best learned on a neurophysiologic basis by grouping them according to cholinergic classification (Table 32–9). There is some variability in parasympathetic nervous system manifestations because they are opposed by the sympathetic nervous system, which has preganglionic cholinergic innervation. Thus, the heart rate may be slow, normal, or fast and the pupils may be small, normal, or large depending on which system predominates. In one large series of organophosphate-poisoned patients, 90% had at least muscarinic manifestations, 40% both muscarinic and nicotinic manifestations, 30% muscarinic and central nervous system manifestations, and 10% had all three. The number of systems involved increases with the severity of intoxication. Mild poisoning is usually manifested by mild muscarinic signs and symptoms only.

The onset of illness after acute overexposure is unpredictable, but is related to dose and route of exposure. Mild symptoms generally precede more severe ones, often for periods of 6–8 hours, but following extreme overexposure, severe symptoms and death can occur within minutes. Absorption through the skin is prolonged, so that onset and progression of symptoms are slower. Because pesticide absorbed at a site near a target organ may directly inhibit acetylcholinesterase without undergoing systemic circulation, that organ may be affected early.

The cause of death in acute organophosphate poisoning is usually respiratory failure. Bronchorrhea or pulmonary edema, bronchoconstriction, and respiratory muscular paralysis all contribute to respiratory failure. Cardiac arrhythmias, such as heart block and cardiac arrest, are less common causes of death. Ventricular arrhythmias have been observed in some of these cases. Seizures are not uncommon in cases of severe poisoning, but rarely persist long enough to require treatment. Severe poisoning from occupational exposure to carbamates is uncommon. Owing to the rapid spontaneous reactivation of acetyl cholinesterase, workers who become ill on the job are often better by the time they are seen at a medical facility.

Organophosphate-induced delayed neuropathy was first identified following two massive outbreaks of paralysis from ingestion of nonpesticidal organophosphate triorthocresyl phosphate. The first occurred in the United States in 1930 as a result of consumption of an adulterated alcoholic extract of ginger root known as Jamaica ginger or Jake; the second occurred in Morocco in 1959 as a result of adulteration of cheap cooking oil with surplus airplane lubricant. A number of other smaller outbreaks have been reported between 1930 and 1978 as a result of contamination of food, and there is one report of exposure in an enclosed space during manufacture of triorthocresylphosphate.

Most of the reported cases of human delayed neuropathy have been manifested initially by signs and symptoms of acute cholinergic excess, although following ingestion these have been predominantly gastrointestinal (nausea, vomiting, stomach cramps, and diarrhea). An asymptomatic period of about 7–21 days generally follows, depending on the size of the dose and the duration of exposure. The first symptoms of neuropathy are usually cramp-like pains in the calves and numbness and tingling in the feet. This is followed by increasing and ascending weakness, initially in the legs, and followed, in many cases, by weakness in the arms. Loss of balance due to weakness is common. Examination reveals symmetric weakness, distal more so than proximal, lower more so than upper, and sensory loss that is generally to a lesser degree than motor loss. Deep tendon reflexes are lost in a pattern corresponding to the degree of weakness (usually ankle, but not knee or wrist).

**B. Laboratory Findings:**

**1. Cholinesterase–**A number of nonspecific laboratory findings may be present in an individual with acute poisoning, including leukocytosis, proteinuria, glucosuria, and hemoconcentration. However, changes in cholinesterase activity, along with the typical signs and symptoms, provide sufficient information for the diagnosis and management of most cases. Red cell cholinesterase is called "true" cholinesterase, since it is the same enzyme present in nerve endings and its activity more closely parallels that in the nervous system than does plasma cholinesterase, particularly in the time course of recovery, after inhibition. However, red cell cholinesterase is more difficult to measure and therefore more susceptible to analytic error than plasma cholinesterase. Organophosphates and carbamates may differentially inhibit one enzyme relative to the other, so that if one and not the other appears depressed, it is conservative to assume that neuronal cholinesterase more closely corresponds to the lower of the two. For example, the commonly used organophosphate chlorpyrifos (Dursban, Lorsban) preferentially depresses plasma cholinesterase, causing illness without significant depression of red cell cholinesterase.

Different types of analytical methods are used to measure both red cell and plasma cholinesterase, with results usually reported in different units. Results obtained by one method cannot usually be compared with results from another, even if the units expressed by each are the same. There is considerable variability in cholinesterase activity in unexposed persons, so that reports of results relative to "normal" are meaningless.

Individuals with a genetic trait for atypical plasma cholinesterase have lowered plasma, but not red cell, cholinesterase. They have prolonged muscular paralysis after administration of succinyl choline and other neuromuscular blocking agents that are normally metabolized by plasma cholinesterase, but they are not more susceptible to cholinesterase-inhibiting pesticides. Plasma cholinesterase will not be a reliable indicator of exposure or poisoning in these individuals, but red cell cholinesterase will remain so.

Plasma cholinesterase production may be lowered as a result of liver disease extensive enough to impair the production of proteins such as albumin. Albumin-losing conditions, such as nephrotic syndrome, may be accompanied by elevated levels of plasma cholinesterase as a result of increased hepatic protein synthesis. The only medical conditions known to influence red cell cholinesterase activity are those associated with reticulocytosis, such as recovery from hemorrhage, pernicious anemia, and some other anemias.

There are two circumstances in which cholinesterase determinations may be useful: (1) routine biological monitoring of exposure to organophosphates; and (2) diagnosis of acute poisoning by organophosphates. In each case, comparison of the current level to a preexposure baseline level is helpful, and for biological monitoring, it is essential. Biological monitoring of exposure consists of determination of preexposure baseline levels followed by periodic determination in intervals based upon the frequency and nature of exposure. If only one test is performed, red cell cholinesterase should be monitored since it is more specific for organophosphate pesticides and is an indicator of cumulative absorption of organophos-

phate over a relatively long period of time. Plasma cholinesterase is more immediately responsive to inhibition by acute doses and may be preferentially inhibited by some organophosphates, such as chlorpyrifos. Cholinesterase levels are of limited value in assessing exposure to carbamates because of the rapid reversal of inhibition, even in a test tube.

The appearance of symptoms is more dependent upon the rate of inactivation of cholinesterase than the absolute level of activity reached. For example, workers may reach a cholinesterase level of 40% of baseline (60% inhibition) over the course of a number of weeks without experiencing symptoms, but a previously unexposed person may develop symptoms at a level of 70% of baseline activity (30% inhibition) following acute exposure.

An individual's baseline red cell cholinesterase activity may vary up to 22% from day to day when measured by the same method by the same laboratory. Therefore, 25–30% inhibition (70–75% of baseline) during periodic monitoring can be taken as a warning level of a biological response to chronic exposure to organophosphate pesticides, approaching a level likely to produce intoxication.

Figure 32–2 shows a set of theoretic values for "Worker 1," monitored routinely every 15 days during exposure by red cell and plasma cholinesterase measurements. In this case, both plasma and red cell cholinesterase levels are progressively declining and in parallel fashion. For Worker 1, both cholinesterase levels have declined to about 70% of baseline on day 60, and removal from exposure on that day was followed by a return toward baseline plasma levels more rapidly than red cell levels. Removal of workers at this level (70% of baseline) and prevention of further exposure until levels return to approximately baseline is likely to prevent the development of clinical signs and symptoms of toxicity. Examination of the workplace situation leading to this level of depression is indicated.

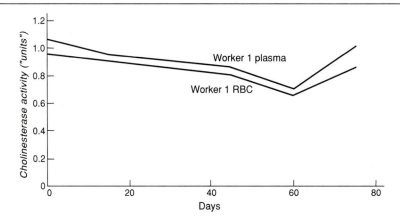

**Figure 32–2.** Cholinesterase monitoring for chronic organophosphate exposure.

Severe poisoning is usually accompanied by cholinesterase levels well below normal for the laboratory. However, patients with mild to moderate poisoning often have cholinesterase levels reported as equivocal, normal, and even above normal. The diagnosis can be confirmed retrospectively by periodic (ie, weekly or biweekly) determinations of cholinesterase until levels fluctuate by no more than 30%. If the average level at this time—the "retrospective baseline"—is more than 30% higher than the level at the time of illness, exposure to cholinesterase-inhibiting pesticides was almost certainly present, and the illness may have been due to that exposure. The rate of recovery of red cell cholinesterase, in the absence of treatment with pralidoxime and of further exposure, depends upon the rate of formation of new red cells, which is about 1% per day. Red blood cell cholinesterase levels will reach a plateau in about 60–70 days and plasma cholinesterase in 30–50 days.

Figure 32–3 shows theoretic values for cholinesterase levels for two workers taken every 15 days following acute organophosphate poisoning on Day 0. "Worker 2" has initial plasma and red cell cholinesterase values within normal, but for both types levels increase to about double the initial values, indicating a probable initial 50% depression from baseline for both. Plasma cholinesterase rises more rapidly and reaches a plateau sooner than red cell cholinesterase. "Worker 3" has an initial red cell cholinesterase value that is below the lower limit of normal and increases to about double the initial value, also indicating a probable initial 50% depression from baseline. Thus, even though Worker 3 has an initial cholinesterase level lower than normal and lower than Worker 2, the actual level of inhibition is similar for both.

**2. Intact Pesticides and Metabolites**–Measurement of the parent organophosphate or carbamate or their metabolites in blood or urine has been investigated to a limited extent. No such measurements are currently likely to be helpful in the diagnosis of acute intoxication. Measurement of alkyl phosphate metabolites in urine has not been of use in biological monitoring of exposure because of its lack of specificity and instability. Measurement of p-nitrophenol in urine can be useful for monitoring exposure to parathion: 0.5 mg/L in a sample collected at the end of an exposure interval corresponds to exposure to parathion at the current TLV. Measurement of 1-naphthol in urine has been used to monitor exposure to carbaryl.

**3. Neurotoxic Esterase**–Laboratory methods to measure neurotoxic esterase (NTE) activity are not available clinically. Limited research has indicated that determination of peripheral lymphocyte NTE may be useful as a biological marker of exposure to a neurotoxic organophosphate pesticide, particularly if its NTE-inhibiting potency is greater than its cholinesterase-inhibiting potency. However, there are at present no specific tests for the diagnosis of organophosphate-induced delayed neuropathy. If, for some reason, exposure to a neurotoxic organophosphate pesticide is uncertain, nerve conduction velocity studies may be of some help in distinguishing organophosphate-induced delayed neuropathy—with little to moderate slowing due to axonal loss—from Guillain-Barré syndrome (idiopathic acute symmetrical polyneuropathy), which is characterized by markedly diminished conduction velocities due to demyelination.

### Differential Diagnosis

Mild acute poisoning from organophosphates or carbamates most closely resembles acute viral influenza, respiratory infections, gastroenteritis, asthma, or psychologic dysfunction. The most significant differential diagnosis is between severe organophosphate poisoning and acute cerebrovascular accident:

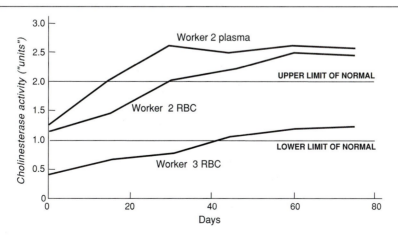

**Figure 32–3.** Cholinesterase monitoring for diagnosis of acute organophosphate exposure.

unequal pupils due to the local effect of an organophosphate in one eye of a comatose patient is a major source of misdiagnosis. Other conditions to be distinguished from acute organophosphate poisoning include heat stroke, heat exhaustion, and infections.

As noted above, the major disorder to be distinguished from organophosphate-induced delayed neuropathy is idiopathic acute symmetric polyneuropathy. Other toxic and disease-related neuropathies are generally insidious in onset and slowly progressive in course.

## Treatment

Treatment that is otherwise indicated should never be delayed, pending determination of cholinesterase levels. The initial diagnosis can be made on clinical grounds alone, samples sent to the laboratory, and a test dose of atropine delivered. Atropine blocks the effects of acetylcholine at muscarinic receptors. A dose of atropine sulfate, 0.5 mg intravenously, produces signs of mild atropinization (dry mouth, dry eyes, increased heart rate, large pupils) in a normal adult; it has no effect in an individual with organophosphate poisoning. A dose of 1–2 mg intravenously will produce marked signs of atropinization in a nonpoisoned adult and may reverse the signs of cholinergic excess in a case of poisoning.

Samples must be sent for cholinesterase measurement before administration of pralidoxime, which will regenerate cholinesterase in red cells and plasma as well as nerves. Atropine has no effect on cholinesterase levels.

Treatment of acute intoxication must be predicated upon assessment of the severity of poisoning, which is largely dependent upon clinical judgment and experience. Assessment of severity should focus primarily on the respiratory system, since it is affected by all three types of cholinergic sites and is the critical one for survival and serious morbidity. The most commonly used severity rating defines mild toxicity as involving only muscarinic signs and symptoms, moderate toxicity as involving more than one system but not requiring assisted breathing, and severe toxicity as requiring ventilatory assistance.

Treatment modalities include the following:

1. Decontamination, including bathing of skin, shampooing of hair, or emptying of stomach, as dictated by route of exposure.
2. Atropine sulfate in a dosage of 1–2 mg intravenously for mild to moderate poisoning, 2–4 mg intravenously for severe poisoning, as often as every 15 minutes, as needed. There is no maximum dosage. Atropine blocks muscarinic activity, but not the nicotinic (muscle paralysis) or central nervous system effects. Patients without evidence of muscle weakness or respiratory depression may be treated with atropine alone until one or more signs of mild atropinization

appear (ie, tachycardia, flushing, dry mucous membranes, or dilated pupils). Multiple doses may need to be administered over a prolonged time.
3. For organophosphate poisoning only, give pralidoxime chloride (2-PAM, Protopam) slowly, 1 g intravenously (no more than 0.5 g/min), repeated once in 1–2 hours, then at 10- to 12-hour intervals, if needed. Pralidoxime acts by breaking the bond between acetylcholinesterase and organophosphate, reactivating the enzyme and restoring acetylcholine activity to normal (Figure 32–1C). Its advantages over atropine include acting at the neuromuscular junction to reverse muscular paralysis and possibly crossing the blood-brain barrier to reverse central nervous system depression. Overdosage is not a problem if the drug is administered slowly to avoid inducing hypotension. The decision to use pralidoxime must be made reasonably soon after diagnosis, since it is not effective once aging has occurred. A high incidence of atropine toxicity may result from the often recommended regimen of first using atropine until primary signs of atropine toxicity appear and then using pralidoxime if necessary. This may be avoided by making the decision to use pralidoxime early.
4. Artificial ventilation, ventilatory assistance, oxygen, and clearance of secretions.

The use of pralidoxime for carbamate poisoning is controversial. Fortunately, it is rarely indicated. There is experimental evidence that pralidoxime may be helpful in the management of poisoning by some rarely used carbamates, but for most of the commonly used carbamates, this drug has not been studied. One animal study indicated that pralidoxime may be harmful in the treatment of carbaryl poisoning.

Morphine, aminophylline, and phenothiazines are contraindicated due to the increased risk of cardiac arrhythmias. Diuretics for pulmonary edema and fluids for hypotension are also contraindicated. It is recommended that atropine be withheld until adequate ventilation has reversed hypoxia, since atropine can be arrhythmogenic in the presence of hypoxia.

By the time the diagnosis of organophosphate-induced delayed peripheral neuropathy is made, the initial manifestations of cholinesterase inhibition, if present, have resolved. Administration of atropine or pralidoxime, initially or later, does not influence the course of neuropathy. Treatment of delayed neuropathy is supportive in a few cases; mechanical ventilation has been required because of respiratory failure due to muscular paralysis.

## Prognosis

If treatment for organophosphate or carbamate poisoning is initiated before hypoxia results in tissue damage, antidotal therapy and respiratory support should ensure complete recovery, even in the most severe cases. Persistence of manifestations beyond 24 hours indicates the possibility of continued absorption of pesticide and the need to carefully consider and examine the skin, fingernails, eyes, and gastrointestinal tract as possible reservoirs.

Sudden death occurs in a small percentage of organophosphate-poisoned patients (2% in one series) 24–48 hours after apparent complete recovery from the acute phase of poisoning, due in at least some cases to ventricular arrhythmia. Sudden relapse of acute signs and symptoms within a few days after apparent recovery has been occasionally reported, perhaps as a result of release of pesticide from fat following mobilization of the patient from bed.

Deaths have been reported as a result of accidental or deliberate ingestion of carbamates, as a result of large doses and prolonged gastrointestinal absorption, and perhaps as a complication of delayed or inadequate treatment. Intoxication from occupational exposure may be serious, but is rarely fatal and usually is of brief duration. Poisoning from contaminated fruits and vegetables with high water content may also be serious, but not persistent.

A number of reports have described persistent central nervous system symptoms in a small percentage of patients following well-documented incidents of acute poisoning from organophosphates, but not carbamates. Typical symptoms include irritability, depression, mood lability, anxiety, fatigue, lethargy, difficulty in concentrating, and short-term memory loss. Limited studies have suggested that neurobehavioral test results and electroencephalograms may be different for such patients, compared with controls. Symptoms may persist for weeks or months after the initial intoxication and are difficult to distinguish from psychologic reactions likely to occur after such an event. Sympathetic counseling and judicious use of antianxiety agents, when appropriate, will generally be more effective than intensive psychotherapy and antipsychotic medicine.

The rate and extent of recovery of delayed neuropathy appears to be related to the severity of the manifestations when they are maximal, usually within a few days to a week after the onset of weakness. At the rate of average axonal regeneration, approximately 1 mm/d, the longest axons affected may take up to a year to recover. Physical therapy appears to strongly influence the rate and perhaps the degree of recovery of strength and function. Long-term follow-up of survivors of Jamaica ginger paralysis indicated the development of an upper motor neuron syndrome that became apparent following recovery of peripheral nerve function. Continued disability was related to spasticity of the lower limbs, though muscle atrophy and weakness were present in some individuals.

# ORGANOCHLORINE INSECTICIDES

## Essentials of Diagnosis

*Acute effects:*
- Central nervous system excitation: irritability, excitability, dizziness, disorientation. paresthesias, tremors, and convulsions.

*Chronic effects:*
- Cancer in animals.
- Aplastic anemia?

## General Considerations

The organochlorine insecticides are chlorinated hydrocarbon compound, of cyclic structure and high molecular weight. In contrast to chlorinated hydrocarbon solvents and fumigants, they are of low volatility and are central nervous stimulants rather than general anesthetics. The prototype organochlorine chlorophenothane (DDT) was discovered in 1939 and until it was banned from most uses in the United States in 1973, over 4 billion pounds were applied, in agriculture and in control programs aimed at mosquitoes and other insects that transmit human disease such as yellow fever and malaria. From 1940 through the 1970s, a number of other organochlorine compounds were widely used as insecticides, but following recognition of their persistence in the environment, bioaccumulation in animals and humans, adverse effects on some wildlife, and carcinogenicity in laboratory animals, most have been deregistered or severely restricted in use. Those compounds still in use in the United States are listed in Table 32–10. Since the acute toxicity of the remaining compounds is low and their use is currently limited, they rarely cause acute intoxication.

## Use

Shortly after the development of DDT, hexachlorocyclohexane, better known as benzene hexa-

Table 32–10. Organochlorine pesticides used in the United States.

| Pesticide | Oral LD50 (mg/kg) | Dermal LD50 (mg/kg) |
|---|---|---|
| Endrin | 5–15 | 10–20 |
| Endosultan | 20–40 | 75–150 |
| Heptachlor | 200 | 100–300 |
| Benzene hexachloride (BHC), gamma BHC lindane | 100–200 | 500–1000 |
| Chlordane | 200–300 | 500–600 |
| Methoxychlor | 5000 | 3000 |

chloride (BHC), was developed and became widely used. Only one isomer, gamma benzene hexachloride, was active, and this was developed into the insecticide lindane. Lindane currently has limited agricultural use, but it is marketed for human use as a scabicide as lindane (Kwell and others) lotion and shampoo. In some European countries, malathion is used instead for scabies.

After 1945, a group of organochlorine insecticides called cyclodienes were developed. These included aldrin, endrin, dieldrin, heptachlor, mirex, chlordecone, endosulfan, and chlordane. Because of environmental persistence and evidence of carcinogenicity of the first six compounds, only endosulfan and chlordane are currently registered and used. Endosulfan is still used in agriculture, while the use of chlordane is restricted to structural termite control. It is available to consumers for this purpose, though recent evidence of evaporation into the inside air of homes may lead to elimination of its use as a termiticide.

## Occupational & Environmental Exposure

There is little information on current occupational exposure to organochlorines. Owing to their persistence and bioaccumulation, environmental exposure to organochlorines will continue for years, even to compounds no longer in use, though there is evidence that levels are decreasing. Most of the world's population has measurable levels of DDT and other organochlorine compounds in fat and blood.

## Pharmacokinetics & Mechanism of Action

The organochlorines are well absorbed by inhalation or ingestion and variably absorbed through the skin. Most are highly fat-soluble and are distributed to adipose tissue, the liver, and the nervous system. Most are metabolized by the liver and excreted in urine as metabolites. For some, this is a slow process, so that accumulation in adipose tissue occurs during chronic exposure. DDT is metabolized and excreted slowly and is found in the fat of most persons; average DDT levels in the fat of Americans has been decreasing since cessation of its use in the United States.

Although the clinical picture of acute intoxication is similar for members of this family of compounds, their precise mechanism of action is unknown, and whether they share a common mechanism is, for that reason, uncertain. These chemicals cause central nervous system excitation and dysfunction with little pathologic change, presumably as a result of changes in the transmission of nerve impulses. They cause hepatocellular necrosis in high doses, hepatocellular hypertrophy, and carcinomas—particularly in mice—at lower doses, and are inducers of hepatic microsomal enzymes.

## Clinical Findings

**A. Symptoms and Signs:** Acute or subacute intoxication from organochlorines produces a picture of generalized nervous system excitability and dysfunction: apprehension, excitability, dizziness, headache, disorientation, confusion, disequilibrium, weakness, paresthesias, muscle twitching, tremor, convulsions, and coma. Nausea and vomiting are common after ingestion, but not after dermal exposure, which is the primary route in the workplace. Most organochlorines are formulated with organic solvents, which may account for central nervous system depression, particularly after ingestion. Fever commonly occurs after seizures, but may be a result of seizure activity rather than an effect of the pesticide. Chlordecone, no longer in use, caused a unique chronic intoxication.

There are a number of case reports and case series suggesting an association between aplastic anemia and exposure to organochlorine insecticides. These reports cannot exclude the possibility of coincidental occurrence of this rare condition with relatively common exposures.

**B. Laboratory Findings:** With the exception of measurement of parent compounds or metabolites in biological samples, laboratory findings are nonspecific. Electroencephalography may show generalized seizure activity. For some compounds, a correlation between biological levels and degree of poisoning is known, but such levels are rarely available in time to assist in management.

## Differential Diagnosis

Severe organochlorine poisoning usually occurs following obvious overexposure and, as a result, does not present a problem in diagnosis. Other causes of central nervous system overactivity or seizures must be considered, particularly drug intoxications. Infections of the nervous system must be considered in the presence of seizures. Pneumonitis may be present as a result of aspiration of organic solvent.

## Treatment

There are no antidotes, so treatment is supportive, directed primarily at maintenance of respiratory function and prompt management of seizures with anticonvulsant medication. Decontamination of the skin, hair, and gut (as appropriate) is important, as in all cases of acute intoxication. Cholestyramine has been shown to accelerate the elimination of chlordecone and recovery from chronic intoxication, but has not been studied for use in management of poisoning with any other organochlorine.

## Prognosis

Uncontrolled seizures may result in anoxic brain or other organ damage. If hypoxia is prevented, recovery should be complete.

# FUMIGANTS & NEMATOCIDES
(Table 32–11)

## Essentials of Diagnosis

*Acute effects:*
- Respiratory tract irritation: burning eyes, nose, throat, cough, shortness of breath, and pulmonary edema.
- Central nervous system depression: headache, nausea, vomiting, dizziness, drowsiness, fatigue, slurred speech, loss of balance, disorientation, loss of consciousness, and respiratory depression.
- Encephalopathy (methyl bromide): tremors, seizures, elevated serum bromide level, late personality changes, and cognitive dysfunction.

*Chronic effects:*
- Liver damage (halogenated hydrocarbons): anorexia, abdominal pain, jaundice, and abnormal liver function tests.

**Table 32–11.** Fumigants and nematocides historically used in the United States.

| Fumigant or Nematocide | Oral LD50 (mg/kg) |
|---|---|
| Halogenated hydrocarbon, Ethylene dibromide | |
| Methyl bromide | 200 ppm vapor inhalation |
| Ethylene dichloride | 700–900 (1000 ppm vapor inhalation) |
| Carbon tetrachloride | 2800 (8000 ppm vapor inhalation) |
| Dibromochloropropane | 150–300 |
| 1,3-Dichloropropene | 250 |
| Chlorpicrin | 250 (150 ppm vapor inhalation) |
| p-Dichlorobenzene | 500 |
| Sulfur and phosphorus compounds, Sulfuryl fluoride | |
| Phosphine (aluminum and zinc phosphide) | |
| Sulfur dioxide | |
| Cyano compounds, Hydrogen cyanide | <0.5 |
| Oxides Ethylene oxide | |
| Propylene oxide | 3000 ppm vapor inhalation |
| Aldehydes, Formaldehyde | 800 |
| Glutaraldehyde | |
| Acrolein | 40–50 |

- Peripheral neuropathy (methyl bromide): progressive distal symmetric sensorimotor neuropathy, ascending paresthesias, numbness, and weakness.

## General Considerations

Most of the fumigants are halogenated hydrocarbons and as such are lipid-soluble anesthetics and often alkylating agents. Most of the nematocides are soil fumigants. Ethylene oxide is a registered pesticide and is used to fumigate spices. However, it is used primarily for the sterilization of medical instruments, a nonagricultural use that is regulated by OSHA (see Chapter 28).

## Use

Fumigants are used to kill insects, insect eggs, and microorganisms. Cultivated crops, herbs and spices, and packaged products such as dried fruits, beans, and medical materials are usually treated in fumigation chambers. Structures such as houses, warehouses, grain elevators, and greenhouses may be sealed, fumigated, and then aerated before being reoccupied. Fumigants are highly penetrating and will pass through most material. Soil is usually treated by application under a tarpaulin that provides a relatively tight seal. The nematocide vapors spread through soil and reach microscopic roundworms in the water that surrounds soil particles.

## Occupational & Environmental Exposure

The fumigants are either gases at ambient temperatures or require heating to generate vapors. Exposure is primarily through inhalation of vapors. Since vapors can penetrate biological tissue and protective clothing and pass through absorbent filters, opportunities for direct exposure must be minimized. Workmen applying fumigants may be exposed when leaks occur in equipment, when buildings are not adequately sealed, and when checking for leaks and entering chambers or buildings before complete aeration without appropriate protective equipment.

Exposure of applicators, field workers, and bystanders to soil fumigant nematocides most commonly occurs when tarpaulins are disturbed, usually by wind. Phosphine is applied in solid formulations of aluminum or zinc phosphide, which liberate phosphine gas when in contact with water in the environment or after ingestion by pests such as rodents.

Zinc phosphide pellets that are ignited and dropped into animal burrows are also available. Poisoning has resulted from accidental ingestion of these preparations and from inhalation of gas following contact of the solid with water while in storage.

The high volatility and rapid environmental degradation of fumigants and nematocides provoked little concern in the past over food residues and water contamination. This changed following the discovery of residues of ethylene dibromide in raw and prepared foods and in water supplies, which led to the phasing out of ethylene dibromide as a pesticide in most countries. The environmental fates of other fumigants and nematocides are of concern as a result, but have been studied to a lesser extent.

## Pharmacokinetics & Mechanism of Action

Most fumigants and nematocides are well absorbed by all routes of exposure and are rapidly excreted without significant bioaccumulation. Inhalation of vapors is the most common route of exposure, though dermal absorption of vapors or liquid can also occur. The vapors and liquids are usually primary irritants, and in some cases are quite potent. Most are general anesthetics (central nervous system depressants), while some, such as methyl bromide, have specific neurotoxic effects. The halogenated hydrocarbon fumigants share most of the effects of the halogenated hydrocarbon solvents, including cardiac sensitization, direct cellular toxicity to the liver and kidneys, and carcinogenicity in laboratory animals. The mechanism of multiple organ toxicity of phosphine and phosphides is unknown. Hydrogen cyanide is a metabolic poison that acts by inactivating cytochrome oxidase.

Most of the halogenated hydrocarbons are carcinogenic in animals. Ethylene dibromide, dibromochloropropane, and methyl bromide are alkylating agents positive in a number of short-term tests of genotoxicity, including mutagenicity. Ethylene dibromide and dibromochloropropane are rodent carcinogens and spermatotoxins and have been banned for most uses for these reasons. Methyl bromide is currently being tested for carcinogenicity. Carbon tetrachloride is an animal carcinogen. Liver cancer has been reported in workers following hepatic necrosis and cirrhosis from acute and chronic exposure.

## Clinical Findings

**A. Symptoms and Signs:** Halogenated hydrocarbon exposure is initially marked by general anesthetic effects: headache, nausea, vomiting, and dizziness, followed by drowsiness, fatigue, slurred speech, loss of balance, disorientation, and, in severe poisoning, loss of consciousness, respiratory depression, and death. Tremors, myoclonus, and generalized seizures may occur, particularly from methyl bromide poisoning. Acute and chronic poisoning from methyl bromide may be followed by prolonged, and in some cases permanent, organic brain damage marked by personality changes and cognitive dysfunction. Workers have been diagnosed as suffering from severe psychologic disorders until a source of methyl bromide exposure was recognized. Direct contact with liquid halogenated hydrocarbons may result in erythema and blisters. Damage to the skin

can be severe if liquid is spilled on clothing and shoes, which retard evaporation.

Chronic exposure to halogenated hydrocarbons may cause liver damage, manifested by anorexia, abdominal pain, nausea, vomiting, jaundice, dark urine, and light stools. Chronic exposure to methyl bromide can result in progressive peripheral neuropathy, with ascending paresthesias, numbness, and weakness, and with or without depressed deep tendon reflexes.

Chloropicrin, formaldehyde, acrolein, and sulfur dioxide are strong mucosal irritants and are water-soluble, affecting exposed surfaces and the upper airway early. Acute exposure causes burning of the eyes, nose, and throat, tearing of the eyes, cough, hoarseness, and sometimes wheezing. Chronic effects other than nosebleeds are unlikely from these potent acute irritants.

The halogenated hydrocarbons and phosphine are less soluble and less potent irritants and are therefore more likely to cause pulmonary edema, which may occur early or late after acute exposure. Many cases of acute phosphine poisoning result in death from pulmonary edema, seizures, and respiratory depression. Nonfatal cases have been marked by liver injury with abdominal pain, nausea, vomiting, jaundice, elevated hepatic enzymes, and coagulopathy with bleeding. The acute and chronic effects of sulfuryl fluoride are uncertain; this compound appears to be an acute irritant and may cause seizures and perhaps liver and kidney damage.

**B. Laboratory Findings:** For the most part, laboratory findings in cases of fumigant poisoning and overexposure are nonspecific and related to the organ affected (eg, abnormal liver function tests). Halogenated hydrocarbons can be measured in blood and exhaled air, but this is rarely helpful except in forensic cases. Methyl bromide is rapidly degraded to inorganic bromide, and measurement of serum bromide may be helpful in diagnosis of methyl bromide toxicity. A level of less than 50 mg/L is usually not associated with symptoms, a level above 50 mg/L is considered indicative of excessive exposure and a need for withdrawal from exposure, and levels above 100 mg/L are usually associated with symptoms and represent a serious threat to health. These levels are based on small numbers of cases in which exposure was both acute and chronic and analysis was performed at variable lengths of time following exposure. They should be used as diagnostic tools for the evaluation of symptomatic individuals and not for routine monitoring of chronic exposure of applicator. They are different from the levels of inorganic bromide associated with poisoning by ingestion of inorganic bromide, a formerly popular sedative, which produces encephalopathy similar to that associated with methyl bromide, but at much higher levels of serum bromide.

## Differential Diagnosis

Anesthesia from halogenated hydrocarbons must be distinguished from exposure to other central nervous system depressants, including drugs and alcohol. The acute irritation produced by chloropicrin, formaldehyde, acrolein, and sulfur dioxide will be marked by the presence of their distinctive odors. Phosphine has a garlic-like odor that can often be detected on a victim's breath. The encephalopathy and peripheral neuropathy from methyl bromide are similar to those from other organic causes of central or peripheral disease, such as alcohol, drugs, and other neurotoxins (see Chapter 24). Toxicity can occur from exposure to levels without a detectable odor, making diagnosis difficult without a history of exposure.

## Treatment

Treatment of all fumigant poisoning except cyanide is symptomatic: respiratory support and anticonvulsants should be provided as indicated. Dimercaprol (BAL) has been used in early methyl bromide poisoning, but without evidence of benefit; given its toxicity, it cannot be recommended. Treatment to increase the excretion of inorganic bromide has no rational basis.

## Prognosis

Toxicity from the irritants chloropicrin, formaldehyde, acrolein, and sulfur dioxide is limited to their acute reversible effects. On the other hand, deaths have been reported from the use of most of the other fumigant and nematocides. Recovery from nonfatal poisoning is usually complete, except for methyl bromide, which has caused permanent organic brain damage and a prolonged, if not permanent, peripheral neuropathy. Acute liver necrosis followed by cirrhosis and liver cancer has been reported from industrial solvent use of carbon tetrachloride, but not from use as an agriculture fumigant

## SUBSTITUTED PHENOLS (Dinitrophenols, Chlorinated Phenols)

## Essentials of Diagnosis

*Acute effects:*
- Uncoupling of oxidative phosphorylation: fever, flushing, sweating, thirst, tachycardia, hypertension, euphoria, anxiety, restlessness, hyperpnea, cyanosis, and seizures.
- Yellow staining of skin, nails, and conjunctiva.

*Chronic effects:*
- Uncoupling of oxidative phosphorylation: weight loss, fatigue, restlessness, anxiety, and thirst.
- Dermatitis.

## General Considerations

The substituted phenols are generally highly toxic compounds used for a variety of agricultural purposes. They act by uncoupling oxidative phosphorylation.

## Use

The dinitrophenols include dinitro-o-cresol (DNOC), dinoseb, dinocap, and binapacryl and are used as insecticides, ovicides, fungicides, and herbicides. The use of dinoseb is being phased out following discovery of its teratogenicity in animals. The chlorinated phenols are represented primarily by pentachlorophenol, which is used principally as a wood preservative and is discussed in Chapter 28.

## Occupational & Environmental Exposure

Pentachlorophenol has been the subject of a relatively large number of occupational and environmental studies. It is known to be present throughout the food chain and can be found in biological samples of most of the population in industrialized societies. In contrast, there is little quantitative information regarding exposure to nitrophenols.

## Pharmacokinetics & Mechanism of Action

The mechanism of action of nitrophenols and chlorinated phenols in human poisoning and in some pests is uncoupling of oxidative phosphorylation, which results in increased oxygen consumption and heat production. The chlorinated phenols are strong irritants, while the nitrophenols are less so. All substituted phenols can directly damage the liver and kidneys by precipitating proteins. There are few chronic toxicity data for most members of these families.

These compounds are well absorbed by all routes of exposure and are primarily excreted in urine unchanged or bound to glucuronide, with a lesser degree of hepatic metabolism. Nitrophenols have been reported to be excreted within 3–4 days, while other substituted phenols may be excreted over longer periods of time due to deposition in fat.

## Clinical Findings

**A. Symptoms and Signs:** Nitrophenols impart a yellow stain to tissues; as a result, yellow skin, nails, and hair are a result of contact and yellow scleras and urine are a sign of systemic absorption. Chlorinated phenols do not produce a stain. Systemic poisoning from any of the substituted phenols consists of a general hypermetabolic state. Profuse sweating, headache, thirst, malaise, and lassitude are common early signs, while fever, flushed skin, apprehension, anxiety, mania, tachycardia, and hypertension occur later, with more serious degrees of intoxication. Altered consciousness, loss of consciousness, seizures, cyanosis, tachypnea, and dyspnea are signs of tissue anoxia, particularly cerebral. Liver and kidney injury are likely to be subclinical. Chronic intoxication is marked by weight loss and low-grade fever.

**B. Laboratory Findings:** The most common findings are nonspecific, due to dehydration and hypermetabolism, such as hemoconcentration and metabolic acidosis. Proteinuria, pyuria, hematuria, glycosuria, and elevated serum urea nitrogen and creatinine reflect renal injury; increased serum AST and bilirubin reflect liver injury. Anemia and leukopenia have been reported after exposure to both chlorinated phenols and nitrophenols and aplastic anemia after chlorinated phenols, though leukocytosis is more commonly seen as a nonspecific response to acute poisoning. Nitrophenols can be measured in blood and urine, but little is known of the relationship of levels to degree of intoxication; more information is available in this regard for pentachlorophenol (see Chapter 28).

### Differential Diagnosis

Other hypermetabolic states to consider include hyperthyroidism, intoxication with stimulant drugs, and aspirin or salicylate poisoning, which also uncouples oxidative phosphorylation.

### Treatment

Specific treatment should be directed at reducing body temperature, restoring fluids and electrolytes, including glucose, and treating seizures or any increase in muscle activity, which contributes to hyperthermia. Reduction of body temperature is similar to the treatment of heat stroke and can often be achieved with sponge baths or a fine spray mist. If this is ineffective, enteric lavage with iced saline solution should be considered. Drugs such as aspirin and other antipyretics and atropine and other anticholinergics should be avoided as they may further increase body temperature with potentially disastrous results. Liberal amounts of glucose should be administered unless marked hyperglycemia is present, since glucose and glycogen stores may be depleted in spite of normal or high blood glucose levels. Hemodialysis and hemoperfusion have not been shown to be of benefit.

### Prognosis

Deaths have occurred from acute intoxication from both nitrophenols and chlorinated phenols. Prolonged seizures and severe renal or liver damage are poor prognostic signs. Following records, reexposure should be avoided until metabolic processes have completely returned to normal and body weight has returned to baseline.

# RODENTICIDES

Rats are the most prevalent pest in many developing countries, and consume up to 20% of stored grain. They represent a significant threat to the food supply in developed countries as well. Other rodents and small mammals such as squirrels, gophers, and rabbits compete for food and act as reservoirs for diseases that affect humans and are considered pests for that reason.

Poisoning with rodenticides is the most widely used method of control of small mammals. To be effective, rodenticides must be attractive to a rat as food, which is difficult since they are fastidious eaters. Rodenticides must also be delayed in action if used as bait, since rats will avoid returning to feed where another rat has died after eating. Unfortunately, what is attractive, edible, and ultimately lethal to a rat is also appealing to pets and other animals and small children. Since application of baits results in negligible exposure to applicators, the primary human health hazard from most rodenticides is childhood poisoning from ingestion, though serious poisoning from single ingestions of warfarin is rare.

Rodenticides in current use are shown in Table 32–12. Yellow phosphorous and Vacor are no longer used because of their extreme human health hazard. Sodium fluoroacetate is similarly hazardous but may have some utility against coyotes and wolves. Strychnine may be useful against rats when anticoagulants are no longer effective, but it is toxic to all warmblooded animals, is not always an effective rodenticide, and its use is controversial. ANTU is rarely used, since rodents quickly develop tolerance to it; it is also a possible bladder carcinogen.

The usefulness of rodenticides is limited primarily by the development of resistance in the target species.

**Table 32–12.** Rodenticides historically used in the United States.

| Rodenticide | Oral LDSO (mg/kg) |
|---|---|
| Alpha-naphthylene thiourea (ANTU) | 6 |
| Coumafuryl | 25 |
| Dicumarol | 550 |
| Diphacinone | 3 |
| Pindone | 280 |
| Strychnine | 1–30 |
| Warfarin | 180 |
| Zinc phosphide | 50 |

Since anticoagulants are usually the only chemical used against rodents, the rest of this discussion will be confined to members of this class.

## Use

The anticoagulants include two classes of closely related compounds: the coumarin, represented by warfarin, and the indandiones, represented by diphacinone. Warfarin is formulated as a dust (10 g of active ingredient per kilogram, or 1%) for use in holes and runs, and as a powder (1 g and 5 g/kg, or 0.1% and 0.5%) for mixing with bait for a final concentration of 50–250 mg/kg (0.000050–0.00025%). Diphacinone is formulated as prepared baits in concentrations of 50–125 mg/kg (0.00005–0.000125%). Both warfarin and diphacinone have been used extensively therapeutically as oral anticoagulant medications.

## Occupational & Environmental Exposure

There are no reports of harmful exposure from the manufacture, formulation, or application of dry anticoagulant rodenticides. There is one report of bleeding in a farmer following extensive and prolonged skin contact with a liquid warfarin solution. Childhood ingestion of these compounds is common, though bleeding as a result is uncommon.

## Pharmacokinetics & Mechanism of Action

Warfarin is well absorbed from the gastrointestinal tract and, to a lesser extent, through the skin. Diphacinone is absorbed following ingestion, but there is no information regarding its dermal absorption. All the anticoagulants act through inhibition of hepatic synthesis of prothrombin (factor II) and factors VII, IX, and X, apparently through formation of an inactive form of vitamin K. In humans and rats, the half-lives of these factors are longer than the half-life of the anticoagulants, so that repeated doses are necessary before significant depression and bleeding occur. The indandiones appear to act in rats faster than the coumarins. Resistance to warfarin in humans and rats appears to be genetic and may be due to rapid metabolism.

The anticoagulants also produce capillary damage through an uncertain mechanism, though this too is reversed by administration of vitamin K. Skin necrosis and dermatitis have been reported as a rare complication of therapeutic use of warfarin, but have not been reported as a result of exposure to rodenticides. The indandiones cause neurologic and cardiovascular toxicity in some animal species, but these effects have not been reported in humans.

## Clinical Findings

**A. Symptoms and Signs:** Most cases of accidental ingestion do not result in evidence of toxicity even without treatment, since doses are usually single and relatively small. Repeated doses could be followed by bleeding, primarily from the mucous membranes such as the gums and nasal passages and into the skin, joints, and gastrointestinal tract. Abdominal, flank, back, and joint pain reflect bleeding into those areas.

**B. Laboratory Findings:** Prolonged prothrombin time may appear 24–48 hours after ingestion of an anticoagulant and is often the only evidence of toxicity following a single exposure. Coagulation time will be increased in cases of significant poisoning, but bleeding time may be normal. Specific factors other than prothrombin may be depressed. Warfarin can be measured in plasma and its metabolites in urine, but these measurements have little utility.

## Differential Diagnosis

Most cases of rodenticide ingestion are observed or reported episodes and do not result in significant toxicity. Failed suicidal or homicidal use may result in otherwise unexplained bleeding and depressed prothrombin time.

## Treatment

Treatment of single acute ingestions is usually unnecessary, but patients should be observed (at home) for 4–5 days following ingestion. Vitamin K (phytonadione, AquaMephyton) may be administered orally in a dosage of 15–25 mg for adults and 5–10 mg for children with a history of ingestion, or intramuscularly in a dosage of 5–10 mg for adults and 1–5 mg (up to 0.6 mg/kg) for children with prolonged prothrombin time or bleeding. Following treatment, prothrombin times should be determined every 6–12 hours and used as the basis for further treatment. If bleeding is severe, slow intravenous infusion may be considered, but carries a risk of adverse reactions including flushing, dizziness, hypotension, dyspnea, cyanosis, and death. Transfusion and iron to replace blood loss should be considered.

## Prognosis

Treatment is usually effective within 3–6 hours. The prognosis is determined by the extent and location of bleeding and is usually good.

# FUNGICIDES
# (Phthalimides, Dithiocarbamates, Benomyl)

Pesticides classified as fungicides are active against fungi and a number of related plant pathogens, including bacteria, viruses, rickettsiae, and others. Most fungicides are distinct from other pesticides, owing to the unique plant characteristics of fungi and the fact that the chemical must kill or inhibit the fungi without adversely affecting the host plant.

About 150 fungicides are available, mostly synthetic organic chemicals of relatively recent development. This discussion will be confined to the most commonly used compounds, the dicarboximides, dithiocarbamates, and benomyl. Others in common use are listed in Table 32–13.

The dicarboximides, or phthalimides, are structurally related to thalidomide but have not been found to share its teratogenicity. Disulfiram (Antabuse), used to treat alcoholism because of its ability to produce an adverse reaction in the presence of alcohol, is a dithiocarbamate and shares a number of properties with these compounds. The dithiocarbamates, which include the ethylenebisdithiocarbamates (EBDCs), are also used as accelerators in the vulcanization of rubber.

These compounds are not acutely toxic: the primary recognized health effect is dermatitis, both irritant and allergic. Animal studies have indicated their potential to cause chronic health effects, though there

**Table 32–13.** Fungicides used in the United States.

| Fungicide | Oral LD50 (mg/kg) |
|---|---|
| **Dicarboximides** | |
| Captan | 9000 |
| Folpet | 10,000 |
| Captafol | 6000 |
| **Dithiocarbamates (ethylenebisdithiocarbamates [EBDCs])** | |
| Ferbam | 1000 |
| Vapam | 1700 |
| Maneb | 7000 |
| Zineb | 5000 |
| Thiram | 800 |
| Ziram | 1500 |
| **Substituted aromatics** | |
| Chlorothalonil | 10,000 |
| Chloroneb | 11,000 |
| Pentachloronitrobenzene (PCNB) | 12,000 |
| Hexachlorobenzene | 10,000 |
| Pentachlorophenot (PCP) | 200 |
| Inorganic Sulfur | None |
| **Copper compounds** | 200–10,000 |
| **Mercury compounds** | 1–200 |

are few studies in humans. The dicarboximides are mutagenic and carcinogenic; the dithiocarbamates are mutagenic, carcinogenic, and teratogenic; and benomyl is teratogenic.

## Use

A broad variety of crops are susceptible to fungi and related diseases. Frequent application of fungicides is often necessary, owing to the rapid replication of many fungi. With the exception of a few systemics, fungicides are only active where they have been left as a residue on a plant, making uniform application necessary. They are applied as sprays or dusts, so that a film of residue is left on the plants. Many seeds are treated with fungicides. A limited number of general purpose lawn and garden fungicides are available for home use.

## Occupational & Environmental Exposure

Field workers and employees in greenhouses and nurseries are more apt to be exposed to fungicides than to other pesticides on a routine basis, since fungicides are only effective as long as a residue is present on plant surfaces and application is often necessary at the same time plants must be handled by these workers. Seed treatment facilities are an important site of exposure to fungicide.

Homeowners are exposed to lawn and garden treatments. Most fruits and vegetables have allowable residues (tolerances) for one or more fungicides.

Water contamination has not been a significant problem to date.

## Pharmacokinetics & Mechanism of Action

Little is known of the pharmacokinetics of the phthalimides in humans; they are rapidly excreted unchanged in urine in animals. They are carcinogenic in animal feeding studies and cause gastrointestinal tumors, but are of uncertain risk via dermal and inhalation exposure. All the dithiocarbamates are metabolized to carbon disulfide (see Chapter 28), which may be the basis for their effects on fungi and the potential for chronic toxicity to humans. The EBDCs are further metabolized to ethylene thiourea, which may account for their antithyroid, mutagenic, carcinogenic, and teratogenic activity. All the dithiocarbamates have the potential to cause a reaction to alcohol (alcohol intolerance) similar to the disulfiram-alcohol reaction, owing to inhibition of alcohol and aldehyde dehydrogenases. Thiram has been shown to potentiate the carcinogenicity of ethylene dibromide as a result of inhibition of alcohol dehydrogenase, which participates in the detoxification of ethylene dibromide. Benomyl is teratogenic in laboratory animals but is believed to be of low human hazard in this regard, owing to limited dermal absorption.

## Clinical Findings

**A. Symptoms and Signs:** The phthalimides, dithiocarbamates, and benomyl all cause allergic contact dermatitis, which is indistinguishable from other contact dermatitises. A few reports indicate that the phthalimides may also cause asthma. An alcohol-dithiocarbamate reaction is marked by headache, nausea, vomiting, flushing, dizziness, confusion, and disorientation.

**B. Laboratory Findings:** Confirmation of a hypersensitivity response to a fungicide is by patch testing for allergic contact dermatitis and inhalation challenge for asthma. Diagnosis of an alcohol dithiocarbamate reaction is based on the history of concurrent exposures.

## Differential Diagnosis

Fungicide-induced allergic contact dermatitis must be distinguished from contact dermatitis due to irritants and allergic contact dermatitis caused by other pesticides or plants. Asthma in a phthalimide manufacturing worker may be due to an intermediate in the manufacturing process.

## Treatment

Allergic contact dermatitis is treated by withdrawal of the offending agent and local steroids. Asthma is treated by removal from exposure and symptomatic treatment as needed.

## Prognosis

Fungicide-related allergies should resolve following cessation of exposure.

# HERBICIDES

## MISCELLANEOUS HERBICIDES OF LOW TOXICITY

Herbicides are pesticides that are intended to prevent or control the growth of unwanted plants or kill them once they have appeared. They have largely replaced mechanical methods of weed control and are currently the largest category of pesticides used in agriculture, accounting for 60% of pesticide sales in the United States and 40% of sales worldwide in 1983. Included here are plant growth regulators that alter plant development, defoliants that cause leaves to drop prematurely, and desiccants that accelerate the drying of plant parts. Nonselective herbicides affect all plants: selective herbicides affect specific target weeds, contact herbicides affect plant parts that touch the chemical, and translocated herbicides are absorbed by the plant and act at distant sites.

The herbicides that have serious recognized or suspected human health effects—the dipyridyls and the chlorophenoxyacetic acids—are considered separately, in following sections. Substituted phenols used as herbicides were discussed above. The organophosphate defoliants are not toxicologically distinct from the organophosphate insecticides. The rest of the organic compounds in this class have few, if any, recognized human health effects. The inorganic herbicides are more hazardous and are being used with decreasing frequency. Some examples of the organic herbicides considered in this class are listed in Table 32–14.

## Use

In addition to agriculture, herbicides are used to clear rights-of-way along roadsides, railroads, power lines, fence lines, and property lines; to reduce competition for seedlings in forests; and for fire prevention

**Table 32–14.** Some herbicides with little or no known acute toxicity to humans.

| Herbicide | Oral LD50 (mg/kg) |
| --- | --- |
| Alachlor | 1000 |
| Amitrole | 1000 |
| Ammonium sulfamate | 4000 |
| Atrazine | 3000 |
| B41enox | 6500 |
| Dalapon | 6500 |
| Dicamba | 1000 |
| Ethafuralin | 10,000 |
| Glyphosphate | 4300 |
| Linuron | 1500 |
| Monuron | 3500 |
| Oryzalin | 10,000 |
| Oturon | 3500 |
| Oxadiazon | 3500 |
| Pictoram | 8000 |
| Prometon | 3000 |
| Pronamide | 5500 |
| Propham | 9000 |
| Propanil | 1500 |
| Simazine | 5000 |
| Terbutryn | 2000 |
| Trifluralin | 3500 |

by reducing the amounts of combustible grasses and brush available as fuel. They are usually sprayed in bands or strips, broadcast over an entire area, or focused on one area or group of weeds (spot or directed treatment). The timing of application may he preplanting (before planting crop), pre-emergence (after planting but before emergence of weeds or crop), and postemergence (after weeds or crops emerge).

## Occupational & Environmental Exposure

Occupational exposure to herbicides occurs as a result of dermal exposure to spray applicators and flaggers, while environmental exposure occurs in the form of residues on crops and food. Although a few studies have suggested the possibility of health effects occurring in populations as a result of spray drift or other environmental contamination from herbicides, with the exception of cases of obvious spray drift with damage to nontarget plants, such exposure is difficult to document.

## Pharmacokinetics & Mechanism of Action

These compounds show little evidence of toxicity to mammals; consequently, there is little information on pharmacokinetics or mechanisms of action in humans. A few of the pesticides shown in Table 32–3 as having some evidence of carcinogenicity in animals are herbicides (most notably alachlor, which is used on grain crops and is one of the most heavily applied pesticides in the United States) may be suspended or canceled as a result.

## Clinical Findings

**A. Symptoms and Signs:** Some formulations of herbicides contain organic solvents, surfactants, emulsifiers, or other vehicles and additives that may cause eye, nose, or throat irritation in applicators exposed to spray mists and dermatitis in mixers and loaders as a result of prolonged skin contact. Otherwise, these compounds have no known human health effects.

**B. Laboratory Findings:** There is little or no information regarding measurement of parent compounds or metabolites in biological media.

## Differential Diagnosis

It is always possible that these compounds have effects not yet appreciated in humans, particularly from accidental or deliberate ingestion. The toxicity of "inert" ingredients should be considered in evaluating persons with symptoms following exposure.

## Treatment

Since these compounds have little or no known human health effects, treatment of any symptoms resulting from their use should be symptomatic only. For evaluation of symptomatic patients, the manufac-

turer should be consulted, particularly for identification of the inert ingredients.

## Prognosis

Acute irritation and dermatitis from herbicide formulations should resolve shortly after cessation of exposure.

## CHLOROPHENOXYACETIC ACIDS

## Essentials of Diagnosis

*Acute effects:*
- Irritation: redness of skin, burning, soreness in throat and chest, and cough.
- Peripheral neuropathy (2,4-D): acute nausea, vomiting, diarrhea, abdominal pain, followed in 7–10 days by rapidly ascending numbness, paresthesias, and weakness, with normal to slightly decreased nerve conduction velocities.

*Chronic effects:*
- None known.

## General Considerations

The principal herbicidal derivatives of phenoxy acetic acid include 2,4-dichlorophenoxvacetic acid (2,4-D), 2,4,5-trichlorophenoxyacetic acid (2,4,5-T), 2-methyl-4-chlorophenoxvacetic acid (MCPA), and their salts and ester derivatives. Silvex, kuron, and fenac are homologues of 2,4,5-T, while 2,4-DB and MCPB, MCPCA, and MCPP are homologues of 2,4-D and MCPA, respectively. They are translocated herbicides relatively selective for broad-leaf plants. 2,4,5-T and its homologues are no longer manufactured or used in the United States because of their combination contamination with 2,3,7,8-tetrachlorodibenzo-p- dioxin (TCDD) and the controversy over its alleged health effects in environmentally exposed populations and Vietnam veterans. While certain batches of 2,4-D have been found to be contaminated with low levels of other lesser chlorinated dioxins such as dichlorodibenzo-p-dioxin, none of its contaminants have been found to be of toxicologic importance. The toxicity of dioxins is discussed in Chapters 28 and 39.

## Use

The chlorophenoxy herbicides have had a wide variety of uses, including control of undesirable perennial hardwood trees and plants for "release" of desirable evergreen softwood trees.

## Occupational & Environmental Exposure

Occupational exposure occurs primarily as direct contact with liquid concentrate during mixing and loading and inhalation and contact with spray mist during application. Although concern has been expressed about environmental exposure of populations living near conifer forests where chlorophenoxy herbicides are applied, in the absence of obvious spray drift with nontarget crop damage, such exposure is difficult to document. 2,4-D is rapidly degraded in the environment, and water contamination has not been a major problem.

## Pharmacokinetics & Mechanism of Action

The herbicidal mechanism of action of chlorophenoxyacetic acids is uncertain but appears to involve a mimicking of plant auxins (growth hormones) and effects on plant metabolism. They are absorbed by inhalation, dermal contact, and ingestion and are excreted rapidly unchanged in urine. The mechanisms of any health effects on humans other than irritation are uncertain. They are weak uncouplers of oxidative phosphorylation and may produce hyperthermia at extremely high doses as a result of increased heat production. A study reported to the EPA indicated that 2,4-D caused an increase in brain tumors in rats given 40 mg/kg/d by mouth. A study of cancer deaths in farmers in Kansas was reported in 1986 to show an association between lymphoma and the use of 2,4-D. 2,4-D is weakly teratogenic in mice.

## Clinical Findings

**A. Symptoms and Signs:** Some formulations produce skin irritation following contact with liquid; irritation of the eyes, nose, throat, and respiratory tract, with burning and cough from exposure to spray mist; and irritation of the gastrointestinal tract, with abdominal pain, nausea, and vomiting following ingestion. Ingestion of chlorophenoxyacetic acid herbicides has resulted in nausea, vomiting, abdominal pain, and diarrhea followed by muscle twitching, myotonia, metabolic acidosis, and a hypermetabolic state with fever, tachycardia, hypertension, sweating, convulsions, and coma.

Approximately six cases of peripheral neuropathy have been reported following relatively large dermal exposures to 2,4-D over the course of a few days. Clinically, these resembled idiopathic acute symmetric polyneuropathy (Guillain-Barré syndrome) and organophosphate-induced delayed neuropathy in their symptoms of an initial influenza-like illness associated with nausea, vomiting, diarrhea, and myalgias, followed by an asymptomatic interval and then, 7–10 days later, by rapidly ascending loss of both motor and sensory nerve function. Respiratory function was spared in most cases.

Chloracne has been reported as a result of exposure to TCDD in 2,4,5-T manufacturing plant workers. A number of epidemiologic studies have suggested an association between exposure to chlorophenoxyacetic acid herbicides and soft tissue sarcomas. A registry of cases of such tumors has been established by NIOSH.

**B. Laboratory Findings:** Exposure to a chlorophenoxyacetic compound can be confirmed through analysis of blood or urine by gas-liquid chromatography. Urine samples should be collected as soon as possible after exposure because the chemical may be excreted completely within 24–72 hours. There is insufficient information to relate a spot urine level precisely to a level of exposure. However, since these compounds are excreted almost entirely unchanged in urine, a dose can be measured by collecting and analyzing all urine, provided collection is begun promptly after exposure. Other laboratory findings in cases of acute intoxication are entirely nonspecific. In the few cases of peripheral neuropathy associated with exposure to 2,4-D where testing was done, nerve conduction velocities have been normal or slightly depressed, and spinal fluid analyses have been unremarkable.

## Differential Diagnosis

Acute irritation following direct exposure or acute intoxication following ingestion present with obvious diagnoses. The differential diagnosis for a patient with peripheral neuropathy following exposure to 2,4-D includes idiopathic acute symmetric polyneuropathy and exposure to other neurotoxic compounds, including organophosphates.

## Treatment

Treatment of acute irritation and peripheral neuropathy are entirely symptomatic. Since chlorophenoxyacetic compounds are weak organic acids, they are preferentially excreted in alkaline urine. In severe poisoning from ingestion of large doses, alkalinization of the urine can hasten elimination of the chemical and may improve the course of intoxication. Administration of large fluid volumes to achieve "forced" diuresis should be avoided, owing to the risk of precipitating pulmonary edema.

## Prognosis

Although death from ingestion of a chlorophenoxyacetic acid has been reported, severe intoxications have apparently been infrequent, and most victims have survived. In cases of peripheral neuropathy following exposure to 2,4-D, maximum paralysis lasted approximately one week or less. Recovery of function was usually prolonged for up to one year following exposure, with some residual weakness in most cases.

## DIPYRIDYLS (Paraquat & Diquat)

### Essentials of Diagnosis

*Acute effects:*
- Contact with skin, eyes, and respiratory tract: irritation and fissuring of skin of hands, cracking and

discoloration of fingernails, conjunctivitis, sore throat, and coughing.

- Ingestion of paraquat: early (1–4 days), oral and abdominal pain, nausea, vomiting, and diarrhea; later (24–72 hours), liver injury, jaundice, elevated hepatocellular enzymes, and renal injury (proteinuria, hematuria, pyuria, elevated serum urea nitrogen and creatinine); late (3–4 days), pulmonary fibrosis (cough, dyspnea, tachypnea, cyanosis, and respiratory failure).
- Ingestion of diquat: same as paraquat without late pulmonary fibrosis.

### General Considerations

Paraquat is used extensively in the United States and worldwide, diquat to a lesser extent. They are nonselective contact herbicides.

### Use

The dipyridyls are used extensively as general purpose herbicides, owing to their ability to kill most plants on contact. They are also used as defoliants and desiccants, since the foliage of plants becomes dry and frostbitten in appearance, resulting in the premature dropping of leaves. Paraquat is used on cotton, potatoes, and soybeans, while diquat is used on alfalfa, clover, and soybeans.

### Occupational & Environmental Exposures

The most important occupational exposures occur by direct contact of the skin with liquid concentrate during mixing and loading and inhalation and skin contact with spray mist during application. A case of acute paraquat intoxication was reported in a flagger who endured extensive dermal exposure to spray mist. Environmental exposure through field residues, food residues, and water contamination has not been a concern. The program of the United States Drug Enforcement Agency to spray marijuana fields with paraquat generated controversy over the possibility of inhalation of paraquat by marijuana smokers. Most of the paraquat probably undergoes thermal decomposition before it is inhaled, but the possibility of adverse effects from paraquat or its decomposition products has not been ruled out.

### Pharmacokinetics & Mechanism of Action

The dipyridyls affect both plants and mammals by damaging tissue through the generation of free oxygen radicals. Their effect on plants requires the presence of sunlight. They are absorbed by inhalation, dermal contact, or ingestion. They damage epithelial tissues such as skin, nails, cornea, gastrointestinal tract, and respiratory tract, and also the liver and kidneys.

Paraquat is more toxic to humans than diquat. A small sip of the liquid concentrate can kill an adult, which accounts for the hundreds of deaths reported worldwide from accidental and deliberate ingestion of this herbicide. An experimental trial that consisted of adding an emetic to formulations of paraquat was recently instituted in an attempt to reduce the frequency of fatal ingestions.

A relatively small number of cases of serious poisoning from paraquat have been reported as a result of large dermal exposures, while none have been reported from inhalation exposure in the absence of significant skin contact. Pulmonary injury from chronic dermal or inhalation exposure has not been reliably reported or found in the few epidemiologic studies performed with applicators. Neither paraquat nor diquat has been adequately tested for carcinogenicity.

### Clinical Findings

**A. Symptoms and Signs:** Direct contact with concentrated liquid dipyridyls results in skin irritation and fissuring and in cracking, discoloration, and sometimes loss of the fingernails. Liquid splashed in the eye can cause conjunctivitis and opacification of the cornea. Inhalation of spray mist can irritate the nose and throat, causing nosebleeds and sore throat.

Ingestion of either paraquat or diquat can result in an early phase (1–4 days) of inflammation of the mouth and gastrointestinal tract, with soreness, ulceration, burning pain, nausea, vomiting, diarrhea, and sometimes hematemesis and melena. These symptoms can range from mild to severe, and their intensity may not predict the severity of the following phases. The second phase begins 24–72 hours after exposure and is marked by evidence of hepatic and renal injury. Hepatocellular injury is indicated by abdominal pain, nausea, and jaundice. Renal injury is usually asymptomatic unless oliguria or anuria develops. Renal and hepatic injury from ingestion of paraquat is common and frequently severe, while that from ingestion of diquat is less common and often milder.

A late phase (> 72–96 hours) of pulmonary fibrosis occurs from paraquat, but not diquat, presumably because paraquat, but not diquat, becomes concentrated in pulmonary epithelial tissue. Pulmonary edema has occasionally occurred following ingestion of either paraquat or diquat. In cases of paraquat poisoning, pulmonary fibrosis is marked by cough, shortness of breath, and tachypnea. Advanced fibrosis is indicated by progressive cyanosis.

**B. Laboratory Findings:** In the early phase of acute poisoning, the findings are nonspecific and are usually related to dehydration from nausea and diarrhea. In the later phase, liver injury is indicated by elevated bilirubin and hepatocellular enzymes. Renal injury, primarily tubular, is indicated by proteinuria, hematuria, pyuria, and elevated serum urea nitrogen and creatinine. Oliguric renal failure typical of acute tubular necrosis may occur. Laboratory evidence of pulmonary fibrosis from paraquat in the form of a progressive decline in arterial oxygen tension and diffusion capacity for carbon monoxide commonly precedes the appearance of pulmonary symptoms. Later, pulmonary function findings are typical of restrictive lung disease.

The diagnosis of acute intoxication from paraquat or diquat can be confirmed by analysis of either compound in blood and urine. Analyses and consultation are available from the Chevron Emergency Information Center (Environmental Health Center, Box 4054, Richmond, CA 94804; 24-hour telephone [415] 233-3737).

### Differential Diagnosis

The early phase of acute intoxication from a dipyridyl may be mild, and in the absence of a history of ingestion may be mistaken for gastroenteritis or ingestion of another irritant chemical. The combination of renal and hepatic injury could occur following exposure to a chlorinated hydrocarbon solvent such as carbon tetrachloride. In the absence of a history of paraquat exposure, the differential diagnosis of the pulmonary injury is the same as for acute pulmonary fibrosis (see Chapter 20).

### Treatment

The primary treatment during any phase of intoxication from paraquat or diquat is supportive, particularly during periods of organ failure. Bentonite and fuller's earth have been found to be more effective absorbents for dipyridyls in the gastrointestinal tract than activated charcoal. If available, they should be administered as a 7 g/dL suspension in normal saline in quantities of at least two liters to any patient suspected of ingesting any quantity of a dipyridyl within the preceding several days. If neither bentonite nor fuller's earth is available, a similar quantity of the usual concentration of activated charcoal should be administered.

Saline catharsis is then recommended, using sodium sulfate rather than magnesium salts because of the risk of magnesium retention in the presence of impaired renal function. This cycle may be repeated for several days. Given the high fatality rate following paraquat ingestion, this extreme degree of gut cleansing is probably worth the risk of fluid and electrolyte imbalance, which must be monitored closely.

The issue of enhanced excretion of dipyridyl is controversial. There is no basis for the recommendation that glucose and electrolyte infusions be given in large quantities to minimize toxicant concentrations in tissues and force diuresis of the compounds. Hemodialysis is clearly ineffective for removal of paraquat. Hemoperfusion with coated charcoal may be effective in removing paraquat from the blood if it is performed before the chemical has been distributed to tissues. However, few patients have a confirmed diagnosis and can be placed in a facility where the

procedure can be performed early (24–48 hours after ingestion). The decision to perform hemoperfusion should be made by a physician with experience in the technique and familiarity with the issues and risks involved.

A number of therapies are available to attempt to retard pulmonary fibrosis from paraquat. Increased levels of alveolar oxygen increase the rate of production of free oxygen radicals and accelerate the process of pulmonary fibrosis. Animal studies have shown increased survival in low oxygen atmospheres, but there are no comparable human studies. Early placement of a patient in an atmosphere of 15% oxygen has been recommended. Supplemental oxygen should be administered only as necessary to maintain minimally acceptable levels of oxygenation. Early experimental results with the free radical scavenger superoxide dismutase have been disappointing. Corticosteroids and cytotoxic agents such as azathioprine have been tried with uncertain results.

### Prognosis

Once pulmonary fibrosis occurs as a result of paraquat ingestion, death from respiratory failure can be expected. Survival with disability from restrictive lung disease may also occur. Occasionally, recovery of lung function may take place over a course of weeks to months. Although death from liver and kidney necrosis may occur following diquat ingestion, recovery is more common than that following paraquat ingestion.

---

# MISCELLANEOUS PESTICIDES

---

### PYRETHRUM & SYNTHETIC PYRETHRIN (Pyrethroid) INSECTICIDES

#### Essentials of Diagnosis

*Acute effects:*
- None known.

*Chronic effects:*
- Allergic contact dermatitis: erythema, vesicles, papules, and itching.
- Allergic rhinitis: nasal congestion and sore throat.
- Asthma: wheezing, cough, chest lightness, and dyspnea.

#### General Considerations

Pyrethrum is a partially refined extract of the chrysanthemum flower and has been used as an insecticide for more than 60 years. There are six known insecticidally active compounds in pyrethrums, two of which are esters known as pyrethrins. Synthetic pyrethrins (pyrethroids) are based structurally on the pyrethrin molecule, but are modified to improve stability.

Chrysanthemum and pyrethrum have long been recognized to be human allergens without other recognized adverse effects in humans. The pyrethroids have not been recognized as having significant human health effects, though a few, such as permethrin and resmethrin, may cause cancer in animals.

## Use

There are several hundred commercial products containing pyrethrum and pyrethroids, usually in combination with a synergist (see below) and often with an additional insecticide, such as a carbamate or organophosphate. Many are available for home use against flies, mosquitoes, and fleas. The usual household formulation contains about 0.5% active ingredient. The greater stability of the synthetic pyrethrins has made them useful in agricultural applications.

## Occupational & Environmental Exposures

Their low toxicity has resulted in little interest in quantifying exposure levels. The application of indoor "bug-bomb" propellants in homes has resulted in some concern about hazards to small children from residues on interior surfaces, particularly with respect to the organophosphates and carbamates.

## Pharmacokinetics & Mechanism of Action

The pyrethrins are apparently poorly absorbed from the gastrointestinal tract and through the skin, hydrolyzed in the gut and tissues, and rapidly excreted. The nervous system toxicity responsible for their efficacy as insecticides is not manifested in mammals. Pyrethrins are active inducers of liver microsomal enzymes, an effect that has not been studied in humans. The allergenicity of pyrethrum to humans has not been replicated in experimental animals.

## Clinical Findings

**A. Symptoms and Signs:** The most common effect of pyrethrum exposure is allergic contact dermatitis, which is manifested by itching and an erythematous vesicular rash. Bullae, edema, and photosensitivity may also occur. Allergic rhinitis is not uncommon, with nasal congestion, sneezing, and sore throat. Asthma and hypersensitivity pneumonitis have been reported but are uncommon. Dyspnea, cough, and wheezing indicate asthma, though these manifestations plus fever, malaise, and pulmonary infiltrates are indicative of hypersensitivity pneumonitis. Anaphylaxis with bronchospasm, laryngeal

edema, and shock have been reported occasionally after inhalation of pyrethrum. These allergic manifestations have not been reported from exposure to synthetic pyrethrins.

**B. Laboratory Findings:** Skin testing can aid in the diagnosis of sensitivity to pyrethrum. There are no biological monitoring methods for exposure to pyrethrum or pyrethroids.

## Differential Diagnosis

Allergy to other pesticides, plants or flowers, insect stings, and household products must be considered in the evaluation of one of the allergic manifestations of pyrethrum.

## Treatment

The key to treatment of any allergy is removal from exposure to the allergen. Allergic contact dermatitis may be treated with application of topical steroid preparations. Allergic rhinitis may be treated with antihistamines, decongestants, and a steroid nasal spray, if needed. Asthma is treated with bronchodilators and steroids as appropriate. Anaphylaxis may require epinephrine, aminophylline, or a parenteral corticosteroid.

## Prognosis

If the diagnosis is correct, treatment prompt, and removal from exposure effective, recovery should be rapid and complete.

## SYNERGISTS (Piperonyl Butoxide)

Although there are a few other examples, by far the most common synergistic insecticide combination is that of piperonyl butoxide with pyrethrins.

## Use

Piperonyl butoxide is used as an insecticide synergist with pyrethrins in ratios of 5:1 or 20:1 in a variety of formulations, many of which are available for home use. They are used primarily for flies, mosquitoes, and fleas, often in combination with a carbamate or organophosphate.

## Occupational & Environmental Exposure

There is no information specifically on exposure to synergists.

## Pharmacokinetics & Mechanism of Action

Piperonyl butoxide is poorly absorbed from the gastrointestinal tract and probably poorly absorbed dermally. It is metabolized but also retained unchanged to an uncertain degree in rodents. Its mechanism of action is inhibition of hepatic mixed function oxidase enzymes.

### Clinical Findings

**A. Symptoms and Signs:** There are no reports of clinical illness occurring as a result of exposure to piperonyl butoxide.

**B. Laboratory Findings:** There is no evidence of enzyme inhibition from piperonyl butoxide in humans. A single oral dose of 50 mg did not change the metabolism of antipyrine in eight volunteers.

### Differential Diagnosis

Any illness occurring in an individual exposed to a formulation containing piperonyl butoxide is probably due to another ingredient, such as allergy to pyrethrum, an effect of a carbamate or organophosphate, or something other than the pesticide.

### Treatment

Treatment, if required, would be symptomatic.

### Prognosis

The outcome depends on the actual diagnosis.

## INORGANIC & ORGANOMETALLIC COMPOUNDS

Included in this group are sulfur, arsenicals, mercurials, cadmium compounds, lead compounds, antimony, and thallium. All of these compounds have been used as insecticides, herbicides, and fungicides. Many, such as the inorganic lead and arsenic compounds and all forms of mercury and cadmium, are of limited use or have been banned because of human and environmental toxicity. Some of these compounds have been discussed elsewhere (see Chapter 27). They will be reviewed only briefly here.

Inorganic sulfur is used in large amounts as a fungicide and acaricide in the form of dusts, wettable powders, and pastes. It has no known systemic toxicity but is a common cause of irritant dermatitis in field workers exposed to residues on foliage. Propargite (Omite) is an organophosphate compound used as a miticide that in some formulations also causes irritant dermatitis. The dermatitis from both sulfur and propargite can be severe and may result in significant lost time from work.

Inorganic arsenicals are no longer used as general insecticides and herbicides. Historically, the use of these compounds in agriculture was associated with skin lesions, skin cancer, and polyneuropathy. Liver toxicity, including hepatitis, cirrhosis, and angiosarcoma in vineyard workers may have been due to ingestion of arsenic-contaminated wine. Remaining uses of inorganic arsenic are the wood preservatives chromate copper arsenate and acetocopper arsenite

(Paris green) and a number of arsenate salts used as ant killers (eg, Antrol). The EPA is considering restrictions for arsenical wood preservatives because of concern over the carcinogenic risk to end-users such as carpenters, who are exposed to arsenic-containing dust. Childhood ingestion of arsenical ant poisons has required treatment with chelating agents such as dimercaprol and penicillamine, but have been reduced in frequency following repackaging into child-resistant containers. Home use of arsenical and chlorinated phenol (pentachlorophenol) wood preservatives has been superseded to some extent by the use of copper-containing preservatives such as copper naphthenate and copper quinolate. Although copper itself has little toxicity unless ingested, these compounds have not been subjected to long-term toxicity testing.

Organotin compounds, particularly tributyltin, are fungicidal and are commonly used in marine antifouling bottom paints. Tributyltin does not show the neurotoxicity displayed by triethyltin, but it is toxic to some marine life and its use may be restricted on this basis. Triphenyltin is used as an agricultural fungicide. It caused marked testicular atrophy in rats fed 20 mg/kg/d for 20 days, and, as a result, its use has been restricted in some locations. There are no reports of systemic toxicity in humans from the pesticidal use of any organotin compounds.

Organomercury compounds were used extensively in the past in the treatment of seeds and as fungicides. These uses were severely curtailed following the disaster of Minimata Bay, Japan, involving alkylmercury compounds. Cadmium once had uses similar to those associated with mercury, but it has largely been replaced by safer fungicides.

## DISINFECTANTS & ALGICIDES

If one includes the use of chlorine and chlorine compounds for water treatment, these are the most heavily used pesticides worldwide. They include the halogens (chlorine, hypochlorites, chloramine, and iodine), the phenols, the aldehydes (formaldehyde and glutaraldehyde), and the detergents.

The use of chlorine in water treatment is generally not a toxic concern, except for accidental releases. The use of hypochlorite in swimming pools has been associated with thinning of dental enamel in people who swim regularly when the acidity produced from the generation of chlorine and hydrochloric acid was not buffered properly. The substitution of chloramine for chlorine has raised concern for dialysis patients and aquarium fish.

The hazards of phenol were discussed in Chapter 29 and those of formaldehyde in Chapter 28. Glutaraldehyde is chemically similar to formaldehyde but has not been tested for carcinogenicity. It is commonly used in hospitals as a disinfectant (Cidex) and causes eye, nose, and throat irritation when an aerosol is created. It has not been reported to cause asthma.

## REPELLENTS

The best known repellents are insect repellents for human application. The most common is deet (diethyl toluamide), used primarily to repel mosquitoes. Its use has generally been without incident, with the exception of a single reported case of an acute neurologic reaction in a young child who underwent heavy aerosol exposure. Some concern has been expressed, however, regarding the heavy use of deet by personnel working outdoors in mosquito-infested areas.

## GROWTH REGULATORS & BIORATIONAL PESTICIDES

Growth regulators are substances that alter the behavior of the target organism, most often a plant, through a physiologic effect, to hasten or retard growth or other biological processes. They are generally without known or suspected adverse human health effects, but the discovery that the breakdown product of the plant growth regulator daminozide (Alar), or unsymmetrical dimethyl hydrazine (UDMH), causes cancer in animals has generated considerable controversy. Daminozide restricts growth of apples so that they remain on the trees longer and become firmer, making them resistant to insects. UDMH is concentrated in processed or cooked apple products, further increasing any cancer risk from daminozide residues. Daminozide was used to a lesser extent on other crops, including fruit, peanut vines, and flower-producing varied growth responses. The manufacturer of daminozide may voluntarily suspend sales in the United States until the risk from residues in apples is resolved.

There are six classes of plant growth regulators. The auxins are plant growth hormones that include indoleacetic acid and the phenoxy acetic acids: the latter is discussed above in the section on herbicides. The giberellins are represented primarily by giberellic acid, which has a variety of beneficial effects on fruit and no known adverse effects on humans. The cytokinins are naturally occurring compounds such as adenine, which are unlikely to affect humans in the amounts used as pesticides. Ethylene generators, including ethylene itself and ethephon, initiate degreening and ripening of many fruits without affecting humans. Inhibitors range from simple organic acids of low toxicity, such as benzoic, gallic, and cinnamic acid, to maleic hydrazide, for which preliminary evidence of carcinogenicity in animals has been reported. Finally, growth retardants include newly developed substances, such as chlorflurenol, that are generally without known human health effects.

A number of insect growth regulator chemical substances that disrupt the action of insect hormones, controlling molting and other stages of development, have been recently developed. Many of these are biorational pesticides, either naturally occurring organisms (such as *Bacillus thuringiensis*), or chemical analogues of naturally occurring biochemical substances (such as the sex attractant pheromones). To date, this class has not produced any evidence causing concern for human health.

## REFERENCES

Ballantyne B, Marrs TC: *Clinical and Experimental Toxicology of Organophosphates and Carbamates.* Butterworth Heinemann, 1992.

Committee on Scientific and Regulatory Issues Underlying Pesticide Use Patterns and Agricultural Innovation, Board of Agriculture, National Research Council: *Regulating Pesticides in Food: The Delaney Paradox.* National Press, 1987.

Coye MJ, Lowe JA: Biological monitoring of agricultural workers exposed to pesticides. I. Cholinesterase activity determinations. II. Monitoring of intact pesticides and their metabolites. J Occup Med 1986;28:619,628.

Farm Chemicals Handbook. Meister Publishing, Published annually.

Hayes, WJ Jr: *Pesticides Studied in Man.* Williams & Wilkins, 1982.

Hayes WJ Jr, Laws ER: *Handbook of Pesticide Toxicology.* Academic Press, 1991.

McConnell R: Pesticides and related compounds. In: Rom WN (editor): *Environmental and Occupational Medicine,* 2nd ed. Little, Brown, 1983.

Morgan DP: *Recognition and Management of Pesticide Poisonings,* 4th ed. US Government Printing Office, 1989.

Moses M: Pesticides. In: Rom WN (editor): *Environmental and Occupational Medicine.* Little, Brown, 1983.

NIOSH: *Criteria for a Recommendrd Standard for Occupational Exposure During the Manufacture and Formulation of Pesticides.* US Government Printing Office, 1978.

# Gases & Other Inhalants

# 33

*Ware G. Kuschner, MD, & Paul D. Blanc, MD, MSPH*

## Definition of Terms

The subject of gases, strictly defined, would include only those substances that are in a gaseous state at normal atmospheric pressure and temperature. In practice, however, the term "gas" is often used generically to subsume a variety of inhalants that are not, in fact, gases. Related terms for inhalants such as fume, mist, aerosol, and vapor each have precise technical meanings, as shown in Table 33–1. This chapter focuses on gaseous inhalants, particularly asphyxiants and respiratory irritants. However, in this context it is also useful to consider certain other exposures that occur in the form of aerosols (eg, acid aerosols), vapors (eg, irritant aldehydes), or complex and heterogeneous mixtures (eg, combustion smoke). The gases and other inhalants that are covered in this chapter fall into three distinct classes: asphyxiants, respiratory irritants, and nonasphyxiant toxicants.

## Route of Exposure & Target Organ Toxicity

By definition, the inhalants discussed here enter the body predominantly, if not exclusively, by route of inhalation. It is, however, important to note that many of these same toxicants may also be encountered in other forms or as the active component or metabolite of nonvolatile materials. For example, cyanide gas, which will be addressed as an archetypical toxic asphyxiant, is frequently encountered when it is generated from cyanide salt solutions that have been inadvertently or inappropriately acidified. Importantly, even at a pH that does not generate significant cyanide gas, cyanide salt solutions are efficiently absorbed through the skin and result in the same toxicity as that caused by cyanide gas. Similarly, ingestion of cyanide salts may result in the same toxic sequelae. Another relevant example is methylene chloride, which can lead to carbon monoxide intoxication after inhalation, ingestion, or skin absorption.

Conversely, there are numerous nongaseous toxicants for which inhalation is an important route of exposure but which are beyond the purview of this chapter. Examples of such inhalants include metal fumes and vapors, solvent vapors, and organic and inorganic dusts.

In toxicology, the concept of **target organ effects** provides a basis for linking mechanisms of action with the pathophysiologic consequences of exposure. While toxicants may have a variety of potential effects, they frequently exert their principal effects on target organs such as the central nervous system, respiratory tract, liver, or kidneys. The toxicology of inhalants can become confusing because it is natural to assume that the lung would be the primary target organ for inhaled toxicants. In fact, as will become clear in this chapter, this is not the case for a number of nonirritant inhalants, particularly the asphyxiants, for which the central nervous system is the primary target organ. In contradistinction to the asphyxiants, the respiratory tract is indeed the principal target organ following irritant gas inhalation.

## Dose Response & Time Course of Effect

Much of occupational and environmental toxicology is concerned with chronic low-level to moderate-level exposures leading to long-term adverse health effects. In contrast, the primary exposure response relationships relevant to gas inhalation are typically short-term, very high-level exposures where initial toxicity is manifest in minutes or hours. These exposures are at an intensity that is at the far end of the dose response curve where most, if not all, exposed individuals will manifest some adverse effect. Under these exposure conditions, issues of susceptible subpopulations are usually not pivotal, although they may impact disease severity. Ambient environmental air pollution is a notable exception in regard to exposure levels and chronicity. The health effects of air pollution are addressed separately (see Chapter 41).

Although toxic inhalants typically exert adverse effects acutely, long-term sequelae of acute exposure can and do occur. Some of these are nonspecific (anoxic brain injury), sporadic (irritant-induced

**Table 33–1.** Definition of terms.

| | |
|---|---|
| **Aerosol** | A dispersion of solid or liquid particles in a gaseous medium, most commonly air. |
| **Gas** | A "fluid" at room temperature and pressure that occupies the space of enclosure; capable of being changed into the solid or liquid phase by both an increase in pressure and a decrease in temperature. |
| **Vapor** | The gaseous phase of a substance normally in the solid or liquid state; capable of being changed to a liquid or solid either by increasing pressure or decreasing temperature. |
| **Mist** | An aerosol of liquid particles, which may be visible, generated by condensation from the gaseous to liquid state or by mechanical dispersion of a liquid. |
| **Fume** | An aerosol of solid particles generated by the condensation of vaporized materials, especially molten metals, often accompanied by oxidation. |
| **Dust** | Solid particles generated by disintegration of organic or inorganic materials such as rocks and minerals, wood and grain; capable of temporary suspension in a gaseous medium such as air. |
| **Smoke** | Aerosols of solids resulting from incomplete combustion. |

asthma), or rare (obliterative bronchiolitis following nitrogen dioxide inhalation). These potential sequelae will be highlighted where relevant in the context of specific exposures.

## Historical Considerations

The hazards of ingested toxicants have been appreciated since antiquity. This is not the case with toxic gases. It was not until 18th century chemistry began to unravel the elemental components of the atmosphere that a parallel perception evolved of "poisons that kill from a distance." These were first recognized (albeit poorly understood) in three circumstances: naturally occurring events (such as geothermal emissions), from the combustion or decomposition of organic matter, and in mining operations, especially underground coal pits.

The naturally occurring toxic gases that were recognized earliest were all asphyxiants. They were first given descriptive names based on the sources from which the toxicants arose. Only later were their chemical structures determined. Sewer gas remains a generic descriptor of hydrogen sulfide, while marsh gas is synonymous with methane. The latter was known as "fire damp" in collieries, while "choke damp" referred to accumulated carbon dioxide in coal mines.

Nineteenth century synthetic chemistry introduced a number of newly produced gases into commerce, especially as industrial intermediates. These included chlorine and anhydrous ammonia. In general, limitations in storage and transportation of these predominantly irritant gases dictated that synthesis on the one

hand and end-use on the other were carried out in close proximity to one another. Industrial point-source releases of these gases were a well-recognized hazard of the 19th century and led to some of the first zoning restrictions on the locations of workshops and factories.

The introduction of poison gas as a weapon of mass destruction in World War I fundamentally changed both scientific and public understanding of the importance of inhalational toxicology. This was followed by air pollution crises in both Europe and North America that illuminated the link between the workplace and the environment beyond the factory door. More recently, the disastrous release of the lethal irritant gas methyl isocyanate in Bhopal, India served to underscore the importance of toxic gases to the field of occupational and environmental medicine.

## SIMPLE ASPHYXIANTS: METHANE, CARBON DIOXIDE, NITROGEN, NITROUS OXIDE, ETHANE, ACETYLENE, NOBLE GASES

### Essentials of Diagnosis

*Acute effects:*
- Rapid loss of consciousness.
- Coma.
- Anoxic brain injury.

*Chronic effects:*
- Residual anoxic injury.

### Exposure Limits

ACGIH TLV: Atmospheric oxygen should > 18% at normal barometric pressure (partial pressure $O_2$ = 135 mm Hg)

### General Considerations

Asphyxiant gases are those inhalants that act predominantly by oxygen deprivation (Table 33–2). This may occur by simply displacing oxygen from inspired air. Other asphyxiants exert toxicity by in-

**Table 33–2.** Common asphyxiant gases.

| **Simple asphyxiant** | |
|---|---|
| Acetylene | Methane |
| Argon | Neon |
| Carbon dioxide | Nitrogen |
| Ethane | Nitrous oxide |
| Ethylene | Propane |
| Helium | Propylene |
| Hydrogen | |
| **Chemical asphyxiants** | |
| Carbon monoxide | |
| Hydrogen cyanide | |
| Hydrogen sulfide | |

terfering with the delivery of oxygen to tissues or by disrupting the utilization of delivered oxygen at the cellular level. A common and useful terminology to differentiate between these two modes of action identifies the former as simple asphyxiants and the latter as toxic asphyxiants.

## Occupational & Environmental Exposure

Simple asphyxiants are potential occupational hazards wherever confined space exposure to these substances occurs (eg, inside storage tanks or mines). Although any inert gas could act as a simple asphyxiant, only a short list of substances is of practical importance. Methane is an endemic hazard in coal mines where, because it is lighter than air, it may accumulate in upper pockets if not properly ventilated. Of historical interest, canaries were brought into mines to provide early warning of the presence of potentially lethal concentrations of methane and other simple asphyxiants. In the presence of hazardous concentrations of these agents, canaries would die, thereby serving as a warning to miners. Of course, in addition to simple asphyxia, methane and other hydrocarbon asphyxiant gases (ethane, acetylene) present an added hazard of explosion and fire. In mines, this could also lead to carbon dioxide and carbon monoxide accumulation post-conflagration ("after damp"). Carbon dioxide is also a product of combustion (although it is usually dwarfed in significance by carbon monoxide production) and fermentation processes. Environmentally, carbon dioxide appears to have been the toxicant responsible for the large scale deaths that occurred from a natural volcanic lake release at Lake Nyos, Cameroon, Africa in 1989. Nitrogen may be encountered in hazardous concentrations in a variety of work settings, including underwater work, mining, metallurgical operations, and pressurizing oil wells.

## Metabolism & Mechanism of Action

By definition, the simple asphyxiants act nonspecifically by oxygen deprivation leading to anoxia. The central nervous system is the organ system most severely affected by hypoxia. Although carbon dioxide is considered a simple asphyxiant, it also acts at high concentrations as a potent central nervous system depressant, which may account for some of its effects as well.

Nitrous oxide is also an anesthetic asphyxiant with direct central nervous system depressant effects not attributable simply to hypoxemia. In chronic exposure, nitrous oxide also has toxic effects on the bone marrow and nerves similar to vitamin $B_{12}$ deficiency.

## Clinical Findings

**A. Symptoms and Signs:** At high exposures, the hallmark of asphyxiant exposure is rapid loss of consciousness and death resulting from acute anoxia. If oxygen deprivation is less severe, symptoms may range from tachycardia, tachypnea, and exercise intolerance (oxygen concentrations 10–16%) progressing to nausea, prostration, and coma (oxygen range reduced to 6–10%).

**B. Laboratory Findings:** There are no specific findings other than the reduction of blood oxygen and associated metabolic derangements.

## Differential Diagnosis

Even a brief occupational history may quickly identify a simple asphyxiant as the likely cause of anoxic injury, especially confined space injury. On clinical grounds alone it may be difficult to differentiate between simple and toxic asphyxia. Specific laboratory findings in the latter conditions are key to the diagnosis. Other causes of collapse, including primary cardiac and CNS events, may need to be excluded depending on the clinical context.

## Prevention

Confined space work should include adequate air supply. It is important to confirm that the air supply intake does not itself entrain other toxins (eg, carbon monoxide from a compressor). Confined space injury often occurs in the setting of inadequate safety training and lack of appropriate supervision.

## Treatment

Immediate removal from further exposure can be life-saving; however, rescuers themselves are often in equal danger without adequate air supply. Post-exposure treatment is supportive and nonspecific, but should include administration of supplemental oxygen.

## Prognosis

Although all of the sequelae of anoxic brain injury can occur, many survivors of simple asphyxiant gas inhalation make a complete and rapid recovery.

# TOXIC ASPHYXIANTS

## CARBON MONOXIDE

### Essentials of Diagnosis

*Acute & subacute effects:*
- Headache.
- Malaise and gastrointestinal distress.
- Cardiac ischemia.
- Coma.
- Anoxic brain injury.

*Chronic effects:*
- Myocardial infarction.
- Residual anoxic injury.

## Exposure Limits
ACGIH TLV: 25 ppm TWA
OSHA PEL: 50 ppm TWA
NIOSH REL: 35 ppm TWA

## General Considerations
Carbon monoxide intoxication is the leading cause of death due to gas inhalation. Most fatalities are due to environmental rather than occupational exposures. In addition to unintentional exposures, carbon monoxide inhalation remains a common method of intentional poisoning.

## Occupational & Environmental Exposure
Carbon monoxide exposure is a potential hazard whenever incomplete combustion occurs. Any source of combustion or industrial process consuming carbon-based fuel may create a source of carbon monoxide release. The internal combustion engine is an important occupational and environmental source of carbon monoxide. Nonelectric fork lifts and other vehicles and gas powered compressors and generators, especially when used indoors, represent important exposure hazards. High-risk carbon monoxide exposure occupations include fire fighters, toll booth workers, and furnace operators. Home heating unit malfunction or misuse, structural fires, automobile exhaust, and cigarette smoke are the most common sources of significant environmental carbon monoxide exposure.

## Metabolism & Mechanism of Action
Carbon monoxide acts by avidly binding to hemoglobin to form carboxyhemoglobin (COHb). This has two adverse effects. First, carbon monoxide competes with oxygen for binding sites on hemoglobin, thereby reducing the oxygen carrying capacity of the blood. Second, the COHb unit interferes with heme-heme interactions such that the oxygen-hemoglobin dissociation curve is shifted to the left, resulting in decreased release of oxygen from hemoglobin carrier sites to the tissues. Carbon monoxide may also bind to other heme-containing moieties besides hemoglobin, but the toxicologic relevance of these effects remains undetermined. In addition to direct inhalation, exposure to carbon monoxide can occur through the metabolism of the common industrial solvent methylene chloride.

## Clinical Findings
**A. Symptoms and Signs:** At high exposures, rapid loss of consciousness, coma, and death occur as with other asphyxiants. In subacute carbon monoxide exposure, symptoms are less marked and can be quite nonspecific, including headache, malaise, and gastrointestinal distress. Cardiac ischemia is a potential risk of carbon monoxide exposure, particularly in individuals with underlying coronary artery disease. Additionally, there are limited experimental animal data suggesting that carbon monoxide exposure may promote the development of atheromatous vascular disease, although this remains controversial. The fetus is at particular risk from carbon monoxide exposure.

**B. Laboratory Findings:** Elevated COHb is confirmed through co-oximeter blood gas analysis. COHb is increased in active cigarette smoking but should not exceed 10% on this account and is usually less than that (typically, 4% to 5%). COHb levels above 30% are associated with moderate to severe symptoms; higher levels (50% and above) approach the lethal range. However, there is a great deal of symptomatic heterogeneity in relation to the absolute COHb level. In pregnancy, a higher fetal level may be reached than that reflected by the maternal COHb level. It is also important to extrapolate back to peak levels, taking into account time since last exposure, the 5–6 hour half life of carbon monoxide, and duration of oxygen therapy prior to the measurement. For example, a COHb level of 15% 5 to 6 hours since last exposure in a person breathing room air since exposure suggests a peak COHb of approximately 30%.

A routine blood gas analysis (not done by co-oximetry) reports a calculated rather than measured oxygen saturation that will be falsely preserved in the setting of carbon monoxide intoxication. Similarly, pulse oximetry is unreliable in the presence of significant COHb. ECG monitoring is useful because myocardial infarction can occur in severe carbon monoxide intoxication even in the absence of typical chest pain symptoms.

## Differential Diagnosis
With severe exposure, the differential diagnosis is that of any anoxic injury. For fire victims, it is often difficult to rule out concomitant cyanide intoxication. The differential diagnosis of subacute carbon monoxide intoxication leading to nonspecific symptoms is quite wide and it is likely that many cases go undiagnosed. A high index of suspicion is needed, particularly in winter months when space heater malfunction is common.

## Prevention
Carbon monoxide is odorless and has no warning properties. Internal combustion engines should not be used in indoor environments unless special precautions are taken. Heating units should be well maintained to ensure proper venting and to avoid partial combustion. Household carbon monoxide alarms are being employed on a widespread basis. Properly used, these may serve to reduce home heating mishaps.

## Treatment

Immediate removal from exposure together with supplemental oxygen (100% by nonrebreathing face mask, or in the comatose patient by endotracheal tube) are the mainstays of treatment for carbon monoxide intoxication. On 100% oxygen, the half-life of COHb is reduced to approximately 60 minutes from 5 to 6 hours on room air alone. Although hyperbaric oxygen reduces the COHb half-life further, this is not an intervention option usually available for immediate initiation. The role of late hyperbaric treatment (ie, after the COHb concentration has been reduced to a level that is no longer an acute threat) remains controversial. A beneficial effect has been argued on theoretical grounds, but this has not been established through controlled clinical trials.

## Prognosis

Anoxic brain injury can occur after severe carbon monoxide exposure (ie, intoxication to the point of loss of consciousness). Injury can be nonfocal and subtle, including neurobehavioral abnormalities. Parkinsonian deficits have been documented as a sequela of carbon monoxide poisoning.

# CYANIDE

## Essentials of Diagnosis

*Acute & subacute effects:*
- Dyspnea.
- Headache.
- Gastrointestinal distress.
- Dizziness.
- Loss of consciousness.
- Anoxic brain injury.

*Chronic effects:*
- Neurotoxicity.

## Exposure Limits

ACGIH TLV: 4.7 ppm ceiling
OSHA PEL: 10 ppm TWA
NIOSH REL: 4.7 ppm STEL

## General Considerations

Cyanide is a important toxic asphyxiant to which exposures occur through ingestion and skin absorption as well as inhalation.

The classic "bitter almond" odor of cyanide cannot be appreciated by a significant proportion of the population, apparently on a genetic basis. Because of its potency and rapidity of action, cyanide has long been important to forensic as well as occupational toxicology.

## Occupational & Environmental Exposure

The major current industrial use of cyanide is as a salt in metal plating operations. As with carbon monoxide, cyanide release is a potential hazard in structural fires, primarily as a thermolysis byproduct of both natural and synthetic polymers. Cyanogenic glycosides are an environmental dietary exposure source in much of the developing world, principally from cassava.

## Metabolism & Mechanism of Action

Cyanide exerts its toxicity by binding to ferrous iron in cytochrome oxidase, blocking oxygen utilization. Cyanide, to a small degree, is generated through normal metabolism, but it is converted enzymatically to thiocyanate, which is excreted in the urine. Certain industrial and consumer product chemicals (acrylonitrile, proprionitrile, acetonitrile), when metabolized yield cyanide, leading to delayed toxicity hours after exposure.

## Clinical Findings

**A. Symptoms and Signs:** With high exposure, rapid loss of consciousness and death rapidly ensue. Lower level exposure leads to dyspnea, dizziness, headache, and gastrointestinal distress, as with other asphyxiants. Low level chronic cyanide exposure in foodstuffs is associated with neuropathy. Cyanide is also present in cigarette smoke and has been theorized to explain the association between cigarette smoking and a rare form of optic neuropathy.

**B. Laboratory Findings:** Cyanide levels are of little use in acute management or surveillance, but frequently are obtained for forensic reasons. Results should be interpreted with caution because of a variety of technical factors that can affect the results, including the contribution of thiocyanate.

## Differential Diagnosis

The differential diagnosis includes other asphyxiants, especially hydrogen sulfide and, in fire victims, carbon monoxide. Cyanide exposure should be suspected when collapse is very sudden after an inhalation or ingestion.

## Prevention

Cyanide gas is released from cyanide salt solutions if the pH falls, as may occur, for example, from inadvertent mixing with an acid. However, absorption following skin contact with salt solutions also occurs, leading to the same toxicity.

## Treatment

The current standard of treatment for cyanide intoxication is induction of methemoglobin with nitrites (to compete for cyanide binding, sparing the cytochrome oxidase) and administration of thiosulfate to promote detoxification of cyanide to thiocyanate. Hydroxocobalamin, shown to be effective as an antidote in animal studies, is used in clinical practice outside of the United States. It has been studied as an "orphan drug" in the United States, but is not used routinely.

## Prognosis

As with other asphyxiants, anoxic brain injury can occur in survivors of severe acute exposure.

## HYDROGEN SULFIDE

### Essentials of Diagnosis

*Acute effects:*
- Mucous membrane and respiratory irritation.
- Loss of consciousness.
- Anoxic brain injury.

### Exposure Limits:

ACGIH TLV: 10 ppm TWA, 15 ppm STEL
OSHA PEL: 20 ppm ceiling, 50 ppm 10-min maximum peak
NIOSH REL: 10 ppm ceiling (10 minutes)

### General Considerations

Hydrogen sulfide is a naturally occurring toxicant generated from the breakdown of organic materials. It is associated with a pungent odor of rotten eggs, although this sense can be rapidly overwhelmed through olfactory fatigue.

### Occupational & Environmental Exposure

Geothermal and fossil fuel energy extraction are the two major occupational sources of industrial hydrogen sulfide exposure, but other occupational risk groups include farmers (manure processing), sewage workers, fish processors, and roofers or surfacers who work with heated tar and asphalt. Hydrogen sulfide is a particular hazard in confined spaces such as fishing ship holds and manure pits.

### Metabolism & Mechanism of Action

Like cyanide, hydrogen sulfide exerts its toxicity by blocking oxygen utilization through the cytochrome oxidase pathway. Unlike cyanide, however, hydrogen sulfide is not metabolized by enzymes facilitated by a sulfur donor such as thiosulfate.

### Clinical Findings

**A. Symptoms and Signs:** High exposure leads to rapid loss of consciousness and death. At lower levels, irritant effects may predominate, including airway irritation and burning eyes. Other findings may include dermatitis, pneumonitis, and pulmonary edema as well as headache, dizziness, and nausea and vomiting.

**B. Laboratory Findings:** There are no direct assays that are specific for the acute diagnosis of hydrogen sulfide poisoning.

### Differential Diagnosis

The differential diagnosis includes other asphyxiants, most importantly cyanide. Signs or symptoms of mucous membrane or respiratory tract irritation would support the diagnosis, since the other toxic asphyxiants are not irritants.

### Prevention

Confined space precautions are particularly relevant to the prevention of hydrogen sulfide injury. The odor warning properties of hydrogen sulfide are not reliable as a protective factor.

### Treatment

The use of nitrites to treat hydrogen sulfide has been argued on theoretical grounds, but is unproved and potentially dangerous as well. Unlike in cyanide toxicity, thiosulfate has no role in the management of hydrogen sulfide toxic exposures. While glucocorticoids are often administered to treat cerebral edema, their efficacy in the setting of hydrogen sulfide toxicity has not been established in controlled clinical trials. Rapid removal from exposure and supportive care remain the principles of treatment.

### Prognosis

Anoxic brain injury can occur. In addition, the sequelae of acute irritant inhalant injury represent a potential adverse outcome (see following section).

---

## IRRITANT INHALANTS

---

### Essentials of Diagnosis

*Acute effects:*
- Mucous membrane irritation.
- Cough.
- Stridor.
- Dyspnea.
- Noncardiogenic pulmonary edema.

### Exposure Limits

See Table 33–3.

### General Considerations

Irritant inhalants represent a heterogeneous group of substances linked by common target organ effects. The majority of these compounds are moderately to highly water soluble, causing potent irritation of all of the mucous membranes with which they come in contact, including the eyes, nose, mouth, and throat. Consequently, exposure to irritants such as chlorine, ammonia, sulfur dioxide, or acid aerosols leads to tearing, rhinorrhea, and burning of the mouth and throat. Greater exposure, either in duration or con-

**Table 33–3.** Major irritant inhalants.

| Substance | Selected Exposure Industries or Occupations | Exposure Limits | | |
| --- | --- | --- | --- | --- |
| | | ACGIH TLV | OSHA PEL | NIOSH REL |
| Chlorine | Plastics industry; water treatment | 0.5 ppm TWA | 1 ppm (C) | 0.5 ppm (C) 15 min. |
| Chlorine dioxide | Paper manufacturing; food preparation | 0.1 ppm TWA | 0.1 ppm TWA | 0.1 ppm TWA 0.3 ppm ST |
| Ammonia | Plastics and fertilizer manufacturing | 25 ppm TWA | 50 ppm ST 35 ppm ST | 25 ppm TWA |
| Sulfur dioxide | Petroleum refining; smelting; cement works; paper manufacturing; refrigerant exposure | 2 ppm TWA | 5 ppm TWA | 2 ppm TWA 5 ppm ST |
| Hydrogen chloride | Chemicals industry; firefighters | 3 ppm (C) | 5 ppm (C) | 5 ppm (C) |
| Hydrogen fluoride | Plastics industry; microelectronics | 3 ppm (C) | 3 ppm TWA | 3 ppm TWA 6 ppm (C) |
| Sulfuric acid | Fertilizer industry; petroleum refining; chemicals manufacturing | 1mg/m$^3$ TWA | 1mg/m$^3$ TWA | 1mg/m$^3$ TWA |
| Ozone | Flight attendants; specialty welding; water treatment | 0.1 ppm (C) | 0.1 ppm | 0.1 ppm (C) |
| Nitrogen dioxide | Gas shielded welding; agricultural workers | 3 ppm TWA | 5 ppm (C) | 1 ppm ST |
| Phosgene | Isocyanate and pesticide manufacturing; welding | 0.1 ppm TWA | 0.1 ppm TWA | 0.1 ppm TWA 0.2 ppm (C) |
| Bromine | Specialty chemical manufacturing | 0.1 ppm TWA | 0.1 ppm TWA | 0.1 ppm TWA 0.3 ppm ST |
| Dibroane | Microelectronics industry | 0.1 ppm TWA | 0.1 ppm TWA | 0.1 ppm TWA |
| Ethylene oxide | Gas sterilizing systems | 1 ppm TWA | 1 ppm TWA | <0.1 ppm TWA 5 ppm (C) |

TWA = time weighted average; TLV = threshold limit value; PEL = permissible exposure limit; REL = recommended exposure limit; C = ceiling; ST = short term exposure limit.

centration, can lead to deeper injury manifested by laryngeal and pulmonary edema. In contradistinction to the more water soluble irritants, several important irritant gases do not produce marked mucous membrane symptomatology, but do cause lower respiratory tract injury, resulting in small airways inflammation and noncardiogenic pulmonary edema. The most important of these low solubility gases are nitrogen dioxide, phosgene, and ozone.

## Occupational & Environmental Exposure

The agent that is the most frequent cause of irritant inhalant injury is chlorine gas (and the related compound, chlorine dioxide). Chlorine gas exposures occur through industrial leaks, especially in textile and pulp bleaching, environmental releases occurring primarily in transport or water purification, swimming pool disinfectant accidents, and household cleaning product misadventures (when chlorine is released from hypochlorite). Potential acid aerosols exposure is also widespread in a variety of industrial processes. Important compounds include hydrochloric, sulfuric, chromic, and hydrofluoric acid. The anhydrous analogues (eg, hydrogen chloride) quickly form acid aerosols in normal atmospheric conditions where humidity is present. Concentrated sulfur dioxide and ammonia exposures result from refrigeration gas leaks; high-level ammonia exposures also occur in agriculture. Important sources of nitrogen dioxide exposure include gas-

shielded electric arc welding, combustion engine exhaust, and silage decomposition. Phosgene, which like chlorine was historically important as a war gas in World War I, is still encountered in chemical synthesis and as an inadvertent byproduct when certain chlorinated hydrocarbons are exposed to heat or ultraviolet light. Other important irritant gases are more limited in their applications, including diborane (microelectronics manufacture), bromine (chemical synthesis, including flame retardants), and methylisocyanate (pesticide manufacture). The pesticide metam sodium breaks down to yield methylisothiocyanate, which can also act as a irritant gas. Formaldehyde, a gas in pure form that also easily vaporizes from solutions (formalin) or off-gases residual monomers from polymers (urea-formaldehyde resins), is an irritant that may be encountered in plastics, textiles, and paper industries, as well as in smoke and photochemical smog.

## Metabolism & Mechanism of Action

The irritants lead to tissue injury through heterogeneous mechanisms that may include free radical or oxidant pathways. In general, these are not substances that require metabolic activation in order to exert their toxic effect.

## Clinical Findings

**A. Symptoms and Signs:** Low to moderate exposure leads to mucous membrane irritation marked by lacrimation, rhinorrhea, and burning of the mouth and face. Higher exposure is associated with cough and respiratory irritation and can also lead to laryngospasm and lower respiratory tract injury. Lower respiratory tract injury may range from mild pulmonary edema to severe injury clinically manifest as Adult Respiratory Distress Syndrome (ARDS). Lower respiratory tract injury becomes evident in the hours immediately following exposure. Exposure to toxic levels of nitrogen dioxide, ozone, or phosgene may also lead to lower respiratory tract injury, which also becomes clinically manifest hours after exposure, but which is not preceded by the immediate mucous membrane irritant symptoms associated with the more water-soluble compounds.

**B. Laboratory Findings:** After significant symptomatic exposure, laboratory evaluation should include pulmonary function testing, chest roentgenogram, and assessment of oxygenation.

### Differential Diagnosis

The exposure history is usually sufficient to identify irritant inhalation as the cause of respiratory compromise. However, nitrogen dioxide or phosgene exposure may sometimes present as occult causes of ARDS for which sepsis would typically be the leading alternative etiology. Lower respiratory tract injury without antecedent mucous membrane irritant symptoms is inconsistent with exposure to a water-soluble irritant such as ammonia or chlorine.

### Prevention

Precautions in the storage and transport of irritant gases are critical to prevention. Household cleaning product misadventures can be prevented by avoiding hypochlorite mixing with other products, especially acid or ammonia-containing cleaners. Nitrogen dioxide injury in agriculture can be prevented by proper silo ventilation. Precautions are particularly important during gas-shielded welding operations (eg, tungsten inert gas or "TIG welding") in confined spaces. Ethylene oxide use in sterilizing systems should be accompanied by adequate venting as well as other engineering controls and specific overexposure monitoring.

### Treatment

The treatment of irritant inhalant injury is supportive and nonspecific and includes supplemental oxygen and bronchodilator therapy. Although corticosteroids are frequently used in the treatment of irritant injury in clinical practice, this has not been studied in a controlled manner. There is no proven role for prophylactic antibiotic use following such exposures.

### Prognosis

In severe exposures leading to ARDS, mortality can be high, but injury of lesser severity resolves without sequelae in most cases. However, irritant-induced asthma (including reactive airways dysfunction syndrome) may result from acute irritant inhalation. The predictors of this adverse outcome have not been identified with certainty. Cigarette smoking may be one risk factor. Other, rare sequelae of irritant inhalation injury include obliterative bronchiolitis (bronchiolitis obliterans), bronchiolitis obliterans organizing pneumonia (BOOP), and bronchiectasis.

## SMOKE

### Essentials of Diagnosis

*Acute effects:*

- Mucous membrane irritation and cough.
- Stridor and dyspnea.
- Noncardiogenic pulmonary edema.
- Loss of consciousness.

### Exposure Limits

See Table 33–4.

### General Considerations

Smoke is a complex mixture of gases and particulates. The components of smoke depend on the material consumed, the temperature of combustion, and the amount of oxygen present. The principal relevant components of smoke include carbon monoxide, hydrogen cyanide, irritant gases and aerosols (particularly hydrogen chloride and acrolein), and carbonaceous particulates (eg, soot).

### Occupational & Environmental Exposure

Firefighters, both urban and wildland, are the largest occupational risk group for smoke inhalation. Environmentally, home cooking and heating with biomass materials is a ubiquitous source of smoke exposure in the developing world.

### Metabolism & Mechanism of Action

Smoke can exert its toxicity through asphyxia (see carbon monoxide and cyanide) or irritant effects. Direct thermal injury is typically not a major sequela of smoke inhalation, in contrast with steam inhalation, where this is a greater problem.

### Clinical Findings

**A. Symptoms and Signs:** Clinical findings in smoke inhalation injury can include features of both asphyxiant and irritant injury. Carbonaceous sputum represents a specific finding.

**B. Laboratory Findings:** Blood co-oximetry should establish the COHb level and document oxygenation status. After significant symptomatic exposure, laboratory evaluation should also include pulmonary function testing and chest roentgenogram.

**Table 33–4.** Common components of smoke from structural fires.

| Substance | Exposure Limits | | |
| --- | --- | --- | --- |
| | ACGIH TLV | OSHA PEL | NIOSH REL |
| Carbon monoxide | 25 ppm TWA | 50 ppm TWA | 35 ppm TWA |
| Acrolein | 0.1 ppm TWA | 0.1 ppm TWA | 0.1 ppm TWA |
| | | | 0.3 ppm ST |
| Formaldehyde | 0.3 ppm TWA | 0.75 ppm TWA | 0.016 ppm TWA |
| | | 2 ppm ST | 0.1 ppm (C) |
| Hydrogen chloride | 3 ppm (C) | 5 ppm (C) | 5 ppm (C) |
| Hydrogen cyanide | 4.7 ppm TWA | 10 ppm TWA | 4.7 ppm ST |
| Particulates (respirable) | 3 mg/m$^3$ | 5 mg/m$^3$ | not specified |
| | 10 mg/m$^3$-inhalable | 15 mg/m$^3$-total | |

## Differential Diagnosis

The differential diagnostic questions following smoke exposure often center on identifying the potential toxicants of greatest concern, especially following chemical fires. Very acrid smoke suggests the presence of hydrochloric acid or other acid aerosols. These are frequently released when polyvinylchloride and other halogenated polymers are burned.

## Prevention

Appropriate use of a self-contained breathing apparatus is the principal preventive measure used for firefighters combating structural fires. Breathing apparatuses appear to be effective in preventing the development of pulmonary symptoms and in reducing both the deterioration in forced expiratory volume in 1 second (FEV$_1$) and the increase in airway responsiveness caused by smoke inhalation.

## Treatment

The treatment of smoke inhalation includes supplemental oxygen, empiric bronchodilator therapy, and supportive care. As with other irritant exposures, corticosteroids are frequently used but have not been studied in a controlled manner.

## Prognosis

Temporary deterioration in pulmonary function and increases in nonspecific airway reactivity have been well-documented in persons exposed to smoke, including fire fighters. In many states, fire fighters can receive workers' compensation on a presumptive basis for lung cancer because of chronic fire smoke exposure. This compensation is based on social policy but does not reflect an established epidemiologic association. Community environmental exposures following conflagrations can lead to widespread concern over possible chronic effects. Acute respiratory symptoms, including aggravation of pre-existing asthma and COPD, can be anticipated. However, long-term sequelae in the absence of clear-cut acute effects would not be anticipated.

# OTHER INHALANT TOXICANTS

## ARSINE

### Essentials of Diagnosis

*Acute effects:*
- Malaise and weakness.
- Gastrointestinal distress and dyspnea.
- Hemolysis.
- Hemoglobinuria.

### Exposure Limits

ACGIH TLV: 0.05 ppm TWA
OSHA PEL: 0.05 ppm TWA
NIOSH REL: 0.002 mg/m$^3$ 15 minute ceiling

### General Considerations

Arsine is highly toxic, but does not cause immediate symptoms in typical low or moderate dose industrial exposures. Features of arsine exposure include hemolysis and multi-organ system dysfunction, which may develop over the 24 hours following exposure. In contrast with the delayed onset of symptoms resulting from lower dose exposure, very high dose exposure can be rapidly lethal.

### Occupational & Environmental Exposure

Arsine gas can be produced de novo in metal refining and other metal working processes when arsenic reacts with an acid in the appropriate environment. Preformed arsine gas, often stored under pressure in large quantities, is widely used as a dopant in the microelectronics industry. In addition to a potential occupational hazard, this also presents an environmental risk to surrounding communities.

### Metabolism & Mechanism of Action

Arsine is toxic to red blood cells, leading to hemolysis. Damage to other tissues may result from secondary damage from hemolysis (eg, kidney deposition of hemoglobin) or from direct toxic effects.

## Clinical Findings

**A. Symptoms and Signs:** The signs and symptoms of arsine toxicity reflect both hemolysis with its sequelae as well as other systemic toxic manifestations. Clinical findings may include malaise, gastrointestinal distress, headache, peripheral neuropathy, renal failure, cerebral edema, intracerebral hemorrhage, dyspnea, cardiovascular collapse, and death.

**B. Laboratory Findings:** The laboratory findings are those of intravascular hemolysis. The blood arsenic level may be elevated, although this is unlikely to be available rapidly enough to aid in the early diagnosis. The free hemoglobin level may help guide management; exchange transfusion has been advocated for free hemoglobin levels greater than 1.2–1.5 g/dL.

## Differential Diagnosis

The principal differential diagnosis includes hemolysis due to other causes. Although chemical oxidant exposures can also cause hemolysis, this would occur in the context of significant methemoglobinemia, which is not present in arsine poisoning. Stibine, or antimony hydride, exposure can also cause massive hemolysis, although it is rarely encountered industrially.

## Prevention

Meticulous control measures and back-up procedures should be in place whenever arsine gas is used. This should include hazardous materials ("HAZMAT") incident planning relevant to community protection.

## Treatment

There is no specific antidote for arsine poisoning. Treatment of massive arsine-caused hemolysis has required exchange transfusion. Alkalinization may reduce hemoglobin precipitation in the kidneys. Interim dialysis may be required if renal failure develops.

## Prognosis

Severe arsine exposure is life-threatening. However, if adequate acute supportive care and transfusion is available, fatalities should be avoidable.

## PHOSPHINE

### Essentials of Diagnosis

*Acute effects:*
- Respiratory distress.
- Headache and dizziness.
- Gastrointestinal distress.
- Coma.

### Exposure Limits

ACGIH TLV: 0.3 ppm TWA, 1 ppm STEL
OSHA PEL: 0.3 ppm TWA
NIOSH REL: 0.3 ppm TWA, 1 ppm STEL

### General Considerations

Phosphine is a systemic toxicant of high potency. It has a strong odor that is described either as "fishy" or "garlicky."

### Occupational & Environmental Exposure

Like arsine, phosphine gas is used in the microelectronics industry. Phosphine is also generated from the hydrolysis of aluminum phosphide and zinc phosphide, which are employed as rodenticides and insecticides, especially in the agriculture industry.

### Metabolism & Mechanism of Action

The toxic mechanism of phosphine is not well understood. A variety of end organs are affected. Pulmonary edema results from phosphine-mediated acute lung injury. Cardiac, hepatic, and renal toxicity can also occur.

### Clinical Findings

**A. Symptoms and Signs:** Multi-system compromise can be anticipated following phosphine exposure with pulmonary, cardiovascular, and central nervous system compromise most notable immediately. With lower level exposure, pulmonary toxicity may be the primary manifestation, marked by dyspnea and delayed-onset pulmonary edema in the hours following exposure.

**B. Laboratory Findings:** There are no specific laboratory findings in phosphine poisoning. Phosphorous levels are not followed in routine practice.

### Differential Diagnosis

Without a history of exposure, it may be difficult to identify phosphine as the cause of the acute multisystem injury this inhalant can induce.

### Prevention

Adequate post-use ventilation and other appropriate re-entry restrictions should prevent overexposure in agricultural settings. In industry, strict engineering controls must be enforced.

### Treatment

There is no specific treatment for phosphine toxicity other than general supportive care. The potential for delayed onset of pulmonary edema should be recognized.

## Prognosis

Potential sequelae related to acute lung injury are a possible problem. There are no data on other chronic effects of phosphine poisoning.

## METHYL BROMIDE

### Essentials of Diagnosis

*Acute effects:*
- Dyspnea and respiratory distress.
- Seizures.
- Coma.

### Exposure Limits

ACGIH TLV: 5 ppm TWA
OSHA PEL: 20 ppm ceiling
NIOSH REL: lowest feasible concentration

### General Considerations

Like phosphine, methyl bromide is a pesticide fumigant. Unlike phosphine, methyl bromide is frequently used in structural pest control in the urban environment. Methyl bromide, which is heavier than air, is a gas at room temperature but does condense at colder temperature ($< 38°$ F).

### Occupational & Environmental Exposure

Pesticide applicators are the principal occupational risk group. Inadvertent environmental exposure occurs following misapplication or inappropriate re-entry to areas treated with methyl bromide.

### Metabolism & Mechanism of Action

Methyl bromide has multiple toxic actions, including alkylation and enzyme inhibition. It has two principal target organ effects in humans: acute lung injury and central nervous system toxicity.

### Clinical Findings

**A. Symptoms and Signs:** Dyspnea and pulmonary edema may coincide with neurologic compromise marked by visual disturbance, tremor, and seizure. In severe cases, status epilepticus ensues.

**B. Laboratory Findings:** Serum bromide may be elevated, but the actual level correlates poorly with symptoms. In some assays, the serum chloride may be falsely elevated due to bromine.

### Differential Diagnosis

Ascertainment of the exposure history is critical. The combination of neurotoxicity and pulmonary injury represents an unusual constellation of symptoms that should suggest methyl bromide inhalation.

### Prevention

Methyl bromide has few warning properties. For this reason, chloropicrin, which is a mucous membrane irritant even at low concentrations, is frequently added to the fumigant.

### Treatment

Treatment is nonspecific. Control of status epilepticus is usually the primary focus of care.

### Prognosis

Neurologic compromise that resolves very slowly or that may be persistent has been well documented following methyl bromide intoxication.

## MILITARY & CROWD CONTROL AGENTS

### Essentials of Diagnosis

*Acute effects:*
- Lacrimation.
- Mucous membrane irritation.
- Dyspnea.

### Exposure Limits of Selected Agents

Zinc chloride
ACGIH TLV: 1 $mg/m^3$ TWA, STEL 2 $mg/m^3$
OSHA PEL: 1 $mg/m^3$ TWA, STEL 2 $mg/m^3$
NIOSH REL: 1 $mg/m^3$ TWA, STEL 2 $mg/m^3$
Chloroacetophenone (mace)
ACGIH TLV: 0.05 ppm TWA
OSHA PEL: 0.05 ppm TWA
NIOSH REL: 0.05 ppm TWA
Orthochlorobenzylidenemalononitrile
ACGIH TLV: 0.05 ppm ceiling
OSHA PEL: 0.05 ppm ceiling
NIOSH REL: 0.05 ppm ceiling

### General Considerations

Tear gases are not actually in gaseous form, but rather are well-dispersed aerosols. Another military agent, the smoke bomb, releases zinc chloride aerosol.

### Occupational & Environmental Exposure

Occupationally, both military and police personnel can be exposed through accidental releases, in training exercises, and in the field. In the latter context, "environmental" exposure may be widespread.

### Metabolism & Mechanism of Action

The precise mechanisms of action of this heterogeneous group of inhalants have not been delineated.

## Clinical Findings

**A. Symptoms and Signs:** The tear gases, principally chloroacetophenone ("CN," Mace) and orthochloro-benzylidenemalononitrile ("CS") are designed to be lacrimators and mucous membrane irritants. Rarely, with severe exposure, lower respiratory injury can also occur. In contrast, zinc chloride, the principal component of smoke bombs, is a severe respiratory irritant.

**B. Laboratory Findings:** There are no specific laboratory findings.

## Differential Diagnosis

All of the lacrimators would be anticipated to have similar effects. Involvement of other organs or systemic toxicity suggests other chemical exposures. Other chemical warfare agents, especially the modern "nerve gases," cause an entirely different presentation, with systemic illness marked by severe cholinesterase inhibition. Another warfare agent, nitrogen mustard, is a vesicant that leads to skin blistering and bone marrow depression in addition to respiratory injury.

## Prevention

Confined space exposures to any of these agents, but most importantly zinc chloride, can be associated with adverse outcomes and should be avoided.

## Treatment

After removal from exposure, treatment is supportive. Lung injury caused by zinc chloride inhalation should be managed as other causes of acute inhalant lung injury would be.

## Prognosis

There are no well-documented common chronic residual health effects of the lacrimators. Smoke bomb inhalation may lead to the sequelae of acute lung injury.

## REFERENCES

### GASES & OTHER IRRITANT INHALANTS: GENERAL PRINCIPLES & REVIEW ARTICLES

Blanc PD et al: Occupational factors in work-related inhalations:inferences for prevention strategy. Am J Ind Med 1994;25:783.

Hryhorczuk DO, Aks SE, Turk JW: Unusual occupational toxins. Occ Med 1992;7:567.

Lees PS: Combustion products and other firefighter exposures. Occup Med 1995;10(4):691.

Olson, KR et al: *Poisoning and Drug Overdose,* 2nd ed. Appleton & Lange, 1994.

Rorison DG, McPherson SJ: Acute toxic inhalations. Emerg Med Clin North Am 1992;10:409.

Scannel CH, Balmes, JR: Pulmonary effects of firefighting. Occup Med 1995;10(4):789.

Taylor AJ: Respiratory irritants encountered at work. Thorax 1996;51(5):541.

### INHALANTS: ACUTE EFFECTS

Blanc P et al: Morbidity following acute irritant inhalation in a population-based study. JAMA 1991;266:664.

Blanc PD et al: Symptoms, lung function and airway responsiveness following irritant inhalation. Chest 1993;103:1699.

Blanc PD, Schwartz DA: Acute pulmonary responses to toxic exposures. Pages 2050–2061 in: Murray JF, Nadel JA (editors): *Textbook of Respiratory Medicine,* 2nd ed. WB Saunders, 1994.

Eckert WG: Mass deaths by gas or chemical poisoning. Am J Foren Med Path 1991.

Weiss SM, Lakshminarayan S: Acute inhaltaion injury. Clin Chest Med 1994;15:103.

### INHALANTS: CHRONIC EFFECTS

Attfield MD, Wagner GR: Chronic occupational respiratory disease. Occup Med 1996;11(3):451.

Blanc PD: Chemical inhalation injury and its sequelae. [Occupational Medicine Epitomes]. West J Med 1994;160.

Kipen HM, Blume R, Hutt D: Asthma experience in an occupational and environmental medicine clinic. Low-dose reactive airways dysfunction syndrome. J Occup Med 1994;36(10):1133.

Schonhofer B, Voshaar T, Kohler D: Long-term lung sequelae following accidental chlorine gas exposure. Respiration 1996;63(3):155.

Rylander R (editor): Endotoxins in the environment. Int J Occup Environ Health 1997;3(Suppl 1).

### SELECTED SPECIFIC INHALANTS

Cook M, Simon PA, Hoffman RE: Unintentional carbon monoxide poisoning in Colorado, 1986 through 1991. Am J Public Health 1995;85(7):988.

Das R, Blanc PD: Chlorine gas exposure and the lung. Toxicol Ind Health 1993;9:439.

Douglas WW, Hepper NG, Colby TV: Silo-filler's disease. Mayo Clin Proc 1989;64:291.

Hertzman J, Cullen MR: Methyl bromide intoxication in four field workers during removal of soil fumigation sheets. Am J Ind Med 1990;17:321.

Mehta PS et al: Bhopal tragedy's health effects. A review of methyl isocyanate. JAMA 1990;264:2781.

Nicholson PJ et al: Time to discontinue the use of solutions A and B as a cyanide 'antidote.' Occup Med 1994;44(3):125.

Snyder RW, Mishel HS, Christensen GC: Pulmonary toxicity following exposure to methylene chloride and its combustion product, phosgene. Chest 1992; 101:860.

Wyatt JP, Allister CA: Occupational phosgene poisoning: A case report and review. J Accid Emerg Med 1995;12(3):212.

# Section V.
# Program Management

# Occupational Stress

# 34

James P. Seward, MD, MPP

Stress is an increasingly important occupational health problem and a significant cause of economic loss. While "stress" remains a broad, somewhat elusive concept, research efforts have led to a clearer understanding of the problem, its causes, and its consequences. Occupational stress may produce both overt psychological and physiologic disability; however, it may also have more subtle manifestations that can affect personal well-being and affect outcomes of organizational importance such as productivity.

Although many of the factors in the workplace that may cause stress have been studied, the ability to predict a stress response in any given individual remains poor. The prevention of occupational stress is best accomplished by creating a healthy work environment according to increasingly recognized organizational principles. It is also important to monitor and control stress by recognizing problem situations as well as early clinical or behavioral signs. Although the treatment of stress in the individual patient depends on the clinical manifestations, rehabilitation must include a consideration both of the work environment and of the patient's coping mechanisms. Organizational solutions for high-stress work units offer promise, but there is relatively little experimental information available to guide these interventions.

## STRESS CONCEPT & MODELS

Hans Selye defined stress in general terms as a syndrome that involves a nonspecific response of the organism to a stimulus from the environment. In framing the concept to make it applicable to the occupational setting, stress might be defined as a *perceived* imbalance between occupational demands and the individual's ability to perform when the consequences of failure are important. The element of individual perception introduces subjectivity into the definition of stress, and this perceptual component has played an important role in the evaluation of stress in the workers' compensation system.

Models of stress attempt to integrate individual and environmental factors into a working scheme of how stress is generated. An ideal model for occupational stress would be useful both in ongoing theoretic research and in practical problem-solving. Such a model would have to meet many criteria. It should offer a clear definition of how stress develops and allow for differentiation of stressful and nonstressful situations. The model should help to explain why certain events produce stress in some individuals but cause no detectable stress in others—and why stress may lead to different degrees of pathologic or even beneficial effects according to the circumstances.

All of the major factors that determine the stress response should be considered in the model. In general terms, these factors would include occupational, social, familial, and individual characteristics. If such a conceptual framework were developed, it would help to integrate the results of past research and suggest new areas for inquiry. It would also allow accurate predictions. Unfortunately, none of the available models meet these stringent criteria.

Several good efforts have been made that reflect different viewpoints on the genesis of occupational stress. Different models or partial models reflect the lack of consensus about weighing the etiologic factors. The main question is whether stress results primarily from the nature of the stimulus, the manner in which the stimulus is perceived, or the way in which the individual responds to the stimulus.

One simple explanatory model has been proposed by McLean (Figure 34–1). Overlapping circles represent the environmental context, individual vulnerability, and the initiating situation or condition, called the stressor. The stressor is able to produce stress only when all circles overlap, indicating a symptomatic response to a concurrence of these factors.

This basic model makes no attempt to weigh environmental versus individual factors in causing stress; however, it implies that favorable individual characteristics (low vulnerability) might prevent a symptomatic stress response when the environmental context and the presence of a stressor would otherwise facilitate one. Similarly, favorable environmental context alone might avoid a stressful outcome.

A more complex paradigm to explain the causa-

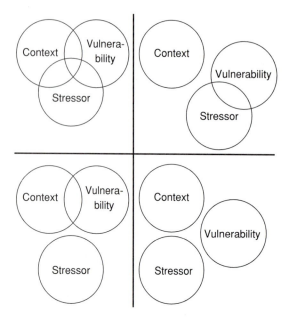

**Figure 34–1.** Symptomatic relationships between context, vulnerability, and stressors. (From McLean AA: *Work Stress.* Addison-Wesley, 1980.)

tion of stress is called the Person-Environment Fit Model (Figure 34–2). In this model, a distinction is made between the objective and subjective evaluations of the individual and the environment. Stress is produced by the subjective Person-Environment Fit, which is mediated ultimately by the individual's perceptions of the self and the environment. In this system, good mental health in the working situation depends on the outcome of four interactions: the objective environment-objective person, the objective environment-subjective environment, the objective person-subjective person, and the subjective environment-subjective person. A simple example will clarify these concepts:

> A garment worker may be expected to produce 40 pieces per hour (objective environment), whereas she believes she is required to produce 50 (subjective environment). She may actually be capable of producing 45 pieces (objective individual), but she thinks she can only produce 40 pieces (subjective individual).

In this case, there is a good match between the objective environmental demands (40 garments) and the objective person's ability (45 garments). However, the worker's perception that 50 garments are demanded (subjective environment) and undervaluation of her own abilities (subjective person) lead to a stressful situation. Given this scenario, the worker might experience stress based on a poor subjective

Person-Environment Fit despite an adequate objective fit.

The Person-Environment Fit Model is fairly comprehensive and clearly places much emphasis on the individual's subjective interaction with the environment. Another model places more emphasis on the work environment and the extent to which it may allow individuals to modify the stress response. The Job Decision Control Model concept holds that stress results from an imbalance between demands on a worker and the worker's ability to modify those demands (Figure 34–3). This model focuses on the adaptive response of the individual to a potentially stressful stimulus. When the worker can modify the response or alter the circumstances, less stress may result. Low decision-making control coupled with high job demands leads to high strain or to a stressful situation. In the Job Decision Control Model, high demands and low control work synergistically to have more impact than either factor alone. Proponents of the Job Decision Control Model have tended to focus on work tasks, but other aspects of the work environment such as organizational features or opportunities for creativity and independent thought might be as important.

The Decision Control Model has received wide attention over the last two decades, and a number of research studies have attempted to validate its predictions. Karasek, a principal proponent of this model, has shown that higher decision latitude is associated with decreased cardiovascular morbidity. The model has also been used to show that workers who participated in company reorganizations and had a resultant increase in job decision control experienced fewer health symptoms than did employees who moved into situations with less decision latitude.

Despite these successes, the Decision Control Model has also been criticized for its inconsistent ability to explain stress outcomes. There are concerns that the model does not apply equally across a range of occupations and social classes and that the relationships are more complex than the model allows. One study has shown that social support is a more powerful predictor of stress outcome than job control.

The research on stress has generated a number of other models that attempt to provide meaningful frameworks for understanding the phenomena. Some emphasize factors such as social support—the amount of positive interpersonal contact and assistance a worker has on or off the job. Research by Kobasa focuses on individual "hardiness" or the extent to which an individual feels challenged, committed, and in control of his or her work life. No model is comprehensive or able to explain the stress experience with great accuracy.

Despite the lack of theoretic consensus regarding occupational stress, a great deal can still be said regarding specific workplace and environmental conditions that produce stress, the effects of stress on the individual and the organization, and methods that

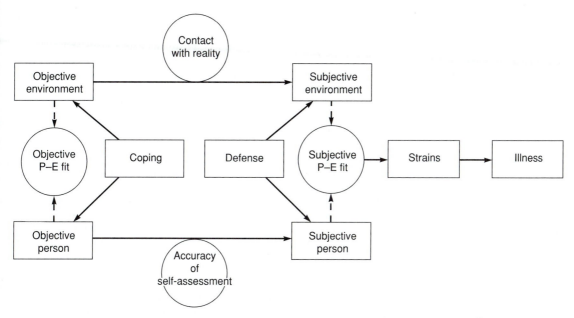

**Figure 34–2.** Effects of psychosocial stress in terms of fit between the person and the environment. Concepts within circles are discrepancies between the two adjoining concepts. Solid lines indicate causal effects. (From Harrison RV: Person-environment fit and job stress. In: Cooper C, Payne R [editors]: *Stress at Work.* Wiley, 1978.)

may control or alleviate stress in the work setting. Subsequent sections will consider these issues.

## WORKPLACE STRESSORS

Various characteristics of working life may contribute to occupational stress (Table 34–1). These characteristics may be grouped with much overlap into five general categories: organization and organizational relationships, career development, role of the individual, job task or assignment, and working environment and conditions. The following sections will discuss the contribution of each of these areas to the genesis of occupational stress.

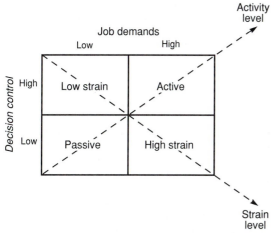

**Figure 34–3.** The job-demand control model indicates the effects of job demands and decision latitude on strain. (From Baker DB: The study of stress at work. Annu Rev Pub Health 1985;6:367.)

**Table 34–1.** Common workplace stressors.

**Organizational**
  Change
  Inadequate communication
  Interpersonal conflict
  Conflict with organizational goals
**Career development**
  Lack of promotional opportunity
  New responsibilities beyond level of training
  Unemployment
**Role**
  Role conflict
  Role ambiguity
  Inadequate resources to accomplish job
  Inadequate authority to accomplish job
**Task**
  Quantitative and qualitative overload
  Quantitative and qualitative underload
  Responsibility for the lives and well-being of others
  Low decision-making latitude
**Work environment**
  Poor aesthetics
  Physical exposures
  Ergonomic problems
  Noise
  Odors
  Safety hazards
**Shift work**

## Organization & Organizational Relationships

Most people in industrialized societies are now employed in some organizational context and are subject to fallout from factors that affect the organization as a whole. Issues inherent in organizational life such as political conflict, communication difficulties, delegation of tasks, decision-making authority, and regulations may be sources of conflict and stress. Relationships with supervisors are particularly important determinants of subjective well-being.

Stressful conditions are often produced when organizations undergo change. The situations encountered in producing new products or services, reorganizing institutional structure, and expanding or contracting operations often challenge the individual's ability to adapt. Increased levels of anxiety and diminished job satisfaction and morale have been shown in companies during the process of introducing new product lines. Thus, the process of change may disrupt an individual's equilibrium within an organization and place him or her at increased risk of a stress response.

Poor communication within organizations and a sense of not being either informed or heard by managers can similarly lead to stress as manifested by low job satisfaction. Conversely, good interpersonal support from colleagues—but especially from supervisors—may alleviate stress. Conflict with a supervisor or coworker is a powerful stressor. Moral or ideologic conflict between the individual and the goals of the organization can also produce psychological strain. The salesperson required to promote what is perceived to be a second-rate or socially irrelevant product and the manager forced to fire a respected older employee will both experience substantial stress.

## Career Development

Many transitions in working life are recognized as stressful situations. A change in jobs, getting a promotion or being passed over, and being laid off or fired are all high-risk events.

Studies of workers undergoing periods of unemployment have shown increased rates of mental illness and alcohol and drug use. There is also a suggestion of increased rates of disease such as peptic ulcer and hypertension.

Retirement as such, on the other hand, does not seem to be the cause of significant mental or physical ill health. Several longitudinal studies of morbidity and mortality rates in retired workers have shown no substantial age-adjusted increase in mortality rates. There is no strong evidence for an overall adverse impact of retirement on mental well-being, with the possible exception of a reduced sense of usefulness.

Promotion is a potential stressor. New job responsibilities, especially when calling for skills not previously exercised, can result in anxiety and psychologi-

cal decompensation. Promotion to a position beyond one's abilities has the potential for inducing behavioral disorders. Frustrated career goals and underpromotion have been associated with increased rates of mental hospitalization, as documented in a study of US Navy enlisted men who achieved officer status. Thus, symptomatic stress may result both from the frustration of thwarted ambition and from the inability to cope with new demands.

## Role in the Organization

Role conflict exists when two or more competing expectations make simultaneous satisfaction of both difficult. Role ambiguity implies insufficient information or guidance on which to base decisions and behavior. In one survey, approximately half of the work force reported having role conflicts and more than a third were disturbed by ambiguous expectations and duties.

Role conflict often occurs at interface positions. For example, a production supervisor occupies a position between management and staff, with an interest in keeping both sides happy without compromising production. Other examples of role conflict include differing opinions over what a given job should entail, contradictory job demands, and managing disputes between colleagues. Correlations have been observed between role conflict and increased heart rate as well as job dissatisfaction.

Role ambiguity may occur as a result of specific ill-defined responsibilities, unclear expectations of personal image, or hazy organizational objectives. The source of stress in these situations may be the lack of clarity itself or the inability to assess one's own performance.

Another type of role-related stress may result when individuals experience discrepancies between their supervisors' expectations and the resources available to meet them. Insufficient time, personnel, or funding puts a strain on the responsible individual who lacks the power to increase the availability of resources or to change expectations.

## Task

Work overload and underload, decision-making ability, and level and type of responsibility are important task-related issues with relevance for occupational stress. Both quantitative overload and qualitative overload have been implicated in stress disorders. In quantitative overload, the individual is overwhelmed by the amount of work. In qualitative overload, the expected functional level is too high—ie, the work is too difficult. High quantitative overload has been associated with coronary artery disease in several studies; there is also a relationship with alcohol and tobacco use, lost work time, poor motivation, and poor self-image.

Qualitative overload also has adverse physiologic effects. Blood cholesterol levels have been shown to rise in medical students under conditions of qualitative overload during an evaluation process. Tax accountants had higher cholesterol levels at deadlines. University professors with personal expectations of very high quality work scored poorly in terms of one stress indicator: self-esteem.

Qualitative and quantitative underload may also cause stress. One study of disease indicators in a large executive population showed higher rates of disease among individuals at the two extremes of the spectrum—the overworked and the underworked. Mental difficulties may be induced by understimulation and excessively routine activities: workers become bored and alienated and lose initiative.

Job responsibilities are significant sources of stress; work that involves responsibility for the lives of others is particularly stressful. Physicians, air traffic controllers, and first-line supervisors who make decisions affecting the lives of others may have higher rates of peptic ulcer; myocardial infarction and hypertension may also be related to work involving responsibility for others.

Several studies have shown a beneficial effect of higher job autonomy on stress indicators. Greater latitude to make basic decisions about the performance of one's work has been associated with fewer myocardial infarctions and fewer job-related injuries. Conversely, low decision-making autonomy has been related to higher levels of stress.

## Work Environment

The physical environment of the workplace may present many potential stressors. Most environmental hazards are identified with specific health effects they may cause, such as hearing loss from noise exposure. However, these exposures may also contribute to stress in a variety of ways. Physical exposures, chemical exposures, crowding, and ergonomic problems may function independently or collectively as stressors.

Noise provides a good example of a multifaceted stressor. In addition to its cumulative effect on the cochlea, noise exposure may acutely raise blood pressure. In addition, high levels of sound isolate workers by preventing conversation and drowning out other auditory cues to events near the workers. In one experiment, many of the physiologic and psychological changes associated with excessive noise were eliminated by providing a button that could be used to control sound levels. The beneficial effect occurred whether or not the control option was used.

Other physical exposures such as excessive heat or cold, extremes of lighting or glare, and vibration may produce ill effects. While the magnitude of these effects may not itself be disabling, the associated discomfort can contribute to mental distress and to secondary physiologic changes characteristic of stress.

Physical comfort and pleasant surroundings have been correlated with mental health. Ergonomic factors in tool and workstation design also play a role in worker frustration, morale, and ultimately productivity.

Research on VDT operators has indicated a complex relationship between workload, ergonomic factors, social factors in the workplace, and stress outcomes. Although the primary focus has been on the ergonomic design of computer workstations, work demands as well as task structure have also been shown to have significant effects on symptoms.

Chemical exposures may also induce stress through a variety of mechanisms. There may be direct irritating or intoxicating effects. Anxiety may arise regarding personal welfare as a result of potentially hazardous exposures. Unpleasant chemical odors—regardless of toxicity—may be powerful stressors by themselves.

Safety hazards inherent in some workplaces, such as risks of explosion or falls, add the element of fear to other work concerns. Welding on a thousand-foot-high tower is clearly more stressful than welding at ground level.

The assumption should be made—even though good documentation is not available—that the effects produced by stressful conditions are additive. Combined environmental stressors may even operate synergistically in some situations. Any given job is likely to have a complex array of potential stressors acting in a variety of ways. More research is needed, specifically on the cumulative effects of environmental stressors.

## Individual & Social Factors in Stress

Both personality traits and stressors from outside the workplace can influence the likelihood of work-induced stress. According to the Person-Environment Fit Model, individual response to a stressor is an important determinant of the outcome. Any comprehensive model of stress must help to explain why workers exposed to the same stressors will exhibit different responses. When attempting to reduce occupational stress, more emphasis should be placed on workplace stressors than on individual predisposition; however, the latter should not be ignored—especially as a precipitating factor.

Many variables may affect individual vulnerability to occupational stress. Personality structure, family life, stage in life, and social support systems are among the most important factors affecting the stress response. Many cases of occupational stress are precipitated by factors in the personal sphere. In addition to a thorough inquiry about stressors at work, physicians should always inquire about events in an individual's nonworking life when evaluating patients with stress symptoms.

The Holmes-Rahe Scale (Table 34–2) of recent life events (both "positive" and "negative") is an effort to rate the difficulty of change and adjustment

**Table 34–2.** The Holmes-Rahe schedule of recent life events.[1]

| Rank | Event | Value |
|------|-------|-------|
| 1 | Death of spouse | 100 |
| 2 | Divorce | 73 |
| 3 | Marital separation | 65 |
| 4 | Jail term | 63 |
| 5 | Death of close family member | 63 |
| 6 | Personal injury or illness | 53 |
| 7 | Marriage | 50 |
| 8 | Being fired from work | 47 |
| 9 | Marital reconciliation | 45 |
| 10 | Retirement | 45 |
| 11 | Change in family member's health | 44 |
| 12 | Pregnancy | 40 |
| 13 | Sex difficulties | 39 |
| 14 | Addition to family | 39 |
| 15 | Business readjustment | 39 |
| 16 | Change in financial status | 38 |
| 17 | Death of close friend | 37 |
| 18 | Change to different line of work | 36 |
| 19 | Change in number of marital arguments | 35 |
| 20 | Mortgage or loan of over $10,000 | 31 |
| 21 | Foreclosure of mortgage or loan | 30 |
| 22 | Change in work responsibilities | 29 |
| 23 | Son or daughter leaving home | 29 |
| 24 | Trouble with in-laws | 29 |
| 25 | Outstanding personal achievement | 28 |
| 26 | Spouse begins or stops work | 26 |
| 27 | Starting or finishing school | 26 |
| 28 | Change in living conditions | 25 |
| 29 | Revision of personal habits | 24 |
| 30 | Trouble with boss | 23 |
| 31 | Change in work hours, conditions | 20 |
| 32 | Change in residence | 20 |
| 33 | Change in schools | 20 |
| 34 | Change in recreational habits | 19 |
| 35 | Change in church activities | 19 |
| 36 | Change in social activities | 18 |
| 37 | Mortgage or loan under $10,000 | 17 |
| 38 | Change in sleeping habits | 16 |
| 39 | Change in number of family gatherings | 15 |
| 40 | Change in eating habits | 15 |
| 41 | Vacation | 13 |
| 42 | Christmas season | 12 |
| 43 | Minor violation of the law | 11 |

[1]Reproduced, with permission, from Holmes TH, Rahe RH: Social readjustments rating scale. J Psychosomat Res 1967; 11:213.

associated with stressful occurrences. In studies of several different groups, there was a correlation between higher total cumulative scores over a 1-year period and higher frequency and severity of illness. It is reasonable to infer that high scores on personal life stressors might also predispose a population to greater impact from workplace stressors.

Personality factors may also predispose certain individuals to a greater risk of stress-related disease. A case has been made for increased incidence of heart disease in individuals with aggressive, achievement-oriented personalities. Individuals with obsessive personality traits may depend on the structure of their jobs and undergo stress when changes occur. Preexisting psychiatric disorders as well as passive-aggressive, antisocial, and other maladaptive personality traits may affect the worker's ability to cooperate and be productive.

Changes in the workplace affect individuals differently according to their age and stage in life. According to the theory of life stages, adults undergo developmental changes that result in new needs and expectations from working life. Phases such as choosing a career, struggling for advancement, and reaching a high level of maturity and experience can be stressful depending on the individual's underlying personality organization and whether the phases are accompanied by appropriate recognition and reward. A transfer to very different job duties may be less taxing to a new employee who is just acquiring skills than to an established one who is trying to gain recognition for accomplishments in a specific area.

Social support by individuals outside the workplace can be an important mitigating factor in development of stress. The spouse is usually the most important person in this regard, but other family members and friends can also play an important role in supporting individuals in stressful occupations. An important concern here is that families often bear the burden of alleviating stress originating in the workplace. The deterioration of family or social support relationships may precede decompensation from stress at work.

With the growth in the number of employed women, more attention and research is needed on their status in relation to occupational stress. Women tend to occupy jobs different from those of men; these are often positions with lower status, fewer benefits, and less opportunity for growth. In addition, women often carry a double burden with substantial child-rearing and homemaking responsibilities. It is relatively common for women to be single mothers. Women in managerial positions may face greater stressors than their male counterparts.

## Shift Work

The rotating work shift is a common stressor that affects a growing proportion of the working population worldwide. Estimates are that between 15–20% of the US workforce do some form of shift or night work. Rotating shifts usually involve regularly changing work hours. Employees' shifts change periodically (eg, every 2–30 days), so that time spent working day, evening, and night shifts will be shared fairly equally by the workforce. These schedule changes have consequences for mental and physical well-being. Much has been learned in recent years about the physiologic effects of shift rotation, and there have been some practical applications (Tables 34–3 and 34–4). Many of the issues faced by shift workers are shared by individuals who have permanent night work schedules.

There have been numerous studies of the physiologic and health consequences of shift work and the

**Table 34–3.** Personal factors influencing possible increased risk from shift work.

Sleep disorders
Gastrointestinal disorders
Cardiovascular disease
Advanced age
Some chronic diseases
Psychological problems
Family and social situations

relationship of shift work to accidents, social well-being, productivity, and absenteeism. Despite these investigations, there is uncertainty about both long-term health effects and the role of personal factors in adaptation to shift work. Some points of general agreement provide the basis for evaluating work schedules and advising shift workers.

## Circadian Rhythms

Many physiologic systems in the human body display a regular circadian rhythm. In a free-running state unregulated by clocks, sunlight, or the regular pattern of daily activity, many of the major human circadian rhythms follow a 25-hour cycle. The usual 24-hour day thus requires a daily adjustment backward of about 1 hour in our "natural" rhythm. In changing our daily schedules, it is generally more difficult to arise progressively earlier than to delay awakening by an hour, since earlier awakening increases the adaptation required (shifting the internal clock back), whereas later awakening is a more natural adjustment. The same theory may explain why adjustment to time zone changes after air travel usually takes longer in the west-east direction; adapting to a more easterly time zone is essentially the same process as awakening earlier.

When this information is applied to rotating shift work, it becomes apparent, from a theoretic standpoint, that successful shift rotation should proceed from day to evening to night shifts rather than the reverse order. By following a "clockwise" progression to later shifts, the rotation order puts less strain on the adaptive ability of the internal clock. Application of the forward-rotation principle to a mining company in the United States resulted in increased productivity and subjective well-being as well as less job turnover.

**Table 34–4.** Factors with special concern or impact for shift workers.

Type of shift schedule
Transportation to work
Physical exposures
Chemical exposures
Safety factors, eg, lighting
Availability of meals
Social environment
Access to medical care

A second issue related to circadian rhythms is incomplete entrainment of the normal diurnal cycle following shift rotation. With change from a day to a night schedule, the various physiologic circadian rhythms begin to readjust; however, each one adapts at its own rate, with resulting dyssynchrony. In theory, all the rhythms would reach a new homeostasis if the new schedule were perfectly maintained. In practice, there is seldom complete readjustment.

Although the human organism has a number of circadian cyclic functions, including the secretion of glucocorticoids, most shift work research has focused on diurnal temperature variations as a surrogate measure for adaptation to new schedules. In a normal daytime-adapted human, the body has a temperature trough in the early morning hours and a temperature peak in the late afternoon. In an individual who becomes adapted to a night work schedule under isolated laboratory conditions, the temperature curve first flattens and then reverses completely.

Under real-life conditions, complete readjustment—or phase-shifting—of the temperature curve fails to occur for several reasons. First, individuals usually revert to daytime schedules on their days off. This causes a partial reversal of any phase-shifting that has occurred. Second, research has shown the importance of light exposure as a synchronizing cue to the human organism; workers on night shift who have exposure to daylight during off-work hours have incomplete readjustment of the temperature curve. Experimental studies of exposure to bright light during the night hours combined with the wearing of dark goggles to avoid light exposure at other times has shown more effective adjustment. Third, the readjustment time required for a complete inversion of the temperature curve is usually several weeks, so that workers on short rotation cycles of days or even a week do not have adequate time to adapt.

There are at least two schools of thought regarding the preferred way to schedule shift work based on a knowledge of circadian rhythms. One approach is to assign shifts that rotate slowly so that workers have at least 5 days and often much longer on a given schedule. In theory, workers have a longer time to adapt to the schedule both physiologically and socially. The other viewpoint advocates a short rotation length of 1–3 days on a given schedule. Proponents of these fast rotations argue that workers never fully adapt to night shifts and that short night rotations cause less chaos with circadian rhythms. Physiology notwithstanding, the acceptability of a shift schedule will depend to a significant extent on environmental, social, and recreational factors.

Proponents of the long-cycle forward shift rotation suggest that humans are able to adapt at least partially to a new schedule, as evidenced by a flattening of the temperature curve, over a period of several weeks. The time recommended for a given shift schedule would be at least 21 days before a rotation forward. Advocates of this approach point out that numerous studies have shown that workers on prolonged or permanent night shifts get more of hours of sleep (average, 6.72 hours) than do workers on weekly rotation schedules (average, 6.30 hours). The latter, in turn, get more sleep than those who rotate more rapidly (average, 5.79 hours).

While there may be physiologic advantages to the long forward shift rotation cycle, the short forward rotation cycle (2–3 days per schedule) is much more acceptable to workers. The principal reason is personal convenience, since the more rapid progression allows more frequent intervals of normal social and family life. Days off between shift rotations appear to offer time for individuals to recoup their sleep. As yet, the evidence regarding performance and accidents does not show a convincing difference between these two alternatives, although one might expect deficits in attention and response time among the workers on rapidly rotating shifts.

The physical and mental exertion involved in the work, the social and family support systems available, and the opportunities to eat well at the workplace should also be considered in scheduling decisions.

## Health Effects of Shift Work

Both short- and long-term health effects have been anticipated as a result of shift work. However, the case for short-term effects is much stronger. One factor influencing the long-term studies is bias through self-selection of individuals who tolerate shift work. The tendency of individuals who experience ill effects to cease shift work may lead to underestimates of the medical consequences.

Among the short-term or immediate problems related to shift work, sleep disorders, cardiovascular disease, gastrointestinal disturbances, and effects on underlying medical problems are of greatest concern.

Sleep is affected in several ways, the major cause being alterations in circadian rhythms. Studies have shown that there is difficulty in maintaining sleep after a night shift and difficulty in initiating sleep (in the early evening) before a morning shift. Sleep may be interrupted by street noise, family activity, the telephone, or other causes. The quality of sleep may also be altered, with changes in the sleep cycles and less REM sleep.

Gastrointestinal complaints are increased in rotating shift workers. There are changes in appetite and increased constipation. Alimentation is often adversely affected by poor availability or poor quality of food for night shift employees. Older studies have shown a high incidence of peptic ulcer among shift workers and an even higher incidence among workers who dropped out of shift work. There have been no good recent studies of this issue, leaving some doubt as to the strength of the association of ulcers with shift work. A contributing factor to the gastrointestinal problems may be the increased consumption of caffeine and tobacco among rotating shift workers.

There is concern and some documentation that rotating shift work exacerbates chronic medical conditions. Insulin-dependent diabetes mellitus may be more difficult to control, in part because of the irregularity of meals. The alteration of the sleep cycle may cause increased seizure frequency in epileptics.

There is conflicting information regarding cardiovascular morbidity and mortality in shift workers. Although older research did not indicate a clear association between shift work and cardiovascular disease, several recent studies do find a link. One investigation showed an increase in ischemic heart disease associated with more years of shift work; the effect was independent of smoking and age. Since there have been additional negative studies, the effect and its magnitude remain uncertain.

While the frequency of psychiatric disorders is not elevated overall, there are clearly social and familial stresses resulting from shift work. A shift worker will often have difficulty maintaining normal social contacts and community involvement. Altered sleep and leisure schedules can result in periods of low interaction with children and spouses. Shift workers tend to have higher scores on stress questionnaires than do non-shift workers.

Despite the wide-ranging impacts on an individual's life and the many ways in which health may be affected, shift work does not appear to change overall mortality. Several studies have examined longevity of rotating-shift workers in relation to daytime workers without showing a significant difference.

Special considerations should be given to concerns of safety for night workers. Especially with boring and repetitive work, there is increased likelihood of reduced attention and increased errors. In situations where safety risk is high, alertness monitors, extra measures to protect against injury, and perhaps shorter shifts should be recommended.

## Medical Advice on Shift Work

Medical evaluation for shift work should include particular attention to a history of cardiovascular disease, gastrointestinal problems, sleep disorders, epilepsy, difficulty with night vision, or other chronic disorders that might be affected by night work and rotating schedules. In shift work, the timing of medication and the quality of nutrition for people with chronic diseases is of concern.

While it is theoretically possible to predict which individuals are well or poorly suited to shift work on the basis of their circadian rhythms or sleep-wake cycles, practical criteria for selection do not yet exist. As a result, an enormous amount of self-selection occurs after experiencing shift work. An important role for the occupational practitioner is to advise shift workers about possible health concerns and how best

**Table 34–5.** Issues in medical evaluation of shift workers.

Health and functioning at work
Sleep quality and quantity
   Sleep environment, noise
   Chronic fatigue, naps
Gastrointestinal disease
Cardiovascular disease
Other chronic diseases
Use of medication
Use of alcohol, caffeine, tobacco, drugs
Accidents on and off the job
Psychological problems
Social and family problems

to adapt to them. It is important to cover social and familial concerns as well as sleeping habits, diet, and use of caffeine and other stimulants (Table 34–5). While routine surveillance of all shift workers is not necessary, the clinician should consider periodic rechecks of individuals with conditions that put them at higher risk for maladaptation or for specific medical problems related to shift work.

In summary, it is best to avoid scheduling shift work and night work when possible. When circumstances dictate, the shifts should rotate forward (day, evening, night). It is best to provide one or more rest days between shifts. Since many individuals have difficulty initiating sleep in the early evening, early-morning shift starts (eg, 4–6 AM) should be avoided. Rapid rotations (2–3 days) are preferred by workers, but there are physiologic grounds for advocating longer rotation cycles. Night work carries a somewhat increased risk of attention lapses and accidents as well as reduced productivity compared with the day shift.

## STRESS & DISEASE

Those who study occupational stress have been attempting to clarify the links between stress and disease. While there is good epidemiologic evidence associating occupational stress with a number of disease states, the pathophysiologic mechanisms often remain obscure. In most situations, a true causal relationship has not been demonstrated.

The question of how stress may produce disease is frequently debated. One theory holds that certain kinds of stress are consistently likely to produce given physiologic responses and, consequently, specific pathologic states. Another viewpoint is that stress is "nonspecific" and that personal factors such as conditioning and heredity determine which organ system, if any, will be affected by a variety of stressors. A given individual may have a specific susceptible organ that will be the target of a variety of stresses; thus, some people are gastrointestinal reactors and others are cardiac or muscle tension reactors. Finally, stress may also be viewed as a non-

specific force that exacerbates existing disease states.

The stress response has been associated with a variety of physiologic changes that may be postulated as mediators in the development of disease. The hypothalamic-pituitary axis, the autonomic nervous system, and the catecholamine response are often cited as stress-sensitive systems. These and other neurologic and endocrine systems may be important actors in the chain of events leading to cardiovascular, gastrointestinal, endocrine, and other stress-related disorders.

## Mental Illness

The mental health effects of stress exist on a continuum ranging from mild subjective symptoms to overt psychiatric disease with significant impairment of functioning (Table 34–6). Subjective reports regarding personal well-being constitute some of the earliest measures of stress. Frequently noted symptoms include anxiety, tension, anger, irritability, poor concentration, apathy, and depression. These manifestations of stress interfere with a sense of well-being and may be precursors of more severe illness.

Behavioral changes may also occur in response to occupational stress. Diminished participation in family activities, increased marital discord, and reduced participation in club activities have been attributed to stress. Rates of substance abuse are often increased. Studies have shown increased rates of alcohol abuse among individuals with high levels of stress and job dissatisfaction. Tobacco consumption is elevated among people with heavy workloads and tends to increase near deadlines. Other behavioral changes may include alterations in appetite and eating behavior, risk-taking (eg, when driving), and reduced interest in recreational activities.

Overt psychological dysfunction is frequently attributed to stress. Examples of such diagnoses include

**Table 34–6.** Examples of mental manifestations of stress.

**Mild subjective**
  Anxiety
  Tension
  Anger
  Depression
  Decreased concentration
  Irritability
**Mild behavioral**
  Decreased participation in family
  Marital discord
  Reduced social activity
  Risk-taking
**Clinical psychiatric disorders**
  Adjustment disorders
  Affective disorders
  Anxiety disorders including posttraumatic stress disorders
  Somatoform disorders and psychophysiologic disorders
  Exacerbation of existing psychiatric conditions
  Substance abuse

clinical depression, anxiety disorders, somatoform disorders (eg, hypochondriasis, psychogenic pain), and exacerbation of existing physical conditions by psychological factors. While these disorders are frequently observed in stressed individuals, no clear model has emerged to adequately explain the genesis of such disorders as related to stress. Rather than being causal, stress may act as a nonspecific promoter of disease. Statistical associations between stressors and overt psychiatric disease have been shown in several instances; unemployment and lack of opportunity for promotion have both been related to increased psychiatric hospitalizations and suicide rates.

There is no good analysis of the specific types of psychiatric disorders that occur most frequently among stressed workers seeking medical attention. The theoretic question again arises whether stress nonspecifically increases the incidence of all psychiatric problems or whether certain diagnoses result with greater frequency. Anxiety disorders (eg, panic disorder, agoraphobia), somatoform disorders, and depression are three types of problems frequently discussed in the literature on stress.

Two specific conditions—posttraumatic stress disorder and mass psychogenic illness—are related to stress and deserve specific mention. Posttraumatic stress disorder usually follows a specific psychologically traumatic episode of significant severity, which, in the occupational setting, is often an accident affecting the patient or a coworker. The patient subsequently reexperiences the traumatic event and develops symptoms of reduced responsiveness to the external world. Anxiety, depression, avoidance of activities that evoke the memory, emotional lability, and other symptoms often accompany the syndrome. This disorder is often a complicating factor in the rehabilitation of injured workers and may be responsive to brief psychotherapy and antianxiety medication.

Mass psychogenic illness is the collective occurrence of physical symptoms among two or more persons without evidence of an identifiable source. Symptoms are usually subjective, such as nausea, headache, dizziness, and neurasthenia. There are usually few, if any, objective findings. The symptoms usually resolve spontaneously with time or supportive care. There is usually a triggering event such as a strange odor or unexplained or rumored illness in one coworker. Factors associated with many industrial outbreaks have included boring, routine work; heavy production demands; physical stressors; poor communication opportunities; and poor labor-management relations. Many of these factors are also implicated in the stress response; it may be theorized that mass psychogenic illness is a particularly dramatic manifestation of occupational stress.

## Cardiovascular Disease

There is growing evidence for the designation of occupational stress as a risk factor for cardiovascular disease. Although causality is difficult to establish, a great number of retrospective and prospective studies have implicated workplace stressors in the etiology of coronary artery disease. Excessive workload has been associated with increased myocardial infarction rates; workers with more than one job or excessively long work hours had more heart disease than a control group with fewer work hours. Role conflict and coronary artery disease are associated for some white-collar workers.

The studies on cardiovascular disease and occupational level are conflicting; some indicate higher rates of disease for high-status employees, whereas others indicate that rates are higher in lower-level employees. This disparity makes it likely that factors other than occupational level will explain the phenomenon better and that future research should examine specific job components.

An inverse relationship between job satisfaction and coronary artery disease has been well demonstrated. This factor seems most strongly predictive for white-collar workers. Self-esteem, which may be related to satisfaction, is also negatively correlated with coronary artery disease. These factors may in turn be related to another proposed predictor of coronary artery disease—job decision-making latitude. Many studies have shown that coronary artery disease mortality and morbidity are increased among individuals with demanding jobs that allow little decision-making latitude.

One of the most widespread concepts relating behavior to heart disease is the "type A personality" hypothesis. In this model, individuals with aggressive, competitive behaviors who also tend to show time urgency are thought to be more prone to coronary artery disease. The type A personality hypothesis has gradually yielded to more complex models of human behavior that move beyond personality predispositions to include other variables such as rewards and frustrations in the workplace, decision latitude, and social support.

Although there is a substantial epidemiologic foundation that strongly suggests an association between stress and cardiovascular disease, there is still considerable doubt regarding the mechanisms through which a causal chain might occur. The first step in the causal process is generally viewed as the link between stress and cardiovascular reactivity. This step may be viewed as the effort to determine the relationships between stress and the physiologic processes that are believed to lead to disease. The next step would be to examine whether this stress-induced cardiovascular reactivity is capable of producing or accelerating coronary artery disease or hypertension.

Research has clearly established a link between stress and cardiovascular reactivity. In studies involving continuous blood pressure monitoring, short-term blood pressure has been shown to increase the stressful conditions on the job. In these studies, the pressures tended to return to normal when the subjects were at rest away from work. There is also evidence for increases in total cholesterol levels and declines in high-density lipoprotein cholesterol levels in workers under stress.

Cardiovascular reactivity appears to be mediated to a significant extent by the sympathetic nervous system and adrenal responsiveness. Catecholamine release is a frequent measure in research studies of the effect. Arterial constriction in response to stressful conditions has been demonstrated. In addition, cardiac arrhythmias, particularly premature ventricular contractions have been noted in stressful situations.

The relationship between stress-induced cardiovascular reactivity and hypertension is not firmly established. One study has shown a threefold increase in the risk of a sustained increase in diastolic blood pressure among workers with job strain. This study also demonstrated an increase in the left ventricular mass index, indicating a chronic effect. However, there is little other evidence from long-term longitudinal studies to corroborate the relationship between work stress and hypertension.

With respect to coronary artery disease, experiments with primate models have shown that the progression of atherosclerotic lesions correlated with experimentally induced psychological stresses over the long term. In one research effort, measures of cardiovascular reactivity to stressful psychological stimuli were better able to predict coronary artery disease than were the traditional cardiologic measures. Overall, there is inadequate research to firmly establish stress-induced cardiovascular reactivity as a cause of coronary artery disease, although the evidence is very suggestive.

Occupational stress may clearly influence behavioral and physiologic risk factors for coronary artery disease. Serum cholesterol levels have been shown to rise in tax accountants near deadlines, students taking exams, and shift workers. Statistically significant rises in blood pressure have been found with some stressful jobs such as telephone switchboard operators and air traffic controllers. Increased serum and urine catecholamine levels have been found in workers in competitive situations or those with high workloads. Tobacco use increases among some stressed workers. Some epidemiologic studies have implicated sedentary work in increasing the risk of coronary artery disease.

## Gastrointestinal Disease

Gastrointestinal disease, particularly peptic ulcer disease, has historically been associated with stress and emotional changes, although there is limited recent epidemiologic information in this area.

While some evidence has pointed to peptic ulcer disease as an ailment of executives and managers, stronger epidemiologic evidence shows an elevated prevalence of peptic ulcer disease among foremen. The explanation for this finding may be that foremen assume responsibility for the behavior and safety of others; they also occupy an interface role between workers and management. Other occupations that involve responsibility for others—physicians and air traffic controllers—are also associated with high rates of peptic ulcer disease. Workers anticipating plant shutdowns also experienced an increase in ulcer disease, as do rotating-shift workers. The incidence of duodenal ulcer—but not gastric ulcer—has also been shown to be related to workload as measured by energy expenditure. The incidence of ulcer disease may be modified by good social support networks both at home and at work.

There are several possible physiologic mechanisms responsible for the relationship of stress to ulcer disease. Autonomic nervous system activity plays a role in gastric acid secretion. Serum pepsinogen levels are often elevated in individuals predisposed to ulcers. Gastric acid secretion in response to catecholamine stimulation may also be a contributing factor. The etiologic importance of these factors should be further explored, in relation both to stress and to the potential causative role of *Helicobacter pylori*.

Other gastrointestinal problems such as eating disorders, ulcerative colitis, functional bowel disease, and constipation have been related to stress. However, there is generally very little information about their association with occupational factors. One exception is rotating shift work, in which appetite disturbances and constipation have frequently been noted.

## Other Diseases

The general model of stress as a stimulus producing a wide variety of physiologic adaptations suggests the possibility that many human diseases are precipitated or aggravated by occupational stress. The great frequency with which some disorders—such as back pain—occur in the work setting makes them logical candidates for study. Although stress may exacerbate muscular spasm and the experience of pain, there is no formal evidence linking stress to this common occupational ailment. However, it has been shown that psychological interventions in workers whose recovery fails to progress normally can speed return to work.

Other diseases such as diabetes, headaches, and asthma, have also been recognized as having a psychophysiologic component in some individuals, and it is probable that occupational stress factors can complicate their control. There is suggestive evidence that air traffic controllers have higher than normal rates of non-insulin-dependent diabetes.

Concern for the effects of stress on reproduction have been raised. Among stressed workers, there is evidence for an increase in cigarette, alcohol, and other substance abuse—each of which can produce ill effects on the fetus. Direct adverse impact of stress on fetal well-being is possible through transplacental hormonal mechanisms; however, there is no clear evidence of poor reproductive outcomes as a result of stress.

The role of occupational stress in the causation of a wide range of diseases from cancer to eczema is not adequately confirmed or defined. Such associations are speculative, and few scientific studies have been done to explore these relationships. Many potential pathophysiologic mechanisms are stimulated by occupational stress. The task remains to study the magnitude and clinical significance of associations between stress and overt disease.

## Accidents

There is a multifactorial relationship between occupational stress and accidents in the workplace. The stress of high workload demands may lead to compromise of safety measures to attain higher productivity. Workers paid on a piecework basis have increased numbers of accidents. Attention span may be altered by low levels of stimulation and long periods without breaks; inattention can lead to accidents. Changes of shift are associated with higher rates of injury on the first days of new shifts. There is mounting evidence to relate shift changes and sleeplessness to airplane pilot and air traffic controller errors. There may also be a relationship between job decision latitude and frequency of injury. The contribution of stress to substance abuse also leads to accidents; a large proportion of motor vehicle accidents on the job involve alcohol.

Some authors have noted a relationship between stressful events in an employee's life and subsequent occupational accidents. The possibility exists that stress from work or personal factors may contribute to the likelihood of an accident. Stressors should be assessed in evaluating injured employees; treatment of the physical impairment alone may not result in successful return to work.

## Sickness, Absence, & Productivity

A clear relationship exists between sickness, absence from work, and lost productivity. Stress may be an independent variable influencing each of these three factors. The case for stress as a contributor to sickness has already been made. However, absence from work is a complex phenomenon involving not just organic disease but also mental health, motivation, satisfaction with employment, and other personal and work-related factors. True malingering probably represents only a small part of the problem. Occupational stress probably contributes to the problem of absence due to illness, but the problem is compounded by sources of stress in the personal sphere.

In most organizations, a small number of employees account for a substantial proportion of the absenteeism. Stressful situations frequently underlie these absences either as a proximate cause or as an exacerbating factor. The illness may provide a justification for escaping the work situation and may be a manifestation of the worker's feelings of alienation from the work environment. Observation in several industries has shown that wage dissatisfaction is not the primary explanation for such absences; pay raises have not altered attendance records in these situations. Stress evaluation and referral for assistance can have an impact on the rate of illness absence.

Productivity on the job is, similarly, a stress-sensitive function. Reduced output, production delays, and poor performance may be manifestations of stress. Declining productivity of an organization or individual should prompt a search for occupational stressors. A stress management program may promote increases in attendance and productivity. This has been demonstrated by experiments that increase employee decision-making participation as well as by revisions of workers' rotating shifts according to psychological principles.

## Stress & Workers' Compensation
## (See also Chapter 3.)

While representing only a small portion of the costs of stress, workers' compensation claims for mental injuries have increased substantially in recent years. Most states in the United States recognize mental stress as a compensable disorder. In California, the number of reported stress claims increased by 500% between 1980 and 1988, although the number has now declined owing to legislative changes.

Several legal developments have permitted the increase in compensated stress cases. In the 1960 case of *Carter v General Motors* (361 Mich 577, 106 NW 2d), the Michigan State Supreme Court awarded workers' compensation benefits to a man with paranoid schizophrenia on the grounds that his illness had been caused by his work with the corporation although no physical injury or single traumatic event was involved. The legal definition of causation used in this and other cases is different from scientific causality. In the legal sense, psychiatric disability may be caused by work if the employment substantially contributed to its development.

Stress-related workers' compensation claims may be loosely divided into three categories for discussion—physical-mental, mental-physical, and mental-mental. Physical-mental claims usually result from well-defined work-related injuries such as crush injuries, amputations, or other sudden, significant, well-defined occurrences, although they may also result from illnesses. The claim is made for mental health effects such as posttraumatic stress, neuroses, or depression resulting from the physical event. Such claims are recognized in all US jurisdictions, although some claim types pose a challenge to the system. For example, mental health effects that an individual claims as a result of a gradually developing occupational disease, such as asbestosis, expand the scope of the physical-mental claim and raise new issues.

The mental-physical category includes instances in which claimants contend that emotional stresses at work have caused physical ailments including a wide variety of disorders such as myocardial infarction and neurologic, dermatologic, and gastrointestinal diseases. The epidemiologic evidence linking emotional stress to the initiation or aggravation of these disorders is variable and often weak. In the United States, most states limit these claims by requiring the presence of an unusual stressor or a close coupling of the events in time.

In recent years, mental-mental claims have drawn the most attention, and the numbers of claims have grown rapidly. Claimants file for compensation on the basis of mental health effects of conditions at work. There are fundamentally three kinds of situations that may precipitate these claims: stress resulting from involvement in sudden emotionally disturbing events, such as witnessing a coworker's death; stress resulting from a continuing situation which is unusual in its demands on the worker (eg, air traffic controllers, some types of police work); and stress arising out of the conditions of everyday work. These claims, particularly the last group, are often difficult to resolve. Many of these cases involve interpersonal conflict, predominantly conflict with supervisors. Both the extent of impairment and the causal factors are difficult to assess objectively. Legal precedent allows the claimant's subjective perception of events to be a factor in determining compensibility in many jurisdictions. As a result of concerns over rising claims, California has legislated that mental stress must be more than 50% occupational in origin to qualify for compensation.

## PREVENTION & MANAGEMENT OF STRESS

The prevention and management of occupational stress is a great challenge. Although there is often insufficient understanding of the genesis of stress in any given situation, it is frequently possible to apply existing knowledge to control this problem. Control begins with recognition—increased awareness on the part of health professionals is essential. Approaches to management and prevention may be organizational or individual in focus.

Historically, stress management programs in the United States have tended to focus on solutions at the individual level by providing instruction in coping and adaptive techniques. Growing evidence and experience point to the need for solutions that improve the relationship of the individual to the workplace. These solutions usually involve organizational changes that health professionals may help to accomplish.

### Role of the Health Professional

Occupational health physicians and other health professionals must monitor their patients and, when possible, the entire organization for signs of adverse consequences of stress. Many possible indicators should be considered. Individuals or clusters of patients may present with symptoms including mild mental distress, frequent absences from work, substance abuse, or severe mental impairment. Productivity may fall. Rates of injury may increase. Physical symptoms may be out of proportion to the type of injury.

Once alerted to the problem, the clinician may take steps to counsel individuals and offer assistance in stress reduction. The availability of programs designed for this purpose is a great asset; however, the clinician must take primary responsibility for helping the patient gain insight into the problem and often for providing concrete advice on its management (see next section).

The role of health professionals in effecting organizational change is often more difficult. Managers will often seek help for the individual employee with stress-related problems. They usually expect the clinician to deal with the situation on an individual level; they do not often expect or welcome intervention at the source of the problem when that involves changes in the workplace. The challenge for occupational health professionals is to bridge the gap from the traditional medical model to a more comprehensive model of stress control as well as to convince employers to cooperate.

Managers may be caught between conflicting objectives of economic gain and employee well-being. Although stress reduction may increase productivity and reduce costs from employee illness, the potential for conflict between these two goals remains an obstacle to many organizational innovations proposed by health professionals.

Ideally, the health professional will not wait for signs of stress to be manifested in the employees; primary prevention of stress-related symptoms is a far more desirable objective. The development of preventive programs requires the commitment of management, access to the work site, and a good understanding of the stressors operating in a given situation. While there is no proof that such efforts are cost-effective, limited positive outcomes have been demonstrated. Improved morale, increased sense of well-being, and less use of sick days have resulted from some interventions. There is a need for controlled studies comparing the impact of different approaches to stress prevention and management.

It is important for the occupational health professional to recognize that organizational stress is not the domain solely of the medical department and that other professionals may also have a significant contribution to make. Human resources specialists, organizational development consultants, employee assistance professionals, and potentially others should have a role in shaping an organization's stress prevention or management program. Given the complexity of the issues, particularly in initiating an organizationally focused program, it is best to think in terms of building interdisciplinary coalitions.

## Individual Approaches

Most stress management approaches focus on the individual and attempt to teach coping skills for the management or reduction of stress. These programs may be offered to all employees of an organization or to targeted groups or individuals.

A great variety of approaches have been developed. Information may be transmitted through methods ranging from simple self-study brochures to intensive individual counseling. Most programs rely on group training sessions. Educational efforts may involve the distribution of written materials, lectures, seminars, poster campaigns, and a variety of other methods.

The objectives of work site stress programs are usually to educate employees about stress and its effects, to increase awareness of stress in their lives and jobs, and to teach coping skills for managing or reducing the problem. These programs aim to identify people in the early stages of stress before it has become a significant health problem.

In recent years, a number of standardized surveys have been developed to assess stress in individuals. Self-assessment questionnaires may help educate employees about stressors and personal levels of stress with respect to a norm. The stress assessment questionnaire may also be a way for clinicians to determine where stress is most prevalent within an organization.

In addition to the self-assessment questionnaires, an important advance in the ability to assess an individual's stress and coping style has been the development of validated surveys that are interpreted by researchers or health professionals. These instruments can be used either in individual counseling or in organizational research and development. One such survey, the Occupational Stress Inventory (OSI), has been the subject of several validation studies. While some issues regarding the validity of one of its scales (the Locus of Control scale) have been raised, it has been used widely and has shown predictive value in a number of situations. Its most appropriate use, however, is to assist in the evaluation of individuals experiencing significant levels of occupational stress. Another survey, called the Occupational Stress Questionnaire, has been developed for research use by the Finnish Institute of Occupational Health.

It is usually insufficient to increase awareness of occupational stress without teaching specific skills to improve the individual's ability to handle the stress-

**Table 34–7.** Relaxation techniques.

Autogenic training
Biofeedback
Deep-breathing exercises
Exercise
Meditation
Progressive relaxation exercise
Yoga

ful situation. Many stress management techniques involve teaching relaxation or meditation exercises (Table 34–7); some emphasize physical activity; and others teach the individual to be aware of emotions related to stressful situations and to discharge them in a safe way. The role of social support from spouses, friends, and coworkers is emphasized in some programs.

Another type of stress-coping program educates the individual to make adaptations to be able to better control the work environment and stress responses (Table 34–8). Some of these stress coping methods involve strategies for dealing with stressful situations; others include time management, priority setting, improved planning abilities, and decision-making skills. These techniques may all be helpful to the individual whose job allows their implementation. Interpersonal skills such as assertiveness training, conflict resolution, and relationship building may also be useful. Another method of stress reduction involves teaching cognitive skills to help individuals recognize what personal beliefs, perceptions, and expectations lead to stress.

Research has been done to identify the characteristics of the stress-resistant individual who remains healthy in stressful circumstances that might produce illness in coworkers. One study of executives found several personal qualities associated with low illness rates under stressful life conditions. Control over one's life, commitment to one's goals and work, and an attitude of challenge when confronted by change distinguished these individuals. While these personal traits may be predictors of resistance to stress, it is unclear whether they can be taught to individuals to prevent or alleviate stress-related problems.

Evaluation of stress-coping efforts in occupational settings is difficult; studies of these programs have tended to show improvements in perceived stress, stress-related symptoms, and a variety of other end points such as muscle tension, use of health services,

**Table 34–8.** Examples of stress-coping techniques.

Assertiveness training
Conflict resolution
Decision-making and problem-solving skills
Goal and priority setting
Interpersonal skills training
Time management

and interference with job performance. However, the benefits of stress management programs have tended to fade with time, and few long-term (1 year or more) follow-up evaluations have been done. There is little information comparing the effectiveness of the various-stress coping techniques.

The potential exists that these stress management programs could result in work site benefits (such as increased productivity) as well; however, few evaluations of these kinds of stress interventions have been done. The role of the programs in stress reduction itself remains to be demonstrated.

By contrast with techniques used for prevention in workers with mild degrees of stress, psychotherapy is usually reserved for individuals with significant stress-related problems who have been identified through employee assistance programs or by health care providers. Personal counseling in these situations may also make use of the other stress management and reduction techniques. One common technique is "stress-scripting" in which an individual is taught to recognize and reframe his or her internal dialog regarding stressful situations. Short-term therapy involving a few sessions may be sufficient to ameliorate the individual's condition; however, periodic follow-up is advised. For some workers, group psychotherapy may be more appropriate and acceptable. Others may experience symptoms of depression or anxiety amenable to a course of antidepressant or antianxiety medication in addition to measures to address the underlying circumstances.

## Organizational Approaches

The development of organizational approaches to stress prevention and control is at the leading edge of occupational stress research. Although a great number of employers have introduced stress management programs directed at individuals, relatively few efforts have been made to focus on the "organization as the patient." However, there is growing theoretic knowledge and practical experience with interventions to protect the workforce against stress through appropriate design of the environment and relationships at work. Similarly, there have been increasing efforts to resolve problems of high stress through institution-wide restructuring or other organizational-level interventions.

The field of organizational-level interventions is relatively new. There have been useful developments both at diagnosing the major stress or within an organization and at designing solutions to the problem. The number of published experimental and "action research" studies has increased, much of it in the organizational development, administrative sciences, or psychology literature.

In the organizational-level approach, the objective is to reduce the stressors arising from with in the organization itself (Table 34–9). Interventions may be directed at altering hierarchical organizational struc-

**Table 34–9.** Examples of potential organizational interventions in stress reduction.

Reducing job overload
Reorganizing job tasks to increase employee decision-making and creativity
Improving organizational communication
Developing employee assistance programs and supervisor awareness of stress
Quality circles and peer support groups
Environmental, ergonomic, and safety improvements at work sites

tures, enhancing communication style, involving employees in decision-making, or clarifying work roles.

Other approaches have included variation of work tasks, improving the physical tasks, improved the physical environment (including ergonomic design), and improved employee training. Increasing attention has also gone into social support systems in the workplace; efforts in this area have usually focused on team-building concepts.

Research done largely in Scandinavian countries has emphasized the development of criteria for a workplace that protects individual physical and psychological well being as well as allowing individual mastery of work skills. The emphasis has been on creating a good work environment, not merely one free of adverse stressors. Clearly, the nature of the industry involved will have a major influence of the relative importance of various aspects of optimal job design. For example, the key factors to avoid in production work are quantitative overload and qualitative overload; by contrast, in the hospital industry, the main tension is created by the conflicting demands of high workload and a need to maintain high standards in the face of qualitatively complex situations.

Apart from a balance of workload and content, other elements of the optimal work environment include a reasonable degree of control over the job task or process, an environment that favors the development of supportive social networks among coworkers, clarity in job roles, and training or other opportunities to learn fully about the job process and how to cope with its variations.

The ability to assess and measure stress in organizations has developed as a result of the application of survey instruments in these settings. While many different surveys exist, there is growing experience with aggregating individual responses to develop an organizational stress profile. The various scales on the survey give an indication of the sources of stress in the organization. This approach has been used successfully to direct the types of interventions needed. For example, an organizational intervention in a hospital as a result, in part, of survey data has led to reduced overall workers' compensation claims.

The survey approach has been applied more commonly in the assessment of the stressors for individuals in a given occupational category. Stress surveys have been done for police officers, schoolteachers, physicians, social workers, and bus operators. The results of these questionnaire studies are only as useful as the questionnaire is valid. However, with a good survey instrument, these studies can be revealing in terms of the underlying dynamics of stress in that profession.

Many organizational-level stress interventions have been attempted, although efforts with managerial or professional employees predominate. Reduced absenteeism and declines in role conflict and ambiguity have been demonstrated in a study of insurance company workers. The intervention consisted of enhanced goal setting and goal clarification. Several studies have shown positive effects from increased levels of employee involvement in decision-making and increased job decision latitude. Increasing perceived time autonomy has also been effective in reducing absenteeism and improving work performance.

Blue-collar interventions have included efforts to improve the work environment, reduce job overload, increase job autonomy, and increase social support. Improved teamwork has been a common theme. Workers have been given more say in the organization of work through Quality Circles and work teams with shared production responsibility. Teamwork has also been seen to increase social support. Job rotation has been a technique to relieve boredom and to increase the workers' understanding of the overall production process.

Organizational stress reduction interventions have often had inadequate evaluations, and there are notably few controlled studies in this area. While this type of intervention offers much promise for the primary and secondary prevention of stress effects on the workforce, much remains to be studied and documented before standard approaches can be recommended.

# REFERENCES

## STRESS CONCEPT & MODELS

Baker E, Israel B, Schurman S: Role of control and support in occupational stress: An integrated model. Soc Sci Med 1996;43(7):1145.

Fletcher B: A refutation of Karasek's demand-discretion model of occupational stress. J Organizational Behav 1993;14:319.

Karasek R: Lower health risk with increased job control among white collar workers. J Organizational Behav 1990;11:171.

Soderfeldt B et al: Psychosocial work environment in human service organizations: A conceptual analysis and development of the demand-control model. Soc Sci Med 1996;42(9):1217.

## ORGANIZATION & ORGANIZATIONAL RELATIONSHIPS

Fenlason K: Social support and occupational stress. J Organizational Behav 1994;15:157.

Fried Y: The main effect model versus buffering model of shop steward social support. J Organizational Behav 1993;14:481.

Huuhtanen P: Stress and change among bank directors and Supervisors. Scand J Work Environ Health 1992; 18:121.

Lindstrom K: Psychosocial criteria for good work organization. Scand J Work Environ Health 1994;20:Spec No:123–33.

## ROLE IN THE ORGANIZATION

Frone M: Intolerance of ambiguity as a moderator of the occupational stress/strain relationship. J Organizational Behav 1990;11:309.

## TASK

Cahill J, Landsbergis PA: Job strain among post office mailhandlers. J Occup Environ Med 1996;26(4):731.

Pietri-Taleb F et al: The role of psychological distress and personality in the incidence of sciatic pain among working men. Am J Public Health 1995;85(4):541.

Uehata T: Long working hours and occupational stress related cardiovascular attacks. J Hum Ergol 1991;20: 147.

## WORK ENVIRONMENT

Arnetz BB, Berg M, Arnetz J: Mental strain and physical symptoms among employees in modern offices. Arch Environ Health 1997;52(1):63.

Arnetz BB: Techno-stress: A prospective psychophysiological study of the impact of a controlled stress-reduction program in advanced telecommunication systems design work. J Occup Environ Med 1996; 38(1):53.

Luczak H: "Good work" design: An ergonomic and industrial engineering perspective. Pages 96–112 in: Quick J (editor): Stress and Well-Being at Work. American Psychiatric Association, 1992.

## INDIVIDUAL & SOCIAL FACTORS IN STRESS

Haines V: Occupational stress, social support and the buffer hypothesis. Work Occup 1991;18:212.

Kushnir T: Major sources of stress among women managers, clerical workers, and working mothers. Public Health Rev 1993;20:215.

Makowska Z: Stress management: Individual differences and determination of situations. Med Pr 1995; 46(4):395.

## SHIFT WORK

Akerstedt T: Psychological and psychophysiological effects of shift work. Scand J Work Environ Health 1990;16(Suppl 1):67.

Eastman C: Light treatment for sleep disorders: Consensus report. VI. Shift work. J Biol Rhythms 1995;10: 157.

Greenwood K (editor): Shiftwork. Int J Occup Environ Health 1997;3(Suppl 3).

Harrington M: Shift work and health—A critical review of the literature on working hours. Ann Acad Med Sing 1994;23:699.

Wilkinson R: Review paper: How fast should the night shift rotate? Ergonomics 1992;35:1425.

## CARDIOVASCULAR DISEASE

Blascovitch J: Cardiovascular reactivity to psychological stress and disease: Conclusions. Pages 225–237 in: Blascovitch J (editor): *Cardiovascular Reactivity to Psychological Stress and Disease.* American Psychiatric Association, 1993.

Hayashi T, Kobayashi Y, Yamaoka K, Yano E: Effect of overtime work on 24-hour ambulatory blood pressure. J Occup Environ Med 1996;38(10):1007.

Lindquist TL, Beilin LJ, Knuiman MW: Influence of lifestyle, coping, and job stress on blood pressure in men and women. Hypertension 1997;29(1):1.

Schnall P: The relationship between job strain, workplace diastolic blood pressure, and left ventricular mass index. JAMA 1990;263:1929.

## STRESS & WORKERS' COMPENSATION

Barth P: Workers compensation for mental stress cases. Behav Sci Law 1990;8:349.

Eliashof B: The role of stress in workers compensation claims. J Occup Med 1992;34:297.

Lippel K: Workers compensation and psychological stress claims in North American law. Int J Law Psychiatry 1989;12:41.

## PREVENTION & MANAGEMENT OF STRESS

Burke R: Organizational-level interventions to reduce occupational stressors. Work Stress 1993;7:77.

Kishnir T, Malkinson R, Ribak J: Teaching stress management skills to occupational and environmental health physicians and practitioners: A graduate-level practicum. J Occup Med 1994;36(12):1335.

Landsbergis P: Evaluation of an occupational stress intervention in a public agency. J Org Behav 1995; 16:29.

Lindstrom K: Psychosocial criteria for good work organization. Scand J Work Environ Health 1994;20 (Suppl):123.

Sauter S: Prevention of work-related psychological disorder: A national strategy proposed by NIOSH. Am Psychol 1990;45:1146.

# 35 Substance Abuse & Employee Assistance Programs

*Kevin Olden, MD*

Dealing with substance abuse in the work place is a challenge for the occupational medicine physician and requires special knowledge of the pharmacology of abusable drugs, knowledge of the legal aspects of urine testing, patient confidentiality, and reporting requirements, and an understanding of the unique clinical presentation of substance abuse syndromes as they appear in the workplace. Identification and proper diagnosis of the substance abusing worker is necessary to preserve the health and safety of the individual. These workers, however, can also pose a direct threat to the safety of coworkers, employers, and the public. The loss of productivity that results from substance abuse-induced impairment exacts an even greater toll. The tendency of the substance-abusing worker to deny and conceal drug usage and the appearance of impairment in the form of decreasing work performance demands that the occupational physician have a thorough understanding of substance abuse and its consequences.

## THE NOMENCLATURE OF SUBSTANCE ABUSE

The definitions of "addiction," "substance abuse," and "dependency" have suffered from a lack of formal nomenclature. In the past, these terms were often used interchangeably. Significant strides in nomenclature have been made over the last few years. The American Psychiatric Association's *Diagnostic and Statistical Manual of Mental Disorders,* 4th edition (DSM-IV), uses a cluster of behavioral, physiological, and cognitive variables to define substance abuse-related conditions such as dependence, abuse, toxicity, and withdrawal. All have specific diagnostic criteria. The basic criteria for substance dependence is a maladaptive pattern of substance use that includes tolerance, withdrawal, and other patterns of use that are maladaptive (Table 35–1). Abuse is a pattern of substance use extending over 12 months that leads to a failure to fulfill major obligations at work, school, or home (Table 35–2). These criteria, although imperfect, serve as a useful common refer-

ence point for the physician attempting to establish a diagnosis of abuse or dependence on a psychoactive substance. Using these standardized criteria can be helpful not only to establish a diagnosis, but to document the need for treatment. Many managed care organizations will not authorize treatment for patients unless they meet the DSM-IV criteria for abuse and/or dependence. These criteria are applicable to the major classes of abusable substances including alcohol, amphetamines, cannabis, cocaine, hallucinogens, nicotine, inhalants, opioids, phencyclidine, and sedative-hypnotics.

## ALCOHOL ABUSE

Alcoholism is by far the most serious chemical dependency problem encountered in the work place. It is estimated that over 200,000 people suffer alcohol-related deaths in the United States annually. One study showed that 71% of industrial-related fractures presenting to an emergency room were associated with on-the-job alcohol usage. In addition, over 50% of all traffic fatalities, murders, rapes, and suicides are directly related to alcohol usage. The impact on traffic safety is enormous. It is estimated that 30–50% of Americans will be involved in an alcohol-related motor vehicle accident during the course of their lifetimes.

The prevalence of alcoholism is difficult to measure precisely due to the lack of standardized diagnostic criteria. However, most studies have suggested that 13% of men and 3% of women are "heavy drinkers" and would likely meet the diagnostic criteria for alcohol dependence. Certain occupations have been associated with an excess prevalence of alcohol dependence as measured by cirrhosis rates. Writers, journalists, longshoremen, bartenders, and waiters are all occupations that have had traditionally high rates of alcohol-related cirrhosis. Accountants, carpenters, and postal workers tend to have lower rates, and physicians are not at an excess risk for development of alcohol dependence. It is difficult to calculate the overall economic impact of alcohol depen-

**Table 35–1.** Diagnostic criteria for substance dependence.

A maladaptive pattern of substance use, leading to clinically significant impairment or distress, as manifested by three (or more) of the following, occurring at any time in the same 12-month period.

1. Tolerance, as defined by either of the following:
   a. A need for markedly increased amounts of the substance to achieve intoxication or desired effect
   b. Markedly diminished effect with continued use of the same amount of the substance
2. Withdrawal, as manifested by either of the following:
   a. The characteristic withdrawal syndrome for the substance (refer to Criteria A and B of the criteria sets for Withdrawal from the specific substances)
   b. The same (or a closely related) substance is taken to relieve or avoid withdrawal symptoms
3. The substance is often taken in larger amounts or over a longer period than was intended.
4. There is a persistent desire or unsuccessful efforts to cut down or control substance use.
5. A great deal of time is spent in activities necessary to obtain the substance (eg, visiting multiple doctors or driving long distances), use the substance (eg, chain-smoking), or recover from its effects.
6. Important social, occupational, or recreational activities are given up or reduced because of substance use.
7. The substance use is continued despite knowledge of a persistent or recurrent physical or psychological problem that is likely to have been caused or exacerbated by the substance (eg, current cocaine use despite recognition of cocaine-induced depression or continued drinking despite recognition that an ulcer was made worse by alcohol consumption).

American Psychiatric Association: *Diagnostic and Statistical Manual of Mental Disorders,* 4th ed. Washington, DC, APA, 1994.

**Table 35–2.** Diagnostic criteria for substance abuse.

A. A maladaptive pattern of substance use leading to clinically significant impairment or distress, as manifested by one or more of the following occurring within a 12-month period:
   1. Recurrent substance use resulting in a failure to fulfill major role obligations at work, school, or home (eg, repeated absences or poor work performance related to substance use; substance-related absences, suspensions or expulsions from school; neglect of children or household).
   2. Recurrent substance use in situations in which it is physically hazardous (eg, driving an automobile or operating a machine when impaired by substance use).
   3. Recurrent substance-related legal problems (eg, arrests for substance-related disorderly conduct).
   4. Continued substance use despite persistent or recurrent social or interpersonal problems caused or exacerbated by the effects of the substance (eg, arguments with spouse about consequences of intoxication, physical fights).
B. The symptoms have never met the criteria for Substance Dependence for this class of substance.

American Psychiatric Association: *Diagnostic and Statistical Manual of Mental Disorders,* 4th ed. Washington, DC, APA, 1994.

dence in the work place. Lost productivity of both alcoholic individuals and coworkers that results from the alcoholic's dysfunctional performance, alcohol-related medical problems requiring sick leave, and work-related injuries and liability incurred by the company for injuries caused by alcoholic workers is staggering. It is estimated that the total cost of alcoholism to the United States economy is $100–150 billion annually. The occupational medicine specialist must be able to recognize the early signs of alcohol-induced impairment and direct employees to appropriate treatment in order to minimize the economic impact that the untreated alcoholic can have on themselves, coworkerss, employers, and the public.

## The Diagnosis of Alcoholism

Physicians have been trained to recognize alcoholism in the context of its medical complications. Most physicians, in the course of their training, see alcoholic patients who are hospitalized for major medical complications related to long-standing alcohol abuse. Alcoholic pancreatitis, alcoholic liver disease, and alcohol-induced dementia are syndromes recognizable to any physician who has trained in a hospital setting. However, it is important for the oc-

cupational medicine physician to recognize that these patients represent cases of end-stage alcoholism and do not accurately reflect the clinical presentation of alcoholism in the work place. Physicians who look for major medical complications of alcoholism will only be able to identify advanced cases. The work place offers an ideal setting for early intervention for alcohol dependence, as many of the subtle behavioral manifestations of alcoholism become apparent in the work place setting long before they are seen at home or in everyday social life. Decreasing work performance in a previously high-functioning employee, excessive absenteeism (particularly on Mondays), and excessive uses of sick leave are all signs of alcohol or other drug impairment. The early identification of the alcoholic patient in the occupational setting can be facilitated by focused history-taking, a carefully focused physical examination, and use of selective laboratory studies.

The physician needs to understand that one of the most prominent symptoms of alcoholism and other chemical dependency is denial of the existence of a problem. Because of this denial, alcoholics tend to have an illusory view of their condition that sometimes takes on extraordinary proportions. In the industrial setting, it is not uncommon to evaluate patients who will state quite calmly and straightforwardly that they have had no alcohol in days or weeks when subsequent determination of blood alcohol shows levels consistent with frank intoxication. Questions about quantity of alcohol drunk, time period of drinking, and choice of beverage are usually not fruitful. Likewise, self-report screening tests such as the Michigan Alcohol Screening Test (MAST) are

**Table 35–3.** The CAGE questionnaire.

1. Have you ever felt you should **C**ut down on your drinking?
2. Have people **A**nnoyed you by criticizing your drinking?
3. Have you ever felt bad or **G**uilty about drinking?
4. Have you ever taken a drink first thing in the morning (**E**ye opener) to steady your nerves or get rid of a hangover?

often not helpful in workplace settings because of the patient's strong tendency to deny or minimize alcohol usage. The most effective strategy for obtaining an alcohol history is to use a validated structured interview and to obtain history from independent sources. The CAGE questionnaire (Table 35–3) is a highly effective tool in establishing a diagnosis of alcohol abuse or dependency. Patients who answer two out of four CAGE questions positively have a score that correlates in excess of 90% the diagnosis of alcohol dependence. The CAGE questionnaire is easy to administer in the context of a work place medical evaluation. Another useful strategy for obtaining an accurate alcohol history is to seek out independent reports of the patient's alcohol (and other drug) history. The importance of obtaining independent reports of an employee's alcohol usage from both coworkers and family members cannot be underestimated. However, it is vital to obtain such history with respect for the patient's confidentiality. It is important for the physician to establish an open dialog and not harbor "secrets" that will only threaten the patient. Reports from supervisors and coworkers on changes in work performance, absenteeism, and observed use of alcohol and drugs can be obtained during a workplace evaluation. Contacting a patient's family or friends outside the workplace, however, needs to be done with the patient's permission. The physician should also inquire about the patient's legal history, including drunk driving arrests, spousal abuse, and credit problems, as they are often associated with substance abuse.

The physical examination can yield subtle clues to alcohol abuse. In many cases, employees abruptly cease alcohol usage when asked to present for a medical evaluation. Temporary cessation of alcohol use will precipitate signs of mild withdrawal, including diaphoresis, tachycardia, mild hypertension, and an upper extremity symmetrical tremor. In addition, signs of trauma, particularly in the lower extremities, associated with falls while intoxicated, can be helpful clues. Fractures, particularly of the ribs, have been associated with alcohol abuse. Signs of frank organ injury such as spider angiomas and organomegaly are also helpful when present, but these injuries represent end organ damage, usually seen only in cases of advanced alcoholism.

The judicious use of laboratory studies can further support the diagnosis of alcohol abuse and dependence. Blood alcohol determinations are usually only helpful if acute intoxication is suspected. Most employees presenting for evaluation will have stopped drinking hours or days prior to the evaluation; subsequently, blood alcohol determinations are often completely negative. Therefore, the determination of a zero blood alcohol level should not be used to conclude that there is no alcohol problem. One exception to this rule is when patients show signs of intoxication in the workplace. In this case, a breathalyzer test or blood alcohol determination can be quite useful. Results from a breathalyzer correlate quite well with blood alcohol levels and can be more convenient to use in the work place.

Chronic alcohol use can induce a wide variety of metabolic changes in a variety of organ systems. Alcohol can also cause direct injury to certain organ systems, such as the liver and bone marrow, which can be reflected in the peripheral blood. A number of studies have shown that the most useful blood studies are the CBC, especially the mean corpuscle volume (MCV), and certain liver enzyme studies, particularly the gamma-glutyl transpeptidase (GGT). A number of studies have shown that elevation of the MCV, particularly when combined with an elevated GGT, can identify over 90% of alcohol abusing-patients. Chronic alcohol use exerts a number of effects on red blood cells, which can cause the appearance of abnormally large numbers of macrocytic cells to appear in the peripheral blood. The first of these effects is alcohol's solvent action on the red cell lipid membrane. This solvent action results in a net increase in red cell permeability, which in turn results in a net influx of fluid, causing the red blood cells to increase in size. Likewise, hypersplenism and hepatomegaly induced by alcohol abuse tend to cause accelerated red cell destruction, which is compensated for by the release of immature red cells from the bone marrow. These immature red cells tend to be larger than mature cells. Finally, nutritional deficiencies, particularly a deficiency of vitamin $B_{12}$ and folate, can also cause a macrocytic picture. Chronic alcohol usage is associated with impaired absorption of folate. This impairment, combined with the poor nutrition commonly seen with chronic alcohol abuse, can lead to a net deficiency of folate, vitamin $B_{12}$, and pyridoxine. The GGT is also commonly elevated with any significant alcohol usage. This test alone, while sensitive, is not very specific. It can be elevated in starvation, obesity, and diseases of the bile ducts or gallbladder as well as alcohol usage. The GGT, in itself, cannot be used as a diagnostic marker for alcohol dependence, nor can the MCV or any other single laboratory test. It is imperative that the physician remember that the diagnosis of alcohol abuse or dependence, like any other diagnosis in medicine, is made on the basis of a careful history and physical examination. In evaluating a patient for any chemical dependency, laboratory studies, including urine testing, should never be used alone, but rather to support findings obtained by careful history taking and a thorough physical examination. Laboratory studies should be used to support a physician's clinical impression and not to establish a diagnosis.

## DRUG ABUSE

The use of psychoactive substances has become an issue of increasing concern in the workplace. Illicit drug use is influenced by a large number of variables, including societal attitudes and fads, availability, and cost. The use of CNS stimulants, depressants, and perceptual substances (hallucinogens) has waxed and waned over the last three decades. The abuse of these substances, along with abuse of prescribed controlled substances, has led increasingly to workplace impairment.

Cannabis is the substance most commonly detected in workplace urine testing. Cannabis is usually smoked and is readily absorbed from the respiratory and intestinal mucosa. Tetrahydrocannabinol (THC) is the active ingredient in marijuana, hashish, and ganja. THC produces a state of emotional and muscular relaxation and euphoria. In susceptible individuals, however, it can produce depression and psychosis. Chronic usage is associated with apathy and impaired judgment and problem-solving ability. Chronic ingestion can lead to respiratory complications, including bronchitis and permanent lung injury. THC is lipid-soluble and tends to remain in body tissues for days to weeks. It can appear in the urine for some time after usage. Whether THC causes permanent brain injury is controversial.

The CNS stimulants include cocaine in its various forms and amphetamines. The leaf of the coca plant contains a potent CNS stimulant that acts on the dopaminergic receptors in the brain. Cocaine is produced as an extract from the coca leaf in the form of pure alkaloid, or "free base," and crystalline hydrochloride salt, which is water-soluble and rapidly absorbed by the respiratory and enteric mucosa. The crystalline version is usually insufflated into the nose or taken orally. Free base cocaine is volatile and is usually smoked with a pipe. This form of ingestion results in rapid absorption, leading to an intense euphoria that lasts about 30–45 minutes. This intense but short-lived effect makes cocaine popular for users who do not desire a prolonged "high." This feature clearly has implications for the workplace, where impairment may be short-lived and intermittent, but quite severe. Cocaine also produces an intense adrenergic discharge, resulting in tachycardia, hypertension, and mydriasis. These syndromes can, in turn, produce acute cardiovascular complications, including myocardial infarction, seizures, cerebral vascular accidents, and cardiac arrhythmias. Sudden death has been associated with cocaine usage. Acute cocaine intoxication can result in acute mania, paranoid psychosis, and impulsive, sometimes severe, vi-

olent behavior. Chronic usage can lead to intense depression, suicidality, and paranoid psychosis. The physical symptoms of cocaine intoxication resolve within days of removal of the drug, but psychiatric complications of cocaine usage can be so intense that acute psychiatric hospitalization is often necessary.

Amphetamines are artificial substances that act in a similar manner to cocaine on the dopaminergic receptors of the CNS. Developed in the 1930s as stimulants to enhance performance, they were quickly shown to be capable of producing intense patterns of dependence associated with psychosis, anorexia, cachexia, and depression. Amphetamines are rapidly absorbed via the respiratory and GI tract and are usually taken orally or intranasally. Methamphetamine is smoked in the same way as "crack" cocaine and is relatively volatile. The amphetamines differ from cocaine in that their half-life is longer and produces a prolonged period of intoxication. In a workplace evaluation, amphetamine-abusing workers are more likely to show acute autonomic signs of intoxication such as tachycardia, hyperemia, and mydriasis. Amphetamines can also produce muscle tremors and, rarely, rhabdomyolysis. Acute amphetamine intoxication is associated with severe toxic psychosis characterized by motor agitation, intense paranoia, and violence.

## OPIOIDS

Opiate problems in the workplace take on two forms. The first type is the worker who is prescribed opiates for a medical reason, including medication prescribed for an industrial injury. Such patients can develop opiate abuse or dependency in the course of their medical treatment and can present a special challenge to the occupational medicine specialist. The challenge is to first diagnose the pattern of abuse or dependence. The occupational medicine physician must then work with the treating physician to develop a shared understanding of the problem. These patients need simultaneous treatment both for their medical condition and the opiate dependence. Often, these patients need a multidisciplinary approach to detoxification, rehabilitation, and workplace re-entry. The second type of opiate abuse is the worker with a primary opiate dependency not associated with a medical condition. These patients are more likely to engage in IV drug use and usually obtain their drugs from illegal sources. These two factors place these patients at high risk for a variety of serious medical complications, including hepatitis B and C, HIV infection, endocarditis, and infections at the injection site (phlebitis and cellulitis).

Naturally occurring narcotics (opiates) and synthetic agents (opioids) act as CNS depressants that bind to MU opiate receptors in the brain. Opiates and opioids produce intense euphoria and feelings of emotional tranquility and sedation. The duration of these effects vary by route of administration and by type of opioid used. The opiates with low protein binding, such as heroin, move into the CNS quickly but are absorbed slowly from the GI tract. This is the reason why addicts, in a attempt to achieve rapid euphoria, tend to use these drugs intravenously. The drugs differ in their half-life and potency. All are excreted in the urine and are readily detectable with urine drug testing. It is important to note that both heroin and codeine are metabolized by the body to morphine. Therefore, patients using either of these agents will test positive only for morphine on urine drug testing. Opiates produce profound mental and psychomotor slowing that will interfere with almost any work task. Depression of cardiopulmonary function is a particular risk for workers in special environments that require the use of respirators or breathing apparatus. The varying strength of street drugs poses the risk of accidental overdose on and off the work site. Detection of opiate abuse, particularly in the nonprescription addict, can be somewhat challenging. Addicts can also be quite covert in their drug usage. Careful history taking, with particular attention to the patient's apathy, depression, and decreased work performance, combined with a focused physical examination, can be quite helpful. Needle tracks, miosis, signs of constipation, weight loss (opiates induce anorexia), and infectious complications of IV drug use can all alert the physician to a covert opiate addiction problem. Urine drug testing can help support the diagnosis.

## SEDATIVE HYPNOTICS

These agents consist mainly of the barbiturates and the benzodiazepines. Early sedative hypnotics such as ethchlorvynol, glutethimide, meprobamate, and methaqualone are rarely used in contemporary medical practice. The typical sedative hypnotic abuser is usually a middle-aged woman who has either a history of previous or concomitant alcohol abuse or a predilection towards alcohol abuse, such as a family history of alcoholism. This profile clearly fits a large number of workers in most industries.

The sedative hypnotics are used to treat anxiety disorders, including panic disorder and insomnia. They have been widely prescribed, although the number of benzodiazepine prescriptions has leveled off in the last few years. Benzodiazepines are, by and large, safe. However, there is a certain profile that can place patients at risk for dependence. These factors include long-term usage of benzodiazepines, previous history of alcohol or sedative hypnotic abuse, and concomitant chronic medical problems or psychiatric problems like dysthymia and borderline or avoidant personality disorder. Clinically, the dosage of benzodiazepines and the type of agent (long versus short-acting) is less important. It is now clear that benzodiazepines can cause cognitive impairment, even with therapeutic dosages. This effect is an important consideration for the occupational medicine specialist who must ensure that employees taking benzodiazepines, even for appropriate conditions and in therapeutic dosages, may need to be excluded from duties that require a high degree of concentration and motor skills. In addition to cognitive impairment, patients who are physically dependent on benzodiazepines can present with seizures and delirium, which can be life threatening. These conditions can be exacerbated when benzodiazepine use is combined with alcohol abuse, and usage is often abruptly discontinued. These patients usually require inpatient detoxification and stabilization before workplace reentry. Consultation with the patient's prescribing physician is extremely helpful to determine benzodiazepine dependency and formulation of a return-to-work treatment plan.

## EMPLOYEE ASSISTANCE PROGRAMS

Because substance abuse disorders are usually accompanied by a steady decline in social and occupational functioning, the workplace has a number of advantages for detecting this decline in an individual's function. First, the average adult spends one-third of his or her daily time at work. Second, the workplace has clearly defined expectations on attendance, work performance, and behavior. Third, the workplace is less influenced by the emotional ties that family and friends of the substance abuser must confront in dealing with a substance abuser's dysfunctional behavior. This combination of factors makes the workplace an ideal venue for the detection of drug and alcohol abuse problems.

Employee assistance programs (EAPs) had their beginning in industries preparing for World War II in the 1940s. The pressure to mobilize industrial production during wartime led to the establishment of workplace alcohol intervention programs. These programs were also influenced by the development of Alcoholics Anonymous (AA). Originally run out of the company's medical department, they would usually involve medical evaluation and referral to AA. The early success of these industrial programs led the National Institutes of Alcoholism and Alcohol Abuse to fund in 1972 occupational program consultants (OPCs) in each state. The OPCs were mental health professionals who facilitated the improvement of workplace substance abuse programs. The introduction of mental health professionals led to the expansion of an EAP's focus to include other mental health problems like depression and other personal and family crises as well as substance abuse problems. Standards for certification of EAP professionals led to creation of the Certified Employee Assistance Professional (CEAPs). Over 4500 professionals have attained EAP certification over the last ten years.

The number of EAP professionals in the workplace has grown tremendously. Access to an EAP professional is usually a function of company size. One study found that while 87% of employees of large companies had access to EAP professionals, only 4% of employees of small companies had the same access. EAP professionals can either be internal employees of a company or external consultants. Within a company, they provide evaluation and referral for treatment that can be supplemented by outside specialists (eg, for psychiatric evaluation). The large overhead of maintaining in-house EAPs usually confines them to large companies. Companies that lack internal EAP departments can contract with an external consultant who provides services as needed. The primary disadvantage is that the EAP professional is located off-site and consequently has less familiarity with the company's culture and employees.

The keys to a successful employee assistance program are as follows: (1) a clear mandate for EAP services from management; (2) a nonpunitive policy on employees seeking the services of an EAP professional; and (3) support of all the constituencies within the company, including management, union officials, supervisors, and the employees themselves. EAP professionals are a major resource for the occupational medicine physician. The EAP professional can help the company retain employees who otherwise would be lost due to substance abuse disorders. In addition, they can train and supervise employees in the recognition of substance abuse-related performance impairment, relieving line staff of these training responsibilities. They also help with appropriate referrals for impaired employees. By functioning as a monitor of workplace impairment and injury, the EAP professional can contribute to lowered medical costs by making appropriate referrals to treatment programs and monitoring services that facilitate employee re-entry into the workplace. One study revealed that 40% of employers see EAPs as a health care cost control tool, and 30% believe that they are helpful in reducing litigation. The data on the effectiveness of EAPs has been generally good. Most studies confirm a trend toward decreased absenteeism and improved work performance.

## ROLE OF THE PSYCHIATRIC CONSULTANT

Both alcohol and other drug dependence are frequently accompanied by significant psychiatric complications. Acute psychiatric syndromes are commonly induced by the substance abuse disorder, and include paranoia, hallucinations induced by CNS stimulants such as cocaine, and depression associated with opiate and alcohol dependency. Anxiety syndromes are commonly associated with alcohol and opiate withdrawal, and severe acute depression is seen in the cessation of CNS stimulant usage.

Co-morbid psychiatric syndromes are often associated with, but are not directly due to, substance abuse. Studies have shown that 50% of opiate addicts have co-morbid major depressive disorder. Ten percent of alcoholics suffer from panic disorder, and another 16% have severe personality disorders. Women alcoholics are likely to have had a preexisting major depressive disorder prior to the initiation of their drinking. Finally, patients with substance abuse disorders, particularly opiate and cocaine dependency, will frequently have co-morbid personality disorders.

Failure to recognize these psychiatric problems in order to properly intervene can lead to treatment failure and a relapse of the substance abuse disorder. In a small number of cases, failure to properly identify psychiatric co-morbidity, particularly in CNS stimulant abuse, can lead to workplace violence. Psychiatric evaluation is beneficial both to help determine a patient's risk to self and others and to make an accurate diagnosis of a specific psychiatric disorder. Treatment plans may need modification upon identification of concomitant psychiatric disorders. The so-called "dual diagnosis" patient is now commonly accepted in chemical dependency treatment units, and many treatment facilities have dual diagnosis tracks—a phenomena that was rare only 10 years ago. The artificial boundary between substance abuse disorders and other behavioral disorders is steadily eroding. A strong alliance with company management, occupational medicine physicians, EAP professionals, and psychiatric consultants contributes strongly to successful diagnosis and treatment.

## URINE DRUG TESTING

Few topics have created more controversy in the workplace than urine drug testing. Urine testing was first adopted by the United States military in the 1980s. It was subsequently used by increasing numbers of employers in certain industries, particularly transportation and nuclear industries, both of which are required by federal statute to test employees. It is estimated that seven million Americans must now participate in mandatory urine drug testing as required by federal law. This requirement, in turn, has led to the accreditation of laboratories by the National Institute on Drug Abuse (NIDA). To acquire certification, laboratories must test for at least five drugs: amphetamines, cannabinoids, cocaine, opioids, and phencyclidine. Drug testing is typically conducted in the following instances: (1) preemployment testing of new employees; (2) random employee drug testing on an ongoing basis; and (3) "for cause" testing to evaluate an employee in the context of an unusual event like an accident on the job or acute behavioral changes.

Preemployment testing is of unclear benefit. One large study of prospective postal employees showed that preemployment test results that were positive for marijuana and cocaine use were associated with adverse employment outcomes as measured by accidents, absences, and turnover rates. The study did not evaluate testing for alcoholism, however. A number of authors have questioned the cost effectiveness of preemployment urine drug testing based on the low prevalence of positive tests. In the study of postal workers, only about 2% tested positive for cocaine and 8% for marijuana. Drug testing of airline employees has yielded less than one-half percent positives in a 1990 study. The true preventative value of preemployment urine drug testing needs to be further evaluated from a safety enhancement and cost/benefit viewpoint. To date, few large studies have been conducted to fully evaluate the effectiveness of these programs.

The rise of drug testing has led to the emergence of a new role as medical review officer (MRO) for physicians. The MRO is charged with reviewing positive urine test results. He or she is responsible for assuring the integrity of the "chain of custody" of the sample from employee to laboratory. The MRO also evaluates the mitigating circumstances related to a positive urine test, (eg, an employee who was taking prescribed medication at the time of the urine test). The MRO needs to be intimately knowledgeable of the pharmacology of the drugs being screened for, the causes of false positives and negatives, the specificity of various laboratory techniques used in drug testing, and the legal issues surrounding drug testing.

These legal issues include federal drug testing regulations, due process, and employee confidentiality. Only time and further research will define the role of drug testing in the workplace. It is clearly an area in which occupational medicine specialists need to be knowledgeable.

## INITIATING TREATMENT FOR SUBSTANCE ABUSE

Once the diagnosis of a substance abuse disorder is made, the employee (patient) needs to be referred for treatment. The level of treatment is determined by the patient's medical and psychological state. Patients with medical complications of substance abuse or those requiring detoxification may need inpatient hospitalization in a chemical dependency unit. This type of treatment is also appropriate for patients whose drug-seeking behavior is chaotic and compulsive. Those patients with acute psychiatric illness will need to be hospitalized in an inpatient unit. However, most patients with a substance abuse disorder can be treated on an outpatient basis. Enrollment in day treatment programs followed by a longer course of less intensive evening treatment is often used. Treatment programs involve education about problem-solving skills, stress and relationship management, and self-help programs like AA and Narcotics Anonymous (NA). Substance abuse and dependence are chronic medical problems that require ongoing treatment. One important role of the occupational medicine physician is to help develop and monitor a return-to-work agreement that outlines the employee's obligation to participate in ongoing care and recovery.

## REFERENCES

American Psychiatric Association: *Diagnostic and Statistical Manual of Mental Disorders,* 4th ed. APA, 1994.

Blum TC, Roman PM: Identifying alcoholics and persons with alcohol-related problems in the workplace: A description of EAP clients. Alcohol, Health and Research World 1992;16:120.

Brewer RD et al: The risk of dying in alcohol-related automobile crashes among habitual drunk drivers. N Engl J Med 1994;331:513.

Institute for Health Policy, Brandeis University: *Substance Abuse: The Nation's Number One Health Problem: Key Indicators for Policy.* Robert Wood Johnson Foundation, 1993.

Lowinson JH, Ruiz P, Millman RB (editors): *Substance Abuse: A Comprehensive Textbook,* 2nd ed. Williams and Wilkins, 1992.

Regier DA et al: Comorbidity of mental disorders with alcohol and other drug abuse: Results from the epidemiologic catchment area (ECA) study. JAMA 1990;264:2511.

Roman PM: Strategic considerations in designing interventions to deal with alcohol problems in the workplace. Pages 235–254 in: Roman PM (editor): *Alcohol Problem Intervention in the Workplace: Employee Assistance Programs and Strategic Alternatives.* Center of Alcohol Studies, Rutgers University, 1991.

Roman PM, Blum TC. Employee assistance and drug screening programs. In: Gerstein DR (editor): *Treating Drug Problems.* Vol 2. National Academy of Sciences Press, 1992.

Walsh DC et al: A randomized trial of treatment options for alcohol-abusing workers. N Engl J Med 1991;325:775.

Warner LA et al: Prevalence and correlates of drug use and dependence in the United States: Results from the national comorbidity survey. Arch Gen Psychiatry 1995; 52:219.

# Occupational Safety

# 36

*Franklyn G. Preiskop, MS, CSP, & Herman Woessner, MS, MA, CSP*

Occupational safety is the professional specialty concerned with the prevention and control of work related injuries, illnesses and other similarly caused harmful events. These events may include property damage and business disruption accidents, environmental incidents that threaten property or public health and safety, and product related injuries and illnesses.

Safety professionals are trained to recognize that all occupational "accidents" and harmful incidents (other than those that result from unpredictable acts of nature) can be anticipated from, and attributed to, substandard work conditions, substandard job practices, or both. These substandard work conditions and job practices are called hazards and are considered the last link in a chain of causation.

The safety professional is primarily concerned with empowering managers, supervisors, and employees with information to identify and control occupational hazards and their enabling factors. A hazard is the proximate cause of an injury or illness. Enabling factors are the underlying deficiencies within the organization's operations that produce or permit the existence of and exposure to a hazard.

The occupational health physician—whether employed directly by a company, retained on a consulting basis, or working in an occupational medicine clinic serving the industrial community—will be called upon to work with safety professionals. In very large organizations, the physician and the safety professional may be part of a loss-control team or may even work in the same department. In smaller organizations, the internal safety professional will often be the point of contact for the outside occupational physician.

The physician's interactions with the safety professional will occur in the following spheres, among others:

- Cooperating in the establishment of emergency medical facilities or services
- Performing individual medical monitoring of employees potentially exposed to occupational health hazards

- Designing and implementing medical screening programs for potential employees
- Participating in employee training programs on health hazards, chemical safety, and the use of personal protective equipment
- Evaluating the effectiveness of personal protective equipment
- Serving on management oversight committees reviewing the safety program's effectiveness
- Assisting in accident investigations or reviews
- Providing medical expertise in the areas of ergonomics or appropriate design of work stations
- Providing consultant services to management to interpret safety analyses

Whatever the level of of contact between the occupational health physician and the safety professional, it will be useful for the physician to understand the safety professional's background, role, and concerns.

## PROFESSIONAL EVOLUTION

Professional safety practice evolved in industrialized countries from the passage of workers' compensation laws in the early decades of the twentieth century and the enactment of employee protection laws and regulations in the decades following World War II.

The workers' compensation laws required employers to compensate injured workers for a portion of their loss wages and medical expenses regardless of fault. The certainty of having to indemnify injured employees led employers to place greater emphasis on accident prevention. Prevention measures mostly consisted of worksite safety inspections, employee hazard awareness training and the installation of guards around hazardous machinery. Gradually, the responsibilities and duties of the "safety engineer" and "safety inspector" became job classifications within many organizations.

The employee protection laws and regulations that have been passed in every industrialized country since World War II have greatly accelerated the growth of the safety profession and expanded its range of activities. In the United States, the Occupational Safety and Health Act of 1970 (OSH Act) created the Occupational Safety and Health Administration (OSHA), an administrative agency within the Department of Labor, and made it responsible for the promulgation and enforcement of safety standards applicable to employers. An increasing number of OSHA standards have recognized certified safety professionals, as well as certified industrial hygienists and physicians, as "qualified" and "competent" to evaluate and control regulated hazards.

## PROFESSIONAL QUALIFICATIONS

The modern safety professional usually has a bachelor's degree but is no longer necessarily an engineer (fewer than 40% have engineering degrees). More valuable today than engineering expertise are degrees in management, business administration, or systems analysis. Several universities offer baccalaureate, masters, and even doctoral degrees specifically in occupational safety and health or safety management, with a few state and community colleges now offering associate degrees or technical certification in the field.

The highest professional designation in the safety profession in the United States is that of Certified Safety Professional (CSP). It is awarded by an independent "Board of Certified Safety Professionals," to practitioners who have passed both a core subject and comprehensive practice examination. To be eligible to take the examinations, safety practitioners must submit two professional references and have 96 units of education and/or professional experience. One month's work experience is equal to one unit and 48 units are allotted for a college degree.

Beginning in 1998, CSP candidates will be required to have a baccalaureate degree or an associates degree in safety from an accredited college or university to be eligible to take the examination, regardless of their number of years of professional experience.

Currently two states, California and Massachusetts, license professional safety engineers. Candidates for the Professional Engineer (PE) in Safety registration must have a bachelor's degree in engineering from an accredited engineering program and five years of professional experience, and must have passed the engineering fundamentals examination and a professional safety practice examination. Many safety practitioners who received their Safety PE registration in California, however, did not obtain their title by meeting these qualifications, but rather were granted registration based on professional experience supported by professional engineering and safety references. Most Safety PEs do not practice solely in the field of safety engineering.

There are any number of other safety certifications

awarded by a wide assortment of professional and academic organizations, but the CSP designation remains the most credible credential for the safety professional.

## FUNCTIONAL RESPONSIBILITIES OF SAFETY PRACTITIONERS

At present, there are well over 20,000 safety practitioners in the United States. Their functional responsibilities vary widely depending on the size and type of organization, the degree of inherent risks within the workplace and the level of safety management expertise. In a small service organization, for example, the "safety person" is often a nonprofessional whose responsibilities are limited to ensuring that the organization complies with applicable OSHA regulations. In a medium size manufacturing company, on the other hand, the safety practitioner may be a trained professional with a wide range of safety and loss control responsibilities. In large, complex organizations, the full scope of safety and loss control responsibilities is usually covered by a staff of certified professionals from among several different departments. The staff may include safety professionals, industrial hygienists, occupational physicians and nurses, engineers, environmental specialists, insurance personnel, security officers and fire protection professionals.

The responsibilities of safety professionals may be grouped into six broad functional categories: (1) safety engineering: the systematic analysis of equipment, tasks, and processes to identify inherent hazards and failure modes, and the development of hazard prevention and control measures based on the findings; (2) safety management: the application of management principles and methods to facilitate and coordinate the establishment and achievement of safety goals and objectives; (3) loss control: the application of safety engineering and safety management methods for the prevention and mitigation of all types of loss-producing events; (4) safety inspection and auditing: observation and evaluation of worksites, job tasks, and policies and procedures to identify deficiencies or omissions that could contribute to an occupational injury or illness; (5) regulatory compliance: communication of applicable safety and health regulations to affected personnel and monitoring of response activities to ensure compliance with the regulatory requirements; (6) education and training: the development, conducting, and/or coordinating of safety training for employees, supervisors and managers.

Many safety practitioners specialize within one or two of the functional categories, and some even concentrate on a subspecialty within a category (eg, traffic safety engineering, electrical safety inspection, hazardous materials training); most, however, perform some duties that fall within each of the broad functions. Some functional specialists and generalists work their entire careers in the same industry and become industry safety specialists. These may include construction safety professionals, chemical safety engineers, and railroad safety inspectors.

## SAFETY & HEALTH MANAGEMENT SYSTEM[1]

One of the principal responsibilities of a safety professional in any organization is to facilitate and coordinate the development and implementation of an effective safety and health management system. The elements of this system are the related policies, goals, plans, programs, procedures, and standards. Their collective purpose is to systematically guide the organization to (1) prevent work related injuries and illnesses (2) comply with applicable health and safety regulations and (3) minimize injury/illness and compliance costs.

Safety professionals seek to make the occupational safety and health management system a self-regulating process by incorporating performance monitoring, feedback, and correction capabilities. These capabilities can be established either as a separate administrative policy/procedure or as an administrative section in each of the organization's hazard control programs and procedures.

The administrative policies and procedures of a safety and health management system are developed to ensure that the system functions properly and consistently. The hazard control programs and procedures are intended to guide affected personnel in the recognition and control of specified hazards.

Some of the system's administrative and hazard control elements may be required by government regulation. The safety professional is usually responsible for ensuring that the safety and health management system includes these required elements. The elements of an organization's safety and health management system are listed in Table 36–1.

## ELEMENTS OF THE SAFETY SYSTEM

### Training

The safety professional is primarily concerned with the prevention of accidents. This can be accomplished to a large extent through proper training of employees. The primary cause of accidents in the workplace is not unsafe machinery or dangerous chemicals—it is the lack of understanding by employees about the nature or severity of the hazards surrounding them.

A prudent employer will provide employees with adequate training to warn them of hazards peculiar to their jobs and instruct them in safe operating practices. The OSH Act required that workers be warned about hazardous materials through the use of warning labels and similar devices, and also that workers be made aware of the relevant symptoms of overexposure and of emergency treatment procedures. But the most important feature of the law is that which requires employers to make workers understand appropriate precautions.

Since the passage of the OSH Act, many other federal and state hazard communications have been promulgated. These require the employer to train workers to understand the labeling of hazardous materials and to use the Material Safety Data Sheets (MSDS) that must be maintained for all chemicals and other hazardous substances to which the worker may be exposed. Various OSH ACT standards also require specialized training for employees operating specific types of equipment (forklifts, cranes, powered punch presses, etc). These laws require that numerous training programs be established for workers in various job categories or working conditions.

### Communication

Safety committees draw together individuals from throughout the work force so they can pool their experience and efforts to achieve greater safety. Several types of safety committees may be formed to fulfill various needs within the organization. The company physician may be asked to serve on an executive committee functioning as an oversight committee for the safety department or on a general planning committee. Other safety committees might include supervisory committees, joint union-management committees, and shop workers committees.

Safety suggestion boxes are a form of communication. To make them effective however, management—often through its delegated representative, the safety professional—must demonstrate that it listens to all serious suggestions and responds in a timely and serious manner.

Safety posters, placards, and signs are also forms of communication. They are effective only insofar as they are kept relevant to the hazards and, in the case of posters, if they are frequently changed to stimulate safety awareness.

### Emergency Response Programs

The safety professional must recognize the need to prepare for a disaster or emergency situation.

**A. Evacuation Planning:** Federal, state, and

---

[1]The safety and health management system of an organization is the same as its safety and health program. The term "management system" was chosen over the word "program" because it is more descriptive and less apt to be confused with its sub-program elements.

**Table 36–1.** Elements of a safety and health management system.

| Administrative Elements | Hazard Control Elements |
|---|---|
| Safety and Health (S&H) Policy Statement | Code of Safe Practices[1] |
| Statement of S&H Responsibilities | Hazard Identification and Control Program |
| Procedure for Communicating S&H Information[1] | Job Safety Analysis Program |
| Process & Criteria for Setting S&H Performance Goals & Indicators | Hazardous Energy Control Procedure[1] (Lockout/Tagout) |
| S&H Program Audit, Feedback and Correction Program | Hazardous Substance Control and Communication Program (Haz/Com)[1] |
| S&H Education and Training Procedure[1] | Confined Space Safety Program[1] |
| Procedure for Development of Annual S&H Plan and Budget | Trenching and Shoring Safety Program[1] |
| Procedure for Establishing and Operating S&H Committees | Vehicle Operation Safety Program |
| S&H Procedure and Standards for Engineering Designs | Laboratory Hygiene Program[1] |
| Contractor S&H Procedure | Ergonomic Hazard Control Program[2] |
| OSHA Compliance Procedure | Indoor Air Quality Program[2] |
| Program for Employee S&H Participation | Personal Protective Equipment Standards[1] |
| Medical Management Program[1] | Respiratory Protection Program[1] |
| S&H Performance Evaluation Criteria Accountability Process | Hearing Conservation Program[1] |
| | Housekeeping Standards |
| | Accident/Incident Investigation Procedure[1] |

[1]OSHA required program, procedure, or activity.
[2]Pending OSHA requirement.

local authorities now require that businesses establish emergency evacuation plans. Items to consider in an evacuation plan include the following:

1. What events might precipitate an evacuation?
2. What other notifications are necessary—medical, fire department, police, etc?
3. What medical facilities are likely to be needed?
4. Will electrical and gas services be shut down also?
5. Are there manufacturing processes that should be shut down in emergencies?
6. Who can authorize evacuation?
7. How will the employees be instructed to evacuate?
8. Who will be responsible to see that evacuation is carried out?
9. Where should evacuated employees go?
10. How will it be determined that all employees, contractor personnel, and visitors been evacuated?
11. Who will do the shutdowns? How? Are they trained?

**B. Chemical Response Teams:** Plants that use large quantities of toxic or dangerous chemicals will often form specialized teams of employees to contain or control exposures to the employees, the general public, or the environment resulting from accidental discharge. The occupational physician will often be asked to help in the planning and training stages when these teams are formed.

**C. Fire Brigades:** Industries or operations located at remote sites or with special fire hazards often require the formation of fire-fighting teams. These trained employees are responsible for ensuring swift reaction to the outbreak of fire and for containing the fire until professional help arrives.

**D. Emergency Medical Facilities:** State regulations now require almost all places of employment to provide a minimum level of emergency medical capability. Depending on the exposures involved, the safety professional, in concert with the occupational physician, might wish to significantly improve on this minimum requirement.

For an office building with no special hazards, the Red Cross Multi-Media training certifications for two or three employees, perhaps with CPR training added, might very well be sufficient. However, a hazardous chemical processing plant would require at least several EMT-1 level trained personnel and perhaps even an occupational health nurse or an on-site occupational physician for each shift.

## Personal Protective Equipment

One method of providing for employee safety in hazardous conditions is the use of personal protective equipment. These devices are intended to protect employees in case an accident occurs or to insulate the employee from a hazardous condition (noise, dusts, fumes, etc) that is part of the normal operation.

The basic problem with personal protective devices is that the individual must understand the need to wear the protection, must wear it properly, and must maintain the device in good working condition. In situations where engineering or administrative controls are not yet effective in eliminating the hazard, protective devices must be issued as a last line of defense to prevent injury to the employee. The occupational health physician may be called on by the safety professional to consult about the appropriateness of the device chosen or to assist in educating employees about the necessity for the device.

Any program that provides personal protective equipment to employees must follow the same basic procedures. First, the hazards must be evaluated to ensure that the equipment will be appropriate. Second, the equipment itself must be checked to see that it meets all applicable government standards of manufacture. Employees must be informed of the hazards involved and be trained in how to wear protective equipment and maintain it properly. Supervisors must be trained to ensure that the protection is worn at all times when it is needed. Warnings must be posted to inform everyone of the need for protection.

## Inspections & Monitoring

The safety professional, especially in the industrial environment, is responsible for numerous inspections and periodic monitoring. The principal monitoring technique is measurement of airborne chemical contamination levels and physical exposure levels to noise, vibration, and ionizing and nonionizing radiation. While monitoring is usually performed by an industrial hygienist, the safety professional is often required to perform some routine monitoring. Individual medical monitoring is also required under certain conditions. Again, while monitoring and testing are usually done under the direction of the occupational health physician, the safety professional is often charged with the administrative and record-keeping details of the program.

Physical inspections are the direct responsibility of the safety professional. Federal and state regulations now require periodic inspections of the work envi-

ronment designed to recognize hazard potentials. Often this type of inspection is actually performed as part of the safety committee's duties, so that various points of view are brought to bear in the attempt to identify accident potentials. However, even when this is the case, the safety professional must review the results and recommendations.

Various pieces of equipment also require periodic inspection to ensure that they are in place, fully functional, certified, and suitable for their intended purposes.

## Chemical Safety

Specific hazards to employees must be recognized and detailed for each chemical or process. Where feasible, engineering controls such as containment, automated processing, or ventilation systems should be installed. Administrative controls such as job rotation or multistationed work processes may be used to control exposures in some circumstances. Where applicable, personal protective equipment must be issued. Periodic monitoring of environmental chemical exposures should be established. Chemical safety training specific to the processes involved must be given to all employees. With certain chemicals, employee health monitoring may be required. Safe chemical handling rules and process instructions must be initiated. Emergency containment or evacuation systems must be initiated. Emergency shutdown and protection equipment must be installed and employees trained in their use. Finally, all of the above procedures and equipment must be periodically reviewed to ensure proper functioning of control measures and to see that controls are adequate. Material safety data sheets must be obtained and reviewed on all chemicals used in the work setting.

## OTHER SAFETY PROGRAM ELEMENTS

### Fire Protection

Safety professionals are usually required to take charge of fire protection activities of the organization as well as employee safety functions. In fact, only organizations with extraordinary casualty exposure will employ a fire protection engineer.

The primary duty is of course to prevent fires. The fire safety program follows much the same pattern as has been outlined for the employee safety program, which was designed to keep injuries from occurring: (1) training, (2) communications, (3) emergency protective equipment, (4) chemical safety, and (5) accident investigation.

The safety professional should be involved in the construction and remodeling of facilities as well as occupancy plans in order to create a relatively fire-protected office or plant environment. Once the facility has been constructed, fire prevention activities are usually limited to monitoring of hazardous areas, fire emergency planning, training, and monitoring of the adequacy of fire suppression equipment.

## Vehicle Fleet Safety

Management usually does not realize the severity of its losses to vehicular accidents unless the company happens to operate an unusually large number of vehicles or is in the transportation industry. The safety professional should gain control of this area of responsibility, as it frequently represents one of the major sources of injury within an organization.

The safety professional would begin with documentation to obtain clear-cut authority for a control program through the company's safety policy and directives.

Employee or applicant screening is probably the major loss control option available to the employer. This is one of the few areas where there is sufficient legal precedent to allow medical and driver-history screening of drivers. Therefore, the safety professional will rely upon the occupational health physician to devise an adequate and responsible medical screening program to meet the employer's needs.

The second element of the fleet vehicle safety program must be a preventive maintenance program on all vehicles. This program must be meticulously documented in order to be of any value in dealing with insurers or the government agencies that monitor them.

The remaining fleet vehicle safety program elements again are training, communications, emergency planning, accident investigation, and inspections or monitoring.

## Product Safety & Product Liability

Manufacturers—especially those whose products end up in the hands of the private consumer or in high-technology systems (eg nuclear reactors, commercial aircraft, or aerospace modules)—are vitally concerned with the safety of their products. It is not uncommon for the organization's safety professional to become involved in product safety or product liability reviews.

A product safety review must consider first the intended uses and foreseeable misuses of the product. The aim of the review is to provide the most painstaking analysis—often using the techniques known as systems safety analysis (see below)—to ensure the product's correct and safe functioning under the most adverse foreseeable usage.

The product liability review is performed to determine how to assess or limit (to the extent possible) the legal liability of any unsafe operation of the product that might occur. From this review, the manufacturer—or its product liability insurance carrier—can determine the probable extent to which the manufacturer may be held liable in litigation for product operations or failures that cause personal injury or property damage.

## MANAGEMENT APPROACHES TO ACCIDENT PREVENTION

### Systems Safety

Systems safety analysis is not a single technique or process but rather a group of analytic techniques wherein operations (such as manufacturing a printed circuit board) or machines (such as punch presses) are viewed as if they were a single system. That system should in turn have each of its discrete parts, steps, or functions analyzed for potential hazards. All of this must be limited by practical considerations of operational effectiveness, time availability, and cost-effectiveness.

The traditional approach to safety is called the "fly-fix-fly" method, wherein an operation is initiated or a machine designed and put into use and then, if the operation or machine breaks down, causes an accident, or generally does not perform as expected, it is redesigned, reengineered, or otherwise changed. The operation or machine is then put back into use again until another problem is found with it. However, there are certain systems for which we cannot afford the first accident, such as the core meltdown of a nuclear reactor, an accidental nuclear weapons explosion, the crash of a commercial airliner, the loss of a manned space shuttle, or the release of a toxic gas cloud in an urban area.

This is not to say that these catastrophes cannot happen but rather that the manufacturers and operators involved must approach these potentials *as if* they cannot be allowed to happen. To guard against such potential safety calamities, the following safety approaches may be used.

**A. Failure Modes and Effects Analysis:** One of the earliest "systems safety" approaches was developed by reliability engineers to identify problems that could arise from machinery malfunctions. The technique analyzes each of the components, sub-assemblies, and subsystems, to find out how each might fail and what effect its failure would have on the system as a whole.

**B. Fault Hazard Analysis:** This refinement of the foregoing considers only those failure modes that could cause an accident, ignoring all other failures or failure modes. This allows analysis of larger systems while not requiring the reviewer to be bogged down in extraneous detail. Criticality ratings are used to see which components or subsystems need design changes, tighter production controls, more comprehensive testing, specialized safeguards, monitoring, shielding, etc.

**C. Fault Tree Analysis:** Unlike the first two techniques, which consider all possible individual failures in order to find out what they would do to the system as a whole, fault tree analysis takes a single undesirable event (such as leakage of a toxic gas from a process) and works backward, trying to establish what could cause leakage to occur. Quantitative values are assigned to individual failure points to show the likelihood that failure will occur. The use of flow-charting clearly demonstrates the relationships between the various components and thus encourages the analyst to consider cumulative failure possibilities (ie, two or more simultaneous component failures that cause the event).

**D. Human Factors Analysis:** This technique was developed to fit the human operator into the system with the maximum safety. Most machinery is designed for the convenience of the work flow or operation, and the operator is required to adapt to the machine's requirements. Because the human being is the most adaptable component in the system, it is relatively easy to make the system fit the "average" physical form. This leads designers and engineers to ignore the human element. Recognition that the "average" human physique and operating limits did not meet all the needs of industry gave emphasis to this discipline.

The most common need is for adjustability of work stations to fit the operator. The occupational health physician can be useful in this systems safety technique by providing consultation and physical data on body mobility, environmental stresses, repetitive motion effects, and sensory inputs.

More challenging still is the fitting of the operator's psychologic and cultural differences into the work environment. The fact that blue instead of red may be the color associated with "stop" or "emergency" in some cultures has cost the lives of workers.

## Employee Operations & Management Reviews

Systems safety analysis was initially concerned only with equipment failures because it grew out of the quality control discipline. Later, it was realized that the operator is more than just a physical element in the system. The human decisions and actions were in fact a major risk factor and therefore had to be considered as part of the system. Finally, systems safety practitioners began applying the techniques of this discipline to human organizations.

**A. Job Safety Analysis:** This technique was developed during World War II when large numbers of inexperienced workers had to be integrated into the work force quickly and safely. By systematic observation and detailed analysis, one uncovers the inherent hazards in the work environment. This task can be performed by supervisors, who in turn gain great understanding and appreciation of the areas under their control. The employees who participate develop a better recognition of the hazards they face. Finally, use of this technique develops an effective

teaching tool and documentation upon which personnel departments may effectively base their physical hiring requirements for certain jobs.

**B. Techniques for Human Error Rate Prediction:** These techniques are primarily methods for quantifying what has been called "pilot error" in the broad sense of that term to determine probabilities of occurrence. Since they are solely directed toward human errors, they are often used in conjunction with fault tree analysis or failure modes and effects analysis.

In this approach, all human tasks are broken down into the smallest possible discrete actions. Each component task is referenced to a set of tables reflecting basic human tasks with the probability of functioning correctly considered for each of nine potential error states. A "basic error rate" can be obtained, expressed as errors per million operations. These values have been obtained through detailed clinical research.

**C. Management Oversight Risk Tree:** This technique was developed to combine the systems safety analysis techniques with modern management techniques. The result was a large analytic diagram or flow chart portraying the operation of a safety management program in a logical and orderly manner, with the actual safety program compared with an idealized system. The evaluator can thus detect omissions, oversights, and ineffective programs. The defects might be as diverse as poor training or employee misconduct, and the effective diagnosis of these problems provides the evaluator with a tool for loss control.

**D. Technique of Operation Review:** This is a system for analyzing the root causes of accidents or other undesired events. The examiner starts with an undesired event and cross-references it on a chart with a large number of organizational processes (training, supervision, management, etc). The technique provides a simplistic but systematic method of examining potential causes of causes within an organization in relation to any specific failure event.

## Root-Cause Identification & Control

Permanent control of unsafe work conditions and unsafe job practices requires elimination of their underlying support system. Correcting hazards without eliminating their "root causes" treats only the symptoms of the problem; the hazards will reappear eventually.

Safety professionals identify the enabling or root causal factors of hazards by systematically analyzing the events, conditions, and values that logic, experience, and training lead them to believe could have contributed to the existence of the hazard. The findings are then evaluated to determine where, how and why the organization's safety and health management system failed to prevent or control the enabling factors. Permanent control of these factors is achieved by correcting identified inconsistencies, contradictions, and omissions in the organization's safety and health policies, programs, and procedures.

## Accident & Incident Investigation

Accidents are defined as unintended events that result in injury, illness, and/or material loss. Unintended events that have the potential to cause human and/or material harm, but which do not only because of chance, are called incidents. Many safety professionals prefer to use the term incident to describe both types of events, because there is a general misconception that accidents are "freak," random occurrences that can not be anticipated. This view can retard an organization's prevention efforts and lead to the recurrence of loss-producing events. Safety professionals regard accidents/incidents as preventable events that indicate correctable deficiencies in the organization's safety and loss control system.

An injury or illness incident occurs when a harmful amount of energy or toxicity is transferred via an unsafe work condition or unsafe job practice to an exposed employee. This transference may occur acutely, as in the case of unprotected contact with a rotating saw blade or with a corrosive chemical, or chronically, from such hazardous exposures as frequent repetitive body motions and long-term inhalation of small amounts of toxic vapors.

Safety professionals conduct and/or coordinate accident/incident investigations to uncover their proximate and enabling causal factors so that measures can be identified and implemented to prevent a recurrence. The investigation process involves the systematic collection, analysis, documentation and communication of relevant information.

Accidents almost never have just one cause but are the result of chains of events and circumstances. Finding the causes of an accident calls for more than simply reviewing the injured employee's actions at the scene; the physical conditions and all equipment must be scrutinized to determine what could be done to prevent recurrences. Such items as work flow patterns, environmental conditions, and stress levels must also be considered. One of the main purposes of accident investigation is to initiate changes or preventive measures to prevent repetitions.

In most routine accidents, it is helpful if the supervisor or manager conducts the accident investigation in order to learn from the experience, though the safety professional will have to instruct the supervisors or managers in how to proceed and should review the results.

Safety professionals often develop a written procedure to systematically guide the investigative process. The procedure typically identifies the types of accidents and incidents that are to be investigated; who is to conduct the investigation, when the investigation is to be commenced and ended, where it is to take place, how it is to be conducted, who is to communicate the findings, and the form in which communications will be made. The accident/incident investigation procedure is an important element of any organization's safety and health management system.

## Safety Performance Goals & Indicators

An important function of safety professionals is to help their organization develop and administer safety performance goals and indicators. There are two types: results-directed and behavior-directed. Results-directed safety goals and indicators focus on the consequences of desired safety behaviors, while behavior-directed safety goals and indicators are concerned with the safety behaviors themselves.

The total injury and illness case rate is the principle results-directed safety performance indicator of most organizations. It can be compared against last year's rate and to the industry average to help determine if current safety performance is acceptable. An annual goal to reduce this rate below the industry average or below last year's total case rate would be examples of a results-directed goal.

The frequency and quality of employee safety meetings are examples of a behavior-directed performance indicator. The greater the frequency and the better the quality of employee safety meeting, the less likely are job errors and unsafe work practices. A behavior-directed goal would be to have qualified trainers hold structured safety meetings every month.

Safety professionals regularly monitor and analyze the safety performance indicators to help identify any significant behavioral or loss trends. This information helps management track the organization's progress toward achievement of its stated performance goals and to implement timely corrections of indicated deficiencies in the safety and loss control system. Key results-directed and behavior-directed performance indicators are listed in Table 36–2.

## OSHA COMPLIANCE

Overseeing the organization's efforts to comply with OSHA regulations is a major responsibility for all safety practitioners. They fulfill this responsibility by analyzing and interpreting the regulations to determine their applicability to the organization, and then communicating the requirements to the affected personnel. They also develop written programs and procedures that are required by the regulations and conduct or arrange mandated training for employees.

If industrial hygiene or medical specialists are employed with the organization, they usually have the lead responsibility for analyzing and interpreting complex health-related regulations. If these special-

**Table 36–2.** Key results-directed and behavior-directed indicators.

| Results-Directed Indicators | Behavior-Directed Indicators |
|---|---|
| Total Case Rate: number of injuries and illnesses × 200,000 hours[1] ÷ number of hours worked | Frequency and quality of workplace safety and loss control inspections |
| Loss Time Case Rate: number of lost time cases × 200,000 hours ÷ number of hours worked | Frequency and quality of job safety observations |
| Lost & Restricted Case Rate: number of lost time and restricted work cases × 200,000 hours ÷ number of hours worked | Frequency and quality of employee safety training |
| Lost & Restricted Day Rate: number of days lost and restricted × 200,000 hours ÷ number of hours worked | Frequency and quality of safety program audits |
| Total Workers Compensation Reserves: the amount of money reserved by the insurance company to pay for current year's injuries/illnesses | Frequency and quality of employee safety meetings |
| Experience Modification Factor: the multiplier based on injury/illness experience used by insurance companies to determine workers compensation premiums. An "ex-mod" factor greater than one is high | Frequency and quality of safety communications to employees |
| Property Damage and Business Interruption Costs: the direct and indirect costs resulting from accidents involving property damage and/or business interruption | Frequency and quality of safety performance appraisals |
| Vehicle Accident Incidence Rate: the number of vehicle accidents × 25,000, 100,000, or 1,000,000 miles ÷ number of miles driven in a year | Frequency and quality of employee safety suggestions |
| Total Vehicle Accident Costs: the direct and indirect costs to pay for accident and to restore vehicles | Timeliness of required responses to employee safety suggestions |
| Annual Number of OSHA Citations: the total number of citations received in a year | Timeliness and quality of accident/incident investigations |
| Cost of OSHA Penalties: annual cost of penalties for OSHA citations | Frequency of personal protection equipment inspections and observations |
| Number and Cost of Product Liability Claims: the annual number and cost of customer injury/illness claims from product defects | Quality and frequency of safety committee meetings |
| Number and Cost of Environmental Accidents/Incidents: the annual number and cost of mishaps that impair the environment, injure members of the public, or both | Frequency and quality of employee involvement in program development and implementation activities |

[1]200,000 hours is the number of hours 100 employees work in 1 year.

ists are not available in the organization, the safety professional will often consult with an external industrial hygienist or occupational physician.

There are many safety and health regulations that directly pertain to occupational physicians. In the United States, OSHA specifically references medical practitioners in regulations covering such subjects as bloodborne pathogens; physical examinations for asbestos, lead, cadmium, arsenic, and other specified toxic substances; biologic monitoring; audiometric and hearing examinations; respiratory protection; pulmonary function testing; laboratory hygiene; regulated carcinogens; sanitation; and hazard communications.

In the outline of the typical OSHA regulation there are four distinct subdivisions:

I. General topic.
  A. Specific sub-topic.
    1. Sub-topic definitions and requirements.
      a. Specifications for sub-topic requirements.

Identifying these subdivisions in the printed regulations will aid clarity and expedite analysis.

The occupational physician who is well informed about OSHA regulations will be better prepared to provide the diagnostic and treatment methods required by government regulations and to work with other safety and health professionals to identify deficiencies in the organization's regulatory compliance efforts that could adversely affect employee health and safety.

## LOSS-CONTROL MANAGEMENT

Safety practitioners like other occupational and safety and health professionals have the well-being of employees as their primary concern, but unlike the other specialists (at least until recently), some safety professionals have the closely related secondary responsibility of loss-control management.

Loss-control management involves planning, organizing, and leading the organization's efforts to prevent all types of loss-producing events and to control the monetary cost when such an event occurs. A loss-producing event is an incident in which either the value of an organizational asset declines or the cost of preserving it increases.

Losses are measured in monetary terms. Accidents and harmful exposures that cause employee injury or illness, property damage, business disruption, environmental impairment, loss worker productivity, adverse public relations, and labor strife are all loss-producing events; they directly or indirectly cost the organization money.

Employees are the most valuable assets of an organization, so the loss control responsibilities of safety practitioners are consistent with and supportive of their injury and illness-prevention interests. Nevertheless, there is a potential for conflict whenever cost considerations may compete with health and safety concerns. This potential for conflict is based on the same kind of issues that characterize the debate over managed health care: physicians wish to deliver the best care to their patients without interference and monetary restrictions from the care-payers (health insurance companies), while the care-payers wish to keep the cost of medical care as low as possible.

In the United States, employers pay for the cost of injury care and workers' compensation through their insurance premiums. They expect, therefore, loss-control managers and health-care providers to protect employee health and safety cost-effectively. To achieve this objective, both prevention and case management efforts are required, with the prevention efforts being the most cost-effective.

## CASE MANAGEMENT

Employers want their loss-control representative and the treating physician to ensure that injured employees receive the proper medical care necessary to return them to full health in the shortest period of time for the least amount of money. The following are ways in which safety professionals and occupational physicians can and should collaborate for better case management.

Safety professionals can provide relevant work history and exposure information to treating physicians as soon as possible after an employee injury and illness is reported. If the safety practitioner fails to provide such information in a timely manner, the physician or an assistant should contact him/her for input prior to completion of the diagnosis.

Nothing can sour the relationship between an employer and a health care provider more quickly than a controversial medical diagnosis that is, or is perceived to be, based on inaccurate or biased information. Physicians can prevent both the reality and perception of an inaccurate or biased diagnosis by obtaining prior input relative to the injured employee's work history and exposure. Information obtained by the occupational physician through annual facility visits and discussions with managers will help to preclude misdiagnoses and misperceptions, and can obviate the need for case input from safety professionals except in unusual cases.

Safety professionals should provide, and medical care providers should seek, information on the organization's modified-duty program and available modified-duty jobs in advance of the determination of a treatment protocol for an injured or ill employee. Insurance data indicates that employees with nondisabling injuries who are placed in a job they are able to perform recover sooner than they would have if they were given time off from work. A lack of a monetary incentive to return to work, insufficient physical and mental exercise and/or the performance of stressful home chores probably account for the slower home healing rates. Safety professionals and occupational physicians can work together on presentations and programs to educate employers about the health and cost benefits of providing modified-duty jobs.

## TOTAL SAFETY MANAGEMENT SYSTEM

The total quality management movement (TQM) was launched by Edward Deming and Joseph Juran in Japan in the 1950s and has spread since then to every advanced country in the world. TQM principles and methods now form the foundation of modern management theory and practice. They provide for continuous organizational improvement through dedicated leadership, a commitment to customer satisfaction, employee empowerment, team management, systems analysis, application of statistical quality controls, extensive training and retraining, and the balancing of cost concerns with quality considerations.

Some safety and health managers have long advocated similar views for improving the quality of safety performance in their organization and many more have adopted the TQM approach in recent years. Their goal is to establish a management system that provides for constant improvement in the quality of all of the organization's safety and loss-control efforts and for continual reduction in the number, frequency, and severity of harmful events.

The safety quality movement has evolved to the point that a technical committee of the International Standards Organization (ISO) has been formed to develop safety and health assessment criteria. Many safety and health professionals wish to have ISO Occupational Safety and Health standards similar to the ones established under ISO 9000 for quality assurance and under the draft ISO 14000 for environmental management. The ultimate goal is to have universally-applicable guidance and assessment documents for quality assurance of the design and performance of an organization's occupational safety and health management system.

## REFERENCES

Bird FE, Germain GL: *Practical Loss Control Leadership*. Institute Publishing, Division of International Loss Control Institute, 1990.

Boylston RP: *Managing Safety and Health Programs*. Van Nostrand Reinhold, 1990.

The Center for Chemical Process Safety: *Hazard Evaluation Procedures*, 2nd ed. American Institute of Chemical Engineers, 1992.

Drucker P: *Managing in a Time of Great Change*. Truman Tally Books, 1995.

Hammer W: *Product Safety Management and Engineering*. ASSE, 1994.

Health E, Ferry TS: *Training in the Workplace*. Aloray, 1990.

Krause TR, Hidley JH, Hodson SJ: *The Behavior-Based Safety Process*. Van Nostrand Reinhold, 1990.

Lack R (editor): *Essentials of Safety and Health Management*. Lewis, 1996.

National Safety Council: Accident Prevention Manual for Industrial Operations, 9th ed. National Safety Council, 1992.

Roland HE, Moriarty B: *System Safety Engineering and Management*. John Wiley & Sons, 1990.

Sashkin M,& Kiser KJ: *Putting Total Quality Management to Work*. Berrett-Koehler, 1993.

Vicoli JW: *Basic Guide to Accident Investigation and Loss Control*. Van Nostrand Reinhold, 1994.

# 37

# Industrial Hygiene

*Douglas P. Fowler, PhD, CIH*

The four definitive elements of industrial hygiene (often called occupational Hygene outside the United States) are the anticipation, recognition, evaluation, and control of health hazards arising in or from the workplace. (*Hazards arising from the workplace include the potential harm that may arise in the community by uncontrolled emissions and such issues as familial exposures from harmful debris taken home on workers' clothing.*) The anticipation and recognition of health hazards have primacy, since they must take place before proper evaluation or control (if needed) can take place. Upon anticipation or recognition of a health hazard, the industrial hygienist should be able to identify measures necessary for proper evaluation. Upon completion of the evaluation, the industrial hygienist then is in a position—in consultation with other members of the occupational health and safety team—to recommend and implement controls needed to reduce risks to within tolerable limits.

## ANTICIPATION OF HEALTH HAZARDS IN THE WORKPLACE

The duty to anticipate health hazards in the workplace is a relatively new addition to the industrial hygienist's traditional responsibilities for recognition, evaluation, and control; and is a heavy, but necessary burden. Anticipation of health hazards may range from a reasonable expectation to mere speculation, but it implies that the industrial hygienist will understand the nature of changes in the processes, products, environments, and workforces of the workplace and how those changes might affect human health or well-being. As an example, transplanting a successful chemical process from a unionized workplace in the US or Canada to another country without understanding important cultural factors or the extent of the industrial experience in that country might cause significant risk of harm to the workers in that new country. As another example, changing weekly work schedules from five 8-hour days to three 12-hour days will almost certainly produce dislocation among

the work force due to the psychosocial and physical effects of shift work, but may also lead to the danger of chemical intoxication, if the chemical exposures are such as to lead to the buildup of excessive body burdens, without the usual 16-hour "rest" period.

An important aspect of anticipation will be an understanding of past exposures and practices, and how that past experience may act to cause injury to those exposed. Such retrospective exposure assessment is, of course, essential to the performance of epidemiological studies in order to come to a sound understanding of risks associated with occupational experience. The industrial hygienist is the person most likely to be able to perform such a retrospective study.

## RECOGNITION OF HEALTH HAZARDS IN THE WORKPLACE

In a workplace where the processes are well established, the recognition of health hazards is the first step in the process that leads to evaluation and control through the identification of materials and processes that have the potential for causing harm to workers. Sources of information about health hazards include clinical data about health problems in exposed populations; information in scientific journals, bulletins of trade associations, and reports of government agencies; conversations with peers; and direct reports from workers, union representatives, supervisors, or employers.

Inspection of the workplace is the best source of directly relevant information about potential health hazards. There is no substitute for observation by an experienced observer of work practices, the use of chemical and physical agents, and the apparent effectiveness of control measures. The physician should be able to recognize major and obvious health hazards, and distinguish those that require formal evaluation by the industrial hygienist.

### The Walk-Through Survey
The "walk-through survey," in the company of the occupational physician, is the first and most impor-

tant technique used to recognize occupational health hazards.

The survey should begin with a proper introduction to plant management, a discussion of the purpose of the survey, and an inquiry about any relevant recent complaints. If appropriate, a simplified process flow diagram should also be prepared at this time.

Following the process flow through the plant is usually most productive. The survey might thus begin at the loading dock, where materials entering the plant can be examined. Warning labels, descriptive language about the chemical composition of materials, and the packaging of incoming materials should be noted. Questions should then be asked regarding the handling of unknown materials or materials about which insufficient information is available. The incoming materials should then be followed into the process flow stream, and each of the processes of interest in the plant should be observed in action. Of interest throughout the survey will be the methods used for materials handling and the labeling of materials, particularly at points where they are transferred from manufacturers' containers into other vessels for use within the plant.

### Observations to Be Made

At each point in the process, the industrial hygienist and physician should observe all handling procedures as well as any protective measures that are employed. Controls that may be appropriate are listed below in the discussion of control of health hazards. Use of respiratory protection and protective clothing should be recorded, as well as other common-sense observations such as the apparent effectiveness of engineering controls—as indicated by absence of characteristic odors, visible dust accumulations, and loud noise. The survey should continue through to the final product produced by the plant and its packaging.

The surveyors should also follow the pathway of any waste materials and determine their disposal sites.

The numbers of employees at each process step should be noted, as well as any relevant data on gender, ethnicity, or age that might affect employees' sensitivity to chemicals in the workplace. It is also important to look for obvious stigmata such as drying and roughening of the skin, as might be expected where exposure to solvents occurs. It is usually appropriate to discuss work practices with the personnel directly involved, since the perception of those practices is often very different on the shop floor from what it is in the executive offices.

Upon completion of the walk-through survey, the industrial hygienist will ordinarily have a closing conference with the plant management, at which time obvious concerns can be discussed and follow-up measures agreed upon. Where the industrial hygienist is a regulatory agency representative, follow-up surveys may require special notices and interaction with

agency officials as well as plant officials. In any case, a report on the walk-through survey, together with conclusions and recommendations, should be completed for the record.

### Data Review

An important part of the industrial hygienist's role in recognition of health hazards in the workplace will be data review. Such data may include reports from physicians on clinical findings that may be related to exposures in the workplace as well as a review of company records on materials coming into the workplace that may represent significant health hazards. The current OSHA "Workers' Right-to-Know" regulation has made explicit (and subject to governmental investigation) the common-sense duty of the employer to inform workers of the nature and hazards of materials to which they may be exposed. Where exposures are to materials purchased from a third party, data on materials and their hazards will usually be derived from Material Safety Data Sheets (MSDSs).

### Value & Limitations of MSDSs

The industrial hygiene review of MSDSs and other information from suppliers, should include attention to identifiable health hazards as well as recommended control measures. While MSDSs have been far more informative recently than in the past, there are still substantial differences between the information provided by different manufacturers for the same (generic) materials. In addition, the MSDSs provided by a manufacturer or distributor may be prepared by people without substantial health science backgrounds and sometimes represent merely a reprinting of data from conventional sources that are often outdated and sometimes inappropriate. The industrial hygienist must therefore compare and balance the recommendations made by various manufacturers in order to provide a unified program for control of materials of similar sorts, regardless of their commercial sources.

As chemical manufacturers become more sophisticated, the available MSDSs have begun to stress protective measures more completely than in the past. This has come about both from manufacturers' concerns that their materials were in some cases being misused and from fear of litigation. In some cases, recommended personal protective measures are unnecessarily complex—particularly where the chemicals are used in very small quantities. The industrial hygienist may be able to recommend less restrictive protection if the combination of quantities used, inherent toxicity, process controls, and other engineering control measures combine to reduce exposures to acceptable levels.

### Materials of Uncertain Toxicity

In some cases, the industrial hygienist must assess the potential for harm of chemicals for which no reliable human toxicologic data are available. This need arises most often in research and development settings but also wherever chemical intermediates are produced. An important consideration is that the worker must be protected at all cost. If uncertainty exists, it should be resolved in favor of a higher standard of concern.

## EVALUATION OF HEALTH HAZARDS IN THE WORKPLACE

Evaluation of health hazards within the plant will include measurement of exposures (and potential exposures), comparison of those exposures to existing standards, and recommmendation of controls if needed.

### Exposure Measurements

Exposure measurements are intended to be surrogates for determinations of doses delivered to the individual. The mere existence of chemicals in the workplace or even in the workplace atmosphere does not necessarily mean that the chemicals are being delivered to a sensitive organ system in quantity sufficient to cause harm. The effective dose will depend upon such things as particle sizes of dusts in the air, the use of protective devices (respirators, protective clothing), and the existence of other contaminants in the workplace. The task of determining the dose delivered to the worker may be further complicated by the existence of multiple pathways of absorption and metabolism. Such contaminants as lead are absorbed through both inhalation and ingestion, and both routes of intake must be considered in evaluation of the potential for harm. Similarly, many solvents are readily absorbed through the skin, and mere determination of airborne levels is not sufficient to determine the complete range of potential exposures.

### Sampling & Analysis of Airborne Contaminants

Inhalation of airborne contaminants is the major route of entry for systemic intoxicants in the workplace. Thus, evaluation and control of airborne contaminants is an important part of any occupational health program.

Sampling and analysis of airborne contaminants is the definitive function of the industrial hygienist. While it is the joint responsibility of the hygienist and physician to interpret the results of such measurements, measurement alone makes a contribution to the awareness of hazards as well as to their evaluation. Recent developments in instrumentation have made it possible to measure very low concentrations, with the result that previously unsuspected contamination is now being discovered.

In some cases, these more sophisticated measurements, coupled with evaluations of the health status of those exposed, have led to discoveries of connections between relatively low levels of airborne contaminants and health effects. The field of "indoor air quality" is one such general case. The determination of exposures to occupants of buildings (office workers) has not received substantial attention in the past, but health effects are now being found at concentrations of contaminants well below established occupational standards.

Maximum acceptable exposure limits have typically been lowered in recent years as both our ability to discern clinical effects and our expectations of no risk of (detectable or undetectable) health effects have increased. A good example, of this phenomenon is concern about asbestos in buildings. A hygienist should attempt to ensure that avoidable exposure to asbestos is eliminated. There is no definitive evidence that there is a threshold dose below which the asbestos-related disease mesothelioma will not occur. In addition, substantial liability may attach to the building owner who permits unnecessary exposure to building employees or tenants. Thus, measurements of asbestos concentrations down to and including ambient levels have become commonplace.

### General Approaches to Air Monitoring

There are two major approaches to air monitoring for determination of airborne contaminant levels. In personal, or breathing zone, sampling, the hygienist places a collection device near to the breathing zone of the worker. The collection device may either be active, requiring that air be drawn through it; or passive, requiring no pump or other suction source (a "dosimeter"). The second approach (area sampling) employs fixed or mobile sampling stations in the work area.

**A. Personal Breathing Zone Monitoring:** Personal breathing zone monitoring is usually preferred since exposures are measured at the point nearest to the actual entry of airborne contaminants and the sampling system moves with the worker. Thus, measurements are more likely to represent actual potential exposures. An example of a worker with a breathing zone (personal) sampler in place is shown in Figure 37–1.

**B. Area Monitoring:** There are disadvantages to the personal breathing zone approach, however. First, the volume of air sampled is limited by the capacity of the battery-operated pumps used (or the diffusion coefficient of a passive collection device), so that trace contaminants may be difficult to measure. Second, where complex evaluations are required, the number of collection devices may be too cumbersome for practical installation in the worker's breathing zone. In these circumstances—or when direct-reading instruments (usually larger and often re-

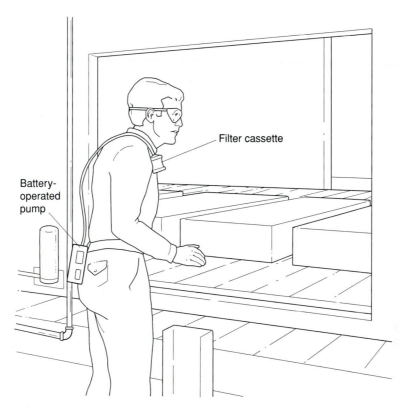

Battery-operated pump

Filter cassette

**Figure 37–1.** Worker wearing personal breathing zone monitor. The monitor samples air near enough to the nose and mouth to catch the same type of air the worker is breathing.

quiring line power) are to be used—area monitoring by means of fixed monitoring stations may be employed. Fixed monitoring stations may also be used to measure emissions from sources; to measure background concentrations; or to measure concentrations in several areas simultaneously in order to evaluate the effectiveness of controls. Figure 37–2 shows the application of both area sampling and personal sampling inside a work area.

## DURATION AND TIMING OF MONITORING

### Determination of Time-Weighted Average Exposures

The time course of exposure potential should be identified before beginning the sampling process, so that all times during which exposure is possible will be appropriately sampled. Time-weighted average exposure determinations should be made for the entire period of work to be evaluated. In a continuous ("assembly line") process, the period of exposure will usually be the entire work shift. In other cases, exposures may only occur for a relatively short time within the work shift. The time-weighted average exposure throughout the workday is usually required for determination of compliance with relevant standards (see below) and may also be useful for comparison of exposures at various points within the plant.

### Determination of the Time Course of Exposure

Although chronic diseases are usually the result of long-continued exposures, peak exposure levels can be important in causing acute effects and may be more directly relevant even in long-term exposures than their relative contribution on a time-weighted average would indicate. In other words, peak exposures may overwhelm such defenses as the mucociliary pathway for removal of contaminants and may occur at times of maximal exertion and maximal intake of airborne contaminants. Peak exposures may be determined by taking an integrated sample for a relatively short period (for performance of a specific operation; or for 10–15 minutes at a time when maximum exposure is expected; or for such other period as may be required by a regulation or standard) or by using direct-reading instruments for real-time measurements.

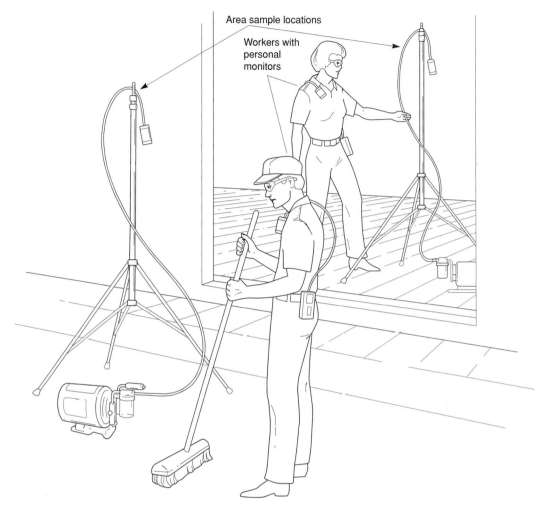

**Figure 37–2.** Worker wearing personal monitor. Industrial hygienist is gaining additional information by installing an area monitoring device.

## SAMPLING FOR SPECIFIC CONTAMINANTS

The general approaches introduced above may be applied to determination of individual agents or groups of agents. In general, sampling and analytic methods are divided into those for gases and vapors and those for airborne particles.

### 1. GAS & VAPOR SAMPLING

Gas and vapor sampling may be accomplished by any of five methods: (1) active collection, by drawing a measured volume of air through a collection system that is then analyzed; (2) passive collection, with a dosimeter that attracts gas or vapor molecules by diffusion from the atmosphere; (3) collection in a color-sensitive medium in a device in which color change is proportionate to concentration of the contaminant and which can be read directly; (4) collection in an evacuated container used to carry a sample of air to a convenient site for analysis; and (5) direct evaluation by direct-reading instruments sensitive to one or several atmospheric gases or vapors.

In general, the first and fourth methods—using active collection devices with subsequent laboratory analysis—are more sensitive and can be used to determine lower concentrations than the other approaches listed. However, the direct-reading devices (both instrumental and color change) provide a more rapid (immediate) result and are useful when an immediate hazard must be assessed. Passive dosimeters offer the advantage of not requiring a suction source to draw air through the collection device and are thus more acceptable to workers since the need for carrying a pump is avoided.

## Collection Media & Analysis

Collection media for gases and vapors may be either solid or liquid.

**A. Solid Sorbents:** The most commonly used solid sorbent is activated charcoal, which can be used for collection of many low-molecular-weight hydrocarbons as well as some inorganic gases and vapors. The most common analytic procedure employed in determining concentrations from the gases and vapors collected on the charcoal is gas-liquid chromatography ("gas chromatography"). The collected sample, with the molecules of gas or vapor adsorbed to the surface of the charcoal, is usually desorbed with a solvent (often carbon disulfide) compatible with those to be determined. The solvent extract of the charcoal is then either injected directly into the gas chromatograph column or the volume of the extract is reduced to provide greater sensitivity, followed by injection.

In some cases, particularly for oxygenated hydrocarbon species, silica gel is used in testing. Desorption is often accomplished with distilled water or oxygenated solvents, again followed by analysis by either gas chromatography or other analytic approaches. Another group of sorbents are less commonly used for routine industrial hygiene sampling but are finding increasing utilization in evaluation of indoor air quality and for collection of samples for analysis of higher molecular weight species. These are the solid sorbents that were initially developed as gas chromatographic column packings. Examples are Tenax and the variously numbered Chromosorb materials. Some of these sorbents can be characterized as "molecular sieves" and find particular use in collection of samples in environments where compounds that may irreversibly bind to charcoal are found. Desorption is often conveniently accomplished by heating the sample collection tube while injecting a carrier gas (nitrogen or other inert gas) through the sample tube during heating. This approach, coupled with analysis of the desorbed gas, by gas chromatography, mass spectrometry, or some other analytic method, is often useful where a complex environment with many trace components is suspected.

**B. Liquid Media:** Cases and vapors may also be effectively collected from the atmosphere using various liquids as the collection media. The air is drawn through the measured volume of the liquid into a device that may be called an "impinger" or "bubbler" or a "gas washing bottle." Sampling in liquid for gases and vapors has several disadvantages when personal breathing zone concentrations are to be determined. Some of the liquids that have been recommended are themselves toxic, and placing a glass vial on a worker's lapel may add to the risk in the workplace. There is a danger also of spillage from any liquid container, and the liquid may evaporate—either of which will complicate evaluation of the results.

**C. Evacuated Containers:** Collection of samples of air in evacuated containers such as inert plastic bags, glass bottles, stainless steel cylinders, or other containers is appropriate only if it is certain that the samples will be analyzed before analytes of interest have had a chance to either degrade or react. In most cases, this limits the utility of the technique to relatively stable gases and vapors. The technique is particularly useful for inorganic and nonreactive gases such as carbon monoxide, although "passivated" stainless steel containers are widely used for collection of ambient air samples for trace hydrocarbon analysis. Reactions may include those with the walls of the container (or simple sorption to the walls) as well as reactions with other airborne contaminants held within the container. In addition, care must be taken to avoid exposure of the collected gas to sunlight or other sources of artificial light that may initiate photochemical reactions. This technique is very useful whenever such analytic procedures as gas-phase infrared spectrometry appear to be useful approaches and a laboratory-based instrument offers advantages in sensitivity or precision over field direct-reading instruments.

## Direct-Reading Instruments

A variety of direct-reading battery-powered instruments is now available, so that direct measurements of "real time" concentrations can be conveniently made in remote or isolated environments. Some of these units measure oxygen concentrations also, making them useful for evaluating the safety of entry into enclosed spaces. Others measure only one or 2 contaminants but are useful where the suspected contamination is relatively well known.

With the recent advent of small portable "data loggers" from which data may be down-loaded to computer systems, it has become feasible to record the real-time output from very small direct-reading instruments. This has made it possible to construct some individual chemical exposure profiles over time, since these units can be as small as a "pack of cigarettes," and are easily carried and not intrusive. An important application of this approach has been in indoor air quality studies, where the relative contributions of various sources to overall exposures to CO and other gases of interest have become much better understood recently.

Other available direct-reading instruments are less portable but may be more accurate and more easily and permanently calibrated. The detection principles employed are often the same as those in the small instruments, but the detection systems and associated electronics may be more reliable. Output may be directed to digital or analog meters, strip chart recorders, or data loggers.

Several kinds of direct reading instruments respond to a wide variety of airborne contaminants, although with differing sensitivity. Each of these must be calibrated for specific chemical mixtures, since each of them may respond differently.

**A. Portable Chromatographs:** A recent development in industrial hygiene instrumentation has been the adaptation of gas chromatographs to portable field use. With these instruments, a bolus of air may be drawn directly into the instrument through a gas sampling valve, or an evacuated container (often a syringe) may he used to collect a small sample of air that is then injected directly into the instrument. These instruments share the advantages (specificity and sensitivity) of laboratory gas chromatographs but have the disadvantage that a relatively extensive calibration effort may be required in order to obtain quantitative results. The detectors used may be selected to measure only the family of airborne contaminants of interest.

**B. Infrared Spectrophotometers:** These instruments (an example of which is the family of MIRAN instruments manufactured by Foxboro-Wilks) can be used to measure concentrations of several hundred gases and vapors at or near the one part per million level. An advantage of the instrument is that corrections for background concentrations of water vapor and other gases and vapors than those of immediate interest can be performed on site.

**C. Direct Reading Instruments With Specialized Detectors:** Some of these instruments may give a single number response to the totality of the atmosphere they are measuring. Such a single number may be imputed to be "total hydrocarbons" or "Volatile Organic Carbon" (VOC), based on the response of the detector. Each such detector has its own characteristic response to the mixture of hydrocarbons present in the air, and comparison of the results from one type of instrument (for example, a photoionization detector) to another (a flame ionization detector) is usually inappropriate.

Other specialized instruments may measure one or several specific individual gases or vapors in the atmosphere, such as carbon monoxide, sulfur dioxide, hydrogen sulfide, or the like. Although these are less likely to be affected by other atmospheric components than those that purport to measure "total hydrocarbons", each of them may have idiosyncratic responses to other atmospheric components and the nature of those responses must be known.

**D. Fixed Monitors:** Any of the direct-reading instruments described above can be made substantially more reliable if installed permanently with line power. Such installations have been used for many years where potential for exposure to highly toxic gases exists.

**E. Colorimetric Indicators:** These may be either passive or active. In the passive type, a "badge," which has a portion that changes color on exposure to specific gases or vapors at a given concentration for a sufficient period of time, may be placed in an area or in the breathing zone of a worker. The system functions by diffusion of the molecules of interest from the atmosphere to the badge. Such devices can be useful to indicate the presence of potentially harmful concentrations of gases without having an industrial hygienist present in the workplace at all times. In the active type, a measured volume of air is drawn through a glass tube containing a reagent (usually adsorbed onto a solid support) that reacts with specified chemicals in the air. The degree of color change in the reagent—either the shade of coloration or the "length of stain" along the tube length—is proportionate to the concentration of contaminant and can be compared to standard charts. The major danger in their use is that they may not be reliable—they should not, generally speaking, be considered any more accurate than about plus or minus half of the indicated value. In addition, their reliable detection limit may be near to the level at which controls should be implemented.

## 2. PARTICULATE MATERIAL SAMPLING

Measurement of airborne particulate contamination can be done either by collection of integrated samples with subsequent analysis or by use of direct-reading instruments. Integrated sample collection and analysis is by far the more common modality of evaluation, both because of certain inherent difficulties associated with direct-reading measurements and because of the greater precision associated with laboratory analysis.

### Filter Sampling

Modern airborne particle sampling is ordinarily done with filters. The filter selected for use must collect and retain the particles of interest; must not offer so much resistance to flow that pumps cannot draw air through it at a useful rate; and must be compatible with the analytic method of choice.

### Size Selective Sampling

Inhalation and retention of particulate material in the lung is dependent upon the "aerodynamic equivalent diameter" (AED) of the particles. That is, only particles within a specific (small) size range (which is also dependent upon the specific gravity and shape of the particles) will both penetrate to and be retained within the alveolar and lower bronchiolar (unciliated) air spaces. Somewhat larger particles may penetrate into the thoracic cavity, while those even larger will be collected in the upper respiratory system (nose and mouth). The very largest particles will only rarely even be carried into the nose or mouth. Thus, sampling to evaluate hazards associated with agents such as crystalline silica is done with the aid of a size-selective sampling device preceding the filter upon which the material is to be collected for analysis. When air is drawn through the sampling system at the proper rate, only particles small enough to both penetrate and be retained within the deep lung space will pass through the selective device and be captured on the filter for analysis. In recent years, general environmental sampling for particles has also used size-selective criteria to define those particles believed to be most likely to cause long-term harm to the respiratory system.

The size selective criteria established, and the devices used to collect the defined range(s) of particles differ from agency to agency, and it is important to verify the current status of regulations and scientific opinion in this rapidly-changing field.

As an example, "respirable dust sampling" using a cyclone (selection device giving a rather broad range of particle sizes with a 50% cut point of 3.5 μm—approximately 50% of the particles passing are less than about 3.5 μm AED) has been the method of choice for evaluation of the pneumoconiosis-causing dusts, with the exception of asbestos. (The respirable fraction is then analyzed to determine the amount of crystalline silica, which is compared to the standard.) All other dusts and particles were typically measured by collection and analysis of total particulate matter. Current opinion favors the adoption of a broader standard (AED ≤ 4 μm), for the pneumoconiosis-causing dusts, as well as particle size-specific standards for other particulate materials, depending on the portion of the respiratory system they may harm or from which they may be absorbed sytemically.

In addition to the cyclone, size-selective devices used in particulate material sampling include direct inertial collectors such as impingers and impactors. The former utilizes a wet collection system, where a jet of air is directed against a collecting surface within a liquid bath. Impingers are now used mainly for gas and vapor collection. While impingers are effective for the collection of large particles, they are not particularly suitable for collection of very small particles owing to the limitations of the inertial forces employed for such collection. They should thus be used with caution when particles less than ~1 μm AED are potentially important in health effects.

Impactors use a dry collection system, wherein particles are directed in a jet of air against a dry (or sometimes greased) collection surface. Impactors are often used in a stacked-plate array, with the plates pierced with holes that decrease in size from inlet to exit. The jets thus formed increase in velocity (as an inverse function of their diameters), and successively smaller particles are removed from the gas stream. The final stage of the impactor is usually a filter, where the remaining (small) particles are collected. Size-selective sampling with greater detail than offered by the cyclone is thus provided.

Special versions of impactors are widely used for the evaluation of viable airborne particles (fungi and bacteria). The devices, having either one or two collection stages, are designed to accomodate petri dishes of conventional microbiological growth media. After air is drawn through the device, and the airborne particles are deposited on the surface of the medium selected, the dishes are taken to a laboratory and the organisms allowed to grow in the usual manner. The dishes are examined by a microbiologist, and the organisms are counted and identified by genus and species, if possible. The number of "colony-forming-units" per cubic meter of air is reported.

## Total Particulate Sampling

In circumstances where a biologically active material may be absorbed readily at many portals of entry, total particulate sampling may be the approach of choice. This is the case, for example, where such biologically active compounds as organophosphorous or carbamate pesticides require evaluation. Such chemicals may be absorbed in the upper respiratory tract, when inhaled into the deep lung, or indeed even upon skin contact. In addition, clearance mechanisms (the mucociliary elevator) may remove the contaminant from the ciliated portion of the respiratory tract and yet not fully clear the contaminant from the body because of the swallowing of saliva. It is therefore important to collect all airborne particles if the full extent of the hazard is to be evaluated.

## Analysis of Particulate Material Samples

Analysis of collected samples may be by any of a variety of techniques appropriate to the analyte of interest.

**A. Microscopy:** In the case of materials such as asbestos, where the numerical concentration of particles is the most important toxicity factor, a sample is taken by drawing air through a filter and the number of particles on the filter is counted by microscopic techniques.

The most common analytic procedure used for evaluation of asbestos is that involving optical phase contrast microscopy as specified by National Institute for Occupational Safety and Health (NIOSH) and Occupational Safety and Health Administration (OSHA). The procedure is relatively simple but has the disadvantages that not all airborne asbestos fibers are visualized or counted and that other (nonasbestos) fibers are counted. However, since the fibers most often considered to be harmful—those longer than 5 μm—are counted, the method gives an index of exposure to all asbestos fibers.

Where more detailed information on the total airborne fiber population is desired, transmission electron microscopy is used. This method, which is capable of visualizing all airborne asbestos fibers (and differentiating asbestos fibers from other fibers) is much more complex and costly. [In the United States in 1996, the analytic cost of the phase-contrast method is typically in the range of $10–25 per sample, while transmission electron microscopy typically costs from $50 to $500 per sample depending upon the level of detail required in the results (and the speed of analysis)].

**B. Other Analytic Approaches:** Other commonly used analytic approaches are atomic absorption or emission spectroscopy for analysis of elements in the particles, x-ray diffraction for identification of crystalline materials, and (where appropriate) any of the aforementioned organic analysis modalities where organic compounds exist in particulate form.

### 3.   COMBINED COLLECTION DEVICES

In some environments. it may be appropriate to use combined particulate and gas or vapor collection devices. This may be the case where a substance exists in particulate form in the atmosphere but has an appreciable vapor pressure, so that substantial amounts may evaporate following collection on a filter. In this case, a vapor-sorbing material would be used behind the filter to ensure complete collection. Such a combined sampling approach is often used for collection of pesticides and polynuclear aromatic hydrocarbons.

### 4.   SURFACE EVALUATION
### (Wipe Sampling)

Evaluation of surface contamination can be a useful supplementary technique to assist in the definition exposure potential and particularly for evaluation of the effectiveness of control measures. Wipe sampling is useful also for identifying contaminated areas where a spill of toxic material has occurred. As an example, wipe sampling is routinely used to evaluate the extent of contamination resulting from spills of such materials as PCBs, pesticides, and other materials for which absorption through the skin may be an important route of entry.

Wipe sampling may also be a useful adjunct to programs used to evaluate the effectiveness of housekeeping measures, particularly in manufacturing facilities where separation of manufacturing areas from cafeterias, offices, or dressing rooms is important. A typical program would call for the wipe sampling of identical areas once a month or quarterly.

Wipe sampling must be done according to a well-defined protocol if it is to have any significant utility for long-term evaluations. Most commonly, a template of a defined size (usually 10 cm × 10 cm) is prepared, and wiping is done within the exposed area of the template for the sake of uniformity. Any suitable substance may be used to perform the wiping. but filter papers (usually the low-ash, "quantitative" type of papers) are most commonly used.

Other methods of surface evaluation are also sometimes useful. For example, the polynuclear aromatic hydrocarbons fluoresce readily when irradiated with ultraviolet light and this characteristic can be used to make qualitative surveys of areas where contamination is feared.

## PHYSICAL AGENT EVALUATION

Evaluation of physical agents requires specialized equipment that is often not routinely available (except for sound level meters). Evaluation of ionizing or nonionizing radiation requires specialized training, but many industrial hygienists have developed expertise in these evaluations.

### Noise Exposure Evaluation

Evaluation of exposures to noise is a traditional industrial hygiene function. The equipment used is of two principal types.

**A.   Sound Level Meters:** Sound level meters consist of a microphone and associated electronic circuitry, with a meter that gives a readout in decibels. The circuitry typically contain filtering circuits that permit evaluation of exposures to components of the noise spectrum weighted in accordance with their effccts upon hearing. The "A weighting" network has been adopted as the standard for determination of occupational noise exposure. In this weighting scheme, the very low and very high frequencies are suppressed, and the middle frequencies (1000–6000 Hz) are slightly accentuated. This gives primacy to the "speech frequencies."

Sound level meters may also be fitted with filtering circuits for determination of noise levels within specified band widths. One octave or one-third octave (less commonly) band width circuits are often employed. With such devices, it is possible to isolate and identify the specific frequencies of occurrence of the noise. This identification of sources is essential to control in complex noise environments.

A sound level meter is shown in use in Figure 37–3. Note that the instrument is used to measure noise intensity in an area, and thus is analogous to area sampling for chemicals.

**B.   Noise Dosimetry:** Noise dosimeters employ a recording circuit consisting of a small microphone placed close to the ear of the worker to record noise exposure. The devices may either give an overall integrated average exposure for the course of the measurement period or a readout showing exposure as a function of time. Dosimetry is the preferred approach, since the exposures measured are specific and unique to the individual, and offers the same advantage over area sampling as indicated above for breathing zone sampling for airborne contaminants. Figure 37–4 shows the use of a dosimeter. Note that the microphone is located close to the worker's ear.

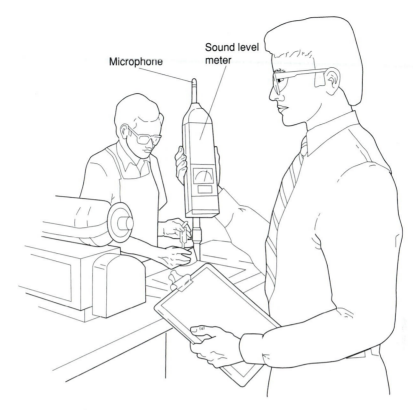

Figure 37–3. Industrial hygienist using a sound level meter in a work area.

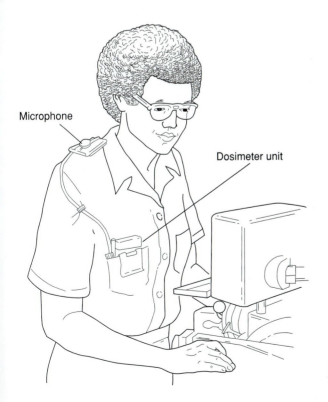

**Figure 37–4.** Worker wearing a noise dosimeter with a microphone located close to the ear.

## Evaluation of Other Physical Agents

Other physical agents ordinarily require specialized equipment for competent evaluation. However, many industrial hygienists are experienced in such evaluations, for such agents as electrical and magnetic fields; microwaves; and ultraviolet and infrared radiation. Similarly, the evaluation of a workplace to determine the extent of hazard due to heat or cold stress can usually be done by an experienced industrial hygienist.

## OBSERVATIONS OF WORK PRACTICES & PROCESS VARIABLES

Exposures often vary substantially from time to time during a day, week, month, or year. The work practices employed by workers whose exposures are measured should be observed during the monitoring period. The description of the workplace must include personal protective devices so that an estimation of "true exposure" (actual intake of chemical into the worker's body) can be derived.

Ventilation equipment and other engineering controls must also be evaluated so that sampling results are placed in a sensible context. Workers and supervisors will ordinarily be able to estimate how closely conditions during the survey period approximate "usual" conditions. General conditions in the workplace, including such things as whether windows and doors are open or closed, must also be evaluated and recorded. The ideal industrial hygiene report will be detailed enough so that another industrial hygienist entering the workplace later will be able to determine whether conditions are the same as or different from those that existed during the survey period. All of the detailed information called for in the Industrial Hygiene Survey Checklist should be obtained and recorded if possible.

## COMPARISON WITH STANDARDS

### Statistical Considerations

The industrial hygienist must determine whether exposures measured are likely to cause harm to those exposed. If such harm seems likely, action must be taken to reduce exposures to tolerable levels. (See Control of Health Hazards, below.) In most cases, the industrial hygienist will refer to a set of standards for various individual chemical contaminants or physical agents. Exposures are usually considered to be "acceptable" (1) if the measured concentrations are less than the allowable upper limit and (2) if exposures are unlikely to rise above that allowable limit under reasonably forseeable circumstances.

Certain precautions are needed in such comparisons. The monitoring process is, in the statistical sense, a "sampling" process. If the systematic biases, and random error (imprecision) in the measurements made are within acceptable limits, it can be presumed that the measurements are "accurate". That is, that the monitoring results are reflective of the true mean of the results that might be obtained if all possible subsets of samples were examined.

However, all industrial hygiene measurements are inaccurate to some degree because of sampling and analytic errors, and cannot be absolutely reflective of all possible workplace conditions, since all possible workplace conditions cannot be evaluated due to cost considerations. Therefore, it is prudent to construct confidence intervals about the sample means, so that the range within which the true average concentration may be expected to fall is known. The upper 95% confidence limit should fall below the allowable exposure limit before it can be stated, with 95% certainty, that the true average concentration is probably below that standard, assuming that the samples taken can be presumed to be otherwise reflective of "typical" conditions in the workplace.

A precautionary note is in order. Because of the inherently great dispersion of environmental data, it should be presumed that the data are log-normally distributed and the logarithmic transformation of individual data points should be performed before the data are evaluated. The "geometric mean" (the inverse log of the average of the logarithms of the data points) is usually an appropriate measure of central tendency when evaluating environmental data, although the conventional arithmetic mean (the average) will more truly represent the exposures of the workforce.

### Occupational Exposure Standards for Airborne Contaminants

Lists of occupational exposure standards for airborne contaminants have been available for over 50 years. The first standards were for a few widely recognized health hazards, such as lead, mercury, and benzene. Currently, hundreds of chemicals and physical agents are either regulated (eg, by federal or state OSHA programs) or have recommended control limits (from NIOSH or voluntary organizations). In the United States, the most important standards are derived from the following sources:

1. The American Conference of Governmental Industrial Hygienists Threshold Limit Values (TLVs) (*Threshold Limit Values and Biological Exposure Indices for 1995–1996*, American Conference of Governmental Industrial Hygienists, 6500 Glenway Avenue, Bldg. D-7. Cincinnati, OH 45211–4438.)

2. The Recommended Exposure Levels (RELS) of the National Institute for Occupational Safety and Health (*NIOSH Recommendations for Occu-*

*pational Safety and Health Standards, 1988, Morbidity and Mortality Weekly Report* (Supplement) August 26, 1988/Vol–37/No. 5–7. Centers for Disease Control, Atlanta, GA 30333.)

3. The Permissible Exposure Limits (PELS) of the Occupational Safety and Health Administration. These are listed at Title 29 of the Code of Federal Regulations, ¶1910, Subpart Z.

Only the OSHA PELs (and similar lists prepared by some state OSHA programs) are legally enforceable by regulatory agencies. The TLVs and RELs should be considered advisory.

All of these standards are typically based on "time-weighted average" (TWA) exposures. That is, concentrations within each day are averaged, with weighting assigned depending on the time period of exposure to each of the concentrations measured. They each may have some upper limit of exposure for shorter periods as well, expressed as a "ceiling" or as a short-term exposure limit (STEL). A ceiling limit will ordinarily be assigned to those substances for which tolerance of overexposure is slight and where the consequences of even modest exceedances for short periods of time of some well-defined limit may be disastrous. (As an example, hydrogen cyanide is most appropriately regulated by a ceiling standard.) A STEL may be assigned to substances for which harmful effects (but not life-threatening or likely to cause permanent disability) may arise at short term exposures to concentrations above the TWA exposure limit, even if there is sufficient time at lower concentrations to bring the TWA within the overall exposure limit. From a practical point of view, it must be recognized that short bursts of intense "peak" exposure to any substance may have harmful effects not anticipated in the usual workplace, and that accumulating the entire exposure sufficient to reach the TWA in, say, an hour, would be unacceptable.

## Threshold Limit Values (TLVs)

Of the sets of standards to which industrial hygienists have reference in this regard, the most important (in the United States) is the table of "Threshold Limit Values" (TLVs) published annually by the Threshold Limit Values Committee of the American Conference of Governmental Industrial Hygienists (ACGIH). This listing has been published annually since the mid 1940s and is used not only in the United States but in other countries as well. In 1970, upon enactment of OSHA, the 1968 TLVs were adopted and given the status of law. In their incarnation as OSHA regulations, they have been named "permissible exposure limits" (PELs). ACGIH also publishes a loose-leaf binder (updated periodically) in which are set forth the data on which the TLVs are based.

The TLVs include values for chemical substances, physical agents (heat, ionizing radiation, lasers, noise and vibration, radio frequency and microwave radiation, ultraviolet and infrared radiation, and visible light). A recently added section sets forth biological exposure indices for a few chemicals for which well-established acceptable levels of the parent chemical or its metabolites in body fluids have been documented. The ACGIH Biological Exposure Indices (BEls) are discussed in Chapter 38.

Despite warnings to the contrary in the ACGIH booklet, many people improperly consider TLVs (and PELs—see below) as "safe levels." However, TLVs have always been intended only as guidelines for control of workplace atmospheres by personnel with adequate training and experience in industrial hygiene. The following is quoted (bold emphasis in the original) from the ACGIH publication, *TLVs: Threshold Limit Values and Biological Exposure Indices for 1995–1996:*

> These limits are intended for use in the practice of industrial hygiene as guidelines or recommendations in the control of potential health hazards and for no other use, eg in the evaluation or control of community air pollution nuisances, in estimating the toxic potential of continuous, uninterrupted exposures or other extended work periods, as proof or disproof of an existing disease or physical condition, or adoption by countries whose working conditions differ from those in the United States of America and where substances and processes differ. These limits *are not* fine lines between safe and dangerous concentrations nor are they a relative index of toxicity, and *should not* be used by anyone untrained in the discipline of industrial hygiene.

Too many personnel (both industrial hygienists and others) interpreting occupational exposure measurements have implied that exposures just beneath the TLVs are acceptable. In fact, it has always been considered good practice to hold exposures to the minimum practically possible—ie, no unnecessary exposure to any toxic material should be tolerated. In some cases it is necessary, because of economic or engineering factors. to expose workers to levels greater than zero (ambient) levels. In such cases, the TLVs should be used as a guide to the *maximum* tolerable exposure levels. (The equivalent German values are in fact entitled, in English translation, Maximum Allowable Concentrations, which was the title of the Threshold Limit Values for several years in the past.) It is emphasized again that the TLVs—or the OSHA PELs and the NIOSH RELS—represent *maximum allowable* exposure levels. The industrial hygienist or physician should attempt to hold exposures to the lowest level practically possible or to a level at which risk is "acceptable," bearing in mind that there is no environment that is risk-free; and that a "safe" environment is one in which the level of risk is acceptable.

Because some of those exposed may develop disease as a consequence of lifetime exposures even at the TLV level, many organizations have adopted a policy of setting standards at some fraction of the TLV. Ten percent, 25%, or 50% of the TLV may be designated the internal control level. Some companies have gone so far as to attempt to remove all contamination from workplace atmospheres. In such cases, any detectable odor or irritation is considered to be unacceptable, and control measures are instituted to reduce exposures when any process effluvia are detected.

## The OSHA Permissible Exposure Limits (PELs)

The OSHA Permissible Exposure Limits were first established in 1970, upon implementation of the Occupational Safety and Health Act, by adopting in toto the 1968 ACGIH TLVs, as well as some other voluntary standards from the American National Standards Institute.

It should be recognized that the OSHA PELs have not been significantly modified since 1970. Industrial experience, new developments in technology, and available scientific data clearly indicate that in many instances those adopted limits are now obsolete and inadequate. Furthermore, many new toxic materials commonly used in the workplace are not covered. These inadequacies are evidenced by the lower allowable exposure limits recommended by many technical, professional, industrial, and government organizations in the United States and elsewhere.

Only a few substances have been added to those regulated, and for a few more the allowable exposures were reduced. Substantial and significant changes were made in the TLVs in that period. Thus, certain exposures that are generally agreed to be potentially harmful are officially acceptable to OSHA. In 1989, OSHA attempted a wholesale upgrade of their PELS, but the attempt was challenged in court by certain industrial interests, and the challengers prevailed. As a result, OSHA must now justify, in extreme detail, each change in each standard. Only a few such changes have been made since 1989.

Many of the individual states have established their own list of allowable exposures, often relying on the TLVs. These may be enforced in lieu of the federal PELs if they are at least as stringent as the PELs.

## NIOSH Recommended Exposure Limits (RELs)

The National Institute for Occupational Safety and Health (NIOSH) has established recommendations for many workplace chemical and physical agents since its establishment in 1970, coincidentally with the establishment of OSHA. In fact, NIOSH was established in the same act with OSHA, with a legal mandate to provide research to support OSHA. A major function of NIOSH in the 1970s was the production of "Criteria Documents" for substances and agents, in which recommendations were made for exposure limits (RELs). In this set of documents, NIOSH has provided an evaluation of the literature, recommended control measures, and recommended upper limits for exposures. Since the early 1980s fewer of these documents have been produced. Many of the allowable exposure recommendations of NIOSH are lower than the recommended TLVs or PELs for the same chemicals. In part, this is due to NIOSH's practice of recommending exposure limits for ten hour workdays, rather than the eight hour workdays assumed by ACGIH and OSHA.

## Other Sources of Standards

Several other sources of recommended exposure limits are available to the industrial hygienist. Among these are the Workplace Environmental Exposure Limits promulgated by the American Industrial Hygiene Association for several chemicals not listed by the TLV Committee. Although many countries outside the United States have adopted the ACGIH TLVs without substantial modification, several have active committees evaluating allowable exposure limits. The International Labor Office has published, in tabular form, the occupational exposure limits for airborne toxic substances from all countries (ILO, 1995). This tabulation is very useful in identifying substances for which exposure limits lower than the TLVs might reasonably be established.

Where no established standards are available for guidance, in-house research may be necessary to establish guidelines. Where a chemical not previously used is being widely adopted in a particular industry, a trade association study of the effects of that chemical may be an appropriate venue for such research. Because of the potential risks associated with subtle health effects not easily foreseen, such control limits should be established only with great caution.

## Exposure Limits for Unusual or Extended Workshifts

As noted above, the usual exposure limits have been established assuming regular workshifts of 8 (ACGIH and OSHA) or 10 (NIOSH) hours. Where the work shifts differ significantly from the usual day, consideration must be given to the effects of more protracted exposures on the workers. A minimum adjustment can be made by simply cutting the allowable exposure limit in inverse proportion to the work day or work week as a fraction of the usual 8-hour day or 40-hour week, depending on the effect of greatest concern and the biological half-life of the chemical. A more conservative general approach is to take into account both the increased workday, and the decreased period away from exposure, but this approach may yield unrealistically low allowable exposures. Finally, detailed physiologically-based pharmacokinetic models may be established. These latter, although they may be the most accurate way to modify general exposure limits, require detailed knowledge of the metabolic pathways of each substance to be so regulated, including information on the biological half-life of each of the substances. DJ Paustenbach (Paustenbach DJ: Occupational exposure limits, pharmacokinetics, and unusual work schedules. In Harris RL, Cralley LJ, Cralley LV (editors): *Patty's Industrial Hygiene and Toxicology,* Vol. IIIA. Wiley, 1994.) has given a good general overview of this difficult topic, as well as providing some worked-out case studies.

## CONTROL OF HEALTH HAZARDS

Upon completion of the evaluation, the industrial hygienist should be in a position to recommend appropriate controls, if needed. Recommendations should take into account not only the conditions found during the survey but also those that may be expected to prevail in the future. Planned process modifications should be taken into account, and recommendations should be adaptable to future needs. Controls should be adequate to prevent unnecessary exposure during accidents and emergencies as well as during normal operating conditions. Consideration must be given to "fail-safe" operation of controls—ie recommended controls should always operate to protect workers regardless of process fluctuations.

### Substitution

All possibilities for substitution of a nontoxic for a toxic material or agent should be explored. If a toxic material can be dispensed with and a less harmful material substituted, that should be done. Substitution can of course only be done if a useful substitute is available—one that is suitable for existing processes or for which the processes can be relatively easily adapted.

This obvious approach must be undertaken with caution, however, since several instances have been known where an apparently harmless substitute for an obvious hazard was later found to be harmful in and of itself.

### Engineering Controls

Engineering controls on toxic exposures consist mainly of enclosure (building structures around the sources of emissions), isolation (placing hazardous process components in areas with limited human contact), and ventilation.

**A. Ventilation:** Ventilation for the control of health hazards may be either local exhaust ventilation or general ventilation.

Local exhaust ventilation conforms to the principle that control should be implemented as near to the source as practically possible. Thus, application of a local exhaust inlet on a specific tool (such as a grinder) would be inherently more desirable than performing the grinding operation in a ventilated hood, which in turn would be more desirable than installing general ventilation in the room where the grinding is performed. In a situation where a very toxic substance is being manipulated in such a way that exposure is possible, all three ventilation systems might be reasonable to use. Thus, the operator would be protected by ventilation of the specific tool, nearby workers (as well as the operator) would be protected by the hood and the remainder of the building would be protected by the general ventilation system. Figure 37–5 is a conceptual model of a "typical" operation, showing the three zones of control required.

On the other hand, where sources are more diffuse or dispersed, or where many people must be protected from relatively low-level contaminants (such as in indoor air quality in an office building), general ventilation alone may be appropriate. Further, for control of comfort, and provision of heating or cooling, general ventilation may be essential. In any case, the general ventilation system must be considered and evaluated for its potential to distribute contaminants throughout a plant or other building.

Design of ventilation systems for contamination control should ordinarily not be left to engineers without specific background or experience. Similarly, an industrial hygienist without engineering training and experience in the processes to be controlled may produce an unsatisfactory design.

ACGIH publishes a biennial document on industrial ventilation that provides guidance on the principles of ventilation control.

**B. Other Engineering Controls:** In addition to ventilation, enclosure, and isolation, some specific engineering controls may be appropriate in the specific process environment. It is, for example, often necessary to design process pipelines and valves to minimize splashes and ejection of toxic chemicals. Control systems that will permit safe and orderly shutdown of the process to avoid runaway reactions may also be of substantial benefit.

### Controls on Human Behavior

These controls on human behavior can be subdivided into the general categories of administrative controls and work practice controls.

**A. Administrative Controls:** Control of behavior patterns within the process environment includes such things as establishment of prohibited areas, areas where smoking and eating are either prohibited or allowed, and safe pathways through the work environment. Administrative controls will also include scheduling of work in such a way that dangerous operations are carried out when the fewest workers are present.

Less desirable is the practice of scheduling indi-

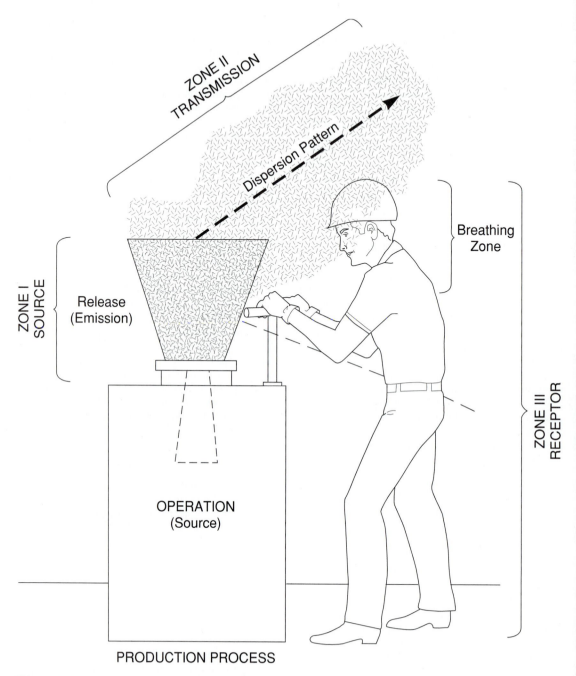

**Figure 37–5.** Conceptual model of the three zones of influence to control workplace hazards. (Reproduced with permission from Corn M: The role of control technologies in preventing occupational disease. Arch Environ Health 1984; 39:235.)

vidual workers to perform tasks for short periods, where excessive exposures would be incurred over an extended period of time. This practice was at one time common in the nuclear power industry, where temporary employees were used to perform maintenance tasks in high radiation environments. These "jumpers" were employed and paid by the day, although their actual work period may have been as short as 15 minutes. Such practices, where exposure to carcinogenic or genotoxic agents is spread across a larger population group although individual exposures are lower, is entirely unacceptable. While the individual risk may be relatively low, the effect of distributing an exposure with potential genetic effects to many members of the population is inherently unsound.

On the other hand, administrative controls that include scheduling are usually essential to control of the work environment. An example is prohibiting personnel who do not have adequate training from entry into spaces where health or safety hazards exist.

**B. Work Practices Control:** Control of work practices implies control over the behavior of individual workers on the job. Such work-related details as handling of contaminated tools and appliances are included in this type of control. Education (on the hazards to be avoided) and training (on the desired practices) are of course required. Close supervision of workers is needed in order to enforce compliance with proper work practices. Controls on work practices are particularly important where engineering controls are either not adequate or not possible and where there is significant potential for generation of airborne contaminants outside of controlled spaces.

## Personal Protection

Personal protective equipment use, though often essential, is less desirable than other approaches because of the difficulty in ensuring that it is both used and it is also effective. For example, on construction sites, personal protective equipment consists of "hard hats" and "safety shoes," and in laboratory environments it consists of protective eyewear and protective garments, such as laboratory coats.

However, there are significant complexities in both design and function of the protective devices used to reduce exposures. A worker who is issued and is wearing a "respirator," for example, may feel adequately protected from all potential hazards in the workplace and may therefore neglect the use of engineering controls, violate administrative control guidelines, and ignore required work practices. In fact, without substantial attention to selection, fitting, training, and maintenance of respirators, exposures during their use may be nearly as high as for those of "unprotected" workers.

Respirators are often handed out without adequate attention to any of these precautions. It is common, for example, to see workers with beards wearing negative pressure air-purifying respirators in areas where contaminants are present in the air. The devices are of course useless unless they fit tightly, which is nearly impossible if the wearer has facial hair.

Similarly, gloves protect against exposure to solvents and other toxicants only if chosen with knowledge of what materials are suitable in each case. (See Table 17–3 for some examples.) In addition, ironically, prolonged wearing of gloves into which skin hazardous materials have either leached or leaked through holes may result in substantial exposure to the worker (sometimes higher than would occur without the gloves).

## Integrated Control

A well-regulated control program in a company with diverse operations will usually employ all of the modes mentioned above plus adequate housekeeping and disposal of waste materials. it is emphasized again that substitution should be the first consideration. Where substitution cannot be rationally adopted, isolation of workers from exposure and enclosure of sources should be next considered. If no substitute material is readily available and if complete isolation and enclosure are not possible, local exhaust ventilation should be next considered. General exhaust ventilation is a useful supplement to local exhaust ventilation and should be part of the ventilation design.

When none of these engineering controls can completely abate the hazard, administrative controls, work practices controls, and personal protection may be necessary.

The controls process must be viewed as a continuing one in which existing controls are continually evaluated for their effectiveness. Equipment ages, personnel change, processes evolve, and the level of management attention to control varies with time. All of these forces act to change the effectiveness of a given control. The evaluation of effectiveness is the province of the industrial hygienist, who must involve physicians, managers, engineers, and workers in the evaluation.

## REFERENCES

### GENERAL INDUSTRIAL HYGIENE

Clayton GD et al (editors): *Patty's Industrial Hygiene and Toxicology*, 4th ed. Vols IA–IB: *General Principles*; Vols IIA–IIF: *Toxicology*; Vol IIIA: *The Work Environment*; Vol IIIB: *Biological Responses*. Wiley, 1991–1995.

Plog BA (editor): *Fundamentals of Industrial Hygiene*, 4th ed. National Safety Council, 1995.

Stellman M (editor): *Encyclopedia of Occupational Health and Safety*, 4th ed. 2 vols. International Labour Office, 1995.

### OCCUPATIONAL EXPOSURE STANDARDS

American Conference of Governmental Industrial Hygienists: *Documentation of the Threshold Limit Val-*

*ues and Biological Exposure Indices*, 6th ed. ACGIH, 1993.

International Labour Office: *Occupational Exposure Limits for Airborne Toxic Substances*, 3rd ed. International Labour Office, 1991.

## SAMPLING & ANALYSIS

American Conference of Governmental Industrial Hygienists: *Air Sampling Instruments*, 8th ed. ACGIH, 1995

United States Department of Health and Human Services, National Institute for Occupational Safety and Health: NIOSH Manual of Analytical Methods, 4th ed. USDHHS (NIOSH) Publication No. 94–113, 1994.

## CHEMICAL PROCESSES

Cralley LV, Cralley LJ (editors): *In-Plant Practices for Job-Related Health Hazards Control*. Vol 1: *Production Processes*; Vol 2: *Engineering Aspects*. MacMillan, 1989.

Grayson M (editor): *Kirk-Othmer Concise Encyclopedia of Chemical Technology*, 4th ed. Wiley, 1995.

# Biological Monitoring

**38**

*Jon Rosenberg, MD, & Robert J. Harrison, MD, MPH*

Biological monitoring is the measurement of a chemical, its metabolite, or a nonadverse biochemical effect in a biological specimen for the purpose of assessing exposure. The term may also be used to denote drug abuse monitoring and other types of medical surveillance, but to avoid confusion it should be restricted to exposure monitoring. Typically, specimens are blood, urine, or exhaled air. For example, exposure to organophosphorus insecticides can be confirmed by measuring the metabolite—alkyl phosphates—in the urine or by measuring a biochemical effect—the activity of the enzyme cholinesterase—in the blood. Most often, however, exposure is assessed by measuring the chemical or its metabolite in a body fluid.

Environmental monitoring is measurement of the ambient (external) exposure of a chemical in the workplace. Typically, samples are taken from the air or from surfaces at the workplace. Environmental monitoring provides information about potential exposure primarily from one route of exposure (eg, air or workplace surfaces), whereas biological monitoring provides a measure of the quantity of a chemical absorbed regardless of the route of absorption (eg, inhalation, skin contact, or ingestion). Total exposure rather than only workplace exposure is measured.

The biological level may not correlate well with environmental measurements (Figure 38–1). This variability occurs for several reasons: (1) Actual work practices vary among employees doing identical work—eg, one worker may have more skin contact or may inhale more of a chemical than another worker; (2) a high respiratory rate can increase pulmonary absorption of solvents by a factor of 3–4; (3) the rate of metabolism and excretion will vary between individuals even when hepatic or renal function is normal; and (4) lipid-soluble chemicals may accumulate to a greater extent in a person with excess adipose tissue.

Workplace exposure to more than 100 different chemicals can be estimated in an individual by measuring the chemical in the blood, urine, or exhaled air. Depending on the pharmacokinetics of the target substance, the body fluid sampled, and the time of sampling, the measured level will reflect the duration of exposure ranging from acute recent exposure or accumulated lifetime exposure (body burden).

The purpose of this chapter is to give the clinician practical information on biological monitoring.

Because some chemicals are rapidly cleared from the blood, interpretation of biological levels depends on accurate timing of sample collection. Because significant errors can be introduced in the sampling process, following standard methods of sample collection will improve the clinician's ability to interpret a biological level.

## HOW TO USE BIOLOGICAL MONITORING

Biological monitoring of workers exposed to toxic agents has gained increasing acceptance as a means of accurately determining exposure. It should be used to augment other sources of exposure assessment, such as occupational history and environmental monitoring. Like environmental monitoring (see Chapter 39), biological monitoring assesses the extent of exposure of workers and thus only indirectly the risk of health effects as a result of that exposure. Moreover, any action arising out of abnormal biological monitoring levels should be based not on a single measurement but on multiple measurements.

It cannot be assumed that a biological level necessarily represents a more accurate reflection of dose than an environmental level. All occurrences of elevated levels judged to be due to excessive workplace exposure should be evaluated with the assistance of an industrial hygienist.

Before a biological monitoring program is instituted, some scientific and practical issues must be considered. The program should be able to produce results that are meaningful, be implemented in a cost-effective fashion, and be used as indicated to reduce worker exposures to levels that cause adverse effects. Tables 38–1 and 38–2 show, respectively, the necessary and sufficient conditions for the consideration of institution of biological monitoring. Ethical and so-

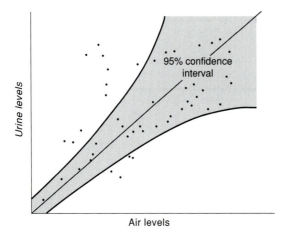

**Figure 38–1.** Relationship of levels of a substance measured in the breathing zone of workers to levels measured in urine.

cial aspects should also be considered: for example, confidentiality of results should be ensured; workers should be encouraged to maintain confidentiality (ie, not share results); and participation should be voluntary. Communication of results and explanation of actions must also be considered.

Table 38–3 summarizes information for chemicals with data sufficient for consideration of biological monitoring. It is useful in two situations. The first is the routine monitoring of a healthy employee who works with a toxic chemical. The clinician must determine whether the exposure is significant and potentially harmful. If the biological level measured is below the "no adverse health effect level" or if it is within the range "levels in unexposed," the exposure is probably not harmful. This situation is analogous to measuring airborne concentrations of a chemical and comparing them with recommended levels. For a few chemicals, biological monitoring of exposed

workers is mandated by law. In the case of an employee who works with lead, if the blood lead concentration is above a certain level, that worker must be transferred to an area where he or she is not exposed to lead.

Table 38–3 is useful also in the clinical assessment of an ill employee who has been exposed to a toxic chemical. Is it possible that the employee's abnormal symptoms, signs, or laboratory tests are due to exposure to that chemical? The "clinical effect level" is one that has been associated with illness typically caused by that chemical. If an employee has signs and symptoms consistent with those caused by the chemical and if the measured level is at or above the "clinical effect level," there is a high probability that the chemical is causing the illness. However, samples from ill individuals are usually taken at variable and often unspecified times following exposure and therefore reflect an uncertain duration of exposure. A biological level—no matter how high—still only reflects exposure and a given probability of illness and is never diagnostic of illness.

Between the "no adverse health effect level" and the "clinical effect level" there often lies a gray zone. These concepts are illustrated in Figure 38–2. If the employee's level falls into this zone, the clinician may repeat the measurement, use other indices of exposure, or do further reading of the primary literature to refine the evaluation.

Individuals differ in their response to chemicals; one worker may develop peripheral neuropathy from n-hexane exposure whereas another worker with the same exposure will not. This difference in sensitivity to a chemical may be due to variable rates of metabolism or excretion, different sensitivity of end organ receptors, different tolerance to discomfort, a preexisting illness, or simultaneous exposure to drugs or other toxins. Because of these differences between individuals, within a group of exposed workers the biological level associated with symptoms will usually follow a bell-shaped distribution.

**Table 38–1.** Necessary conditions to consider biological monitoring (all must be present).

| Item | Condition |
|---|---|
| A. Determinant (substance, metabolite, reaction product, nonadverse biochemical effect) | 1. Present in media (blood, urine, exhaled air)<br>2. Suitable for sampling<br>3. Sampling method acceptable to population to be monitored |
| B. Method of analysis | 1. Practical<br>2. Produces valid reproducible results over the range of concentrations present |
| C. Strategy of sample collection | Produces representative samples |
| D. Results | Can be interpreted in a meaningful fashion |
| E. Action for responding to aberrant results | Established prior to monitoring |

**Table 38–2.** Sufficient conditions to consider biological monitoring (one or more must be present).

| Item | Condition |
|---|---|
| A. Environmental monitoring or other workplace exposure assessment | Conducted to complement biological monitoring |
| B. Exposure routes to substance being monitored | Other than or in addition to workplace inhalation (skin, gastrointestinal, nonoccupational) |
| C. Environmental monitoring | 1. Not adequate to assess exposure<br>  a. Respirators or other personal protection is used<br>  b. Absorption is uncertain because of particle size and/or solubility<br>  c. Individual variability in respiratory volume or work practices is extreme<br>  d. Exposure fluctuates rapidly over time<br>2. Not feasible<br>  a. Plants or sites are in multiple locations<br>  b. Physical constraints such as work in a closed space or protective clothing are present |
| D. Substances to be monitored | 1. Cumulative toxicants<br>  a. Metals bound to tissues (Pb, Cd, Hg)<br>  b. Organics that are fat soluble and/or poorly metabolized (PCBs, dioxin)<br>2. Multiple agents with shared biochemical effects<br>  a. Cholinesterase for organophosphate pesticides<br>  b. Methemoglobin for multiple inducers<br>  c. DNA adducts for antineoplastic drugs |

## METHODOLOGY

Ideally, the biological level of a chemical is determined by its rate of absorption, elimination, and metabolism. Unfortunately, many other factors affect the measured level and are potential sources of error.

### Timing of Collection

The timing of the sample collection relative to the exposure is usually the most critical methodologic factor and may be the greatest source of error. For chemicals with a short half-time, the difference between sampling 15 minutes versus 1 hour after the end of exposure may alter the results by as much as a factor of 10.

### Collection Methods

Before taking a specimen, it is advisable to consult the laboratory about proper collection methods. Errors in sampling will occur if standard collection methods are not followed. Once collected, chemicals may deteriorate if not analyzed rapidly. The specimens often must be centrifuged or frozen soon after collection. An improper container may bind (adsorb) the chemical of interest or contaminate the specimen (eg, lead-free glass tubes should be used for measuring blood lead levels). A urine collection can be contaminated from unwashed hands or clothing.

### Body Site Sampled

The most frequent sites sampled are blood, urine, and exhaled air. Other body sites that are sampled but for which there is little scientific information about are hair and adipose tissue. The utility of hair analysis is limited by the unpredictable absorption of many chemicals by the hair root.

**A. Blood:** Blood is usually considered to provide the most accurate assessment of exposure. However, for volatile substances with short half-times, the variation in blood level can be considerable.

Unless otherwise indicated, blood sampling calls for whole venous blood. If the plasma-erythrocyte distribution ratio is not near unity, sampling may call for a serum specimen. The venous sample of a chemical that easily penetrates the skin—eg, nitroglyc-

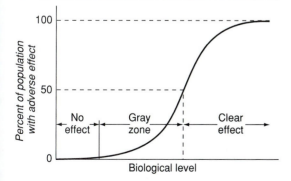

**Figure 38–2.** Percentage of population demonstrating adverse clinical effects from increasing biological levels of the chemical.

**Table 38–3.** Chemicals for which there are reliable data for determining reference biological monitoring levels.

| Chemical Determinant[1] | Media (units) | Levels Without Occupational Exposure | No Adverse Effect Level | Clinical Effect Level | Timing of Sample[2] | Terminal Half-Time ($t_{1/2}$) | Comments |
|---|---|---|---|---|---|---|---|
| **Inorganics: Metals** <br> Arsenic | Urine ($\mu$g/L) | <30 | 500–300 | >300 | EWW | 1–2 d | No seafood for 48 hours before collection. |
| Cadmium | Urine ($\mu$g/g Cr) | 0.02–4 | 5–10 | 20 | NC | 10–30 y | Reflects chronic exposure (years) after 1 year of exposure. |
| | Blood ($\mu$g/L) | 0.4–1 | 5–10 | 20 | NC | 10–15 y | Reflects recent exposure (months). Smokers may have blood levels of 1.4–4.5 $\mu$g/L. |
| Chromium | Urine ($\mu$g/g Cr) | <5 | 30 | . . . | EOS, EWW | 15–40 h | Exposure from welding stainless steel. |
| Lead | Blood ($\mu$g/dL) | 2–9 | 25 | 80 | NC | . . . | Use lead-free needles and tubes, BEI, blood 50 $\mu$g/dL. |
| | Urine ($\mu$g/g Cr) | 10–65 | 150 | . . . | NC | . . . | $t_{1/2}$ for soft tissue is 1 month; for skeleton, 20 years. |
| *Zinc protopor-phyrin(ZPP)* | Blood ($\mu$g/dL) | 16–35 | 100 | . . . | NC | 2–4 wk | Useful after 1 month of exposure. Reflects total body burden. Free erythrocyte protoporphyrin (FEP) is interpreted similarly to ZPP. |
| Mercury (inorganic) | Urine ($\mu$g/L) | <20 | 35–50 | 200 | PNS | 60 d | Reflects prior 2–4 months' exposure. |
| Nickel | Urine ($\mu$g/L) | <5 | 70 | . . . | EOS | 17–39 h | Corrected to SG of 1,018. Measures only soluble nickel. |
| | Plasma ($\mu$g/dL) | 0.2–0.4 | 0.7 | . . . | EOS | . . . | |
| Selenium | Plasma ($\mu$g/dL) | 5–18 | . . . | . . . | . . . | . . . | |
| | Urine ($\mu$g/g Cr) | 7–79 | 25 | . . . | . . . | 100–150 d | |
| Vanadium | Urine ($\mu$g/g Cr) | <1 | 50 | . . . | EOS, EWW | 20–40 h | |
| **Inorganics: Other** <br> Carbon disulfide <br> *TTCA* | Urine (mg/g Cr) | 0 | 5 | . . . | EOS | 2–3 d | TTCA is 2-thiothiazolidine-4-carboxylic acid. Carbon disulfide is a metabolite of disulfiram (Antabuse) and dithiocarbamates. |
| Carbon monoxide <br> *COHb* | Blood (%) | 0.4–0.7 | 3.5 | 10 | EOS | 1–8 h | Blood COHb following: Cigarettes 1 ppd = 5–6% <br> 2–3 ppd = 7–9% <br> Driving on urban highways = 5% |
| Cyanide <br> *Thiocyanate* | Urine (mg/24 h) | 0.11 | 6.5 | . . . | . . . | . . . | |
| Fluorides | Urine (mg/L) | <0.4 | 3 | . . . | PNS | 4–7 h | In unexposed persons, varies with drinking water fluoride, use of dental products. |
| | | . . . | 10 | . . . | EWW | . . . | |
| **Organics: Aliphatics and alicyclics** <br> Acetone | Urine (mg/g Cr) | <2 | 20 | 46 | DS | . . . | |
| | Blood (mg/dL) | <0.2 | 2 | . . . | DS | 6 h | Elevated during diabetic or fasting ketoacidosis. |
| | Alveolar air (mg/m$^3$) | . . . | 53 | . . . | DS | 4 h | |
| Cyclohexane <br> *Cyclohexanol* | Urine (mg/L | . . . | 3.2–5.5 | . . . | L4H | . . . | |

*(continued)*

**Table 38–3.** Chemicals for which there are reliable data for determining reference biological monitoring levels. (continued)

| Chemical Determinant[1] | Media (units) | Levels Without Occupational Exposure | No Adverse Effect Level | Clinical Effect Level | Timing of Sample[2] | Terminal Half-Time ($t_{1/2}$) | Comments |
|---|---|---|---|---|---|---|---|
| Cyclohexanol | Blood (µg/dL) | . . . | 46–52 | . . . | DS | . . . | |
| Cyclohexane | End-exhaled air (mg/m$^3$) | . . . | 780–880 | . . . | DS | . . . | |
| Dioxane β-Hydroxyeth- oxyacetic acid | Urine (mg/L) | . . . | 36.5 | . . . | EOS | 1 h | |
| Dioxane | Blood (mg/L) | . . . | 12 | . . . | DS | . . . | |
| Ethylene glycol Oxalic acid | Urine (mg/g Cr) | <100 | . . . | 0.3–4.3 g/L | . . . | 2–6 h | |
| Ethylene glycol monoethyl ether Ethoxyacetic acid | Urine (mg/L) | <0.07 | 6 | . . . | PNS | 21–24 h | |
| | | | 100 | . . . | EOS, EWW | | |
| n-Hexane 2,5-Hexanedione | Urine (mg/L) | 0.1–0.8 | 5 | . . . | EOS | . . . | Large individual variability. Correlates best with air con- centration. |
| n-Hexane | End-exhaled air (ppm) | . . . | 40 | . . . | DS | 1–2 h | Large individual variability. |
| Methanol | Urine (mg/L) | 0.3–2.6 | 15 | . . . | EOS | 1.5–2 h | |
| Formic acid | Urine (mg/g Cr) | 5–50 | 80 | . . . | PNS, EWW | . . . | |
| Methyl ethyl ketone | Urine (mg/L) | . . . | 2–5 | . . . | EOS | . . . | Large individual variability. |
| 2-Methyl pentane 2-Methyl-2- pentanol | Urine (mg/L) | . . . | <0.1–5.5 | . . . | EOS | . . . | |
| 3-Methylpentane 3-Methyl-3- pentanol | Urine (mg/L) | 0 | <0.1–1 | . . . | EOS | . . . | |
| Propylene glycol monoethyl air ether (PGME) | End-exhaled air (ppm) | 0 | 4 | . . . | EOS | . . . | |
| **Organics: Aromatic** Benzene Total phenol | Urine (mg/L) | 0–20 | 50 | . . . | EOS | 28 h | Large individual variability. |
| Benzene | Mixed- exhaled air (ppm) | <0.03 | 0.06 | . . . | PNS | 30 h | |
| | End-exhaled air (ppm) | <0.03 | 0.12 | . . . | PNS | 30 h | |
| | Blood (µg/dL) | . . . | . . . | 1–20 | PNS | 1–3 h | |
| Ethyl benzene Mandelic acid | Urine (g/g Cr) | <0.005 | 1.5 | . . . | EOS | 5 h | Large individual variability. |
| Ethyl benzene | End-exhaled air (ppm) | <0.03 | 2 | . . . | PNS, EWW | 2 d | |
| Phenol | Urine (mg/g Cr) | 0–20 | 250 | . . . | EOS | 3.5 h | Large individual variability. |
| | Urine (mg/h) | . . . | 15 | . . . | L2H | | |
| Styrene Mandelic acid | Urine (g/g Cr) | <0.005 | 0.8 | . . . | EOS | 25 h | Large individual variability. |

(continued)

**Table 38–3.** Chemicals for which there are reliable data for determining reference biological monitoring levels. (continued)

| Chemical Determinant[1] | Media (units) | Levels Without Occupational Exposure | No Adverse Effect Level | Clinical Effect Level | Timing of Sample[2] | Terminal Half-Time ($t_{1/2}$) | Comments |
|---|---|---|---|---|---|---|---|
| Styrene | Mid-exhaled air (ppm) | 0 | 0.04 | ... | PNS | 3 d | Large individual variability |
| | | 0 | 18 | ... | DS | | |
| | Blood (mg/L) | 0 | 0.55 | ... | EOS | 3 d | |
| | | 0 | 0.02 | ... | PNS | | |
| Penylglyoxylic acid | Urine (mg/g Cr) | ... | 240 | ... | EOS | 7–10 h | |
| Toluene Hippuric acid | Urine (g/g Cr) | <1.5 | 2.5 | ... | EOS | 1–2 h | Large individual variability. |
| | Urine (mg/min) | <0.4 | 3 | ... | L4H | | |
| Toluene | Blood (mg/L) | <0.015 | 1 | >1 | EOS | 3–4 h | |
| | End-exhaled air (ppm) | 0 | <20 | ... | DS | 3.7 h | |
| Xylene Total methylhippuric acid | Urine (g/g Cr) | 0 | 1.5 | ... | EOS | 30 h | |
| | Urine (mg/min) | 0 | 2 | ... | L4H | | |
| Xylene | Blood (mg/L) | 0 | ... | 3–40 | EOS | 20–30 h | Fatalities reported at 3–40. |
| **Organics: Halogenated** Methyl bromide Bromide | Blood (mg/dL) | 0.05–0.2 | 1.1 | 5 | ... | ... | |
| Methylene chloride Carboxyhemoglobin | Blood (%) | 0.4–0.7 | 2.5 | >10 | EOS | 10–12 h | Smoking and CO exposure additive in COHb levels. Longer $t_{1/2}$ than with CO exposure. |
| | | | 1 | ... | PNS | ... | |
| | End-exhaled air (ppm) | <2 | 3–6 | 8–13 | EOS | 10–12 h | |
| Methylene chloride | Blood (mg/dL) | 0 | 0.08 | 0.3–1.2 | EOS | ... | |
| Perchloroethylene | End-exhaled air (ppm) | 0 | 18 | 30 | EOS | ... | |
| | | | 5–10 | ... | PNS, EWW | 64 h | |
| | Blood (mg/dL) | 0 | 0.5–1 | ... | PNS, EWW | ... | |
| Trichloroacetic acid | Urine (mg/g Cr) | 0 | 3.5–7 | ... | EOS | 80 h | |
| Polychlorinated biphenyl Total chlorobiphenyl | Blood (µg/L) | 0–30 | 150 | 600 | NC | 3–7 y | Method of analysis critical. Results differ depending on specific PCB isomer. |
| 1,1,1-Trichloroethane | End-exhaled air (ppm) | 0 | 40 | ... | PNS, EWW | ... | |
| | Blood (mg/dL) | 0 | 0.5 | ... | EOS | ... | |
| Trichloroethanol | Urine (mg/L) | 0 | 30 | ... | EOS, EWW | 10–15 h | |
| | Blood (mg/L) | 0 | 1 | ... | EOS, EWW | | |

(continued)

**Table 38–3.** Chemicals for which there are reliable data for determining reference biological monitoring levels. (continued)

| Chemical Determinant[1] | Media (units) | Levels Without Occupational Exposure | No Adverse Effect Level | Clinical Effect Level | Timing of Sample[2] | Terminal Half-Time ($t_{1/2}$) | Comments |
|---|---|---|---|---|---|---|---|
| *Trichloracetic acid* | Urine (µg/L) | 0 | 10 | . . . | EWW | 70–100 h | |
| Trichloroethylene *Free trichloro-ethanol* | Blood (mg/L) | 0 | 4 | . . . | EOS, EWW | 12 h | |
| Trichloroethylene | End-exhaled air (ppm) | 0 | 0.5 | . . . | PNS, EWW | 30 h | |
| *Trichloroacetic acid* | Urine (mg/L) | 0 | 100 | 200 | EWW | 50–100 h | Large individual variability. |
| *Trichloroacetic acid and trichloroethanol* | Urine (mg/L) | 0 | 300 | . . . | EOS, EWW | . . . | |
| **Organics: Nitrogen-containing** Aniline *p-Aminophenol* | Urine (mg/L) | 0 | 50 | . . . | EOS | . . . | Large individual variability. |
| *Methemoglobin* | Blood (%) | 1–2 | 5 | . . . | EOS | . . . | |
| Dimethylformamide *N-Methylform-amide* | Urine (mg/g Cr) | 0 | 20–40 | . . . | EOS | 12 h | |
| Dinitrobenzene *Methemoglobin* | Blood (%) | 1–2 | 5 | . . . | EOS | . . . | |
| Ethylene glycol dinitrate | Blood (µg/L) | 0 | 0.2 | . . . | DS | 30 min | |
| Nitrobenzene *p-Nitrophenol and p-aminophenol* | Urine (mg/g Cr) | 0 | 5 | . . . | EOS | 60 h | |
| *Methemoglobin* | Blood (%) | 1–2 | 1.5 | . . . | EOS | . . . | |
| **Organics: Pesticides** Organophosphates *RBC cholinesterase* | Blood (% depression) | <20 | <30 | >40 | NC | 20–30 d | Levels are % depression from baseline. Symptoms depend on rate of decline in addition to absolute level. |
| Parathion *RBC cholines-terase* | Blood (% depression) | <20 | <30 | >40 | NC | 20–30 d | Reflects chronic exposure. |
| *p-Nitrophenol* | Urine (mg/L) | 0.01–0.03 | 0.5 | 2 | EOS | 4 h | Reflects recent exposure. |
| Carbamates *RBC cholines-terase* | Blood (% depression) | <20 | <30 | >40 | EOS | 1–2 h | Cholinesterase is reactivated very quickly. |
| Carbaryl *RBC cholines-terase* | Blood (% depression) | <20 | <30 | >40 | EOS | 1–2 h | Cholinesterase is reactivated very quickly. |
| *1-Naphthol* | Urine (mg/g Cr) | 1.5–4 | 10 | . . . | EOS | . . . | |
| Chlordane | Blood (µg/L) | 0 | 6 | 3000 | . . . | . . . | |
| Dieldrin | Blood (µg/L) | . . . | 150 | 200–1000 | . . . | . . . | |
| Endrin | Blood (µg/L) | 0 | 50 | | EOS | . . . | |
| *Anti-12-hydroxy-endrin* | Urine (mg/g Cr) | 0 | 130 | . . . | EOS | . . . | |
| Hexachloroben-zene | Blood (mg/L) | . . . | 3 | . . . | NC | 2 y | |
| Lindane | Serum (µg/L) | 0 | 20–30 | 500 | . . . | 20 h | |

[1]If the laboratory determinant is other than the material itself, it is listed below it in italics.
[2]NC = not critical; DS = during shift; EOS = end of shift; EWW = end of work week; L2H = last 2 hours of shift; L4H = last 4 hours of shift; PNS = prior to next shift; · · · = insufficient data.

erin—may reflect skin absorption distal to the sampling site and not total body exposure.

**B. Urine:** Urine is the easiest fluid to sample. A 24-hour urine collection provides the most accurate assessment of exposure, but for practical reasons in the workplace setting the sample usually collected is the spot urine—a single sample collected at a specified time relative to exposure. Unfortunately, significant variation can occur in spot urine levels owing to fluctuation in urine concentrations. This variability may be reduced by adjusting levels to urine specific gravity (SG 1.014) or urine creatinine (1 g of creatinine). This type of standardization should be done on a case-by-case basis. For example, while correcting for urinary creatinine will decrease variability in the assessment of mercury exposure, it appears to have no effect on variability when one is assessing cadmium exposure. In Table 38–3, urine values refer to spot urine levels and where appropriate are corrected for specific gravity or creatinine. Highly concentrated (SG > 1.030 or Cr > 3 g/L) or highly dilute spot urine specimens (SG < 1.010 or Cr < 0.3–0.5 g/L) are usually not suitable for monitoring, and a new specimen should be collected. Urine monitoring may not be appropriate for workers with advanced renal disease.

**C. Exhaled Air:** Measurements of chemicals in exhaled air are noted in the "comments" column of Table 38–3 to be either mid-exhaled or end-exhaled air. In general, the concentrations in end-exhaled air during exposure are smaller than in mixed-exhaled air, and during postexposure the concentrations in mixed-exhaled are smaller than in end-exhaled air. Workers with emphysema should not be monitored by exhaled air sampling. Sampling must be performed in an area free of the chemical being measured. The process usually involves breathing into a Saran bag that is then exhausted through a charcoal-containing tube.

## Selecting a Laboratory

Selection of a laboratory for analysis of specimens is generally the responsibility of the medical supervisor of a biological monitoring program. Selection should be on the basis of analytic accuracy, convenience, turnaround time, and cost. Analytic accuracy is the most important factor but is often difficult if not impossible to assess. The only true assessment of accuracy is an independent intralaboratory and interlaboratory program of quality assurance. This is accomplished by submitting blind samples to laboratories and comparing the results with those of a reference laboratory, followed by certification of laboratories meeting minimum standards. Certification in this way has been implemented on a national basis in the United States only for blood lead determinations.

Determination of cholinesterase levels for state-mandated monitoring of pesticide handlers must be done by state-certified laboratories in California, the only state with such a program. The World Health Organization recently conducted an international quality assurance program for blood lead and urine cadmium determinations.

Initial feedback from these testing and certification programs indicates that even the most experienced laboratories can fail to meet minimum standards and that without a regular quality assurance program, analytic quality cannot be ensured. The practitioner responsible for a monitoring program should request data on the laboratory's testing and certification status. It is more common, however, for the practitioner to rely on the use of "experienced" laboratories to produce reliable monitoring results. Analysis of a random sample of "split" specimens by another—preferably a reference—laboratory is an alternative to an internal quality assurance program.

For a number of compounds, the use of specific collection equipment is critical. Many laboratories provide such equipment as a service and may deliver and pick up samples on site. The laboratory should provide information on methods of sample collection, containers, and sources of contamination. Some laboratories have collected biological specimens from unexposed populations and generated a range of "normal" or "background" levels. Careful attention must be paid to the definition of "normal," which may be different for workers than for nonoccupational populations. The amount of assistance and accuracy of information provided should help to indicate the level of experience and expertise of the laboratory in analyzing the compounds of interest.

## HOW TO USE TABLE 38–3

### Selection of Chemicals

Only agents for which there have been adequate biological monitoring studies to date have been included in Table 38–3. Chemicals are arranged in the table first by major chemical group (metals, other inorganics, organics, etc). Within each major group, the chemicals are arranged alphabetically.

Under each chemical name are listed the body media (blood, urine, breath) in which the chemical or its metabolite can be measured and in what units. Only those media that have been adequately studied are included. The body fluids to be sampled are ranked so that the one with the greatest scientific validity is listed first. For practical reasons, the one ranked highest may not always be the measurement of choice.

### Levels in Unexposed Populations

Biological levels in populations without occupational exposure to that agent usually follow a Poisson distribution (skewed bell shape). The ranges listed in this column will include the majority, or 90%, of the unexposed population. The 5% of the population with the highest levels would be expected to be above this range.

## No Adverse Health Effect Level

This is the level at which almost all workers will be free of symptoms, signs, and adverse clinical laboratory test results. An adverse result is one that reflects end organ damage. For example, an elevated serum AST would be considered an adverse laboratory result, whereas an abnormal serum ALA synthetase level would not. A very small number of people with biological levels below the "no adverse health effect" level may have clinical findings. Unless otherwise noted, reproductive or carcinogenic effects of chemicals are not considered in calculating this level.

Only a limited number of chemicals have been studied for the purpose of determining the biological level associated with absence of adverse health effects. If such data do not exist, the "no adverse health level" may be based on extrapolation from limit values of environmental monitoring recommended by ACGIH or NIOSH. For example, almost all workers exposed to perchloroethylene (a cleaning solvent) below ambient air levels of 100 ppm will fail to experience the irritant and central nervous system depressant properties of perchloroethylene. The corresponding perchloroethylene blood or exhaled air level would be the biological "no adverse health effect" level. This does not take into account the theoretic risk of cancer from animal cancer data. "No adverse health effect" levels that have been arrived at by extrapolation from recommended environmental levels are identified with an asterisk.

Biological exposure indices (BEI) are reference biologic monitoring levels established by the ACGIH. A BEI is a level that corresponds to the level measured in a worker exposed to a substance at the threshold limit value-time weighted average (TLV-TWA) (see Chapter 37). Where a BEI has been established, it is in essential agreement with Table 38–3 unless otherwise noted in the comments to that table.

## Clinical Effect Level

This is the level that is commonly associated with symptoms, signs, or abnormal laboratory tests. This level is most useful for diagnostic purposes, ie, for evaluating a worker with an abnormal clinical presentation whose degree of exposure is uncertain. For example, the differential diagnosis of a worker exposed to pentachlorophenol includes salicylate poisoning, hyperthyroidism, and pentachlorophenol poisoning. The latter would be confirmed by a blood pentachlorophenol level near or above the "clinical effect" level.

## Timing of Sample Collection

The interpretation of a biological level is critically dependent on the timing of sample collection. The following abbreviations are standard times for biological sample collections and should be considered relative to standard work days and work weeks. For example, PNS ("prior to next shift") means sampling 16 hours after the last shift, and EOS ("end of shift") means sampling 15–30 minutes after the last exposure. The time recommendations are most important for the number that appears in the "no adverse health effect level" column.

> **NC** not critical
> **DS** during shift
> **L2H** last 2 hours of shift
> **L4H** last 4 hours of shift
> **EOS** end of shift
> **PNS** prior to next shift
> **EWW** end of work week

## Terminal Half-time

The rate of elimination of an agent—its terminal half-time—is useful for interpreting measured levels relative to the timing of sample collection. If the half-time is short (minutes to hours), the timing of collection is critical. If the half-time is long (days to weeks), the timing of collection is not critical.

Most organic chemicals have two half-times—an initial short half-time and a terminal longer one. The short half-time is usually a measure of the rate at which the solvent equilibrates from the blood to other tissues (fat, muscle, brain) and may be very rapid. The terminal half-time more accurately reflects the rate of elimination of the bulk of the chemical from the body.

Biological levels of chemicals with short half-times should be interpreted with caution when they are evaluated by using an average elimination half-time. The rates of metabolism and elimination may vary significantly between individuals. For example, the average half-time of carboxyhemoglobin is about 5 hours, with a range of 1–8 hours. A carboxyhemoglobin level obtained 1 hour after exposure will therefore represent somewhere between 50% and 95% of the end-of-shift level depending on the individual's elimination half-time.

## REFERENCES

Aitio A et al: Biologic monitoring. In: Zenz C, Dickerson OB, Horvath EP (editors): *Occupational Medicine,* 3rd ed. Mosby, 1994.

American Conference of Governmental Industrial Hygienists: *Documentation of the Threshold Limit Values and Biological Exposure Indices,* 6th ed. Vol III: Documentation of the Biological Exposure Indices. ACGIH, 1991.

American Conference of Governmental Industrial Hygienists: *1995–1996 Threshold Limit Values (TLVs) for Chemical Substances and Physical Agents and Biological Exposure Indices (BEIs).* ACGIH, 1995.

Ashford NA: *Monitoring the Worker for Exposure or Disease: Scientific, Legal, and Ethical Considerations in the Use of Biomarkers.* Johns Hopkins, 1990.

Boeniger MF, Lowry LK, Rosenberg J: Interpretation of urine results used to assess chemical exposure with emphasis on creatinine adjustments: A review. Am Ind Hyg Assoc J 1993;54:615.

Deutsche Forschungsgemeinschaft: *MAK- und BAT-Werte-Liste 1992.* VCH Verglagsgesellschaft, 1992.

Dillon HK: *Biological Monitoring of Exposure to Chemicals: Metals.* Wiley, 1991.

Droz PO, Fiserova-Bergerova V: Biological monitoring IV. Pharmacokinetic models used in setting biological exposure indices. Appl Occup Environ Hyg 1992;7:574.

Fiserova-Bergerova V: Biological monitoring VIII. Interference of alcoholic beverage consumption with biological monitoring of occupational exposure to industrial chemicals. Appl Occup Environ Hyg 1993;8:757.

Fiserova-Bergerova V, Ogata M (editors): *Biological Monitoring of Exposure to Industrial Chemicals. Proceedings of the United States-Japan Cooperative Seminar on Biological Monitoring.* ACGIH, 1990.

Health and Safety Executive, Occupational Medicine and Hygiene Laboratory: *Guidance on Laboratory Techniques in Occupational Medicine.* Her Majesty's Stationery Office, 1991.

Lauwerys RR: *Industrial Chemical Exposure: Guidelines for Biological Monitoring, Second Edition.* CRC Press, 1993.

Murthy LI, Halperin WE: Medical screening and biological monitoring: A guide to the literature for physicians. J Occup Environ Med 1995;37(2):170.

Ogata M, Fiserova-Bergerova V, Droz PO: Biological monitoring VII. Occupational exposure to mixtures of industrial chemicals. Appl Occup Environ Hyg 1993;8: 609.

Rosenberg J: Biological monitoring IX. Concomitant exposure to medications and industrial chemicals. Appl Occup Environ Hyg 1994;9:341.

Rosenberg J, Rempel D: Biological monitoring. In: Medical monitoring in the workplace. Occup Med State Of Art Rev 1990;5:491.

Travis CC: *Use of Biomarkers in Assessing Health and Environmental Impact of Chemical Pollutants.* Plenum Press, 1993.

# Section VI.
# Environmental Health

# Environmental Exposures & Controls

# 39

*Joseph LaDou, MD, Richard J. Jackson, MD, MPH,*
*& John Howard, MD, JD*

Beginning with the industrial revolution in England in the late 18th century, environmental contamination has increased steadily throughout the world—and radically so since World War II. The technologic advances of the past 40 years have resulted in toxic hazards that proliferate each year as new materials and new methods of production are introduced.

Government at all levels, as well as the public, are becoming increasingly concerned about contamination of the environment. Widely publicized disasters such as those at Minamata Bay, Chernobyl, and Bhopal, have emphasized these concerns, and similar events not so widely publicized are equally important.

Occupational physicians are today increasingly concerned with problems of environmental health. The physician must be concerned with contamination outside the workplace as well as within and must be knowledgeable about disposal of toxic wastes emanating from the workplace. All physicians must understand the effects of toxic environmental exposures, and the requirement for greater awareness in this area extends also to public health officials, and to many other levels of government.

To control all naturally occurring contaminants in the environment would be an impossible task. To control the toxic hazards we ourselves introduce into the environment is at least theoretically possible given sufficient resources and the will to do so.

United States there are more than 500,000 sites where hazardous waste has been discarded, along with contaminated pits, ponds, and lagoons. Very few of these sites have been adequately remediated.

The air in urban areas is heavily polluted by the annual release of hundreds of millions of pounds of xylene and more than 1 billion lb of toluene as automotive exhaust gases. Water systems used by the majority of people now contain volatile organic compounds. The effectiveness of water treatment for purposes of infection control may be declining as chemical contamination of drinking water increases. Water contamination is becoming a major public health problem all over the world.

Rural areas become contaminated because of the injudicious use of pesticides and herbicides in agriculture. Forests and fisheries are decimated by sulfur and nitrogen emissions carried by wind and rain from highly populated areas and industrial centers.

The vast size of the subject population and the proliferation of new materials with unknown effects introduced by advancing technology have made it critical that we find some means of controlling the possible deleterious health effects of environmental contaminants. Unfortunately, we know little about what these effects will be, particularly over the long term, and epidemiologic studies—our primary source of information—cannot answer many of our questions.

## THE MAGNITUDE OF ENVIRONMENTAL CONTAMINATION

All industrialized nations are faced with serious problems of environmental contamination, and the developing countries are beginning to realize the extent of these difficulties as their industrialization progresses. US industries produce more than 300 million tons of hazardous wastes each year, or more than 1 ton per person. To compound the problem, in the

## PRIMARY SOURCES OF CONTAMINATION

Chemical manufacturing is one of the main sources of environmental contamination. Others include pulp and paper milling, petroleum production, textile manufacturing, mining and metal smelting. All these activities produce chemical byproducts, particulates or dusts that contaminate air, land and water.

Federal and state restrictions on automotive output of particulates have reduced the problem somewhat, but there are still older motor vehicles in use, so that contaminants continue to be discharged into the environment in unacceptable quantities.

Population growth and rising standards of living are invariably accompanied by increases in energy generation. The burning of coal, oil and wood add to the global burden of pollution, and provide a ready explanation for the greenhouse effect now recognized as an ecological disaster in the making.

Agriculture is a major contributor to environmental contamination through the extensive use of pesticides and herbicides. As insects adapt to survive contact with currently used pesticides, new and more potent ones are produced. These substances contaminate not only surface and underground waters, but also the land itself as well as the food it produces.

## MAJOR ENVIRONMENTAL CONTAMINANTS

Of all the contaminants that human commercial ingenuity has introduced into the environment, probably the most publicized are asbestos, lead, dioxins, and polychlorinated biphenyls (PCBs). All are highly toxic and persist for long periods in the environment.

### Asbestos

The mineral asbestos is a family of fibrous hydrated silicates that is one of the most pervasive environmental hazards in the world. Asbestos fibers in ores are not respirable until released and made airborne during mining and processing. The family of asbestos minerals can be subdivided into serpentine and amphibole fibers. Chrysotile, which accounts for over 90% of the world's production of asbestos, is the most common fibrous serpentine whereas the amphiboles, a chemically diverse group of less industrially important minerals, include the fibrous minerals and crocidolite, amosite, anthophyllite asbestos, actinolite asbestos, and tremolite asbestos. Tremolite, actinolite and anthophyllite, which occur in both fibrous and nonfibrous forms, have been only rarely mined for use as commercial asbestos. Both the fibrous and nonfibrous forms of these amphibole minerals are sometimes found as contaminants of commercial deposits of chrysotile, talc, vermiculite, and other minerals.

Asbestos is present in more than 3000 manufactured products, and more than 30 million tons of asbestos in its various forms have been mined since the turn of the century. To some, its perceived benefits outweigh the importance of preventing further asbestos contamination of the environment. Many countries have considered a ban on the mining and uses of asbestos only to begin a long process of granting exceptions to maintain competitive positions in world trade. Asbestos manufacturing is moving rapidly to developing countries where it is already a major cause of occupational illness.

The advantages of asbestos products are the result of its resistance to heat and chemicals, high tensile strength, and lower cost compared to man-made materials. The United States and many European countries have banned the use of spray-on asbestos as a fire-proofing material or insulation. Nonetheless, asbestos is incorporated currently into cement construction materials (roofing, shingles, and cement pipes), friction materials (brake linings and clutch pads), jointing and gaskets, asphalt coats and sealants, and many other similar products.

Asbestos is associated with the development of pulmonary interstitial fibrosis (asbestosis), lung cancer, and malignant mesothelioma in occupationally exposed workers. The pathogenicity of different forms of asbestos varies—long thin amphibole fibers are most pathogenic, particularly in the induction of mesothelioma. The concentration of asbestos fibers in air, type of asbestos, and size of fibers are important factors in the evaluation of potential health risks.

Because asbestos has been implicated in the development of gastrointestinal cancers, its presence in more than 100,000 miles of water mains and sewage pipes in the United States is being studied. Asbestos contaminates drinking water both through the natural erosion of surface rock formations and by the breakdown of asbestos-containing products made by humans. Asbestos is found in the drinking water of most Americans, usually less than 1 million fibers per liter. Some water supplies contain over 1 billion fibers per liter, and where water flows through natural areas of asbestos, the concentrations in drinking water are over 10 billion fibers per liter.

**A. Major Health Effects:** Asbestos is inhaled in dust particles that lodge in the lungs and usually remain there. It can result in asbestosis, a chronic reaction of the lungs accompanied by fibroid induration; lung cancer; and mesothelioma, a tumor arising in the membranes lining the pleural and peritoneal cavities. By the 1930s, asbestosis was generally regarded as a hazard to persons working with asbestos fibers in manufacturing. Although the risk of lung cancer was suspected at that time, it was not until the mid 1950s that the causal link was firmly established. Mesothelioma resulting from asbestos exposure was not demonstrated until 1960. The danger of this mineral is exemplified by the experience of 8–11 million shipyard workers from World War II into the 1960s. Approximately 50% of all deaths among this group resulted from lung cancer or other asbestos-related diseases. At present, there are questions about whether cancer of the gastrointestinal or genitourinary tract may result from ingestion of asbestos fibers. Nonetheless, by the year 2000, an estimated 300,000 US workers will have died of the diseases known to be caused by asbestos. It is anticipated that deaths will continue to occur well into the next century. With the global spread of asbestos manufacture and asbestos-containing building materials, the pandemic is now extending to the Third World.

**B. Sources of Exposure:** Asbestos fibers enter the body either by inhalation or by ingestion. Not only are asbestos workers at risk from inhaling the fibers, but a large proportion of the population is at some risk from the breakdown of the many products in which it has been incorporated.

Ingestion of the fibers comes primarily from drinking water contaminated either from natural sources or from asbestos-reinforced concrete water pipes as they gradually deteriorate. Asbestos fibers are present in a number of foods—particularly processed foods—and other ingestible items. Sizable numbers of fibers have been found in everything from aspirin tablets to chewing gum. They occur also in mayonnaise, lard, catsup, sticky rice, and many other foods that have been shown to contribute more than a million fibers a day to the typical diet.

Epidemiologic studies to date that compare populations drinking high concentrations of asbestos in water with low-exposure groups have failed to demonstrate an increased rate of gastrointestinal and genitourinary cancers in the high exposure groups. But the studies are flawed because the fibers in foods were not taken into account. Future studies will be difficult to conduct because there is no readily available technique for assaying the asbestos content of various foods. Asbestos in drinking water and foods may be a carcinogen of major significance, but in the absence of a control group, it will be difficult to measure the effects in humans.

The level of exposure that produces asbestosis can be determined with relative reliability, but it has not been possible to determine a dose level that produces a finite risk of cancer in humans. It is known, however, that a far smaller dose is required for developing cancer than for developing asbestosis. Unfortunately, occupational standards for asbestos exposure have until very recently dealt only with risk estimates for asbestosis. Examples of variation in state and federal protection standards for workers reflect this inherent problem.

**C. Controlling the Problem:** It may not ever be possible to fully control asbestos exposure. Asbestos is ubiquitous in our environment, and there is no way in which the enormous quantities already used can be removed. In many instances, experts agree that methods of containment are far more practical than efforts at removal.

An estimated 20% of buildings have asbestos-containing materials. Asbestos in buildings does not spontaneously shed fibers, but physical damage to asbestos-containing materials by decay, renovation, or demolition can cause release of airborne fibers. The discovery that asbestos-containing materials were used in schools, buildings, and hospitals, led to the Asbestos Hazard Emergency Response Act (AHERA), a mandate from the Environmental Protection Agency (EPA) that requires inspection of the nation's public and private schools for asbestos. This, in turn, resulted in the appearance of a large number of asbestos identification and removal companies. Remediative efforts to control airborne asbestos at approximately 733,000 public and commercial buildings that contain asbestos will cost more than $100 billion over the next 30 years.

Asbestos exposure in the ambient air of many urban areas is higher than it is in buildings containing asbestos products. One study of the risk to students exposed to an average asbestos concentration of 0.001 fiber/mL of school room air for an average enrollment period of 6 school years is about 5 lifetime excess cancers per million students.

## Lead

Lead is a highly toxic heavy metal that contaminates all of the environment but especially urban centers. Lead is used in the manufacture of storage batteries, gasoline additives, printing, radiation shielding, cable covering, solder, foil, paint, and numerous alloys. One estimate is that the average city dweller discards into the trash over 40 lb of lead annually. Little progress is being made in the reduction of lead from smelting emissions. Worldwide, atmospheric lead emissions have increased 2000-fold since the pre-Roman era, when lead was already being mined.

Lead serves as an excellent example of the complexity of dealing with environmental issues on a global basis. The economic impact of dealing with lead as a public health problem is greater than the world will bear. There are political repercussions and human considerations inherent in any attempt to control the use of lead. The simple fact is that lead has been damaging to the public health for thousands of years, and will continue to be a serious public health problem even if extreme measures are undertaken to control its global use.

Lead is not biodegradable. It is indestructible and cannot be transformed into a nontoxic form. About half of the 300 million metric tons of lead ever removed from the earth was released as contamination and is available to human exposure. Current lead production is about 3.4 million metric tons per year, and current lead release to the environment is about 1.6 million metric tons per year. Lead contamination of the Northern Hemisphere and surrounding waters has increased since the Industrial Revolution by at least one order of magnitude. Lead in the atmosphere is now 100 times natural concentrations. Consequently, we have total body burdens of lead 100–1000 times those of our pre-Columbian ancestors.

**A. Major Health Effects:** Lead is highly toxic by inhalation or ingestion of either dust or fumes. The toxicology of occupational lead exposure is discussed in Chapter 27.

Children are particularly susceptible to the toxic effects of lead. Excessive absorption of lead dust is one of the most prevalent and preventable of debilitating childhood health problems. The US Public Health Service and the Centers for Disease Control designate the maximum permissible concentration of blood lead as 10 micrograms per deciliter to protect the health of children, and 20 micrograms per deciliter as the level for medical intervention. About 6 million children and fetuses in the United States are estimated to exceed the protective blood lead level, with the worst exposures taking place in disadvantaged neighborhoods. Prenatal lead exposure increases the risk of preterm delivery, and is associated with reduced birth weight. In young children, blood lead levels as low as 10 micrograms per deciliter cause a constellation of adverse neurotoxic and biochemical effects manifested as depression of neurological and psychological function, effects that appear to be permanent. Lead is associated with disturbances in cognition, behavior, and attention at levels below those that cause frank symptoms. Chronic lead exposure in childhood may result in obesity that persists into adulthood.

Although the detrimental CNS effects of low to moderate exposure to lead is well documented in children, such an effect remains controversial in adults. Animal studies have demonstrated that relatively low doses of lead can produce modest elevations in blood pressure. Epidemiologic studies of both the occupational and general population do not provide conclusive evidence that lead exposure is positively associated with hypertension. The evidence is most convincing in adult men aged 40–59 years old and for systolic rather than diastolic pressure. In middle aged men, a mean increase in systolic blood pressure of 1.0–2.0 mm Hg appears to occur for every doubling in blood lead levels, with the increase being somewhat less in adult women. A recent study found that mean levels of lead in blood and bone were signficantly higher in hypertensive subjects suggesting that long-term lead accumulation may be a risk factor for developing hypertension in men in the general population.

**B. Sources of Exposure:** There are many sources of lead exposure in the home and environment. Homes built before 1940 contain lead in a variety of construction products including insulation, paint, interior woodwork, and wallpaper. Many common household items also contain significant quantities of lead. Because lead is found in so many inks and dyes, brightly colored magazine pages may be significantly contaminated with lead. Printed food wrappers, handles of kitchen utensils, and the seals on bottles of wine may serve as exposure opportunities for both adults and children. Acid foods and beverages dissolve lead from improperly glazed earthenware pottery. Copper pipes conveying drinking water through lead-soldered joints are a common source of lead exposure. The EPA estimates that about 20% of the US population (including 3.8 million children) consumes drinking water with lead levels above 20 μg/dL. The FDA has estimated that about 20% of all dietary lead comes from canned food; about two-thirds of that amount results from lead solder in cans.

**C. Controlling the Problem:** The control of lead dusts and fumes in the environment is a large undertaking. To date, some important steps have been taken in that direction, notably (1) the concerted effort to restrict lead-containing emissions from motor vehicle exhausts, (2) the restriction on use of lead in paint and in tin can lid soldering, and (3) the requirement that smelters and refiners and other lead-related industries install equipment to control their emissions. Companies that work with lead are also required to install exhaust equipment that will protect workers from exposure to hazardous lead levels. Furthermore, because of known reproductive effects, women of child-bearing age are no longer permitted to work in lead products operations without proper engineering controls. Workers should be required to shower and change clothes after their shifts so as not to carry lead dust out of the workplace.

There are circumstances that tend to frustrate control efforts. The nation has thousands of older homes where lead is inherent in the structure, in paint, woodwork, insulation, and water systems that contain lead pipe. In addition, the emission control devices used on smelters and other industrial emitters of lead dusts and fumes are not totally effective. It is unfortunately true also that not all lead industries are committed to the idea of controlling the problem.

Lead is far from necessary for many of its current industrial applications. The predominant use of lead is in large rechargeable batteries. Substitutes for lead in certain products are being sought in only a few developed countries. Yet, almost without exception, regulation of lead exposure is the sole method by which the countries of the world deal with the hazards of lead. Source reduction is seldom if ever discussed, primarily because so many countries profit from lead mining and smelting. Realistically, source reduction is the only reliable long-term answer to the global crisis in lead exposure. As economically painful and socially disruptive as this fact may be, a global ban on lead mining and smelting should be at the center of international environmental discussion.

It is surprising that, with all that we have learned about lead and all that we have done to combat lead exposure, there is so little movement toward global source reduction. Lead is mined at ever-increasing quantities in the world today. Australia and the United States lead the world in lead production. Russia and China are large miners of lead ore, as are Canada and Peru. Few areas of the world do not profit from lead mining, smelting, and refining. If lead mining and smelting were to be banned worldwide, the short term economic impact would likely be severe.

An international ban on lead mining and primary smelting would cause the cost of lead to rise. This, in turn, would stimulate efforts to find substitute products and to develop new industrial processes. An increase in the value of lead would enhance efforts to recover lead released from other mining and smelting operations. Continued demand for lead products would increase the use of secondary smelting (recycling already accounts for almost half of world refined lead production).

The use of lead should be phased out all over the world. The first focus of the endeavor will be lead in gasoline because it is the fastest growing segment of lead use outside of the United States. Later efforts will address lead acid battery recycling, lead in paints and food cans, and lead in plumbing. Phaseout activities such as these can be complimented by efforts at source reduction. US phaseout programs may find application in some other countries, but not in most developing countries. Source reduction through a global ban on lead mining and smelting is the only reliable approach to the global crisis in lead exposure.

**D. International Dimensions:** Lead exposure is a worldwide environmental problem. Lead is quietly moved in prodigious quantities between countries to redistribute the hazards involved in smelting, refining and manufacture. Estimates of lead exposure and surveys of blood lead in populous countries such as India and China indicate that most of the world's children are already at risk from the effects of environmental lead exposure. Preliminary studies show that blood lead levels of children in Africa and Latin America virtually all exceed 10 μg/dL. Pregnant women in developing countries are much more likely to exceed the protective blood lead level than pregnant women in the developed countries, and workers exposed to lead in countries such as Thailand, Mexico, and Romania represent a greater public health problem than any perceived in the developed countries.

The reduction in lead exposure in the United States masks a shameful record of the export of lead to other countries, most of which are unaware of the extent of lead's impact on the public health. Regions of Taiwan are stacked high with waste lead acid batteries exported by the United States for recycling at a healthy distance. Mexico is also a major source of lead recycled for US industry from our exported waste lead.

## Dioxin

Dioxin (see 2,3,7,8-TCDD in Chapter 28) is a trace contaminant of the chlorinated hydrocarbon 2,4,5-trichlorophenoxyacetic acid (2,4,5-T). After the neurotoxin botulin and some nerve gases and other weapons of chemical warfare, it is arguably the most toxic substance known. Moreover, it is highly stable in the environment. It has been widely distributed in herbicides throughout the United States and was a contaminant of the defoliant Agent Orange (a mixture of equal parts of 2,4-D and 2,4,5-T), used on rice paddies, trails, and jungles during the Vietnam War. Dioxin's contamination of products used in this country to control weeds in lawns, along highways, and in utility and railroad right-of-ways and in commercial forests, may have caused adverse health effects. Anthropogenic production of dioxin has decreased during the past two decades, and is smaller by far than the amount produced by natural fires. Nonetheless, annual industrial emissions total about 26,000 tons, and in some instances they affect communities in higher concentrations, such as that produced from wood pulp bleaching operations, than from natural emissions.

**A. Major Health Effects:** The known near-term effect of exposure to dioxin is chloracne, a severe form of acne that persists for long periods. In 1976, an explosion at a chemical factory in Seveso, Italy, exposed the nearby town to a cloud of dioxin and other contaminants. Four percent of the population, including many children, suffered chloracne. Persons residing in three zones of decreasing TCDD contamination and a reference population were followed up for cancer occurrence in 1977–1986. The most exposed subgroup was small, and only 14 cancer cases were observed. In the next most exposed subgroup, hepatobiliary cancer was elevated, especially for those living in the area for more than 5 years (RR = 2.8; 95% CI = 1.2–6.3). Men exhibited an increase in hematologic neoplasms, most notably lymphoreticulosarcoma (RR = 5.7; 95% CI = 1.7–19.0). Women experienced an increased incidence of multiple myeloma (RR = 5.3; 95% CI = 1.2–22.6) and myeloid leukemia (RR = 3.7; 95% CI = 1.9–15.7). In the least exposed subgroup, the incidence of soft tissue tumors and non-Hodgkin's lymphomas was elevated.

Although dioxin has been found to produce carcinogenic and teratogenic effects in some laboratory animals at uniformly low doses and has been lethal to some species at doses of less than 1 μg/kg of body weight, little has been determined about the long-term effects in humans. The lowest dose of dioxin in the pregnant rat necessary to cause reproductive outcomes in the offspring (64 ng/kg) is not far from the current average background dose of dioxin and related chemicals that has accumulated in humans (5–10 ng/kg). The fact that dioxin produces adverse developmental and reproductive effects in fish, birds, and mammals suggests that it could do so in humans.

In a case-control study including 237 cases with soft tissue sarcoma and 237 controls, previous jobs and exposures to different agents, including pesticides, were assessed. Exposure to phenoxyacetic acids or chlorophenols gave a statistically significant increased rate ratio (RR) of 1.80 for soft tissue sarcoma. The increased risk was attributed to dioxin-contamination.

The many Vietnamese exposed to dioxin from Agent Orange would be an excellent subject population for epidemiologic studies, but the difficulty of conducting such studies is obvious. However, thousands of US service personnel were also exposed and are currently the subject of numerous studies. Skin conditions, hepatic, cardiovascular, and immune profiles are similar for Vietnam veterans and controls. The veterans do have a significantly increased incidence of basal cell carcinomas, but no difference with respect to melanoma and most all systemic cancer. Vietnam veterans have a higher risk of non-Hodgkin's lymphoma, but exposure to Agent Orange does not appear to increase the risk. Nonetheless, a National Academy of Sciences panel agrees that there is sufficient evidence of an association between Agent Orange exposure and three cancers: soft tissue sarcoma, non-Hodgkin's lymphoma, and Hodgkin's disease. The panel is unable to verify a link to other cancers or problems such as birth defects and immune disorders.

**B. Sources of Exposure:** Exposure to dioxin is possible wherever the substance has been indiscriminately used as a herbicide. In Times Beach, Missouri, for example, 10 years before the danger of dioxin was fully recognized, waste oils containing dioxin were sprayed on roads to control dust. This created such outrage in the community—with extensive media coverage—that the EPA ordered the area closed and the federal government actually paid for the deserted houses in the evacuated area.

Aside from areas of large accidental release or deliberate spraying, as in Seveso and Vietnam, the most important source of exposure is in the use or manufacture of herbicides, in the bleaching of paper pulp, and in the combustion products of low-temperature incineration. Many older incinerators in Europe and the United States have been closed because of dioxin emissions even though there is no American standard for incinerator emissions or human exposure. The major environmental exposure hazard for humans is with fish consumption. Bioconcentration of dioxin by fish is similar to that of PCBs (discussed below).

**C. Controlling the Problem:** The only means of controlling the problem of dioxin contamination of the environment is to outlaw its further presence in plant hormones, herbicides, and defoliants and to control its emissions in waste burning operations. Fish assays and inspections may lead to greater regulation of fish consumption.

## Polychlorinated Biphenyls

Polychlorinated biphenyls (PCBs) are biphenyls extracted from petroleum and chlorinated in the presence of a catalyst, usually iron. PCBs were manufactured in the United States between 1929 and 1977.

Because of their stability, high boiling point, and low electrical conductivity, they were used primarily as coolants for electrical transformers; as dielectrics for electrical capacitors; and in stone-cutting oils, hydraulic fluids, and heat transfer fluids. They were also used as plasticizers, in carbonless multicopy office forms, and as constituents of paints and objective immersion oils for microscopes. Although their manufacture is no longer permitted, total PCBs currently in the environment exceed 500 million lb, and 750 million lb are still in use in capacitors and transformers. PCBs are thus a continuing danger in the environment.

**A. Health Effects:** PCBs are stored in body fat, and it is believed that exposure has been widespread in industrialized nations. In the United States, almost everyone has detectable amounts of PCBs in the body.

Pregnant women working in low-exposure areas produce premature infants of significantly lower birth weight. Newborn infants whose mothers consumed moderate quantities of lake fish contaminated with PCBs had lower birth weights and smaller head circumferences. Lactating mothers transmit the toxicants in milk.

PCBs cause hepatocellular carcinoma in rats. Although carcinogenic effects to date have not been established in humans, numerous other deleterious health effects have been determined. Much of what is known about the toxicity of PCBs in humans resulted from an incident in Japan in 1968, when an accidental leak in a rice oil processing plant caused high levels of PCBs (and furans) in the cooking oil. In a matter of weeks, consumers of the oil were ill and exhibited mild to severe chloracne; hyperpigmentation of the skin, nails, conjunctiva, and mucous membranes; liver disease, including necrosis; fatigue; headache; menstrual disorders; palpebral edema and meibomian gland hypersecretion; and birth defects, usually hyperpigmentation. Nursing infants who had not ingested the oil also showed symptoms, indicating that the mother's milk may have transmitted the toxicant.

A similar event occurred in Taiwan in 1979. Rice cooking oil was contaminated by polychlorinated dibenzofurans and PCBs as well as a wide variety of other chemicals and their isomers. By the end of 1980, there were a reported 1843 cases of PCB poisoning from four counties in central Taiwan. The latent period from time of ingestion to the manifestation of clinical symptoms was approximately 3–4 months. After 3.5 years, 2061 persons were determined to have PCB poisoning. Thirty-nine infants born to PCB-exposed mothers showed hyperpigmentation. In the Taiwan case, the fatality rate was relatively high. By the end of 1980, eight of the exposed group had died; and by the end of 1983, 24 more had died. Almost half had died from hepatomas, liver cirrhosis, or liver disease with hepatomegaly.

Children born to affected women were shorter and lighter than controls. Delays of developmental milestones were observed, along with abnormalities noted on behavioral and developmental testing. The findings of growth abnormalities and hyperpigmentation, persistent conjunctival swelling, and abnormalities of nails, hair, teeth, and gums are generally consistent with an acquired neuroectodermal dysplasia.

It is not yet known whether the health effects of such major exposures are similar to those of long-term, low-level exposures that are occurring in many areas. Over prolonged periods, the moderate consumption of contaminated fish may show similar effects. Sport fish consumption has been estimated to deliver a dose of PCBs that is 4300 times greater than background exposure from inhalation or drinking water. The potential mechanisms by which PCBs may impair human health and reproduction are poorly understood. Placental transport of PCBs and other organochlorine compounds has been demonstrated. Placental tissue from women exposed to PCBs has been found to display markedly elevated induction of microsomal benzo($a$)pyrene despite nondetectable concentrations of placental aryl hydrocarbon receptors (AhRs). PCBs and other organochlorine contaminants have been associated with endocrine disruption, neurotoxicity, and developmental delay in humans, and may be harmful to testicular function. Because PCBs can induce cytrochrome P450, it has been suggested that the effect of PCBs on the reproductive system could be related to alterations in steroid hormones. Moreover, PCBs have been found to be mutagenic, with dose-related chromosome breakage in human white blood cell lines at low levels of exposure.

A rapidly increasing number of chemicals, or their degradation products, are being recognized as weakly estrogenic. Hormonally active xenobiotics can come from the diet, such as the phytoestrogens coumestrol and genestein, or from the environment (eg, DDT and PCBs). Among the environmental chemicals that may be able to disrupt the endocrine systems of animals and humans, PCBs are of considerable concern. One possible mechanism by which PCBs may interfere with endocrine function is their ability to mimic natural hormones. These actions reflect a close relationship between the physicochemical properties encoded in the PCB moleculear structure and the responses they evoke in biological systems.

An association between estrogen exposure and breast cancer has been a topic of debate for a number of years. It is not understood whether estrogens act as initiators, promoters, or both, in breast cancer. Many breast cancers, as well as nonmalignant reproductive tract conditions such as endometriosis, are hormonally responsive, which makes estrogenic exposure an important component of their etiology. The possibility of human exposure to environmental chemicals possessing estrogenic activity is of understandable concern. Recent reports have hypothesized a link between the observed increase in testicular tumors and lower sperm counts in humans and possible prenatal and neonatal estrogen exposure. In addition to the possible cancer and noncancer effects of environmental estrogen on humans, there are reported estrogenic effects on wildlife populations related to fertility and sexual development. The current evidence is far from conclusive about the association of organochlorine exposure and breat cancer risk. The connection to male reproduction, including sperm counts, is highly speculative.

**B. Sources of Exposure:** Accidental leaks of PCBs are the primary source of acute exposures. Such leaks can contaminate surface and groundwaters and contaminate freshwater fish. Devastating health effects resulted from PCB contaminations of food in Japan and Taiwan. More subtle health problems are being monitored because of the ubiquitous contamination of fish, particularly shellfish. This is the major source of chlorinated hydrocarbon exposure in humans.

**C. Controlling the Problem:** Solving the problem of PCB contamination of the environment will require the efforts of both the government and the electrical utilities—the government in locating the dangerous discarded PCB sources, and the utilities in carefully monitoring units still in use and discarding others properly. Further study will be needed on health effects of PCBs and on safe and effective means of disposing of these contaminants. In some localities, the level of fish contamination with PCBs is leading to regulation and recommendations to women of child-bearing age or those breast feeding to eat a diet containing no fish or fish oils.

## Agricultural Contamination: Pesticides & Fertilizers

The agricultural use of pesticides (including herbicides) and fertilizers is treated separately here because it contaminates more than one aspect of the environment. Both materials run off or leach into the soil through the action of rain and irrigation. As a result, they contaminate the soil itself, enter the food chain, and poison both surface water and groundwater, destroying natural resources and endangering human health.

Since the introduction of DDT in 1939 and its successful use against mites, ticks, and mosquitoes during World War II, the production and number of pesticides has proliferated in the United States. Faced with a continuing problem of insects and weeds that became resistant to current products, the chemical industry has concentrated on developing more and more new products. Between 1945 and 1995, pesticide production (including herbicides) in the United States rose from 100 million lb to over 3 billion lb. Herbicide use is increasing dramatically as the savings in fuel costs for plowing and cultivating is added to the savings in human labor costs. Herbicides are used in greater quantities than insecticides in the United States. The United States is the largest producer and user of these products in the world. The federal Office of Technology Assessment reports that 260,000 tons of active ingredients in pesticides and 42 million tons of fertilizer are annually spread over the equivalent of 280 million acres across the United States. Moreover, homeowners use 10 times more chemical pesticides per acre than farmers do. Of the 34 major pesticides commonly used on lawns, 32 have not been tested for their long-term effects on humans and the environment.

**A. Health Effects:** The impact of toxic agricultural agents on human health has become a growing concern as their residues increasingly enter drinking water sources and the food chain. Continuing exposure to low levels of pesticides places farm workers at risk of cancer, reproductive disorders, birth defects, and many long-term illnesses. Especially disturbing are the residues of pesticides that affect infants and children. Organochlorine pesticide residues, despite their replacement in agriculture with organophosphate pesticides, will continue in the food chain and be concentrated in the fatty tissues of almost all Americans for the foreseeable future. One recent study found that imported fruits and vegetables contained twice the levels of residual pesticides found in domestic foods.

Illness from legal residues in food is difficult to document. This is so because the clinical diagnosis is difficult to determine, and because many of the health effects of pesticides are not acute. Pesticide health effects may not be manifest for long periods of time. An example of this is found with the clinical diagnosis of low dose exposures to organophospate insecticides. Low doses are likely to cause diarrhea and possible mood and other neurological symptoms. These nonspecific symptoms would not lead an individual to seek medical care and a clinician to order an expensive and nonspecific screening of food for one of the more than 300 pesticide compounds used on food. Human illnesses from consuming pesticides in food have been recognized in episodes where highly toxic compounds in foods led to acute manifestations. Two dramatic examples are the contamination of watermelons in the Western United States because of the illegal use of the pesticide aldicarb; and the second was a probable food tampering episode of a frozen food with the organochlorine insecticide endrin. In both episodes, the public health problem was first identified by an alert individual who notified public health officials.

In the past, pesticide food tolerances (legal pesticide residue limits) were set at levels based on the availability of a laboratory measurement of the compound and, of greater importance, the need to maintain agricultural production. New pesticide tolerances are set to offer margins of safety for human health for most healthy adults. Tolerances constitute the single, most important mechanism by which EPA limits levels of pesticide residues in foods. A tolerance must be established for any pesticide used on any food crop. Tolerance concentrations are based primarily on the results of field trials conducted by pesticide manufacturers and are designed to reflect the highest residue concentrations likely under normal conditions of agricultural use. Tolerances are not based primarily on health considerations. The determination of what might be a safe level of residue exposure is made by considering the results of toxicological studies of the pesticide's effects on animals and, when data are available, on humans. Both acute and chronic effects, including cancer, are considered, although acute effects are treated separately. These data are used to establish human exposure guidelines (ie, a reference dose [RfD]) against which one can compare the expected exposure.

Children may be more sensitive or less sensitive than adults, depending on the pesticide to which they are exposed. Current testing protocols do not, for the most part, adequately address the toxicity and metabolism of pesticides in neonates and adolescent animals or the effects of exposure during early developmental stages and their sequelae in later life. Both government and industry data on residue concentrations in foods reflect the current regulatory emphasis on average adult consumption patterns. Estimates of expected total exposure to pesticide residues should reflect the unique characteristics of the diets of infants and children and should account also for all nondietary intake of pesticides. Determinations of safe levels of exposure should take into consideration the physiological factors that can place infants and children at greater risk of harm than adults.

**B. Controlling the Problem:** The use of pesticides has significantly altered agricultural processes that previously helped control pests. First, crop rotation—a method for ensuring that more pest-resistant crops would alternate with less resistant ones—no longer appeals to farmers, who would rather use the readily available chemical controls. Second, tilling agricultural waste acreage to eliminate out-of-season support of pests has decreased considerably. Third, the use of natural predators of the pests has declined.

However, the ever-growing resistance of pests has led to research to determine whether the former methods should not be combined with the use of less toxic chemical agents to solve the problem. This outcome would be preferable to deluging the environment with a continuous flow of newer and ever more toxic chemicals.

Finally, restrictions on chemical agricultural products will need to be more stringent, and black markets for these chemicals will have to be eliminated.

Controlling the problem will not be easy in a contracting agricultural economy.

## Ionizing Radiation

Ionizing radiation is electromagnetic radiation that has sufficient energy to separate electrons from their atomic or molecular orbits. Exposure to ionizing radiation poses a severe threat to humans and animals.

Although natural background radiation from both cosmic and terrestrial sources has always been part of the environment, technology has added numerous other potential sources of exposure to ionizing radiation, particularly in the field of medicine. Moreover, humans also carry internally trace amounts of radioactive isotopes, such as carbon 14 and potassium 40.

**A. Health Effects:** From the beginning of this century, cases have been seen of severe radiation burns in physicists and medical personnel working with unshielded x-ray tubes and with radionuclides, especially radium. After appropriate latency periods, an unusual incidence of various cancers was also observed among these early researchers and practitioners. Very early, it was recognized that radiation exposure caused eye irritations, cataracts, dermatitis, loss of hair, and cancerous ulcers. Laboratory animals also exhibited—in addition to the effects seen in humans—evidence of bone growth inhibition, bone abnormalities, and sterility. Later findings in both humans and animals have identified additional effects, including cell death, genetic defects, cancer, impairment of the immune system, and shortening of life.

A number of factors affect the severity of radiation damage, including age, individual physiologic variations, and differences between species. The usually long latency period of cancer development may mask other health effects when research objectives concentrate strictly on carcinogenic effects. For example, when the immune repair mechanism is damaged by radiation, exposed individuals may die much earlier from infectious diseases, particularly pneumonia, so that the cancer indigence would appear only in the strongest individuals.

Present knowledge of the health effects of radiation has been derived from 2 primary sources: atomic bomb survivors in Japan and medical patients who have undergone radiation diagnostic studies or radiation therapy. Both of these groups received high-level exposure. Consequently, the health risk level of low-dose exposure is not entirely clear and remains a major issue of environmental protection today.

Evidence of the hazards of radiation exposure continue to mount. Evaluations of cancer risk from ionizing radiation have undergone significant upward revisions compared to those published about a decade earlier. Those revisions were necessitated primarily by considerable differential increases in cancer deaths among the low-dose subcohorts of the A-bomb survivors, and far-reaching revisions of the individual dose estimates for the survivors. Both the A-bomb survivor cancer mortality and incidence data fail to suggest the existence of a threshold for cancer induction down to very low doses. Doses less than 5 cGy and probably as low as 1.6 cGy have been associated with excess cases of leukemia among A-bomb survivors. Doses in the range from less than one to a few cGy have been associated with brain damage in prenatally exposed children of A-bomb survivors. Mortality for solid cancers in the 6–19 cGy dose group is significantly higher than it is in the 0–5 cGy dose group.

In recent studies, significant increases in specific types of cancer among exposed workers were found; for example, lung, bladder, and prostatic cancers, multiple myeloma, lymphatic and hematopoietic neoplasms, and leukemia. A cancer mortality and incidence study among about 900 Canadian male pilots showed significant excess rates for several cancers, including Hodgkin's disease and nonmelanoma skin cancer. Leukemia clusters have been found near nuclear plants, several demonstrating an increased risk for leukemia in young people. The risk factor for prenatal x-ray examinations of the fetus during the first trimester is about nine times that of the general population. The most recent data suggest an excess relative risk associated with an intrauterine x-ray examination of about 40%. There are conflicting studies of thyroid neoplasms and leukemia in populations near nuclear facilities. Reproductive outcome measures are demonstrated with elevated background levels of radiation.

**B. Sources of Exposure:**

**1. Natural Background Radiation—**Levels of natural background radiation differ with geographic location. The type of soil in the area and the radionuclides present in soil affect the exposure rate, or dose-equivalent rate. For example, the Colorado Plateau area has a higher dose-equivalent rate (75–140 mrem/y) than do either the Atlantic and Gulf Coastal plains (15–35 mrem/y) or the remainder of the coterminous United States (35–75 mrem/y).

Cosmic radiation that descends to earth consists of extraterrestrial particles that pass through the earth's atmosphere and additional particles created by the passage. The dose-equivalent rate increases as the earth's atmospheric shield becomes thinner. The dose-equivalent rate from extraterrestrial sources is higher at higher altitudes, being twice as high at 1800 m as it is at sea level. It is also affected by solar changes. Overall, the dose-equivalent rate for the US population is estimated to be approximately 31 mrem/y.

**2. Radon—**Uranium is a common constituent of rocks and soils throughout the United States. During the radioactive decay process, uranium decays to radium which in turn decays to radon, a noble gas. Radon then diffuses out of the rocks and soils in which it is formed and undergoes further decay (with a half-life of 3.82 days) into a series of short-lived solid isotopes which are commonly called "radon daughters."

These radon-decay products, either free or attached to airborne particles, are inhaled and undergo further radioactive decay in lung tissue. During this radon decay process in the lungs, high-energy alpha emissions penetrate the cells of the epithelium lining the bronchi and alveoli. Energy deposited in these cells during alpha radiation is believed to initiate the process of carcinogenesis. The US Environmental Protection Agency, the National Cancer Institute, and the Centers for Disease Control and Prevention estimate that as many as 14,400 lung cancer deaths a year are attributable to radon, based on animal studies and data from epidemiologic studies of uranium and other underground miners. This represents about 10% of US lung cancer victims.

Radon is recognized as the second leading cause of lung cancer, following tobacco smoking. Tobacco smoke in combination with radon exposure has a synergistic effect. Smokers and recent former smokers are believed to be at especially high risk. Estimates are that the increased risk of lung cancer to smokers from radon exposure is ten to twenty times higher than to people who have never smoked. However, about 20% of the lifetime risk of lung cancer in nonsmokers may be associated with radon exposure. Lung cancer is presently the commonly accepted disease risk associated with radon exposure. Radon in water is discussed in Chapter 44.

While the occupational risks, of lung cancer from radon exposure in uranium and other underground miners has been known since the late 1960s, the environmental risk from radon exposure in indoor air spaces has only been documented since the 1970s. The EPA estimates that as many as six million homes throughout the United States have radon levels at or above the 4 pCi/l action level of radon as a result of the concentration of uranium-containing rocks, sometimes far beneath the surface on which the structure is built. Since 1988, EPA and the Office of the Surgeon General have recommended that homes below the third floor be tested for radon. Some 2000–4000 US lung cancer deaths per year may be prevented if all homes with radon levels exceeding the EPA's action level were repaired.

EPA advises that short term testing is the quickest way to determine if a potential problem exists, taking anywhere from two to ninety days to complete. Low-cost radon test kits are available by mail order, in hardware stores, and through other retail outlets. Measurement devices should be state-certified or display the phrase, "Meets EPA Requirements."

Trained contractors who meet EPA's requirements can also provide testing services. The most com-

monly used devices are charcoal canisters, electretion detectors, alpha-track detectors, and continuous monitors placed by contractors.

Short-term testing should be conducted in the least occupied area of the home, with the doors and windows shut. Long-term testing can take up to a full year, but is more likely to reflect the home's year-round average radon level than short-term testing. Alpha track detectors and electretion detectors are the most common long-term testing devices. Corrective steps include sealing foundation cracks and holes, and venting radon-laden air from beneath the foundation.

Physicians should keep in mind that, in addition to tobacco smoking, occupational and environmental exposure to radon can contribute to the development of lung cancer. Effective measures to prevent lung cancer in smokers and nonsmokers alike should include assessment of radon exposure.

**3. Radiation Generated by Health Services–** The Bureau of Radiological Health has determined that x-rays used in patient diagnosis or treatment are the chief source of radiation exposure of the US population. More than 300,000 x-ray units exist in the various health services, and an estimated 150 million people are exposed annually through medical and dental x-rays. Those most at risk are the people who work with the equipment daily. The EPA has estimated that these people receive about 50 mrem/y.

Another important source of radiation exposure in health services is the use of radiopharmaceuticals, which more than 10,000 physicians in the United States are licensed to administer. Ten to 12 million doses of the radionuclides are administered annually for diagnosis or treatment involving the brain, liver, bone, lung, thyroid, kidney, and heart. According to EPA estimates, this represents about 20% of the total radiation resulting from health services.

**4. Exposure from Nuclear Weapons Tests–** Prior to 1963, when most nuclear tests were performed in the atmosphere, large amounts of radioactive material were released to be carried by the wind and brought to earth by rains. The first explosion at Bikini Atoll in 1954 exposed many in the area to radioactive fallout, including the inhabitants of surrounding islands and 23 Japanese fishermen who were downwind. It was estimated that the fishermen themselves received an average of approximately 200 R of total body radiation, and all suffered from acute radiation syndrome. One subsequently died from a transfusion complication. The catch of tuna was also severely contaminated, and other catches contaminated via the waterborne route were detected intermittently over several months. Among the Marshall Islanders, an unusual incidence of benign and malignant thyroid nodules, hypothyroidism, and growth retardation has been documented secondary to radioiodine exposure. Both groups suffered from acute beta irradiation burns to the skin.

This and related episodes indicate that significant harmful exposure occurs outside the prescribed "danger area," in part because of the unpredictability of atmospheric dispersion. Moreover, radionuclides can enter the food chain by means of rainfall on croplands as well as via contaminated fish and drinking water. Atmospheric tests conducted in Nevada during the 1950s and 1960s produced excessive levels of radioactivity in food and dairy products in many parts of the United States.

**5. Radiation Exposure from Nuclear Power–** Several hundred nuclear reactors now exist in the United States for power production, scientific study, and other uses. Because of public indignation over the Three Mile Island and Chernobyl accidents and because of the accelerating costs involved, the building of additional nuclear reactors remains in question. However, the existing reactors pose a risk not only to their workers but also to populations in the area. Short of a full-scale "meltdown" with breach of the containment vessel, the major concern with possible reactor accidents relates to the emission of radioactive isotopes of iodine and their potential effect on the thyroid. Radioiodines, particularly $^{131}$I, are the major public health risks following a reactor accident, because they are readily volatilized and dispersed and rapidly taken up by the thyroid gland.

The mining and milling of uranium to feed the reactors pose a steady-state risk to the inhabitants of several southwestern states in the United States, where 140 million tons of radon-emitting uranium mill tailings lie exposed to the atmosphere. Further risks are related to the disposal of radioactive wastes and to the flow of cooling water containing tritium, carbon 14, and krypton 85 into streams and rivers. These elements are nearly impossible to contain or remove and are capable of contaminating fish, drinking water, and the crops used for human consumption or animal feed that are irrigated with the water.

**6. Other Sources of Radiation–**Additional sources of potential radiation include a number of products, some of which are in widespread use. Products that either contain radioactive materials or generate x-rays during operation include luminous dial watches, dental prostheses, smoke detectors, cardiac pacemakers, tobacco products, fossil fuels, and some building materials. Air flight also is a source of radiation from the x-ray inspection systems at airports to cosmic radiation exposure during flight. Further exposure may occur if the flight is transporting radioactive materials.

**C. Controlling the Problem:** Since all possibilities cannot be included in any radiation research project, no reliable permissible dose equivalent has yet been established. Rather, the problem has been approached from risk-benefit considerations: ie, How much radiation exposure are we willing to accept to achieve the benefits of nuclear energy? Most scientists would agree that no level of ionizing radiation is entirely safe or can ever be made so. Man-made radiation sources have already doubled the level of exposure in the past hundred years.

## THE GLOBAL MIGRATION OF INDUSTRY

Foreign companies and investors from developed countries today account for almost two-thirds of industrial investment and development in the Third World. For many nations such investment is the primary source of new jobs. The low cost of labor is the principal reason for the rapid growth of industry in the developing world. Unfortunately, the Third World's lack of health and safety standards and of pollution control regulations provide another powerful incentive for industry to migrate to these developing countries. Examples of problems and abuses abound, from the exposure of women workers in the semiconductor industry in Malaysia to an unexplained reproductive risk, to the high incidence of lead poisoning and asbestosis in China. Solutions to these problems will involve the establishment of environmental and workplace regulations and enforcement in the developing world, and of a legal framework for dealing with abuses.

Most investment in developing countries goes to Asia. Japanese companies and investments are found in almost every country in the world. With limited land and great population density, Japan has a pressing need to export its waste-producing industries. Both Japan and the United States have significantly realigned their investment strategies toward Asia in recent years. Western European nations have exported hazardous and environmentally outmoded industries to Africa and the Middle East, and are now beginning to export them to Central Europe. Western European corporations are the largest investors in Bangladesh, India, Pakistan, Singapore, and Sri Lanka.

China and India, with the world's largest populations, have had dramatic policy reversals in recent years, and as a result have welcomed industries from many countries. US corporations are dominant in China, Hong Kong, Indonesia, the Philippines, Taiwan, and Thailand.

In the developed countries, industry provides jobs, pays taxes that support community services, and is subject to environmental and occupational health laws. As industrialized nations enact laws to limit the environmental hazards associated with many industrial operations, production costs rise and undermine competitive advantages. To offset this problem, manufacturers move many of their hazardous operations to the newly industrialized countries. They are welcomed because the creation of an infrastructure in many developing nations relies on industrial expansion by foreigners. When industry migrates to developing nations, companies not only take advantage of lower wages, but also benefit from the low tax rates in communities that are not spending much on such things as sewage systems, water treatment plants, schools, and public transportation. When companies establish plants in developing countries, their tax burden is a small fraction of what it would be in most developed countries.

Developing countries seldom have enforceable occupational and environmental regulations. They are concerned with overwhelming problems of unemployment, malnutrition, and infectious diseases, often to the exclusion of environmental hazards. About 450 million people live in extreme poverty and malnutrition, while another 880 million live in what can only be described as absolute poverty. Newly industrialized countries are eager for the financial benefits that foreign companies and foreign investors bring them. However, these benefits bring profound social and ecological problems.

The positive economic and social results of industrial activity in Third World nations are accompanied by serious environmental degradation. The major cities of developing nations are now reeling with the impact of air pollution, the absence of sewage treatment and water purification, and the growing quantities of hazardous waste buried in or left on the soil or dumped into rivers or the oceans. In many of the world's countries, there are no environmental regulations, or if they exist at all, there is little or no enforcement.

According to a World Bank Report, the amount of sulfur dioxide, nitrogen dioxide, and total suspended particulates in the air—three of the most dangerous industrial pollutants—increased by a factor of ten in Thailand, eight in the Philippines and five in Indonesia during the past decade. Five of the seven cities in the world with the worst air pollution are in Asia. With energy demand doubling in Asia every 12 years, Asian countries will produce in the next ten years more sulfur dioxide than Europe and America combined.

The workforce of developing nations is accustomed to working in small industry settings. Generally, the smaller the industry, the higher the rate of workplace injury and illness. These workplaces are characterized by unsafe buildings and other structures; old machinery; poor ventilation; noise; workers of limited education, skill, and training; and employers with limited financial resources. Protective clothing, respirators, gloves, hearing protectors, and safety glasses are seldom available. The companies are often inaccessible to inspection by government health and safety enforcement agencies. In many instances, they operate as an "underground industry" of companies not even registered with the government for tax purposes. Many investors in foreign plants allow no spending on occupational health and safety training and equipment and virtually no attention to

the environment until the investment returns a profit. For most new companies, this takes years.

Developed countries account for three quarters of all shipments of "dirty" products, with almost 40% of world exports coming from the EEC. In the past 20 years, there was a drop of over 6% in shipments of dirty products originating in North America, and a more than doubling of the share originating in Southeast Asia. If one looks at the share of dirty goods in total exports from each region, Eastern Europe, followed by the Latin American-Caribbean area, are the two regions with the highest concentration of dirty products. In these vast regions of developing countries, dirty products account for over one fifth of total exports (28% in the case of Eastern Europe). Such figures indicate a relative decline in the importance of these exports in developed countries, while Eastern Europe, Latin America, and West Asia show an increasing and alarming reliance on the export value of dirty products.

Migrating industries, including virtually all the transnationals, conform to the inadequate environmental and occupational health and safety standards of the host country. Consequently, worker fatality rates are much higher in newly industrialized countries than in the developed nations, and workplace injuries occur with rates common to the developed nations during the early years of the Industrial Revolution. In this regard, the Industrial Revolution is taking place all over again, but with much larger populations of workers and in many more countries.

There is no worldwide effort to maintain occupational safety records. The International Labour Office (ILO) estimates that 180,000 worker fatalities and 110 million workplace injuries occur each year. If the developing countries continue their current rate of industrial growth, these figures will double by the year 2025.

Virtually all of the world's population growth is occurring in the Third World. At present, the labor force in developing countries totals around 1.76 billion, but it will rise to more than 3.1 billion in 2025—implying a need for 38–40 million new jobs every year. This being the case, worker demands for better working conditions are not likely to occur.

## Women Workers

Both absolute and relative rates of labor force participation among women in the manufacturing sector have increased substantially. The overall participation rate for women in the industrial labor force increased significantly in those nations where development strategies focused on export processing. The availability of low-wage women workers is a major ingredient in the success of such places as Taiwan. Women workers are largely young and unmarried, and work in waged rather than salaried positions, and are paid less, on average, than men working in equivalent jobs. Most of the positions are unskilled, monotonous, and dead-end, offering few benefits to those who hold them—and are unattractive to men seeking work with opportunities for advancement. Industrialization in Taiwan was, and continues to be, fueled by a large reserve of women who are willing to work at tedious jobs for low wages. Nonetheless, most women are still relegated to the service sectors and the overall participation rates in the manufacturing sector of developing countries remain low.

The University of California, the Johns Hopkins School of Public Health and Hygiene, and the University of Massachusetts have all studied the health of US semiconductor workers. The studies collectively demonstrate that women have a major increase in the risk of miscarriage when they work in semiconductor cleanrooms where a broad array of chemicals is necessary to the manufacture of integrated circuits. Neither the semiconductor industry nor the US government has responded with the funding of further studies. The cause of the reproductive hazard is not known at this time. The semiconductor industry has been rapidly migrating to the developing nations of Southeast Asia.

The migration of American and Japanese semiconductor companies to Southeast Asia is dramatically demonstrated in the newly industrialized country of Malaysia. Over the past 20 years Malaysia became the world's third largest semiconductor manufacturer, and the world's largest exporter of semiconductors. It is very unlikely that foreign companies will continue to fund research on occupational and environmental health in a distant country with foreign workers. The savings realized by foreign manufacture of semiconductors will be enhanced by the ability of these companies to neglect health and safety as do many of their international rivals. The miscarriage rate of semiconductor workers will be ignored by governments and by industry in newly industrialized countries. Workers, for the most part, will not recognize the association between work and miscarriage.

### Child Labor

Children account for up to 11% of the workforce in some countries in Asia, up to 17% in Africa, and up to a quarter in Latin America. The condition of child workers has worsened dramatically in recent years (ILO, 1992). A conservative estimate is that at least 200 million children under the age of 14 are working fulltime in the world today. Children are the most easily exploited of all workers, and in the developing world, their numbers are ever increasing. Few countries have developed comprehensive plans to deal with child labor.

### Occupational Diseases

The incidence of occupational diseases has never been greater than it is today. The United Nations estimates that 10 million occupational disease cases occur each year worldwide. Occupational diseases occur with greater frequency in the developing countries, accompanied with greater severity.

Among miners, construction workers, and asbestos workers in some developing countries, asbestos is the major cause of disability and ill health, and by some counts, the major cause of death. The occupational and environmental hazards posed by asbestos products do not discourage the asbestos industry from promoting asbestos in the Third World where demand for low-cost building materials outweighs health concerns.

One-third of the urban Chinese population reports a history of occupational dust exposure. This is reflected by the fact that more than one million Chinese have silicosis. Silicosis is rare in developed countries, but is the most common occupational disease in China, the most populated country in the world. In Malaysia, silicosis occurs in one-quarter of the quarry workers.

When developed countries boast of accomplishments in the area of lead recycling, almost invariably the lead is recycled in developing countries and returned to the developed countries as finished products. This is the comfortable arrangement the United States enjoys with Mexico, Taiwan, and a number of other poorer countries.

In developing countries, governments and industries accept the transfer of hazardous materials knowing that reasonable exposure levels will not likely be legislated or enforced. Many products containing lead, such as gasoline, batteries, paints, inks and dyes are produced in developing countries by companies that are foreign-owned and the products are then sold internationally by the controlling interests.

### Pesticide Poisoning

In developing countries, where the majority of workers are in agriculture, pesticides are often applied by hand, or without proper protection of workers who use spray equipment. Three million pesticide poisonings occur each year in Southeast Asia alone. The use of pesticides in the developing countries is growing rapidly as they learn the advantages that such chemicals offer to the agricultural industry and as they gain the capability to produce the pesticides in their own countries.

Pesticides such as DDT and DBCP, which are banned in most developed countries, are widely sold and used without restrictions in the Third World. It is entirely legal for a US company to manufacture and distribute a chemical that is banned for use in the United States, so long as the sale and distribution are in another country whose laws are not violated by the transfer. For example, the insecticides chlordane and heptachlor were banned for agricultural uses in the United States in the 1970s. Yet between 1987 and 1989, the US manufacturer of these chemicals produced and exported nearly 5 million lb of the insecticides to some 25 countries.

## Conclusion

The experience of industrialized countries with the costs of occupational health and safety and environmental programs is that a very substantial financial burden is being shifted to newly industrialized nations. The World Bank estimates that ill health caused by pollution costs as much as $3 billion per year in lost productivity in Bangkok alone. The cost of pollution in the big cities of Asia is nearing 10% of urban GDP. The cost of clean-up is perhaps 1–2% of GDP. Postponing the investment will raise costs later. The cost of future accidents such as Bhopal, mitigation of environmental damage, and effects on the public health are not often discussed with candor in the Third World. The consequences of global industry may produce widespread international conflicts when the long-term economic realities of industrial migration become more apparent.

## INTERNATIONAL ENVIRONMENTAL LAW

In a global trade economy, many occupational and environmental health problems have taken on an international dimension. This is reflected in the increasing concern about the migration of air and water pollutants across national boundaries and the effect that those pollutants can have on the public health and the environment of the affected country.

Concern about transboundary air and water pollution has led to several different international agreements to regulate such environmental degradation and its possible adverse health effects. These agreements have been spearheaded by the efforts of the United Nations, the World Health Organization (WHO), the International Labor Organization (ILO), the European Community, the Organization for Economic Cooperation and Development (OECD), and by the trade provisions of the North American Free Trade Agreement (NAFTA) and the General Agreement on Tariffs and Trade (GATT).

The movement of hazardous waste across national boundaries has attracted special international attention. In 1989, the Basel Convention on the Control of Transboundary Movement of Hazardous Wastes and Their Disposal was adopted at a conference of more than 115 countries and went into effect in 1992.[1] The Basel Convention permits movement and disposal of hazardous waste only if all involved countries—including any transit countries—give their written consent.

In addition to specific environmental problems like the movement of hazardous waste across national boundaries, efforts are underway to harmonize the multitude of different occupational and environmental health and safety regulations which exist among the world's economies. However, harmonization may prove elusive. The GATT views stringent health and safety regulations as nontariff barriers, while others—concerned about exploited workers—view lax regulations as a subsidy to production. Another hurdle is that enforcement of environmental regulations is nonexistent in some countries and differs markedly even among industrialized countries. For instance, while American regulatory systems carry the threat of fines and jail, European regulatory systems are in large part only advisory.

Nevertheless, international trade may improve rather than compromise occupational and environmental health. If a superior technology, designed in an industrialized country, was deployed and perfected first in a developing country, then such a technology could eventually compete with the older, less-desirable technologies in both the donor and the recipient countries. The receiving country could then be given an equity share in subsequent sales both back to the exporting country and to other developing countries. But as some point out, such an approach requires a deliberate industrial policy for the environment, not the current collection of laissez-faire trade practices.

Lastly, occupational and environmental risk management has received increasing attention as a tool that product manufacturers can use to protect the public health and environment. Federal OSHA's Process Safety Management Standard (29 CFR 1910.109) is an example of a occupational regulatory mandate on manufacturers of hazardous chemicals to engage in environmental risk analysis and management on a periodic basis.

In the environmental arena, EPA has promoted the use of environmental auditing as a systematic way for manufacturers to evaluate the effectiveness of their environmental management systems already in place, to verify compliance with environmental requirements and to assess risks from regulated and unregulated materials and practices. However, environmental auditing remains a little used environmental risk management tool in the United States. This is so largely because manufacturers are concerned that they cannot protect the confidentiality of their audit results when disclosure of those audit results is demanded in legal proceedings.

On the international level, efforts are underway to "internationalize" product quality standards through voluntary, multi-national agencies such as the International Standards Organization (ISO). ISO 9000 and 14000 standards are beginning to be used as benchmarks for the selling of products in the international marketplace. Structurally, the ISO 14000 series of Environmental Management Standards (EMS) are a

---

[1] Fed. Reg. 20,602 (May 13, 1992).

set of voluntary standards and guideline reference documents which include environmental management systems, environmental audits, eco-labeling, environmental performance evaluations, life cycle assessment, and environmental aspects in product standards. The EMS do not directly establish requirements for environmental compliance nor specific levels of environmental performance. Rather, the emphasis is on management standards, much like the ISO 9000 Quality Management Standards (QMS) series. However, the EMS specification document addresses compliance indirectly through a commitment to both compliance with environmental laws and prevention of pollution.

The increasing emphasis on international environmental standards is the result of (1) foreign facilities becoming subject to foreign environmental laws with potential sanctions for noncompliance, particularly in the United States and Europe; and (2) the adoption of GATT by most of the trading countries in the world has raised the specter of potential trade sanctions against those countries or regions that have adopted stringent environmental laws which might be construed as trade barriers to importing countries with less rigorous environmental laws. Many companies based in the United States and Europe perceive that the development of international environmental management standards might be the only mechanism for avoiding or minimizing arbitration before the World Trade Organization.

# REFERENCES

## ASBESTOS

Gamble JF: Asbestos and colon cancer: a weight-of-evidence review. Environ Health Perspect 1994;102(12): 1038.

Kishimoto T: Cancer due to asbestos exposure. Chest 1992;101(1):58.

Landrigan PJ, Kazemi H, Selikoff IJ (editors): The third wave of asbestos disease: exposure to asbestos in place. Public Health Control. Ann NY Acad Sci 1991; Special issue.

Mossman BT et al: Asbestos: Scientific developments and implications for public policy. Science 1990;247: 294.

Stayner LT, Dankovic DA, Lemen RA: Occupational exposure to chrysotile asbestos and cancer risk: A review of the amphibole hypothesis. Am J Public Health 1996;86(2):179.

## LEAD

Allen D: Electric cars and lead. Science 1995;269:741.

Andrews KW, Savitz DA, Hertz-Picciotto I: Prenatal lead exposure in relation to gestational age and birth weight: A review of epidemiologic studies. Amer J Ind Med 1994;26:13.

Balbus-Kornfeld JM et al: Cumulative exposure to inorganic lead and neurobehavioural test performance in adults: An epidemiological review. Occ and Envir Med 1995;52:2.

Centers for Disease Control: Guidelines for the Prevention of Lead Poisoning in Children. US Public Health Service,1991.

Hu H et al: The relationship of bone and blood lead to hypertension. JAMA 1996;275(15):1171.

Kim R et al: A longitudinal study of chronic lead exposure and physical growth in Boston children. Environmental Health Perspectives 1995;103(10):952.

Needleman HL (editor): *Human Lead Toxicity.* CRC Press, 1991.

Needleman HL et al: The Long-term effects of exposure to low doses of lead in childhood. N Engl J Med 1990; 322:83.

National Research Council: *Measuring Lead Exposure in Infants, Children, and Other Sensitive Populations.* National Academy Press, 1993.

Pirkle JL et al: The decline in blood lead levels in the US JAMA. 1994;272:284.

Rosen JF: Adverse health effects of lead at low exposure levels: Trends in the management of childhood lead poisoning. Toxicology 1995;97:11.

Schwartz J: Lead, Blood pressure, and cardiovascular disease in men. Arch Environ Health 1995;50(1):31.

Silbergeld EK: The international dimensions of lead exposure. Int J Occup Environ Health 1995;1(4):336.

Todd AC et al: Unraveling the chronic toxicity of lead: An essential priority for environmental health. Environ Health Perspect 1996;104(Suppl 1):141.

Wu TN et al: Occupational lead exposure and blood pressure. Int J Epidemiol 1996;25(4):791.

## DIOXIN

Beck H, Dross A, Mathar W: PCDD and PCDF exposure and levels in humans in Germany. Environ Health Perspect 1994;102:173.

Bertazzi PA et al: Cancer incidence in a population accidentally exposed to 2,3,7,8-tetrachlorordibenzo-para-dioxin. Epidemiology 1993;4(5):398.

Birnbaum LS: Developmental effects of dioxins. Environ Health Perspect 1995;103(Suppl 7):89.

Fletcher CL, McKay WA: Polychlorinated dibenzo-p-dioxins (PCDDs) and dibenzofurans (PCDFs) in the aquatic environment—a literature review. Chemosphere 1993;26:1041.

National Academy of Sciences, Institute of Medicine. *Veterans and Agent Orange Update 1996.* National Academy Press, 1996.

Patterson DG et al: Levels of non-ortho-substituted polychlorinated biphenyls, dibenzo-p-dioxins, and dibenzofurans in human serum and adipose tissue. Environ Health Perspect 1994;102(Suppl l):195.

The Selected Cancers Cooperative Study Group: The association of selected cancers with service in the US military in Vietnam. II. Soft tissue and other sarcomas. Arch Intern Med 1990;l50:2485.

Svensson B-G et al: Exposure to dioxins and dibenzofurans through the consumption of fish. New Engl J Med 1991;324(1):8.

Wolff MS, Toniolo PG: Environmental organochlorine exposure as a potential etiologic factor in breast cancer. Environ Health Perspect 1995;103 (Suppl)7: 141.

## PCBS

Brown JF Jr et al: PCB metabolism, persistence, and health effects after occupational exposure: Implicatons for risk assessment. Chemoshphere 1994;29 (9–11):2287.

Chen YCJ et al: A 6-year follow-up of behavior and activity disorders in the Taiwan Yu-cheng children. Am J Public Health 1994;84:415.

Hsieh SF et al: A cohort study of mortality and exposure to polychlorinated biphenyls. Archives of Environ Health 1996;51(6):417.

Jacobson JL, Jacobson SW: Intellectual impairment in children exposed to polychlorinated biphenyls in utero. N Engl J Med 1996;335:783.

McKinney JD, Waller CL: Polychlorinated biphenyls as hormonally active structural analogues. Environmental Health Perspectives 1995;102(3):290.

Mendola P et al: Consumption of PCB-contaminated sport fish and risk of spontaneous fetal death. Environmental Health Perspectives 1995;103(5):498.

Rogan WJ, Gladen BC: Neurotoxicology of PCBs and related compounds. Neurotoxicology 1992;13(1):27.

Safe SH: Environmental and dietary estrogens and human health: Is there a problem? Environmental Health Perspectives 1995;103(4):346.

Sauer PJ et al: Effects of polychlorinated biphenyls (PCBs) and dioxins on growth and development. Hum Exp Toxicol 1994;13(12):900.

Swanson GM, Ratcliffe HE, Fischer LJ: Human exposure to polychlorinated biphenyls (PCBs): A critical assessment of the evidence for adverse health effects. Regul Toxicol Pharmacol 1995;21(1):136.

## AGRICULTURAL CONTAMINATION

Benbrook CM et al: *Pest Management at the Crossroads*. Consumers Union, 1996.

Goldman LR, Beller M, Jackson RJ: Alcicarb food poisoning in California, 1985–1988: Toxicity estimates for humans. Arch Environ Health 1990;45:141.

Goldman LR et al: Pesticide food poisoning from contaminated watermelons in California, 1985. Arch Environ Health 1990;45(4):229.

Fenske RA et al: Potential exposure and health risks of infants following indoor residential pesticide applications. Am J Public Health 1990;80:689.

National Research Council, Committee on Pesticides in the Diets of Infants and Children. *Pesticides in the Diets of Infants and Children*. National Academy Press, 1993.

Romero P, Barnett PG, Midtling JE: Congenital anomalies associated with maternal exposure to oxydemetonmethyl. Environ Res 1989;50:256.

Simonich SL, Hites RA: Global distribution of persistent organochlorine compounds. Science 1995;269:1851.

Waller K et al: Seizures after eating a snack food contaminated with the pesticide edrin: The tale of the toxic taquitos. West J Med 1992;157:648.

Wargo J: Our Children's Toxic Legacy: *How Science and Law Fail to Protect Us from Pesticides*. Yale University Press, 1996.

Zweiner RJ, Ginsberg CM: Organophosphate and carbamate poisoning in infants and children. Pediatrics 1988;81:121.

## IONIZING RADIATION

Balter M: Chernobyl's thyroid cancer toll. Science 1995; 270:1758.

Band PR et al: Mortality and cancer incidence in a cohort of commercial airline pilots. Space Environ Med 1990;61:299.

Committee on the Biological Effects of Ionizing Radiation. *Health Effects of Exposure to Low Levels of Ionizing Radiation, BEIR V*. National Research Council. National Academy Press 1990.

International Commission on Radiological Protection. *Recommendations of the ICRP*. Publication 60. Permagon Press, 1991.

Lubin J: Mining the radon studies. Environmental Helth Perspectives 1995;103(10):895.

National Research Council: *Health Risks of Radon and Other Internally Deposited Alpha-emitters*. National Academy Press, 1992.

Neel JV: Update on the genetic effects of ionizing radiation. J Am Med Assoc 1991;266:698.

Neuberger JS: Residential radon exposure and lung cancer: An overview of published studies. Cancer Detect Prevent 1991;15:435.

Nussbaum RH, Kohnlein W: Inconsistencies and open questions regarding low-dose health effects of ionizing radiation. Environ Health Perspect 1995;102(8): 656.

Upton AC, Shore RE, Harley NH: The health effects of low-Level ionizing radiation. Ann Rev Publ Health 1992;13:127.

United Nations Scientific Committee on the Effects of Atomic Radiation. Sources and Effects of Ionizing Radiation. United Nations, 1994.

US EPA: Technical Support Document for the 1992 Citizen's Guide to Radon. EPA 400-R-92-011. Environmental Protection Agency, 1992.

Wakeford R: The risk of childhood cancer from intrauterine and preconceptional expousre to ioninizing radiation. Environ Health Perspect 1995;103(11): 1018.

## INTERNATIONAL ENVIRONMENTAL HEALTH

Casto K, Ellison EP: ISO 14000: Origin, structure, and potential barriers to implementation. Intl J Occup Environ Heatlh 1996;2(2).

Cohen JE: Population growth and earth's human carrying capacity. Science 1995;269:341.

Fleming LE, Herzstein JH, Bunn B (editors): *Issues in Occupational and Environmental Medicine*. OEM Press 1996.

Goldemberg J: Energy needs in developing countries and sustainability. Science 1995;269:1058.

Holland HD, Petersen U: *Living Dangerously.* Princeton University Press, 1995.

Jamall IS, Davis B: Chemicals and environmentally caused diseases in developing countries. Infectious Disease Clinics of North America 1991;5(2):365.

LaDou J: International occupational and environmental health. In: Rom WN (editor): *Environmental and Occupational Medicine,* 3rd ed, Lippincott-Raven, 1997.

LaDou J, Levy B (editors): International issues in occupational health. Int J Occup & Environ Health 1995; 1(2):Special Issue.

Low P, Yeats A: Do "Dirty" Industries Migrate? Chapter 6 in: Patrick L (editor): *International Trade and the Environment.* The World Bank, 1992.

Shahi G et al (editors): *International Perspectives in Environment, Develoopment, and Health: Toward a Sustainable World.* Springer, 1996.

# 40 Routine Industrial Emissions, Accidental Releases, & Hazardous Waste

*Rupali Das, MD, MPH, Melanie Marty, PhD, & Marilyn Underwood, PhD** *

The worldwide publicity that followed the 1984 accidental release of methyl isocyanate in Bhopal, India, resulted in increased public awareness of the effects of chemicals released into the environment and sparked a host of regulations aimed at preventing a recurrence of a similar tragedy. Smaller, less known releases of hazardous chemicals continue to occur today. Interest in toxic hazards has increased in some sections of the medical community, but not until recently has education about toxic environmental hazards been emphasized. It is essential for occupational and environmental health care professionals to become familiar with both legal and medical issues relating to environmental pollution so that they may adequately respond to concerns in their communities.

The United States has the most comprehensive and adversarial system for the regulation of pollution in the world. United States environmental law is complex and encompasses both state and federal statutes. This is a growing field in other countries, as well. Substances that are potentially hazardous to health may be released into the air, water, or soil. The risks to human health and environmental integrity vary according to the media into which the release occurs, the amount released, and the duration over which exposure occurs. Environmental laws have traditionally been grouped according to both environmental media and the nature of pollutants: air pollution, water pollution, noise pollution, hazardous waste, hazardous materials management, remediation of contaminated soil and groundwater, and registration of toxic substances and pesticides.

This chapter covers environmental health hazards resulting from routine and accidental releases of hazardous chemicals and waste material into the environment and the laws that are intended to regulate polluting industries and prevent adverse health effects from occurring. The chapter is divided into three sections: routine industrial emissions, accidental releases, and hazardous waste. Each section will cover relevant health-based environmental regulations and the evaluation of potential health effects, termed risk assessment.

## ROUTINE INDUSTRIAL EMISSIONS

In our modern technologic society, industries produce an enormous variety of products using vast amounts of chemicals and numerous physical processes. All industrial processes are associated with emissions of chemicals into the air, water, or land. It was not until very recently that society has sought information on the impacts of these emissions on human and ecologic health. This section focuses on available information on the extent and public health impacts of emissions into air.

The earliest form of anthropogenic airborne emissions was woodsmoke. Humans have required sources of warmth and cooking fuel for millenia. Coal smoke contributed greatly to air pollution problems in the early days of the industrial revolution and continues to do so in some parts of the world. Currently, industrial emissions include a vast array of familiar and unfamiliar chemicals. Few airborne chemicals are well-characterized toxicologically. In addition, information about the toxicity of chemicals derived from animal studies generally involves exposure of a genetically homogeneous population of rodents to one chemical at a time. Thus, little knowledge exists about the interactions of chemicals or consequences of exposure to many chemicals simultaneously. Sources of airborne emissions are varied and range from large facilities like oil refineries to small sources such as gas stations, auto body shops, and dry cleaning operations. Emissions are somewhat characteristic for specific processes and source types.

*The views expressed in this chapter are those of the authors and do not necessarily represent those of the Office of Environmental Health Hazard Assessment, the California Environmental Protection Agency, the California Department of Health Services, or the State of California.

## TYPES OF SOURCES AND EMISSIONS TO THE AIR

Air pollutants have been characterized for regulatory purposes into two basic categories: criteria air pollutants (CAP) and toxic air contaminants (TAC). The distinction is somewhat arbitrary in that both types of emissions are toxic.

### Criteria Air Pollutants

Criteria air pollutants are typical components of smog and include chemicals emitted in large quantities and from many sources such as carbon monoxide (CO), sulfur oxides ($SO_x$), and nitrogen oxides ($NO_x$). The descriptor "criteria" refers to those chemicals for which there are regulatory standards determined by the United States Environmental Protection Agency (EPA), or, in some states, by state regulatory bodies. The standards are air concentrations that are designed to protect public health and which are not to be exceeded if an area is to be in compliance with the Clean Air Act at the federal level or state regulations, where they apply. The federal ambient air quality standards are depicted in Table 40–1. These pollutants are subject to regulation under state and federal statutes and are the pollutants originally identified by environmental scientists as posing public health risks.

### Toxic Air Contaminants

TACs are essentially everything else emitted into the air that is not a CAP and for which there is some regulatory concern. There are legal definitions for TAC in both state and federal statutes, and the federal government and the state of California have lists of chemicals that have been formally identified as TAC or candidate TAC. Substances may be listed by EPA as TAC for specific regulations. The EPA also has a list of Hazardous Air Pollutants (HAPs) that are subject to specific regulatory requirements. Similarly, California has listed TACs (Table 40–2) that are subject to stationary source emissions controls. Cancer potency factors or unit risk factors generated by EPA or the state of California for some of the carcinogens can be used in risk assessments to estimate the public health impacts of TAC emissions. The EPA has reference concentrations (RfC) and the state of California has Reference Exposure Levels (REL) for some of these compounds that are useful in estimating public health impacts for noncancer toxicologic end points. Both RfC and REL can be viewed as exposure levels at or below which adverse health

**Table 40–1.** Ambient air quality standards.

| Pollutant | Averaging[1] Time | National Standards Primary[2,3] |
|---|---|---|
| Ozone | 1 hour | 0.12 ppm (235 µg/m$^3$) |
| Carbon monoxide | 8 hour<br>1 hour | 9 ppm (10 mg/m$^3$)<br>35 ppm (40 mg/m$^3$) |
| Nitrogen dioxide | Annual average<br>1 hour | 0.053 ppm (100 µg/m$^3$) |
| Sulfur dioxide | Annual average<br>24 hour<br>1 hour | 0.03 ppm (80 µg/m$^3$)<br>0.14 ppm (365 µg/m$^3$) |
| Suspended particulate matter (PM$_{10}$) | Annual geometric mean<br>24 hour<br>Annual arithmetic mean | 150 µg/m$^3$<br>50 mg/m$^3$ |
| Lead | 30 day average<br>Calendar quarter | 1.5 µg/m$^3$ |

[1]National standards, other than ozone and those based on annual averages or annual arithmetic means, are not to be exceeded more than once a year. The ozone standard is attained when the expected number of days per calendar year with maximum hourly average concentrations above the standard is equal to or less than one.

[2]Concentration expressed first in units in which it was promulgated. Equivalent units given in parentheses are based upon a reference temperature of 25 °C and a reference pressure of 760 mm of mercury. All measurements of air quality are to be corrected to a reference temperature of 25 °C and a reference pressure of 760 mm of mercury (1,013.2 millibar); ppm in this table refers to ppm by volume, or micromoles of pollutant per mole of gas.

[3]National Primary Standards: The levels of air quality necessary, with an adequate margin of safety to protect the public health. Each state must attain the primary standards no later than three years after that state's implementation plan is approved by the Environmental Protection Agency.

Source: ARB Fact Sheet 39; (Revised 1/1/91) AAA/RBB/RD.

**Table 40–2.** Toxic air contaminants identified in California.

Acetaldehyde
Arsenic
Asbestos
Benzene
Benzo(*a*)pyrene (and related PAH)
Butadiene
Cadmium
Carbon tetrachloride
Chloroform
Chromium (+6)
Ethylene dibromide
Ethylene dichloride
Ethylene oxide
Formaldehyde
Lead
Methylene chloride
Nickel
2,3,7,8-Tetrachlorodibenzo-*p*-dioxin (and related 2,3,7,8-chlorinated congeners)
Tetrachloroethylene
Trichloroethylene
Vinyl chloride
United States EPA's 189 hazardous air pollutants (HAPs)

impacts are not anticipated. For the most part, however, there are not enforceable ambient air quality standards for TAC.

## Types of Sources

There are a great number of sources of airborne chemicals in the United States. For regulatory purposes, these sources have been divided into mobile sources (primarily cars, trucks, and buses) and stationary sources. The remainder of this section adresses stationary sources of airborne industrial emissions. Stationary sources are traditionally referred to as major and minor sources. Major sources include large industrial complexes such as refineries, aerospace manufacturing, chemical manufacturing facilities, etc. Major sources usually have large energy requirements and fulfill these demands via combustion of a wide variety of fuels, resulting in significant CAP emissions. Major combustion products include carbon monoxide and oxides of nitrogen and sulfur. Particulate matter is also emitted from combustion sources, particularly those that are poorly controlled. Refineries are some of the largest emitters of CAP, releasing hundreds of tons per day of sulfur oxides and nitrogen oxides. Oxides of nitrogen react with hydrocarbons emitted into the air to produce ozone on hot, sunny days. Thus, ozone, a major component of photochemical smog, is not emitted directly but represents one reaction product of atmospheric transformation of air pollutants.

Minor sources are usually associated with lower emissions of criteria air pollutants than major sources. Yet, minor sources can be important emitters of TAC, which are process-dependent. Specific industrial processes tend to use the same chemicals

and result in similar emissions. Small dry cleaning sources emit tetrachloroethylene, an animal carcinogen and possible human carcinogen. Incinerators tend to emit an array of products of incomplete combustion ranging from carbon monoxide to complex chlorinated compounds such as the carcinogenic 2,3,7,8-tetrachlorodibenzodioxin and related congeners, as well as metals and acid gases. Polycyclic aromatic hydrocarbons, some of which are carcinogens, are also large complex products of incomplete combustion emitted by incinerators and combustion processes. Both large and small sources can have incinerators as emitting devices. Metal finishing operations are usually small sources, but may be associated with potentially significant public health impacts. The known human carcinogens hexavalent chromium and nickel are used extensively in metal finishing operations, which are frequently associated with relatively high estimated cancer risks in an environmental context (eg, ten to one hundred in a million). Typically, regulatory agencies consider an excess individual cancer risk of one in one million for lifetime exposure to be *de minimis*. Regulatory activities, such as clean-up of hazardous waste sites or required air emissions controls, generally occur above this estimated level of cancer risk.

## EMISSIONS DATABASES

There are currently few emissions databases that reflect emissions inventories from individual facilities. The EPA maintains the Toxic Release Inventory (TRI), a database of stationary source emissions to air, water, and land, for specified compounds. In addition, the state of California maintains a database of emissions of toxic chemicals (excluding the criteria air pollutants) to the air from stationary sources. A separate database exists for emissions of criteria air pollutants from stationary sources in California. These databases are described below.

### National Toxics Release Inventory

In 1986, Congress enacted the Superfund Amendments and Reauthorization Act (SARA) and added Title III, known as the Emergency Planning and Community Right-to-Know Act. Section 313 of SARA Title III created the Toxics Release Inventory and gave the EPA authority to collect information on emissions of over 300 chemicals and chemical classes emitted by industrial sources. The chemicals on the TRI list include those listed as "extremely hazardous substances" by the EPA; substances covered by the Comprehensive Environmental Response, Compensation, and Liability Act (CERCLA); hazardous chemicals subject to Occupational Safety and Health Administration (OSHA) standards; and chemicals listed by the EPA on the basis of known or reasonably anticipated acute or chronic health effects or adverse environmental effects. SARA Title III's passage was stimulated by the tragedy in Bhopal, India, which resulted in death and injury to many thousands of people following the release of deadly methyl isocyanate gas from a Union Carbide plant. Part of the premise for the statute is that citizens have a right-to-know about toxic materials used, stored, and released into the environment in their communities. The statute also mandates emergency planning for chemical accidents (discussed elsewhere in this chapter).

Facilities that need to report emissions to the EPA are those that produce, import, or process 25,000 pounds or more of a listed substance, or use in any manner 10,000 pounds or more of a listed substance in a given reporting year. The facility must have a Standard Industrial Code (SIC) 20 to 39, which are the SIC for facilities engaged in manufacturing. In addition, the facility must have 10 or more full-time employees. As a result, only manufacturing facilities are required to report releases. For chemicals used exclusively in manufacturing processes, TRI probably captures the majority of releases. However, for some chemicals, only a small fraction of actual releases are captured in the TRI database. Even some large facilities who use and release chemicals extensively do not report under TRI.

Emissions to air, wastewater discharges, disposal into on-site landfills, injection of liquid wastes into underground wells, transfer of wastes to publicly owned wastewater treatment works, and transfers of chemicals to off-site facilities for treatment, storage, or disposal must all be reported. Both routine releases and accidental spills are covered in the emissions reports. The Pollution Prevention Act of 1990 added further reporting requirements to SARA Title III that result in an ability to compare years by percent change and requires the facility to estimate emissions for future years. In addition, the amended act allows information to be gathered regarding on-site or off-site recycling of chemical wastes and source reduction practices and opportunities.

The EPA has made great efforts to make the information available on a variety of media. The TRI database is available on-line through the National Library of Medicine's TOXNET computer system. In addition, the EPA publishes an annual report and printed lists, desktop diskettes with county-level data, CD-ROM and magnetic tapes of the entire database, and microfiche records in public libraries. In addition, there is an EPA Hotline ([800] 535-0202) for information.

TRI data have been used for a variety of purposes. State agencies have used the data to compare to operating permits and to help in source reduction efforts. Public interest groups have used the data to help educate the public about toxics in their communities, to pressure industry into reducing toxic emissions, and to lobby the government to change policies. Industries have used the information to help in source reduction efforts and to educate themselves about the costs of wasting raw product.

The initial reports for the year 1987 indicated a total release from all reporting manufacturing facilities of 5.11 billion pounds, including 2.65 billion pounds to the air, 411 million pounds discharged to water, 736 million pounds released to land, and 1.32 billion pounds injected underground. Total transfers of toxic materials included 1.29 billion pounds transferred to other off-site locations and 621 million pounds "transferred" to publicly owned wastewater treatment plants (ie, sent down the drain).

Emissions from facilities reporting to TRI appear to have decreased over time. This is partly due to increasing familiarity with the process of estimating emissions, resulting in better reporting. However, the TRI program motivates facilities to decrease their emissions. Poor public relations associated with being an emitter and a desire to waste less raw product combine to result in more efficient operations, more recovery and recycling of raw product, and a decrease in overall emissions from the manufacturing sector. Emissions for 1993, summarized in Table 40–3 and Table 40–4, reflect these changes.

Table 40–3 summarizes the information in the TRI database for 1993 on the 15 most common chemicals released into the air in the United States. Those carcinogens with reported releases into the air totaling over 100,000 pounds are depicted in Table 40–4. Many of the 15 most common chemicals have toxicity criteria developed by either the EPA or state agencies. These criteria are useful for estimating public health hazards through a risk assessment process. Of the 23 carcinogens in Table 40–4, ben-

**Table 40–3.** Top 15 TRI chemicals with the largest emissions to air, 1993.

| CAS Number | Chemical | Reported Total Air Emissions (Pounds) |
|---|---|---|
| 108-88-3 | Toluene | 177,301,671 |
| 67-56-1 | Methanol | 172,292,981 |
| 7664-41-7 | Ammonia | 138,057,165 |
| 67-64-1 | Acetone | 125,152,462 |
| 1330-20-7 | Xylene (mixed isomers) | 111,189,613 |
| 75-15-0 | Carbon disulfide | 93,307,339 |
| 78-93-3 | Methyl ethyl ketone | 84,814,923 |
| 7647-01-0 | Hydrochloric acid | 79,073,655 |
| 7782-50-5 | Chlorine | 75,410,108 |
| 75-09-2 | Dichloromethane | 64,313,211 |
| 71-55-6 | 1,1,1-Trichlorethane | 64,066,031 |
| — | Glycol ethers | 45,292,417 |
| 74-85-1 | Ethylene | 33,306,026 |
| 100-42-5 | Styrene | 32,570,591 |
| 79-01-6 | Trichlorethylene | 30,114,113 |
| | Subtotal | 1,326,262,306 |
| | Total for all TRI chemicals | 1,672,127,735 |

**Table 40–4.** TRI carcinogens emitted into air in quantities of 100,000 pounds or greater in 1993.

| CAS Number | Chemical | Reported Total Air Emissions (Pounds) |
|---|---|---|
| 75-09-2 | Dichloromethane | 64,313,211 |
| 100-42-5 | Styrene | 32,570,591 |
| 67-66-3 | Chloroform | 13,808,692 |
| 50-00-0 | Formaldehyde | 11,371,021 |
| 127-18-4 | Tetrachlorothylene | 10,942,019 |
| 71-43-2 | Benzene | 10,799,125 |
| 75-07-0 | Acetaldehyde | 6,507,137 |
| 106-99-0 | 1,3-Butadiene | 3,274,316 |
| 05-06-2 | 1,2-Dichloroethane | 2,304,877 |
| 56-23-5 | Carbon tetrachloride | 2,228,909 |
| 107-13-1 | Acrylonitrile | 1,393,618 |
| 8001-58-9 | Creosote | 1,152,129 |
| 75-21-8 | Ethylene oxide | 1,147,222 |
| 75-56-9 | Propylene oxide | 1,123,896 |
| 75-01-4 | Vinyl chloride | 1,013,962 |
| 7439-92-1 | Lead | 695,904 |
| 117-81-7 | Di-(2-ethylhexyl) phthalate | 578,940 |
| 7440-02-0 | Nickle and nickle compounds | 500,806 |
| 123-91-1 | 1,4-Dioxane | 434,017 |
| 7440-47-3 | Chromium | 426,198 |
| 106-89-8 | Epichlorohydrin | 384,132 |
| 106-46-7 | 1,4-Dichlorobenzene | 357,891 |
| 140-88-5 | Ethyl acrylate | 186,391 |

zene, hexavalent chromium, nickel, and vinyl chloride are known human carcinogens.

The TRI data provide a large amount of information regarding industrial releases into the environment. However, its limited scope results in overall underreporting of total environmental releases. Only large manufacturing facilities are required to report. As shown in California's emissions database for air, small facilities can be major contributors when their emissions are summed. Moreover, many large facilities emit substances into the environment, but are not required to report because they are not classified as manufacturing facilities. In addition, mobile sources contribute a great deal to airborne toxic chemicals but are not targeted by SARA Title III. For example, benzene and 1,3-butadiene emissions reported in TRI really represent a relatively small fraction of total emissions into the air of these two chemicals because nonmanufacturing sources and mobile sources contribute a significant amount. Finally, the toxic chemicals released from use of consumer products are not considered in any database, including the TRI. In the authors' opinion, the amount of chemicals released into the environment by use of consumer products is likely to be equivalent to or possibly greater than the amounts released in manufacturing for some compounds (eg, volatile organic compounds and chemicals in cleaning products). Many air emissions of compounds used in manufacture represents wasted raw product, while most of the chemical goes into a product that is then used by the consumer and released into the environment.

## California's Air Toxics Hot Spots Inventory

The California legislature passed the Air Toxics Hot Spots Information and Assessment Act in 1987 (Health and Safety Code Sections 44300 et seq), partially in response to the Bhopal tragedy. The Act provides the California Air Resources Board (CARB) with a means of generating a comprehensive inventory of emissions of over 400 chemicals from stationary sources in the state, and has a community right-to-know provision as well. The intent of the act was twofold: to gather information for cost-effective statewide toxics risk reduction and to provide citizens with information on toxics emitted into the air in their communities. A third objective was added in a later amendment; namely, to require emissions reductions from facilities posing significant public health risks. Facilities were phased into the program according to the extent of criteria air pollutant emissions, which are generally an indicator of energy use and size.

Emissions inventories are generated by the facilities and submitted to the local air pollution control district and the CARB. The districts prioritize facilities into categories of high, medium, or low concern based on the amount of pollutant emitted, toxic potency of pollutants, and proximity to populations. Facilities in the high priority category are required to conduct a quantitative risk assessment of their airborne toxic emissions, which includes a comprehensive analysis of the dispersion of hazardous substances into the environment, the potential for human exposure, and a quantitative assessment of both the individual and population-wide health risks associated with those levels of exposure. If the facility is deemed by the district to pose significant risk, the facility must notify the community and engage in risk reduction activity. This differs from the TRI in that there is a large risk assessment and public notification component to this state program.

The reporting requirements are quite different than those for the TRI database. The reporting triggers are considerably lower; none is above 100 pounds per year. In addition, all types of facilities report their emissions, not just those classified as manufacturing facilities. In that respect, the Air Toxics Hot Spots Inventory is quite comprehensive. Data are available for emissions from small facilities (eg, dry cleaners) as well as from large complex facilities such as refineries. However, unlike the TRI, the California program focuses only on airborne emissions, and there is no comparable database for land or water emissions in California. In addition, the TRI facilities are required to report yearly, while the California program only requires reporting every four years.

Of 307 chemicals actually reported as emitted to the air in California as of December 1995, 92 are emitted in amounts greater than 10,000 pounds per

**Table 40–5.** Top 25 chemicals by volume of emissions in California's air toxics inventory.

| CAS Number | Chemical | Reported Total Air Emissions (Pounds) |
|---|---|---|
| 71-55-6 | 1,1,1-Trichlorethane | 23,718,886 |
| 7664-41-7 | Ammonia | 21,040,109 |
| — | Chlorofluorocarbons | 12,333,493 |
| 75-09-2 | Dichloromethane | 7,420,307 |
| 127-18-4 | Tetrachloroethylene | 6,756,022 |
| 7783-06-4 | Hydrogen sulfide | 5,842,524 |
| — | Gasoline vapors (including benzene) | 5,191,727 |
| 108-88-3 | Toluene | 5,155,024 |
| — | o,m,p-Xylenes | 4,149,621 |
| — | Glycol ethers and their acetates | 3,785,200 |
| 67-56-1 | Methanol | 3,761,244 |
| 7647-01-0 | Hydrogen chloride | 3,192,245 |
| — | Crystalline silica | 2,916,158 |
| 100-42-5 | Styrene | 2,627,770 |
| 50-00-0 | Formaldehyde | 2,013,091 |
| — | Carbon black extracts | 1,572,803 |
| 71-43-2 | Benzene | 1,183,527 |
| 74-90-8 | Hydrogen cyanide | 1,107,731 |
| 1310-73-2 | Sodium hydroxide | 796,978 |
| 75-56-9 | Propylene oxide | 727,909 |
| 108-95-2 | Phenol | 515,164 |
| 7782-50-5 | Chlorine | 467,360 |
| 75-00-3 | Ethyl chloride | 291,051 |
| 7440-66-6 | Zinc | 283,294 |
| 75-21-8 | Ethylene oxide | 273,754 |

**Table 40–6.** Top 25 carcinogens by volume emitted in the California Air Toxics Hot Spots Database.

| CAS Number | Chemical | Reported Total Air Emissions (Pounds) |
|---|---|---|
| 75-09-2 | Dichloromethane | 7,420,308 |
| 127-18-4 | Tetrachloroethylene | 6,756,022 |
| — | Crystalline silica | 2,916,158 |
| 100-42-5 | Styrene | 2,627,771 |
| 50-00-0 | Formaldehyde | 2,013,091 |
| — | Carbon black extracts | 1,572,803 |
| 71-43-2 | Benzene | 1,183,527 |
| 75-56-9 | Propylene oxide | 727,909 |
| 75-21-8 | Ethylene oxide | 273,754 |
| 123-91-1 | 1,4-Dioxane | 238,635 |
| 79-01-6 | Trichloroethylene | 223,628 |
| — | Nickel and compounds | 228,651 |
| 67-66-3 | Chloroform | 125,201 |
| 117-81-7 | Di-2-ethylhexylphthalate | 112,818 |
| — | Polycyclic aromatic hydro-carbons | 74,922 |
| — | Creosotes | 59,568 |
| 7439-92-1 | Lead | 40,227 |
| 584-84-9 | Toluene-2,4-diisocyanate | 32,650 |
| 106-46-7 | p-Dichlorobenzene | 30,161 |
| 106-99-0 | 1,3-Butadiene | 22,357 |
| — | Diesel exhaust PM | 19,312 |
| 75-01-4 | Vinylchloride | 17,161 |
| 56-23-5 | Carbon tetrachloride | 15,447 |
| 7440-38-2 | Arsenic | 12,905 |

year. The 25 most common chemicals by volume of emissions are summarized in Table 40–5; these are emitted in amounts greater than 467,000 pounds per year. The 25 most common carcinogens are summarized in Table 40–6. Most of this information comes from reporting years 1989–1993. Of the 25 most common carcinogens listed, arsenic, vinyl chloride, nickel, benzene, and ethylene oxide are known human carcinogens. It is interesting to note that the most troublesome chemicals may not be those with a large volume of emissions. For example, emissions in pounds per year for hexavalent chromium are relatively small (6500 pounds per year). Yet, because of the potency estimates for this known human carcinogen, the public health risk estimates are large for airborne hexavalent chromium. Similarly, emissions of polychlorinated dibenzodioxins and dibenzofurans are quite small. But chemicals in this class of compounds are potent carcinogens, and risk estimates for facilities emitting very small amounts can be relatively large. Compared to the California database, tetrachloroethylene emissions to air appear to be grossly underreported in TRI. This is undoubtedly because many smaller operations use tetrachloroethylene and emit more overall than those facilities required to report in TRI.

Over 700 risk assessments conducted by facility operators have been reviewed by the state of California's Office of Environmental Health Hazard Assessment. Cancer risks estimated for high priority facilities ranged from one in one million to one in one thousand for lifetime exposures to modeled airborne concentrations. Figure 40–1 depicts the numbers of facilities in a particular risk range. These risks are based primarily on 1989 emissions. This program demonstrates that a large number of facilities have risks greater than one in one million, the traditional de minimis level for regulatory agencies. About 44% pose estimated cancer risk over ten in one million.

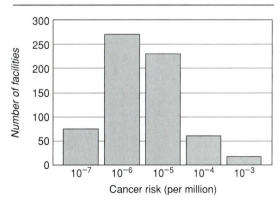

**Figure 40–1.** "Hot spots" risk assessment review findings.

Key chemicals that are drivers of cancer risk estimates in facilities posing cancer risks greater than ten in one million include benzene, hexavalent chromium, tetrachloroethylene, polycyclic aromatic hydrocarbons, methylene chloride, arsenic, and formaldehyde. Many of these facilities have taken steps to reduce their emissions. Thus, the program is a successful motivating force for facilities to reduce emissions, partly because of the public notification provisions and partly because of the recognition by industries that much of their air emissions represents wasted raw product and inefficient industrial processes.

Facilities with relatively small emissions may pose high risks to a small number of people if the dispersion characteristics are poor. For example, cancer risk estimates for dry cleaning facilities are, in some cases, large for nearby residents because the dry cleaner is located in close proximity to housing, and the tetrachloroethylene emissions are not vented through a tall stack, resulting in poor dispersion. Measures taken in California to reduce risks from tetrachloroethylene emissions include requiring solvent-recycling equipment and better ventilation and dispersion systems.

Large facilities such as refineries may emit tremendous quantities of material, but in some cases have lower individual excess cancer risk estimates than many smaller facilities because residences are usually located further away from the source than other sources, and the materials are emitted from tall stacks, resulting in better dispersion. However, the number of persons exposed to that estimated cancer risk may be considerable.

## California's Criteria Air Pollutant Emissions Inventory

California maintains an inventory of emissions of the criteria air pollutants: CO, $NO_x$, $SO_x$, and particulate matter less than 10 μm in diameter (PM10), as well as emissions of total suspended particulate matter (TSP), reactive organic gases (ROG), and total organic gases (TOG). ROG and $NO_x$ combine to form ozone; tracking these two categories of emissions is useful in predicting ozone concentrations. The inventory for 1993 is summarized in Table 40–7. The category "stationary sources" represents a variety of industrial sources including manufacturing, petroleum refining, food and agricultural processing, utilities, cleaning and surface coating, and chemical manufacturing. Industrial emissions account for a significant proportion of total emissions of these pollutants into the air in the state. Emissions listed under "areawide" sources are dominated by consumer products use, architectural coatings, use of pesticides and fertilizers, residential heating, farming operations, and waste burning and disposal. While some of these processes are industrial, others are clearly related to domestic upkeep and maintenance. Included in the table for comparison are both mobile source (cars, planes,

Table 40–7. Statewide 1993 emissions of major components of smog in California (tons per day).

| | Stationary[a] Sources | Areawide[b] Sources | Mobile[c] Sources | Natural[d] Sources | Total Statewide |
|---|---|---|---|---|---|
| TOG | 3,400 | 1,300 | 1,900 | 350 | 6,900 |
| ROG | 820 | 920 | 1,800 | 240 | 3,800 |
| CO | 400 | 2,300 | 14,000 | 240 | 17,000 |
| $NO_x$ | 690 | 91 | 2,500 | 3.6 | 3,300 |
| $SO_x$ | 150 | 5.9 | 200 | — | 360 |
| PM | 440 | 9,800 | 310 | 320 | 11,000 |
| $PM_{10}$ | 220 | 5,100 | 200 | 230 | 5,800 |

[a]Stationary sources include: industrial processes, fuel combustion, and waste disposal from industrial sources; cleaning and surface coatings operations; petroleum production and marketing.
[b]Areawide sources include: solvent evaporation from consumer products, architectural coatings, pesticides/fertilizers, asphalt paving, refrigerants, residential fuel combustion, farming, construction, road dust, fires, waste burning and disposal, utility equipment, and miscellaneous other.
[c]Mobile sources include: on-road motor vehicles, off-road recreational vehicles, aircraft, trains, ships, recreational boats, commercial mobile equipment, farm equipment.
[d]Natural sources include: biogenic sources, geogenic sources, wildfires, windblown dust.

trucks, trains) and natural sources (biogenic, geogenic, wildfires, windblown dust). Mobile sources are a major source of all these pollutants because of the combustion of petroleum products used to generate energy for locomotion. Natural sources account for less than 10% of most pollutants with the exception of particulate matter, where natural sources contribute roughly 30% of TSP.

In addition to tracking emissions of criteria air pollutants, ROG, and TOG, the CARB also maintains a monitoring network to measure ambient air concentrations of these substances. This helps regulators evaluate air quality, particularly in metropolitan areas of the state, and the effectiveness of pollution control efforts. Data on air quality are published both quarterly and annually and are available from CARB in the publication entitled California Air Quality Data, Air Resources Board, California Environmental Protection Agency.

## IMPORTANCE TO HEALTH CARE PERSONNEL

Epidemiologic studies of adverse health effects of air pollution have focused primarily on the major components of smog, such as ozone, particulate matter, nitrogen oxides, and carbon monoxide. A detailed description of studies is presented in another chapter of this book. Recent studies indicate that children growing up in high pollution areas of the United States (eg, the Los Angeles basin) suffer from reduced lung function, increased respiratory infections, and exacerbations of asthma. Ozone is a critical component of Los Angeles–type smog and contributes to respiratory and eye irritation in the Los Angeles basin on smoggy days. Studies have shown that ozone and particulate matter at levels typical for Los Angeles exacerbate asthma in children. Acidic aerosols may also contribute to transient decreases in lung function in children. Particulate matter has recently been associated in a number of studies with increased morbidity and mortality from respiratory and cardiac conditions. The association is consistent across studies, despite the differing chemical composition of particles in different cities. The association is not likely to be due to weather related changes such as temperature.

To date, smaller emphasis has been placed on epidemiologic studies of adverse health effects attributable to toxic air contaminants. In large part, this is due to the difficulty of such studies, including a lack of exposure data. Although one study has indicated an association between exposure to volatile organic compounds in ambient air and increased rates of respiratory symptoms in children characteristic of reactive airways, most of the health impacts of air pollutants other than CAP have been inferred from occupational epidemiologic studies and toxicologic studies in experimental animals. Exposure to toxic chemicals in air may contribute to respiratory disease and injury as well as result in systemic toxicity.

Medical consequences of either acute or chronic exposure to pollutants other than the CAP are poorly documented. Patients may have respiratory or other system complaints due to acute or chronic exposure to substances. However, few studies exist that study the effect of routine industrial emissions. Such studies need to be done on a case-by-case basis. Currently, public health agencies extrapolate potential health problems from occupational exposure studies and animal toxicology studies.

Risk assessments conducted for stationary sources in California under the Air Toxics Hot Spots program have indicated relatively high (in an environmental context) excess individual cancer risks for people living near some facilities. As stated earlier, regulatory agencies traditionally view cancer risk of one in one million as a *de minimis* level not requiring any regulatory action. Some of the estimated cancer risks from stationary source emissions are as high as one in one thousand. The cancer incidence rate is about one in four in the United States. There are a large number of causative agents of cancer in the United States and elsewhere. Chemical carcinogens emitted into the environment represent one source of these causal agents. Airborne carcinogens contribute to the total exposure to carcinogens, and presumably to the total cancer burden experienced by a population. In addition, risk assessments have indicated that certain industrial processes may contribute to respiratory or systemic adverse health impacts that are non-neoplastic in nature.

## REGULATION OF STATIONARY SOURCES

### State Regulations—California

The Toxic Air Contaminants Identification and Control Act (1983) created California's program to reduce health risks from air toxics. This was the first comprehensive state air toxics program to evaluate chemicals in the air and control sources of air toxics. CARB lists about 200 chemicals as toxic air contaminants. ARB considers a number of factors in evaluating exposures to TACs. Emissions from many source types are identified via the Air Toxics Hot Spots emissions inventory database and by a program that tests motor vehicle emissions. There are also statewide ambient air monitors that collect data on over 50 chemicals. After formally identifying a substance as a TAC, CARB investigates the need, feasibility, and cost of reducing emissions of that substance. This process has resulted in 11 air toxics control measures to reduce emissions from the following sources: gasoline service stations (benzene, other volatiles); chrome plating and anodizing shops (hexavalent chromium); cooling towers (hexavalent chromium); sterilizers and aerators (ethylene oxide); medical waste incinerators (polychlorinated dibenzo-dioxins and dibenzofurans); serpentine rock in surfacing applications (asbestos); dry cleaning (tetra-chloroethylene); metal melting (cadmium, nickel, arsenic); low emission vehicle/clean fuels regulations (benzene, 1,3-butadiene); and reformulated diesel fuel (diesel exhaust).

At the local level, new and modified sources of air pollution are required to obtain operating permits from local air pollution control agencies. The goal is to ensure that new and modified devices are able to meet all air quality standards and not exacerbate air pollution problems in an area.

## Federal Regulations

The Federal Clean Air Act of 1990 represents a comprehensive statutory framework designed to reduce overall exposure to TAC, protect the stratospheric ozone layer, and reduce deposition of acidic constituents of air pollution (eg, acid rain and acid snow). The Act provides for use of market-based principles and other innovative approaches to reducing air pollution. Under Title III of the Clean Air Act, the EPA established a list of 189 Hazardous Air Pollutants (HAPs). These HAPs are frequently referred to as "air toxics". Technology-based standards are being promulgated by the EPA to control emissions of HAPs from major sources and "area" sources (defined by the EPA in this instance as minor sources). In later years of the program, residual risks (cancer and noncancer risks remaining after control devices have been put in place) will be assessed following the implementation of the technology-based standards of air pollution control. Further control measures may be developed if residual risks are considered by the EPA to be unreasonable.

## WORLDWIDE PERSPECTIVE

The concept of the EPA's Toxic Release Inventory (TRI) has attracted the attention of other countries. The Canadian government established a National Pollutant Release Inventory with many similarities to the US TRI. The European Commission is currently establishing a registry for pollutant emissions from industries. In addition, the Organization for Economic Cooperation and Development is also working on a Pollutant Release and Transfer Register at the request of the United Nations' International Program on Chemical Safety. Developments on the international level will facilitate pollution control efforts on a global scale.

# ACCIDENTAL RELEASES

On July 26, 1993, a valve on a rail tank car ruptured during an illegal unloading procedure at a chemical plant in Richmond, California. The release continued for four hours, unleashing a 15-mile-long cloud of oleum, a respiratory irritant. A computerized telephone warning system failed to notify most households in the community that the release was occurring. Over the next week, hospitals and clinics were overwhelmed as over 20,000 people sought medical care. Individuals complained of respiratory and ocular symptoms and gastrointestinal distress. Only 5% of these patients had objective signs related to their complaints. Twenty-two people were hospitalized, most with preexisting cardiovascular or respiratory conditions. The response to this accident involved a multitude of individuals and organizations, including hospitals, health care personnel, local and state health departments, and state and federal agencies regulating health, environment, and transportation. As a result of this accident: (1) monetary penalties exceeding $1 million were imposed on the company responsible for the accident; (2) the company contributed funds towards the construction of a health clinic to serve the community affected by the release; (3) thousands of personal injury claims were filed against the company; (4) the design of the type of tank car involved in the accident was altered; and (5) more stringent air pollution regulations and penalties were proposed in the state of California.

## Accidental Chemical Releases & the Role of Health Care Providers

An accidental chemical release may result in health consequences for multiple organ systems (Table 40–8). However, it is often difficult to relate exposure from a release to alleged injury. Much of the information about the public health effects of chemical spills is based on reviews of medical records from initial clinic visits or medical consultations. Appropriate recording of medical information immediately following exposure is essential to gaining an accurate understanding of the immediate and delayed health effects of accidental releases. In addition to recording subjective complaints and the results of physical examination and laboratory tests, health care personnel should record information that will help to assess the extent of exposure to the released compound and the relationship of exposure to disease. The following details should be documented in the medical database:

**Table 40–8.** Types of health effects reported following accidental releases of hazardous substances.[1]

| Health Effect | No. of Injuries[2] (%) |
|---|---|
| Respiratory irritation | 1367 (35.9) |
| Eye irritation | 654 (17.2) |
| Headache | 422 (11.1) |
| Nausea | 405 (10.6) |
| Dizziness or other central nervous system symptoms or signs | 279 (7.3) |
| Skin irritation | 206 (5.4) |
| Vomiting | 102 (2.7) |
| Trauma | 89 (2.4) |
| Chemical burns | 88 (2.3) |
| Thermal burns | 20 (0.5) |
| Heat stress | 12 (0.3) |
| Other | 164 (4.3) |

[1]Based on 4244 events analyzed in 1994 by ATSDR's Hazardous Substances Emergency Events Surveillance system.
[2]Since a person may have more than one type of health effect, the number of injuries exceeds the number of victims.

- a general medical history, including the presence of preexisting medical conditions such as asthma, and a history of smoking
- an occupational history, including potential exposures that might contribute to health complaints
- the results of specific laboratory tests, such as spirometry, if the history and symptoms warrant
- the geographic and physical location of the individual relative to the site of the release
- during the incident, the estimated length of time spent at any given location relative to the release
- activities that may have affected the dose of chemical received, such as strenuous exercise in the area of the chemical release or consumption of contaminated water or food
- the timing of onset of symptoms relative to potential exposure to accidentally released chemicals
- the identity of the substance(s) released
- whether fires or explosions occurred as a result of the accident, which could involve exposure to combustion or pyrolysis products

## The Larger Perspective

Although emergency planning and management have not traditionally involved many health care professionals, the example at the beginning of this section illustrates that physicians and nurses, as well as other medical personnel, may be called upon in the event of an accidental release of hazardous chemicals. This response usually consists of medical as-

sessment and treatment of first responders (firefighters, police, paramedics, etc), workers, and members of the public exposed to potentially toxic substances. The information gathered by physicians during their assessment of potentially exposed persons may be essential in the public health assessment of the effects of the release as well as in planning for prevention of future releases. Consequently, it is important for health care personnel to be aware of the relevant regulations, health data, and reporting requirements as well as the steps involved in the public health assessment of accidental releases. It is also important to be aware of the hazards surrounding accidents involving radioactive materials, although they occur less frequently than those involving nonradioactive hazardous chemicals.

As a result of increased consumer demand for products such as motor vehicles, new homes, and furnishings, chemical production in the United States and the world is rising. Of the 60,000 chemicals produced and commonly used in the United States, approximately 2000 are subject to reporting requirements in the event of a release. Even fewer have adequate toxicity information. The increase in the United States has resulted in an increased likelihood of adverse health impacts due to accidental chemical releases for two reasons. First, accidental chemical releases are increasingly occurring near homes or businesses. In California, the state reporting the highest number of accidental releases, incidents occurred predominantly in residential neighborhoods, increasing from 24% in 1988 to 28% in 1991. Industrial or business areas were the second most frequent locations of hazardous chemical accidents (16%). Second, in spite of improved control measures at production facilities and improved storage and transport container design, the number of accidental chemical releases reported to the US Environmental Protection Agency (EPA) due to accidents, including both stationary facilities (eg, utility and chemical production plants) and transportation-related events, has increased steadily over the past decade. Although partly accounted for by stricter enforcement of reporting requirements, this may actually represent a true increase in the number of unplanned releases. This trend suggests that management measures have not adequately controlled the occurrence of accidents and underscores the need for preventive planning.

## ACCIDENT STATISTICS

### Prevalence and Causes of Accidental Releases

Both worldwide and in the United States, chemical production has risen nearly 30% over the last decade. In 1994, the US output of the 50 chemicals manufactured in the greatest quantities totalled more than

720 billion pounds. Sulfuric acid topped the production list with more than 89 billion pounds.

The storage and transportation patterns of hazardous chemicals contribute to the high potential for accidental releases. It is estimated that more than 10 billion pounds of hazardous chemicals are stored at manufacturing plants around the United States. In 1992, the largest amount of hazardous materials was stored in Louisiana, followed by Texas; South Dakota had the lowest amount. On average, 43 pounds of hazardous materials per person are stored in the United States. More than 1.5 billion tons of hazardous materials (excluding pipeline transport) are transported annually in the United States, about 60% by truck. Ten percent of all trucks on the road at any time, and more than 10% of railroad tank cars, carry hazardous materials. The materials most often transported by rail are liquified petroleum gas, chlorine, anhydrous ammonia, and vinyl chloride.

From 1987 to 1995, more than 180,000 accidents involving hazardous substances were reported to the National Response Center (see Sources of Data, below); of these, over 4000 resulted in evacuations, injuries, or deaths. During this period, the highest number of accidents occurred in California, with Texas a close second, and Louisiana third. A breakdown of accidents by state is shown in Figure 40–2. National Response Center reports show that accidental releases occur more commonly at fixed facilities than during transport (Table 40–9). The most frequent cause of stationary facility accidents is equipment failure. Overall, marine and offshore incidents are the most common causes of transportation accidents because petroleum products, which account for the majority of accidental releases, are most often spilled in this setting. Transportation accidents involving nonpetroleum hazardous substances most commonly occur on highways. Transportation events are more likely to result in injury and death than are stationary source accidents; most deaths or injuries are due to truck accidents.

Table 40–9 provides a nationwide summary of accidental releases reported to the National Response Center. The reported releases are divided into two categories: oils and hazardous substances as defined under the Comprehensive Environmental Response, Compensation, and Liability Act of 1980 (CERCLA) (see Federal Regulations, below). Sixty percent of releases reported to the National Response Center are due to oil products; petroleum accounts for 39% of total spills. The five most frequently released petroleum products are, in decreasing order, crude oil, diesel oil, automotive gasoline, waste oil, and hydraulic oil. Nonpetroleum oil products account for 20% of total releases, and include relatively nonhazardous substances such as palm, sunflower, and fish oils. CERCLA hazardous substances account for approximately 19% of releases reported. The 10 most frequently released CERCLA hazardous substances are listed in Table 40–10.

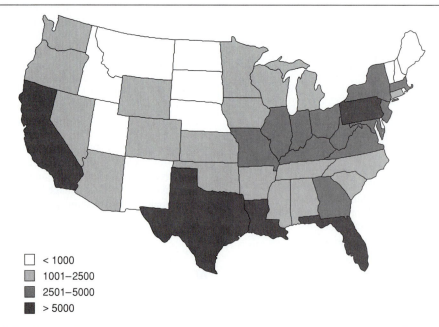

□ < 1000
▨ 1001–2500
▦ 2501–5000
■ > 5000

**Figure 40–2.** Number of CERCLA hazardous waste substances and oil releases reported to the Emergency Release Notification System (ERNS) from January 1990 to September 1995. The information is based on initial notification and may contain duplicate reports (see text).

**Table 40–9.** Summary of accidental releases involving CERCLA hazardous materials and petroleum compounds, 1987–1995.[1]

| Factor Associated With Release | CERCLA | Petroleum |
|---|---|---|
| Number of reports (% total) | 58,546 (19%) | 120,739 (39%) |
| | **% of Reported Information[2]** | |
| **Cause of accidental release** | | |
| Equipment failure | 41 | 39 |
| Operator Error | 13 | 15 |
| Natural Phenomenon | 2 | 2 |
| Dumping | 10 | 8 |
| Transportation accident | 6 | 10 |
| Other | 12 | 9 |
| Unknown | 16 | 18 |
| **Transportation mode** | | |
| Fixed facility | 71 | 42 |
| Highway | 10 | 17 |
| Rail | 4 | 3 |
| Marine/offshore | <1 | 7 |
| Pipeline | 2 | 14 |
| Air transport | <1 | 2 |
| Storage tank | 3 | 5 |
| Unknown | 9 | 11 |
| **Media into which release occurred** | | |
| Land | 46 | 36 |
| Air | 34 | 5 |
| Water | 14 | 54 |
| Facility | 3 | 2 |
| Groundwater | 1 | 2 |
| Other | 2 | 1 |

[1]Information based on U.S. EPA's ERNS database, 1987–November, 1995.
[2]Only 33% of reports list the cause of accident and media of release.

## Public Health Consequences of Releases

The Agency for Toxic Substances and Disease Registry (ATSDR) has implemented an active, state-based Hazardous Substances Emergency Event Surveillance system to describe the public health outcome of accidental releases. Information is actively collected and verified, using several different data sources. In 1994, 12 state health departments participated in this surveillance system and reported over 4000 events.

In 1994, 80% of the accidents reported to the ATSDR surveillance system occurred at stationary facilities and 20% during transportation. In 90% of the reported incidents, only one substance was released. Ten percent of reported events resulted in injuries, with stationary facility events accounting for 84% of victims. Five nonpetroleum substance categories accounted for over 80% of injuries. In decreasing order, they were: acids, ammonia, bases, chlorine, and other inorganic substances. The most frequent cause of injury was chlorine, which was released in only 3% of accidents, but was responsible for 33% of injuries. Ammonia was the second most common cause of injury, with 6% of releases accounting for 17% of victims (Table 40–11).

According to data gathered by the ATSDR surveillance system, the most commonly reported immediate adverse health effect following accidental releases at fixed facilities is respiratory irritation. Trauma is more common following transportation-related incidents. Most victims of hazardous materials incidents are transported to and treated at a hospital. Less than 5% of affected individuals are admitted to a hospital. When fatalities occur as the result of a hazardous materials release, employees are most often the victims, followed by members of the public. Death is often the result of transportation-related trauma.

Following accidental releases of hazardous materials, workers are injured most frequently, followed by the general public, and then emergency response personnel (eg, firefighters, police). In part, this is because workers (and members of the public) wear less protective equipment than emergency responders at the scene of a release. Most employees and 50% of emergency responders who are injured do not wear any personal protective equipment. Emergency re-

**Table 40–10.** Ten most frequently accidentally released CERCLA hazardous substances.[1]

| Substance | Most Common Mode of Transportation Accidents[2] |
|---|---|
| 1. Ethylene glycol | Highway |
| 2. Ammonia | Highway |
| 3. Polychlorinated biphenyls | Highway |
| 4. Sulfuric acid | Rail |
| 5. Chlorine | Rail |
| 6. Benzene | Pipeline |
| 7. Hydrochloric acid | Highway |
| 8. Hydrogen sulfide | Pipeline |
| 9. Vinyl chloride | Pipeline |
| 10. *n*-Hexane | Rail |

[1]Based on US EPA's ERNS database for 1990–September, 1995.
[2]Most spills occur at stationary facilities.

**Table 40–11.** Accidentally released chemical categories: percentage of total accidents and resulting injuries.[1]

| Substance Category | Percentage of Injuries Caused by Substances[2] | Percentage of Total Accidents Involving Substances |
|---|---|---|
| Chlorine | 33.1 | 2.9 |
| Ammonia | 16.8 | 6.0 |
| Acids | 16.1 | 9.8 |
| Other inorganic substances | 10.6 | 16.2 |
| Pesticides | 9.3 | 9.1 |
| Bases | 8.6 | 4.5 |
| Other | 8.0 | 27.6 |
| Volatile organic compounds | 6.6 | 19.3 |
| Paints and dyes | 6.0 | 2.0 |
| Polychlorinated biphenyls | 2.2 | 2.6 |

[1]Based on data collected from 12 states by ATSDR's Hazardous Substances Emergency Events Surveillance system (1992).
[2]The sum of this column is greater than 100 because an accident may involve more than one substance.

sponders are more often injured in transportation-related events than in fixed facility releases; the opposite is the case for workers.

## RESPONSE TO ACCIDENTAL RELEASES

### Medical Response

**A. Health Care Provider Role:** In addition to providing medical information during a release and treating exposed victims, health care providers can act as reliable spokespersons on the potential health threat of toxic chemicals being used or stored at facilities in the community. When evaluating individuals for potential exposure to accidentally released chemicals, health care personnel must first identify the compound, consider decontaminating the individual, and decide on appropriate treatment measures. Computer databases, material safety data sheets, and regional poison control centers should be consulted for substance identification and medical treatment options. Occasionally, the preceding sources will not have the appropriate toxicity information and it may be necessary to contact the manufacturer directly. While manufacturers are allowed to withhold trade secrets about hazardous chemicals from the public, they are required by Title III of the Superfund Amendments and Reauthorization Act to provide this information to physicians or nurses who require it for the purpose of treating victims of exposure. While the person receiving this information must sign confidentiality agreements with the facility, this clause assures that specific information can be legally obtained in order to render appropriate medical care.

**B. Hospital Role:** Following major chemical incidents, local hospitals are often overwhelmed by the volume of patients seeking acute care. To optimize response to these emergencies, it is necessary for hospitals to have a community-based plan for response to accidental releases and to establish policies specifying the scope and conduct of patient care to be provided at the facility. This includes determining methods to be used to triage patients into mild, moderate, and severe injury categories; establishing treatment protocols; and specifying decontamination methods to be used. In addition, there should be ready availability of current toxicologic reference materials that contain treatment and antidote information, including on-line databases and telephone numbers of the regional poison control center (Table 40–12). A listing of referral and consultation services, including local, state, and governmental agencies, should be readily available.

Although hospitals and other helath care providers perform essential functions, they are part of a statewide emergency medical care system that coordinates patient distribution and hospital and other medical resource monitoring during a mass casualty incident. The emergency medical care system also assists in planning and training as well as certifying certain response personnel, such as paramedics. It is essential for hospitals and emergency responders to coordinate drills and simulations to ensure optimal response during a large-scale emergency.

**Table 40–12.** Resources for planning for and response to accidental releases of hazardous materials.

| | |
|---|---|
| **SUBSTANCE IDENTIFICATION**<br>• National Fire Protection Agency labels<br>• U.S. DOT placards | • Labeling system for describing chemical hazards<br>• Warning placards for vehicles carrying hazardous materials |
| **TOXICITY & RESPONSE INFORMATION**<br>**Databases**<br>• Chemical Hazard Response Information System (CHRIS)<br><br>• Integrated Risk Information System (IRIS)<br><br>• New Jersey Hazardous Substance Fact Sheets<br><br><br>• Oil and Hazardous Materials/Technical Assistance Data System (OHM/TADS)<br><br>• Registry of Toxic Effects of Chemical Substances (RTECS®)<br><br>• Toxicology, Occupational Medicine, and Environment Series (TOMES) Plus ® System | • Online information from the United States Coast Guard for emergency response for transportation accidents involving hazardous chemicals<br>• Online health risk assessment information on chemicals from the United States EPA<br>• CD-ROM provides summarized information on hazards, safe storage, control, first aid, and emergency procedures for common chemicals<br>• On-line assistance from the United States EPA for responding to emergencies involving substances designated as oils or hazardous materials<br>• Online toxicity data from NIOSH for potentially toxic chemicals, including NTP test status<br>• CD-ROM product that brings together 14 different databases containing toxicity data, information for safe handling of chemicals, responding to hazardous chemical spills, and evaluation and treatment of persons acutely exposed |
| **Manuals**<br>• Managing Hazardous Materials Incidents. Volumes I–III. ATSDR, 1991. | • Planning guides for emergency medical services, hospital emergency departments, and emergency department physicians |
| **Telephone Resources**<br>• CHEMTREC [(800) 424-9300]<br><br><br><br>• Regional poison control center (consult local listing) | • 24-hour hotline operated by Chemical Manufacturer's Association; provides information on identity and hazardous properties of chemicals; can put caller in touch with industry representatives and medical toxicologists<br>• Provides information on immediate health effects, need for decontamination, protective gear, and specific treatment |
| **REPORTING INFORMATION**<br>• National Response Center [(800) 424-8802] | • 24-hour reporting system staffed by the United States Coast Guard which handles all significant hazardous materials spills under agreements with DOT and the United States EPA; relays calls to relevant response agencies |

## Treatment

Following most cases of accidental exposure, symptomatic treatment will suffice. For severe exposures, ensuring the integrity of cardiovascular function is critical. For inhalation exposures, special attention should be given to assessing the respiratory system. Symptoms due to anxiety should be distinguished from those caused by direct chemical effects. For some chemicals, clinical effects may not be immediately obvious, and delayed toxicity may need to be considered. For example, following phosgene inhalation exposures, patients should be monitored for 24 hours for onset of pulmonary edema (see Chapters 19 and 20 for more detailed information on acute upper airway and pulmonary injury). Occasionally, chemical-specific medications or antidotes will be required. For example, following inhalation or dermal exposure to hydrofluoric acid, treatment options may include nebulized or subcutaneous calcium gluconate in addition to corticosteroids.

## Decontamination

To minimize contamination of response personnel and most efficiently treat exposed individuals, the incident commander at a hazardous materials incident should establish a command post and create hazard zones (Figure 40–3). The hot zone, also known as the "exclusion" zone, is closest to the spill and only responders wearing personal protective equipment should be allowed to enter. Entry and exit must be carefully controlled through an entry point and a separate point of exit. Only rudimentary first aid should be provided in this area. The warm zone provides a systematic way to lessen the exposure to the chemical hazard for those who have been in the hot zone and also serves to control the spread of contamination into the cold zone. Decontamination takes place in the warm zone and may extend into the cold zone. The cold zone is also termed the support zone; this area is theoretically safe from the chemical hazard and is usually set up a considerable distance upwind of the spill. Command and control activities, first aid,

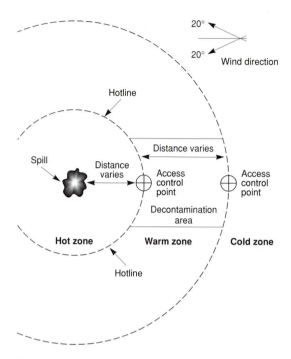

**Figure 40–3.** Schematic represenation of hot, warm, and cold zones at a hazardous materials spill site. (Adapted from Olson KR, Mycroft FJ: Emergency medical response to hazardous materials incidents. In: Olson KR (editor): *Poisoning & Drug Overdose,* 2nd ed. Appleton & Lange, 1994.)

and planning take place in the cold zone. Plume modeling may be used to map expected chemical concentrations to determine the different zones.

Many local jurisdictions have developed Hazardous Materials (HAZMAT) teams, trained to identify and respond to hazardous materials incidents. Decontamination in the field is most likely to be performed by these teams. Guidelines, such as those developed by ATSDR (1992), exist for the decontamination of potentially exposed emergency responders. OSHA has issued requirements for emergency medical technicians and any other health care providers who may be required to respond to a hazardous materials spill. OSHA also requires that employers provide the necessary protective equipment and training to any employee who may encounter a situation involving hazardous materials.

Guidelines for decontamination of the public also exist, but there is no uniform procedure that is followed by all agencies. Because the level of exposure is often unknown, it is considered good management to decontaminate at or near the site of the release. Decontamination, whether in the field or at the medical treatment facility, involves removing the clothes and copiously rinsing the skin and eyes with water to remove chemical contaminants. Spills involving oily materials

such as petroleum products may require the use of soap. Run-off water should be contained, if possible, to prevent the contamination of water sources.

An additional issue of occasional concern is that of secondary contamination of health care facilities and workers with toxic materials on the skin or clothes of accident victims or from toxic vomitus, in the case of ingestion. An example of a substance that is of low risk for toxicity from secondary contamination is a gas, such as chlorine. Substances of high risk for toxicity for secondary contamination require protection of both treatment facilities and medical personnel and include concentrated acids and bases and potent chemical carcinogens (Table 40–13).

## Sheltering in Place Versus Evacuation

In addition to controlling the spill, responses to unintentional chemical releases may include protection of the affected community, decontamination following exposure, and medical assessment and treatment of exposed victims. In general, a decision to institute protective actions immediately following a spill is made by the emergency response incident commander, such as a fire chief, police officer, or coast guard officer, in conjunction with local health personnel and elected officials. Providing reliable toxicity information to first responders and the community in a timely manner should be one of the main goals of health professionals responding to a release.

Few options are available for the protection of community residents after accidental releases. In the case of a release into water, residents may be cautioned to avoid contact with or consumption of the contaminated source. Following releases into air, the two alternatives for protective action are sheltering-in-place or evacuation. Little objective data exist to

**Table 40–13.** Examples of substances that present low and high probability for secondary contamination of health care facilities and providers.

| Probability of Secondary Contamination | Chemical or Substance Category |
|---|---|
| Low | Gases: chlorine, ethylene oxide<br>Vapors: sulfuric acid mist; (unless there has been significant exposure)<br>Weak acids and bases: sodium hydroxide<br>Most hydrocarbon products: gasoline |
| High | Strong acids and bases: hydrofluoric acid<br>Volatile liquids: isocyanates, formaldehyde<br>Potent pesticides<br>Potent chemical carcinogens<br>Radioactive materials<br>Biologic agents |

definitively support one choice over the other in a given release situation, although several theoretical guidelines are available. The decision to evacuate or shelter-in-place involves weighing many factors. For example, the characteristics of the chemical, the estimated concentration as a function of time, the source, size, and duration of the release, meteorologic conditions and the intactness and infiltration rates of the structures used for protection must all be considered. Finally, the proximity of institutions that might require special attention during both evacuation and sheltering-in-place, such as schools, hospitals, and prisons, should be considered.

Theoretical research suggests that in-place protection is nearly always better than evacuation. It is of greatest benefit when the chemical's peak concentration, rather than its cumulative dose, presents the greater toxicity. Sheltering-in-place should be the initial response while any situation is being assessed. Buildings with ventilation systems turned off and with intact doors and windows closed may reduce exposure to half compared to unprotected outdoor exposures. Evacuation may be the preferred choice when there is the threat of a release, though none has yet occurred, or when the release may create an explosion or fire hazard. Evacuation is usually a time-consuming and confusing process and is the safest alternative only when it can be completed prior to the time when a toxic cloud reaches a populated area.

Both in-place protection and evacuation are most effective in protecting individuals from toxic exposure when the local population has received prior education about the proper procedures to follow in the event of an accidental release. Education about toxic incidents is best coordinated with instruction on planning for and response to other natural and man-made disasters. Depending on the community, notification about an impending or ongoing accident may take place by an automated telephoning system or by siren. The community should be actively involved in the decision to implement either system; educational and practice sessions should be held with the full participation of all agencies that might respond to an actual event. Chemical emergency planning is most effective when industry, government, the medical community, local community organizations, and public interest groups have established working relationships and coordinate their efforts to mitigate the effects of an accident.

## PUBLIC HEALTH RISK ASSESSMENT AFTER ACCIDENTAL RELEASES

### The Four Steps of Risk Assessment

During an actual release of a hazardous material, the health care provider must be prepared to assess the attendant risks and assist with the response. In general, the assessment of health risk following any toxic exposure can be divided into four distinct steps. These are: (1) hazard identification; (2) exposure assessment; (3) toxicologic and dose-response evaluation; and (4) risk characterization. Risk assessment is discussed in greater detail in Chapter 47. In theory, risk assessment is separated from risk management decisions made during an accidental release. In practice, however, because time constraints are imposed by the emergent nature of accidental releases, there is no clear separation of these four steps and risk assessors may play a part in influencing management decisions based on the incomplete data available. Public health officials may act as either risk assessors or as risk managers, and multidisciplinary and interagency involvement is customary, even during small-scale chemical accidents. A large-scale accident may involve physicians, toxicologists, epidemiologists, emergency responders, and other staff from local, state, and federal agencies. The response to the oleum release in Richmond, California (described at the beginning of this chapter) will be used to illustrate the use of the four steps of risk assessment during an accidental release.

**A. Hazard Identification:** The first step in health risk assessment is hazard identification. This involves describing the released chemicals and determining their relative hazards in order to ascertain the immediate, delayed, and longer-term health risks posed by the release. The parent compound, as well as the breakdown products and other major ingredients in the formulation, must be identified, using on-line government and chemical manufacturer databases. However, identification of the spilled compound may not always be easy as rail tank car placards may be missing or inadequate toxicity testing may lead to failure to accurately categorize a chemical as hazardous. For new chemicals, the necessary health effects data may be classified as confidential business information and may not be readily accessible. Information on breakdown products, chemical interactions, and nontoxicologic hazards, such as flammability, should be sought. In addition to causing thermal injury, explosions or fires may result in the release of a variety of toxic products of incomplete combustion, such as benzene, phosgene, or sulfur dioxide.

When more than one substance has spilled, additional exposures may result from chemical interactions in the environment; the biological effects of simultaneous exposure to multiple substances should also be taken into account, although scientific data specific to these situations may often be lacking. During the Richmond release, government officials were easily able to identify the spilled oleum as sulfur trioxide, which is rapidly converted to sulfuric acid in the presence of atmospheric moisture, on the basis of information supplied by the responsible company.

**B. Exposure Assessment:** The second step, exposure assessment, entails the characterization of the source and location of the release, the potential pathways of human exposure, the population at risk, and the level of exposure. Exposures must be evaluated immediately following the release and levels predicted until the source is contained. In most cases, public health officials will need to rely on emergency responders for information on the exact location of the release, the time of the accident, whether the release has been contained, and the total amount spilled. During the oleum release, it was initially assumed that the entire contents of the 100 gallon tank car had spilled; much later, the company involved calculated that four tons of oleum had actually been released. However, this was never confirmed by a regulatory agency.

The route of exposure to a hazardous substance often determines the types of health effects observed following its accidental release. After characterizing the release, the potential human exposure pathways should be identified. Inhalation is more common than oral or dermal exposure. Dermal exposures are of most concern to workers and emergency responders. Although routes of exposure are often obvious, as when inhalation exposure follows a massive release into the air, this may not always be the case. For any particular spill, multiple routes of exposure may need to be considered. Dermal, as well as inhalation, exposure may have followed the release of oleum into the air; oral exposure to the parent compound or to neutralized breakdown products was a possible, though unproved, route of exposure following consumption of garden vegetables in the affected area.

The 1991 release of the 19,000 gallons of the nonvolatile herbicide metam sodium from a tank car into the Sacramento River in California illustrates how the most important route of exposure may not be immediately obvious. This spill resulted in extensive killing of fish and other aquatic life downstream. Health officials were concerned about the most obvious routes of exposure, ingestion of, and contact with contaminated water. However, due to the rapid environmental conversion of metam to its volatile and more toxic breakdown product, methyl isothiocyanate (MITC), inhalation was the most significant source of exposure for residents along the river.

Geographic information systems (GIS) that take into account terrain, weather, and residential locations may be used to map spills and predict the path of the chemical plume to better characterize potential exposures and identify the population at risk. Often, however, in the confusion that follows an accidental release, GIS does not provide accurate, timely information to guide risk management decisions. Environmental monitoring of the released chemical and its breakdown products or other *de novo* toxicants is important to accurately determine the level of exposure; monitoring is essential in the case of a dynamic exposure source. During the oleum release, dispersion modeling was used to predict the spread of the sulfuric acid cloud and the concentrations were compared to existing exposure standards. An initial model, based on the first estimates of the amount released and available meteorologic data, was available within hours. The model was subsequently revised to reflect more accurate information when it became available. Air monitoring of ambient sulfate levels supported the predictions of the dispersion model.

The population at risk of exposure includes employees of the facility or transport mode responsible for the release; people at nearby facilities, residences, and businesses; and people in transit in their vehicles in the area of the release or in the path of the chemical plume. During the oleum spill, the chemical cloud passed over a major transportation route during the morning hours, resulting in exposure to many thousands of commuters. Although emergency responders are most likely to wear personal protective equipment, they are also at risk of exposure.

**C. Dose-Response Evaluation:** The third step in health risk assessment is toxicologic and dose-response evaluation. This involves: (1) identifying the toxicologic end points of concern from the published literature as well as unpublished documents, if available; and (2) characterizing the relationship between the exposure dose and the adverse health effects. In the case of a pesticide spill, information in the EPA's pesticide registration database may be considered confidential by the manufacturer. Legal permission to access the data may be required. Both animal and human data should be consulted, as human testing is often inadequate. The results of acute, subchronic, chronic carcinogenicity and reproductive toxicity testing should be obtained. When quantitative human data are unavailable, animal data are related to an equivalent human dose on a body weight or surface area basis. Dose-response evaluation following the oleum release, was facilitated by the availability of many animal and human data, including experimental studies in asthmatics.

**D. Risk Characterization:** The final phase of risk assessment, risk characterization, involves: (1) identification of health effects that may be expected from the release and of individuals or institutions at greatest risk of adverse health effects; and (2) institution of emergency response action levels to protect individuals from further exposure or to prevent injury.

**1. Health Effects**–Health effects following accidental releases may be categorized into immediate, delayed, and carcinogenic. Table 40–8 lists the immediate health effects most commonly reported as a result of spills. Short-term, immediate health effects, such as skin or eye irritation or exacerbation of asthma, and delayed effects, such as birth defects or other effects on a pregnancy and cancer, are of most concern to the community and to public health officials following an accidental release of a chemical into the environment. While most health care providers evaluate and treat exposed persons for immediate effects, persistent or delayed conditions following exposure to accidentally-released compounds may occur. For example, various reports exist in which reactive airways dysfunction syndrome has been described in police officers following a single exposure during transportation accidents. For the majority of hazardous substances releases, however, inadequate information is available on the long-term effects of acute exposures.

After a short-term exposure (up to two weeks), a quantitative evaluation can be made of certain potential long-term effects such as cancer, based on the inherent toxicity of the compound, the exposure level, and the dose-response assessment. For most compounds, a short-term exposure would result in a negligible risk of cancer. If an accidental release results in chronic environmental or occupational exposures to relatively low levels of a contaminant, however, it is prudent to estimate risks of cancer or other long-term effects to guide surveillance and other response measures.

In addition to physical consequences of accidental chemical exposure, the psychological impact of accidental releases is an important factor to consider. Depression, anger, and anxiety are common in communities immediately following, and as prolonged consequences of, accidental releases. Health care providers and public health officials should recognize that exposed persons may need evaluation for and treatment of psychological problems. Additionally, anxiety about the possible effects of released chemicals may increase health care utilization by the "worried well" as well as by individuals considering litigation. For example, in the five days following the Richmond, California oleum release, 20,000 people sought medical attention; a review of 14,000 medical records revealed that 15% had no health complaints. A class action suit was filed by thousands of individuals alleging personal injury as a result of this release.

Persons who may be predisposed to adverse effects following exposure to accidentally-released chemicals are termed "sensitive individuals," some of whom are identified in Table 40–14. Institutions housing such individuals, such as schools, hospitals, or elderly care facilities that are in the vicinity of an accidental release may warrant special mitigation measures. Public health officials may need to notify the public that certain sensitive subpopulations may be at an increased risk of specified health consequences.

**2. Emergency Response Standards**–Officials may use emergency response action levels to guide shelter-in-place or evacuation decisions; if evacuation has taken place, these levels may be used to determine when it is safe for community members to reenter the area. In general, a level defines the concentration and duration to which most individuals may be exposed without suffering from a designated health effect (for example, mild, severe, or life-threatening). To derive an emergency response level, the EPA recommends dividing the highest exposure dose that does not result in the health effect of interest (the no adverse or lowest adverse effect level) by uncertainty factors ranging from 1 to 10 to account for inadequacies in the database, incomplete scientific knowledge, and protection of sensitive subpopulations. The use of uncertainty factors offers a margin of safety for officials to consider when recommending responses to accidental releases. During the Richmond release, several emergency exposure standards were identified for sulfuric acid because it is such a commonly used, and accidentally released, chemical.

In the event of an accidental release, a variety of exposure reference levels may be used. These standards vary considerably in their use of accurate scientific methods and intent to protect public health. The EPA offers rough guidelines for "safe" one-hour exposures for most members of a community. If standards have not been developed by the local or state responding agency, the EPA recommends that emergency planning be based on specific one-hour airborne concentrations chosen for their theoretical abil-

**Table 40–14.** Examples of "sensitive individuals" with conditions predisposing toward adverse health effects following exposure to chemicals.

| Sensitive Subpopulation | Proposed Reason for Increased Sensitivity | Chemical Examples |
|---|---|---|
| Infants and children | Age-related differences in anatomy & physiology, organ susceptibility, exposure | Pesticides; lead |
| Developing fetuses | Critically timed organogenesis extremely susceptible to disruption of normal events | Toluene |
| Asthmatics | Increased sensitivity to end-organ effects of substances | Ozone |
| Individuals with coronary artery disease | Increased sensitivity to end-organ effects of substances | Carbon monoxide |

**Table 40–15.** The United States EPA's recommended hierarchy of emergency response (one-hour) action standards for guiding actions during and after accidental releases.[1]

| Name of Standard | Agency |
| --- | --- |
| **Preexisting Levels (Preferred):** | |
| 1. Levels based on comprehensive review of literature | State or local governmental agency |
| 2. Short-term Public Emergency Guidance Levels | National Academy of Sciences |
| 3. Emergency Response Planning Guidelines-2 | American Industrial Hygiene Association |
| **Levels Developed During Accident (if Above Are Not Available):** | |
| 4. Levels based on brief toxicity review | Government toxicologists |
| **If Nothing Else Is Available:** | |
| 5. Threshold Limit Value-Short Term Exposure Limit | NIOSH |
| 6. Threshold Limit-Time Weighted Average multiplied by 3 | NIOSH |
| 7. Immediately Dangerous to Life and Health values divided by 10 | NIOSH |

[1]From the United States Environmental Protection Agency: Handbook of Chemical Hazard Analysis Procedures. Federal Emergency Management Agency, 1989.

ity to prevent adverse health consequences in the event of an accidental release (Table 40–15). The preferred one-hour levels on which to base emergency response actions are the Short-Term Public Emergency Guidance Levels developed by the National Academy of Sciences or the Emergency Response and Planning Guidelines-2 (ERPG-2) (there are three ERPG levels available) developed by the American Industrial Hygiene Association. Although relatively few substances have been addressed by these organizations to date, guidance levels are available for some of the most commonly released substances (eg, chlorine, ammonia, sulfuric acid).

If these levels are not available for a spilled chemical, the EPA recommends consultation with toxicologists (working in regulatory agencies) for advice based on a review of the toxicity of the material of concern. For example, even on an emergent basis, toxicologists may be able to derive exposure guidance levels based on literature review, utilizing uncertainty factors to account for data gaps such as interspecies and intraspecies differences. If this is not possible, the EPA recommends that the highest among the following existing values be used: the Threshold Limit Value Short-Term Exposure Limit, the Threshold Limit-Time Weighted Average multiplied by three, and NIOSH's Immediately Dangerous to Life and Health (IDLH) values divided by 10. The EPA offers no specific justification for these recommendations. These latter values may not be based solely on scientific data and are recommended for use

during emergencies only because they may be more readily available than other levels that are specifically derived for use during accidental releases. IDLH values are currently undergoing revision to more accurately reflect the available scientific literature.

The EPA's focus on events with the potential for outcomes similar in severity to the accident in Bhopal is reflected in its emphasis on incidents that have high acute hazard potential. Incidents resulting in deaths, injuries, or evacuations are given the highest priority. This emphasis is reflected in the accident definitions that guide emergency planning activities. The EPA defines minor accidents as those having low potential for serious human injuries and no potential for human fatalities. Moderately severe accidents are defined as having the potential to result in up to 10 fatalities, 100 injuries, and evacuation of up to 2000 people. In recommending the use of the exposure standards summarized above, the EPA does not claim that these levels protect identifiable subpopulations who may be particularly susceptible to the adverse health effects of hazardous substances, such as asthmatics and persons with coronary artery disease (Table 40–14).

The EPA is in the process of developing Acute Exposure Guideline Levels (AEGLs) that will serve as biological reference values for use during the planning and response phases of accidental releases of hazardous substances. For each chemical, up to three levels (AEGL-1, AEGL-2, and AEGL-3), referring to increasing levels of severity of health effects, will be proposed. In addition, some state agencies, such as the California Environmental Protection Agency, are developing exposure standards that may similarly be used as biological reference values for emergency planning and that are geared toward the protection of identifiable sensitive subpopulations.

## Coordination of Multi-Agency Response

The preceding discussion suggests that a number of different governmental agencies and professional specialties may be involved in the response to an accidental chemical release. For example, following the oleum release, the agencies responding to the event included the United States EPA, the United States Coast Guard, the California EPA, the California Department of Health Services, the local air quality enforcement agency, the local health department, and the local fire department. Responses such as this one may be confusing, frustrating, and duplicative. To streamline response to major incidents, some local and state agencies have coordinated efforts to establish joint plans.

For example, California has instituted two such plans: the Standardized Emergency Management System (SEMS) and the Railroad Accident Prevention and Immediate Deployment (RAPID) plan. SEMS operates under all kinds of emergencies, including earthquakes and fires, and provides for five-levels of response, activated as needed, to deliver effective aid to multi-agency and multi-jurisdiction emergencies. These levels are: (1) field, (2) local government, (3) county, (4) region, and (5) state. RAPID, which coordinates 17 state governmental agencies under an incident command system, is activated when a hazardous materials release overwhelms local authorities or involves more than one local jurisdiction. As of this writing, the future of RAPID is uncertain because of decreased funding for this state program.

## REGULATIONS

### General

Physicians who may be involved in the planning for or response to accidental releases should be aware of the complex regulations governing this area of environmental health and the sources of data for hazardous substance releases.

**A. Definition of Hazardous Materials:** In the United States, the transport of hazardous materials is regulated by the Department of Transportation (DOT) under the Hazardous Materials Transportation Act of 1975. Hazardous materials are defined as materials or substances in forms or quantities that, if released, may pose an unreasonable risk to health and safety or property. Approximately 2400 materials have been listed and classified broadly into categories such as explosives, flammables, corrosives,

combustibles, poisons, oxidizers, biological agents, and radioactive materials. These substances have been designated as hazardous materials because of their adverse effects on health or the environment.

Hazardous substances are a subset of hazardous materials regulated by the EPA under the Comprehensive Environmental Response, Compensation, and Liability Act of 1980 (CERCLA). All CERCLA substances are also automatically listed and regulated by the DOT as hazardous materials.

**B. Types of Hazardous Materials Accidents:** Unplanned releases of hazardous materials are categorized as either stationary source or transportation accidents. For the most part, these two categories are regulated separately, with stationary source accidental release planning and response under the jurisdiction of the EPA and transportation accidents under the DOT. Both types of accidents have similar requirements for reporting (see below). The distinction between stationary source and transportation issues becomes blurred on occasion, as discussed below in the section on transportation accidents.

### Stationary Source Accidents

**A. Federal Regulations:** Mandatory emergency planning and reporting requirements for the manufacture, storage, and transportation of hazardous materials are determined by two major federal regulations, CERCLA, commonly known as "Superfund," and Title III of the Superfund Amendments and Reauthorization Act of 1986 (SARA). CERCLA allows the EPA to respond to releases or threatened releases of hazardous substances, pollutants, or contaminants that may present an imminent and substantial danger to the public health or welfare. Title III of SARA, also known as the Emergency Planning and Community Right-to-Know Act of 1986, requires states to establish state-wide and local emergency planning groups to develop chemical emergency response plans for each community. It also requires facilities to provide material safety data sheets (MSDSs) or a list of hazardous materials on site to states, local planners, and fire departments, and through them, the public. In theory, SARA Title III builds the foundation of the community emergency response plan and public/industry dialogue on accidental release risk and risk reduction. In practice, the information contained in MSDSs typically does not provide accurate or adequate toxicity information on potential health effects resulting from exposure.

As required by SARA Title III and CERCLA, for each hazardous substance, the EPA has established "threshold" quantities based on its physical, chemical, and toxicological properties, including aquatic and mammalian toxicity, ignitablity, and reactivity, among other factors. Any person in charge of a facility at which there is a release of a CERCLA hazardous substance equal to or in excess of the threshold quantity must report immediately to the National

Response Center as well as to state and local emergency response officials. Failure to report accidental releases to the National Response Center can include civil and criminal penalties, including monetary fines, imprisonment, or both. Under CERCLA, this notification is required for transportation incidents and releases from vessels as well as stationary source emergencies. There is no requirement to report non-CERCLA substances. The latter category includes chemicals for which there is inadequate toxicity information for characterization as hazardous materials. For example, there was little toxicity data on methyl isocyanate prior to its release in Bhopal.

In addition, even if a release does not occur, Title III requires facility operators to notify the state emergency response commission (or its equivalent) of the type and quantity of hazardous materials stored in quantities equal to or in excess of the threshold amount. These regulations and their resultant penalties have resulted in increased notification of local, state, and federal governments about hazardous materials stored at facilities and improved knowledge of the patterns of accidental releases from both fixed and mobile sources. However, local governments still lack information about transportation of these substances through their jurisdictions.

To fill a gap left by the two regulations described above, the Clean Air Act Amendments of 1990 (Section 112r) added regulations aimed at preventing accidental releases of regulated materials and other extremely hazardous substances to the air and minimizing the consequences of releases by focusing preventive measures on those chemicals that pose the greatest risk. It requires facilities to identify hazards resulting from releases, to design and maintain safe facilities, and to minimize the consequences of releases when they occur.

In addition, the Clean Air Act Amendments of 1990 are unique among environmental regulations in that they aim to protect not only the environment and the health of the public, but the health and safety of workers, as well. To fulfill the latter requirement, OSHA has promulgated a chemical process safety standard to protect workers from chemical accidents at facilities using highly toxic, reactive, flammable, or explosive substances (57 Code of Federal Regulations Part 6536). To fulfill the former requirement, the EPA finalized a rule in 1996 governing Risk Management Programs for Accidental Release Prevention (40 Code of Federal Regulations Part 68). Starting in 1999, the latter rule will require facilities to prepare hazard assessments evaluating potential effects of an accidental release of any regulated substance. Based on these hazard assessments, facilities must develop programs aimed at prevention of emergency response to accidental releases. The Clean Air Act Amendments also required the establishment of an independent Chemical and Hazard Investigation Board. The purpose of this board would have been to investigate and report the cause of major accidents and to recommend methods to reduce their occurrence. However, funding for this board was never established. Consequently, the EPA has attempted to fulfill some of these responsibilities, but only in a limited manner.

Several states already have notification and accident prevention programs in place similar to the proposed federal requirements (see below). State and federal governments have been working together to streamline the risk management process to prevent confusing and duplicative requirements for reporting to different government agencies.

**B. State Regulations:** Four states—New Jersey, California, Delaware, and Nevada—have regulations requiring facilities to prepare and implement plans for the prevention of chemical accidents and emergency response in the event of a release. The current programs of the first two states will be briefly described.

New Jersey's Toxic Catastrophe Prevention Act of 1987 is one of the best examples of an effective accident prevention program. Facilities that have "extraordinarily hazardous substances" equal to or in excess of a threshold quantity must prepare a risk reduction program similar to that described above for the federal risk management program. One hundred and ten extraordinarily hazardous substances are defined and regulated, based on their volatility and toxicity. In the 10 years since its inception, the Toxic Catastrophe Prevention Act has resulted in major reductions in registered inventories of extraordinarily hazardous substances through the substitution of less hazardous substances.

Another example of a state accident prevention plan is California's Risk Management and Prevention Program, enacted in 1986. The goal of this program is to prevent accidental releases by anticipating their occurrence and requiring that preemptive actions be taken. This program requires the managers of a facility that handles a certain quantity of "acutely hazardous materials" to prepare documents reviewing its design and operations to determine potential sources of a chemical accident and the consequences such an accident could have on neighboring communities (an off-site consequence analysis). These documents are to be submitted for review to local "administering agencies" (eg, fire departments, county health departments). The effectiveness of this program is limited by the technical expertise available in the local administering agencies, resulting in uneven review of such documents.

## Transportation Accidents

The safe interstate transport of hazardous materials is regulated by the DOT through Hazardous Materials Regulations and the Hazardous Materials Transportation Act. Hazardous Materials Regulations regulate the safe transportation of hazardous materials through requirements for the appropriate labeling of containers and the thickness and materials used in packaging and testing for intactness of containers when damaged. In addition to federal regulations, there may be local rules for the safe transportation of hazardous materials.

Approximately 2400 substances are listed in the Hazardous Materials Regulations. But there are many chemicals not included on this list that exhibit properties that meet the definition of one or more "hazard class" and so are subject to the rule. This law covers the loading, unloading, "storage incidental to movement," and transport of hazardous materials during commerce. It is often a challenge to determine whether a material being transported meets the hazardous materials definition, and if so by which law it is governed. Indeed, it is not always clear whether the material is being "transported."

The latter point is illustrated by the "30-day Rule." Under this rule, a transport vessel, such as a rail tank car, that remains on the premises of a facility for less than 30 days is subject to DOT jurisdiction; after 30 days, it is considered to be a part of the facility and subject to local and EPA regulations. The Richmond oleum release occurred from a tank car that was being used for storage on company property. Because it was unclear how long the tank car had been stored on the facility grounds, there was confusion as to which agency had the responsibility for regulating violations that led to the spill.

The National Transportation Safety Board is the federal agency responsible for investigating and determining probable causes of transportation accidents and in recommending remedial public safety measures. For example, the National Transportation Safety Board has long been active in investigating railroad tank car accidents involving hazardous materials and recommending changes in tank car design. These changes have resulted in a marked decline in fatal tank car incidents since the 1980s. However, accidents still occur and are cause for concern. Since the early 1980s, there have been more than 10,000 accidental releases of hazardous materials involving tank cars. The National Transportation Safety Board and other agencies investigating these accidents have been critical of the DOT for not taking a more proactive approach to ensure the shipment of hazardous materials in safe containers. As a result, the National Research Council (1994) has recently issued recommendations for improving the safety performance of tank cars as well as for improving the regulatory process in the DOT and the Coast Guard.

The Federal Railroad Administration enforces the rules governing tank cars used for transporting hazardous materials. The relationship of the National Transportation Safety Board and the Federal Railroad Administration and the reactive nature of interventions is illustrated in the following example. In May 1991, the National Transportation Safety Board found that a certain type of tank car was inadequate for transporting hazardous materials, as evidenced by a several-year accident history. However, the Federal Railroad Administration did not ban the use of this tank car for carrying these products until a subsequent release occurred from the same type of car being used to store oleum in Richmond, California in 1993.

## SOURCES OF DATA

Because no single source of information is comprehensive, several databases need to be consulted to determine the true magnitude and severity of accidental releases. Several national databases have been used to characterize the public health consequences of hazardous substance releases. These include the Hazardous Materials Information System, a DOT database that contains reports of transportation accidents involving hazardous materials, and the Emergency Release Notification System (ERNS), a database of accident reports made to the National Response Center and managed by the EPA. Each has its advantages and shortcomings. With the exception of ATSDR's Hazardous Substances Emergency Event Surveillance system described earlier, none of these databases contain detailed information about the health effects of accidental releases.

In spite of its limitations, ERNS is the preferred information system with nationwide statistics on accidental releases from both stationary and transportation sources. Accidental release data reported to the National Response Center, the EPA, and the United States Coast Guard from 1987 to the present are catalogued in ERNS. This reporting system is updated quarterly, is available to researchers for analysis, and covers CERCLA hazardous substances and petroleum and nonpetroleum oil products (see Accident Statistics above for examples of these products). Information gathered by ERNS includes the amount of material released, the location and cause of the accident, the origin of the release (fixed facility or transportation), and the number of persons injured, killed, or evacuated. Limitations of this database include inadequate health data and the potential for duplicate reporting. In addition, because reports are made during the initial phases of an accident, are not verified, and are not subsequently modified after more thorough investigation, the information may not be entirely accurate or complete.

In addition to the federal system, accurate information on accidental releases may be collected and utilized effectively by some states. For example, since 1988, any spill of a hazardous material in California must be reported to the Office of Emergency Services and detailed information is compiled into the California Hazardous Material Incident Reporting System. This reporting system allows the examination of the factors most commonly associated with accidental chemical releases and facilitates planning for preventive measures to reduce their occurrence.

## WORLDWIDE PERSPECTIVE

Although it is clear that both major and minor chemical accidents are widespread, it is difficult to gain an accurate perspective of the magnitude of these incidents, because reporting requirements and record keeping vary so widely between countries. The approach of industrialized countries, particularly Europe, to accidental releases is the closest to that of the United States, while that of developing countries is still in its infancy. The following information aims to familiarize readers with situations in various countries, but it is not meant to be a detailed accounting of their programs.

### Industrialized Countries

In 1982, following accidents in Flixborough, United Kingdom, in 1974 and Seveso, Italy, in 1976, the European Community (EC) initiated a directive (the Seveso Directive) on the major accident hazards involving dangerous substances. The Directive provides guidelines on risk management and emergency planning for the prevention of chemical accidents. The purpose of the legislation is two-fold. The first is to incorporate control and safety measures into the design of a plant or process and to prepare emergency plans. The second is to inform the general public about the following information regarding their facilities: the substances on site that have the potential to cause a hazardous incident, possible harmful effects on humans and the environment, details regarding hazardous incident warning systems, and recommendations for actions to be taken in the event of a hazardous incident. In addition, it provides for notification of authorities if dangerous materials are stored, transported, used in operations, or released in an accident. The requirements regarding storage of hazardous materials, their potential risks, and on-site emergency plans for dealing with accidents apply to approximately 200 substances that are extremely toxic, carcinogenic, or explosive and whose amounts exceed specified thresholds.

An amendment to the Directive in 1988 replaced the passive transfer of information on a "need-to-know" basis with a requirement for active provision of information to the public on a "right-to-know" basis. The most recent revision of this directive (Seveso II) went into effect in January 1997. In addition to mandatory public notification, this document requires safety reports, accident prevention, and emergency response plans.

There are several differences between the United States and Europe in planning for accidental releases. First, the terms of European directives are binding but leave member states free to choose forms and methods of implementations. Community directives become effective only when they become a part of national laws. Not all EC member states have incorporated the directives into their national legislation. Next, lists of hazardous substances that are subject to requirements contain different chemicals than those in the United States. Finally, the threshold amounts that trigger public notification and emergency planning are higher in Europe than in the United States.

One of the main differences between Europe and other nations is the physical planning required for plants near large housing districts. For example, in both the United Kingdom and in the Netherlands, no new housing is allowed within a certain distance of plants that are considered hazardous. As attested to by the Bhopal release, this is a marked contrast from developing nations such as India.

Several separate systems exist for hazardous materials incidents reporting in Europe. The Major Accident Reporting System database, maintained in Ispra, Italy, contains reports of accidental releases from all EC states. Member nations are required to report incidents, but enforcement is variable and the information is incomplete. The hazardous materials accident database maintained by The Netherlands since 1977 is the most complete. In the United Kingdom, the Major Hazard Incident Database Service records hazardous materials incidents worldwide, with most information coming from North America and Europe. Information on transportation accidents in the United Kingdom is also included in general accident statistics maintained by the Department of Transport. Canada's Hazardous Material Incidents Reporting System and National Analysis of Trends in Emergencies System database have been in place since 1973 and are similar to those in the United States. More recently, Australia has instituted its System For Hazardous Material Incident Reporting.

### Developing Countries: Asia

**A. General:** Exposures to hazardous materials as a result of both routine and accidental releases pose a large risk to public health and environmental integrity in some Asian countries. In countries such as China and Taiwan, economic reforms and rapid industrialization have taken precedence over the setting and enforcement of environmental standards. In contrast, industrially developed countries with greater resources, such as Japan and Singapore, have paid more attention to controlling damage to the environment, including that caused by accidental releases.

China's key agency for promulgating and implementing environmental policy is the National Environmental Protection Agency. Numerous regulations and orders have been promulgated to deal with air and water pollution and natural resources deterioration, among other environmental concerns. In reality, these regulations are often violated by government agencies as well as by joint ventures with foreign companies. Lack of standards and enforcement regulations also plague Taiwan's Environmental Protection Administration, which was created in 1987 to ameliorate that country's highly polluted air and water.

**B. India:** In the years following the Bhopal accident, the Indian government enacted a wide array of legislative and regulatory changes aimed at controlling pollution, protecting the environment, conserving natural resources, and improving safety-management practices in hazardous industrial facilities. For example, the Environment Protection Act requires firms to disclose detailed information on hazardous materials on site, air, and water pollution and investments in environmental protection and pollution control. The Public Liability Insurance Act requires plant owners to carry insurance to cover death, injury, or property damage resulting from an accident.

Other rules obligate plant managers to ensure the safety of all industrial activities, to prepare emergency response plans, and to report "major accidents" to the "concerned authority." Managers are also required to report on-site storage of hazardous chemicals that are on a list of over 400 substances defined on the basis of their acute toxicity, flammability, and explosiveness.

The effectiveness of this extensive legislation is dampened by the lack of compliance by industry. For example, the National Safety Council of India reports that there are over 1000 factories with hazardous chemicals on site. Less than 75% of these plants (722) have prepared emergency response plans.

Like other developing nations, India does not maintain a nationwide database of accidental chemical releases. Instead, the high morbidity and mortality rate of such incidents can be gleaned from newspaper reports. In 1994, over 60 major accidents were reported by the press. Over 400 persons, including 30 children, were killed and over 1000 were injured as a result of these incidents. Most of the deaths occurred in workers. The actual number of accidents and resulting morbidity and mortality rate is likely to be much higher.

### International Programs

The Organization for Economic Cooperation and Development (OECD), an organization of 24 industrialized countries from North America, Western Europe, and the Pacific, which meets to compare, coordinate, and harmonize national policies, recorded 74 major accidents worldwide in the 8 years preceding the the Bhopal accident and 106 incidents in the 8 years following. As a result of the incidents leading up to and shortly after the Bhopal accident, the United Nations Environment Program (UNEP) suggested a series of measures to help governments, particularly in developing countries, minimize the occurrence and

harmful effects of chemical accidents. Released in 1988 as the Handbook on Awareness and Preparedness for Emergencies at Local Level (APELL), this publication is designed to increase community awareness about local risks and hazards related to industrial operations, including accidental releases of hazardous substances and, based on this information, to develop emergency response plans. Although the UNEP recommendations are nearly a decade old, they have not changed.

To complement the APELL program, the OECD Environment Committee, with the United States EPA, prepared voluntary guidelines to provide a foundation to prevent, prepare for, and respond to chemical accidents throughout the world. Published in 1993, the "Guiding Principles for Chemical Accident Prevention" was developed in cooperation with the International Labor Organization, UNEP, the World Health Organization, and the World Bank. The document describes the roles of industry, public authorities, employees, the public, and organizations to prevent and mitigate the effects of hazardous materials accidents (Table 40–16). It is suggested that safety programs be aimed toward completely preventing harm to human health, environment, and property ("zero-risk"), while recognizing that accidents will still occur. Although transportation is not specifically addressed, the principles described may be applicable to this accident category. The "Guiding Principles" are notable for their statement that industries from OECD countries should operate with these same guidelines in their plants located in non-OECD (developing) nations.

### NUCLEAR ACCIDENTS

In spite of such well-known radiation accidents as Three Mile Island, Pennsylvania, in 1979 and Chernobyl, Ukraine, in 1986, emergency preparedness for nuclear accidents is often overlooked by public health professionals. Although the detailed consideration of unintentional releases of radiologic material into the environment is beyond the scope of this chapter, the topic of accidental releases would not be complete without at least a brief mention of planning for and response to nuclear accidents.

Nuclear accidents may occur anywhere radioactive materials are in use but may be more likely in countries with covert nuclear programs, where safety and early warning systems may be inadequately tested or nonexistent. While large-scale accidents are well-publicized, numerous small accidental exposures, including military and hospital over-exposures, may not be publicly reported for several years after their occurrence. Unlike the multiple reporting systems for accidental chemical releases, reporting systems for radiologic accidents in the United States are not standardized or easily accessible.

**Table 40–16.** Summary of roles of interested parties involved in planning and response to accidental chemical releases internationally, as described in Guiding Principles for Chemical Accident Prevention, Preparedness and Response (OECD, 1993).

| Interested Party | Role |
|---|---|
| Public authorities | 1. Motivate sectors of society to recognize need for accident prevention and response<br>2. Establish safety objectives: notification & information requirements, enforcement actions, inspection systems<br>3. Investigate and report accidents; publish results<br>4. Notify community of risks<br>5. Establish emergency preparedness programs<br>6. Provide guidance to industry |
| Management of hazardous installations | 1. Design and operate safe facilities, with goal of "zero incidents"<br>2. Rank hazards in terms of risk for harm, release<br>3. Cooperate with public authorities<br>4. Conduct emergency planning on- and off-site |
| Employee | 1. Follow established procedures, taking reasonable care of his/her personal safety and that of others<br>2. Should have right to refuse any task he/she believes may create unwarranted risk of hazardous material accident<br>3. Adverse consequences should not result if employee brings up safety issues |
| Industry in general | 1. Larger industries should offer assistance to small enterprises in meeting safety objectives<br>2. Bears primary responsibility for carrying out safety-related research |
| Other | 1. Polluter-Pays Principle<br>2. Media should be provided with information for communication to public |
| Investments, technology transfer, aid programs in non-OECD facilities | 1. Facilities from OECD countries should operate on same principles in non-OECD nations<br>2. Technology transfer to non-OECD countries should take place only when assurance is received that operating conditions are safe; especially applies to accident prevention |

As mentioned above for chemical accidents, planning for response to nuclear accidents must include arrangement for medical services for contaminated victims. Hospitals should be prepared to assess, triage, and treat exposed individuals. Policies for triage of victims should be in place. The medical consequences of exposure to ionizing radiation and treatment options are summarized in Chapter 12.

## Regulation in the United States
### A. Agencies Involved in Accident Response:
Accidental exposure to radiologic material may be due to situations as varied as nuclear reactor or nuclear power plant accidents, transport incidents involving radioactive material, space-craft reentry, or fallout from atmospheric testing of nuclear devices. In the event of a radiologic accident, various federal agencies coordinate their efforts at the accident scene under the umbrella of the Federal Radiological Emergency Response Plan. The Federal Emergency Management Agency coordinates federal and state activities. The Nuclear Regulatory Commission is the lead federal agency in an emergency at a licensed nuclear facility. The Department of Energy is the lead agency in an emergency at one its nuclear facilities or in a transportation accident involving radiologic material in its custody. The EPA is the lead agency in an emergency involving radioactivity originating in a foreign country or in a domestic accident involving unregulated radioactive material. State and local gov-

ernments are responsible for the health and welfare of the general public during an emergency.

The EPA has developed a system of Protective Action Guides (PAGs) to help officials make critical decisions. These guidelines identify the radiation levels at which state and local officials should take actions to safeguard human health during an accident and direct the development of emergency response plans. The PAGs identify three phases of an emergency: early, intermediate, and late. In the early phase, which usually lasts from several hours to several days, evacuation and sheltering are the principal actions to insulate the public from exposure to direct radiation and inhalation of airborne radioactive material. In the intermediate phase, which can last from weeks to months, actions may include limiting food and water consumption to decrease ingestion of radioactive material and relocating people to minimize radiation exposure. In the late phase, which can last from months to years, the PAGs address the decontamination of property. In an actual emergency, in addition to those addressed by the PAGs, other protective actions may be needed.

### B. Nuclear Reactor Accidents:
There are currently over 100 licensed reactors in the United States and formal approval of emergency response plans are a condition for obtaining and maintaining operating licenses of these facilities. The NRC coordinates all offsite radiologic emergency preparedness efforts and evaluates state and local plans. Current regulations require that emergency planning be conducted

at the facility with provisions for off-site emergency response, including arrangements for medical services for injured or radiologic contaminated individuals and training for those who may be called on to assist in an emergency.

The NRC has a nuclear plant emergency preparedness goal that sets health objectives in terms of probability of occurrence compared to other events. For example, the goal for severe accident prevention is a frequency of occurrence of less than one in a million per reactor per year; the risk to an average individual in the vicinity of a nuclear power plant of prompt fatalities that might result from reactor accidents should not exceed 0.1% of the sum of prompt fatality risks resulting from other accidents; and the risk to the population in the area near a nuclear power plant of cancer fatalities that might result from nuclear power plant operation should not exceed 0.1% of the sum of cancer fatality risks resulting from all other causes.

### International Coordination

There are some efforts to institute international safety standards for nuclear reactors. Accident management activities exist in OECD countries, although there is significant variation among member countries as to what should be classified as severe accident management. The Nuclear Energy Agency, a panel of the OECD, has outlined existing programs in member countries and has encouraged further efforts at emergency preparedness. Differences may exist even within countries. For example, the lack of uniformity found in older Soviet-designed reactors currently poses problems in the international safety regulatory arena.

There are separate regulations for emergency response planning for transport accidents involving radioactive material. It is estimated that over 40 million shipments of packages containing radioactive material are made each year throughout the world, although there have been no reported transport accidents with serious radiologic consequences to date. The International Atomic Energy Agency has issued guidelines that have served for years as the basis for regulating the safe transport of radiologic materials worldwide. These universal recommendations are implemented by local authorities, taking into account the specific legislative structures and actual shipments.

# HAZARDOUS WASTE

After hearing that the groundwater in their neighborhood is contaminated with chemicals coming from a nearby landfill, a couple went to their doctor. They were having trouble conceiving a baby and were sure that it was due to the contaminated water. The doctor discovered that the man had an extremely low sperm count.

Several children are referred to a pediatrician by the school nurse. These children have been singled out by the teacher for hyperactivity and inattentiveness. When the nurse speaks with their parent, they voice concern about the mercury-containing mine tailings that their homes are built on.

Concern about hazardous waste typically ranks at the top of the list when the public is polled about environmental concerns. The public is increasingly turning to physicians for advice and answers to problems such as the ones posed above. A physician should have a working understanding of the health risks created by hazardous waste and be able to take an exposure history. The ability to recognize when an exposure may be occurring is critical since environmental medicine, like occupational medicine, is prevention-oriented.

The following section on hazardous waste will include an overview of the nature and magnitude of the problem, the use of exposure assessment and health studies for studying the impact of hazardous waste facilities, and a synopsis of hazardous waste regulation and management. The focus will be on chemical waste; however, radioactive waste and medical waste will also be addressed. The last part provides a glimpse into hazardous waste issues at the international level.

## DEFINING THE PROBLEM

The term hazardous waste is ambiguous. It more accurately should refer to hazardous chemicals since it is unclear when a hazardous chemical becomes a hazardous waste. For the most part, in US regulation, there is control over the storage, treatment, and disposal of hazardous waste, not hazardous chemicals. The single exception is the regulation of underground storage tanks. There are as many possible types of hazardous wastes as there are possible combinations of hazardous and toxic chemicals. These are the byproducts of industry, home, agriculture, or the environment. Over 11 million chemical substances are known; 60,000 to 70,000 chemicals are in regular use. Of those, approximately 3,000 account for 90% of total commercial and other uses. Only a tiny fraction of chemicals in use have adequate toxicologic data. Data on interactions between different chemicals is even more sparse.

Hazardous waste as defined by US legislation is a subset of solid waste and can include solids, sludges, liquids, and containerized gases. These broad definitions have a myriad of exceptions, many being a result of the political influence of those who create the waste. The following materials are not considered solid waste and, as a result, are not listed as hazardous waste: domestic sewage, certain nuclear waste, in-situ mining waste, and pulping liquors used in the production of paper in the Kraft paper process. Household chemicals are also excluded from hazardous waste categorization, although there are many toxic chemicals in today's commercial products. Other hazardous waste exclusions include agricultural wastes used as fertilizers, mining overburden, discarded wood treated with arsenic, chromium wastes, petroleum-contaminated media from tank cleanup, specific ore processing wastes, specific utility wastes, oil and gas exploration, development and production waste, and cement kiln waste.

It is important to note that hazardous waste also excludes chemicals discharged directly into the air or water (ie, releases allowed by permits under other federal pollution control statutes such as the Clean Air Act and the Clean Water Act). Firms that generate small quantities of hazardous wastes can escape management requirements. Hazardous wastes mixed with fuel oils can be burned and released into the environment without adequate controls.

Americans are the largest producers of hazardous waste per capita; however, it should be noted that despite all the exceptions mentioned above, the definition of hazardous waste in the United States encompasses much more than that of any other country. In 1993, 24,632 large quantity generators produced 258 million tons of hazardous waste, which is more than one ton for each person. Chemical and petrochemical companies were responsible for more than 70% of all hazardous waste generation. Metal industries accounted for approximately 22%. The states generating the most hazardous waste were Texas, Tennessee, Louisiana, Michigan, and New Jersey, accounting for 65% of the national total quantity generated.

It has been estimated that as many as 425,000 abandoned hazardous waste sites exist in the United States, though the EPA has inventoried only 31,000 at this time. As of October 1995, 1,233 sites were on the EPA's National Priorities List (NPL). The EPA proposes sites for the NPL by applying a Hazard Ranking System, which is an assessment of the relative public health, environmental, and ecologic threat posed by a given site. There are 155 sites owned by the federal government, primarily the Department of Energy and the Department of Defense, on the NPL. These federal sites pose significant concern because of their large geographic areas and the complex mixture of waste that is contaminating them.

## Medical Waste

Medical waste is composed of waste that is generated or produced as a result of any of the following: diagnosis, treatment, or immunization of human beings or animals; research dealing with infectious agents; serums, vaccines, antigens, and antitoxins; waste that is biohazardous; or "sharps"—devices having acute rigid corners, edges, or protuberances capable of cutting or piercing, including hypodermic needles, syringes, blades, needles, and broken glass. Medical waste is generated by a variety of health-care-related facilities, including physician and dentist offices, clinics, hospitals, skilled nursing facilities, research facilities, research laboratories, clinical laboratories, and other health care facilities, or by illicit drug use and in homes by diabetics and others who depend upon injections for health reasons.

Medical facilities generate half a million tons of infectious medical waste every year. Hospitals, which comprise only 2% of the total number of generators, produce approximately 77% of the total. The quantity of medical and infectious waste is increasing due to the increasing dependence in the medical community on disposable items.

## Radioactive Waste

The production of nuclear power and weapons creates hazardous waste from remnants left from uranium mining, routine radioactive waste at nuclear power facilities, weapons production facilities, nuclear bomb testing locations, and cleanup at decommissioned nuclear power plants and military sites.

Low-level radioactive waste (approximately 0.5 curies per cubic yard) results from radiologic uses at more than 20,000 facilities nationwide such as hospitals, universities, biomedical research, pharmaceutical development, and other industrial sources. Civilian nuclear waste also arises from the 109 nuclear reactors in the United States. These reactors produce low-level waste (approximately 1 curie per cubic yard) that includes contaminated trash, sludges and resins from the reactor, and irradiated reactor parts. Spent fuel from nuclear reactors has a high level of radioactivity (689,999 curies per cubic yard of waste).

In addition, there are 12 nuclear reactors that are currently in shutdown mode and are being decommissioned. The decommissioning of these facilities produces spent fuel and low-level waste (approximately 76 curies per yard).

The other major source of radioactive waste is from the production of nuclear weapons by the Department of Energy for the Department of Defense. Defense waste is divided into low-level waste (1 curie per cubic yard), transuranic waste (4 curies per cubic yard), and high-level waste (approximately 780 curies per cubic yard).

In 1993, about 800,000 cubic yards of civilian low-level radioactive waste and 10,000,000 cubic yards of military low-level radioactive waste were produced. That same year, commercial nuclear reactors produced 28,000 metric tons of high-level waste (spent fuel) that accounted for 96% of the total radioactivity of all nuclear waste generated. The military produced 1,500,000 cubic feet of high-level and 1,110,000 cubic yards of transuranic waste. In addition to these wastes produced as a result of typical operating practices, the decommissioning of civilian reactors and military bases resulted in an additional amount of nuclear waste, primarily low-level waste.

## EXPOSURE AND RISK ASSESSMENT

Exposure assessment is the process of identifying all individuals or population subgroups that have been exposed to a chemical or chemicals. Based on demographic data available in the 1980s, the EPA estimated that approximately 41 million people live within four mile radii of the 1,134 NPL sites at the time. Of course, residence near a hazardous waste site or a facility that handles hazardous waste does not necessarily translate to actual exposure to substances released from the site. For instance, completed exposure pathways were identified at only 39% of the NPL hazardous waste sites. A completed exposure pathway consists of the following five elements: a source of contamination, an environmental medium, a point of exposure, route(s) of exposure, and a receptor population. Some of the exposure pathways that should be considered are listed in Table 40–17.

At 91% of the NPL hazardous waste sites with completed exposure pathways, the exposure occurred through contaminated groundwater; at 46% of the sites exposure occurred from contaminated soil; at 14% of the sites exposure was via contaminated biota. However, these data need to be understood in the context of how they are collected by regulatory agencies. When hazardous waste sites are evaluated, the soil and groundwater are almost always sampled; however, air monitoring and sampling of biota are not usually conducted. Additionally, most environmental data is collected from the land immediately comprising the site and not from the surrounding

**Table 40–18.** Top 10 most hazardous substances and the 10 substances found most often in completed exposure pathways at CERCLA sites.

| Rank | Hazardous Substance | Completed Exposure Pathways (% of 1,328 Sites) |
|---|---|---|
| 1. | Lead | Lead (59%) |
| 2. | Arsenic | Trichloroethylene (53%) |
| 3. | Mercury, metallic | Chromium (47%) |
| 4. | Benzene | Benzene (46%) |
| 5. | Vinyl chloride | Arsenic (45%) |
| 6. | Cadmium | Tetrachloroethylene (41%) |
| 7. | Polychlorinated biphenyls | Cadmium (39%) |
| 8. | Benzo(a)pyrene | Toluene (39%) |
| 9. | Chloroform | 1,1,1-Trichloroethane (32%) |
| 10. | Benzo(b)fluoranthene | Methylene chloride (31%) |

neighborhood where potential exposed populations may be living. It is typical that community exposure is evaluated using models to estimate the fate and transport of chemicals from on-site to the neighborhood.

There are more than 2,000 unique substances found at waste sites in the United States; the top 10 substances are presented in Table 40–18. The prioritization of the substances is based on three criteria: frequency of occurrence of a toxic substance at NPL sites, the substance's toxicity, and the potential for human exposure. Table 40–18 also lists the 10 contaminants most often found in completed exposure pathways at 1,328 hazardous waste sites and the percentage of sites at which each substance was released. Most hazardous waste sites are contaminated with a mixture of chemicals rather than a single chemical, and very little toxicologic information is known about mixtures.

People in communities are very suspicious of the modelled exposure and risk estimates used to assess the health impact. Communities that live around hazardous waste sites are increasingly asking for biological monitoring investigations to ascertain their exposure.

Biological monitoring measures exposure by monitoring body fluids (typically blood or urine) for the chemicals of interest. Biological monitoring provides the best evidence of exposure and avoids many of the exposure assumptions and animal-to-human extrapolations that are used in traditional exposure/risk assessment. However, depending on the pharmacokinetics of the chemical, biological monitoring may not provide the needed information about chronic exposure to chemicals from a hazardous waste site. For instance, volatile organic compounds like vinyl chloride have very short half-lives (two to four hours) in the blood, and thus a discrete blood sample analyzed for vinyl chloride may not reflect chronic, residential exposure. Unlike public health standards for allow-

**Table 40–17.** Exposure pathways investigated at hazardous waste sites.

Direct ingestion of contaminated groundwater
Direct ingestion of contaminated surface water
Incidental ingestion of contaminated soil and dust
Ingestion of contaminated fruits and vegetables
Ingestion of contaminated meat, poultry, and dairy products
Ingestion of contaminated fin fish and shellfish
Ingestion of contaminated breast milk
Inhalation of contaminants that volatilize from water
Inhalation of contaminants that volatilize from soil
Dermal absorption from contaminated water
Dermal absorption from contaminated soil
Dermal absorption from contaminated air

able concentrations of a chemical in drinking water or soil, there are no accepted guidelines for the interpretation of biological monitoring levels. Laboratories that conduct this type of testing define "normal," but these numbers have not been rigorously reviewed and are typically abstracted from one published study or from a straw poll of laboratory workers. Finally, if the chemical is detected above the "normal," interpretation of the results to the community member or patient as a short- or long-term health impact is a huge unknown at this time.

Interpretation of biological monitoring for individuals or communities surrounding a hazardous waste facility is greatly facilitated by the availability of large databases on the levels of chemicals in the "population," essentially "historical controls." As a part of the Second National Health and Nutrition Survey (NHANES), conducted from 1980–82, the serum and urine from 21,000 individuals was analyzed for 38 pesticides and toxic substances. The National Human Adipose Tissue Survey (NHATS) sampled 785 tissue samples in 1978.

> Concern for polychlorinated biphenyl (PCB) exposure to a residential community located next to the Monsanto plant in Anniston, Alabama led to monitoring for PCBs in the serum. Typical was defined using the NHANES data where 95% of individuals had levels less than 20 ppb. Of the 103 residents who volunteered for the investigation, 28 had a level of PCBs in their blood above 20 ppb, though only 5 would have been expected to have an elevated level. PCB soil levels in the residents' backyards were weakly correlated to the corresponding residents' PCB blood levels. PCB blood levels increased with the length of time that a person lived at his or her current residence. Eating locally-caught fish and game was not a risk marker. Eating homegrown vegetables was a significant risk marker for having elevated PCB blood levels.

## HEALTH IMPACT OF HAZARDOUS WASTE

In general, little is known about long-term exposure to low-levels of contamination in the environment. Various techniques have been used and are being used to study the health impact. However, the world of small-area epidemiology has all of the usual problems of an uncontrolled or multivariable study, as well as several more. In addition, this aspect of hazardous waste has not been adequately funded. For example, approximately 4.2 billion dollars is spent each year on hazardous waste sites in the United States, yet less than 1% has been devoted to the study of health risks at these sites.

Reviewing existing health outcome data is often the first step taken at a site. Data may be drawn from morbidity and mortality databases, birth statistics, medical records, tumor and disease registries, and surveillance databases.

> An underground waste storage tank at a semiconductor plant in Santa Clara County, California leaked solvent into the groundwater. State health scientists found an increased prevalence of cardiac defects and spontaneous abortions among women who resided in the census tract that received contaminated water compared to the rest of the county. However, further studies showed no association.

Many disease- and symptom-prevalence studies have been conducted in response to community concerns about living next to hazardous waste sites. Many of these studies do not show statistically significant increases in adverse health effects. However, these studies are often plagued by inadequate study sample size, insufficient information about the level of exposure, and bias in self-reporting. Several investigations at specific sites have documented a variety of symptoms of ill health in exposed persons, including low birthweight, cardiac anomalies, headache, fatigue, and a constellation of neurobehavioral problems. It is more difficult to find an association with exposure and disease for those health outcomes that are delayed in appearance, especially cancer.

> Many health studies have been conducted on the community that lived near Love Canal, New York since 1978. Study approaches have included ecologic studies using birth, cancer, and death registry or certificate information, small research studies of chromosomal changes in exposed individuals, a large telephone survey of self-reported symptoms, and retrospective reproductive outcome studies. Generally speaking, the studies have had a mixture of conclusions and criticisms. The strongest link occurs with low birth weight and maternal residence in the potentially affected neighborhood.

Biomarkers of effect may be used to make comparisons of preclinical events rather than frank disease. This is an improvement over long-term, equivocal cancer cluster or other end point studies. Biological markers of effect are indicators of change or variation in cellular or biochemical components or processes, structures, or functions that are measurable in humans and, depending on the magnitude, are recognized as an established or potential health impairment or disease. One major limitation of the usefulness of biomarkers of effect to ascertain the health impact of hazardous waste sites exposures is that they are often not substance specific; therefore, the adverse effect might be caused by factors other than the exposure of concern.

A cross-sectional study was conducted of a Native American population in Idaho to investigate health concerns, particulary respiratory effects, that might be attributed to two nearby phosphate-processing plants. The prevalence of self-reported pneumonia and chronic bronchitis was statistically significant among the 229 cases as compared to the 286 controls. In order to follow-up the self-reported respiratory problems, pulmonary function tests were performed on 100 residents from each group. Results of pulmonary function tests showed decreased air flow in the cases, but these differences were not significant.

Lack of good exposure information is common to most health studies of hazardous waste sites. This flaw reflects historical tendencies to collect data to conform to remediation efforts rather than health impact concerns. Site investigations historically have determined the extent of soil and groundwater contamination on the hazardous waste site only. Community exposure information may then be modelled or surrogates for exposure may be used. In ecologic studies, exposure may equate to residency within a census tract or zip code. In symptom-prevalence studies, distance from the site or self-reported odor detection may be used. Exposure from groundwater contamination has probably been the most quantifiable, though this information is also based on several assumptions.

In 1979, a large open dump in Woburn, Massachusetts, was discovered to have contaminated two municipal wells with chlorinated organic compounds. Using water distribution system information, contaminant levels in individual residences were estimated by modeling the percentage of water that came from the contaminated wells. The health outcomes were identified by a telephone survey conducted of 4936 pregnancies and 5018 residents of Woburn aged 18 or younger. The investigators reported that increased use of water from contaminated municipal wells was associated with newborn deaths, eye and ear birth defects, other environmentally-linked birth defects, and childhood leukemia, lung/respiratory disorders, and kidney and urinary-tract disorders.

Most hazardous waste sites studies are restricted by the small size of the exposed community, which does not allow for an adequate study size. Use of meta-analyses to pool similar studies and the creation of exposure registries are two approaches that may help to deal with this problem.

Meta-analysis is a quantitative review and pooling of similar studies. The combination of studies of small populations into meta-analyses might generate sufficient power to reach conclusions, provided that the basic measures involved are comparable and that sound methods are used in all separate studies. The interpretation of meta-analyses is tempered by the awareness that reporting and publication biases can distort the sample of studies available for pooling. Meta-analyses have not yet been used for hazardous waste epidemiology as they have for clinical trials, but they may be useful in the future if there is consistency in environmental studies.

The federal Agency for Toxic Substances and Disease Registry (ATSDR) was established, in part, to create registries of populations exposed to hazardous wastes and follow these populations over time to observe associated health effects. ATSDR has developed several specialized registries to study the long-term health effects of exposure to specific chemicals at hazardous waste sites, with the intention of combining data from several sites where similar exposures have occurred to achieve populations large enough that the associated health effects can be detected. Four hazardous substances have been selected for the chemical-specific registries: trichloroethylene (TCE), 2,3,7,8-tetrachlorodibenzo-p-dioxin (dioxin), benzene, and trichloroethane.

After reviewing over 280 sites where TCE was a contaminant in drinking water, 14 sites with over 5,000 exposed people were chosen for inclusion in the registry. Exposure to the TCE-contaminated water occurred at these sites from 1970 to 1990 with an exposure period varying from 7 to 18 years. Maximum concentrations of TCE at the sites ranged from 3 to 19,380 ppb. An initial interview with the participants took place in 1989 and consisted of a self-reported health questionnaire. Compared to national survey data (The National Health Interview Survey and The National Household Survey on Drug Abuse), the TCE registry participants reported more adverse health outcomes. The adverse health outcomes reported in excess of those reported by the national sample, for all or specific age groups, included speech impairment, hearing impairment, hypertension, stroke, liver disease, anemia and other blood disorders, diabetes, kidney disease, urinary tract disorders, heart disease, and skin rashes. There also appeared to be an excess number of deaths after 1985 among TCE participants, but additional information is needed before firm conclusions can be reached. Conclusions are limited by comparability of the questions from the initial interview and the national surveys, recall bias, non-confirmed reporting of medical diagnoses, and inconclusive dose-response calculations. Longitudinal following of the TCE registry participants will continue on a routine basis.

An emerging condition reported from communities living next to hazardous waste sites is "sensitivity to chemicals." This condition, frequently called multiple chemical sensitivity (MCS), is characterized by a wide variety of symptoms to extremely low levels of chemically unrelated, everyday substances. The most common symptoms appear to be fatigue, mood changes, memory and concentration difficulties, followed by various muscular, airway, headache-related and eye irritation complaints. Over 120 substances ranging from barbecue smoke and public restroom deodorizers to detergents, newspaper print, and marking pens have been said to trigger these symptoms. There are no generally recognized physical signs or laboratory tests to describe this condition, thus MCS as a medical diagnosis is very controversial. MCS is, in essence, in the research phase with many models and mechanistic hypotheses being put forward to explain it.

Psychological health effects are some of the most important effects observed in those living next to a hazardous waste site or a large facility that handles hazardous waste. While there has been some effort to scientifically study the physical health effects from living next to hazardous waste facilities, the psychological effects are unquantified and unsubstantiated except for anecdotal description. Research on the psychological impact of man-made disasters such as the effects of the Exxon Valdez disaster have shown that members of the high-exposure group were 3.6 times more likely to have generalized anxiety disorder and 2.9 times more likely to have post-traumatic stress disorder (PTSD). This acute environmental incident resembles a natural disaster more than the long-term stress impact from living next to a permanent potential or real health problem of an abandoned hazardous waste site.

Communities that experience chronic stress from living near a hazardous waste site suffer even more uncertainty than those involved in an acute disaster due to the fact that there are so many more unknowns about how health will be impacted in the future. There is also the feeling of a complete loss of control over the environment and their homes that were once a haven and are subsequently felt to be unsafe. In addition, unlike with a natural disaster, these communities are seen as hypersensitive because the outside world cannot see the devastation that natural or man-made acute disasters incur. Documentation of the chronic psychosocial effects of living near a hazardous waste site is not yet available. Therefore, these communities are overlooked. Rather than joining as a community to react to an acute disaster, these communities tend to fragment and those individuals who are not directly affected view those who are suffering symptoms as overreacting. Built-in community support systems often break down in these situations.

Federal and most state laws do not provide a mechanism for compensating individuals who have developed illnesses from environmental exposures to hazardous waste sites. Instead, individuals must bring personal injury actions against firms shown to have caused disposal of the waste and must prove that a particular waste caused the illness. Despite the fact that these suits are difficult to win, thousands of plaintiffs are pressing such claims in the United States and in many other countries.

## Medical Waste

The primary health risks associated with medical wastes are due to occupational exposure for those who handle it and not for the general population. Treated medical wastes disposed of in a landfill pose some of the same potential impacts as solid waste if the landfill is not properly maintained. Untreated medical waste that is disposed of in a landfill poses little risk because the likelihood of pathogens surviving and migrating from a landfill is considered highly improbable. Air contamination could arise if the incinerators burning medical waste are not operated properly, and surface water may be affected from sewer discharge that is untreated.

The spread of hepatitis B virus (HBV) and the human immunodeficiency virus (HIV) through medical waste has become a public fear. Due to the extremely limited viability of HIV outside a living host, the potential for developing HIV infection from medical waste is remote. HBV has a more lengthy viability in the environment, and therefore presents a slightly higher risk of infection from medical waste. Sharp objects pose the greatest concern, due to their ability to puncture the skin and provide a portal of entry for disease transmission.

## Radioactive Waste

For communities living next to nuclear waste facilities involved in nuclear power, disposal, or weapons production, the primary routes of exposure come as a result of using contaminated water for drinking, showering, or recreation; eating fish harvested as food habituating in the contaminated water; or consuming edible plants that were irrigated with the contaminated water and absorbed some of the radioactive substances. Additionally, there are low releases of radioactivity in the air emissions from most nuclear waste-generating facilities.

The main health effect associated with radiation exposure is cancer. In general, tissues with a high rate of turnover are more susceptible to the effects of ionizing radiation. Thus the thyroid, lung, breast, stomach, colon, and bone marrow have high sensitivity.

Another group of fast-growing cells susceptible to ionizing radiation is the germ cells. There is some evidence showing that parental exposure to ionizing radiation may result in increased cancer for offspring. In utero exposure to ionizing radiation has also been associated with spontaneous abortion, growth retardation, and congenital defects.

Further information on the health impact of radiation may be found in another chapter of this book.

## HAZARDOUS WASTE REGULATION

The recognition of environmental problems in the United States has historically been a reactionary process.

Reaction to the hospitalization of several people in 1972 in Minnesota resulting from drinking well water that had been contaminated with arsenic wastes resulted in the first legislation to address hazardous waste: the Resource Conservation and Recovery Act (RCRA, 1976). RCRA requires that hazardous waste is identified and tracked as it is generated, ensures that it is properly contained and transported, and regulates the storage, disposal, and/or treatment of hazardous waste. This has been termed "cradle to grave" hazardous waste tracking.

In 1993, 2,584 treatment, storage, or disposal facilities subject to RCRA permitting standards managed 235 million tons of hazardous waste. Ninety-four percent of the national total was wastewater management (ie, management in aqueous treatment units, neutralization tanks, underground injection wells, or other wastewater management systems). Land disposal accounted for 11.6% of the management total. Nationwide, 234 million tons of hazardous wastes were disposed in underground injection wells, 2 million tons were disposed in landfills, 276 thousand tons were managed in surface impoundments, and 159 thousand tons were managed by land treatment (land farming). Recovery (recycling) operations, including waste oil, solvent, and metals recovery, accounted for 3.5% of the national management total, and thermal treatment accounted for 1.6% of the national management total.

As a result of the discovery of the Love Canal dumpsite in 1975, the public became concerned about the past mismanagement of hazardous waste. Public pressure came to bear on the federal government to take regulatory action to protect public health. Health authorities and public health professionals were pressured to identify the actual and potential health problems that were associated with abandoned hazardous waste sites. A law referred to as CERCLA, or Superfund, was created in 1980 to address inactive or abandoned waste sites. The Superfund derives its name from a large federal trust fund capitalized with a special tax on chemical and petroleum feedstocks, federal appropriations, penalties collected from firms found responsible for contamination, and interest earned on the fund balance.

While RCRA is a regulatory program that addresses current hazardous waste storage, treatment, and disposal, CERCLA deals with abandoned, hazardous waste sites. The bulk of the CERCLA program requires private parties to remediate existing waste sites. CERCLA also causes hazardous waste producers to exercise great care in disposing of hazardous wastes to avoid the creation of a future Superfund site.

Many states have developed their own superfund programs frequently by creating new environmental protection agencies. State hazardous waste site programs were largely modeled after the Superfund program.

### Medical Waste

In the late summer of 1987, a 30–40 mile stretch of beaches on Long Island and New Jersey was affected by trash washing ashore. The appearance of syringes and other medical wastes on the shore caused great alarm and resulted in the closure of some beaches. Even though the EPA, the National Institutes of Health (NIH), and the Centers for Disease Control and Prevention (CDC) argued that medical waste constituted no more of a health hazard than any other form of municipally generated solid waste, the Medical Waste Tracking Act of 1988 was passed by Congress in less than two months. The legislation consisted of a demonstration tracking system for medical waste, of limited duration and with voluntary state participation. The Act was aimed at large generators of medical waste and as a result did not affect the homecare services or illegal drug activities that had been responsible for the "needles on the beach." Medical waste disposal has since been delegated to state authority.

### Radioactive Waste

Following the Three Mile Island accident in 1979, the public became very concerned about radioactivity. Nuclear waste disposal became a liability for the few states that had been accepting waste from other states. In late 1979, two of the three low-level waste facilities in the United States announced their intention to close their doors to nuclear waste from other states. In response to the impending nuclear waste backlog, the Low-Level Radioactive Waste Act, a federal mandate that defined the states' responsibility for the low-level wastes produced within their borders, was passed by Congress in 1980. Since there was little progress toward the states acting independently, the Low-Level Radioactive Waste Amendment Act of 1985 placed the states in regional compacts for the purpose of sharing the burden of disposal and set milestones for the construction of regional repositories. There are 10 compacts currently active, with the final compact waiting to be approved by Congress. Within each state, there must be at least one site developed for disposal of low-level waste.

At this time, there are only three active licensed low-level disposal sites: Barnwell, South Carolina, Hanford, Washington, and Clive, Utah, serving three compacts. Ward Valley in California was licensed in 1993, conditioned upon future ownership but the opening of this site is still not settled. Three compact sites' licenses are currently being reviewed.

The Nuclear Waste Policy Act of 1982 specifies a detailed approach for high-level radioactive waste disposal, with the Department of Energy having operational responsibility and the Nuclear Regulatory Commission having regulatory responsibility for the transportation, storage, and geologic disposal of the waste. This legislation requires that the health and environmental impact of a high-level disposal site be acceptable for thousands of years. The waste site must be in a solid form in a licensed deep, stable geologic structure. The Nuclear Waste Policy Amendments Act of 1987 designated a candidate site for a high-level waste repository at Yucca Mountain, Nevada. The DOE is determining the site suitability.

## HAZARDOUS WASTE PUBLIC HEALTH

Toxicologic animal studies that examine the mechanism, pharmacokinetics, and cell and organ impact of hazardous waste have typically been carried out within academic research institutions usually funded by the National Institute of Environmental Health Sciences (NIEHS) or the EPA. On the other hand, human-based studies of hazardous waste are carried out in the public health arena, historically by state health departments. The roles of the various public health levels of government in responding to the concern over the impact of hazardous waste on the health of the citizenry will be described in this section. Hazardous waste epidemiologic research is also now being conducted by environmental and occupational health clinics within academic institutions.

Local health departments are on the frontline, along with physicians, in responding to environmental and public health concerns raised by citizens. The environmental and public health response at the local level is multifaceted, with hazardous waste issues being one aspect. Addressing the underground storage issues, tracking medical waste, and permitting and inspecting RCRA facilities are some of the responsibilities that are generally mandated for the local health departments to regulate. Additionally, these same organizations often must not only be regulators but public health officials, as well. For questions and problems beyond its expertise or funding abilities, the local health department staff then refer issues to the state health department.

Many state health departments have specialized staff to deal with hazardous waste issues such as environmental toxicologists, epidemiologists, health educators, community coordinators, and physicians. State health departments play a supportive role for local health departments in addition to investigating alleged cancer and other disease clusters around hazardous waste sites.

Beginning in 1987, the Agency for Toxic Substances and Disease Registry has supported staff within the states to provide public health oversight at the hazardous waste sites, primarily the Superfund sites, in those states. This funding has greatly enhanced state efforts to address the health issues that confront them at Superfund sites.

At the federal government level, there are several groups that are concerned with the health effects of hazardous waste. These include the National Institute of Environmental Health Science (NIEHS), the Center for Environmental Health (CEH), and the Agency for Toxic Substances and Disease Registry (ATSDR). The Superfund legislation (CERCLA) created ATSDR to address the health issues of hazardous waste to complement the regulatory mandate given to the EPA for overseeing clean-up. This pairing of a nonregulatory, scientific fact-finding agency with a regulatory agency had previously been done with the pairing of NIOSH and OSHA.

ATSDR's multi-pronged approach to dealing with hazardous waste sites includes reviewing and assessing the real health impact of each site, conducting or sponsoring epidemiologic and health studies of exposed communities, educating the community and the health care providers about hazardous waste exposure and potential health impact, and reviewing the literature and identifying gaps in the toxicologic information about hazardous waste chemicals (Table 40–19).

## DATA SOURCES

Information sources concerned with hazardous waste usually fall into two categories: those that deal with facilities or sites and those that deal with chemicals considered hazardous (Table 40–20). In order to evaluate whether a site may be causing health effects in an individual living near a facility, it is necessary to first establish what chemicals may be stored, treated, or disposed of on the site and whether there is the possibility that these chemicals have migrated off-site. Site exposure information may be obtained from databases generated from government reporting systems that are available to the public. These databases include the Hazardous Substance Release Effects Database, the Toxic Release Inventory, the Biennial Reporting System, the CERCLIS list, and the Nuclear Reactor List. Once exposure to chemicals of concern has been established, it may be necessary to research the toxicologic information about those chemicals. While basic toxicologic information may

**Table 40–19.** Public health activities carried out by the Agency for Toxic Substances and Disease Registry (ATSDR).

| ATSDR Activity | Description of Activity | ATSDR's Accomplishments |
|---|---|---|
| Prepares toxicologic profiles | In the profiles, ATSDR summarizes the literature and interprets available toxicologic information and epidemiologic evaluations to determine levels of significant human exposure. | ATSDR created a priority list of 275 substances found at NPL sites and believed to be most hazardous. Profiles are available to the public and some of the information is available on the Internet. |
| Identifies and fills toxicity information gaps for the priority substances | In the profiles, ATSDR assesses the information that is available to determine levels of exposure to the chemicals that pose a significant health risk to human health. | ATSDR is working with NIEHS and EPA to ensure that the substance-specific research needed to fill some of the data gaps is undertaken by other parts of the federal government, by the private sector, or by directly supporting research. |
| Prepares health assessments for site on the National Priority List, at RCRA sites upon EPA's request, and for other sites upon request by the public or the states | In the health assessment, there is a review of the nature and extent of contamination, pathways of exposure, the size and susceptibility of communities within the likely pathways, and a comparison of expected human exposure levels to short- and long-term exposure health standards associated with the chemicals. The health assessment is intended to provide the public with qualitative information on the public health implications of a site and to identify the need for further action to protect the community or to research the health effects associated with current or past releases from the site. | ATSDR and the 22 state health departments that are funded by ATSDR to carry out their mission have written 1,719 health assessments: 3% pose an urgent public health hazard and 40% pose a non-urgent health hazard. The health assessments are available to the public and some of the information is available on the Internet. |
| Conducts health studies, when appropriate | Health studies have included self-reported illnesses and symptoms, organ system evaluation through biomedical testing, and, whenever possible, determining a biologic dose.<br><br>ATSDR has completed reports on immune function, lung and respiratory, and neurologic biomedical test batteries for environmental field studies.<br><br>ATSDR established four chemical subregistries to study the long-term health consequences of trichloroethylene, dioxin, benzene, and chromium. | ATSDR or the state health departments or academic institutions that ATSDR has supported have conducted pilot health studies, full-scale epidemiologic studies, registries of exposed persons, and/or other health surveillance programs. |
| Provides health consultations | ATSDR provides consultations on health issues related to exposure to hazardous or toxic substances. Consultations are often needed during emergency releases or threatened releases of hazardous substance. | ATSDR has a response team to respond to hazardous waste emergencies anywhere in the United States. During 1994, ATSDR emergency response personnel came on-site at seven emergencies. They also responded to requests for information related to 51 other acute events. |

be found using Medline or by reading medical journals, there are several information sources that have compiled toxicologic and other chemical-specific information into a readily accessible and well-organized format. These toxicologic databases include the Hazardous Substance Release Effects Database and the Hazardous Substances Database (Table 40–20).

## HAZARDOUS WASTE MANAGEMENT PRACTICES

Hazardous waste management is an attempt to achieve a balance between minimizing the environmental and health impact and costs of an industrial society and the economic and social costs involved in achieving these objectives. Management of hazardous waste involves recycling, treating the waste to reduce its volume or hazardous level, or disposal. All of these activities are regulated, but there may still be some potential health risk posed. In addition, there is still the continued disposal mismanagement or accidental release by a few hazardous waste users.

Hazardous waste laws are based on the legal concept that generators of hazardous waste are liable for the long-term impact of their waste management practices, including their past practices. As a result, there has been an impetus for change in the waste management arena. One estimate puts the cost of cleaning up a hazardous waste site at 10–100 times

**Table 40–20.** Hazardous waste databases.

| Database Name/Location | General Description of Database | Specific Fields in Database |
|---|---|---|
| Hazardous Substance Release Effects Database (HazDat)<br><br>http://atsdr1.atsdr.cdc.gov | A scientific and administrative database developed by ATSDR that provides information on the release of hazardous substances from Superfund sites or from emergency events<br><br>and | Site characteristics, activities and site events, contaminants found, contaminant media and maximum concentration levels, impact on population, community health concerns, ATSDR public health threat categorization, ATSDR recommendations, environmental fate of hazardous substances, exposure routes, physical hazards |
| | Substance-specific information for ATSDR's Priority List of Hazardous Substances (currently 150 hazardous substances) | Health effects by route and duration of exposure, metabolites, interactions of substances, susceptible populations, and biomarkers of exposure and effects |
| Toxic Release Inventory (TRI)<br><br>http://www.epa.gov | Self-reported annual releases both accidental and permitted from industrial facilities to the air, water, land, or underground injection of over 300 chemicals and chemical categories. TRI is built and maintained by EPA and is authorized under the Emergency Planning and Community Right-to-Know Act of 1986 | Facility name and address; latitude-longitude; parent company; description of chemical manufacturing, processing, or usage that occur at the facility; the quantity and type of chemical releases to the air, land, underground injection, surface water discharge, a publicly-owned treatment facility (sewer system), or transfer off-site for disposal or treatment; description of on-site treatment method including air emission treatment and biological, chemical, physical, or thermal treatments |
| Hazardous Substances Database (HSDB)<br><br>Toxnet/National Library of Medicine | Toxicity information for over 4,300 chemicals. Database also contains other chemical-specific information. File is fully referenced and peer-reviewed. File is built and maintained by the National Library of Medicine and co-supported by ATSDR | Contains 150 data fields arranged in broad categories: substance identification; manufacturing/use information; chemical and physical properties; safety and handling; toxicity/biomedical effects; pharmacology; environmental fate/exposure potential/exposure standards and regulations; monitoring and analysis methods |
| Biennial Reporting System (BRS)<br><br>http://www.epa.gov | EPA's database of information on large quantity generators (24,362 in 1993) that are permitted to store, treat, or dispose of hazardous waste | Facility name, waste type produced, tonnage of RCRA managed waste, exempt managed waste, and state managed waste |
| Comprehensive Environmental Response, Compensation, and Liability Inventory System (CERCLIS)<br>http://www.epa.gov | EPA's database of hazardous waste sites that are recommended for further study and for eventual inclusion on the NPL. Currently there are 11,000 sites on CERCLIS. | Site summary and location; EPA enforcement activities, events, and financial expenditures |
| Nuclear Reactor List<br><br>http://www.nrc.gov | The Nuclear Regulatory Commission's database containing information on the 111 nuclear energy reactors and the 45 nonpower reactors located in the United States. | Facility statistics, emergency response information, plant description summary, simplified plant system diagrams, detailed plant system data |

greater than the cost of originally treating the wastes in the most efficient fashion. Now, most generators endeavor to minimize waste, and many manufacturers even factor waste management into the life cycle of their products (from research through manufacturing to use by the consumer and eventually ultimate disposition).

Reduction, reusing, and recycling of industrial waste are being actively pursued by many companies. This holistic approach to hazardous waste management is termed "industrial ecology". Waste reduction requires changes such as product formulation, process modification, equipment redesign, recovery of waste materials for reuse, and waste separation for exchange or resale. Waste reduction may involve material substitution, process modification, equipment modification, or retraining personnel to get rid of wasteful habits and other housekeeping practices. Recycling consists of recovering and treating waste, and reuse means the recovery, without additional treatment, of hazardous waste that can then be used by the industry generating the waste or by another industry. Recycling of waste water, solvents, and used oil are commonplace now. As the costs of raw materials, waste treatment, and disposal rise, so has the popularity of industrial ecology. Waste exchanges, regional clearinghouses that facilitate the effective utilization of waste between various industries, began appearing in the late 1980s.

## Treatment of Hazardous Waste

Treatment of hazardous waste that cannot be reused or recycled and remediation of contaminated hazardous waste sites involves a variety of methods: physical, chemical, biological, and thermal treatment. Physical treatment does not reduce the toxicity of the waste but does transfer the waste into another media or prevents the waste from migrating. Air stripping is one of the most common physical processes used for remediating groundwater contaminated with volatile organic compounds. Air stripping is a mass transfer process that enhances the volatilization of compounds from water by passing air through water to improve the transfer between the air and water phases. The vapor may be released without treatment or may be passed through activated carbon before release. Similarly, contaminated soils may be cleaned using soil vapor extraction. Soil vapor extraction consists of passing an air stream through soil contaminated with volatile organic compounds, thereby transferring the contaminants from the soil matrix to the air stream.

Chemical treatment is used to alter the chemical structure of the waste constituents, thereby reducing the material's toxicity. The simplest example of this is the neutralization of an acidic or alkaline waste stream. Chemical oxidation using ozone, hydrogen peroxide, and chlorine is capable of destroying a wide range of organic molecules, including volatile organic compounds, mercaptans, phenols, and inorganics such as cyanide. Other chemical treatment methods include precipitation, ion exchange, and chemical dechlorination.

Stabilization, solidification, and fixation are physiochemical methods used to stabilize waste prior to disposal so that it is easier to handle and also as a remedy at abandoned, hazardous waste sites that primarily keeps the material from migrating and decreases the permeability, thereby reducing leaching.

Biological treatment is the degradation of organic waste by the action of microorganisms with the aim of changing the molecular structure to create less toxic metabolites or completely breaking down the molecule to carbon dioxide, water, and inert inorganic residuals. Biological treatment of almost any organic material can be accomplished since virtually all organic compounds can be degraded if the proper microbial communities are established, maintained, and controlled. Biological treatment has been used for many years with municipal and industrial wastestreams. *In situ* bioremediation means that biological treatment is used to clean-up contaminated groundwater and subsurface contaminants where

they are found without excavating the overlying soil. This technique is receiving a lot of attention but is still in the developmental stages.

Thermal methods such as incineration and thermal desorption involves the use of heat to clean up contaminated soil. Incineration uses very high temperatures (1400–1800 °F) to alter the molecular structure to ideally reduce the toxicity. The soil typically becomes an ash. Incineration changes hydrocarbon molecules into carbon dioxide and water vapor. The combustion of wastes containing sulfur produces sulfur dioxide and sulfur trioxide. Halogen-containing wastes produce the corresponding acid halogen gas (eg, hydrogen chloride, hydrogen bromide, etc). Metals cannot be destroyed and are oxidized. The volatility of oxidized arsenic, antimony, cadmium, and mercury can create problems in the flue gas. Due to the tight regulations on incineration air emissions and concern from communities, incinerators are rarely chosen as a remedy selection at hazardous waste sites.

Thermal desorption uses temperatures between 200–1000 °F to drive low volatile compounds from contaminated soil. The compounds are then trapped, cooled, and recovered for proper disposal. Unlike incineration, the soil remains intact with thermal desorption.

## Disposal of Hazardous Waste

Disposal means long-term storage in landfills, underground injection wells, or ocean dumping. Surface impoundments such as pits, ponds, and lagoons are not land disposal facilities but storage facilities.

In the past, it was cheap and simple to dig a hole in the ground, fill it with untreated waste and cover the waste with clay to keep the rain out. However, chemicals in the waste leached from the fill, resulting in the contamination of groundwater and drinking water throughout the United States. Landfills are still the most popular method for disposal, but there are now strict guidelines for their construction. Federal regulation requires landfills to be double-lined, a leachate collection system to collect the inevitable migration of liquid through the liner, and a groundwater monitoring system to check for failure of the leachate collection system. Additionally, waste may be disposed of in a landfill if it meets certain criteria related to corrosivity, reactivity, flammability, and toxicity. Thus, waste may often be treated prior to its deposit in a landfill. The treatment method may also generate a byproduct that must be disposed as hazardous waste (ie, incineration dust). As a result, even though landfilling of hazardous waste is discouraged, there will always be the need for some landfills.

Injection of waste into deep, underground wells is also used for disposal of hazardous waste. Injection usually occurs below the deepest drinking water aquifer, 1,000 to 10,000 feet down. Modern deep wells use such safety features as double or triple casings and leak detection systems. However, even if a leak is detected, remedying the problem may be impossible. Injection of waste into deep, underground injection wells is being discouraged at this time.

Ocean dumping has been a method of choice for disposal of dredge spoils, industrial waste, sludge from wastewater treatment plants, and radioactive waste, but is currently being discouraged because of concern for ecologic damage and contamination of marine food chains.

## Medical Waste

Previously, every hospital had an incinerator in which it burned the infectious and noninfectious waste that was generated within the hospital. However, these incinerators had only rudimentary air-pollution control devices, and heavy metals, acid gases, and dioxins release may have resulted. With the advent of stricter air pollution laws, many hospital incinerators were shut down. For instance, in California in 1985, there were 146 medical waste incinerators, and in 1995 there were only four.

To replace on-site incineration, many medical waste generators are utilizing steam sterilization. Steam sterilization renders medical waste noninfectious by exposing wastes to saturated steam at no less than 121 °C for a minimum of 30 minutes. Another method that is quite popular for dealing with needles and other medical waste capable of puncturing is the solidification of sharp medical objects within a disinfecting polymer. Either the steam sterilized or the polymerized material is then disposed of as a solid waste.

## Radioactive Waste

Radioactive wastes do not respond sufficiently to stabilization by chemical, physical, or biological processes. Only time can render radioactive wastes inactive. At present, storage appears to be the only means of successfully solving the disposal problem.

Spent fuel from nuclear reactors can be reprocessed. This involves extracting the uranium and the plutonium, but this method results in concentrated fission process product wastes that also require disposal. In addition, because of the concern that plutonium, a by-product of reprocessing, could be diverted to produce nuclear weapons, reprocessing of nuclear fuel elements has been discontinued in the United States.

Radioactive wastes require confinement for shorter or longer periods of time, depending on the characteristics of the radionuclides contained within them. The radioactivity of low-level waste will decline to safe levels in approximately 200–300 years, while intermediate-level waste will need safe containment for thousands of years. High-level waste, with half-lives of millions of years, requires special treatment.

Storage for radioactive wastes can broadly be categorized into two groups: near-surface disposal facilities and deep disposal facilities. Low-level waste disposal typically involves near-surface disposal facilities. Near-surface disposal facilities are required to be topped with an impermeable cover that will not allow air emissions and will keep rainwater from filtering through the waste. Still, the most likely mechanism for the release of radionuclides to the environment is transport in groundwater.

There are not yet any high-level or spent fuel facilities in the licensing process or in operation (worldwide). The relatively small quantities produced so far are temporarily being stored where they have been generated.

## INTERNATIONAL PERSPECTIVES

Other countries are also dealing with hazardous waste issues. The kind and size of each country's response to these concerns varies according to the social, political, and economic policies of the nation's government and people. Examining each country's approach to hazardous waste is beyond the scope of this chapter; however, the responses may be crudely reviewed according to developed, democratized countries, developing central and eastern European countries, and other developing countries.

The status quo of hazardous waste regulation and public health protection for these country groupings are likely to change tremendously in the coming years with globalization of the commercial enterprise and trade liberalization. It is unclear how the recently-signed North American Free Trade Agreement (NAFTA) or the latest round of the General Agreement on Tariffs and Trades (GATT) will impact hazardous waste and other environmental issues in the world.

Some people are concerned that trade liberalization under GATT may encourage countries to set low levels of environmental protection, standards, and enforcement to reduce production costs and encourage foreign investment. In essence, lax regulations could be viewed as a production subsidy. Others see health and environmental protection as nontariff barriers.

Unlike any previous trade agreement, the North American Free Trade Agreement (NAFTA) does allude to environmental standards in its text and a side agreement focuses on environmental issues. NAFTA, which was passed in 1993, encourages free trade between the signers: Mexico, the United States, and Canada. Because of the pollution problem along the border between Mexico and the United States, there was tremendous pressure by nongovernmental and governmental organizations in the United States to address environmental issues that go along with industrial development in NAFTA. NAFTA provides that obligations of international environmental agreements on hazardous wastes and other concerns take precedence over NAFTA obligations, subject to certain conditions. Time will tell whether these nonenforceable aspects of NAFTA will have any impact.

Efforts to deal with transboundary hazardous waste and other pollution have been spearheaded by the efforts of the United Nations, the World Health Organization, the International Labor Organization, the European Economic Community, and the Organization for Economic Cooperation and Development.

## Developed, Democratized Nations

Most industrialized nations have established a national regulatory program that is aimed at protecting human health and the environment from the mismanagement of hazardous waste. The major elements in a national control system for hazardous waste management are:

- developing an administrative definition for identifying and classifying hazardous waste to the particular level of detail necessary to support its legal procedures
- defining the responsibilities placed on the waste generator
- registering or licensing those involved in collection, transport, intermediate storage, treatment, and disposal of hazardous wastes
- controlling transport, including importing and exporting, using a "cradle to grave" theory involving a manifest system
- permitting of treatment or disposal facilities
- developing a national strategy or plan for establishing facilities
- addressing old or abandoned sites

In most developed countries, the responsibility for managing the national control system is shared among the national, regional, and local governments. While the details differ from country to country, the national government is generally responsible for establishing national standards, guidelines, or codes of practice. Regional and local governments are often responsible for enforcement and licensing activities.

Although most industrialized/developed nations have created hazardous waste management systems that include the elements mentioned above, there are differences in how these elements are implemented. Without examining each country's system in detail, the essence of the various differences can be represented by listing examples.

- From 1979 to 1984, European countries incinerated some 100,000 tons of waste at sea.
- Shallow sea dumping is utilized in a number of countries; the United Kingdom dumped 260,000 tons at sea in 1985.
- Every national system differs in the detailed

method for defining hazardous waste and in the breadth of waste included. For instance, "specifically controlled waste" is the term used for hazardous waste in Japan. Japan classifies fewer items as hazardous waste than any other developed country.
- Sewage sludge is specifically excluded in some countries' hazardous waste definition, but not in others.
- Effluents are excluded from waste statistics in many countries, but partially included in the United States. As a result, the United States appears to produce a much greater amount of waste than any other industrialized/developed country.
- It is extremely difficult to compare quantities of industrial or hazardous waste in different countries not only because of the various definitions but also because of inconsistent collection of statistics.
- Unlike many developed countries, the United States has not developed a national strategy for dealing with nonradioactive hazardous waste.
- In most developed countries, collection and transport of hazardous waste is carried out by private industry. In Sweden, collection and transportation of hazardous waste are handled through local utility companies run by the municipality.
- Hazardous waste in most developed countries is generally transported by road. The main exception is Denmark, where waste is transported primarily by rail.
- In most developed countries, hazardous waste may move freely across internal boundaries within the country. In Germany, a special permit is required before a shipment of hazardous waste is allowed to cross state boundaries.
- The United Kingdom is well-known for its advocacy of co-disposal of hazardous waste in municipal waste landfill sites.
- The Netherlands has an almost total absence of suitable sites for landfilling; thus, landfilling of hazardous waste is prohibited unless specific exemption is granted.
- In most developed countries, the primary means of encouraging waste avoidance or recycling is imposition of strict controls on hazardous waste disposal, accompanied by the charging of a stiff fee.
- Most countries have developed a national inventory and clean-up program of old or abandoned hazardous waste sites. One of the exceptions is Japan, where there is no general law governing the identification, assessment, and cleanup of contaminated soil, although many cases of such pollution have been identified.

## Developing Countries

It has been estimated that developing countries generate 20 million tons per year of hazardous waste.

Of this amount, roughly 15 million tons are produced by the Central and Eastern European countries. Three primary sources of hazardous waste in developing countries are: wastes generated by foreign-owned, state-owned, or joint-venture firms; wastes generated by small entrepreneurs, farmers, and householders; and wastes imported from other, usually more developed, countries. On the whole, major corporations have assumed responsibility for their own wastes. However, in cases where the industries are small or locally-owned, adequate responsibility for treatment and disposal has not been assumed. Developing countries do not have resources to deal effectively with any of these sources.

Training, technical expertise, facility development, legislation, and the necessary governmental institutions, all in varying degrees, are inadequate in developing countries. Multinational companies may be expected to help, but they have a vested interest that would be expected to interfere with their dealing effectively with the full problem. Much assistance will need to be provided by developed countries.

To begin to fill the organizational void in these countries, information exchanges have been created by developed nations and international organizations. For instance, the United Nations Environmental Programme has developed an International Register of Potentially Toxic Chemicals to identify all chemicals that have been banned or severely restricted by five or more countries and is currently preparing guidelines to assist countries in developing environmental protection legislation.

Democratization and the end of one-party rule in most of Eastern Europe are considered to have an important impact on hazardous waste issues in these developing countries. Most of the former socialized countries have well-developed occupational health services and rather poorly developed environmental health services and hazardous waste management programs. The ideology of the previous Communist governments may explain this pattern: worker well-being was valued more than environmental quality and most of the industry was owned and operated by the national governments. Toxicology, clinical occupational medicine, and some aspects of industrial hygiene have been relatively strong in many Eastern European countries, while epidemiology, environmental engineering, risk assessment, and risk communication have not.

Unlike the industrialized, developing countries of Eastern Europe, hazardous waste concerns are a relatively new phenomenon in the developing countries of Africa, Asia, and Central and South America. However, this is changing, primarily due to exportation of hazardous waste and the transfer of hazardous industries from developed countries to the developing world. Environmental exposure to hazardous chemicals is increasing in developing countries. The major cities of developing nations are now reeling with the impact of air pollution, the absence of sewage treatment and water purification, and the growing quantities of hazardous waste buried in or left on the soil or dumped into rivers or oceans. In many of the world's countries, there are no environmental regulations for hazardous waste, or, if they do exist, there is little or no enforcement. The daily struggles for survival are the primary focus. Political agreements between developing and industrialized countries are critical to ensure that environmental and human health protection take place in developing countries. Efforts at the international level have centered on controlling hazardous industries and hazardous wastes.

Thousands of tons of hazardous waste are shipped internationally each year. In 1990, more than 100 countries agreed to the Basel Treaty, the first step to regulate international transportation of hazardous waste. This treaty requires notification of intent of international hazardous waste transport and prior informed consent (PIC) by receiving parties; it also allows hazardous waste transport to continue. In response, a coalition of countries in Africa in 1991 adopted more stringent hazardous waste transportation laws in the Bamako Convention; the Lome IV convention also banned hazardous waste export among more than 80 countries in Africa, the Caribbean, Europe, and the Pacific. As of March 1994, industrialized countries agreed to an immediate ban on exporting hazardous wastes to developing countries for incineration or burial; export of hazardous wastes for "recycling" will be banned as of December 31, 1997.

Such international cooperation may be elusive. Various reports of countries redefining hazardous waste in order to avoid complying with the Basel Agreement are already surfacing. This is another reason that efforts such as those underway by the Organization for Economic Cooperation and Development (OECD) to harmonize "hazardous waste" definitions into an international standard are so critical.

The transfer of hazardous waste technologies to developing countries is a consequence of stringent industrial and environmental regulations and increasing labor costs in the industrialized world. Alternatively, developing countries are attractive because of cheap labor and lack of (or poor implementation of) labor, environmental, and industrial regulations. Efforts to affect ethical behavior in the exporting of hazardous technologies to developing countries have also been attempted by international organizations: the Organization for Economic Cooperation and Development (OCED) Guidelines for Multinational Enterprises, the United Nations Code of Conduct on Transnational Corporations, and the International Labor Organizations Tripartitie Declaration of Principles Concerning Multinational Enterprises and Social Policy.

## Radioactive Waste

According to the International Atomic Energy Agency, about 10,000 cubic meters of high-level radioactive waste accumulate each year in 11 countries with 65 nuclear reactors. This massive amount of radioactive material has no permanent home. Not a single country has implemented a long-term plan for its disposal; each relies on interim measures. Most countries are hoping to dispose of the high-level waste deep underground in geologically stable areas. Other considerations have been permanent subterranean storage, entombment under the sea, and nuclear transmutation.

Historically, the primary mechanism of disposing of low-level radioactive waste had been sea dumping, which depends on delayed dispersal and subsequent extreme dilution. However, the practice was discontinued in 1983, in part because of widespread public opposition and a nonbinding resolution passed by the signatories to the London Dumping Convention, which placed a *de facto* moratorium on sea dumping.

# REFERENCES

### ROUTINE INDUSTRIAL EMISSIONS

California Air Resources Board: California's Air Toxics Program. California Environmental Protection Agency, 1994.

Doa MJ: The Toxics Release Inventory. Hazard Waste Hazard Mater 1992;9:61.

Lynn FM, Kartez JD: Environmental democracy in action: The toxics release inventory. Environ Management 1994;18:511.

Neas LM et al: The association of ambient air pollution with twice daily peak expiratory flow rate measurements in children. Am J Epidemiol 1995;141:111.

Ostro B: The association of air pollution and mortality: Examining the case for inference. Archiv Environ Health 1995;48:336.

Ostro B et al: Air pollution and asthma exacerbations among African-American children in Los Angeles. Inhal Toxicol 1995;7:711.

State and Territorial Air Pollution Program Administrators and the Association of Local Air Pollution Control Officials: Summary of the Clean Air Act Amendments of 1990, 1990.

US Environmental Protection Agency: 1993 Toxics Release Inventory. Public Data Release. Office of Pollution Prevention and Toxics. EPA 745-R-95-010, 1995.

Ware JH et al: Respiratory and irritant health effects of ambient volatile organic compounds. The Kanawha County Health Study. Am J Epidemiol 1993;137:1287.

### ACCIDENTAL RELEASES

Agency for Toxic Substances and Disease Registry: Hazardous Substances Emergency Events Surveillance (HSEES):Annual Report. US Department of Health and Human Services, 1994.

Agency for Toxic Substances and Disease Registry: Managing hazardous materials incidents Volumes I–III. US Department of Health & Human Services, 1992.

Alexeeff G, Lewis D, Lipsett M: Use of toxicity information in risk assessment for accidental releases of toxic gases. J Hazard Mater 1992;29:387.

Baxter PJ: Major chemical disasters. Br Med J 1991; 302:61.

Casto K: International environmental auditing and site assessment. Occup Environ Health 1995;1:158.

Cox RD: Decontamination and management of hazardous materials exposure victims in the emergency department. Ann Emerg Med 1994;23:761.

DiBartolomeis MJ et al: Regulatory approach to assessing health risks of toxic chemical releases following transportation accidents. J Hazard Mater 1994;39: 193.

European Community: Council Directive 96/82/EC of 9 December 1996 on the Control of Major-Accident Hazards Involving Dangerous Substances. Off J Eur Commun, L, Legis 1997;40:13–33.

Glickman TS, Ujihara AM: Deciding between in-place protection and evacuation in toxic vapor cloud emergencies. J Hazard Mater 1990;23:57.

Golding D et al: *Managing Nuclear Accidents: A Model Emergency Response Plan*. Westview Press, 1992.

Guzelian PS, Henry CJ, Olin SS (editors): *Similarities And Differences Between Children And Adults: Implications For Risk Assessment*. International Life Sciences Institute, 1992.

Hall HI et al: Surveillance of hazardous substance releases and related health effects. Arch Environ Health 1994;49:45.

Jasanoff S (editor): *Learning From Disaster: Risk management after Bhopal*. University of Pennsylvania Press, 1994.

Leonard RB: Hazardous materials accidents: Initial scene assessment and patient care. Aviat Space Environ Med 1993;64:546.

Mahoney MA, Kubota C: Electronic resources for toxicology and environmental health. In: Fan AM, Chang LW (editors): *Toxicology and Risk Assessment*. Marcel Dekker, 1996.

Makris J: A digest report: Chemical emergency planning and the medical community. Health Environ Dig 1992; 5:1.

National Research Council: *Ensuring Railroad Tank Car Safety*. National Academy Press, 1994.

Nuclear Energy Agency: Severe Accident Management: Prevention And Mitigation. Report By An NEA Group Of Experts. Organisation for Economic Co-operation and Development, 1992.

Olson K, Mycroft F: Emergency medical response to hazardous materials incidents. In: Olson KR (editor): *Poisoning & Drug Overdose*. Appleton & Lange, 1994.

Organization for Economic Cooperation and Development: Guiding Principles for Chemical Accident Prevention, Preparedness and Response. United States Environmental Protection Agency Office of Solid Waste and Emergency Response, 1993.

Porter SW Jr: Planning for and management of radiation accidents. In: Miller KL (editor): *CRC Handbook of Management of Radiation Protection Programs*. CRC Press, 1992.

Quarantelli EL: Disaster planning for transportation accidents involving hazardous materials. J Hazard Mater 1991;27:49.

Steen JJ: Chemical Spills: Where does the hot zone end and the warm begin? Safety and Health 1994;150:84.

United Nations Environment Program: APELL, Awareness And Preparedness For Emergencies At Local Level: A Process For Responding To Technological Accidents. Industry & Environment Office. United Nations Environment Program, 1988.

United States Environmental Protection Agency: Emergency Response Notification System (ERNS) Database. United States Environmental Protection Agency Office of Solid Waste and Emergency Response, 1995.

United States Department of Energy: Federal Radiological Monitoring and Assessment Center (FRMAC), Overview of FRMAC Operations, DOE/NV-358. Nevada Field Office, 1992.

## HAZARDOUS WASTE

Baller J, Carlo GL, Sund KG: The Agency for Toxic Substances and Disease Registry: An emerging power in the hazardous waste arena. Environ Reporter 1991:1951.

Burg JR et al: The National Exposure Registry: Morbidity analyses of noncancer outcomes from the trichloroethylene subregistry baseline data. Int J Occ Med & Toxicol 1995;4:237.

Forester WS, Skinner JH (editors): *International Perspectives on Hazardous Waste Management*. Academic Press, 1987.

Frumkin H, Hernandez-Avila M, Torres FE: Maquiladoras: A Case Study of Free Trade Zones. Intl J Occ Environ Health 1995;1:96.

Gershey EL et al: *Low-Level Radioactive Waste: From Cradle to Grave*. Van Nostrand Reinhold, 1990.

Graedel TE, Allenby BR: *Industrial Ecology*. Prentice-Hall, 1995.

Hall EJ: *Radiation and Life,* 3rd ed. McGraw-Hill, 1992.

Hendee WR: Disposal of low-level radioactive waste: Problems and implications for physicians. JAMA 1993;269:2403.

Hird JA: Superfund: *The Political Economy of Environmental Risk*. The Johns Hopkins University Press, 1994.

Johnson BL: Nature, extent, and impact of Superfund hazardous waste sites. Chemosphere 1995;31:2415.

Johnson BL: ATSDR's information databases to support human health risk assessment of hazardous substances. Toxicol Lett 1995;79:11.

Kemp R: The Politics of Radioactive Waste Disposal. Manchester University Press, 1992.

LaGrega MD, Buckingham PL, Evans JC: *Hazardous Waste Management*. McGraw-Hill, 1994.

Louka E: *Overcoming National Barriers to International Trade: A New Perspective on the Transnational Movements of Hazardous and Radioactive Wastes*. Graham & Trotman/Martinus Nijhoff, 1994.

MacKnight KT: The problems of medical and infectious waste. Environ Law 1993;23:785.

National Research Council: Environmental Epidemiology Vol. 1 Public Health and Hazardous Waste. National Academy Press, 1991.

Shulman S: *The Threat at Home: Confronting the Toxic Legacy of the US Military*. Beacon Press, 1992.

US Department of Health and Human Services, Agency for Toxic Substances and Disease Registry: Fort Hall Air Emissions Study, Fort Hall Indian Reservation. National Technical Information Services, 1995.

US Department of Health and Human Services, Agency for Toxic Substances and Disease Registry: Priority Health Conditions: An Integrated Strategy to Evaluate the Relationship Between Illness and Exposure to Hazardous Substances. National Technical Information Service, 1993.

US Environmental Protection Agency: Handbook of Chemical Hazard Analysis Procedures. Federal Emergency Management Agency, 1989.

US Environmental Protection Agency, Solid Waste and Emergency Response: National Analysis: the National Biennial RCRA Hazardous Waste Report. National Technical Information Service, 1995.

Uzych L: Medical waste management: Regulatory issues and current legal requirements. J Environ Health 1990;52:233.

Wagner TP: *The Complete Guide to the Hazardous Waste Regulations*. Van Nostrand Reinhold, 1991.

Wolf, SM: *Pollution Law Handbook*. Greenwood Press, 1988.

# Outdoor Air Pollution

# 41

*Cornelius H. Scannell, MD, MPH, & John R. Balmes, MD*

The dramatic air pollution episodes that occurred in the early part of the twentieth century in the Meuse Valley of Belgium, Donora, Pennsylvania, and London, England are not likely to occur in the world today. These episodes were due to the large scale burning of coal in the presence of "ideal" meteorologic conditions—atmospheric inversion leading to a stagnant air mass. A clearly evident excess mortality was observed during and after these episodes. Current air quality standards in North America preclude the development of episodes of this magnitude today. However, certain environmental air pollutants, such as ozone and respirable particles, do reach levels that may cause acute and chronic respiratory effects. Furthermore, in some Eastern European countries where sulfur-containing fuels are burned without adequate air-quality regulations, air pollution levels may be attained similar to those that were associated with excess mortality.

## REGULATION OF OUTDOOR AIR POLLUTANTS

The Clean Air Act (CAA) was passed by the United States Congress in 1970 and last amended in 1990. It is the principal federal standard addressing outdoor air quality. It requires the Environmental Protection Agency (EPA) to list those pollutants for which there is sufficient scientific evidence documenting the risk to public health from unregulated exposure. To achieve this, the EPA periodically reviews a large body of scientific research dealing with the adverse health effects of pollutants. The subsequently produced documents are used in the development of a National Ambient Air Quality Standard (NAAQS) for each of the so-called criteria pollutants. Table 41–1 lists the six criteria air pollutants, their NAAQSs, and their principal adverse health effects.

The CAA mandates that the primary NAAQS be set to protect the health of all sensitive groups within the population. The EPA has identified children, people with chronic respiratory disease such as asthma, and people with ischemic heart disease as constituting sensitive groups (ie, that demonstrate a response to a pollutant at a lower level or to a greater degree than the average response of the general population).

## TYPES & SOURCES OF EXPOSURE

Outdoor air contains an array of naturally occurring pollutants including soil, dust, pollens, and fungi. In addition, human activity generates complex mixtures of pollutants. Much of the regulatory effort and scientific research has concentrated on the individual components of these complex mixtures. This chapter discusses the criteria pollutants (Table 41–1) and acidic aerosols, a yet unregulated pollutant. It does not discuss highly toxic air pollutants, so called "air toxics," that are emitted from point sources and that are present in low concentrations in the environment (see Chapter 40).

The sources of outdoor air pollution are usually categorized as stationary or mobile. Stationary sources are primarily power or manufacturing plants and are responsible for most sulfur dioxide ($SO_2$) emissions as well as considerable amounts of nitrogen oxides ($NO_x$) and particulate matter. In the eastern United States and Canada, atmospheric acidity is largely due to the oxidation of $SO_2$ to sulfuric acid ($H_2SO_4$) and other acid sulfate species. The combustion of fossil fuel is the most important cause of stationary source emissions, although release of volatile organic compounds (VOCs) by various industrial facilities can contribute to the generation of ozone ($O_3$) in the atmosphere.

In contrast to the pollution from stationary sources that characterizes eastern North America, southern California "smog" is primarily derived from automotive, or mobile source, emissions. A large fraction of ambient $O_3$ is the product of complex photochemical reactions involving $NO_x$ and VOCs emitted from automotive tailpipes. Nitric acid ($HNO_3$) is a more important contributor to atmospheric acidity than

**Table 41–1.** Criteria air pollutants.

| Air Pollutant | Standard | Principal Adverse Health Effect |
|---|---|---|
| Ozone | 0.12 ppm as a 1 hour maximum concentration not to be exceeded more than 3 times in a 3-year period | Increased respiratory symptoms<br>Decreased lung function<br>Airway inflammation<br>Increased airway responsiveness to nonspecific stimuli |
| Nitrogen dioxide | 0.053 ppm as an annual arithmetic mean concentration | ? Increased airway responsiveness<br>Increased respiratory symptoms and illnesses in children |
| Particulate matter ($PM_{10}$) | 50 $\mu g/m^3$ as an annual arithmetic mean<br>150 $\mu g/m^3$ as a 24-hour standard | Increased respiratory symptoms<br>Increased respiratory illnesses<br>Increased respiratory morbidity in asthmatics and mortality in persons with COPD |
| Sulfur dioxide | **Primary:** 0.03 ppm as an annual arithmetic mean concentration and 0.14 ppm as a 24-hour max. concentration<br>**Secondary:** 0.5 ppm as a 3-hour max. concentration | Increased respiratory symptoms<br>Increased respiratory morbidity and mortality<br>Decreased lung function in asthmatics |
| Lead | 1.5 $\mu g/m^3$ as a maximum quarterly average | Hypertension in adults<br>Neurobehavioral alteration in children |
| Carbon monoxide | 9 ppm as an 8-hour average not to be exceeded more than one time per year<br>35 ppm as a 1-hour average not to be exceeded more than one time per year | Decreased exercise capacity in healthy adults<br>Shorter duration to onset and increased duration of angina in people with CAD |

$H_2SO_4$ in southern California and is formed in the atmosphere from the reaction of $NO_x$ with the hydroxyl radical (OH–). Motor vehicle emissions are also responsible for much carbon monoxide and particulate pollution. A major success story in the control of the criteria pollutants involves the markedly decreased concentrations of lead in the ambient air of United States cities achieved as a result of the removal of tetra ethyl lead from gasoline.

## PERSONAL EXPOSURE

Central stations monitor the ambient air for concentrations of the criteria pollutants. However, the regional average concentrations measured at such stations may not adequately characterize personal exposures. For example, local conditions will affect $O_3$ concentration to the extent that areas downwind from major traffic congestion may have higher levels than those in the immediate vicinity of the congestion. How much time is spent outdoors is an important determinant of personal exposure. Most people spend most of their time indoors, where the concentrations of pollutants are generally lower than in the outdoor air. The concentration of $NO_2$, however, may be higher in indoor air, largely as a result of natural gas-burning stoves. Individuals who spend a lot of time outdoors, especially if they are increasing their effective dose by means of increased minute ventilation from exercise, may sustain relatively high exposures to pollutants such as $O_3$ and particulate matter. Therefore, total personal exposure should be considered; this is estimated by the summation of the products of the concentrations of the pollutant in various microenvironments with the duration spent in each.

## PRINCIPLES OF INHALATIONAL INJURY

For any one individual, the total potential dose to a pollutant can vary depending on the above described factors. Furthermore, pollutants in inhaled air are either gases or aerosols—droplets of liquid or particles suspended in gas—and their site of deposition after inhalation is largely determined by their water solubility. Gases that are extremely water-soluble, such as $SO_2$ and $HNO_3$ vapor, will be deposited and removed primarily by the upper respiratory tract. Therefore, these water-soluble gases will mainly induce toxic effects on the proximal airways and will only damage the distal lung when inhaled in high concentrations. In contrast, gases that are of relatively low water solubility, such as $NO_x$ and $O_3$, may predominantly injure the distal lung. The less soluble the gas, the greater the potential for damage at the level of the terminal respiratory unit.

The deposition of aerosols is determined by a number of factors, including the size and chemical characteristics of the aerosol, the anatomy of the respiratory tract, and the breathing pattern of the exposed person. The size of the droplet or particle is usually the primary factor affecting deposition, although the chemical nature of the inhaled pollutant can be important, especially if it is a water-soluble acid aerosol that can be neutralized by oral ammonia, such as a $H_2SO_4$ mist. The majority of inhaled particles with a mass median aerodynamic diameter (MMAD) $\geq$ 10 μm are deposited in the nasopharynx and will not penetrate below the larynx. Particles in the range of 2.5–6 μm will deposit primarily in the conducting airways below the larynx and particles in the range of 0.5–2.5 μm will deposit primarily in the distal airways and alveoli.

Particles with a MMAD < 0.5 μm are exhaled without significant deposition. The site of particle deposition is also influenced by hygroscopic growth in the humidified environment of the airways, the shape and dimensions of the respiratory tree, ventilatory pattern (respiratory rate and tidal volume), oral versus nasal breathing, and the amount and nature of respiratory tract secretions. Respiratory tract disease can affect particle deposition by altering airway dimension, airflow pattern, or respiratory secretions. Exercise increases oral breathing, bypassing the nasal scrubbing mechanism, and increases minute ventilation, thereby increasing particle velocity and inertial impaction. Both of these changes result in greater particle deposition in the lower airways.

Clearance of inhaled pollutants occurs by several mechanisms. In general, highly water-soluble particles and gases are absorbed through the epithelial layer into the bloodstream near where they have been deposited. The clearance of insoluble particles is dependent on where they impact. Those deposited in the anterior nasal cavity are expelled by sneezing or rhinorrhea, while the remainder of particles deposited in the nose are cleared posteriorly to the pharynx. Particles deposited in the trachea, bronchi, or bronchioles, where there is ciliated epithelium and a layer of mucus, are transported up the mucociliary escalator to be expelled by coughing or swallowing. Particles deposited distal to the terminal bronchioles are cleared by alveolar macrophages and/or dissolution. Alveolar macrophages will ingest particles and migrate to the mucociliary escalator or into lymphatics. A small fraction of particles deposited in the alveoli will migrate through the alveolar epithelial layer directly into the lymphatic circulation.

## SPECIFIC OUTDOOR AIR POLLUTANTS

In 1991, about 86 million people lived in counties in the United States with measured air quality above the primary NAAQSs. Therefore, from a clinical and public health perspective, such exposures continue to be of relevance. The health effects of the outdoor air pollutants have been compiled by the interpretation of toxicologic studies (ie, animal studies, in vitro studies, and controlled human exposure studies) and epidemiologic studies (ie, ecologic, cross-sectional, and case control designs). The following section discusses each of the major air pollutants individually; however, it should be understood that exposures often occur to a mixture of pollutants and separating out the individual contribution of each pollutant is frequently not possible.

## Ozone

Ozone ($O_3$) is a colorless, pungent, relatively water insoluble gas that occurs with other photochemical oxidants and fine particles to form "smog." Tropospheric $O_3$, or ground level $O_3$, is an environmental air pollutant and is distinct from the stratospheric $O_3$ that occurs at altitudes of greater than 10 km above the earth's surface. $O_3$ is generated by a series of sunlight-driven reactions involving $NO_x$ and VOCs from predominantly mobile (ie, motor vehicle), but sometimes stationary sources. The meteorological conditions that tend to foster the generation of ozone are typically present from late spring to early fall. Peak concentrations of $O_3$ typically occur in mid-afternoon, after both the morning rush hour and several hours of bright sunlight. Indoor sources of $O_3$ include office equipment with electric motors or ultraviolet light such as photocopy machines and electrostatic devices such as air purifiers and ion generators.

While $O_3$ has long been associated with southern California smog, many other areas of North America also experience high concentrations of this pollutant, especially Mexico City and cities in the eastern United States and Canada during the summer months. In 1991, 69 million people in the United States resided in counties where the current NAAQS for $O_3$ was not attained. In some southern California communities, there were over 90 days in 1993 during which the standard was exceeded. During the particularly hot summer of 1988, rates of $O_3$ generation increased and violations of the NAAQS occurred in counties with a population totaling 135 million. Thus, the adequacy of the current NAAQS for $O_3$ for the prevention of adverse respiratory effects is of considerable public health importance.

Ozone is a potent oxidant and is capable of reacting with a variety of extracellular and intracellular molecules. When these molecules are unsaturated lipids, free radicals and toxic intermediate products, such as hydrogen peroxide and aldehydes, are generated and can lead to cellular damage or cell death. Although direct cytotoxicity is clearly a necessary mechanism of $O_3$-induced tissue injury, secondary damage from the inflammatory response may also play a role.

Dosimetric studies indicate that much of the inhaled $O_3$ is deposited in the upper and proximal lower airways. However, because of its relative water insolubility, a considerable fraction does penetrate to the distal airways and alveoli. Increased inspiratory flow, such as with exercise, may overcome the upper airway "scrubbing mechanisms" and cause greater deposition of $O_3$ in the distal lung.

Most of the research on the health effects of $O_3$ has focused on short-term exposure. $O_3$ inhalation by healthy subjects causes mean decrements in forced expiratory volume in 1 second ($FEV_1$) and forced vital capacity (FVC) that correlate with concentration, exposure duration, and minute ventilation. These decrements in lung function are due primarily to decreased inspiratory capacity rather than airways obstruction. The mechanism of the decreased inspiratory capacity appears to be neurally-mediated involuntary inhibition of inspiratory effort involving stimulation of C-fibers in the lungs. Somewhat surprisingly, older subjects and those who are cigarette smokers demonstrate lower $O_3$-induced decrements in pulmonary function than healthy subjects. The acute decrements in pulmonary function induced by $O_3$ usually resolve within 24 hours.

Respiratory symptoms appear to be associated with these mean decrements in pulmonary function. There is a correlation between the decline in $FEV_1$ and the probability of developing lower respiratory tract symptoms (eg, substernal chest discomfort, cough, wheeze, and dyspnea). These symptoms have been observed while at or below the current NAAQS.

Another adverse effect of short-term exposure to $O_3$ is enhanced airway responsiveness to nonspecific stimuli such as methacholine and histamine. This effect may persist longer than the acute decrements in lung function and may occur in individuals who do not experience a decline in their $FEV_1$.

Nasal inflammatory changes, Type I alveolar and ciliated airway epithelial cell injury, infiltration of the airway mucosa by neutrophils, and increased bronchoalveolar lavage (BAL) fluid neutrophils and inflammatory mediators have also been observed after exposure.

The effects of chronic $O_3$ exposure in humans have not been adequately defined. It has been hypothesized that chronic exposure would lead to emphysematous or fibrotic parenchymal changes; however, to date, animal toxicologic studies have failed to substantiate the induction of diffuse disease after long-term exposure to ambient concentrations.

Because of their tendency to experience bronchoconstriction upon inhalation of noxious stimuli, persons with asthma are usually more sensitive to inhaled irritants. Although studies of asthmatic and atopic subjects have failed to show enhanced spirometric responses to short-term $O_3$ inhalation, there are indications that asthmatics may experience a greater inflammatory response to exposure. Furthermore, there are several epidemiologic studies that show that high ambient $O_3$ concentrations are associated with an increased rate of asthma attacks and increased hospital admissions/emergency department visits for respiratory disease, including asthma.

Ozone toxicity may be enhanced by coexposure to other pollutants such as other oxidants, particulates,

and atmospheric acidity commonly seen in urban smog. The mechanisms by which these cofactors may potentiate $O_3$ toxicity are poorly understood.

In summary, tens of millions of persons in the United States are exposed to levels of $O_3$ above the current NAAQS. This exposure is capable of inducing both acute decrements in lung function and respiratory symptoms. Although these effects are transient, acute respiratory tract inflammation can also be induced by short-term exposure to ambient concentrations of $O_3$ with exercise. The long-term consequences of this type of acute inflammatory response are not well understood. Chronic exposure to ambient levels does not cause emphysema or diffuse fibrosis in animal studies. Because $O_3$ inhalation can induce both airway inflammation and enhanced airway responsiveness, it is reasonable to expect persons with asthma to have greater susceptibility to this pollutant. Ozone is rarely the sole pollutant of concern in urban smog, and it is likely that environmental cofactors enhance its toxicity.

### Nitrogen Dioxide

Most ambient nitrogen dioxide ($NO_2$) is generated by the burning of fossil-derived fuels, during which oxygen and nitrogen react to form nitrogen oxide (NO), which further reacts to form $NO_2$ and other $NO_x$. The principal source of $NO_2$ in outdoor air is motor vehicle emissions, but power plants and fossil fuel-burning industrial facilities also contribute. In most US urban areas, ambient levels of $NO_2$ vary with traffic intensity. Annual average concentrations range from 0.015–0.035 ppm. Of all regions in the United States reporting $NO_2$ monitoring data in recent years, only the Los Angeles basin exceeded the current NAAQS.

In contrast to other criteria pollutants, $NO_2$ is a common contaminant of indoor air, and indoor levels often exceed those found outdoors. Indoor sources of $NO_2$ include gas cooking stoves, gas furnaces, and kerosene space heaters. Because the majority of homes in the United States have gas cooking stoves and Americans spend a large proportion of time in their homes, the home environment is usually the most important contributor to total $NO_2$ exposure. High concentrations may be generated in a kitchen with a gas stove in use. Nitrous acid (HONO) and other $NO_x$ are emitted by gas stoves, so health effects associated with the use of such appliances may not be due to $NO_2$ alone.

Nitrogen dioxide, like $O_3$, is an oxidant, but it is less chemically reactant and is therefore usually considered less potent. Although both pollutants are relatively insoluble in water, the solubility of $NO_2$ is somewhat higher. When $NO_2$ is absorbed onto the moist surfaces of the respiratory tract, it can be hydrolyzed to evolve acidic species such as HONO and $HNO_3$. The potential for $NO_2$ to cause the local generation of hydrogen ions in the airways may be an important feature of its toxicity. Nitrogen dioxide and $O_3$ are frequent copollutants in Southern California smog.

The annual averaging time of the NAAQS for $NO_2$ (as opposed to the 1-hour maximum for $O_3$) reflects an assessment that the health effects of this pollutant are determined more by chronic, low-level exposure than by transient, high-level exposures. Whether this assessment is correct or not has important consequences for individuals in the population with preexisting respiratory disease, such as those with asthma or chronic obstructive pulmonary disease (COPD) who are susceptible to the development of acute exacerbations. The lack of a short-term averaging time in the current NAAQS means that asthmatic persons are not felt to be at risk of developing acute exacerbations after brief exposures to $NO_2$.

The results of controlled human exposure studies have demonstrated no significant decrements in pulmonary function in normal, healthy subjects after exposure to $NO_2$ at low concentrations. Controlled exposure studies of subjects with asthma, however, have produced inconsistent results. Low-level $NO_2$ exposure was reported to have enhanced airway responsiveness after exposure. Unfortunately, subsequent studies produced conflicting results, so this issue has yet to be resolved.

The toxic effects of $NO_2$ exposure have been extensively studied. There are abundant animal toxicologic data and reports of accidental human exposure that indicate that short-term inhalation of high concentrations of $NO_2$ can produce terminal bronchiolar and diffuse alveolar injury; exposure of humans to very high concentrations (ie, > 150 ppm $NO_2$) typically results in death. However, in contrast to what is seen with $O_3$, short-term exposure to $NO_2$ at concentrations in the ambient range does not induce airways inflammation.

Chronic exposure of animals to high concentrations of $NO_2$ has been shown to cause structural damage to alveoli with airspace enlargement, which is somewhat analogous to human emphysema. The terminal lung unit is the site of greatest $NO_2$-induced injury. Animal infectivity studies after $NO_2$ exposure have shown that high concentrations may impair respiratory tract defenses against some bacteria and viruses. The mechanism(s) of $NO_2$-induced enhanced microbial infectivity are not clearly understood, but is likely due to alveolar macrophage dysfunction. However, this finding has not been consistently observed in humans.

Numerous epidemiologic studies have studied the relationship between ambient levels of $NO_2$ and respiratory illnesses. While some studies have shown a positive association between these two factors, others have failed to demonstrate this finding. However, a recent meta-analysis using 11 cross-sectional and prospective studies of residential $NO_2$ concentrations in children estimated a 20% increase in risk of respiratory illnesses per 15 ppb increments in long-term $NO_2$ exposure. A more recent study of indoor $NO_2$ levels and respiratory symptoms failed to show an association between these factors. The inconsistency of this association in epidemiologic studies may be due in part to methodological factors such as different statistical power, confounding, and misclassification.

As was noted for $O_3$, environmental exposures to $NO_2$ do not occur without coexposure to other pollutants. Somewhat surprisingly, given that both pollutants are oxidants, studies of combined exposure to $NO_2$ and $O_3$ in human subjects generally have not demonstrated enhanced toxicity.

In summary, $NO_2$ is a pollutant that is a ubiquitous component of urban smog. It is generated by combustion of fossil-derived fuels from both mobile and stationary sources. Indoor concentrations often exceed those outdoors, primarily due to the use of gas stoves. Inhaled $NO_2$ penetrates to the deep lung because of the relatively low water-solubility of the gas. Studies to date have shown conflicting evidence of $NO_2$-induced health effects at ambient levels of exposure. Chronic exposure of experimental animals to high concentrations of $NO_2$ has caused emphysema-like changes and decreased resistance to bacterial infection. The applicability of these findings to ambient exposure of humans is not straightforward. Epidemiologic studies have shown inconsistent associations between respiratory symptoms and illnesses and outdoor/residential $NO_2$ levels. Indoor $NO_2$ exposure is of greater concern regarding potential adverse respiratory health effects than outdoor exposure. Nevertheless, $NO_2$ remains an important air pollutant because of its role in the generation of tropospheric $O_3$.

## Particles, Sulfur Dioxide, & Acid Aerosols

Particles, sulfur oxide(s), and acid aerosols are discussed as a group, as they usually occur together as components of a complex pollutant mixture. Their production is primarily a result of fossil fuel combustion. Particles and sulfur dioxide ($SO_2$) are the primary products of combustion, and acid aerosols are formed by subsequent atmospheric chemical reactions. This mixture of solid and liquid particles suspended in the air is termed "particulate air pollution;" the constituent particles differ in size and composition. Particles with an aerodynamic diameter of ≤10 μm ($PM_{10}$) are the focus of regulatory interest because particles of this diameter may penetrate into and be deposited in the airways of the lower respiratory tract and the gas exchanging portions of the lung. Acid aerosols are usually a complex and variable mixture and include dissolved gaseous pollutants.

Sulfur dioxide is a major air pollutant in many urban areas. The gas is emitted by coal and oil-fired power plants and by industrial processes involving fossil fuel combustion. It leads to the secondary formation of acid aerosols. Because high sulfur-content coal has remained a relatively cheap fuel in regions where it is mined, $SO_2$ emissions have generally been more of a problem in the Eastern United States than in Southern California, where smog is primarily a result of photochemical reactions involving motor vehicle emissions. Unfortunately, the building of tall smokestacks to reduce the local concentrations of $SO_2$ around Midwestern and Eastern United States power plants has led to the long-distance transport of sulfur oxide pollutants and their progeny, acid sulfates, to New England and Canada (so-called "acid rain").

Sulfur oxide emissions in the United States increased steadily during the 20th century to a peak of 32 million tons in 1970. Exposure to high concentrations of $SO_2$ is highly localized to the vicinity (within 20 km) of major stationary sources. The initial clues that $SO_2$ might be an air pollutant capable of causing adverse respiratory effects came from the severe pollution episodes occurring earlier in this century. During these episodes, high ambient concentrations of $SO_2$, particles, and acid aerosols occurred and were clearly associated with increased mortality, primarily among persons with preexisting cardiopulmonary disease. During the 1952 air pollution episode in London, there were an estimated 4000 excess deaths. More recently, multiple epidemiologic studies have demonstrated an association between lower levels of particulate pollution and increased daily mortality from cardiopulmonary disease. The consistent finding of this association in studies conducted at various times and diverse geographic locations makes it likely that there is a true causal relationship between respirable particulate pollution and daily mortality. However, the biologic mechanism underlying this association remains obscure, especially given the lack of toxicity of ambient levels of particulate matter in animal studies.

Acute morbidity associated with lower level particulate pollution has been examined using a variety of indicators, including measures of health care utilization by exposed populations, health status of exposed individuals, symptom questionnaires, and lung function tests. Use of these indicators has demonstrated that particle exposure has been associated with increased emergency room visits for respiratory illness, such as asthma and pneumonia, and higher rates of hospital admissions for respiratory and cardiovascular illnesses.

Studies in adults have also shown associations between exposure to particles and reports of respiratory symptoms severe enough to restrict activity. In smokers with chronic obstructive pulmonary disease (COPD), declines in pulmonary function and daily emergency room visits for acute exacerbations have been positively associated with particulate air pollution. In children, studies have shown associations with particulate concentrations at levels commonly encountered today with respiratory illnesses, declines in pulmonary function, and aggravation of asthmatic attacks.

The chronic health effects of particulate air pollution are a more difficult end point to study. Despite this, a number of studies have shown an association between air pollution levels and the following: reports of bronchitis, chronic cough, and lower respiratory illnesses; increased symptoms of COPD; doctor's diagnosis of asthma, and a diagnosis of emphysema with shortness of breath; and, in the Harvard Six Cities study, an increase in city-specific mortality rates.

From a toxicologic viewpoint, $SO_2$, particles, and acid aerosols have different mechanisms of action. Sulfur dioxide is highly soluble in water and is mostly absorbed in the upper airways. Although the nose effectively removes much of the inhaled gas, significant amounts may penetrate to the large airways. Here, the irritant molecules may act directly on smooth muscle or via sensory afferent nerve fibers to cause reflex bronchoconstriction. At high concentrations, $SO_2$ can cause epithelial sloughing in the trachea and proximal airways, leading to a bronchitis-like pathology. Despite the irritant potential of $SO_2$, studies have failed to demonstrate effects on respiratory mechanics (at levels up to 1.0 ppm) in healthy people. However, in asthmatics, low-level exposure has been shown to cause bronchoconstriction. This acute bronchoconstriction is observed within minutes of exposure and resolves within 1 hour after exposure ceases. While the mechanism of $SO_2$-induced bronchoconstriction is not fully understood, a reflex mechanism involving vagal afferent and cholinergic efferent nerves has been postulated.

The toxicity of inhaled particles is determined by the physical and chemical nature of the particles, the physics of their deposition and distribution in the respiratory tract, and the biologic effect(s) of exposure. Particle toxicity is often complicated by the presence of other air pollutants that may cause interactive effects. Particle size is thought to be a critical determinant of toxicity. After inhalation of ultrafine particles (those with a diameter in the region of 0.2 μm), acute interstitial inflammation has been noted. In vitro studies of the cytotoxicity of particles collected from polluted urban air have also demonstrated that such particles can be highly toxic to alveolar macrophages. The relative toxicity of the particles studied was dependent on both the metal and combustion-derived organic content of the particles.

Acid aerosols consist predominantly of sulfate ($SO_4^{2-}$) and bisulfate ($HSO_4^-$) ions that coexist with ammonium ($NH_4^+$) ions. In some areas where combustion of sulfur-containing fuels is not common, such as Los Angeles, nitric acid ($HNO_3$) is a major cause of atmospheric acidity. Because of its high vapor pressure, $HNO_3$ is often in vapor form in the atmosphere. While formic and acetic acids are also found in the atmosphere, their contribution to overall acidity is negligible. The toxicity of the acid aerosols is related to their acidity, which can cause airway irritation. Reduction of tracheobronchial clearance rates through alteration in mucociliary function and increased nonspecific airway responsiveness has been noted in human, as well as animal, studies. Airway inflammation does not appear to occur at ambient levels of exposure. The data are conflicting about whether asthmatics are more sensitive to the effects of acid aerosols than healthy people; it is likely that only a subgroup of asthmatics have increased sensitivity.

In summary, particles, $SO_2$, and acid aerosols are a complex group of air pollutants that share a common origin. Epidemiologic studies have consistently shown that they exert adverse health effects on both respiratory morbidity and mortality. In vitro and in vivo studies have attempted to study the mechanism(s) of these effects, but their interpretation is complicated by the difficulty in separating out the individual contributions and the potential synergistic interactions of the components.

## Lead

Lead continues to be recognized as a significant toxicant and is known to have adverse health effects on humans of all ages (see Chapter 39). However, the phase-out of the additive tetra ethyl lead from gasoline in the United States as a result of the CAA has been associated with declines in ambient lead concentrations and blood lead levels in the population. Thus, widespread airborne exposure to lead has ceased to be a major health problem in the United States.

## Carbon Monoxide

Carbon monoxide (CO) is a colorless, odorless, nonirritating gas that is generated by the incomplete combustion of carbon-containing fuels, such as oils, gasoline, coal, and wood. Because of these described properties, exposure to CO may be insidious; in fact, exposure to high levels of CO is the leading cause of poisoning deaths in the United States. Ambient environmental air pollution levels are unlikely to cause acute toxicity and death, although low-dose exposure may be associated with adverse health effects. The most common source of exposure in nonsmoking individuals is from vehicle emissions. Engine exhaust may cause local accumulation of CO, especially during periods of heavy traffic. In transit exposure assessments, commuting individuals have been shown to be exposed to high levels. In fact, in one study of commuters, levels as high as 50 ppm with mean values of 10–12 ppm were recorded. Emissions from

nonvehicular sources such as lawn mowers, chain saws, space heaters, and charcoal briquettes also contribute to ambient CO exposure.

The toxicity of CO lies in its ability to strongly bind to hemoglobin and interfere with the transport of oxygen from the alveoli to tissues. The gas rapidly diffuses across the alveolar-capillary membrane after inhalation. Here, it binds with an affinity greater than 200 times that of oxygen to hemoglobin to form carboxyhemoglobin (COHb). This COHb complex interferes with oxygen delivery to the tissues by two major mechanisms. It reduces the number of available sites for oxygen binding and it induces an allosteric change in the hemoglobin proteins, which slows the dissociation of oxygen from the heme binding sites. An additional route of toxicity may be through the ability of CO to bind to myoglobin and reduced cytochromes, thereby impairing oxidative metabolism through disruption of the electron transport chain. The degree of exposure to CO may be determined by measuring the blood COHb level. Normal levels in nonsmokers range from 0.3% to 0.7%. The NAAQS is 9 ppm as an 8-hour average, not to be exceeded more than once a year.

Because CO has no direct effect on the lungs, its principal adverse health effects are through its ability to cause or exacerbate diseases associated with impaired oxygen delivery. Effects on fetal development, cardiovascular disease, chronic respiratory diseases, and nervous system disease have been described.

Animal studies have shown that low-level CO exposure during pregnancy may have developmental effects on the fetus. The findings of low birthrate, fewer successful pregnancies, and increased fetal and neonatal mortality have been observed. However, a case-control study has failed to duplicate these findings in humans.

In healthy human subjects, controlled exposure studies have shown that low-level CO exposure decreases exercise capacity. In individuals with ischemic heart disease, a shorter duration to onset and an increased duration of angina, as well as earlier ST-T changes (an objective measure of myocardial ischemia), have been observed with low-level CO exposure. Ambient levels of CO have not been consistently shown to cause ventricular arrhythmias. Several epidemiologic studies have shown an association between high ambient levels of CO and cardiorespiratory hospital admissions and cardiac deaths.

Because the principal pathophysiologic effect of CO is the impairment of oxygen delivery to tissues, exposure to the gas may increase the symptoms of dyspnea and decrease the exercise tolerance of individuals with COPD. It is not known to produce pulmonary inflammation or exacerbate airway disease.

Multiple studies have failed to demonstrate an effect of CO on motor skills at ambient levels of exposure. A single community study did show an association between headaches and daily ambient CO levels in the Los Angles area.

In summary, CO at ambient levels of exposure may exacerbate ischemic heart disease, worsen respiratory symptoms in individuals with COPD, increase cardiorespiratory morbidity and cardiac mortality, and lead to an increase in headaches in exposed individuals. However, no significant effects on fetal development and the central nervous system have been consistently demonstrated.

## REFERENCES

### GENERAL

Devlin R: Air pollutants: Human health studies. In: Rom WN (editor): *Environmental and Occupational Medicine,* 3rd ed. Lippincott-Raven, 1997.

Harber, Schenker, Balmes JR: *Occupational and Environmental Respiratory Disease.* Mosby-Year Book, 1996.

Health Effects of Outdoor Air Pollution. State of the Art. I and II. Am J Respir Crit Care Med 1996;153:3,477.

Samet JM: Community air pollution. In: Rom WN (editor): *Environmental and Occupational Medicine,* 3rd ed. Lippincott-Raven, 1997.

### OZONE

Aris RM et al: Ozone-induced airway inflammation in human subjects as determined by airway lavage and biopsy. Am Rev Respir Dis 1993;148:1363.

Balmes JR et al: Ozone-induced decrements in FEV1 and FVC do not correlate with airway inflammation in human subjects. Am J Respir Crit Care Med 1996; 153:904.

Balmes JR: The role of ozone exposure in the epidemiology of asthma. Environ Health Perspect 1993;101 (Suppl 4):219.

Graham DE, Koren HS: Biomarkers of inflammation in ozone-exposed humans. Am Rev Respir Dis 1990; 142:152.

Molfino NA et al: Effect of low concentrations of ozone on inhaled allergen responses in asthmatic subjects. Lancet 1991;338:199.

Scannell C et al: Greater ozone-induced inflammatory responses in subjects with asthma. Am J Respir Crit Care Med 1996;154:24.

Spektor DM et al: Effects of single- and multi-day ozone exposures on respiratory function in active normal children. Environ Res 1991;55:107.

### NITROGEN DIOXIDE

Hasselbad V, Kotchmar DJ, Eddy DM: Synthesis of environmental evidence: Nitrogen dioxide epidemiology studies. J Air Waste Management Assoc 1992; 42:662.

Hazucha MJ et al: Lung function response of healthy women after sequential exposures to $NO_2$ and $O_3$. Am J Respir Crit Care Med 1994;150:642.

Neas LM et al: Association of indoor nitrogen dioxide with respiratory symptoms and pulmonary function in children. Am J Epidemiol 1991;134:204.

Schlesinger RB: Nitrogen dioxide. In: Rom WN (editor): *Environmental and Occupational Medicine,* 3rd ed. Lippincott-Raven, 1997.

### PARTICLES, SULFUR DIOXIDE, & ACID AEROSOLS

Aris R et al: Effects of nitric acid gas alone or in combination with ozone on healthy volunteers. Am Rev Respir Dis 1993;148:965.

Aris R et al: Lack of bronchoconstrictor response to sulfuric acid aerosols and fogs. Am Rev Respir Dis 1991; 143:744.

Dockery DW et al: An association between air pollution and mortality in six US cities. N Engl J Med 1993; 329:1753.

Frampton MW et al: Sulfuric acid aerosol exposure in humans assessed by bronchoalveolar lavage. Am Rev Respir Dis 1992;146:626.

Ostro BD et al: Asthmatic responses to airborne acid aerosols. Am J Public Health 1991;81:694.

Pope CA, Dockery DW: Acute health effects of PM10 pollution on symptomatic and asymptomatic children. Am Rev Respir Dis 1992;145:1123.

Schwartz J: Air pollution and daily mortality: A review and meta-analysis. Environ Res 1994;64:36.

Schwartz J et al: Acute effects of summer air pollution on respiratory symptom reporting in children. Am J Respir Crit Care Med 1994;150:1234.

Thurston GD et al: Respiratory hospital admissions and summertime haze air pollution in Toronto, Ontario: Consideration of the role of acid aerosols. Environ Res 1994;65:271.

### CARBON MONOXIDE

Beckett W: Chemical asphyxiants. In: Rom WN (editor): *Environmental and Occupational Medicine,* 3rd ed. Lippincott-Raven, 1997.

Cook M, Simon PA, Hoffman RE: Unintentional carbon monoxide poisoning in Colorado, 1986 through 1991. Am J Public Health 1995;85(7):988.

Sheps DS et al: Production of arrhythmias by elevated carboxyhemoglobin in patients with coronary artery disease. Ann Intern Med 1990;113:343.

# Smoking & Occupational Health   **42**

*Neal L. Benowitz, MD*

## CIGARETTE SMOKING & DISEASE

The smoking of cigarettes and other tobacco products is the most significant preventable cause of sickness and death in civilized countries. In the United States, it is estimated that more than 400,000 deaths a year are a consequence of cigarette smoking. The major immediate causes of death attributable to cigarette smoking are coronary heart disease, lung cancer, and chronic obstructive lung disease. Other diseases related to cigarette smoking are listed in Table 42–1.

### Cigarette Smoking as a Form of Drug Dependency

Cigarette smoking is a form of drug dependency that appears to be motivated by the desire to partake of the pharmacologic actions of nicotine. Nicotine has multiple psychological effects, including euphoria, reduction of anxiety or tension, suppression of appetite, mood stimulation or relaxation, and improvement in performance and memory. The stimulant effects of tobacco use may be particularly useful for workers who perform repetitive tasks but need to remain vigilant. Smokers tend to regulate nicotine intake to maintain consistent levels from day to day.

Smokers often find it extremely difficult to quit smoking, even when the motivation to do so, such as illness or social pressure, is high.

### Components & Toxicology of Tobacco Smoke

Tobacco smoke is a complex mixture of chemical substances in the form of gases and particulates (Table 42–2). Toxic gases include carbon monoxide, which binds hemoglobin preferentially to oxygen and results in reduced oxygen delivery to tissues (see Chapter 33). Other gases such as nitrogen oxides are oxidizing agents or irritants and may contribute to chronic obstructive lung disease. Hydrogen cyanide impairs ciliary function in the lung, which may predispose to pulmonary infection. Volatile nitrosamines and other gaseous substances such as formaldehyde may contribute to cancer formation.

The particulate phase of tobacco smoke includes the alkaloids—chiefly nicotine—and tar. Aside from its central nervous system actions, nicotine is a sympathetic nervous system stimulant that increases heart rate, blood pressure, and myocardial contractility and causes release of free fatty acids. Nicotine causes release of stress hormones such as cortisol and growth hormone as well as vasopressin and b-endorphin. As a consequence of the cardiovascular effects of nicotine, myocardial oxygen demand increases. Exposure to nicotine and carbon monoxide results in reduced exercise tolerance in patients with angina pectoris and enhances the risk of acute myocardial infarction and sudden death in persons with coronary heart disease. Nicotine induces vasoconstriction and may contribute to coronary spasm as well.

Tar is a complex mixture of chemicals that includes most of the suspected carcinogens, cocarcinogens, and tumor promoters in tobacco smoke. These include benzo*(a)*pyrene and other polynuclear aromatic hydrocarbons, nicotine-derived nitrosamines, β-naphthylamine, polonium-210, and metals such as nickel, arsenic, and cadmium.

## OCCUPATION & SMOKING BEHAVIOR

Currently in the United States, about 25% of adults smoke cigarettes. The distribution of smokers within various occupations is not homogeneous. Persons who are better educated and have white-collar jobs are less likely to smoke. Blue-collar workers (not including farmers) are most likely to smoke, and their cigarettes are more likely to be high-tar cigarettes.

Rates of smoking in particular industries have been as high as 80% in some studies. In the United States today, about 45% of blue-collar workers smoke. Unfortunately, this group is also the one most likely to be exposed to occupational chemical carcinogens.

Men were at one time considerably more likely to

**Table 42–1.** Diseases related to cigarette smoking.

Chronic bronchitis and emphysema
Coronary heart disease
Peripheral arterial occlusive disease
Stroke
Aortic aneurysm
Cancer, many types (see Table 42–3)
Peptic ulcer disease
Esophageal reflux
Reproductive disorders: Reduced fertility, spontaneous
  abortions, low-birth-weight deliveries, increased neonatal
  mortality rates
Osteoporosis
Cataract
Fire injuries

be smokers than women. By the early 1980s, this difference had all but disappeared.

The higher rate of smoking among blue-collar workers is a potential confounding factor in understanding the relationship between smoking, occupation, and disease. Smoking as a marker for lower socioeconomic class may be associated with dietary differences, greater consumption of alcohol, and greater air pollution in the home environment—due both to industrial pollution related to geographic location of housing and higher probability of exposure to tobacco smoke in the home.

## INTERACTIONS BETWEEN SMOKING & OCCUPATION

Cigarette smoking can interact with occupational exposures to cause disease in several ways:

(1) Contamination of tobacco products with toxic substances in the workplace. For example, toxic exposures might occur when cigarettes become contaminated with pesticides, lead, or other chemicals.

(2) Pyrolysis of workplace chemicals into toxic chemicals, which are then inhaled by the smoker. An example is polymer fume fever in workers who inhale fumes from heated Teflon in contaminated cigarettes. The syndrome can be quite severe, causing pulmonary edema and even death. Prevention of such

diseases requires prohibiting smoking at work and encouraging hand washing before smoking.

(3) Additive exposures to toxic agents found both in the workplace and in tobacco smoke. Most of the chemicals in tobacco smoke, with the exception of nicotine, may be found in work environments, particularly where there is combustion of organic material. Carbon monoxide is an example of a toxin for which there may be additive contributions of workplace and smoking. Habitual heavy smokers have blood carboxyhemoglobin concentrations of 5–10%. Similar increments may follow occupational carbon monoxide exposure owing to the presence of combustion engines or furnaces or to exposure to methylene chloride (which is metabolized in the body to carbon monoxide). A blood level of 5–10% occurring after either smoking or occupational exposure may be well tolerated, but a level of 10–20% resulting from combined exposure can cause headache, impair psychomotor function, and, in high-risk patients, aggravate ischemic vascular disease.

(4) Additive or synergistic (multiplicative) effects of workplace and tobacco smoke toxins. Effects of pulmonary irritants and carcinogenic compounds from cigarettes and the workplace may increase the risks of chronic obstructive lung disease or cancer. Synergistic interactions, such as the increased risk of lung cancer with exposure to cigarette smoke and asbestos, are particularly important because most cancers result from combined exposures to smoking and occupational toxins. Control of smoking would prevent most such cancers.

(5) Accidental injury related to tobacco smoking. This includes injuries from fires produced from cigarettes as well as vehicular, machinery, and other accidents occurring at a higher rate in smokers than in nonsmokers.

In addition to specific interactions, as discussed above, smokers are also less well able to tolerate respiratory tract infections, such as influenza. Smokers have more severe illnesses and prolonged disability after such infections. From all causes, smokers have 50% more work loss days than nonsmokers.

It has been estimated—considering excess health insurance, fire loss, worker's compensation claims and workplace accidents, absenteeism, loss of productivity, and the health consequences of passive smoking—that each smoking employee costs the employer $485–880 a year (in 1986 dollars).

## SMOKING & OCCUPATIONAL CANCER

Smoking is believed to be responsible for 30% of cases of cancer in the United States today. Eighty to 90% of lung cancers, 75% of oral, laryngeal, and esophageal cancers, 30–40% of bladder and kidney cancers, and 15–30% of leukemia and myeloma

**Table 42–2.** Major toxic components of cigarette smoke.

| | |
|---|---|
| Nicotine | Carbon monoxide[1] |
| Catechols | Acetaldehyde[1] |
| N′-Nitrosonornicotine | Nitrogen oxides[1] |
| Phenol[1] | Hydrogen cyanide[1] |
| Polynuclear aromatic hydrocarbons[1] | Acrolein[1] |
| β-Naphthylamine[1] | Ammonia[1] |
| Nickel (carbonyl)[1] | Formaldehyde[1] |
| Cadmium[1] | Urethane[1] |
| Arsenic[1] | Hydrazine[1] |
| Polonium-210[1] | Nitrosamines |

[1]Potential occupational and environmental exposures.

**Table 42–3.** Cancers related to cigarette smoking.[1]

| Site or Type | Relative Risk (Men, Women) | % of Deaths Attributable (Men, Women) |
|---|---|---|
| Lung | 22, 12 | 90, 79 |
| Throat | 10, 18[2] | 81, 87 |
| Mouth | 28, 6[2] | 92, 61 |
| Esophagus | 8, 10[2] | 78, 75 |
| Bladder | 2.9, 2.6 | 47, 37 |
| Kidney | 3.0, 1.4 | 48, 12 |
| Pancreas | 2.1, 2.3 | 29, 34 |
| Leukemia | 2.0, 2.0 | 2.0, 2.0 |
| Stomach | 1.5, 1.5 | 17, 25 |
| Uterus | —, 2.1 | —, 31 |

[1]Data from Newcombe PA, Carbone, PP: The health consequences of smoking. Med Clin North Am 1992;76:305.
[2]Alcohol acts synergistically.

cases have been attributed to smoking (Table 42–3). Lung cancer incidence data most clearly illustrate the smoking-cancer connection. The incidence of most types of cancer has been relatively constant in the United States since 1900, but the lung cancer rate has been steadily rising. The rise in lung cancer rate parallels the average per capita consumption of cigarettes, with a lag of 20–30 years. Smoking prevalence for men peaked in 1950–1960, but because of the lag, the lung cancer rate reached its peak in the 1980s. Women began smoking later than men, and as a result lung cancer rates have more recently begun to increase for women.

Lung cancer has now overtaken breast cancer as the leading cause of cancer deaths in American women.

## How Does Cigarette Smoking Cause Cancer?

Tobacco smoke and smoke condensates produce cancer in experimental animals. The greatest contributors to the carcinogenesis of tobacco condensate appear to be the polycyclic aromatic hydrocarbons, the most potent of which is benzo(*a*)pyrene.

Carcinogenesis is most likely when tumor initiators are delivered in high concentration to a target organ in the presence of tumor promoters. Tobacco smoking is an ideal model for carcinogenesis. Carcinogens and cocarcinogens are effectively delivered to the airways via inhaled cigarette smoke. A number of tumor promoters are also supplied to permit completion of the carcinogenesis process. Nonspecific pulmonary effects, including chronic inflammation with generation of free radicals of oxygen and impaired pulmonary clearance of carcinogens, may also contribute. Autopsy studies have shown that dysplastic lesions occur at the site of chronic inflammation. These dysplastic lesions are thought to be premalignant, preceding the development of squamous cell carcinoma. Inflammation may predispose to development of lung cancer; nitrogen oxides, acrolein, and

other irritants are thought to contribute to carcinogenesis also.

Tobacco smoke carcinogens and occupational toxins may interact synergistically. If, as is currently thought to be the case, carcinogenesis depends on exposure to both initiators and promoters, smoking may provide the cocarcinogen or tumor promoter needed to compliment the actions of occupational carcinogens. Tobacco smoke may also be the vehicle for transmission of occupational carcinogens into the lung. Finally, cigarette smokers may be more tolerant to noxious substances in the air, allowing greater exposure to environmental carcinogens.

## Asbestos, Smoking, & Lung Cancer

Lung cancer is a major type of cancer in asbestos workers. The interaction between smoking, asbestos exposure, and lung cancer is the best-studied example of the influence of smoking on occupational disease.

Studies of asbestos workers have indicated a substantially increased risk of lung cancer, but most lung cancers occur in persons exposed to both asbestos and cigarette smoke. For example, in analysis of data from a cohort of 12,051 asbestos installation workers with 450 cancer deaths, it appears that had there been no smoking but the same asbestos exposure, the cancer rate would have been only 10% of that observed (Table 42–4). Workers with lower levels of asbestos exposure have a correspondingly lower risk of lung cancer.

Several mechanisms of interaction between asbestos and smoking have been proposed: (1) Asbestos may act as a foreign body, resulting in chronic inflammation, with cell injury and repair. (2) Tobacco smoke acting as a tumor promoter might impair the capacity of cells to repair injury, leading instead to cancer. (3) Asbestos in the lung may attract pulmonary alveolar macrophages, which are capable of metabolizing polycyclic hydrocarbons to carcinogenic metabolites. (4) Asbestos fibers may adsorb, concentrate, and slowly release carcinogens from tobacco smoke.

The latency for lung cancer in asbestos workers is about 20 years. Although control of asbestos expo-

**Table 42–4.** Attributable risk of death of lung cancer from smoking and asbestos exposure.[1]

| | |
|---|---|
| Total deaths | 1946 |
| Lung cancer deaths | 450 |
| Deaths attributable to: | |
| Cigarette smoking alone | 94 |
| Asbestos exposure alone | 44 |
| Smoking and asbestos | 303 |
| Deaths unrelated to smoking or asbestos | 9 |

[1]Modified from Selikoff IJ: Two comments on smoking and the workplace. (Letter.) Am J Public Health 1981;71:92.

sure has improved considerably in recent years, many workers have large body burdens of asbestos. The multiple-step carcinogenesis model strongly points toward smoking cessation as an intervention that could reduce the cancer risk prior to development of cancer. Thus, for workers already exposed to asbestos, the single most important way to decrease the risk of lung cancer is to stop smoking.

## Smoking, Uranium Mining, & Cancer

Studies have shown a relationship between cumulative radiation exposure and the risk of bronchogenic cancer. Cigarette smoking substantially amplifies lung cancer rates, particularly at high radiation levels (Figure 42–1).

Uranium and other metal ores release radon gas, which decays to daughters, two of which are alpha radiation emitters. The alpha-ray radiation, when present in close proximity to bronchial cells, causes local damage and ultimately neoplasm formation. Radioactive gases may adsorb onto particles which are then inhaled and deposited in the lung. Cigarette smoke may be an important source of particles for delivery of radiation to the lung. Tobacco itself is also a source of polonium-210. Therefore, smokers could have an additive radiation risk in addition to the risk from other sources of radiation. The carcinogenic effect of radiation is believed to be promoted

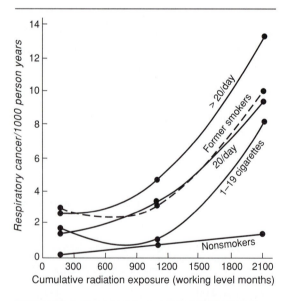

**Figure 42–1.** Dose-response relationship between cumulative radiation exposure (working level months) and respiratory cancer rate in uranium miners. Cigarette smoking amplifies the cancer rate, particularly at higher radiation exposure levels. (From Archer VE, Gillam JD, Wagoner JK: Respiratory disease mortality among uranium miners. Ann N Y Acad Sci 1976;271:280.)

by toxic materials in tobacco smoke, which would explain shorter onset and latency times to cancer development in uranium miners who are smokers.

## Chloromethyl Ethers: Can Smoking Protect Against Occupational Cancer?

Chloromethyl ether and bischloromethyl ether (a contaminant) are known to be carcinogenic in animals and humans. Chemical production workers exposed to chloromethyl ether experience a higher than normal incidence of respiratory cancer, characterized by a short latency interval and a small cell histologic type. In a prospective study of 125 production workers, cancer was associated in a dose-related fashion to chloromethyl ether exposure but inversely related to the number of cigarettes smoked.

Chloromethyl ether and bischloromethyl ether are alkylating chemicals that are believed to produce cancer by actions on DNA. It is hypothesized that the presence of bronchorrhea due to smoking-related chronic bronchitis dilutes, degrades, or accelerates clearance of chloromethyl ethers.

An alternative explanation for the "protective" effect of smoking is self-selection, such that workers heavily exposed to chloromethyl ether, which produces respiratory irritation and dyspnea, are less likely to smoke.

## Lung Cancer in Workers: Occupation Versus Smoking

There is convincing evidence in asbestos workers and uranium ore miners that smoking shifts the dose-response curve for occupational exposure, resulting in many more occupational cancers. Pastorino and coworkers (1984) attempted to determine the relative importance of occupation and smoking in causing lung cancer in a general population. In a study of all men in an industrial region of northern Italy, they identified 204 cases of lung cancer and 351 controls in whom occupational histories could be obtained. Subjects were classified as occupationally exposed if they worked with any of the following suspected respiratory carcinogens: asbestos, polycyclic aromatic hydrocarbons, arsenic, nickel, chromium, bischloromethyl ether, chloromethyl ether, and vinyl chloride. About 80% of the population were cigarette smokers. The relative risk of lung cancer was increased in workers with occupational exposure—and in a dose-dependent manner for cigarette smokers (Figure 42–2). At all smoking levels, the risk for exposed workers was twofold, indicating a multiplicative effect. Overall, 33% (95% confidence interval, 19.1–46.9%) of cases were attributable to occupational exposure (without modifying tobacco exposure) and 81% (95% confidence interval, 68.8–93.2%) to smoking (without modifying occupation).

This study indicates that in a general industrial

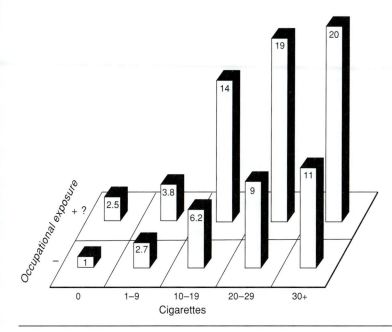

**Figure 42–2.** Risk of lung cancer in men in the Lombardy region of Italy as a function of occupational exposure (to chemicals known to cause lung cancer in humans) and daily cigarette consumption. Risks of occupational exposure and smoking are multiplicative. (Data from Pastorino V et al: Proportion of lung cancers due to occupational exposure. Int J Cancer 1984;33:231.)

worker population, occupational exposure to chemicals is a significant cause of cancer but that most of it would be prevented by smoking control. It also illustrates how an association between occupational chemical exposure and lung cancer risk might easily be missed where there is a high proportion of cigarette smokers in the work force unless very large worker populations are studied.

## SMOKING & OCCUPATIONAL LUNG DISEASE

The major occupational chronic lung diseases are bronchitis, pneumoconiosis (fibrotic disease of the lung parenchyma), and occupational asthma. Cigarette smoking is clearly the major cause of chronic bronchitis and chronic obstructive lung disease and may also produce airway constriction in asthmatics. The net impairment of pulmonary function in workers is the sum of the influences of cigarette smoking, occupational exposures, and other factors such as genetic deficiency of $\alpha_1$-antitrypsin.

### Pathology & Pathophysiology of Smoking-Related Lung Disease

Chronic bronchitis—characterized by increased size of mucous glands, increased numbers of goblet cells, and mucus hypersecretion—is a nonspecific response to chronic irritant exposure. It may result either from cigarette smoking or from exposure to a variety of chemicals or dusts. The risks of chronic bronchitis from smoking and occupational exposure to dusts are additive in most studies, with the largest

percentages of cases today attributable to cigarette smoking. Chronic bronchitis may be associated with reduced airflow at high lung volumes, consistent with large airway disease.

Chronic obstructive lung disease is the lung disease most specific for cigarette smoking. Small-airway injury is common in smokers even without symptoms. Pulmonary function tests in smokers commonly reveal reduction of maximum midexpiratory flow rates, a manifestation of small-airway disease.

Emphysema is a more advanced stage of smoking-related chronic lung disease in which destruction of alveolar walls results in airflow obstruction, increased lung compliance and total lung capacity, and decreased diffusing capacity for carbon monoxide. The pathophysiology of smoking-related emphysema is believed to involve exposure to oxidant gases with concomitant impairment of antioxidant protective mechanisms such as $\alpha_1$-antitrypsin activity. Migration of neutrophils into the lung, which may be mediated in part by the effects of nicotine, may contribute to oxidant injury of membranes. Typically, the pattern of smoking-related emphysema is centrilobular.

Exposure to mineral dusts, such as coal or silica, may also produce small airway disease, with fibrosis of small airways and, later, focal emphysema. Typically, such disease is asymptomatic. Parenchymal lung disease with diffuse fibrosis may occur with asbestosis, silicosis, or coal miner's pneumoconiosis. Chest x-rays usually show parenchymal opacities ranging in size from less than 1 cm to massive fibrosis that involves large portions of the lung, and pulmonary function tests reveal severe restrictive disease, though there may be an element of obstructive disease as well. Findings of advanced pneumoconiosis are generally distinguishable from those associated with tobacco-related emphysema.

Cigarette smoking, including passive smoke exposure, may increase the degree of airway obstruction in asthmatics. Smoking increases the risk of sensitization to occupational allergies and would be expected to aggravate occupational asthma from any cause. Specific examples of interactions between occupational exposures and cigarette exposures in causing disease are shown in Table 42–5.

A good example of the interaction between smoking and occupation in causing acute respiratory disease is byssinosis in textile workers exposed to cotton dust. Some workers develop bronchitis or chest tightness after exposure to cotton dust, typically following a weekend or holiday when they have not been exposed. Pulmonary function tests indicate acute bronchoconstriction resembling asthma. The severity of symptoms is related both to the magnitude of cotton dust exposure and to whether or not the worker is a cigarette smoker. The symptoms and the magnitude of the pulmonary function test abnor-

malities are greatest in workers with higher dust exposure. Symptoms and manifestations are much more severe with the same level of cotton dust in smokers.

Although controversial, there are also reports of chronic airway disease in cotton textile workers, most severe in smokers but occurring also in nonsmokers. The interaction between smoking and cotton dust exposure has provoked debate concerning workers' compensation and regulatory issues; clearly, control of both risk factors should be goals of occupational health programs.

## PASSIVE SMOKING

### Mainstream Versus Sidestream Cigarette Smoke

On average, 75% of the smoke generated in smoking a cigarette is released into the environment. Sidestream smoke—that which is released into the environment—comes from tobacco burned at a higher temperature with less oxygen compared to mainstream smoke. Concentrations of various toxic chemicals, including polycyclic aromatic hydrocarbons,

**Table 42–5.** Interactions between occupation and cigarette smoking in causing disease.

| Occupation | Exposure | Disease | Smoking-Occupation Interaction |
|---|---|---|---|
| Asbestos workers | Asbestos | Lung cancer | Multiplicative |
| | | Chronic lung disease (restrictive, obstructive) | Additive |
| Aluminum smelter workers | Polynuclear hydrocarbons | Bladder cancer | Additive or multiplicative |
| Cement workers | Cement dust | Chronic bronchitis, obstructive lung disease | Additive |
| Chlorine manufacturing | Chlorine | Chronic obstructive lung disease | Additive |
| Coal miners | Coal dust | Chronic obstructive lung disease | Additive |
| Copper smelter workers | Sulfur dioxide | Chronic obstructive lung disease | Additive |
| | Arsenic | Lung cancer | Additive or multiplicative |
| Grain workers | Grain dust | Chronic bronchitis, obstructive lung disease | Additive |
| Rock cutters, foundry workers | Silica dust | Obstructive lung disease | Additive |
| Textile workers | Cotton, hemp, flax dust | Acute airway obstruction (byssinosis) | Possibly multiplicative |
| | | Chronic bronchitis | Additive |
| Uranium miners | Alpha radiation | Lung cancer | Additive or multiplicative |
| Welders | Irritant gases, metal fumes, dusts | Chronic bronchitis, obstructive lung disease | Additive |

are higher in sidestream compared to mainstream smoke. Sidestream smoke condensate is more carcinogenic than mainstream smoke condensate. Irritant gases such as formaldehyde, ammonia, and volatile nitrosamines are present in far greater concentration in sidestream than in mainstream smoke.

## Evidence That Nonsmokers Inhale Cigarette Smoke

Several studies have provided evidence of tobacco smoke components in the environment and in biological fluids of nonsmokers. Biochemical measures have included plasma, saliva, and urinary nicotine and cotinine (the latter a metabolite of nicotine). Cotinine excretion in the urine of nonsmokers exposed to other cigarette smokers in the home and in the urine of those exposed in the workplace are equivalent. Exposure in both places results in an additive increase in cotinine excretion (Figure 42–3). From urinary cotinine data, it is estimated that nonsmokers

with exposure to environmental tobacco smoke (ETS) typically absorb a dose of nicotine equivalent to one sixth to one third of a cigarette; however, with heavy ETS exposure, the amount of nicotine may be equivalent to as much as one to two cigarettes per day. There is overlap in the intake of heavily passively exposed nonsmokers and light primary smokers.

## Health Hazards of Passive Smoking

A number of studies have indicated that passive cigarette smoke exposure may present health hazards. Exposure of a nonsmoker to cigarette smoke is well known to be a source of annoyance, primarily because of eye irritation, nose irritation, and malodor. That passive smoking may affect pulmonary function is supported by observations in children whose mothers smoke, ie, a higher incidence of respiratory infection during the first year of life, exacerbation of asthma, and evidence of reduced pulmonary function. In adults, passive smoke exposure may aggravate angina pectoris or asthma and may result in mild impairment of small-airway pulmonary function, although the lifelong significance of the latter is unclear. Several epidemiologic studies have found an association between ETS exposure and an increased risk of myocardial infarction in nonsmokers with spouses who smoke. On average, ETS exposure has been associated with a 30% increase in the risk of coronary heart disease, which has been estimated to cause as many as 37,000 premature deaths in the United States annually.

## Cancer & Passive Smoke Exposure

Many studies have reported an increased risk of lung cancer in nonsmokers who are passively exposed to cigarette smoke. The first report was of a study of 142,800 women in Tokyo, of whom 91,500 were nonsmoking wives. In a 14-year follow-up prospective study, there were 346 cases of lung cancer, including 174 in nonsmoking wives. The relative risk for lung cancer in women who were smokers compared with women who neither smoked nor had a spouse who smoked was 3.8. The relative risk of lung cancer in nonsmoking wives with husbands who smoke was 1.6 if husbands smoked less than 20 cigarettes a day and 2.1 if husbands smoked more than 20 cigarettes a day. Since most men in Japan at the time of the study smoked cigarettes and most women did not, passive smoke exposure appeared to be the most important cause of lung cancer in Japanese women.

A number of criticisms of the Japanese study have been voiced, including questions about statistical methods and comments about cultural differences between Japanese and American wives, raising a question about relevance of the results for American

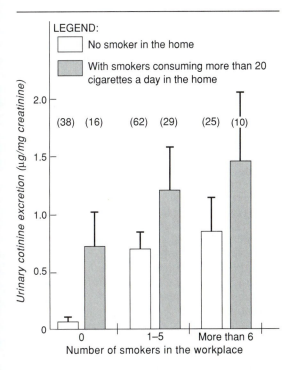

**Figure 42–3.** Intake of environmental tobacco smoke by nonsmokers as a function of number of smokers in the workplace. Cotinine is a metabolite of nicotine. Urinary cotinine is an indicator of nicotine intake. Intake after workplace and home exposures are additive. Figures in parentheses indicate numbers of subjects in each group. Bars indicate SEM. (Data from Matsukura S et al: Effects of environmental tobacco smoke on urinary cotinine excretion in nonsmokers: Evidence for passive smoking. N Engl J Med 1984;311:828.)

women. Subsequently, more than 30 cohort or case-control studies from many countries have been published. Most studies have found an increased risk of lung cancer in nonsmokers married to smokers compared with those not married to smokers, including several studies showing a risk that is proportional to the number of cigarettes that the spouse smoked.

A problem in many of these studies is the difficulty of measuring the extent of passive smoke exposure. The studies also suffer from the absence of occupational and other environmental tobacco smoke exposure data. This is a more significant problem in the American studies because a larger percentage of American women—compared with women from other countries where studies were conducted—work outside the home, where they might be exposed to tobacco smoke or other chemical toxins.

Recently, the US Environmental Protection Agency (EPA) has reviewed the world literature and has concluded that environmental tobacco smoke is a class A carcinogen, meaning that it has been shown to cause cancer in humans. The relative risk was estimated to be about 1.2, accounting for an estimated 3000 lung cancer deaths annually in the United States.

In addition to lung cancer, there are reports indicating an increased risk of cervical and other smoking-related cancers in nonsmoking spouses of smokers.

## Passive Smoking & Workplace Illness

Workplace exposure to cigarette smoke can result in significant smoke intake, and passive smoke exposure may be related to impaired respiratory function and an increased risk of lung cancer in nonsmokers. For nonsmokers sharing a work environment with cigarette smokers, the workplace must be considered hazardous independently of any specific industrial toxic exposure. This risk is particularly important when a high percentage of the workers smoke or where smokers and nonsmokers work in poorly ventilated areas.

Another concern is that passive smoke exposure may act synergistically—as does primary smoking—with toxic industrial materials to amplify the dose-response curve for those substances. Although there is no empiric evidence to support this hypothesis at present, the possibility must be considered.

Asthma in adults has been reported to be aggravated by ETS, although research is conflicting. When exposed to ETS, nonsmokers often complain of eye irritation, nasal congestion, headaches, and coughing. Although these symptoms are prevalent in nonsmokers with exposure to ETS, they are more severe in people who have a history of allergies. The increased risk of respiratory tract infection, asthma, and middle ear effusion in infants and children exposed to ETS

provides a basis for mandating that child-care facilities be smoke free.

## CONTROL OF SMOKING IN THE WORKPLACE

If the goal of an occupational health program is to prevent illness and disability, the most effective way to do so is by control of cigarette smoking. The importance of controlling exposure to potentially toxic industrial chemicals is obvious, but total elimination of exposure is often impossible. An optimal employee health program should include simultaneous control of toxic exposures and smoking. A smoking control program should include both programs to encourage smoking cessation and environmental control measures to protect nonsmokers from tobacco smoke of their colleagues.

### Smoking Cessation Strategies

Three general strategies are available for control of workplace smoking. The first is development of programs to encourage employees to quit smoking by physician counseling, educational activities, and either offering smoking cessation programs on the job or by paid referral of workers to outside smoking cessation programs such as those made available through the American Cancer Society or the American Lung Association. Some businesses also offer various incentives for employees to quit smoking. Optimally, smoking cessation programs should be sponsored jointly by management and labor.

A second strategy is restricting or prohibiting smoking in the workplace. Most large US companies now restrict smoking in common work areas. However, many small businesses do not have such restrictions. Of note, smoking restrictions in the workplace result in smokers smoking fewer cigarettes each day and increase the likelihood that smokers will quit.

A third strategy is not to hire cigarette smokers. When the risks of smoking and occupational exposure are clearly synergistic, such as with asbestos exposure or uranium mining, not hiring smokers seems quite sensible.

### Control of Passive Smoke Exposure

The concentration of tobacco smoke in a room depends upon the size of the room, the number of smokers, the extent of ventilation, and other factors such as the nature of wall surfaces. Ventilation with outside air or the use of high-efficiency filtration systems substantially reduces smoke concentrations and is required at a minimum for workplace control of cigarette smoke. But even with good ventilation, such as with central air conditioning systems, substantial concentrations of carbon monoxide and particulates are found in the workplace. Ventilation alone is not adequate.

Segregation of smokers and nonsmokers by space alone is partially effective, but primarily for particulates. The greater the ratio of smoking to nonsmoking areas, the less effective the segregation. Placing physical barriers between smoking and nonsmoking areas may be more effective, but the effectiveness depends on the air flow between the segregated areas. If it is not possible to place smokers and nonsmokers in separate rooms, barriers are better than nothing.

Prohibition of smoking at the work site is the most effective way to reduce environmental smoke concentrations. Restricting workplace smoking so as to provide a smoke-free workplace for nonsmokers has been mandated legislatively in a number of communities. Compliance with such local ordinances has been good, and enforcement has not been a major problem.

Air quality standards and permissible occupational exposure levels relevant to tobacco smoke components should be developed, monitored, and enforced. This may be an important area of activity for the Occupational Safety and Health Administration (OSHA).

Finally, where there is not adequate environmental control of cigarette smoke, nonsmoking workers should be advised of and given the opportunity to accept or reject the health risks of passive smoke exposure, as would be the case for workers in other hazardous environments.

# REFERENCES

## CIGARETTE SMOKING & DISEASE: GENERAL CONSIDERATIONS

Benowitz NL: Cigarette smoking and nicotine addiction. Med Clin North Am 1992;76:415.

Centers for Disease Control: The health benefits of smoking cessation. *A Report of the Surgeon General, 1990.* DHHS Publication no. (CDC) 90-8416. US Department of Health and Human Services, 1990.

MacKenzie TD et al: The human costs of tobacco use (first of two parts). N Engl J Med 1994;330:907.

MacKenzie TD et al: The human costs of tobacco use (second of two parts). N Engl J Med 1994;330:975.

Peto R et al: Mortality from tobacco in developed countries: Indirect estimation from national vital statistics. Lancet 1992;339:1268.

Surgeon General of the United States: *Smoking and Health in the Americas: A Report of the Surgeon General.* US Department of Health and Human Services, 1992.

Surgeon General of the United States: *The Health Benefits of Smoking Cessation: A Report of the Surgeon General.* US Department of Health and Human Services, 1990.

## GENERAL RESOURCE

Office on Smoking and Health (OSH)
National Center for Chronic Disease Prevention and Health Promotion
Centers for Disease Control and Prevention
Mailstop K-50
4770 Buford Highway, N.E.
Atlanta, GA 30341-3724
(770) 488-5705

## OCCUPATION & SMOKING BEHAVIOR

Covey et al: Cigarette smoking and occupational status: 1970 to 1990. Am J Public Health 1992;82:230.

## INTERACTIONS BETWEEN SMOKING & OCCUPATION

Penner M, Penner S: Excess insured health care costs from tobacco-using employees in a large group plan. J Occup Med 1990;32:521.

Ryan R, Zwerling C, Orav J: Occupational risks associated with cigarette smoking: A prospective study. Am J Public Health 1992;82:29.

## SMOKING & OCCUPATIONAL CANCER

Jarup L, Pershagen G: Arsenic exposure, smoking, and lung cancer in smelter workers—A case-control study. Am J Epidemiol 1991;134:545.

Newcomb PA, Carbone PP: The health consequences of smoking. Med Clin North Am 1992;76:305.

## SMOKING & OCCUPATIONAL LUNG DISEASE OTHER THAN CANCER

Bates DV et al: Prevention of occupational lung disease. Chest 1992;102(Suppl):257S.

## PASSIVE SMOKING

Byrd J: Environmental tobacco smoke: Medical and legal issues. Med Clin North Am 1992;76:377.

Chilmonczyk BA et al: Association between exposure to environmental tobacco smoke and exacerbations of asthma in children. N Engl J Med 1993;328:1665.

Environmental Protection Agency: *Respiratory Health Effects of Passive Smoking: Lung Cancer and Other Disorders.* US Environmental Protection Agency Document No. EPA/600/6-90/006F. US Environmental Protection Agency, 1992.

Siegel M: Involuntary smoking in the restaurant workplace—A review of employee exposure and health effects. JAMA 1993;270:490.

Steenland K: Passive smoking and the risk of heart disease. JAMA 1992;267:94.

## CONTROL OF SMOKING
## IN THE WORKPLACE

Betera RL: The effects of behavioral risks on absenteeism and health-care costs in the workplace. J Occup Med 1991:33:1119.

Brigham J et al: Effects of a restricted work-site smoking policy on employees who smoke. Am J Public Health 1994;84:773.

Hocking B et al: A total ban on workplace smoking is acceptable and effective. J Occup Med 1991;33:163.

Lewitt EM: Responses among New Jersey's largest employers to legislation restricting smoking at the work site. Am J Ind Med 1992;22:385.

Sorensen G et al: Effects of a worksite nonsmoking policy: evidence for increased cessation. Am J Public Health 1991;81:202.

Sorensen G et al: Work-site smoking policies in small businesses. J Occup Med 1991;33:980.

Wakefield MA et al: Workplace smoking restrictions, occupational status, and reduced cigarette consumption. J Occup Med 1992;34:693.

# Building-Associated Illnesses

43

*Michael L. Fischman, MD, MPH*

The Clean Air Act, passed in the mid 1960s, focused national attention on cleaning up outdoor air but directed little interest toward improving the quality of indoor air—although people spend only 10–20% of their time out-of-doors and the rest of their time indoors at home or at work. Until recently, buildings and homes were thought to pose to occupants little hazards from pollutants trapped inside structures. Recent studies confirm that concentrations of pollutants inside buildings may greatly exceed standards established for outdoor concentrations.

Indoor air contamination has been linked to a wide variety of building materials and consumer products. The problem is exacerbated by concerns about energy conservation that have led to decreasing air turnover in homes, offices, and other buildings.

## TYPES OF BUILDING-ASSOCIATED ILLNESSES & HEALTH CONCERNS

It is possible to divide building-associated illnesses into two categories: (1) acute short-latency illnesses and (2) potential chronic long-latency illnesses. The nature of the exposures that may give rise to each type differs substantially. The term building-associated illnesses is reserved for health problems that develop in settings customarily considered nonhazardous (eg, homes and offices). A classification scheme for building-associated illness is presented in Table 43–1.

Short-latency illnesses include sick building syndrome, mass psychogenic illness, specific illnesses resulting from identifiable sources of noxious materials, certain infectious diseases, and building-associated hypersensitivity pneumonitis. In 1987, a committee on indoor air quality for the National Research Council defined building-related illnesses as those specific clinical syndromes that result from exposure to indoor air contaminants (eg, hypersensitivity pneumonitis or Legionnaires' disease). In contrast, sick building syndrome refers to the occurrence, in more than 20% of the work population, of a variety of nonspecific symptoms, wherein it is not possible to make

a specific diagnosis. These conditions are characterized by a relatively acute onset, closely related in time to the individual's presence within the building and often relieved by removal from further exposure. Some of the building-related illnesses do not resolve promptly upon leaving the building.

In contrast, the long-latency illnesses include cancer and chronic pulmonary diseases, which may result from long-term, low-level exposure to contaminants of indoor air. Because of the long induction-latency periods for these conditions and their multifactorial origin, it is much more difficult to establish a causal link to the building exposure. Agents in indoor air that may be responsible for such illnesses include cigarette smoke, asbestos, radon gas, oxides of nitrogen, polycyclic aromatic hydrocarbons, and chlorinated hydrocarbon insecticides.

The relationship of these long-latency illnesses to indoor air pollution is generally speculative. Estimates of incidence are predicated often on the basis of mathematical extrapolations from high-dose industrial or animal experimental exposures to substances encountered in lower doses in building environments.

There are more data suggesting a problem with cigarette smoke than with any other agents (see Chapter 42). Indoor asbestos exposure occurs at very low levels unless the insulation materials are disturbed or improperly removed. Exposure to low levels of radioactivity occurs in the form of radon gas from building materials and soil underlying basements or foundations. Polycyclic aromatic hydrocarbons are released into indoor air from wood-burning fireplaces and other sources. Based on the increased risk of lung cancer in much more heavily exposed asbestos workers, uranium miners, and coke oven workers, respectively, there is some concern about the impact of these agents on lung cancer incidence in the general population.

Certain products of combustion, such as oxides of nitrogen from unvented gas appliances, may pose long-term health risks. There is limited epidemiologic evidence suggesting increased respiratory infections and reduced performance on pulmonary

**Table 43–1.** Types of building-associated illness.

**Short-latency illnesses**
  Sick building syndrome
  Mass psychogenic illness
  Building-associated hypersensitivity pneumonitis
  Building-associated infections
    Legionnaires' disease
    Pontiac fever
    Q fever
  Illnesses associated with specific contaminants
**Possible long-latency illnesses**
  Lung cancer
  Chronic nonmalignant respiratory disease

function testing associated with exposure to gas stove emissions.

## NATURE, SOURCES, & CONCENTRATIONS OF EXPOSURES

Potential sources of indoor air contaminants can be classified as follows: (1) contaminants released from the building or its contents, including asbestos, formaldehyde, and radon; (2) contaminants generated by such diverse human activities as cooking, heating, cigarette smoking, and cleaning; and (3) infiltrated contaminants—agents that enter the house or building along with the outside air, but in lower concentration (typically 25–75%).

The concentration of contaminants is influenced not only by the source of exposure but also by the exchange rate between indoor and outdoor air. The introduction of outdoor air into a home or building occurs either by implemented ventilation or by infiltration. Infiltration occurs through cracks or other leaks in the structure or through open doors or windows. The amount of infiltration is dependent on the type of building, the amount of insulation and other weather-proofing, and climatic conditions. Implemented ventilation (eg, forced-air heating or air conditioning systems) may provide substantial amounts of outdoor air but may also be designed to recirculate preconditioned air with minimal fresh air intake.

The amount of fresh air exchange is often expressed in air changes per hour (ACH). ACH may vary from 0.2 in tightly sealed homes to 0.7 in an average home to 60 or more in some industrial settings with implemented ventilation. Alternatively, with implemented ventilation, the amount of outdoor air supplied may be expressed in cubic feet per minute (cfm) or cfm per occupant. The concentration of contaminants at any location within a building will be influenced by the location of the source and the degree of air mixing. In the case of reactive or particulate contaminants, the concentration will be affected by the rate of chemical reaction or the rate of deposition, respectively.

## EVALUATION OF BUILDING-ASSOCIATED ILLNESS

Proper assessment of illnesses relating to indoor air quality involves both evaluation of the symptoms, usually by a physician, and assessment of the work environment, usually by an industrial hygienist. A symptom questionnaire may be helpful in establishing the nature, chronology, and frequency of complaints, the locations at which complaints arise, any incidents or activities that preceded the complaints, and the coexistence of any medical problems or risk factors that might account for some of the symptoms. Alternatively or in addition, personal interviews and targeted physical examinations of affected employees may be useful. Analysis of the symptom data, with grouping of symptoms into categories and searching for factors associated with symptom occurrence across the population, is essential.

Industrial hygiene evaluation should begin with gathering of background information on the building, such as its age, type of construction, ventilation system design, and history of renovations and repairs. A walk-through survey will permit an appreciation of the floor plan and the physical locations at which symptoms have occurred as well as inspection of the ventilation system and any possible point sources of air contaminants (eg, blueprint machines, cleaning supplies, and cafeteria equipment).

Guidelines for temperature and humidity control to achieve a comfort zone for the majority of occupants have been issued by the American Society of Heating, Refrigeration, and Air Conditioning Engineers (ASHRAE). For slightly active or sedentary individuals in office buildings, this zone lies between 73 and 77° F and between 30% and 60% relative humidity. Relative humidity levels below 20% often result in drying of mucous membranes, with associated discomfort. Depending upon the ventilation system design, there may be localized areas with within buildings that fall outside the comfort zone even though the rest of the building is adequately controlled.

ASHRAE has also issued guidelines for provision of adequate amounts of fresh outside air. For office areas, outside air should be provided at a rate of 20 cubic feet per minute (cfm) per occupant (no less than 15 cfm per person for certain other nonresidential buildings).

Limited environmental monitoring may be helpful in assessing the adequacy of ventilation, including the extent of fresh versus recirculated air, temperature, and humidity control. Minimal equipment is required for this monitoring—a room thermometer and relative humidity meter, smoke tubes to assess air movement, and direct-reading carbon dioxide colorimetric detector tubes.

Because carbon dioxide is a product of respiratory metabolism, its accumulation in office buildings reflects a balance between generation by building occupants and removal through ventilation and introduction of fresh outdoor air. Measurement of $CO_2$ levels aids in evaluating whether sufficient quantities of fresh air are being introduced into the building. The outdoor concentration of $CO_2$ varies typically from 250 to 350 ppm. The presence of $CO_2$ in concentrations above 1000 ppm inside the building suggests inadequate fresh air ventilation. In prior building investigations, levels above 1000 ppm of $CO_2$ are often associated with complaints of headache and mucous membrane irritation. Though the $CO_2$ itself is clearly not responsible for these symptoms, a high concentration suggests that other air contaminant levels are likely to be increased; in other words, the $CO_2$ level serves as a surrogate measure for the presence of other as yet unidentified contaminants likely to be the cause of these symptoms. A ventilation rate of 15 cfm per person will generally keep $CO_2$ levels below 1000 ppm. Ellenbecker indicated that indoor air quality complaints occur occasionally with concentrations of $CO_2$ as low as 700–800 ppm. Increasing the fresh air ventilation rate to 25 cfm per person will reduce the $CO_2$ concentration below this level, often resulting in a subsidence of symptoms. Table 43–2 lists some guidelines for factors impacting indoor air quality.

Further and more specific air sampling should be performed if significant sources of air contaminants are identified or suspected. In the absence of such point sources, however, it is quite unlikely that extensive untargeted industrial hygiene sampling will identify an unrecognized contaminant in concentrations sufficient to cause symptoms. Such sampling will typically be quite expensive. Moreover, in part because of the very high sensitivity of available ana-

lytical methodology, sampling will invariably detect some contaminants. Daisey et al studied 12 buildings with three types of building ventilation (naturally ventilated, mechanically ventilated with operable windows and no air conditioning, and mechanically ventilated with sealed windows and air conditioning) in the San Francisco Bay area, only one of which was a sick building. Excluding the two buildings with liquid-process photocopiers (known sources of volatile organic compounds), the median total volatile organic compound (TVOC concentration was 410 $mcg/m^3$. The level of TVOC did not vary appreciably with the three types of building ventilation, nor were the levels higher in the problem building. Geometric mean (GM) concentrations of individual volatile organic compounds were less than 5 ppb, with the exception of ethanol (19 ppb GM). There was considerable variability in the chemical composition of the volatile organic compound (VOC) mixtures in the different buildings. Oxidized hydrocarbons, including ethanol, accounted for the largest proportion of the VOCs in almost all of the buildings. A variety of chlorinated hydrocarbons, alkanes, and aromatic hydrocarbons were also detected; the latter two groups being predominantly of outdoor origin from motor vehicle emissions.

## RESULTS OBTAINED FROM BUILDING INVESTIGATIONS

Investigators at the National Institute for Occupational Safety and Health have reported the results of their evaluations, through December, 1986, of 446 buildings with indoor air quality problems. Although

**Table 43–2.** Relevant guidelines for indoor air quality.

| Factor | Guideline/Study Finding | Comment |
|---|---|---|
| Temperature | 73–77° F<br><72°[a] | ASHRAE guideline<br>Reduced prevalence of SBS symptoms[a] |
| Relative humidity | 30–60%<br>>35%[a] | ASHRAE guideline<br>Reduced prevalence of SBS symptoms[a] |
| Fresh outside air | 20 cfm per occupant | ASHRAE guideline |
| Carbon dioxide | 1,000 ppm<br>650 ppm | Japanese standard/consensus[b]<br>Massachusetts (recommended)[b] |
| Total volatile organic compounds (TVOC) | No guideline | |
| Formaldehyde | 0.1 ppm | ASHRAE guideline[b] |

[a]See text for relevant study.
[b]Source: Spengler and Samet.

they recognized that some of the problems may have had multiple causes, they were able to classify the results by the primary identified cause. In 32% of the evaluations, building ventilation was found to be inadequate, as evidenced by inadequate fresh air intake, poor air distribution and mixing, draftiness, poor temperature and humidity control, pressure differences between office spaces, or air filtration problems. Inside sources accounted for 17% of the problems, and included contaminants from various types of wet copiers, improper pesticide application, improper use of cleaning agents such as rug shampoo, tobacco smoke, and combustion gases (eg, from cafeterias). Such contaminants were present at levels above the normal background but far below any permissible exposure limits. Outside contamination sources were the primary factor in 11% of the investigations, generally due to entrainment of contaminated outside air as a result of improperly located exhaust and intake vents or contaminant generation near intake vents. One of the most common identified sources was the entrainment of vehicle exhaust fumes from parking garages into the air intake vent. Other contaminants included boiler gases, previously exhausted air, and asphalt from roofing operations. Microbiologic contamination accounted for 3% of the problems, resulting from standing water in ventilation system components or from water damage to carpets or other furnishings. A variety of disorders—hypersensitivity pneumonitis, humidifier fever, allergic rhinitis and possibly allergic asthma, infrequently, and conjunctivitis—can arise from microbial contaminants. Building materials were the source of contaminants in 3% of the investigations, including materials such as particle board, plywood, urea-formaldehyde foam insulation, and some glues and adhesives. In 12% of the investigations, the factor or factors involved remained unknown.

Though they did not list it as a primary cause, the NIOSH investigators indicated that tobacco smoke may be a major contributor to indoor air quality problems, largely because it contains numerous irritant compounds. The significance of environmental tobacco smoke in the induction of closed-building syndrome or other building-related illness remains a hotly debated subject. There is no question that heavy cigarette use, when combined with poor ventilation, can result in high levels of environmental tobacco smoke that may result in irritant symptoms in crowded areas such as cafeterias or lobbies. In the more typical office building environment, the extent to which tobacco smoke contributes to indoor air quality problems is less clear and probably depends on ventilation and fresh air intake rates as well as on smoker density. Some investigators have demonstrated significant increases in respirable particulate concentrations in buildings where smoking is permitted relative to comparable nonsmoking buildings. Urinary levels of cotinine, a metabolite of nicotine,

increase in a clear dose-response relationship with increasing exposure to environmental tobacco smoke in a variety of settings.

Survey results indicate that many office workers feel that smoke generated by coworkers impairs their productivity. Other surveys suggest that contact lens wearers and allergic individuals may be more susceptible to irritant effects of tobacco smoke. Because of nonsmoking policies implemented in many workplaces in recent years, environmental tobacco smoke is now a less frequent contributor to indoor air quality problems in nonresidential buildings.

# SHORT-LATENCY ILLNESSES

## SICK BUILDING SYNDROME

The term sick building syndrome (previously referred to as closed building syndrome or tight building syndrome) denotes a characteristic set of symptoms, typically headache and mucous membrane irritation, recognized among occupants of nonindustrial buildings, such as offices and schools. In most cases, the syndrome has occurred in relatively new buildings with centrally controlled ventilation systems and without operable windows. In many cases, the buildings were tightly sealed to prevent the infiltration of outside air, hence the concept of closed or tight building syndrome. Many sealed structures were built in the 1970s and 1980s in accordance with ventilation engineering standards designed to conserve energy.

### Occurrence & Etiology
The incidence of sick building syndrome is unknown, but reported outbreaks of illnesses consistent with this diagnosis have increased dramatically in recent years. Thirteen percent of requests to NIOSH for health hazard evaluations were to investigate health complaints attributed to the building (in nonindustrial workplaces). Outbreaks have occurred chiefly in government offices, business offices, and schools or colleges.

The contaminants responsible for this syndrome have not been identified. Despite extensive measurements for a wide variety of possible contaminants, no substances have been found to be consistently present in concentrations judged sufficient to induce symptoms. One common feature present in virtually all afflicted buildings is a central ventilation system that depends on a significant proportion of recirculated air. Once of the more widely held theories is that this ventilation design permits the accumulation of low levels of many contaminants—volatile organic, compounds, aldehydes, cigarette smoke, etc—which together induce the symptoms. In five published experimental or cross-sectional studies, as pointed out by Mendell and Fine, the prevalence of symptoms of sick building syndrome was significantly higher at lower outdoor air ventilation rate (when one or both of the compared rates was at or below 21 cfm per person). In contrast, when both rates were above 21 cfm per occupant, there was no difference in symptom prevalence between the two ventilation rates. These findings tend to support the above hypothesis. However, in a recent blinded cross-over study by Jaakkola et al, symptom scores did not differ between the two phases (70% recirculated air, 13 cfm per person of outdoor air compared to 0% recirculated air, 42 cfm per person of outdoor air). This inconsistency probably reflects the substantial differences between buildings and the multitude of factors, in addition to outdoor air ventilation rate, which may affect indoor air quality.

There are a number of potential sources for air contaminants in the office environment. Formaldehyde is present in and evaporates from resins in particleboard and plywood (used in furniture and construction materials) and furnishings (including carpets and draperies). Other sources include cigarette smoke and unvented gas appliances. Volatile organic compounds may evaporate from carpet glues and drying paints. Releases from photocopiers and other office equipment may also contribute to the symptoms.

Dryness of indoor air may contribute to some of the symptoms of sick building syndrome. Blinded experimental studies of office workers and hospital workers have demonstrated a reduction in symptoms of dryness of mucous membranes (eye and throat dryness or irritation) and skin (dryness, irritation, and itching) with air humidification of up to 35–45% compared to control conditions of about 25–35%. There was also a reduction in perceived air dryness. An allergic symptom score (considering nasal congestion and excretion and sneezing) was also significantly reduced during humidification for the office workers. Given that relative humidity often falls in indoor environments during the heating season, low humidity may play a significant role in the induction of symptoms of sick building syndrome in some situations. Jaakkola et al also point out that two studies have suggested that room temperatures greater than 22 °C (about 72 °F) may be associated with increased prevalence of the symptoms of sick building syndrome.

Skov and Valbjorn et al, in their Danish Town Hall Study, have reported a variety of factors that are associated with the occurrence of the symptoms of sick building syndrome in a study of 2369 office workers in 14 buildings in Copenhagen. The buildings were chosen based upon their location in the region around Copenhagen, not because of recognized indoor air quality problems. The authors studied two groups of work-related symptoms: work-related irritation of the mucous membranes and work-related general symptoms (headache, abnormal fatigue, or malaise). Symptoms of mucosal irritation were significantly correlated with area of the office, number of workplaces in the office, floor dust, organic floor dust, floor covering (carpets versus bare floor), and the fleece and shelf factor. The fleece factor is the area of all textile floor coverings, curtains, and seats divided by the volume of the room. The shelf factor is the length of all open, filled shelves and cupboards divided by the volume of the room. General symptoms were significantly correlated with area of the office, volume of the office, number of workplaces in the office, organic floor dust, and the fleece and shelf factor. The report postulates that dust accumulation and perhaps the accumulation of contaminants in fleecy materials might account for these associations. In a separate publication, Skov, Valbjorn et al reported that women had a higher prevalence of both mucosal irritation and general symptoms. Individuals with hay fever had a higher risk for work-related mucosal irritation, while individuals with a history of migraine headaches were more likely to report general symptoms. Moreover, they found that a variety of psychosocial work characteristics, including absence of varied work, dissatisfaction with the supervisor, job satisfaction diminished by the quantity of work, little influence on the organization, and high work speed, were associated with the prevalence of symptoms, both mucosal irritation and general symptoms. However, these psychosocial factors could not fully account for the differences observed in the reporting of symptoms; the indoor climate factors noted above remained strongly associated with the symptoms.

Jaakkola et al studied the impact of textile and other soft fiber wall materials (SWM) by evaluating the occurrence of symptoms in two similar buildings, one of which did not use textile wall materials. Using logistic regression analyses, they found that workers in offices with SWM reported significantly more mucosal irritation symptoms (eye symptoms, nasal dryness, nasal congestion, pharyngeal irritation) than those workers in the reference offices, with an odds ratio of 2.46 (for any of the symptoms) in the high exposure group and 1.82 in the low exposure group. Symptoms considered to reflect an allergic reaction (nasal excretion and sneezing) were also more prevalent in the exposed group. The study postulates that it may be the capability of these materials to adsorb (and release) volatile organic compounds and to accumulate (and release) organic and inorganic particulates that may lead to an influence on indoor air quality.

Incidences in which the occupants relate symptoms to the building are common, even in buildings without recognized problems. Nelson et al studied four nonproblem buildings in Washington State, using a self-administered questionnaire. Environmental measurements demonstrated low levels of volatile organic compounds, fungi and bacteria, and acceptable levels of carbon dioxide (mean of 618 ppm, range of 541–792 ppm). Fifty-five percent of the 646 respondents reported recent upper respiratory symptoms, including dry eyes, nasal symptoms, dry or sore throat, and cough, which were temporally related to being at work. In multivariate analyses, the upper respiratory symptoms were significantly associated with contact lens use, perception of the air as too dry, perception of too little air movement, perception of the workspace as too noisy, and, to a lesser extent, dissatisfaction with the overall physical environment, perception of high sensitivity to chemicals in the workplace, and job stress. Forty-eight percent reported central nervous system symptoms, including headache (24%), unusual tiredness (24.8%), tension (23.4%), and mental fatigue (16.2%). These symptoms were most strongly associated with female gender, perception of too little air movement, perception of the workspace as too noisy, and, to a lesser extent, dissatisfaction with the overall physical environment and job stress. Symptoms were not correlated with measured air contaminant levels.

While these studies have revealed a number of building, work, and occupant factors that are statistically associated with the occurrence of symptoms of sick building syndrome, they have not, as yet, established causal relationships. For example, relative to the consistent excess of symptoms observed in women, Ryan and Morrow point out that women are more likely to work in clerical jobs with little control over their job and work environment and possibly greater exposure to VOCs and other contaminants (from photocopiers, correction fluid, perhaps from textile partitions, etc). Thus, some significant associations may not be causal, because of the inter-relationships between the many variables. Table 43–3 lists possible causative factors for the sick building syndrome. In any case, these studies do support the prevalent view that most episodes of sick building syndrome are multifactorial in etiology. They certainly provide some basis for a multi-pronged, multidisciplinary approach to evaluation and management in the individual problem building.

## Clinical Findings

The most common symptoms are those associated with mucous membrane irritation and headaches. Eye irritation, difficulty in wearing contact lenses, nasal and sinus irritation and congestion, throat irritation, chest tightness or burning, nausea, headache, dizziness, and fatigue are common complaints. Some symptoms may be psychophysiologic in origin.

**Table 43–3.** Postulated causative or contributing factors to sick building syndrome.

| Category | Factor |
| --- | --- |
| Building factors | Contaminants<br>    Volatile organic compounds<br>    Formaldehyde<br>    Odors<br>    Organic dust<br>    Inorganic dust<br>    Microbial agents<br>    Other contaminants<br>Inadequate fresh air ventilation<br>Central ventilation system with no operable windows<br>Low relative humidity<br>High temperature<br>Fleece factor<br>Carpeting<br>Textile wall materials<br>Shelf factor<br>Noise |
| Host factors | Atopy (hayfever/asthma)<br>History of migraine headaches<br>Female gender<br>Psychological conditions |
| Work factors | Job stress<br>Lack of control of work/environment<br>Dissatisfaction with the supervisor<br>Absence of varied work<br>Job satisfaction diminished by quantity of work<br>High work speed<br>Little influence on the organization |

Symptoms typically occur shortly after entering the building and are relieved soon after leaving. Physical findings are nonexistent or minimal, consisting perhaps of mild injection of the oropharyngeal or conjunctival mucous membranes. Laboratory studies, including spirometry and chest x-rays, are normal. Atopic subjects, with a history or findings consistent with allergic rhinitis or asthma, seem in general to be more prone to develop symptoms in association with indoor air quality problems.

## Treatment & Prevention

For the individual patient, treatment consists of reassurance, with explanation of the apparent source and benign nature of symptoms, and temporary removal from the environment, if necessary. Fear about potential exposures, uncertainty about their health significance, and rumors about serious illnesses, alleged to be related to the building, in a population that is often medically and toxicologically unsophisticated, may lead to considerable anxiety, which, in turn, may amplify or prolong symptoms. Since a group of workers is typically affected, meetings with the group as a whole may be useful, providing ample opportunity for discussing the findings and questioning the investigators. Successful treatment of the building often involves increasing the ventilation rate, particularly the fresh air intake. Such alterations, even without prior knowledge by building occupants, have often resulted in resolution or diminution of symptoms. There is some empirical support for an approach sometimes referred to as "baking out" the building, by raising indoor temperatures with the ventilation system set for maximum fresh air intake when the building is unoccupied. Dependent upon the nature of the problem identified, other changes may be necessary also, such as relocation of air intake vents or alteration in cleaning or pesticide application practices. Prevention would appear to require balancing energy conservation concerns with the need to provide adequate fresh air intake rates when designing ventilation systems.

## MASS PSYCHOGENIC ILLNESS

Mass psychogenic illness is an illness of psychophysiologic origin occurring simultaneously in a group of individuals. Less satisfactory terms include "mass hysteria" and "behavioral contagion."

## Occurrence & Etiology

Episodes felt to represent building-associated mass psychogenic illness have occurred in office buildings, light industrial facilities, and electronics plants. The incidence of these illnesses is unknown. The precise cause, though unknown, would appear to involve the occurrence of an appropriate stimulus or trigger in a psychologically susceptible population. The trigger is often an unexplained odor, concern about which may initiate psychophysiologic symptoms in some individuals. Since the trigger may be low levels of a respiratory irritant or an irritating odor, symptoms of sick building syndrome may occur concurrently. Thus, sick building syndrome and mass psychogenic illness may occur simultaneously or sequentially in the same building incident. While sick building syndrome symptoms tend to occur in those individuals who appear to be most exposed to the suspected environmental causal factors, Ryan and Morrow describe the transmission of building-associated mass psychogenic illness within specific social networks in the workplace. In other words, friends of the initially affected individuals (index cases) are more likely to be affected.

Episodes of mass psychogenic illness have occurred in groups of workers in low-paying jobs they perceive as stressful, often with repetitive work and physical stress from such factors as poor lighting. Ryan and Morrow indicate that available evidence suggests that there is a psychological vulnerability to the development of mass psychogenic illness, affecting individuals who have lived and worked under high levels of stress and anxiety long prior to the illness outbreak. These individuals then incorrectly attribute their symptoms of psychologic and psychophysiologic origin to the problem building.

## Clinical Findings

Symptoms commonly reported in NIOSH investigations of outbreaks felt to represent mass psychogenic illness have included headache; dizziness; lightheadedness; drowsiness; nausea; dry mouth and throat; eye, nose, and throat irritation; chest tightness; and weakness, numbness, and tingling. It may be difficult to attribute particular symptoms in any given incident to mass psychogenic illness as opposed to sick building syndrome. Headache, dizziness, nausea, and numbness tend to predominate over symptoms of mucous membrane irritation in mass psychogenic illness when compared with symptom profiles in sick building syndrome. In mass psychogenic illness, symptoms are diverse in individuals in the group and occur or recur when the group is together, both inside and outside the building. The attack rate is generally higher among women than among men. There are few or no physical or laboratory findings. Some subjects may be observed to hyperventilate. In contrast to sick building syndrome, symptoms usually do not resolve promptly when the individual leaves the building.

Certain features strongly suggest the diagnosis of mass psychogenic illness. The symptoms are difficult to explain on an organic basis and are not consistent with the toxicologic properties of any suspected contaminants. There is a visual or auditory chain of transmission. In other words, subjects typically do not become ill unless they see or hear that others are becoming ill. The illness in the index cases may be due to actual exposure to an unpleasant odor or noxious substance or to a nonoccupational cause (eg, a viral syndrome). Despite severity and sudden onset of illness, the illnesses are consistently benign without sequelae.

## Treatment

Treatment primarily involves reassurance in a supportive environment away from the site at which symptoms developed. As in the management of groups suffering from sick building syndrome, emphasis should be placed on the lack of physical findings and other abnormalities and the absence of evidence suggesting a significant toxic exposure. Some investigation of the building is indicated to exclude the presence of significant contaminants. The scope of such an investigation will depend upon the potential sources of exposure, which are limited in an office setting. An exhaustive search for every measurable chemical substance is a costly, low-yield effort. Early intervention with the group is essential, reporting to them the absence of significant exposures or hazards and the benign nature of the symptoms.

## BUILDING-ASSOCIATED HYPERSENSITIVITY PNEUMONITIS

Hypersensitivity pneumonitis is a form of interstitial lung disease characterized pathologically by lymphocyte and granulomatous infiltration of alveolar walls that results from inhalation of a variety of organic dusts. The prototype of this disease is farmer's lung, which results from inhalation of bacterial spores and antigens from stored moist hay. However, hypersensitivity pneumonitis has been described in a variety of occupational and avocational settings.

Recently, hypersensitivity pneumonitis has been reported in a number of individual homes or offices where mold has been allowed to grow on humidifiers or air conditioners. Attack rates in such outbreaks have varied from 1% to 71% of the exposed population.

## Occurrence & Etiology

Hypersensitivity pneumonitis is an immunologic disorder triggered by repeated inhalation exposures to a foreign antigen, which probably results from a combination of immunopathogenic mechanism. There is evidence to suggest a type III immunologic (immune complex-mediated) reaction with precipitating or complement-fixing antibodies to the offending antigen. Some antigens may be capable of direct complement activation. Type IV T cell-mediated immune responses probably play a role in disease development, particularly in chronic hypersensitivity pneumonitis. In building-associated hypersensitivity pneumonitis, a number of agents and antigens have been implicated, including bacteria (thermophilic actinomycetes such as *Thermoactinomyces vulgaris* or *Micropolyspora faeni*), fungi (*Aspergillus*, *Penicillium*, *Alternaria*, and others) and perhaps amebas (*Naegleria* and *Acanthameba*). The source of antigens has usually been contaminated ventilation systems. Less commonly, carpets, furnishings, and surfaces persistently moist from water leaks in occupied areas have been implicated.

## Clinical Findings

There are both acute and chronic forms of hypersensitivity pneumonitis. The acute form typically presents with fever, chills, shortness of breath, nausea, myalgia, malaise, and cough without wheezing, usually developing 4–6 hours after exposure to the antigen. Symptoms may erroneously be attributed to an influenza-like illness. With the acute form, avoidance of exposure results in resolution of symptoms, and reexposure will result in recurrence of symptoms.

The chronic form of hypersensitivity pneumonitis is typically manifested by the insidious onset of fatigue, progressive dyspnea, nonproductive cough, and weight loss. A history of acute bouts of illness, as described above, may not be present. Physical findings may include fever, tachypnea, dyspnea, and bibasilar rales.

## Diagnosis

Laboratory features may include leukocytosis with a leftward shift in acute bouts and chest x-ray and pulmonary function test abnormalities. Chest x-rays may be normal or may show increased interstitial markings or patchy ill-defined densities. Pulmonary function tests may reveal a restrictive pattern, with reductions in vital capacity and total lung capacity. However, ventilatory abnormalities are not always present. The most consistent pulmonary function abnormality is reduction of diffusing capacity for carbon monoxide.

The presence of serum precipitating antibodies to suspected antigens is of limited usefulness in that it documents intense and extensive exposure but does not indicate the presence of clinical pulmonary disease. Such antibodies may be seen in asymptomatic individuals, and some individuals with hypersensitivity pneumonitis may have negative precipitin tests. Gallium lung scans, bronchoalveolar lavage (demonstrating a predominance of lymphocytes), inhalation provocation studies, and ultimately lung biopsy may be useful in confirming a diagnosis.

In a study of hypersensitivity pneumonitis in office workers exposed to a contaminated air cooling system, a respiratory questionnaire was found to be the most sensitive method by which to detect possible cases among the large group of potentially exposed workers. Shortness of breath and fever were present in all of the affected individuals. If the onset of these two symptoms was in close temporal association with exposure to the workplace, these findings were even more suggestive of hypersensitivity pneumonitis. Chest x-rays and assays for precipitin were of limited value, while preexposure and postexposure measurements of $FEV_1$, FVC, and diffusing capacity were quite helpful in confirming a diagnosis.

## Treatment

Avoidance of further exposure by removal from the environment usually results in resolution of symptoms and abnormalities. If symptoms fail to resolve following removal, a short course of corticosteroids (typically Prednisone in high doses) is indicated. In some outbreaks, extensive clean-up efforts, including removal of contaminated items and alteration of ventilation systems, have allowed the return of affected workers without recurrence of symptoms.

## OTHER BUILDING-ASSOCIATED ILLNESSES

Certain noncommunicable infectious diseases may be transmitted in indoor air. Legionnaires' disease, a multisystem disease dominated by pneumonia, is caused by the bacterial organism *Legionella pneumophila*. Most commonly, building-associated outbreaks have resulted from contaminated aerosols, usually disseminated in the ventilation system, from cooling towers, evaporative condensers, decorative fountains, humidifiers, and air-conditioning systems. *Legionella* species can be cultured in up to 40% of cooling towers, although infections stemming from exposure to the aerosols are uncommon. Proper cleaning and maintenance of these potential sources is critical in preventing outbreaks of Legionnaires' disease. Pontiac fever, also caused by *Legionella pneumophila*, is an influenza-like illness characterized by fever, chills, headache, myalgias, and occasionally cough and sore throat. Again, the sources are typically contaminated air-conditioning systems.

Finally, Q fever, caused by the rickettsial organism *Coxiella burnetii*, has been responsible for several building-associated outbreaks. The animal reservoirs for this infection are sheep, goats, and cattle. Airborne transmission of organisms from animal excreta to humans has occurred via ventilation systems in animal handling and medical research facilities.

Certain hazardous materials not routinely suspected in nonindustrial buildings have been linked to building-associated symptoms or illnesses. Elevated levels of formaldehyde have been found in mobile homes and trailers—in which large quantities of urea-formaldehyde wood products are used—and in conventional homes to which urea-formaldehyde foam insulation has been applied. One study of residences whose occupants had reported symptoms found median levels of 0.35 ppm of formaldehyde, with some levels as high as 2–4 ppm (the ACGIH threshold limit value for 8-hour occupational exposures is 1 ppm TWA). Commonly reported symptoms included eye irritation and burning, runny nose, dry or sore throat, headache, and cough.

Carbon monoxide in buildings may be the cause of mild symptoms, such as headache and nausea, or more severe, potentially life-threatening intoxication. Incomplete combustion in defective gas furnaces or unvented gas stoves and other appliances, typically in residences, may occasionally be the source of significant indoor emissions of carbon monoxide. Less commonly, carbon monoxide may be entrained from the outside via air intakes in the vicinity of vehicle loading docks.

In a questionnaire-based study, Jaakkola and Heinonen demonstrated an increased risk of the common cold significantly associated with shared office space. They used logistic regression analysis to control for factors that were significantly associated with the risk for colds, such as being a parent of young children and having hay fever. They found that sharing a room with coworkers at the workplace had an adjusted odds ratio of 1.35 (95% CI, 1–1.82) for experiencing more than two episodes of the common cold in the preceding 12 months, compared with the reference group who had no colleagues in their work area. These findings, if supported by further studies, have potential implications regarding the frequent complaint of employees in problem buildings that they suffer from colds more frequently.

## REFERENCES

Daisey J et al: Volatile organic compounds in twelve California office buildings: Classes, concentrations and sources. Atmospheric Environment 1994;28:3557.

Ellenbecker MJ: Engineering controls for clean air in the office environment. Clin Chest Med 1992;13:193.

Hoffman RE, Wood RC, Kreiss K: Building-related asthma in Denver office workers. Am J Public Health 1993; 83(1):89.

Jaakkola JJ, Heinonen OP: Shared office space and the risk of the common cold. Eur J Epidemiol 1995;11:213.

Jaakkola JJ, Tuomaala P, Seppanen O: Air recirculation and sick building syndrome: A blinded crossover trial. Am J Public Health 1994;84:422.

Jaakkola JJ, Tuomaala P, Seppanen O: Textile wall materials and sick building syndrome. Arch Environ Health 1994;49:175.

Kaltreider HB: Hypersensitivity pneumonitis. West J Med 1993;159:570.

Gecewicz TE, et al: Legionnaires' disease associated with cooling towers—Massachusetts, Michigan, and Rhode Island, 1993. MMWR Morb Mortal Wkly Rep 1994;43:491.

Marbury M, Woods J: Building-related illnesses. Pages 307–308 in: Samet J, Spengler J (editors): *Indoor Air Pollution: A Health Perspective*. Johns Hopkins University Press, 1991.

Mendell MJ, Fine L: Building ventilation and symptoms—Where do we go from here? Am J Public Health 1994; 84:346.

National Institute for Occupational Safety and Health: Guidance for Indoor Air Quality Investigations. NIOSH, 1987.

Nelson NA et al: Health symptoms and the work environment in four nonproblem United States office buildings. Scand J Work Environ Health 1995;21:51.

Nordstrom K, Norback D, Akselsson R: Effect of air humidification on the sick building syndrome and perceived air quality in hospitals: A four month long longitudinal study. Occup Environ Med 1994;51:683.

Reinikainen LM, Jaakkola JJ, Seppanen O: The effect of air humidification on symptoms and perception of indoor air quality in office workers: a six-period cross-over trial. Arch Environ Health 1992;47:8.

Ryan CM, Morrow LA: Dysfunctional buildings or dysfunctional people: An examination of the sick building syndrome and allied disorders. J Consult Clin Psychol 1992;60:220.

Skov P, Valbjorn O, Pedersen B: Influence of indoor climate on the sick building syndrome in an office environment. Scand J Work Environ Health 1990;16:363.

Spengler JD, Samet JM: A perspective on indoor and outdoor air pollution. Pages 1–29 in: *Indoor Air Pollution: A Health Perspective*. Johns Hopkins University Press: Baltimore, 1991.

# Water Pollution

# 44

*Daniel T. Teitelbaum, MD*

Access to adequate quantities of a safe and reliable water supply is the most fundamental requirement of human life. Without adequate water, human existence is impossible. When water supplies are limited or otherwise compromised, sustainable development of agriculture or industry is not tenable. History records the rise and fall of civilizations because of changes in their water supply. Wars have been fought over access to water. In some areas of the world—the Middle East, the Indian subcontinent, and in Africa—future conflict over the ownership and distribution of water supplies seems inevitable. Because of the finite quantity of potable water available, the unequal distribution of water over the earth's surface, and its vulnerability to contamination by natural chemicals and minerals, pathogens, and anthropogenic biological and chemical wastes, water may be the most threatened resource on the planet.

The Resolution of the United Nations Water Conference in 1981 declared that access to a sufficient and safe water supply is a right of all peoples:

> All peoples, whatever their stage of development and their social and economic conditions, have the right to access to drinking water in quantities and of a quality equal to their basic needs.

Whether such a declaration is feasible or enforceable is uncertain. However, without active commitment to the protection of earth's finite water supply, the goal of world-wide access to ample, safe water cannot be achieved. Unfortunately, in many developed and developing areas of the world, commitment to "clean water" is not universal. Individual countries have legislated rules and regulations to protect portions of their potable water. Some regions of the world have begun to cooperate in the cleanup of mutually critical sources of water. None the less, the NIMBY syndrome *(not in my backyard)* is still rampant in water resource development and control. Although slow progress has been made in the remediation of local water pollution problems associated with human endeavor, transborder and supranational

water pollution problems continue to exist on every continent. In North America, the Canadian-American acid precipitation problem and its consequences to the water supply and biota of the Northeastern United States, as well as the saline water and agricultural waste problems in the Rio Grande and Colorado Rivers basins on the United States-Mexico border are relevant examples of transnational water pollution issues. In Europe, the contamination of the Rhine River basin by anthropogenic wastes, and, in South America, pollution of the Amazon River and its outfall are similar issues of concern.

## BIOCONTAMINATION OF WATER SUPPLIES

Biocontamination of water supplies used or intended for human drinking water represents the most immediate water-borne threat to human health. In 1855, Dr. John Snow proved that the City of London's potable water supply at the Broad Street Pump was contaminated with sewage, and was the source of the London cholera epidemic of that year. Since then, public health authorities have accepted the role of biocontaminated water as a cause of human disease. A growing understanding of the epidemiologic characteristics and patterns of disease associated with human pathogens distributed in drinking water has led to the development of a competent infrastructure of potable and wastewater collection, storage, treatment, disinfection, and distribution in the urban areas of most developed countries. As the microbiological integrity of the supply of potable water has improved, a significant reduction in human disease due to water-borne pathogens has occurred. Nonetheless, recent experience has demonstrated that the potable water supply throughout the world is always at risk. Serious water-borne disease epidemics with recognized and new pathogens continue to occur in immunocompetent and immunocompromised humans in both developed and developing areas of the world. The cost of these epidemics has not been fully evaluated in monetary or human terms. However, a recent

Danish epidemic of water-borne gastrointestinal disease in which 1455 people were affected has been studied. This epidemic, which was due to an unidentified agent conveyed to the potable water supply by unusual rainfall that caused sewage overflows, resulted in the loss of close to $500,000 in sick leave costs, and a total of 1658 lost workdays.

Acute diarrheal diseases characterized by loose or watery stools are often accompanied by vomiting and fever. Many of these diarrheal episodes are the result of water-borne infection with bacteria, viruses, or parasites, or the ingestion of their enterotoxins. Cholera, shigellosis, salmonellosis, coliforms, yersiniosis, giardiasis, *Campylobacter* iosis, cryptosporidiosis, and viral gastroenteropathies produce diarrheal signs and symptoms. Careful evaluation of the patient and the water supply using newer laboratory tests permits the correct etiological diagnosis of diarrhea in more than 70% of cases that are adequately evaluated in developing countries. Unfortunately, the resources and equipment for such evaluations are often not available. Paradoxically, in industrialized countries, fewer cases can be etiologically defined. Forty-five percent of cases of diarrhea in industrialized countries are etiologically identifiable, except in the winter months and in infants. According to the American Public Health Association, 50–70% of the incident cases of infant diarrhea are caused by rotavirus alone.

Effective methods of microbiological and chemical treatment and surveillance of water supplies are in place in most public water supplies in developed countries. In less developed and developing countries, and in rural areas of developed countries where raw or untreated water from surface or groundwater sources is used as potable water, effective control of microbiological water contamination is not always assured. In spite of the technological sophistication of civil engineering of water and wastewater supplies, outbreaks of water-borne disease occur frequently in both developed and developing countries. On most occasions, epidemics of water-borne disease in developed countries are the result of technical flaws or unusual and unforeseen climatological events that disrupt the normal potable water supplies. In less developed countries, the ordinary juxtaposition of human residence, agriculture, animal husbandry, and unprotected potable water sources are typically the cause of epidemic water-borne disease. In some areas, the use of wastewater containing human excreta as agricultural irrigation water greatly increases the risk of contamination of local drinking water supplies and the transmission of enteric and other diseases through the consumption of food crops contaminated with pathogens by this process.

The use of wastewater for irrigation purposes was and is recommended in certain areas of the world where water resources are very limited. Originally developed in Europe and North America in the nineteenth century, sewage farming was conceived as an efficient and economical way to dispose of urban wastewater. Rainwater was allowed to enter the rivers from which drinking water was traditionally drawn, and wastewater was applied to the fields where natural biological processes were expected to purify the water before it reached the rivers and reentered the potable water resources. As long as there was enough agricultural land in close proximity to large urban centers, this system was useful. However, as the proximity of agriculture and urban life diminished, the usefulness of the sewage farming techniques also decreased. However, in arid lands, the economic advantages of wastewater farming remain. Properly employed, wastewater farming can be both safe and economically attractive. The World Bank has studied sewage farming extensively, and finds it to be both practical and safe when specific guidelines for the use of wastewater for irrigation are followed. The Engelberg Guidelines for the microbiological quality of treated wastewater used for crop irrigation were developed by the World Health Organization (WHO) for use in developing areas where the scarcity of water dictates the reuse of wastewater for agricultural purposes. They are based on extensively studied use of wastewater in agriculture. They utilize new coliform content guidelines that are higher than the coliform counts recommended in the California guidelines, which were developed in the 1940s by the California Health Department. Based on a "zero risk" concept, the California guidelines permitted only 2 fecal coliforms per 100 mL of irrigation water used on crops eaten raw. Their concept was that the mere presence of coliforms in the irrigation water presented an unacceptable risk of disease. However, these guidelines were not based on epidemiologic studies of outcome of use of these salad crops. The Engelberg guidelines suggest that a geometric mean of 1000 coliforms per 100 mL of irrigation water for unrestricted crop use is safe, based on epidemiologic outcome studies. This level is still less than half of that permitted in bathing water in Europe (< 2000 fecal coliforms/100 mL). The guidelines also create, for the first time, appropriate controls on the presence of helminth eggs in irrigation water.

If the Engelberg Guidelines are adhered to, the increased pathogen counts that are permitted are considered to be of little significance. No adverse health effects or drinking water impacts are expected to result from the use of wastewater, sewage, septage, or sediment for agricultural irrigation. If they are not followed, the use of contaminated water and human excreta for food or subsistence crops will lead to human disease and may adversely impact drinking water quality.

Throughout the world, catastrophic events such as political upheaval, revolution, and war, with their consequent disruption of human life and public health, often lead to biocontamination of water and epidemics of human disease. Furthermore, the spectrum of infectious diseases appears to be changing. Worldwide, explosive population growth, expanding poverty, urban migration, and increased international travel affect the risk of exposure to water-borne infectious disease. These emerging diseases include water-borne cryptosporidial diarrheal disease and cholera, as well as hemorrhagic fevers, tuberculosis, and hantavirus infections.

Major climatologic changes such as drought and flooding also contribute to disruption of the normal supply of water in all countries. Abnormal events such as earthquakes, hurricanes, tornadoes, snowstorms, and similar phenomena cause disruption of normal potable water supplies and may result in epidemic disease in humans. In all such events, increased surveillance of water supplies and rapid response with appropriate public health measures are indicated. Such responses include "boil water" advisories, temporary shift of water supplies to uncontaminated resources, and microbiologic assessment of the supply for viral, bacteriologic, parasitologic, and helminthic contamination. In addition, facilities and supplies for the immediate assessment and treatment of victims of water-borne epidemics, which may include typhoid, cholera, hepatitis, and other diseases, should be prepared and put in place. General measures for public health action in emergencies caused by epidemics are reviewed in a WHO publication of 1986.

## CONTROL OF MICROBIOLOGIC WATER CONTAMINATION

### BOD, COD, TOC, & TSS

Conventional management of potable water and wastewater supplies involves separation of the flow of the two fluid streams and the protection of the potable water supply from contamination with the contents of the wastewater stream. Conventional wastewater treatment systems are developed to remove organic matter from wastewater on the basis of their biochemical oxygen demand (BOD) or chemical oxygen demand (COD). The BOD is a measure of the load placed on the oxygen resources of the receiving waters, usually as a result of microbiologic growth. Treatment efficiency is evaluated on the basis of BOD removal by the treatment facility. Unless otherwise stated, BOD signifies the biochemical oxygen demand for five days at 20 °C.

The BOD is useful to determine the extent to which oxygen can be utilized by a supply of microbial life. The test is most important in the management of wastewater and in food manufacturing and drinking water preparation facilities. High concentrations of dissolved oxygen predict that oxygen uptake by microorganisms is low, and that the breakdown of nutrient resources in the water by microorganisms is

also low. Low concentrations of dissolved oxygen signify high microorganism demands and imply contamination of the water.

COD, chemical oxygen demand, is also employed in the assessment of water quality. This test determines the quantity of oxidizable material in the water. It varies with the composition of the water, temperature, concentration of the reagent, period of contact, and other factors. Generally speaking, the COD, BOD, and the total organic carbon (TOC), a quick method of estimating organic contamination of water, are correlated. A full explanation of the theory, methods, and implication of these tests and parameters may be found in the 18th edition of *Standard Methods for the Examination of Water and Wastewater,* the analytical bible for water resource management.

Treatment facilities are also designed to remove total suspended solids (TSS) to a level that is both microbiologically and esthetically acceptable. Recently, tertiary treatment facilities have been designed that improve pathogen removal to produce finished water with very low pathogen counts.

### Water & Wastewater Treatment

Conventional wastewater treatment systems that employ sedimentation, activated sludge, biofiltration, aeration, and oxidation, combined with chemical disinfection, produce water with coliform counts that are very low. In the absence of a disinfection step, low coliform counts may not be achieved. Without slow sand filtration of water and wastewater, protozoa, viruses, and other pathogens may also remain in the finished water. Tables of pathogen significance and persistence in public water supplies may be found in the second edition of the WHO Guidelines for Drinking-Water Quality. The use of slow sand filtration should control the water-borne spread of the various hepatitis viruses, including hepatitis E, which is currently a major problem in many parts of the world.

The intensity of water treatment for a particular supply and distribution area must depend on the nature and quality of the source. The degree of contamination will determine the required treatment. *Multiple treatment barriers* are recommended by the WHO for contaminated water sources to prevent the spread of pathogens. The fundamental purpose of water treatment is to protect the consumer from pathogens and impurities in the water that may be unacceptable from a health or esthetic point of view.

Typical treatment processes for urban water drawn from lowland sources include impoundment and reservoir storage. If needed, predisinfection is applied during impoundment. Impoundment and storage in reservoirs may result in a 99% reduction in fecal indicator bacteria, salmonella, and enteroviruses. During storage and impoundment, the microbiologic environment changes as a result of natural sedimentation, the lethal effect of ultraviolet light on the surface layers of the water, the deprivation of nutrients required by the organisms, and predation. Following impoundment and storage, coagulation, flocculation, and further sedimentation or flotation to remove solids are employed. Filtration and disinfection complete the cycle of typical urban water treatment. Aeration to improve the aesthetic quality of the final product may also be used. This typical system meets the multiple barrier requirements of WHO's Water Quality Guidelines of 1993.

In rural and remote areas, multiple barrier concepts may also be used. Typical protocols dictate impoundment and protection of the water, sedimentation and screening, gravel prefiltration and slow-sand filtration, and a final disinfection step.

The efficacy of these treatment protocols may be expected to be high, and the quality of the finished water is likely to be excellent. Monitoring of the results of urban water treatment is required under the Safe Drinking Water Act in the United States and under various state and local regulations. In other countries, specific guidelines for monitoring treated water have been adopted. WHO recommends that monthly sampling of public water supplies be performed. The number of recommended samples varies with the size of the water system.

## PATHOGEN-CAUSED WATER-BORNE DISEASE

Water-borne bacterial disease includes the most classic infections of large populations: enterocolitis due to coliforms, cholera, typhoid and paratyphoid fevers, shigellosis, and salmonellosis. *Campylobacter* infections have also become significant in recent years.

The most recent surveillance of water-borne diseases in the United States, published by the Centers for Disease Control and Prevention (CDC) in 1996, demonstrated that for the last complete survey years of 1993–1994, there were 405,366 persons who became ill as a result of reported water-borne disease in the United States. During this period, 17 states reported 30 outbreaks of water-borne disease. Twenty-nine of these outbreaks involved 2366 cases of disease, and one, the outbreak of cyptosporidiosis in Milwaukee, Wisconsin, involved 403,000 cases. This was the largest water-borne disease outbreak reported in the United States.

The 1991–1992 CDC surveillance reported 34 outbreaks of water-borne disease in 17 states. 17,464 persons became ill in these episodes. Of the 11 episodes involving swimming-associated gastroenteritis, giardiasis and cryptosporidiosis were the cause in 6 outbreaks. The most frequently reported illness in this period was whirlpool or hot tub associated pseudomonas dermatitis. This illness is only reported in developed countries. During 1991–1992, the first reported water-borne outbreak of *Escherichia coli* 0157:H7 infection associated with recreational exposure was also reported.

### *Campylobacter* Diarrhea

*Campylobacter jejuni* was responsible for 3 documented outbreaks of water-borne diarrheal disease in the United States during the 1993–1994 period. This organism, and closely related species, includes several biotypes and serotypes. *Campylobacter* species are believed to cause 5–14% of cases of diarrhea worldwide. In developed countries, the American Public Health Association reports that children and young adults have the highest frequency of disease. Several *Campylobacter* species have been associated with infection in homosexual men. In developing countries, the illness occurs primarily in children under 2 years of age. The use of unchlorinated drinking water is highly associated with *Campylobacter* infection.

### Cholera

Cholera remains a threat throughout the world. A major epidemic of cholera has been in progress in South and Central America for more than five years. Recent reports of cholera in Guatemala, the country with the third highest number of cholera cases in the Western Hemisphere, have identified a newly introduced, toxigenic *Vibrio cholerae 01* strain in a food-borne/water-borne outbreak of cholera spread by street vendors in contaminated noncarbonated beverages and other comestibles. The outbreak was not associated with municipal drinking water. This strain of *Vibrio cholerae* was resistant to several antibiotics. It differed substantially from the dominant Latin American strain present in the hemisphere since 1991.

Recent outbreaks of cholera in Ecuador in 1991 with characteristic acute massive diarrhea were demonstrated to be highly associated with the drinking of unboiled water, the drinking of beverages supplied by street vendors, and eating raw seafood. Always drinking boiled water at home was protective against the illness, as was the presence of soap in either the kitchen or the bathroom of the home. The cholera strain identified in this outbreak also demonstrated multiple antibiotic resistance. A recent large outbreak of cholera in Riohacha, Colombia was directly associated with contamination of the municipal water supply. This outbreak was highly associated with the consumption of unchlorinated and unboiled water from the piped municipal water system.

An epidemic of cholera was recently reported in the mountainous region of Daghestan. The source of this epidemic was traced to consumption of raw river water massively contaminated with *V cholerae* from wastewater effluents. A significant failure in sanitary engineering that permitted the mixing of wastewater from the cholera hospital in the region with the river that supplied the potable water for the area led to many secondary cases and the prolongation of the epidemic to over 40 days after its identification.

A major cholera outbreak occurred during the recent civil war and population upheaval in Rwanda. Explosive epidemic diarrhea due to *V cholerae* and *E coli* was associated with death rates of 20–35 per 10,000 per day at the height of the epidemic. More than 50,000 refugees died in this epidemic. Health relief, correction of malnutrition, and public health intervention reduced the death rates to 5–8 per 10,000 per day by the second month of the crisis. In the emergency phase, only low technology interventions were used, which included bucket chlorination disinfection of water and designated defecation areas, active case identification, and emergency oral rehydration of cases.

In 1993–1994, only one case of *non 01 V cholerae* infection was reported in the United States, and no cases were reported in the previous reporting period. The single cholera case was associated with commercially bottled water.

Management of cholera cases requires strict oral-fecal precautions and other measures designed to confine the spread and mitigate the illness. Oral rehydration is effective in most cases. Rehydration with polyelectrolyte solution that contains glucose is effective. Volume for volume replacement should be undertaken, once existing losses at presentation have been corrected. Antibiotic treatment or mass prophylaxis is generally not useful. However, some experienced physicians recommend the use of tetracycline prophylaxis or cotrimoxazole prophylaxis in family outbreaks. Immunization of contacts is not indicated in epidemic situation. The value of the currently available vaccine is not high. It provides protection only for a brief period, not more than 90–120 days. Some countries where cholera is endemic continue to require vaccination, but the protective value of the procedure is uncertain. Prophylaxis must rest on the avoidance of water, food, and contact, as in any oral-fecal transmitted disease.

## Typhoid Fever & Paratyphoid Infections

Disease due to water-borne *Salmonella typhi* is quite rare in developed countries. It can usually be associated with a particular food-borne event. In the United States, no more than 200–500 cases are reported annually. Prior to 1950, several thousand cases occurred annually in the United States. Recent reports of outbreaks of typhoid fever in Spain have demonstrated that despite the important progress in water engineering that has occurred since 1985 in that country, the threat of typhoid fever remains. A major outbreak of typhoid occurred in Bages County, in Catalonia, in the City of Barcelona in 1994. This epidemic was traced to a break in sewer pipes near a drinking fountain. Epidemiologic study of water and biologic markers confirmed the common source outbreak and identified the organism.

In endemic areas where sanitation is poor, many cases occur annually. The disease has a case fatality rate of 10%, although appropriate treatment with antibiotics results in a case fatality rate of less than 1%. Ten percent of patients discharge the bacterium for up to 3 months after infection. A chronic carrier state may be established among 2% of cases who become infected in middle age. Women with a history of gall bladder disease seem most likely to develop the carrier state. Available laboratory tests permit identification of the responsible organism and permit distinction between typhoid and paratyphoid disease.

Vaccination against typhoid is not generally employed in developed countries. Currently, it is recommended that travelers to endemic areas who have significant potential for exposure due to their occupation be vaccinated. The primary series of inoculations requires two injections, several weeks apart. Booster doses every 3 years are also recommended. An oral vaccine is available that causes considerably less reaction than the traditional injectable vaccine. It appears effective for standard doses of the bacterium, but may not protect against massive ingestions of contaminated water or food.

Treatment of most cases of typhoid fever is readily accomplished with fluid replacement and several antibiotic regimens, including amoxicillin, cotrimoxazole, or tetracyclines. The emergence of some resistant strains of *S typhi* is a continuing challenge. Usual and customary management may not be effective in cases of typhoid fever due to resistant organisms. In that instance, and for the carrier state, chloramphenicol may be indicated. The use of chloramphenicol carries a significant risk of irreversible aplastic anemia and the drug should be employed only when no other antibiotic is suitable. Pang et al have reviewed the use of various antibiotic regimens in treatment of typhoid fever, including the resistant cases.

Systemic paratyphoid fever occurs frequently, but may not be reported. The case fatality rate is much lower than in typhoid fever. Epidemiologic parameters are similar to typhoid fever. The infection may be due to several different organisms and many phage types. When the infection is confined to the gastrointestinal tract, the illness is more properly called salmonellosis. Chronic carrier states do not occur. No vaccination is available for paratyphoid fever.

## Nontyphoidal Salmonellosis

Disease due to nontyphoidal salmonella strains occurs frequently but is rarely reported unless very large numbers of people are involved. Industrial cattle and chicken breeding and food production facilitate the water-borne spread of nontyphoidal salmonella. In immunocompromised patients, these disorders can be life-threatening, although most patients recover fully without treatment. The 1993–1994 CDC reports contained data on a single outbreak of *Salmonella typhimurium* in the United States, which resulted in seven deaths.

## Shigella & Other Pathogenic Bacteria

*Shigella sonnei* and other related shigella strains are often responsible for diarrheal diseases that occur under adverse conditions. On the Navajo Reservation in the Southwestern United States, families who live outside of organized settlements and use well water or surface water sources for potable water have frequent episodes of shigella-induced diarrhea. These episodes are rarely reported.

In 1993–1994, *Shigella sonnei* and *Shigella flexneri* were reported to have caused one outbreak each in the United States. Elsewhere in the world, *Shigella dysenteriae* Type 1 causes large numbers of cases of diarrhea in children who live under crowded and unsanitary conditions and drink water from ad hoc and untreated water supplies. The case fatality rate in *S dysenteriae* infection is particularly high in children.

## *Escherichia Coli* Diarrhea

*E coli* are frequently responsible for diarrheal episodes. "Traveler's diarrhea" is often the result of *E coli* infection. Most episodes are not etiologically identified, although abnormal coliform counts in water supply during such episodes are the rule rather than the exception. *E coli* can cause a variety of syndromes. Water and food are common vehicles of transmission of *E coli*. The gastrointestinal and systemic disease may present in one of five forms:

1. Enterotoxigenic (ETEC).
2. Enteroinvasive (EIEC).
3. Enteropathogenic (EPEC).
4. Enterohemorrhagic (EHEC).
5. Enteroaggregative (EAggEC).

Recent reports have identified the enterotoxigenic strain of *E coli* 0157:H7, which was responsible for a disastrous food-borne epidemic from undercooked hamburger in the Northwestern United States as the cause of an outbreak of water-borne diarrheal disease.

Prophylaxis of "traveler's diarrhea" can be accomplished with bismuth subsalicylate taken orally for several days prior to travel, through the period of travel, and then for 2–3 days after travel is completed. The only complication of this regimen is black stool from the bismuth. Adequate fluid intake must be maintained during the use of this medication because of the salicylate load. Prophylaxis with norfloxacin, 400 mg daily, is also effective. Most often, hydration alone is indicated for treatment of the infection and diarrhea that results. In severe cases, particularly in children, early treatment of infection with cotrimoxazole is also indicated. No vaccines are available.

## Water-borne *Legionella* Illness

*Legionella* species have repeatedly been identified as the cause of outbreaks of the respiratory disease known as Legionnaires' disease. The disease is transmitted by water droplets contaminated with the organism. Hot tubs, cooling tower aerosols, air conditioning systems, and other water-facilitated machinery have been the source of the aerosol that carries the pathogen.

Recent reports of major outbreaks of Legionnaires' disease among cruise ship passengers who favored the use of the whirlpool spa, either by immersing themselves in the spa or sitting beside it, have suggested a need to alter the management of water resources aboard cruise ships. In this outbreak, a clear dose-response curve was demonstrated, which associated hours at the spa with risk of Legionnaires' disease.

## Cyclospora (Cyanobacteria [Blue-Green Algae-Like] Enteritis)

Recent reports have associated cyclospora species with outbreaks of food-borne enteritis. The food that carries this emerging bacterial pathogen has variously been identified as strawberries and raspberries. Outbreaks along the US East Coast and in Texas have puzzled public health authorities. So far, no clear epidemiologic information on the organism, its survival, and its pathogenicity has been collected. A major problem with the delineation of the pattern of disease associated with this cyanobacterium relative is the delay commonly noted to occur between ingestion of the putative carrier food and the onset of the disease. As much as a week may pass before the severe repetitive and troublesome diarrhea develops. To date, fatalities have not been reported. Epidemiologists are currently involved in a nationwide food supply study using PCR (polymerase chain reaction) studies to trace the source of this organism in the food supply.

One outbreak of diarrheal illness in the United States due to cyclospora was traced to the tap water in a physicians' dormitory in Chicago. Whether the organism was locally introduced or entered the tap water from the municipal water supply is unknown.

An outbreak of cyanobacterial illness occurred in Brazil during impoundment of water in a dam building project. It is not clear whether this outbreak was due to the cyclospora organism. Another outbreak of cyclospora-caused disease associated with chlorinated drinking water in Nepal was briefly reported in 1994.

## PROTOZOA-CAUSED WATER-BORNE DISEASE

Among the traditional and emerging water-borne diseases, protozoan-induced illness has become the major threat to human health. While amebiasis, which was once a major cause of diarrheal and systemic disease, is now rare in developed countries, other organisms such as *Cryptosporidium parvum* and *Giardia lamblia* now exact a heavy toll.

### Amebiasis

Amebic dysentery and systemic amebiasis is ubiquitous. Fortunately, it is now rarely detected in developed countries. Slow sand filtration or its equivalent is required to remove infectious amebic cysts from potable water.

Most infections with ameba are asymptomatic, although severe enterocolitis and systemic disease may occur. *Entameba histolytica* is the usual cause of the disease, although other pathogenic ameba are recognized. *Acanthameba* and *Leptomyxida* have been noted to cause progressive granulomatous encephalitis in immunosuppressed hosts. Five cases of disseminated cutaneous amebiasis without CNS findings were recently noted in AIDS patients. One case of amebic keratitis was reported in a nonimmunosuppressed individual who wore disposable contact lenses. The pathogens in this cases were not the usual *Acanthameba* species, but rather *Vahlkampfia* and *Hartmanella* species, two other free-living ameba.

Other nonpathogenic ameba may be found in the intestine and should not be confused with the pathogenic species. The disease is always water-borne. Acutely ill individuals are only of limited danger to others because they do not excrete the infectious cysts and the live trophozooite does not survive for a long period in stools, water, or food. Chronic carriers of amebic cysts may pass the cysts for years and are infectious throughout this period.

### Cryptosporidium Parvum Diarrhea

Many outbreaks of cryptosporidiosis have been reported in developed countries. The most dramatic epidemic occurred in Milwaukee, Wisconsin, during March and April of 1993 and affected almost half a million people. Both primary and secondary cases of the disease occurred. The source of this epidemic was fecal contamination of the drinking water, which is river drawn from areas in which cow manure entered the river. Inadequate sand filtration probably allowed the protozoan pathogen to enter the drinking water supply. Unfamiliarity with the disease and its transmission probably contributed to the delay in recognition of the epidemic and prolonged its persistence.

Other epidemics of cyptosporidiosis have been reported in Clark County, Nevada, where water treatment is considered to be state-of-the-art. Water quality in this community exceeds US federal guidelines.

The outbreak involved both immunocompromised and immunocompetent persons. Twenty of 32 immunocompromised adults who died during this epidemic had cryptosporidiosis listed on their death certificates. Persons who drank any unboiled municipal water had a four-fold greater likelihood of infection than those who drank only bottled water. No coliforms and no oocysts of cryptosporidium were found in the potable water source, Lake Mead, during the epidemic. However, presumptive oocysts were found intermittently in samples of source water, filter backwash, and finished water.

An outbreak of cryptosporidial disease occurred in Washington, DC, in December 1993. Early in the month, water treatment plant operators noted that the performance of the municipal filtration system had declined and that turbidity levels had increased. Small suspended particles exceeded the USEPA permitted level. A "boil water" advisory was instituted, although adequate chlorination was maintained throughout this period. However, *Cryptosporidium parvum* is highly resistant to chlorination and must be filtered out of the water.

Other cryptosporidial outbreaks have been reported in Warrington, in Bradford, England, in Florida, and elsewhere. In each case, the likely source of the original pathogen appears to have been cattle feces from which infective oocysts reached the potable water supply because of a breakdown in filtration procedures or because of their absence in the multiple barriers system.

### Giardiasis

Giardiasis is a major water-borne protozoal disease. Often reported in cold countries, outbreaks have occurred in Vail, Colorado and Zermatt, Switzerland. Both of these towns are high altitude, winter resorts where water was drawn from cold surface mountain sources believed to be pure. Prior to these outbreaks of disease in the 1970s, the survival of the protozoan in cold mountain streams was not recognized. Outbreaks have also been experienced in Saint Petersburg, Russia, and other large cities with older wastewater disposal systems. In 1993–1994 in the United States, 75% of the water-borne gastrointestinal disease outbreaks were due either to *Giardia* or *Cryptosporidium*.

Recent outbreaks of giardiasis in Canada were shown to be water-borne. Contaminated community drinking water was identified as the source in a community in British Columbia where two successive outbreaks were traced to the same strain of *Giardia* by ELISA (enzyme linked immunoabsorbent assay) techniques.

Campers and backpackers who use surface water sources for potable water during their travels should be particularly careful to use filters and treatment systems that are now commercially available to remove *Giardia* organisms from drinking water. Treatment of giardiasis is effectively accomplished with metronidazole, although the diagnosis is sometimes difficult to confirm by stool examination. Severe diarrhea in a camper or backpacker who has been using surface water for drinking should alert the physician to the possibility of giardiasis. Empiric treatment with metronidazole may then be appropriate.

## Toxoplasmosis

Toxoplasmosis has occasionally been demonstrated to have been transmitted through a waterborne route. A report from British Columbia identified the source of an outbreak of toxoplasmosis as a municipal drinking water supply.

## WATER-BORNE VIRAL DISEASE

### Enterovirus (Picornovirus)
### Hepatitis A

Water-borne hepatitis epidemics are common throughout the world. In developed countries, hepatitis A is frequently spread from a single case through food-borne means; however, water-borne transmission is reported. Most often, water-borne transmission of hepatitis A in developed countries occurs as a result of sewage contamination of potable water supplies. In less developed countries and in the rural areas of developed countries, water-borne transmission of the hepatitis A virus is common. In countries where environmental sanitation is poor, infants and children frequently contract hepatitis A and the survivors become immune. In more developed areas, where environmental sanitation is better, a reservoir of nonimmune adults is found, and epidemic disease in adults may be seen. In the United States, epidemic hepatitis A occurred in waves during the 1980s. Large epidemics are now infrequent, but may occur from time to time. Outbreaks in nurseries and day care centers and as a result of food and water contamination occur sporadically.

Identification of the disease is helpful in order to distinguish it from hepatitis E, which has a similar course and indistinguishable epidemiologic pattern. Serologic diagnosis is available, which uses either ELISA or radioimmunoassay (RIA) techniques. Positivity may linger for months. Most young persons recover with little or no sequelae. However, a case fatality rate of 0.6% is noted. Most fatalities occur in adults who have fulminant disease. No specific treatment is available for hepatitis A. Hyperimmune globulin has usually been given as prophylaxis if knowledge of an exposure to hepatitis A becomes known and the disease is not yet symptomatic. The current availability of a well-tested and effective anti-hepatitis A vaccine throughout the world should help reduce the remaining pool of susceptible persons and limit the epidemic nature of the disease. Travelers and workers who plan to work in areas with high rates of endemic hepatitis A should be vaccinated in accord with CDC recommendations long enough in advance of the trip to allow buildup of adequate antibody before departure to the endemic area.

## Hepatitis E

Like hepatitis A, hepatitis E is an enterically transmitted viral infection of the liver. The causative organism has not been fully characterized, although recent studies identify it as a single strand polyadenylated RNA virus. Hepatitis E disease is often called enterically transmitted non-A, non-B hepatitis to distinguish it from hepatitis A and from the bloodborne hepatitis B. It has also been called fecal-oral non-A, non-B hepatitis.

Hepatitis E is an acute infection that causes mild to severe disease with varying case fatality rates. It commonly occurs in the 15–40 year age group in developing countries where it is an important cause of morbidity and mortality. In the general population, case fatality rates of 0.5–3.0% are noted. Pregnant women appear to be particularly sensitive to the effects of hepatitis E infection. In several reported studies, case fatality rates as high as 20% have been reported among pregnant women, although overall mortality in the same epidemic is very much lower. Transmission of hepatitis E is almost invariably through contaminated water, although person-to-person transmission may also occur.

In Somalia, during the recent war, an epidemic of hepatitis E was temporally related to the rise of the river during a period of heavy rain. The peak of the epidemic coincided with the peak of the river during the rainy season. The attack rate was higher in villages supplied with drinking water from the river (6.0%) than it was in villages that relied on wells (1.2%) and ponds (1.7%) for their water supply.

A serologic test to determine the presence of hepatitis E is available. Recent studies have indicated that 2–3% of blood donors in the United States and in Northern Europe are positive for hepatitis E antibodies. 6.8% of blood donors in Spain carry antihepatitis E antibodies, and 70% of blood donors in Thailand carry the antibody. In India, during identified outbreaks of hepatitis E, 85% of the affected individuals lacked evidence of antibodies either to hepatitis A or B and 84% were positive for antibodies to hepatitis E virus.

No specific treatment is available for hepatitis E and no vaccine is yet available. Immune globulin is not currently indicated for prophylaxis of the disease. Chlorination of water cannot be relied upon to reduce the risk of water-borne hepatitis virus. Slow sand filtration is required to remove the causal organisms.

### Other Water-borne Viral Infections

Other viruses have been associated with waterborne epidemics from time to time. Poliovirus, the cause of poliomyelitis, has long been suspect as transmissible through water routes, but little credible evidence has been found to support this view. In 1988, contamination of the drinking water supply of the City of Haifa, Israel with poliovirus was suspected. This led to an immunization campaign but no cases. In the developed world, where wild type poliomyelitis is now virtually eradicated, spontaneous cases of polio are usually associated with vaccines.

Norwalk virus has been identified as a cause of epidemic enteritis in New South Wales, Australia. From time to time, many other water-borne epidemics of viral disease occur. The sporadic episodes are usually due to breakdown of the multiple barriers system in developed countries, and the use of fecally contaminated water in less developed areas for the potable water supply.

## WATER-BORNE TREMATODE & HELMINTH INFECTIONS

### Schistosomiasis (Bilharziasis)

Schistosomiasis due to *S hematobium* is a major problem throughout Africa. *S mansoni* causes the disease in the Arabian Peninsula, South America, some of the Caribbean Islands, and in areas of the Middle East. *S japonicum* is endemic in Asia. A number of other schistosomes are found regionally and locally. A blood fluke (trematode), the schistosome lives in blood vessels of the host for long periods of time.

Three forms of schistosomiasis are recognized: swimmer's itch or cercarial dermatitis, acute schistosomiasis, and chronic schistosomiasis. Chronic schistosomiasis causes severe illness in the host. Bladder, kidney, and other infections have been reported. Fibrosis, granulomas, obstructive uropathy, and bladder cancer may result from schistosomiasis. Bilharziasis, an older name for the same disease, is favored as the disease designation in South America and in other parts of the world.

The schistosomal infection is acquired from water containing the free swimming larval form, the cercariae. The life cycle is complex, but in most mammals, the eggs leave the host in the urine, hatch in the water, and are then carried in snail hosts. From the snail host, the cercariae are released into water, from which they penetrate the skin of human waders or swimmers and the cycle progresses.

Schistosomiasis is not transmissible from person to person, but infected persons are able to transmit the disease through excretion of infective eggs in urine for a lifetime. Prophylaxis is dependent on avoiding exposure to contaminated water.

Praziquantel is the drug of choice for treatment of all species of schistosome infection. Other drugs are also available and are sometimes effective in treating the disease.

### Ascariasis

Roundworm, or *Ascaris lumbricoides*, generally causes an asymptomatic infection of the intestinal tract. The organism is ubiquitous. In tropical countries, infection rates of up to 50% have been noted. Some patients develop pulmonary ascariasis and are symptomatic. Fever, cough, wheezing, and other pulmonary symptoms may occur. Ascariasis may contribute to nutritional deficiency.

Although soil contaminated with the eggs of the worm is the usual mode of transmission, water-borne transmission has also been reported. Effective treatment is available with mebendazole, although reinfection commonly occurs. Mebendazole is contraindicated during pregnancy. Pyrantel has also been reported to be effective in single doses against Ascariasis. A number of other drugs are also reported to be safe and effective in treatment of the infestation.

## CHEMICAL WATER CONTAMINATION

Chemical contamination of water is a worldwide problem. The prospect for remediation of extant chemical water pollution problems is not hopeful in the near term. For example, studies of trout and perch in Scandinavia, performed by Norheim et al have shown that decreases in mercury tissue concentration since the 1970 ban on the use of phenyl mercury in pulp and paper production has been very slow. They estimate that even though a river habitat is involved in their studies, 15 years is required for mercury levels in trout in the mercury polluted waters downstream from a pulp and paper plant to fall to a level equal to that in the trout upstream of the plant. Similar long delays in the remediation of water quality have been noted for arsenic, chromium, and other metals and persistent organics.

The opportunity for primary prevention of further deterioration in the universal water supply by intervention in agricultural and industrial activities that contribute to the load of biologically unacceptable materials in water is significant. Occupational and environmental health professionals who understand the processes conducted in the industrial facilities that they serve and the biological consequences of the materials used in the processes with which their patients work can intervene in the processes of facilities and practices designed to minimize or eliminate the release of toxic material or harmful biota to the external water supply. Such a preventive approach will substantially mitigate the problems of the future in the control of water pollution. This approach must be adopted both in developed and developing societies, if the impact on the limited supply of potable water in the world is to be significant.

## HUMAN DRINKING
## WATER REQUIREMENTS

Human drinking water requirements are well-defined. Studies in temperate conditions have demonstrated that acclimatized adults consume approximately 2 L of water per day. Under more extreme conditions, such as desert environments or under heavy work, human water consumption and water loss may rise precipitously. Adolph and colleagues first defined the effects of extreme temperatures and low humidity on human function in the Southwestern US deserts during World War II. Other physiologists have further elucidated the range of water consumption that is associated with variations in environmental conditions and work load. According to Weitzman and Kleeman, the average acclimatized 70 kg human, living in a temperate climate and at rest, consumes 800–1000 mL of water per day as water in food, and generates 300–400 mL of water from oxidation of food. One to 2 L per day are consumed as liquid, some of which may reasonably be expected to be tap water. To balance this intake, 800–1000 mL of water are insensibly lost in exhaled air and approximately 200 mL are evaporated as sweat. One hundred to 200 mL of water are lost in the feces and 1–2 L of urine are produced per day. Thus, a balance at 2100–3400 mL of water intake and output is normal.

Under desert conditions and heavy work, an extreme increase in the water intake is to be expected. The physiologists of the Israeli army have estimated that a fit, acclimatized young soldier marching in the desert at noon and carrying a 25-kg pack may sweat 3 L/h. In heavy military operations in the desert, the Israeli defense forces allocate 18 L of water or more per day for each soldier for drinking and light hygiene purposes.

In water utilization dosage calculations performed by various agencies of the US Government including the Environmental Protection Agency (EPA) and the US Agency for Toxic Substances and Disease Registry (ATSDR), daily water doses are assumed to be 2 liters per adult. Adjustments are made for age and size of children. Regrettably, no adjustment is made for the environmental conditions under which the subjects live. Estimates of toxicity from the ingestion of water-borne chemicals are often incorrect. The use of unadjusted EPA or ATSDR water-borne toxic dosage calculations without a critical review of the environmental conditions that exist in the area under study is likely to result in a substantial underestimation of the dose of absorbed toxic materials.

In addition to the dosage of water that is ingested daily, humans are exposed to water vapor, aerosols, and mists of water on a continuous basis. While this exposure to atmospheric water vapor and aerosols may contribute little to the water balance of the exposed humans, soluble organics and inorganics in this inhaled water may substantially increase the dose of toxic material that is absorbed through the respiratory system. In addition, water that is on the skin may contain dissolved material that can penetrate the epidermis and dermis and thus be absorbed. Dermally absorbed organics may also contribute significantly to the total dose of toxic substances delivered to humans from contaminated water sources. The ATSDR estimates that in circumstances where humans use water contaminated with partially soluble organic materials such as halogenated hydrocarbons for all ordinary domestic purposes, consumption, cooking, and hygiene, one-third of the absorbed dose of toxic materials comes from the water they drink, one-third from inhaled water vapor and aerosol, and one-third from dermal contact. McKone and colleagues have shown that the dose of hydrocarbons absorbed by inhalation of contaminated water used for showering and bathing may exceed the dose consumed by the same individuals by an order of magnitude. In view of these observations, assessment of human water-borne exposure to toxic materials must be very carefully evaluated for environmental conditions and work loads and for the utilization of water for purposes other than consumption by the population under study.

## THE WATER CYCLE & SOURCES
## OF HUMAN DRINKING WATER

The earth's water is constantly in a cycle of evaporation and precipitation. Once deposited on the earth's surface, water may run off, be impounded, or percolate through various layers of soil, sand, and rock to become free-flowing water or confined water. Deep aquifers are often confined. They do not participate in the evaporation and precipitation cycle unless the confining zone above them has been penetrated and fluids extracted from them. Evaporation from saline water sources, the oceans, and large salt marshes also contributes to the total airborne water vapor that may eventually precipitate to the earth's surface. The process of evaporation and precipitation has the potential to cleanse water of organic and inorganic contaminants, as does percolation of water through sand and soil and the action of humic bacteria and other mechanisms. Unfortunately, soluble organics that may escape the soil/sand adsorption process or that may be resistant to bacterial degradation may be evaporated with water, separately and at different rates, only to redissolve in the water/air mass. While much of this organic load is the result of industrial and agricultural activity, a very significant portion may be volatile halomethanes of several different structures produced in finished drinking water that has been chemically disinfected with chlorine- or bromine-based disinfection systems. The most prominent of these halomethanes is chloroform, a proved animal and probable human carcinogen. Other closely related halo-organic species also occur in finished water and in the air as a result of water disinfection processes. Bromomethanes, chloramines, and other closely related chemicals have been identified in finished disinfected water.

Airborne particulate matter, which is produced by the combustion of fossil fuels, may carry high loads of oxides of sulfur. These sulfur compounds are either adsorbed to the particulate's core or are dissolved in the aerosols that oxidative combustion produces. Acid particulates contribute an acid load to atmospheric water, which may become acid precipitation. Since these acidic materials are quite stable in water, they progressively acidify the surface and groundwater into which they are mixed. Smokes, aerosols, mists, and vapors may all contribute organic materials and inorganic substances of varying toxicologic significance to the air. In the vicinity of some coal-fired power plants and some other solid or beneficiated fuel-fired facilities, alkaline fly ash is deposited, which produces paradoxical alkalinization of the soil and adjacent surface and ground waters. Much of the particulate-bound load is partially water-soluble. It will reprecipitate to the earth's surface as atmospheric conditions change and rain falls. Oxynitrogenated organics, partially-soluble polynuclear organics, and metallo-organics may participate in the evaporation/precipitation cycle to contaminate surface and subsurface waters.

## SIGNIFICANT POLLUTANT SOURCES & INPUT TO SURFACE & GROUNDWATER SOURCES

Surface waters and groundwater are particularly vulnerable to pollution by the direct influence of anthropogenic wastes. Figure 44–1 demonstrates many of the inputs and outputs of the water cycle. Agricultural chemicals, industrial chemicals, mining wastes, septic tank and landfill leakage, and direct sewage discharge to surface or groundwater may contaminate drinking water resources. Small scale inputs of agricultural chemicals from domestic lawn and garden care with herbicides such as 2,4-D can pollute large quantities of drinking water. In the early 1970s, 2,4,5-T, a phenoxy herbicide closely related to 2,4-D, which was a component of Agent Orange, the defoliant used in Vietnam by American military forces, was deregistered for domestic lawn care purposes because of its potential to contaminate water in or around homes with materials that were believed teratogenic or embryotoxic to humans.

Halogenated solvents, paints and varnishes, carburetor cleaners, and gasoline may become troublesome if released to the groundwater or surface waters in quantities below those which are regulated and reportable. These chemicals are a significant source of local and regional surface and groundwater pollution. Large scale contaminant discharges are often sudden and are clearly recognized by those responsible for the release. Large releases must be reported to state and federal EPAs when the discharge is recognized. However, smaller scale backyard and garage contamination sources may be equally dangerous. Though unrecognized and unreported, these releases will quite soon afterwards appear in the water supply of the local districts.

Surface water and groundwater contamination from industrial disposal practices was common until the passage of the Clean Water Act and its amendments in the aftermath of Rachel Carson's publication of *Silent Spring,* in 1962. Prior to the early 1960s there was rampant disposal of many persistent organic compounds into surface and groundwater supplies. In recent years, massive-scale dumping of agricultural and industrial chemicals has been greatly reduced. In the future, new major pollution problems may not occur as a result of deliberate disposal practices in the United States because of enforcement of the Clean Water Act.

The right to discharge materials into the environment is granted under a permitting process that is administered by state, local and federal authorities. The permits that are granted specify the quantities of pollutants that may be discharged, the conditions under which they may be discharged, and the time of discharge. They also establish the monitoring and other activities that must be carried out to assure compliance with the permit. These NPDES permits are designed to keep information flowing about environmental contamination. They help to assure that a responsible standard is applied uniformly to all who discharge hazardous materials and who contaminate water resources, soil, or air.

## SPECIFIC SOURCES OF WATER POLLUTANTS

### Pulp & Paper Industry

There are some permitted specific industrial sources of water pollutants that are still worrisome. Among these are the river and stream discharges of the pulp and paper manufacturing industry. This industry discharges large quantities of toxic persistent and complex organics directly into surface waters, albeit with fully permitted facilities that generally operate close to or within their permitted limits. In addition to abietic acids, lignins, and other organic extracts, chlorine-based pulp bleaching plants discharge tetrachlorodibenzoparadioxin (2,3,7,8–TCDD) and its congeners to streams and rivers throughout the United States. These highly persistent organics are transferred to silt, sediment, and biota. From the silt, toxics are transferred to fish in the stream

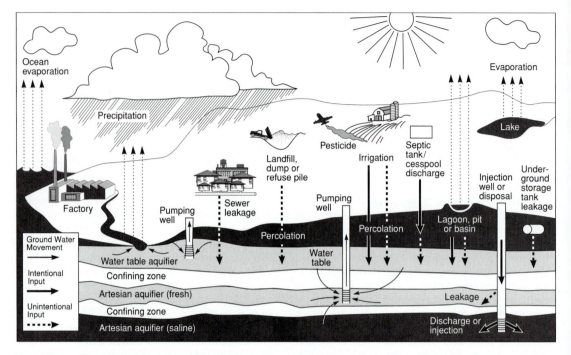

**Figure 44–1.** How waste-disposal practices can contaminate the groundwater system. (Reproduced, with permission, from Chivian E, McCally M, Hu H, Haines A [editors]: *Critical Condition: Human Health and the Environment.* MIT Press, 1993, page 33.)

ecosystem. The pollutants may be concentrated many-fold within the fish before they are consumed by humans or animals. When sportsmen or subsistence fishermen consume contaminated fish, they may further concentrate the toxins. The fishermen and their families may subsequently develop illnesses caused by the chemical of interest.

Bioconcentration of lipophilic organics, metals, and other substances has been well-studied. Tables of bioconcentration values may be found in most environmental ecology texts. The Hazardous Substances Databank of the National Library of Medicine, which may be accessed by computer users of the TOXNET database, contains information on the bioconcentration of various toxins in the food chain. Bioconcentration of toxins that are present in very low concentrations in water supplies from which humans draw agricultural or drinking water, or which are used for subsistence, commercial, or sport fishing is a major cause of water pollutant derived risk of disease to humans.

## Petrochemical Exploration, Refining, & Distribution

Large-scale chemical disposal problems with prominent water pollution components arise in the petrochemical industries. Both surface contamination and groundwater pollution occur as a result of losses and spills in petrochemical extraction, refining, dis-

tribution, and utilization. Control of production and distribution wastes has improved in the petrochemical industry. However, wetlands in the South Central and Southwestern United States in Texas, Louisiana, California, and elsewhere have both brackish and sweet water resources contaminated with oil production and refining wastes. At the oil field level, abandoned drilling mud, a complex semifluid material that may contain barium, chromium, asbestos, and many other substances, may be found. Many of these substances, including the hexavalent chromium used in the ferrochrome component of the drilling fluid, are water-soluble. They may enter the human drinking water supply. Waste crude oil and well head condensate were often dumped on-site at drilling locations. Such materials have penetrated to drinking water in some areas of the "oil patch."

During petrochemical refining and transport, spills of intermediates and final product occur. The Exxon Valdez crude oil spill in Alaskan coastal waters is one dramatic example of the problem. More common are the small spills from barges, trains, trucks, and other transport vehicles reported in the media around the world on an almost daily basis.

Leakage of gasoline products from underground storage facilities continuously inputs significant quantities of toxic and carcinogenic hydrocarbons such as benzene, toluene, and xylene, as well as the newer and relatively poorly understood MTBE (methyl-tert-butyl ether) into groundwater and surface waters that become the human drinking water supply. These volatile hydrocarbons are also released into the air of the homes of persons who live above contaminated groundwater plumes. Contaminant plumes may be the cause of human illnesses such as immunologic impairment, neurologic and cognitive deficits, birth defects, and cancers characteristic of exposure to these substances. Careful analysis of gasoline storage tanks and gasoline service station leakage problems has been carried out by NESCAUM, the Northeast States for Coordinated Air Use Management. Their models and scenarios of groundwater releases of gasoline products from service stations are very helpful to understand the potential toxic consequences of releases of organics to groundwater.

Current regulations prohibit the disposal of oily wastes to groundwater or surface water sources or the placement of these materials in landfill or municipal-controlled solid waste sites. Impoundment and cleanup/purification and treatment of oily and sour water wastes are required before these materials may be released to sewage systems. However, past practices and current breaches of operating rules in the petrochemicals industry continue to contribute significant levels of hydrocarbons to the drinking water supplies of residents who use well water that is collected in the vicinity of these operating units.

## Land Farming & Sludge Applications

The practice of land farming or sludge disposal from industrial and municipal waste plants continues to be common. In the petrochemicals industry, contaminated sludge from sumps, separators, and other sources is applied to uncontaminated soil. This sludge is exposed to environmental conditions that promotes the movement of these materials from the sludge to groundwater. Municipal treatment plant sludge, which is high in both organic and inorganic materials as well as in semi-dry biological products and bacterial contaminants, is similarly applied to soil. Sludge frequently contains dioxins and related products, metals, and other persistent toxins. Land farming practices are permitted by the USEPA and by state and local environmental authorities because of their potential for soil beneficiation. Most companies and municipalities try to operate within the limits of their permits for sludge application. However, the wisdom of land farming as a waste disposal method for sludge, which contains persistently toxic, partially soluble organics, metals, and bacterial contaminants of significant long-term toxicity, even at quite low concentrations, remains questionable.

## Deep Well Injection of Toxic Materials

Direct injection of waste chemical materials into deep saline aquifers continues to be a permitted method of disposal of hazardous chemicals in some areas of the United States and elsewhere in the world. This process of injection of materials into the deepest saline water resources was acceptable for many years. Unfortunately, penetrations into the deep artesian sources for petroleum exploration purposes has made this practice unwise, since the waste materials do not remain inaccessible. They may be pumped for various purposes. Thus, saline water may be moved to fresh water aquifers that provide drinking water supplies. In a recent review performed for the State of Texas in Mitchell County, a proposed hazardous waste site with deep water injection wells was rejected because the proposed well was to be placed in a stratum previously explored and abandoned for oil. There were many abandoned penetrations that would have permitted the injected material to return to the free flowing ground water strata.

In the late 1960s, deep water injection wells at the Rocky Mountain Arsenal in Denver were in active use for the disposal of military chemical biological warfare wastes. These wells were regularly used until it became apparent that the material was being injected into the Derby Fault, a geological formation that underlies the Denver Metropolitan region. Each time the water wells were used, a minor earthquake resulted. When the association between the use of the wells and the tremors was demonstrated by local geologists, the use of the wells was abandoned. The consequences of the injection have never been fully evaluated.

## Mining & Minerals Production

On a global basis, mining and minerals production and the processing and fabrication of the final metallic products is one of the largest sources of water pollutants. Exploitation of mineral resources results in the transfer of large volumes of metals from relatively protected deep mineral deposits to surface areas. Natural migration and solvation of metals from mineral deposits to drinking water can result in human poisoning. This process is responsible for areas of endemic blackfoot disease due to arsenic in well water in Taiwan. In these areas, liver, kidney, lung, and bladder cancer appear to be elevated. Extrapolation of the Taiwanese data to the concentrations of arsenic present in drinking water supplies in the United States suggests that the risk of cancer due to arsenic may be comparable to that due to environmental tobacco smoke and radon.

Acute arsenic poisoning from environmental sources in the United States has also occurred. However, most metal pollution of water resources is the result of working mineral deposits. Extraction of the minerals of interest and preparation of the economic product introduces large volumes of metals and the chemicals used to extract them to the surface and groundwater resources.

Not only does the direct extraction of metals produce water pollutants, acid mine drainage also contributes significantly to water pollution in the downstream areas. In southern Ohio, acid mine drainage has significantly affected stream ecosystems, contaminated fish populations, and increased stream mineral loads. Aluminum at toxic levels has also been detected in surface waters draining acid-sensitive watersheds. The source of this aluminum may be mine wastes or may occur naturally. The acid load is derived both from mine drainage and from acid rain precipitation from fossil fuel burning.

Lead, zinc, copper, nickel, vanadium, manganese, and iron compounds at toxic concentrations have been demonstrated in surface and groundwater adjacent to and downstream from mines and minerals extraction facilities. Drinking water wells in mining areas or highly mineralized areas should be tested for metal content as well as for extraction chemicals such as phosphates, nitrates, and cyanides, because these materials readily enter the water table from leaky extraction facilities. Tailing ponds, tailing piles, slag heaps, and other abandoned mineral rich waste collections often weather under the influence of rain and other water flows and relatively insoluble mineral forms such as galena (lead sulfide) are converted to lead carbonate, which then migrates into drinking water wells. Other mining-associated materials that have been identified in surface and groundwater sources for drinking water include polychlorinated biphenyls and sulfuric acid.

Asbestos and other mineral fibers that contaminated Great Lakes water from taconite (iron ore) mining operations in the Minnesota iron range have also been ingested in drinking water in Duluth, Minnesota and in other cities that draw their water supply from Lake Superior. Ongoing studies of the effect of asbestos contamination of the Great Lakes water found associations between asbestos fibers in drinking water and cancer incidence or mortality at many body sites, including the esophagus, stomach, small intestine, colon, and other organs. While there are methodological problems with all of the epidemiological studies of the association between ingested asbestos fibers and human disease, the problem is a real one. It needs to be followed with concern.

In the Balkan states, Balkan nephropathy has been identified and associated with mineral nitrogen, which probably arises in the course of minerals extraction. Studies of nitrite water contamination in the former Yugoslavia and its associated interstitial nephritis have raised concerns about the effect of these compounds on renal health. In Belgium, cadmium-induced nephropathies have been reported by Lauwrys and Roel. Itai itai, or "ouch-ouch" cadmium-induced systemic disease, occurred in Japan as a result of the contamination of estuarine waters that provided most of the dietary fish to a large population.

## Radionuclides

Radioactive minerals extraction used during Cold War military activities and for the purposes of fueling nuclear power plants has led to surface and groundwater contamination with radionuclides. These radioactive materials include radium, uranium, and their decay products. The water may release radon gas. In a number of areas, water has been significantly contaminated with tritium and alpha emitters as a result of these activities. In some localities, these elevated concentrations of water-borne radionuclides are believed to be responsible for elevated childhood leukemia rates.

Many countries are currently attempting to develop water standards for radionuclides, but the state of the art is somewhat uncertain. Only limited success in reaching a consensus on water standards for radionuclides has been reached.

Natural radioactivity also leads to contamination of groundwater and drinking water sources. Drinking water contaminated by naturally radioactive derivatives of the uranium and thorium decay series accounts only for a very small portion of the total annual dose of radiation for most humans. In some situations, the risk of leukemia and other cancers is elevated for those who live above, or drink from, groundwater sources that contain higher than normal radionuclide decay products. The products include radon and thoron.

Extensive study of the quantitative cancer risk associated with radon in groundwater and drinking water has been undertaken. In some studies, the risk is considered to be formidable. Regulations to limit radon concentrations in drinking water have been proposed in the United States, but formal adoption of these rules has not yet been completed.

## High Technology Industries

High technology industries such as semiconductor manufacturing plants, which are now proliferating in both the developed and developing areas of the world, are water intensive. Each facility uses large quantities of water. It may then return large quantities of potentially contaminated water to the sewage systems. The materials used in these facilities have included large quantities of halogenated organics such as trichlorethylene, trichloroethane, perchloroethylene, and carbon tetrachloride. Many complex organics are used as photoactive agents in photoresists. Metals and metalloids such arsenic, selenium, beryllium, cadmium, and lead are also in use in these plants. All semiconductor facilities have plating sections where cyanides and metallic plating solutions containing hexavalent chromium and other carcinogenic metals are in use. Many of the materials are in water-soluble formulations. They may enter the waste water discharge systems of the facilities either by design or in error. Although on-site treatment is required in the United States and other western countries, it is not so effectively enforced to prevent the accidental contamination of groundwater. In less developed countries, a far more serious problem exists. The costs of treatment on site must be borne by the manufacturers. In the absence of rigorous enforcement, it is probable that releases of semiconductor manufacturing chemicals to the environment will occur.

Groundwater and drinking water contamination from high technology industries has occurred in areas where groundwater sources are important contributors to drinking water supplies. In Phoenix, Chandler, and Mesa, Arizona, there is widespread groundwater contamination with as many as 37 different solvents from acetone to xylene leaching from leaking underground storage tanks, from the use of "French drains," and from leaching fields used for organic chemical disposal in the 1950s and 1960s.

In Tucson, Arizona, an aircraft manufacturing facility caused widespread trichloroethylene contamination of the drinking water supply for a portion of the city. Thousands of residents used this water as their source of drinking and domestic water. Epidemiologic assessment of this population has demonstrated a statistically significant increase of cardiac anomalies in children born to mothers who consumed the contaminated water. As a result of this water contamination episode, extensive litigation has taken place in Tucson and has resulted in large monetary settlements. Some of the settlement proceeds are to be used to compensate those injured by the contamination and some for cleanup of the problem.

Similar groundwater contamination problems have occurred in the Silicon Valley communities of Mountain View and Milpitas, California as a result of semiconductor industry chemical use in the 1950s and 1960s. These identified problems represent only a portion of the contaminated groundwater problems that exist in the United States. No inventory of actual contamination exists.

Simple loss of hazardous materials from the waste water systems of industrial facilities through leaky pipes and other problems continues to occur. Recently built treatment facilities and remediation of existing contaminated sites under and adjacent to these and many other high technology plants may eventually provide a source of clean water to the contaminated communities. At the present time, however, many people are drinking water contaminated with halocarbons and other materials that probably originated in these plants.

The current situation is worrisome because the majority of the chemicals that have been leaked by these plants are of the same general type as the halohydrocarbons produced in the disinfection of drinking water. Thus, the concern about long-term carcinogenic and other effects from disinfectant chemical residues, which at this time are inevitably present in community water supplies, is accentuated by the consumption of this high technology chemical cocktail.

The greatest concern must be directed towards bladder and colon cancer, which are increased in communities where there is long-term consumption of water with elevated concentrations of halo-hydrocarbons. Research done by Cantor of the USEPA in 1975 and by Wilkins and colleagues in 1979, as well as more recent studies by Gottlieb and Mangione et al, contribute to the rising concern that lifetime or long-term consumption of water contaminated with halo-hydrocarbons increases cancer rates in a meaningful fashion. Since it appears that water disinfection technology is not sufficiently developed to permit abandonment of the chlorination procedures currently in use, the added burden of halo-hydrocarbons in the drinking water supply from industrial sources is very worrisome.

## Power Plants & Cooling Towers

Thirty-eight percent of all water used in the United States is employed to cool machinery used in the production of electrical power. Much of this water is used as cooling water for coal and other fossil fuel-fired plants. Some is used for cooling water for nuclear power facilities. Many of these electrical power facilities are private plants developed by large industrial facilities such as refineries, chemical plants, heavy manufacturing facilities, and municipalities. In countries other than the United States, such local power facilities are the rule rather than the exception. In Eastern and Central Europe, every large and many smaller industrial facilities have their own on-site power generation facility.

Each of these facilities must treat its water to prevent corrosion of the cooling towers and to arrest growth of bacteria, such as the *Legionella* genus and fungi in the cooling water. For many years, the principal materials used to prevent cooling tower corrosion were hexavalent chromium compounds. Organic mercurials were the rule for cooling tower biocides. These materials are no longer in use in the United States for these purposes in cooling system. Elsewhere in the world, hexavalent chromium corrosion inhibitors continue to be used, as do mercurial biocides. These highly toxic materials may be disposed of directly to the water systems. At best, they are impounded and evaporated. From impoundment ponds they may reach the groundwater after subsequent leaching caused by rain and runoff. In California, at least one community groundwater supply was severely contaminated by the practice of disposal of cooling tower wastes from a natural gas compression plant containing hexavalent chromium into waste water ponds. The hexavalent chromium, a class one human carcinogen, later leached into the domestic wells of the surrounding residences. Concentrations of chromium hundreds of times above California's standards were measured in some of the wells. It may be hoped that in these situations the hexavalent chromium will eventually be transformed to trivalent chromium by natural reductive processes. However, local conditions are so variable that there is substantial risk that carcinogenic chromium will be distributed in the drinking water, along with organic mercurial biocides and other substances from cooling system chemicals from any such use and disposal practice.

### Agricultural Chemicals

Agriculture is the largest user of water resources around the world. It is also the industry with the most direct access to surface and groundwater resources. Because agriculture is universally chemically intensive, and the chemicals are generally applied in solution, suspension, or as wettable concentrates and powders, agricultural chemicals have the greatest potential to produce serious water pollution problems. In every large study that has been conducted, it has become apparent that no area of the world is free of agricultural chemical contamination of surface and groundwater resources.

In the past 50 years, the development of a chemically intensive agricultural pattern in every country has led to the contamination of water supplies with many evanescent and persistent chemicals of considerable acute and chronic toxicity. In the latter half of the 20th century, contamination of individual and community water supplies with every agricultural chemical that has been introduced has occurred.

In the 1960s, water pollution from organomercurial seed coating fungicides used on the Indian subcontinent led to the contamination of deep sea tuna with levels of mercury that were unacceptable to the Western Countries. The source of this organic mercury was the fungicidal substances that were applied to rice seed. Since the use of organomercurials produced an 1800% increase in rice yield per acre, it was inevitable that those countries in the Indian subcontinent that depend on rice to prevent starvation would continue to use the mercurials. Only recently have run-offs from the rivers of Asia had reduced levels of mercury.

Organic mercury contamination from seed coating fungicides, paper pulp fungicides, and cooling tower biocides has been a major cause of water pollution in Japan, the Indian Ocean, and Scandinavia.

The Minimata Bay ecosystem in Japan was contaminated with industrial mercury runoff in the 1950s. Consumption of mercury-contaminated fish from this region resulted in many children being born with neurological birth defects. The impact of this tragedy was graphically portrayed by W. Eugene Smith in his photographic essay, *Minimata*. It is most poignantly depicted in the photograph "Tomoko in her Bath" (Figure 44–2). This photograph of a severely deformed, neurologically damaged child being bathed in her mother's arms tells far more effectively than any other icon might the tragedy that mercurial

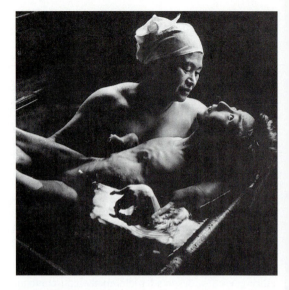

**Figure 44–2.** "Tomoko in her Bath," 1972. Photograph by W. Eugene Smith. Collection of the Center for Creative Photography. ©1982 Aileen M. Smith.

water pollution can produce. Litigation over this incident, which began in the 1950s, was concluded in Japan in 1996. No apology was ever received from the Government or the industry responsible for this mass poisoning episode, much to the consternation of the affected population in Japan.

Perhaps of greater significance than organic mercurial or halogenated hydrocarbon exposure in the past is the current widespread contamination of drinking and ground water supplies of wells and rivers throughout Europe, Asia, and North America with herbicide chemicals of every structure. Reports from the United States, Europe, and Asia confirm the contamination of rural, suburban, and urban water supplies with every agricultural chemical. The most widely used chemicals lead the contaminant list. Atrazine, a triazine herbicide used for preemergence weed control, appears in virtually every well in every United States area where it has been used. Other materials have similar widespread distribution. Chlorophenols, fluorinated compounds, chlorothalonil, dinoseb, metribuzin, linuron and monuron, glyphosate, and others have all been identified in public and private drinking water supplies.

Sheila Hoar Zahm and colleagues at the National Cancer Institute have suggested that the widespread contamination of agricultural water resources with herbicides such as 2,4-D and atrazine, among many others, may be causally associated with the world wide epidemic of non-Hodgkin's lymphoma that has been underway for several years. Roloff and colleagues have demonstrated abnormalities of human lymphocytes at concentrations of atrazine and linuron similar to those found in drinking water supplies. In California, groundwater contamination with aldicarb, a powerful carbamate insecticide, has resulted in statistically significant lymphocyte cd2/cd8 ratio changes in women who consumed this water.

In many parts of the world, dibromochloropropane (DBCP) contamination of ground water has occurred as result of the direct injection of this carcinogenic compound into the soil for the control of nematodes in bananas, pineapples, and sugar beets. Dibromochloropropane causes male sterility in agricultural and manufacturing workers who make or apply this material. The widespread contamination of groundwater with this reproductive toxin in Costa Rica, Honduras, Philippines, Ivory Coast, and in Fresno County, California, is very serious. Recent out-of-court settlements were negotiated between the City of Fresno, California, and the manufacturers of dibromochloropropane in lawsuits filed by the city to recover large sums of money that must be spent to upgrade the city's capacity to purify drinking water so that the DBCP concentration in finished water meets California's drinking water standards.

Contamination of surface and groundwater with nitrates used as fertilizers has led to serious and even fatal acute illness in children who consumed this water in infant formula. Recent studies in Eastern and Central Europe and earlier work performed in the United States has confirmed that agricultural nitrate runoff has reached levels that are capable of causing methemoglobinemia in children. In addition, these nitrates are the substrate for further biological alteration to nitrosamines, which are carcinogenic.

Other persistent and transient elevations of water pollutants in groundwater and drinking water makes imperative the development of newer techniques to control water-borne exposure to chemicals in agriculture.

## DRINKING WATER
## REGULATORY CONSIDERATIONS

Estimates are that close to 350 billion gallons of water are used in the United States each day. This total of about 1400 gallons of water per capita is the highest in the world. Only 10% of the total water usage in the United States each day is for drinking water purposes. Eleven percent is for industrial purposes, 38% is used to cool electric power generating plants, and 41% is used for agricultural purposes. The Bureau of the Census reported that the largest user state for water resources in 1985 was Idaho, at more than 275 million gallons of water each day. Most of this water is for agricultural purposes. Each of the major water-consuming segments contributes significant waste water to the United States water supply. Many contribute substantial contaminant loads to it, as well.

Public drinking water systems supply much of the drinking water in the United States and elsewhere around the world. The sources for these drinking water systems vary widely. Surface waters such as rivers, streams, lakes, and reservoirs and shallow and deep groundwater aquifers may be used. These water systems are generally regulated by local or national regulatory bodies, which set specific standards for water quality. Standards include treatment requirements and the concentration of contaminants and pathogens that are allowed in the finished drinking water. In the United States, local governments are most often responsible for the provision of finished drinking water. The quality of the water is defined by local regulation, which must be at least as strict as that required by the Federal Safe Drinking Water Act of 1974 and by the amendments to that Act, which were passed in 1986. The Safe Drinking Water Act applies to all water systems that serve more than 15 connected customers or more than 25 people. Currently, the Act and its amendments are under heavy attack as overly costly for the protection that it achieves. The outcome of this debate is not known.

The Safe Drinking Water Act limits total halomethanes in finished, disinfected drinking water to 100 ppb. This is a performance-based standard that does not take into account the health effects of the halomethanes. Rather, it considers the technological and economic infeasiblity of water engineering systems and practices to achieve a lower level of disinfectant byproducts at the present time. Other water contaminants are limited in finished drinking water by the Safe Drinking Water Act. Metals such as arsenic, lead, and barium; pesticides such as aldicarb, 2,4-D, and chlorinated organics; and non halogenated substances such as benzene and other aromatic and aliphatic compounds are regulated. In addition, radioactivity in water supplies is also regulated by the Safe Drinking Water Act. Certain inorganic ions such as cyanide and nitrate, and pathogenic organism counts are regulated as well.

Enforcement of the Safe Drinking Water Act is in the hands of the US EPA. The EPA sets two standards for each regulated pollutant. The first standard, called a Maximum Contaminant Level Goal (MCLG), is set at a concentration that is not expected to cause adverse health effects over a lifetime of consumption of water at that concentration. A substantial safety margin for this MCLG is included in each unenforceable standard. There is no penalty assessed for violation of the MCLG concentration by a public water supply system. In addition to the MCLG, the EPA has promulgated enforceable standards called Maximum Contaminant Levels (MCLs) for each regulated contaminant. Regulated suppliers of drinking water must comply with the MCLs. By law, the EPA must attempt to set the MCL as close to the MCLG as is technologically and economically feasible. In almost all cases, the enforceable MCL is higher than the

MCLG. The 1986 Safe Drinking Water Act amendments also banned the use of lead pipe or soldered connections in any public drinking water system in order to reduce lead contamination of water that may affect the intellectual development of infants and children. Suppliers of public drinking water must comply with these regulations, as well.

MCLs apply only to public drinking water supplies in the United States. MCLs for noncarcinogenic compounds are believed to be protective of the most sensitive human populations that may be exposed to them. Details of the protective factors and diseases or effects protected against may be found for each substance in the US EPA Integrated Risk Information System (IRIS) database, which is accessible through the National Library of Medicine's online TOXNET database. Only two current MCLs, those for bacteria and nitrate, would cause acute illness if they were exceeded. All others consider chronic or long-term adverse effects.

MCLs for carcinogens are considered by US EPA to be protective to a level where the allowed concentration of the regulated contaminant in water would not cause a human population risk of cancer greater than 1 in 100,000. Details of the carcinogenesis decision-making bases for each MCLG and MCL are also found in the IRIS online data base. The decisions for short and long-term water standards are based on calculations of NOAEL (no adverse effect levels) and LOAEL (low adverse effect levels) from which ADI or Acceptable Daily Intakes are developed by the Office of Drinking Water of the EPA. The process has a high level of uncertainty, which is adjusted for to some degree in the calculations. The regulations are often based on indirect evidence of questionable relevance. From the available data, the EPA calculates 1-day health advisories for noncarcinogenic effects for children, 10-day health advisories for children,

and 1-day, 10-day, and lifetime health advisory (HA) levels for 70-kg adults. These calculations are used as informal guidelines to municipalities and other institutions in the event of emergency chemical spills and in other contamination situations.

MCLs do not apply to private drinking water wells, which estimates suggest supply 15% of the US population, or 40 million people, with their daily drinking water supplies. Neither MCLGs nor MCLs apply to bottled water, which is often used as a substitute for contaminated public drinking water supplies. If the bottled water is drawn from private wells or springs, as is often the case, only the supplier's goodwill protects the ultimate consumer of the water from consumption of contaminants that would not be permitted in a public water supply. No contaminant concentration limits exist for the use of groundwater, recreational water, springs, streams, lakes, or ponds, as drinking water supplies.

Additional regulatory proposals have been made for materials for which no enforceable MCLG or MCL exist. These proposals are not legally enforceable. They are often health-, rather than performance-, based guidelines. Because of the limited toxicologic database on which these suggested guidelines are based, or for other economic and regulatory considerations, MCLs have not been officially adopted as binding for many known toxic water contaminants. The EPA is actively developing data on water pollutants, which is published in its Drinking Water Criteria Documents. These documents provide detailed assessments of the contaminants and their toxic profiles. Unfortunately, the information that is available on many water contaminants is incomplete and inconclusive. Uncertainty limits the ability to regulate the chemicals in water, even though the evidence is suggestive that chronic consumption of these materials produces disease in animals and humans.

## REFERENCES

### BIOCONTAMINATION OF WATER SUPPLIES

Anonymous: Addressing emerging infectious disease threats: A prevention strategy for the United States. Executive summary. MMWR Morb Mortal Wkly Rep 1994;43:1.

Benenson AS (editor): *Control of Communicable Diseases in Man,* 15th ed. American Public Health Association, 1990.

Berkelman RL: Emerging infectious diseases in the United States, 1993. J Infect Dis 1994;170:272.

Mara D, Cairncross S: *Guidelines for the Safe Use of Wastewater and Excreta in Agriculture and Aquaculture: Measures for Public Health Protection.* World Health Organization, 1989.

### CONTROL OF MICROBIOLOGICAL WATER CONTAMINATION

Greenberg AE, Clesceri LS, Eaton AD: *Standard Methods for the Examination of Water and Wastewater,* 18th ed. American Public Health Association, 1992.

World Health Organization: *Guidelines for Drinking Water Quality,* 2nd ed. Vol. 1, 1993.

### PATHOGEN-CAUSED WATER-BORNE DISEASE

Desenclos JC et al: Large outbreak of *Salmonella enterica* serotype paratyphi B infection caused by a goats' milk cheese, France, 1993: A case finding and epidemiological study. BMJ 1996;312:91.

Huang P et al: The first reported outbreak of diarrheal illness associated with Cyclospora in the United States. Ann Intern Med 1995;123:409.

Koo D et al: Epidemic cholera in Guatemala: Transmission of a newly introduced epidemic strain by street vendors. Epidemiol Infect 1996;116:121.

Pang T et al: Typhoid fever and other salmonellosis: A continuing challenge. Trends Microbiol 1995;3:253.

Rabold JG et al: Cyclospora outbreak associated with chlorinated drinking water. Lancet 1994;344:1360.

## PROTOZOAN-CAUSED WATER-BORNE DISEASE

Bell A et al: Outbreak of toxoplasmosis associated with municipal drinking water—British Columbia. Can Commun Dis Rep 1995;21:161.

Goldstein ST et al: Cryptosporidiosis: An outbreak associated with drinking water despite state-of-the-art water treatment. Ann Intern Med 1996;124:459.

Isaac-Renton JL. Characterization of Giardia duodenalis isolates from a waterborne outbreak. J Infect Dis 1993;167:431.

Mac Kenzie WR: A massive outbreak in Milwaukee of cryptosporidium infection transmitted through the public water supply. N Engl J Med 1994;331:161.

## WATER-BORNE VIRAL DISEASE

Dilawari JB: Hepatitis E virus: Epidemiological, clinical and serological studies of north Indian epidemic. Indian J Gastroenterol 1994;13:44.

## WATER-BORNE TREMATODE & HELMINTH INFECTIONS

Kightlinger LK, Seed JR, Kightlinger MB: Ascaris lumbricoides aggregation in relation to child growth status, delayed cutaneous hypersensitivity, and plant anthelmintic use in Madagascar. J Parasitol 1996;82:25.

## SPECIFIC SOURCES OF WATER POLLUTANTS

Angle CR: If the tap water smells foul, think MTBE. JAMA 1991;266:2985.

Collman GW, Loomis DP, Sandler DP: Childhood cancer mortality and radon concentration in drinking water in North Carolina. Br J Cancer 1991;63:626.

Goldberg SJ et al: Cardiac teratogenesis in mammals produced by dichloroethylene and trichloroethylene. Pediatr Cardiol 1990;11:244.

Hoar Zahm S et al: A Role of the herbicide atrazine in the development of non-Hodgkin's lymphoma. Scand J Work Environ Health 1993;19:108.

Hoffmann W, Kranefeld A, Schmitz-Feuerhake I: Radium-226-contaminated drinking water: Hypothesis on an exposure pathway in a population with elevated childhood leukemia. Environ Health Perspect 1993; 101(Suppl 3):113.

Kross BC, Ayebo AD, Fuortes LJ: Methemoglobinemia: Nitrate toxicity in rural America. Am Fam Physician 1992;46:183.

Mao Y et al: Inorganic components of drinking water and microalbuminuria. Environ Res 1995;71(2):135.

McGeehin MA: Case-control study of bladder cancer and water disinfection methods in Colorado. Am J Epidemiol 1993;138:492.

Roloff BD, Belluck DA, Meisner LF: Cytogenetic studies of herbicide interactions in vitro and in vivo using atrazine and linuron. Arch Environ Contam Toxicol 1992;22:267.

Smith AH et al: Cancer risks from arsenic in drinking water. Environ Health Perspect 1992;97:259.

Staessen JA et al: Public health implications of environmental exposure to cadmium and lead: An overview of epidemiological studies in Belgium. J Cardiovasc Risk 1996;3(1);26.

# 45      Multiple Chemical Sensitivity

*Robert Harrison MD, MPH*

Clinicians have been increasingly challenged by the individual with multiple complaints relating to low-level occupational or environmental exposures. Patients report respiratory, central nervous system, musculoskeletal, gastrointestinal and systemic symptoms after exposure to common environmental irritants such as perfumes, cigarette smoke, home or office furnishings, household cleaners, and a host of other petrochemical products. Upper respiratory (nasal congestion, dryness, or burning), central nervous system (concentration problems, memory difficulties, insomnia, drowsiness, irritability, depression) and vegetative (fatigue, headache, arthralgias, myalgias) symptoms predominate. Symptoms occur with exposures well below thresholds accepted by federal or state agencies as causing adverse effects in humans, resulting in significant impairment, lost work time, complete job loss, or major alterations in social and family functions. Individuals may report symptom onset following acute or chronic low-level occupational or environmental exposures, with persistent symptoms that are triggered by subsequent environmental irritants. Other individuals report these symptoms without obvious occupational or environmental etiology but are concerned that *potential* exposure to environmental toxicants may trigger or aggravate their symptoms. Patients seek help from multiple health care providers who suggest psychiatric etiologies or treatment, obtain toxicologic or immunologic test batteries, or initiate a variety of empirical treatments. Workers' compensation or disability claims are often disputed, and employers often have difficulty accepting or accommodating clinician or patient requests for alternative work environments. As a result, frustration, anger, hostility and suspicion may confront the clinician when significant impairment continues despite lengthy and expensive consultations.

Considerable controversy continues to surround the etiology, case definition, diagnosis and treatment of individuals with Multiple Chemical Sensitivity (MCS). Many authors believe that etiologic theories, diagnosis, and the clinical management of MCS are not consistent with sound medical science. The spe-

cialty of clinical ecology that emerged in the 1960s adopted theories of causation that differ from those of traditional allergy, immunology, and toxicology, thereby laying the basis for medical and legal disputes regarding legitimate or acceptable forms of treatment, medical or workers' compensation insurance reimbursement, and disability benefits. In order to guide the clinical evaluation of individuals with this disorder or respond to requests for epidemiological investigation, the health care practitioner should be aware of these current controversies, including knowledge gaps and the need for further research.

## EPIDEMIOLOGY & CASE DEFINITIONS

There is no single term or universally accepted case definition for individuals with this disorder (Table 45–1). "Environmental hypersensitivity" has been defined as a chronic (ie, continuing for more than three months) multisystem disorder, usually involving symptoms of the central nervous system and at least one other system. Affected persons are frequently intolerant to some foods and react adversely to some chemicals and to environmental agents, singly or in combination, at levels generally tolerated by the majority. Affected persons have varying degrees of morbidity, from mild discomfort to total disability. On physical examination, the patient is usually free from any abnormal objective findings. Improvement is associated with avoidance of suspected agents and symptoms recur with reexposure. The term "environmental illness" has been described as an acquired disease characterized by a series of symptoms caused and/or exacerbated by exposure to environmental agents. Symptoms involve multiple organs in the neurologic, endocrine, genitourinary and immunologic systems. The term "multiple chemical sensitivity" has been defined as an acquired disorder characterized by recurrent symptoms, referable to multiple organ systems, occurring in response to demonstrable exposure to many chemically unrelated compounds at doses far below those established in

**Table 45–1.** Terms used to describe syndrome of symptoms in association with low-level occupational or irritant exposures.

Environmental illness
Multiple chemical sensitivity
Chemical hypersensitivity syndrome
Ecological illness
Universal allergy
20th century illness
Environmental allergy
Cerebral allergy
Chemically associated immune dysfunction
Multiorgan dysesthesia
Idiopathic environmental illness

the general population to cause harmful effects. No single widely accepted test of physiologic function can be shown to correlate with symptoms. Seven criteria are included in one definition of MCS:

1. The disorder is acquired in relation to some documentable environmental exposure(s), insult(s) or illness(es).
2. Symptoms involve more than one organ system.
3. Symptoms recur and abate in response to predictable stimuli.
4. Symptoms are elicited by exposures to chemicals of diverse structural classes and toxicologic modes of action.
5. Symptoms are elicited by exposures that are demonstrable (albeit at low level).
6. Exposures that elicit symptoms must be very low, by which is meant standard deviations below "average" exposures known to cause adverse human responses.
7. No single widely available test of organ function can explain the symptoms.

A practical limitation of this case definition is the lack of objective testing to confirm symptoms following demonstrable or predictable exposures. Patients with MCS are distinguished from those indi-viduals with acute occupational diseases (eg, acute solvent intoxication, occupational asthma) and psychiatric disorders (eg, post-traumatic stress disorder, somatoform disorder, mass psychogenic illness). Other criteria have been proposed for MCS, including those based on a survey of occupational physicians, clinical ecologists and internal medicine and otolaryngology specialists. These criteria differ from those proposed by the National Research Council, and the Agency for Toxic Substances and Disease Registry Working Groups (Table 45–2).

An operational definition of multiple chemical sensitivity has also been proposed based on the concept of "adaptation." With this operational definition, the patient with multiple chemical sensitivities can be discovered by removing the person from the suspected offending agents and by re-challenge, after an appropriate interval, under strictly controlled environmental conditions. Causality is inferred by the clearing of symptoms with removal from the offending environment and recurrence of symptoms with specific challenge. "Adaptation" refers to a sequence of stages (known as preadaptive, addictive and postadaptive) along with stimulatory and withdrawal levels of reaction, by which an individual manifests symptoms as a result of cumulative environmental exposures. A "stimulatory effect" from foods or chemicals is followed by "withdrawal" symptoms; eventually the individual becomes "addicted" or adapted to chronic environmental or food exposures. Clinical manifestations of adaptation are highly individualized and variable, with a broad range of gastrointestinal, cardiopulmonary and central nervous system symptoms. It is only by "withdrawing" the individual to an environment free from chemicals and food "incitants" that the illness can then be "unmasked." Likewise, a variety of intradermal and sublingual tests are used as diagnostic tools to provoke symptoms. These concepts were initially formulated in relation to food allergies, and then were extended to chemical exposures. "Ecologic" or "environmental control" units have been established to provide

**Table 45–2.** Proposed case definitions for multiple chemical sensitivity.

| Cullen | National Research Council | ATSDR | Nethercott |
| --- | --- | --- | --- |
| Documentable environmental exposures | Symptoms elicited by low level exposures | Change in health status | Symptoms reproducible with exposure |
| Symptoms in more than one organ system | Symptoms in more than one organ system | Symptoms triggered by multiple stimuli | Condition is chronic |
| Symptoms recur and abate to predictable stimuli | Symptoms and signs wax and wane with exposures | Symptoms for at least 6 months | Symptoms with low level exposure |
| Symptoms elicited by diverse chemicals | | Defined set of reported symptoms | Symptoms improve with avoidance |
| Symptoms elicited by demonstrable exposures | | Symptoms in three or more organ systems | Responses to multiple substances |
| Symptoms elicited by very low exposures | | Exclusion of other medical conditions | |
| No single test to explain symptoms | | | |

chemically-free environments where these diagnostic and therapeutic techniques are employed.

The field of clinical ecology emerged in the mid 1960s based on the proposal that chronic adverse reactions to low level chemical or food exposures cause or exacerbate symptoms in susceptible individuals, and that changes in the frequency of and intervals between exposures can mask the clinical manifestations of or alter the sensitivity to those substances. Ecologic illness is defined as a polysymptomatic, multisystem, chronic disorder manifested by adverse reactions to environmental incitants, as they are modified by individual susceptibility in terms of specific adaptations. The incitants are present in air, water, drugs, and in our habitats. The controversy over these theories and clinical application have resulted in several reviews from professional medical organizations rejecting both the theoretical basis for ecologic illness as well as controversial diagnostic and treatment methods. Some authors have concluded that no credible evidence exists that permits acceptance of MCS-related disorders or demonstrates the validity of treatments used by clinical ecology practitioners, while others advocate for greater acceptance of the MCS patient and new, as yet untested theories.

Little epidemiologic evidence exists regarding this syndrome. Limited population-based data exist regarding the prevalence of MCS, or occupational or demographic characteristics of this syndrome. Over 15% of the general population reported unusual sensitivity to everyday chemicals in a population-based survey in California. A disproportionate number of patients in studies of MCS are women, ranging from 70% to 85% in case series and case-control studies. A questionnaire for use in population studies shows that patients with MCS report significantly more substances that elicit symptoms than other medical or occupational clinic patients. Several populations have been identified that may develop symptoms of MCS, including industrial workers, occupants of "tight buildings" such as office workers and school children, residents of communities whose air or water is contaminated by chemicals, and individuals with unique, personal exposures to various chemicals in domestic indoor air, pesticides, drugs, or consumer products. Workplace exposures to poor indoor air quality, pesticide exposure and remodeling have been associated with the onset of MCS. Other diagnostic subsets have been reported among individuals with solvent-associated psycho-organic syndrome, chemical headaches, and intolerance to solvents. Records-based reports from an allergy practice, academic occupational medicine clinic, and environmental health center suggest that individuals with MCS are predominantly women in the 30- to 40-year age range, with a disproportionate number from service industries. MCS patients in these reports tend to be of higher socioeconomic status, and had a diversity of

both occupational and environmental exposures. The most commonly reported symptoms in one survey were headache, fatigue, confusion, shortness of breath, and arthralgias; another survey found that previous psychological difficulties (depression, anxiety, somatization, stress, and stress-related functional illness) were prominent among MCS patients.

Symptoms of MCS also resemble those of sick-building syndrome, a constellation of excessive work-related symptoms related to an indoor office environment (headache, eye, nose and throat irritation, fatigue, dizziness) without an identifiable etiology. Multiple chemical sensitivities has been reported to follow pesticide exposure among employees in a casino and among several office workers following a large-scale outbreak of sick-building syndrome. Several symptoms included in the Centers for Disease Control case definition of chronic fatigue syndrome (fatigue, confusion, memory loss, sleep difficulties, myalgias, headaches) are also common among individuals with MCS, and affected individuals may be concerned about occupational or environmental etiologies for chronic fatigue syndrome. Aside from symptom overlap, there is currently no evidence linking chronic fatigue syndrome to occupational or environmental chemical exposures.

## ETIOLOGY

Lack of a uniform case definition for individuals with MCS has hampered investigation of etiology, and the criteria for study eligibility have varied depending on the target population. Etiologic hypotheses have focused on either psychiatric or physiologic mechanisms. Symptoms in MCS patients are not consistent with toxicologic effects, because workplace or environmental exposures in this population are considerably lower than those expected to cause end-organ toxicity based on dose-response relationships, consistency, and predictability of clinical responses, or animal models.

Symptoms of individuals with thrombophlebitis, vasculitis, and cardiac disease have been reported in uncontrolled case series to have been reproduced with specific chemical challenges. Symptoms have improved following withdrawal in a chemical-free environment. Signs and symptoms of chemical sensitivity have been assessed using low-dose chemical inhalant challenges and placebos in an environmental control unit, but these studies have not been duplicated using more rigorous scientific methods, and they fail to shed any light on the mechanism by which symptoms are produced. Carefully controlled, double-blinded, placebo-controlled, inhalation challenge studies have not been performed.

### Psychiatric Hypotheses

Individuals with MCS have been described as a

medical subculture with a long history of pre-existing psychological symptoms and recurring physical complaints unsupported by objective physical findings, who seek physicians to confirm their own convictions about their symptoms, and who organize their lifestyle around their illness. In this view, a society with a heightened awareness of toxic hazards, physicians with a ready explanation of symptoms based on physiologic theories, a favorable workers' compensation system, and medical, legal, and patient advocacy supports contribute to the emergence of MCS as a self-described medical disorder.

Other psychological factors, such as the attribution of normal changes of aging to toxic exposure, traumatic neurosis, psychosis, work stress, and conflicts, secondary gain from the sick role, and the need for vindication, also contribute to what has been described as a somatoform disorder. Practitioners of clinical ecology become a last resort for many patients when traditional practitioners fail to explain the cause of bodily symptoms. Symptom reports may be the result of a perceived toxic exposure, with a variety of perceptual biases and conscious or unconscious reporting biases determined in part by media influences, influence of other coworkers, monetary self-interest, and the forensic environment.

The majority of patients with MCS are reported to have psychiatric conditions (psychoses, affective or anxiety disorders, or somatoform disorders-somatization, conversion, and hypochondriases), many with symptoms well before their diagnosis of environmentally related illness. Some patients with persistent or recurrent medically unexplained symptoms may have an atypical posttraumatic stress disorder, where specific and recurrent somatic symptoms follow acute or chronic chemical exposures, with subsequent experience of symptoms repeatedly triggered by low-level environmental irritants.

Individuals with MCS may have a heterogeneous group of other psychiatric disorders, either causally related or secondary to MCS, with depression, anxiety, and a variety of somatoform disorders (hypochondriases, conversion disorder, somatization disorder). Prolonged physical symptoms and sensitivity to common environmental irritants have been described as a behavioral conditioned response or an "odor-triggered panic attack." Specific cognitive and behavioral interventions such as systematic desensitization, relaxation techniques, self-hypnosis, or biofeedback have been suggested as treatment strategies. Some MCS patients have been described as primarily ideational (obsessive/compulsive) or phobic in character, requiring a different psychotherapeutic approach focusing on the effect of physical symptoms on psychological function, stress associated with physical and interpersonal isolation, or the frustration of multiple physician consultations.

Neuropsychologic measures (EEG, scalp EMG, skin resistance) during relaxation in individuals who attribute medical and psychological symptoms to chemical exposures have been compared with subjects with primary psychological disorders and with a control group. MCS patients did not differ from psychologic subjects, and both were significantly different from controls, suggesting that individuals with MCS may have primary emotional, anxiety, attentional, or personality disorders. The MCS group had a higher somatization score on a standard self-report symptom inventory, and a subset of these patients had a history of early childhood sexual abuse.

Other studies have compared subjects with MCS with matched controls using a variety of standardized psychological interview schedules and self-administered symptom questionnaires. Subjects with a diagnosis of environmental illness had a higher prevalence of affective disorders (particularly major depression), anxiety, and somatoform disorders compared with controls, and more environmental illness subjects met lifetime criteria for a major mental disorder. Individuals with environmental illness filing workers' compensation claims had a greater prevalence of prior psychiatric morbidity (anxiety, depression, somatization trait) and higher self-reported measures of somatization and hypochondriasis.

Psychiatric and psychological disorders may be a consequence, rather than a cause, of MCS. Among subjects referred to an occupational medicine clinic who met the case definition for MCS, psychiatric evaluation did not suggest any premorbid psychiatric diagnosis or a premorbid tendency toward somatization. Clinically significant psychiatric symptoms of depression and anxiety were present among most subjects, with a subset performing poorly on tests of verbal performance. Despite a preponderance of psychiatric symptoms among MCS patients, psychiatric diagnoses were uncommon and most did not suffer from diagnosable psychiatric disease. Patients recruited from the practice of a community allergist with a reported diagnosis of chemical sensitivity were compared with control patients from a university-based occupational musculoskeletal and back-injury clinic. Cases of MCS reported a higher prevalence of current psychological distress (depression, anxiety, somatization) and somatization symptoms preceding the onset of sensitivity symptoms. Neuropsychologic performance did not differ when adjusted for the level of psychological distress.

## Immunologic Hypotheses

Environmental and occupational chemical exposures may affect the immune system, with a variety of cellular and cell-mediated immunologic effects established in both animals and humans. Xenobiotics may produce immunosuppression and alter host resistance in experimental animals following acute or subchronic exposure, and immunologic effects in humans have been reported in association with dusts (silica, asbestos), polyhalogenated aromatic hydrocarbons (dioxins, furans, polychlorinated biphenyls), pesticides, metals (lead, cadmium, arsenic, methyl mercury), and solvents. However, neither experimental immune dysfunction nor epidemiological evidence of altered immunity have been correlated with clinical disease.

Environmental illness has been postulated to be an immunologic disorder, with generalized immune dysregulation as a result of free radical generation and alkylation, structural alteration of antigens, or hapten/carrier reactions. Chemicals are hypothesized to alter immune responses, triggering lymphokines leading to clinical symptoms of cell-mediated immune response. Chemically sensitive patients are reported to have altered T and B lymphocyte counts, abnormal helper/suppresser ratios, and antibodies to a variety of chemicals. Patients with building-related illness have been reported to have an abnormal antibody response and altered cellular immunity to formaldehyde, although these findings have not been confirmed using controls, and clinical correlation is absent. MCS has also been hypothesized to be the result of an interaction between the immune and nervous systems.

Studies of patients with environmental illness or MCS have found no consistent abnormalities in immunoglobulins, complement, lymphocytes, or B-cell or T-cell subsets. A study of patients with MCS found no evidence of increased autoantibodies, lymphocyte count, helper or suppresser cells, B or T cells, or TAI+ or interleukin-2+ cells compared with control subjects. Absence of objective evidence for immunologic abnormality distinguishes patients with MCS from those with other allergic disorders, autoimmune diseases, and congenital or acquired immunodeficiencies. There is no convincing evidence that MCS is an immunologic disorder.

### Respiratory Hypotheses

Many individuals with MCS report a heightened sense of smell or develop symptoms at low levels of environmental irritant exposure. MCS has been hypothesized to represent an amplification of the nonspecific immune response to low-level irritants. Altered function of c-fibers, respiratory epithelium, or neuroepithelial interaction is postulated to result in increased symptom reporting correlated with physiologic abnormality. Neurogenic inflammation mediated by cell-surface enzymes could play a role in upper respiratory symptoms reported by MCS patients. Subjects with MCS are reported to have higher nasal resistance and respiration rates, and patients with MCS were found with rhinolaryngoscopy to have marked cobblestoning of the posterior pharynx, base of the tongue, or both. The relevance of these findings to the etiology of MCS remains to be determined.

### Olfactory-limbic Hypotheses

MCS has been postulated to be the result of environmental chemical exposure, with the triggering or perpetuation of affective and cognitive disorders as well as somatic dysfunction in vulnerable individuals via kindling mechanisms. Kindling is a type of time-dependent sensitization of olfactory-limbic neurons by drug or non-drug stimuli, with activation of neural structures such as the amygdala and hypothalamus. In this model of MCS, sensitization to food or chemicals parallels the phenomenon of time-dependent sensitization from drugs or non-drug stressors, with heightened sensitivity to stimuli, gradual improvement following withdrawal, and reactivation of symptoms following reexposure. Time-dependent sensitization has been studied as a possible model for cacosmia (subjective sense of feeling ill from odors) among nonpatient populations, which may have relevance to similar symptoms reported by MCS patients. It has been hypothesized that shy individuals may have hyperreactive limbic systems and may self-report greater symptoms of illness due to chemical exposures. Further research is needed to determine whether the olfactory-limbic model may explain symptoms in patients with MCS.

## CLINICAL MANAGEMENT

### History & Physical Examination

A careful, thoughtful, and compassionate exposure and psychosocial history is critical. Although the etiology of MCS is controversial, the patient may be suffering from disabling symptoms, frustrated by the lack of definitive answers from clinicians, and is sometimes desperately seeking advice and counsel regarding treatment. Approaching the history with the suspicion that the patient with MCS is suffering from a psychiatric disorder, is malingering, or is seeking monetary benefits, is not helpful in establishing a therapeutic relationship. Acknowledgment of symptoms and the establishment of a trusting relationship should not necessarily be avoided because the etiology is uncertain or patient motivation is suspect.

A history should be obtained of symptom onset in relationship to acute or chronic exposures. Attention should be paid to respiratory, dermal, neurologic, and systemic symptoms. Duration and severity of symptoms should be recorded, particularly in relationship to repeated exposures in the workplace or environment (eg, improvement away from work, or on weekends/vacations, with worsening symptoms at work). An occupational history should be obtained, including past employment and exposure to chemicals, dusts, or fumes. Recent and past chemical exposures should be identified by product names or Material Safety Data Sheets, and any environmental monitoring data reviewed if available.

The individual with MCS typically reports symptoms after exposure to common environmental irritants such as gasoline, perfumes, or household cleaners. Symptoms of headache, fatigue, lethargy, myalgias, and trouble concentrating, may persist for hours to days or even weeks, with typical "reactions" reported after these common exposures. Often the individual with MCS will have already identified a variety of irritants that result in symptoms and will have initiated an avoidance regimen. Varying degrees of restrictions in social and work activities may be reported, including problems driving an automobile, grocery shopping, wearing certain types of clothing, or staying away from office buildings or other workplaces.

Individuals with MCS usually do not have concurrent presence of other obvious occupational or environmental diseases such as asthma or contact-allergic dermatitis. It is essential to rule out other non-occupational diseases through a comprehensive history, review of previous records, and appropriate diagnostic studies. A few patients may have hyperreactive airway disease and develop symptoms of chest tightness or shortness of breath on exposure to low-level environmental irritants. Nonspecific airway challenge testing or patch testing may be useful in selected patients. The physical examination is almost always normal in patients with MCS, but particular attention should be paid to examination of the lungs for the presence of wheezing that may indicate asthma.

Additional psychological evaluation should be considered if the history suggests the presence of significant psychiatric disorder. Psychiatric consultation, treatment, or both, may be advised regardless of the etiology of MCS, as many patients may have significant psychiatric morbidity with this disorder.

### Diagnostic Tests

Several controversial techniques have been employed for the diagnosis of MCS, including provocation-neutralization testing, chemical and food challenges, immunologic testing, inhalant challenges, serologic testing for Epstein-Barr virus antibodies, various autoantibodies, blood testing for organic hydrocarbon and pesticides, and hair testing for heavy metals. Many of these tests have no diagnostic utility. There is no evidence linking MCS to past infection with the Epstein-Barr virus. There is no association between MCS and levels of organic hydrocarbons or pesticides in blood or fatty tissue, and knowledge of minute residues of these chemicals may only serve to mislead and alarm the patient. The use of biomarkers (eg, detailed profiles in serum of lipid-soluble toxins and their metabolites, or heavy metals in the hair matrix) have no role in the diagnosis of patients with MCS. These tests have not been correlated with any pathological consequences in MCS or control groups.

Routine laboratory evaluations do not reveal any consistent diagnostic abnormalities. Laboratory testing to rule out other medical conditions, or diagnostic tests (such as nonspecific airways challenge with methacholine or histamine) that are suggested by clinical complaints may be useful. Neuropsychologic testing may be helpful with a history of exposure to a known neurotoxin and symptoms of cognitive impairment. Blinded provocation testing has been employed in research studies, but has not been rigorously evaluated as a useful diagnostic technique for individual patients.

Single photon emission computed tomography (SPECT) or positron emission tomography (PET) studies of brain perfusion, computerized EEG analysis, or visual evoked response (VER) and brain stem auditory evoked response (BAER) have not been evaluated in controlled studies, and should not be performed as a diagnostic clinical tool outside of a research setting. Likewise, results of tests for porphyrin metabolism in blood, urine or stool specimens have not been correlated with clinical symptoms and should not be obtained unless part of a research protocol.

In the absence of other concurrent medical conditions suggested by history, physical examination, or routine lab testing, the diagnosis of MCS relies on the patient's history of multiple symptoms triggered by low-level chemical exposures.

### Treatment

A variety of controversial methods have been utilized for the treatment of MCS, including elimination or rotary diversified diets, vitamins or nutritional supplements, oxygen, antifungal and antiviral agents, thyroid hormone supplement, supplemental estrogen or testosterone, transfer factor, chemical detoxification through exercise and sauna treatment, intravenous gamma-globulin, and intracutaneous or subcutaneous neutralization. A specially designed chemical-free environmental control unit has been advocated as a method to decrease blood pesticide levels and improve symptoms as well as intellectual and cognitive function. Controversial treatment methods offer hope of improvement to many individuals with MCS, and some patients report symptom improvement over time. Many of these treatment methods are expensive and are rarely covered by health insurance. These treatment methods have not been validated through carefully designed, controlled trials, may have unwanted side effects, and may serve to reinforce counterproductive behaviors. Patients should be advised that such treatments are controversial, have not been subject to controlled clinical trials, and are not recommended by most medical professional organizations.

Avoidance of those low-level environmental irritants that provoke symptoms is often already implemented by many patients, but some clinicians are reluctant to recommend specific changes in the home environment, work restrictions, or a trial away from work. Elimination of exposures at home, workplace, or school through a variety of strategies (including room air filters) has been suggested. Avoidance of low-level irritants has not been tested in controlled scientific studies. In some patients, avoidance may reinforce the notion of disability and lead to further isolation, powerlessness, and discouragement. In one case series of MCS patients from an occupational health practice, improvement in symptoms was associated with self-reported avoidance of specific substances or materials.

Education regarding general principles of toxicology (for example, routes of exposure of toxic chemicals, routes of elimination) may be reassuring to the patient concerned about long-term storage of chemicals in the body and the fear of ongoing damage.

Although it is not clear whether psychological symptoms are the cause of MCS or simply accompany the diagnosis, specific cognitive and behavioral interventions may be useful in the treatment of MCS. A biopsychosocial model of illness conceptualizes a close correlation between physical and psychologic diseases. MCS may be a heterogeneous disorder with more than one causal mechanism. Significant psycho-physiologic symptoms may occur after exposure to low-level volatile compounds, in persons with and without coexisting or preexisting psychiatric illness. Cognitive techniques or behavioral desensitization of the individual through relaxation techniques, breath-control exercises, and visualization or other hypnotic techniques may be useful, along with a structured plan to increase overall physical and social activity. Improving the patients understanding of the role of stress on illness, and enhancing coping mechanisms for the impact on daily life may be helpful. Biofeedback-assisted relaxation training and cognitive restructuring has been reported with some success in case reports. Pharmacologic treatment for specific symptoms suggestive of depression or anxiety, in conjunction with other behavioral techniques, may offer some relief as part of an overall treatment program.

MCS is considered a disability under the Americans with Disabilities Act, MCS patients may seek protection under federal housing discrimination laws, and MCS is considered a handicap under several state employment discrimination statutes. Patients with MCS should be advised that, as with a chronic illness, treatment is not directed at a "cure" but rather at accommodation. Care should emphasize relief of symptoms and a return to active work and home life. These treatment strategies entail a treatment alliance between patient and clinician, without judgment regarding the etiology of MCS. Regardless of etiology, psychological symptoms play a prominent role in this disorder, and behavioral techniques appear to be the most promising treatment approach. Limited follow-up studies indicate that up to half of MCS patients may improve over a period of years, but the majority continue to note a major impact on career, marriage or family, and other common daily activities.

## REFERENCES

American College of Physicians: Clinical ecology (position paper.) Am Intern Med 1989;111:168.

Ashford NA, Miller CS: *Chemical Exposures: Low Levels and High Stakes*, Van Nostrand Reinhold, 1991.

Cullen MR: The worker with multiple chemical sensitivities: an overview. Occup Med 1987;2:655.

Mitchell FL (editor): *Multiple Chemical Sensitivity: A Scientific Overview*. US Department of Health and Human Services, Agency for Toxic Substances and Disease Registry. Princeton Scientific, 1995.

National Research Council: *Addendum to Biologic Markers in Immunotoxicology*. National Research Council, 1992.

Nethercott JR et al: Multiple chemical sensitivities syndrome: toward a working case definition. Arch Env Health 1993;48:19.

Report of the Council on Scientific Affairs, American Medical Association: Clinical ecology. JAMA 1992;268:3465.

Rest KM: Advancing the understanding of multiple chemical sensitivity (MCS): (overview and recommmendations from an AOEC workshop). Toxicol Ind Health 1992;8:1.

Sparks PJ et al: Multiple chemical sensitivity: a clinical perspective. I. Case definition, theories of pathogenesis, and research needs; II. Evaluation, diagnostic testing, treatment, and social considerations. J Occ Med 1994; 36:718,731.

Terr AI: Multiple chemical sensitivities. Ann Intern Med 1993;119:163.

# Population-Based Disease Registries

# 46

*Peggy Reynolds, PhD, MPH*

The use of population-based disease registries has become an increasingly cost-effective means for investigating initial concerns about human health effects of workplace or environmental sources of toxicants, or for initial identification of unusual patterns of morbidity or mortality. The various kinds of disease registries currently available offer a wide variety of opportunities to both better understand the patterns of disease occurrence and plan for primary and secondary disease control measures.

## TYPES OF DISEASE REGISTRIES

Various sources of health outcome information that could be characterized as disease registries exist. These sources are not all necessarily population-based, nor do all of them offer complete information on the diseases of interest. There are many sources of health outcome information that, while designed to serve a different purpose, may also serve as important source information in environmental or occupational health investigations. Particularly salient features of data from various types of registries include the degree of diagnostic confirmation associated with a specific disease classification and information regarding the registries' representativeness of all of the events for a population of interest. Examples of types of registries classified by these features is summarized in Table 46–1.

### Vital Records

The most prevalent source of health outcome information is vital records. Registration of basic birth and death information is available for local, national, and international populations. Information on causes of death is categorized by a general coding system, the International Classification of Diseases (ICD). Basic demographic information is collected on newborns and their parents and on decedents.

These data have the advantage of being population-based and standardized within certain minimum parameters, and in summary form can provide valuable initial impressions on regional variations and secular trends in patterns of population change and mortality. They can be useful for looking at broad measures of adverse reproductive outcomes or cause-specific mortality. Although they have the advantage of broad coverage, vital records data typically have the disadvantage of a lack of detailed information on diseases of interest and provide rather indirect evidence for the actual incidence of most disease endpoints. Although some vital records systems contain information on multiple causes of death, most are restricted to underlying cause of death information. As such, they provide a good indirect tool for measuring incidence trends in diseases with high case fatality rates (such as lung cancer), but do not provide good descriptive information on incidence for diseases associated with good survival.

### Hospital-Based or Occupational Surveillance Systems

Institutional sources of targeted morbidity information are commonly available for special purposes. Hospitals typically maintain a diagnostic index or discharge summary that reflects the census of inpatients by presenting conditions for a particular period of time. In some cases, this information is aggregated for a broad geographic area to reflect the pattern of hospitalizations across institutions. Similarly, some employers maintain medical surveillance information on their employees. This information reflects anything from voluntary use of in-house medical services for minor ailments to mandatory accident reporting for certain events of interest for the industry. Some employers also offer screening programs for various conditions that may be motivated by special occupational risks, or simply as part of a larger workplace wellness program. More specialized occupational surveillance programs have also been initiated for employers in some states, as in California's Lead Poisoning Registry and Pesticide Illness Reporting System.

Information from such sources serves as a valuable planning tool for within-institution resource allocation, or for characterizing some between-institution differences. This information may also serve as

**Table 46–1.** Types of disease registries.

| Diagnostic Confirmation Rate | Population-Based | |
| --- | --- | --- |
| | **No** | **Yes** |
| Low | • Workplace medical surveillance<br>• Lead screening programs | • Vital records<br>• Health administrative data bases<br>• Pesticide illness reporting |
| High | • Hospital discharge data/diagnostic index<br>• Screening programs | • Communicable disease reporting<br>• Cancer registries<br>• AIDS registries<br>• Birth defects registries |

an indicator, or early warning sign, for health outcomes of special concern. It does not, however, provide a broad view of morbidity for the population of interest. Hospital discharge data may provide valuable insights into the profile of clientele and service needs. For many conditions, however, discharge data tend to represent the extremes, or episodes of illness severe enough to require hospital admission. This information may also be duplicated by person, representing episodes of illness rather than individuals with a condition. As such, these data may better reflect the urgent care needs of a small subgroup than the incidence or prevalence of diseases of interest.

## Other Administrative Data Sources

In addition to hospital discharge data or a hospital's diagnostic index, there are a number of other sources of administrative data that can facilitate health studies. These include pharmacy data bases, health care maintenance organization records, and other large scale medical care programs that serve targeted populations such as the US Federal Health Care Financing for the Aged (HCFA) or California's MediCare program. Although these programs are designed for medical delivery rather than research, they can also serve as valuable resources for both health care research and epidemiologic investigation. To a limited extent, and for specific subgroups, such sources of information approximate the integrated socialized care health information for some European countries. Even though health outcome information is limited, because some of these programs are virtually population-based for identified groups, they can form the basis for preliminary indicators of health patterns, or for selection into more in-depth studies. For example, in case-control studies of cancer, the HCFA files (which include individuals over age 64) have been commonly used to identify potential population-based controls in older age groups much more cost-efficiently than other procedures such as ran-

dom-digit dialing. These data bases can also be used to examine purely ecologic associations as well. Information on trends for sales of the conjugated estrogen Premarin in the 1970s were temporally associated with an epidemic of endometrial cancer in postmenopausal women in California. Increased use of screening mammography during the late 1980s was associated with an increased incidence of early stage breast cancer. Both of these ecologic associations were later demonstrated to be consistent with the evidence from case-control and cohort studies of these disease outcomes.

## Population-Based Disease Surveillance Systems

The "gold standard" for disease registration is a population-based disease surveillance program. Early concerns about basic public health disease control gave rise to legally mandated population-based reporting requirements for targeted infectious diseases. For noninfectious diseases, the best established model for such systems has come from population-based cancer registries. At one time, these were primarily voluntary reporting systems, but in recent years, many local governments have enacted mandatory cancer reporting requirements similar to those for infectious diseases. In the United States, population-based cancer registration dates back to 1935 when the Connecticut Tumor Registry initiated a surveillance system for all newly diagnosed malignancies among residents of the state. The Connecticut Tumor Registry has been operating continuously since then, and has been one of the most valuable, and one of the only, sources of information for long-term cancer incidence trends.

Up until the 1970s the National Cancer Institute (NCI) conducted a series of national cancer surveys in targeted areas of the United States to assess patterns of incidence. During the same time, the NCI collected patient treatment and follow-up information from a series of hospitals throughout the country. These hospitals volunteered to contribute to the End Results program, which formed the basis for information on differences in expected survival for various types of cancer. Following the Third National Cancer Survey (for the years 1969–1971), the NCI initiated an ongoing surveillance system that integrated elements of both the national surveys and the End Results program. This program, called the Surveillance, Epidemiology and End Results (SEER) program, collects and maintains an integrated system of information on newly diagnosed cancers as well as basic treatment and follow-up (survival). Operating in several designated areas of the United States, the SEER system was designed not to be representative of the total population, but rather to reflect the population diversity of the United States. The SEER program today represents roughly 10% of the US population and is the primary basis for national statistics on cancer incidence and survival.

The United States is not unique in supporting population-based cancer registration systems. Many countries throughout the world have done likewise, although many of those cancer reporting systems are not as old and not as detailed as various US registration systems. The International Agency for Research on Cancer (IARC) (formed in 1965 by the World Health Organization) has published a series of monographs of international incidence data called Cancer Incidence in Five Continents, which began in 1966 and was published by a predecessor organization, the International Union against Cancer. The most recent monograph (Volume VI) was published in 1992, and contains cancer information from 50 areas of the world. These monographs are designed to be representative, rather than comprehensive, of the world's populations, and include data from registries that meet the IARC's standards of data quality. Over the last several decades, they have been the single most valuable source of information on international variations in cancer incidence.

In the 1980s, there was a great deal of local interest in developing legislation to mandate statewide cancer registries throughout the United States and Canada. During this time, there was a rapid proliferation of population-based cancer reporting. By the late 1980s, the American Association of Central Cancer Registries, an organization of state and local cancer registries in the United States was formed. This organization, now called the North American Association of Central Cancer Registries, plays an active role in setting data standards and establishing a minimal data set across registries, and has also begun to generate summary data for its 36 United States and 12 Canadian registry members.

Broad-based population-based registries are rare for other chronic disease health outcomes, although more recently a number of areas have developed birth defect registries. One of the largest of these is in California. Combined with birth registration data (which provides the denominator for rates of birth defects), this registry has provided important descriptive and analytic information on the occurrence of a wide spectrum of birth defects. Similarly, as acquired immune deficiency syndrome (AIDS) became more common in the United States in the 1980s, a number of geographic areas developed population-based AIDS registries. These have served to enhance our understanding of changes in the demographic profile of the AIDS epidemic in the United States over the last decade.

## LINKAGE TO ENVIRONMENTAL OR OCCUPATIONAL COHORTS

By themselves, disease registries serve an important function in providing descriptive information on the geographic/demographic scope and temporal changes in the occurrence of diseases of interest. In combination with other sources of information on population groups defined geographically, occupationally, or with respect to some other common characteristics, registries also offer a powerful tool for better understanding the causes or course of disease.

### Geographic

Disease registry information has been an important resource for better understanding spatial patterns of disease, and has served as an important planning tool for secondary prevention programs. Population-based registries typically collect address information that can be geocoded to various levels of detail with geographic coverage ranging from state, county, zip code, census tract, or block group to actual x, y ("real world") coordinates, which can provide information on the exact location of an event within a city block. The increasing availability of geographic-based reference information based on census characteristics of the population, environmental exposure measures, or physical geography, along with increasingly sophisticated geographic information system (GIS) technology, provide opportunities to evaluate patterns of disease in the context of a wide range of factors.

These tools provide the basis for "ecologic" studies of disease. These include studies that correlate differences in disease rates with such population characteristics as socioeconomic status, or with environmental characteristics such as land use. Well known examples of these are general studies of the association of skin cancer rates with "sunny" climates or specific studies of various cancer types by the proportion of petrochemical industries by county in the United States. Such studies do not in themselves make a case for disease causation, but such observations can provide valuable evidence for developing hypotheses that can be tested in other study designs. Likewise, these tools have proved to be a valuable adjunct to the difficult enterprise of studies of "disease clusters," or in evaluating the potential health impact of identified environmental toxicants on the health of a community.

Ecologic studies are not new. They date back at least as far as John Snow's classic observations about the eight- to nine-fold higher rate of cholera deaths among London residents served by the Southwark and Vauxhall water company in the mid-1800s. Inferences drawn from that observation led to swift public health intervention, removal of the Broad Street Pump handle, and the introduction of legislation requiring London water companies to filter their water. Notably, this occurred nearly 20 years *before* the identification of the cholera vibrio by Koch. Some of the simplest geographic studies, those which merely examine rate differences associated with other area differences, have served to stimulate active areas of epidemiologic enquiry. Studies that have reported the correlation of higher heart disease and breast cancer mortality rates in countries with higher levels of dietary fat consumption have provoked more sophisticated assessments of these associations. Studies that have noted striking international differences in stomach and colon cancer rates between Japan and the United States, with intermediate rates evident for migrant populations, have served as the basis for studies of the influence of diet and other cultural differences as possible risk factors for these gastrointestinal malignancies.

## Occupational or Environmental

Occupational cohorts, or other defined cohorts, can also be linked to disease outcome registries. Such linked data sets have proved to be a valuable source of hypothesis generation for a variety of suspected exposure-disease relationships. One of the more widely reported examples is the Swedish Cancer Environment Registry, which has linked individual information on occupation and residence from the national 1960 Census to twenty years of follow-up information from the population-based cancer registry, and has provided fruitful information on environmental, socioeconomic, and occupational risk factors for a variety of cancers. Sweden also maintains a linked registry between the national census data and its medical birth registry, which has formed the basis for studies of adverse reproductive outcomes among certain employment groups. A recent report from this linked registry suggested that infants born to mothers working in chemical industries experienced higher rates of several adverse outcomes, including low birth weight, short gestational age, and infant mortality.

Similarly linked national registers have been reported from Denmark and from Great Britain. The Danish registry has additionally linked its census-cancer registry to more detailed work history information from a variety of Danish industries, providing valuable background information for such major international efforts as the IARC's monograph series on the Evaluation of Carcinogenic Risk to Humans.

Linkage efforts such as these, which represent the full universe of a population at risk linked to a system of completely ascertained disease reporting, represent an ideal resource for preliminary evaluations of suspected risk associations. As a result, they are a first step in the search for causality. Provocative risk associations can be followed up in nested case-control studies, with study subjects selected from a well-defined and well-characterized universe.

Although not all places offer such universal opportunity for evaluation, similar approaches have proved useful in the evaluation of cancer risks in cohorts of individuals selected in other ways, particularly in a wide spectrum of occupational cohorts in the United States. Such an approach was taken in the late 1970s, when clinicians in the small California community of Livermore noted an apparently high frequency of

malignant melanoma of the skin occurring in patients who were employees of the Lawrence Livermore National Laboratory (LLNL), a US Department of Energy high-energy physics research facility in Livermore and one of the primary local employers. The LLNL medical staff was aware of some of the melanoma cases, but was not sure how many additional cases there might have been, nor how many might have been expected in the lab work force, which consisted primarily of white men. Because the San Francisco Bay Area, including Livermore, was covered by population-based cancer registration, it was possible to use computerized linkage methods to match the historical LLNL employee roster to the cancer files to fully ascertain the number of melanomas occurring among members of the LLNL work force. The number of observed cases was roughly four times that which would have been expected, compared to the same age, race, sex, and areas of residence of the lab employees. Furthermore, an analysis of adult melanoma rates in Livermore suggested that they were slightly higher than might be expected based on prevailing rates for the county, but that when LLNL employees were removed from the numerator and denominator of the community rates they were indistinguishable from rates elsewhere in the county. This initial evaluation was conducted reasonably quickly because of the availability of the population-based cancer registry. Subsequent studies have been undertaken to evaluate the degree to which workplace, or other factors, may explain this apparent disease excess.

The most widely reported health outcomes in these studies have been cancers of various types. This is because population-based cancer registries are more common than registries for other chronic disease outcomes, and incidence data are considered somewhat more reliable and relevant than mortality data. Nonetheless, similar approaches have also been reported for various adverse birth outcomes and, in some Scandinavian countries, even for registration of cardiovascular events.

## LIMITATIONS OF DISEASE REGISTRIES

### Behavioral Risk Factors

One of the most important limitations of studies based on record linkage between a cohort and disease registries, or surveillance systems themselves, is the lack of individual risk factors that may mediate the apparent association between a suspected occupational risk factor and a specific disease outcome. For example, numerous studies have suggested that a variety of blue-collar occupations are associated with a higher risk for lung cancer. But unless such studies are designed to adjust for the effect of active smoking, the apparent occupational associations are less convincing. Typically, behavioral risk factors are either unavailable or not available in sufficient detail, in either cohort or disease registry files, to be able to assess the role of such factors in record linkage studies. The influence of some of these factors can be indirectly assessed by using external information sources. One approach, especially for geographic studies, is to use group attributes available at the census tract or block group level to indirectly adjust for such effects. A similar approach can be used by applying group summary information to other identifiable groups, such as an occupational cohort. This latter approach was used in a study of occupational mortality in California, in which standardized mortality ratios were estimated for broad occupational categories indirectly adjusting for smoking, alcohol consumption, and socioeconomic status. In addition, a linked exposure-outcome file can be used as the basis for selecting cases and controls from whom to collect additional risk factor information for follow-up studies.

In some areas, cancer registry programs have initiated a complementary risk factor surveillance program to enhance the ability to evaluate potential risk associations for various cancers. The general approach is one of a random-digit dialing population survey for targeted risk factors of interest that can serve as a comparison group for specially collected information on cases in the registry. One well known model for this type of program is from the Detroit Cancer Registry, which instituted a system of collecting occupational information from a community survey that could then be compared to occupational data from the registry. This occupational risk factor surveillance system, in combination with occupational data collected by the cancer registration process, has provided some provocative evidence for higher risks for certain cancers in several occupational groups, including observations of elevations among certain types of workers in Detroit's automotive industry. This is a cost-effective way to generate hypotheses that can be pursued in more in-depth studies of occupational risks for cancer.

## Temporal/Geographic Associations

While the availability of computerized cohort and disease outcome registries offer a marvelous opportunity for hypothesis generation about disease causation, or for identification of high-risk subgroups, inferences from such studies need to be interpreted cautiously with respect to the temporal association between exposure and disease. Because of the relative recency of most computerized population-based disease registries, particularly for long latency diseases such as cancer, it has not been possible to evaluate apparent occupational or environmental associations with disease over as long a time period as may be desirable.

Similarly, because address information in disease registries typically represents address at the time of diagnosis, admission, or death, geographic information from such sources is limited and does not necessarily represent an individual's long-term residence. Importantly, address at the time of a health event, particularly in increasingly mobile populations, may be unlikely to represent locations associated with exposures of interest.

An important exception to these constraints is offered by the model of cancer-environment registries developed in some of the Scandinavian countries. In the case of the Swedish cancer-environment registry, in which 1960 census information on individuals was linked to persons diagnosed with cancer during a follow-up period (1961–1979), it was possible to evaluate differences in disease rates by occupational affiliation. This has been the source of a number of studies of occupational associations and cancer. Interestingly, it has also provided the basis for evaluating the degree to which childhood socioeconomic status (as defined by father's occupation) is a predictor of cancer risk in later life.

## Confidentiality Concerns

Though the use of disease registries, especially those that involve linkage between a cohort and outcome file, provides the opportunity to better understand disease-association risks, it raises special concerns about the confidentiality of the identity of individuals in each record system. These are nontrivial concerns, as the enabling legislation for most population-based disease registration includes provisions for maintaining confidentiality. Because of the possibility of breach of confidentiality, many Scandinavian countries, which are among the richest resources for such studies, have recently enacted strict restrictions on these uses of registry data that virtually preclude access to many potential investigators.

With the increasing sophistication of geographic information system technology, the potential to identify individuals from characteristics associated with rare events at smaller levels of geographic detail also has raised confidentiality concerns about mapped data presentation even when individual identities are unknown.

## Diagnostic/Treatment Detail

Typically, disease registries are designed to provide information that can guide primary treatment decisions and profile the incidence of disease occurrence. To do this, data must be collected with sufficient detail and accuracy to fully characterize the heterogeneity of broad classes of disease. Cancer registries, for example, collect detailed information on the anatomic subsite, cell type, laterality, and staging for most tumors. Quality control procedures generally require a high percentage of histologic confirmation for diagnosis. Studies that have compared death certificate information on cancer type to that from registry data for decedents suggest that death certificates provide less reliable information on the type of cancer that may have been the underlying cause of death. For some cancers in particular, death certificate information may systematically misrepresent the distribution of underlying disease. Unfortunately, with the need for large scale standardization, registries sometimes fall behind in the ability to characterize what may be considered state-of-the-art specific disease markers. For cancer, these include such important site-specific information as microstaging for malignant melanoma or estrogen receptor status for breast malignancies.

## ADVANTAGES OF DISEASE REGISTRIES

### Completeness of Ascertainment

One of the primary advantages of disease registries is that unlike the perceptions that may be developed based on clientele from a given clinical practice, they provide an opportunity to evaluate the full spectrum of specific disease outcomes. Particularly in the case of population-based disease registration, great emphasis is placed on the ability to collect and maintain health outcome information for all members of a temporally and geographically defined population at risk.

### Definition of Disease

Another advantage of disease registries is that they use explicit decision rules for disease classification, constant from institution to institution. Cause of death information is typically coded centrally by a nosologist trained to use standard decision criteria for underlying and contributing causes of death noted on the death certificate. Cancer registries use specially-trained tumor registrars to abstract and code diagnostic detail on newly identified cases, using standard criteria for malignancy, subsite distribution, and multiple primaries. While there may be many gray areas of definition within the medical community, disease registries use documented consensus criteria that allow for comparisons across treatment facilities, states, or countries.

### Secular Trends

Because disease registries use standard procedures for identifying and classifying a disease in a defined population, it is possible to examine changes in incidence, mortality, prevalence, or survival over time.

Changes in the observed occurrence of various disease outcomes in hospital settings, for example, could easily be a function of changes in the institutional catchment area, referral patterns, or reimbursement criteria rather than changes in the underlying disease experience of the population. While changes in diagnostic conventions can affect both kinds of reporting systems, temporal correction factors can be applied to registry data.

### Comparison Groups

Another particularly valuable contribution of population-based disease registries is the ability to compare health outcomes in subgroups of interest. Disease registries are a valuable tool in secondary prevention (disease control) and can provide an important early warning signal when subgroups defined by age, race, sex, geography, or time demonstrate a disproportionate disease burden compared to normal levels in the general population. A study that first linked records from local AIDS and cancer surveillance systems in San Francisco provided valuable information on concerns about the trends in Kaposi's Sarcoma incidence among the city's residents. This study also identified Hodgkin's Disease as another sentinel cancer for AIDS in young men.

## SUMMARY

Disease registration is not a new concept. Some idea of a defined population at risk and the incidence of disease in that population dates back to the earliest efforts to control the spread of infectious diseases. In more recent years, similar tools have been applied to understanding the scope of noninfectious diseases, particularly cancer. Vital records provide the most basic model for population-based disease registration. While hospital based, or occupationally based, surveillance systems provide similarly useful information, population-based disease registries used in conjunction with geographic, occupational, or environmental information on defined cohorts of interest provide a less biased view of their underlying disease experience. Disease registries are somewhat limited by the breadth and depth of information on diagnostic detail and relevant risk factors. By virtue of their standards for completeness and consistency, however, they offer a valuable means for assessing important population variations in disease that can be used as the basis for designing substantive studies of disease etiology or intervention efforts for disease control.

# REFERENCES

## GENERAL

Hansen J et al: Availability of data on humans potentially exposed to suspected carcinogens in the Danish working environment. Pharmacology and Toxicology 1993;72(Suppl):77.

Lepantalo M, Salenius JP, Ylonen K: Introduction of a population-based vascular registry: Validity of data and limitations of registration. British Journal of Surgery 1994;81:979.

Lynge E: Danish cancer registry as a resource for occupational research. Journal of Occupational Medicine 1994;36:1169.

Scherer K et al: Using administrative health data to monitor potential adverse health effects in environmental studies. Environmental Research 1994;66:143.

## EXAMPLES

Chow WH et al: Occupational risks for colon cancer in Sweden. J Occup Med 1994;36(6):647.

Coogan PF et al: Variation in female breast cancer risk by occupation. Am J Ind Med 1996;30(4):430.

Demers PA et al: Cancer incidence among firefighters in Seattle and Tacoma, Washington. Cancer Causes Control 1994;5(2):129.

Ekbom A et al: Intrauterine environment and breast cancer risk in women: A population-based study. J Natl Cancer Inst 1997;1(89):71.

Goodman KJ, Bible ML, London S, Mack TM: Proportional melanoma incidence and occupation among white males in Los Angeles County. Cancer Causes Control 1995;6(5):451.

Kallen B, Landgren O: Delivery outcome in pregnancies when either parent worked in the chemical industry: A study with central registries. Journal of Occupational Medicine 1994;36:563.

Kristensen P et al: Cancer in offspring of parents engaged in agricultural activities in Norway: Incidence and risk factors in the farm environment. Int J Cancer 1996;65(1):39.

Reynolds P et al: The spectrum of AIDS-associated malignancies in San Francisco: 1980–1987. American Journal of Epidemiology 1993;137:19.

Starzynski Z, Marek K, Kujawska A, Szymczak W: Mortality among different occupational groups of workers with pneumoconiosis: Results from a registry-based cohort study. Am J Ind Med 1996;30(6):718.

# 47

# Health Risk Assessment

*Dennis J. Paustenbach, PhD, DABT, CIH*

It is clear that the actions of nearly any country have the potential to adversely affect the health of people and their environment in other nations. For example, the destruction of the rain forests in South America or changes in the ozone layer in Antarctica are alleged to influence the climate in North America and Europe. Because of potential distribution of toxics among the various nations, it would be useful for all countries to have a consistent approach to assessing environmental risks and using the information to set their priorities. In 1996, the United States spent nearly $190 billion on environmental issues. This figure is expected to increase at a rate of about 7% annually until the turn of the century. Elsewhere, another approximately $400 billion was spent in 1994 by countries who were tackling similar environmental problems. Yet, even these resources are generally considered inadequate to address the concerns levied by citizens of virtually every nation. Due to competing pressures for limited funds, most nations are giving serious consideration to the use of risk assessment techniques to prioritize their environmental agendas. In the United States, for example, nearly 15 different proposals regarding the proper use of health risk assessment are currently being debated in Congress.

Risk assessment has been broadly defined as the methodology to predict the likelihood of numerous unwanted events, including industrial explosions, workplace injuries, failures of machine parts, natural catastrophes (eg, earthquake, tidal waves, hurricanes, volcanic eruptions, tornadoes, blizzards), injury or death due to an array of voluntary activities (eg, skiing, football, sky diving, flying, hunting), diseases (eg, cancer, developmental toxicity caused by chemical exposures), death due to natural causes (eg, heart attack, cancer, diabetes), death due to lifestyle (eg, smoking, alcoholism, diet), and others (Paustenbach, 1989).

Health risk assessment is the process through which toxicology data collected from animal studies and human epidemiology are combined with information about the degree of exposure to quantitatively predict the likelihood that a particular adverse response will be seen in a specific human population.

The risk assessment process has been used by regulatory agencies for almost 40 years, most notably within the US Food and Drug Administration (USFDA). However, the difference between assessments performed in the 1950s and 1960s versus those performed in the 1980s and 1990s is the incorporation of complex and quantitative exposure assessment (Finley and Paustenbach, 1994). With the emergence of quantitative methods, current risk assessment models are now better able to estimate the probability of the likelihood that a specific adverse effect will occur over a wide range of doses (Reitzetal, 1996). Since 1980, many environmental regulations and some occupational health standards have, at least in part, been based on the results of low-dose extrapolation models and exposure assessments. For example, risk assessment methodologies have been used to set standards for pesticide residues, drinking water guidelines, and ambient air standards, as well as exposure limits for contaminants found in indoor air, consumer products, and other media. Risk managers increasingly rely on risk assessment to decide whether a broad array of risks are significant or trivial; an important task, since more than 300 of the approximately 5000 chemicals routinely used in industry have been labeled carcinogens in various animal studies.

In the United States, the popularity of human and environmental risk assessment as a policy instrument has been due, in large part, to public concern regarding the relationship between cancer and chemical exposure, as well as other adverse health effects, and frustration with the perceived inability of government to regulate these chemicals. Further, industry has insisted that an adequate scientific rationale be provided to support potentially restrictive regulatory decisions. Risk assessment has generally been successful in satisfying both demands. As a result, over the past decade, quantitative risk assessments have become an accepted methodology in the United States and elsewhere for identifying a range of options, each having specific cost and benefit information important to risk managers, policy makers, and the public.

# HEALTH RISK ASSESSMENT

The emergence of modern health risk assessment can be traced to about 1975 (Crump et al, 1976). Nearly three dozen guidance documents (about 5,000 pages) on how risk assessments should be conducted have been written by the US Environmental Protection Agency in the past 10 years. Unfortunately, when the United States standardized the process through regulation, risk assessments often became too inflexible to properly characterize the true or most likely risks. Specifically, most attempts by regulatory approaches to standardize health risk assessment methods introduced a significant level of conservatism because such assessments, for the sake of public safety, rely upon default assumptions, which have overestimated rather than underestimated the true risks.

Risk assessment, by its very nature, is a process whereby the magnitude of a specific risk is characterized so that decision makers can conclude whether the potential hazard is sufficiently great that it needs to be managed or regulated. Therefore, before deciding to conduct such analyses, one must concede that some level of risk can be deemed acceptable; that is, a risk-benefit balance can be found.

Although many in society are concerned about the uncertainty of the scientific precision of today's environmental decisions, the public can take solace in the fact that new and better information on toxicology, fate and transport, and knowledge of the degree of exposure is being continually developed. Because chemical hazards are not completely eliminated when decisions are based on a risk assessment, Germany and some other highly developed countries, have traditionally elected to regulate chemicals to the lowest level achievable or to impose a ban. In the latter case, imposing a ban can sometimes necessitate complete removal of a chemical from contaminated soil, water, or air; which raises yet another set of risk and technology issues.

Although it is true that reducing health risks to levels that are "as low as reasonably achievable" (ALARA) or requiring the use of the "best available technology" (BAT) can produce significant reductions in the degree of exposure, there are two possible shortcomings in adopting such a policy. First, adopting an ALARA or BAT approach can be costly and may not result in an overall benefit (reduction of risk) to society. Second, a reliance on banning may not ensure that a significant or even measurable level of risk reduction has occurred. History demonstrates that banning chemicals may well eliminate one risk, but often this hazard is replaced by another and the financial sacrifice is often not to the overall benefit of society (Tengs et al, 1995). In an ideal world, the costs of decisions concerning risk reduction should be weighed against the benefits of applying the same resources to reduce other important risks such as adequate medical care for all citizens or immunization (Breyer, 1994).

Health risk assessments are separated into four parts or sections: hazard identification, dose-response assessment, exposure assessment, and risk characterization (Figure 47–1). Hazard identification is the first and most easily recognized step in risk assessment. It is the process of determining whether exposure to an agent could (at any dose) cause an increase in the incidence of adverse health effects (cancer, birth defects, etc) in humans or wildlife. Dose-response evaluations define the relationship between the dose of an agent and the probability of a specific adverse effect in laboratory animals. Exposure assessment estimates the magnitude and probability of uptake from the environment by any combination of oral, inhalation, and dermal routes of exposure. The most important part of an assessment, risk characterization, summarizes and interprets the information collected during the previous activities and identifies the limitations in the risk estimates.

## Hazard Identification

During the first 20 years of health risk assessment, it has become clear that most animal carcinogens (at some dose) will generally pose a human cancer hazard; however, the risk at very low doses continues to be debated (Aylward et al, 1996). The criteria by which a risk assessor determines that a chemical could pose a significant carcinogenic or developmental threat to humans based on animal studies involves consideration of at least six factors. For carcinogens, these factors include the number of animal species affected, the number and types of tumors occurring in the animals, the dose (relative to the acute toxic dose) at which the animals are affected, the dose/response relationship, and the genotoxicity of the chemical. For developmental toxicants, the key issues in the hazard identification step are similar to those for carcinogens and include the number of species affected, the severity of the effect, and the relationship between the dose that affects the mother compared to that which affects the offspring, etc.

Regulatory agencies are aware that they cannot place equal weight on all data reported in the literature since some are more reliable than others. Agencies have generally learned to resist the tendency to place an emphasis on any piece of data that suggests that a chemical might pose a carcinogenic or developmental hazard, and little weight on data that suggest that the chemical failed to cause these effects. This approach has heretofore been considered both prudent and health protective from a public policy standpoint, but it is not scientific nor is it necessarily in the best public interest (Breyer, 1994).

Frequently, extraordinary confidence has been placed on studies that suggest that a chemical may pose a particular hazard with often only modest consideration given to the study's quality. The scientific

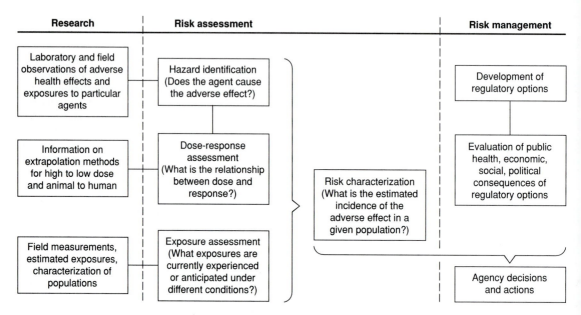

**Figure 47–1.** Elements of risk assessment and risk management. (From: National Academy of Sciences, 1983.)

community and most regulatory agencies have come to accept that not all data are equal, and that only data of similar quality should be judged equally. In the United States, this is known as the "weight of evidence" approach. It represents an important refinement and is applicable not only to the hazard identification segment of risk assessment, but also the exposure and dose-response evaluations. The benefit of using a "weight-of-evidence" approach is that it minimizes the possibility that huge sums of money will be spent to conduct several high quality toxicity studies simply to refute the results of one or two poorly conducted ones.

## Dose-Response Assessments

A dose-response evaluation usually requires an extrapolation from the generally high doses administered to experimental animals, or exposures reported in occupational studies, to the exposures expected from human contact with the agent in the environment (Figure 47–2). A model is used to estimate the response at doses below those tested (NAS, 1994).

It is clear that the most uncertain portion in the assessment of chemicals, especially carcinogens, is the low-dose extrapolation. Most toxicologists agree that they have a limited ability to estimate the risks associated with typical levels of environmental exposure based on the results of the standard rodent bioassay. There are many reasons why this is so. First, we do not fully understand all of the various possible mechanisms of action for carcinogens and many other classes of chemicals. Second, the doses under which we conduct the animal tests are so high that they often produce effects that would not occur at the doses

to which humans are exposed. Third, there are usually significant differences between animals and humans with respect to the rate at which chemicals are metabolized, distributed, and excreted. Fourth, the delivered dose to specific target tissues in animals will frequently be relatively different and it may produce a different response in human tissue. Accordingly, scientists must rely on a model or theory to es-

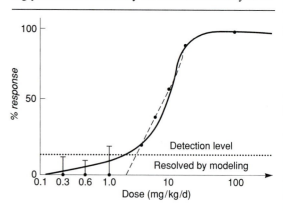

**Figure 47–2.** A dose-response curve from a carcinogenicity study. The solid line is a best fit of the eight data points identified in the test. The three lowest data points indicate that at these doses, no increased incidence in tumors was observed in the test animals. The error bars on the three lowest doses indicate the statistical uncertainty in the test results, since a limited number of animals were tested (n = 100). In an effort to derive risk estimates that are unlikely to underestimate the risk, nearly all low dose extrapolation models derive risk estimates based on the estimated upper bound of the plausible response, rather than the best estimate (Crump et al, 1976).

**Table 47–1.** PB-PK models have been developed for the following chemicals (Leung and Paustenbach, 1995).

| | |
|---|---|
| Benzene | Methanol |
| Benzo(*a*)pyrene | Methoxyethanol |
| Butoxyethanol | Methylethylketone |
| Carbon tetrachloride | Nickel |
| Chlorfenvinphos | Nicotine |
| Chloroalkanes | Parathion |
| Chloroform | Physostigmine |
| Chloropentafluorobenzene | PPBs |
| Chromium | PCBs |
| *Cis*-dichlorodiammine platinum | Styrene |
| Dichloroethane | Toluene |
| Dichloroethylene | TCDF |
| Dichloromethane | TCDD |
| Dieldrin | Tetrachloroethylene |
| Diisopropylfluorophosphate | Trichloroethane |
| Dimethyloxazolidine dione | Trichloroethylene |
| Dioxane | Trichlorotrifluoroethane |
| Ethylene oxide | Vinyl chloride |
| Hexane | Vinylidene fluoride |
| Kepone | Xylene |
| Lead | |

timate the human response at doses often 1000-fold below the lowest animal dose tested (Figure 47–1). The most scientifically rigorous (and likely most valid) models for estimating safe level of human exposure based on animal data are the physiologically based pharmacokinetic (PB-PK) models (Table 47–1) (Paustenbach, 1995; Leung and Paustenbach, 1995).

Low-dose extrapolation models (sometimes called quantitative risk assessment [QRA]) have become the backbone of dose-response assessments for carcinogens. Because these models play such a dominant role in the regulatory process, it is useful to understand some of their characteristics. First, the six most routinely used models will usually fit the rodent data in the dose region used in the animal tests. Second, the different models usually yield very different results at the doses to which humans are exposed, as exemplified by the analysis of dichlorodiphenyltrichloroethane (DDT) (Figure 47–3, Table 47–2). Third, the results of these six models usually vary in a predictable manner because they use different mathematical equations for predicting the chemical's carcinogenic potency. Although not in all cases, the one hit and linearized multi-stage models will usually predict the highest risk and the probit model will predict the lowest. To date, most regulatory actions in the United States regarding acceptable levels of exposure to air, water, and soil contaminants have been based on statistical rather than biologically based models like the PB-PK analyses or the MVK model (Moolgavkar et al, 1988). In the not-so-distant future, it can be expected that much greater weight will be placed on those assessments that attempt to quantitatively account for biological phenomenon.

It is noteworthy that rodent studies now used to predict the magnitude of the human risk were never intended for that purpose. These studies were de-signed to qualitatively identify potential human hazards, not to quantitatively estimate the human risk at low levels of exposure. Like in the hazard identification step, whenever adherence to strict regulatory guidance requires that dose-response assessments must use a single mathematical model, as is the case in most agencies, the assessment can become so constrained that valuable biological information (which could dramatically alter the results) is not fully accounted for.

We have learned a good deal about the biology of cancer during risk assessment's formative years and this information should be considered in the dose-response assessment. For example, we now know that there are at least three broad classes of mechanisms by which chemicals may produce a carcinogenic response in rodents: repeated cytotoxicity, promotion, and initiation. Some have suggested that there may be at least eight different classes of carcinogens. These distinctions are important since the appropriate method for estimating the cancer risk for humans exposed to low doses of a cytotoxicant or promoter should be different than that for an initiator. Because at relatively high doses nongenotoxicants may produce repeated cytotoxicity, the primary reason for excessive cell turnover, many scientists expect them to possess a threshold dose below which no cancer hazard would be present. This is in contrast with genotoxicants, which may pose some risk, albeit small, even at very low doses.

In general, the scientific underpinnings of the dose-response models used for assessing carcinogens are based on our understanding of ionizing radiation and genotoxic chemicals. Both types of agents may well have a linear, or a nearly linear, response in the low dose region. In contrast to radiation and chemical initiators, promoters and cytotoxicants should not have a linear dose-response curve. Scientific data increasingly suggest that they would be expected to be very nonlinear at low doses and, as importantly, probably have a genuine or practical threshold. The increased acceptance of this postulate is evidenced by EPA's position that the linearized multi-stage model is inappropriate for dioxin, thyroid type carcinogens, nitrilotriaceticacid (NTA), trimethyl pentane, and presumably, similar nongenotoxic chemicals.

When presenting the results of the dose response assessment, we should not only present the upper bound risk from the cancer models but also identify the best estimates as well as the upper and lower bounds of the risk. The objective of the bounding techniques is to attempt to account for the statistical uncertainty in the results of the animal tests, however, we have rarely presented the degree of potential conservatism within the bounding procedure. The shortcoming is that the risk manager is often not fully aware of the breadth of equally plausible risk estimates (Figure 47–4). For example, the cancer risk as-

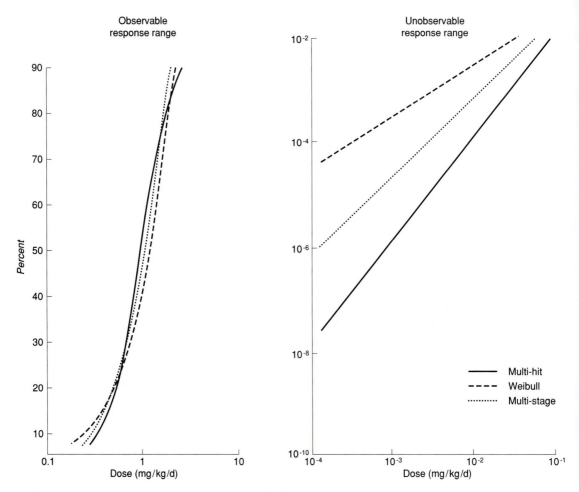

**Figure 47–3.** The fit of most dose-response models to data in the observable range is generally similar *(left plot)*. However, due to the differences in assumptions upon which the equations are based, the risk estimates at low doses can vary dramatically between the different models *(right plot)*.

sociated with exposure to chloroform in drinking water has been reported to be as high as one in ten thousand using the upper bound risk estimate of the multi-stage model; however, using the same model, the best or maximum likelihood estimate (MLE) of the risk is about one in a million and the lower bound estimate is virtually zero (about 1 in 10,000,000). Therefore, the plausible range of risk is as high as one in ten thousand and as low as zero. When biological factors such as its weak genotoxicity and pharmacokinetics are consider, the carcinogenic risk associated with low concentrations of chloroform in chlorinated drinking water is most likely to be quite small or negligible.

One mathematical model alone should not be relied upon. There are at least six different models that may need to be considered when estimating the risks at low doses (Figure 47–3). Each of them can yield results that are plausible, depending on the mechanism of action and pharmacokinetics of the chemical,

as well as the characteristics of the dose-response curve. Due to our better understanding of carcinogenesis and the shortcomings of statistical models, regulatory agencies have recently become more willing to consider models that can quantitatively account for chemical-specific mechanisms of action. However, support for flexibility in risk estimation has been criticized on the grounds that our knowledge about carcinogenesis is insufficient to regulate in other than a very conservative manner.

Greater weight should be given to the results of epidemiology studies. It is usually claimed that these studies are almost never as statistically robust as the animal studies and, therefore, are not very useful. However, total acceptance of this assertion is inappropriate because epidemiological studies can, at the least, establish the degree of confidence that should be placed in the results of low-dose extrapolation models. Often, even less-than-perfect epidemiology studies coupled with retrospective exposure assess-

**Table 47–2.** Estimates of lifetime risk to humans from exposures to methylene chloride based on salivary gland region sarcomas in male rats derived from four different models[1] (95% Upper Confidence Limit of Additional Risks).

| Air Concentration on $\mu g/m^3$ | Multistage Model | One-hit Model | Weibull Model | Log-probit Model |
|---|---|---|---|---|
| 1 | $1.8 \times 10^{-7}$ | $2.0 \times 10^{-7}$ | $4.8 \times 10^{-10}$ | $3.5 \times 10^{-31}$ |
| 10 | $1.8 \times 10^{-6}$ | $2.0 \times 10^{-6}$ | $1.7 \times 10^{-8}$ | $1.6 \times 10^{-22}$ |
| 100 | $1.8 \times 10^{-5}$ | $2.0 \times 10^{-5}$ | $6.1 \times 10^{-6}$ | $2.5 \times 10^{-15}$ |
| 1,000 | $1.8 \times 10^{-4}$ | $2.0 \times 10^{-4}$ | $2.0 \times 10^{-5}$ | $1.3 \times 10^{-9}$ |
| 10,000 | $1.8 \times 10^{-5}$ | $2.0 \times 10^{-3}$ | $6.1 \times 10^{-4}$ | $2.4 \times 10^{-1}$ |

[1]U.S. Environmental Protection Agency (USEPA). Health Assessment Document for Dichloromethane (Methylene Chloride). Final Report. February 1985. EPA/600/8-82/004F.

ments can yield much more defensible estimates of the likely human health hazard than statistical models based on animal studies.

Quantitatively scale-up data from rodents to predict the human response. For example, when evaluating most toxicologic effects, statisticians and biologists have generally assumed that at a given dose (mg/kg/d) the rodent response to a chemical will be nearly identical to the human response. This approach is usually reasonably accurate for chemicals with a short biologic half-life and for noncarcinogenic effects. In contrast, for carcinogens, several factors need to be considered when trying to predict how humans will respond compared to rodents. First, the biologic half-life between rodents and humans can be expected to be different for virtually all chemicals. Often, for a given chemical, these differences will vary in a predictable manner based simply on the body weight to surface area ratio and/or life span. This may also be valid for those chemical carcinogens that require activation. Consequently, for regulatory purposes, surface area corrections have been used in an attempt to adjust for the pharmacokinetics differences between rodents and humans. Other dose metrics should also be considered for those chemicals with a long biologic half-life (Aylward et al, 1996).

The most promising method for predicting the human response from rodent data is the physiologically based pharmacokinetic model (PB-PK) (Reitz et al, 1996). These models quantitatively account for the various differences between the test species and humans by considering body weight, metabolic capacity and products, respiration rate, blood flow, fat content, and a number of other parameters (Figure 47–5). Although complete confidence in the results of PB-PK models often relies on some frequently untestable assumptions, such as the delivered dose of an unstable metabolite to a target organ, it represents one of the most important advances in toxicology and health risk assessment of the past 40 years. The variability in predicting the results can be significant and some of these have been evaluated. To date, PB-PK models have been developed and validated for carbon tetrachloride, styrene, methylene chloride, chloroform, trichloroethane, dioxane, tetrachlorodibenzo-p-furan, tetrchlorodibenzo-p-dioxin (TCDD), benzene, trichloroethylene, vinyl-chloride, and others (see Table 47–1) (Leung and Paustenbach, 1995). The benefits of this approach have been so impressive that two major symposia have been held to encourage its use; one by the National Academy of Science in 1987 and the other by the US EPA in 1994.

Low-dose models are only useful for objectively ranking classes of carcinogens, but they cannot precisely predict the cancer risk because most do not account for biological information such as the types of

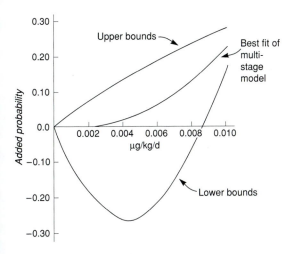

**Figure 47–4.** The range of plausible risks using the bounding technique inherent in the multi-stage model. The specific depiction is based on the application of the linearized multistage model to the doses observed in the CIIT Inhalation Study of Formaldehyde. (Reprinted, with permission, from Robert Sielken, Jr. 1987. The capabilities, sensitivity, pitfalls, and future of quantitative risk assessment in *Environmental Health Risks: Assessment and Management.* McColl RS [editor]. University of Waterloo, Waterloo, Ontario. Copyright 1987, by the Institute for Risk Research, University of Waterloo.)

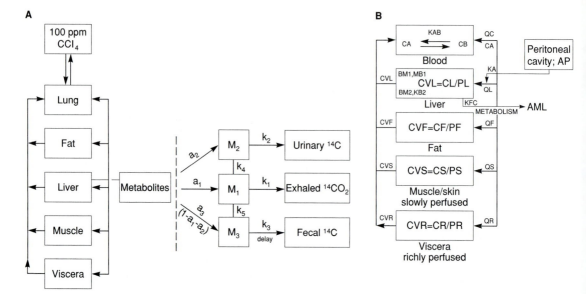

**Figure 47–5.** A physiologically based pharmaceutic (PB-PK) model for inhalation exposure to carbon tetrachloride **(A)** (Paustenbach et al, 1988) and a PB-PK model for uptake following IP dosing **(B)** of a nonvolatile chemical. These types of models allow scientists to quantitatively predict how humans will respond to a chemical based on data collected in rodents. Basically, the movement and transformation of the test chemical within the rodent is described by two mathematical equations. The same is done for the human. When there is evidence that the rodent model can accurately predict the behavior of the chemical in humans, one can quantitatively predict the response of humans with a high level of confidence. This method has been used by toxicologists only since about 1984, but became widely accepted by 1996. These methods are now routinely considered in regulatory decision-making.

tumor, time to onset, and its genotoxicity. Perhaps the most promising approach to incorporating biological factors into risk estimates is the use of biologically based models such as the one by Moolgavkar-Knudson-Venzon (MKV). This model accounts for the number of mutations required for malignancy and the role of target cell birth and death processes in the accumulation of these mutations. A key element is a quantitative description of how the carcinogen affects the cellular birth, death, and mutation rates. Because most of the information needed to perform these analyses is not yet available, it holds limited promise in the near future.

Thus far, the low dose models for carcinogens recommended by the EPA frequently do not respond to the characteristics of the dose-response curve. As such, it does not seem appropriate to base important regulatory decisions on the results of models if they are minimally "responsive" to the very costly information collected in standard lifetime rodent studies. Another way to look at the issue is to understand the fragility or sturdiness of these models not only when interpreting bioassay data but also when selecting the dosing regimen to be used in new bioassays. If one conducts only one statistical test for selecting the form of the model, we limit our ability to learn all we can from the rodent data. One way to avoid this shortcoming is to conduct simulations of the model's responsiveness to alterna-

tive, but similar, data sets to ensure that the extrapolation is reasonable (Paustenbach, 1995).

## Exposure Assessment

In general, exposure assessment will contain less uncertainty than other steps in the risk assessment. Admittedly, there are a large number of factors to consider when estimating exposure and it is a complicated procedure to understand the transport and distribution of a chemical that has been released into the environment. Nonetheless, the available data indicate that scientists can do an adequate job of quantifying the concentration of the chemicals in the various media and the resulting uptake by exposed persons if they account for all the factors that should be considered. For some chemicals, the actual uptake of a chemical by exposed persons need not be estimated using models and assumptions; instead, these can often be measured directly in body fluids, excrement, or hair.

The primary routes of exposure to chemicals in the environment are inhalation of dusts and vapors, dermal contact with contaminated soils or dusts, and ingestion of contaminated foods, water, or soil. Initial efforts to quantitatively estimate the uptake of environmental contaminants by humans were first conducted by scientists in the field of radiological health (Baes et al, 1985) and their work can be a source of valuable information when conducting assessments of chemical contaminants. Numerous methodologies for estimating the human uptake of contaminants have been proposed and refined in recent years.

The experience in the United States has shown that in our attempts to be prudent, or highly protective of the public health, we placed too much emphasis on the "so-called" maximally exposed individual (MEI). Often, the results of those analyses were misinterpreted by the public and/or misrepresented by some scientists or lawyers. For example, some assessments only addressed the MEI. Such an approach presented only a small part of the story. The current USEPA exposure guidelines and guidance from the National Academy of Science acknowledge this deficiency and note that a worst-case or MEI analysis should be used only to decide if an exposure is insignificant, and should not be used to characterize the actual or likely plausible human health risks. In short, most MEI analyses should only be used in screening assessments, although some have noted that so-called reasonable person assessments fail to characterize certain portions of the population.

As we have learned how to accurately characterize the risks of exposure for about 95% of the population, more emphasis has been placed on evaluating the various special groups (eg, Eskimos, subsistence fisherman, dairy farmers). Although the risk for these populations, which can be exposed to particularly high doses (the 95–99.9% group), needs to be understood, the typical levels of exposure for the majority of the population should be the initial focus of the assessment. For example, if a regulatory agency bases their decision on the results of an assessment assuming that a person eats about 100 g of fish every day of his or her lifetime (99th percentile), yet the average American eats only 6 g of fish per day (lifetime average), the analysis should reflect the fact that 99 of 100 persons are not represented by the corresponding risk estimate. To help minimize the potential for misunderstanding, we have found that it is important to describe the number of exposed persons at each of the anticipated dose levels, along with the most likely and upper estimates of exposure and the associated plausible risk. With this information, risk managers are equipped with enough information to decide whether large or small sums of money are warranted to reduce the health hazard (NAS, 1994).

The repeated use of conservative assumptions should not be allowed to dictate the results of the assessment. The problem can be illustrated by one assessment of the dioxin hazard posed by a municipal waste incinerator. Before deciding to issue a permit, the USEPA conducted a screening level assessment, so they evaluated the theoretical cancer risk for a child who lived within a short distance (0.8 km) from the hypothetical incinerator. They assumed that a child could eat as much as 2000 mg of dirt each day, that his house was down-wind of the stack, that he

ate fish from a pond near the incinerator, that his fish consumption was at the 95th percentile level, that he drank contaminated water from the pond, that he ate food grown primarily from the family garden, and that he drank milk from a cow that grazed at the farm. Not surprisingly, it was predicted that siting the incinerator could plausibility increase the child's lifetime cancer risk by 1 in 100; but he could hardly be portrayed as a typical person living near a municipal incinerator. Regrettably, the associated upper-estimate of the risk was the only one reported by the press. Certainly, it would have been more appropriate to have studied and presented the number of persons likely to be exposed to this amount of contaminant, as well as the level of exposure for the typical person living within 10 miles of the facility. It may also have been useful to note that few farms are located near most incinerators, since operators try to minimize transportation costs from urban areas.

Fortunately, the problems associated with the repeated use of overly conservative assumptions and the need to properly account for small (but highly exposed) populations can now be overcome through the use of Monte Carlo techniques (Thompson et al, 1992). The probabilistic, or Monte Carlo, technique addresses the main deficiencies of the point estimate approach because it imparts a great deal more information to the risk manager (Figure 47–6). Instead of presenting a single point estimate of risk, probabilistic analyses characterize a range of potential risks and their likelihood of occurrence. In addition, those factors that most affect the results can be easily identified. For example, in a probabilistic analysis, one can present the risk manager with the following type of information: "the plausible increased cancer risks for the 50th, 95th, and 99th percentiles of the exposed population are $1 \times 10^{-8}$, $5 \times 10^{-7}$, and $1 \times 10^{-6}$, respectively."

Risk managers and the public want to know of the statistical confidence in our estimates of risk. Sensitivity analyses can yield important information about the critical exposure variables and the degree of confidence. For example, we can now make the following kind of statement if a thorough risk assessment is conducted: "our understanding of the concentration of DDT in the edible portion of small mouth bass is based on high quality, reliable data, therefore, our confidence in the risk estimates is high. Our analysis indicates that 90% of the increased cancer risk could be eliminated if there were a ban on catching carp or catfish in the river and that little additional reduction in risk would be achieved if bass and trout fishing were banned." This type of characterization provides the kind of information risk managers need in order to make informed decisions regarding the necessary magnitude of regulatory action, the cost/benefit analyses, and whether a range of risk reduction alternatives should be considered.

One of the other advances in risk assessment is

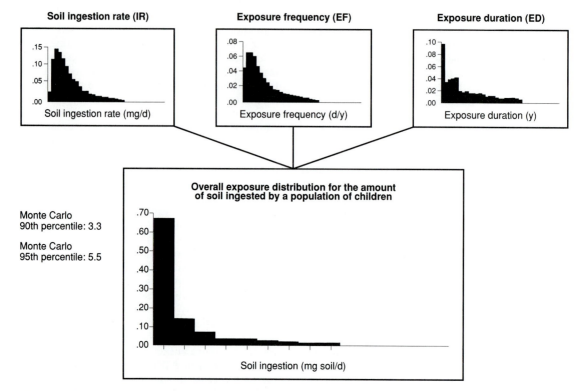

**Figure 47–6.** An example of how probability density functions (distributions) for three different related exposure factors are combined to form a distribution for the amount of soil ingested by a population of children. The Monte Carlo technique allows the risk assessor to account for the variability in many exposure parameters within a population and then to produce a distribution that characterizes the entire population.

that we now recognize the importance of accounting for the log-normal distributions and other statistical issues. As has been shown repeatedly, most environmental and occupational data are log-normally distributed rather than conform to a Gaussian distribution, but few environmental scientists were aware of the significance. As noted in the recently proposed EPA guidelines for exposure assessment, inappropriate statistical analysis of environmental data represents one of the most easily corrected of the common errors in exposure analysis.

We have also learned how to better statistically handle samples having no detectable amount of a contaminant. Frequently, regulatory agencies have used the limit of detection (LOD) of the analysis in the exposure calculations relying on the premise that the contaminant might be present at that level. Some agencies have suggested that 50% of the LOD should be used to calculate the plausible degree of human exposure, others have suggested that the LOD divided by the square root of two, and much more complex approaches should be considered. When such an approach is used on a site that may only be 2–10% contaminated (based on surface area), the predicted severity of the average level of contamination will be much higher than what is likely.

In exposure assessment, the environmental fate of the chemical needs to be accounted for. Many factors such as degradation by sunlight, soil and water microbes, and evaporation can dramatically influence the degree of human exposure, yet assessments have frequently assumed concentrations measured today will exist for 30–50 years in the future. For instance, the public health hazard posed by the potential release of dioxin vapors from incinerators was recently evaluated. It was alleged that the vapors posed a serious health hazard to surrounding residents. Consequently, a risk assessment was conducted. It was soon recognized that the environmental half-life of dioxin (as a vapor) was a critical factor in this analysis since it has a half-life of only 90 minutes. In contrast, TCDD in deep soil or fly-ash may have an environmental half-life of 50–500 years. What had been portrayed as a potentially serious health hazard was shown to be relatively insignificant when its photolytic half-life was considered.

Although, in the past, the sampling and analytical procedures were inadequate to measure the low concentrations of toxicants found in the environment, better techniques have become available. As field measurement techniques are further refined, less reliance should be placed on mathematical models for predicting the distribution of chemicals in the environment.

Perhaps the most significant advance in the exposure assessment of airborne contaminants involves accounting for indirect pathways of exposure. For example, the uptake of a contaminant in water by humans due to ingestion is obvious (and direct), but the uptake of the same contaminant by garden vegetables due to deposition or uptake via the inhalation of volatile contaminants while showering are indirect pathways that have not always been evaluated in assessments. Perhaps the most important indirect route of exposure, which had not been considered before 1986 when regulating airborne nonvolatile chemicals, is the ingestion of particulate emissions that have deposited into soil and plants and are subsequently eaten by grazing animals. The ingestion of the meat and milk from these animals can produce, depending on the chemical and conditions of exposure, risks 100–500 fold greater than the risk due to inhalation. Methods for estimating uptake through virtually all indirect routes have been developed and continue to be refined.

Over the past 5–10 years, analytical chemists have increased their ability to detect very small quantities of nonnatural chemicals in blood, urine, hair, feces, breath, and fat. Measurement of parts per trillion and parts per quadrillion is now possible. For many chemicals, the results represent a direct indicator of either recent or chronic exposure to a chemical. Often, direct measurement is far superior for predicting the possible health risks than a series of mathematical formulas. For example, the uptake of dioxin by Vietnam veterans exposed to 2,4,5-T was recently evaluated by analyzing the amount of dioxin in their blood. This study, conducted almost 15–20 years after the last day of service in Vietnam, allowed epidemiologists to conclude that the vast majority of veterans had only a modest degree of exposure to this chemical, which has been alleged to produce numerous adverse health effects in field soldiers. These data were much more valuable than mathematical predictions.

## Risk Characterization

Characterizing risk has consistently been the weakest component of a risk assessment because it requires the assessor to draw on numerous aspects of science and regulatory policy to properly describe whether a significant human health hazard exists in a specific setting. A thorough characterization should discuss background concentrations of the chemical in the environment and in human tissue, pharmacokinetic differences between the animal test species and humans, the impact of using a PB-PK or biologically based model, the effect of selecting specific exposure parameters (a sensitivity analyses), uncertainty and statistical sensitivity analyses, as well as other factors that can influence the magnitude of the estimated risks (Figure 47–7).

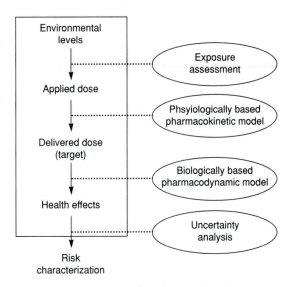

**Figure 47–7.** A general description of the issues that need to be addressed in a high-quality risk characterization.

Procedures designed to develop upper bounds on risk are routinely treated as generating best estimates, and rarely are key assumptions and uncertainties in risk assessment fully acknowledged. The important role of choice of data or the low-dose extrapolation model, for example, is rarely discussed, especially in a quantitative manner. Thus, a risk manager cannot know the scientific plausibility or certainty of the estimate of risk.

The biggest problem with the current risk characterization, from a scientific perspective, is that the default assumptions and methods are more scientifically plausible for some chemicals than for others. This means that "plausible upper bounds" of carcinogenic potency may be reasonable estimates for some compounds and wild overestimates for others.

The default, conservative, methods of risk assessment sometimes used by EPA and other regulatory agencies assume a dose-response function that is linear in the low-dose region and has no threshold. There is evidence that some agents, like certain types of radiation and directly mutagenic chemicals, may indeed have this type of dose-response relationship. However, many scientists believe the linear, no-threshold approach to risk estimation is inappropriate for many other chemicals, such as some that are not direct mutagens.

This means that when EPA applies standard procedures to all chemicals, regardless of how appropriate they might be for a given substance, the amount of conservatism in a risk estimate varies greatly. A risk estimate for a powerful direct mutagen may be quite close to the calculated "plausible upper bound," while for a nonmutagenic compound the estimate may be an extreme overestimate of plausible risk.

Two "plausible upper bound" risk estimates that are generated through consistent procedures may have very different levels of scientific plausibility. This needs to be discussed in the risk characterization.

Comparison and prioritization of the many public health risks facing our country is another reason for the need for a complete risk characterization. Since statistics for many other public health threats, such as motorcycle accidents or AIDS cases, are not deliberately inflated, environmental risk assessment must go beyond single "plausible upper bound" risk characterization to ensure that public health officials can make meaningful comparisons.

In the risk characterization, presentation of multiple estimates of risk will help to avoid the trap of false precision. It can also help combat false consistency. It can be expected that in the coming years choices made by the risk assessor will no longer be hidden, because risk estimates will be presented using all plausible choices, not picking and choosing just one. Much of the risk assessment process contains some degree of scientific uncertainty and disagreement, and this is exactly what risk characterization should convey.

The risk characterization portion offers numerous opportunities to fail to describe the "big picture" to the risk manager or the public. Depicting the theoretical increase in cancer risk of one in a million or even 1 in 10,000 as a serious public health risk should be avoided. One reason is that the risks predicted in most assessments usually represent the upper estimate of the potential risks, not a best estimate of risk. Second, nearly every risk assessment conducted in the United States by a regulatory agency states that risk estimates represent an upper bound of the plausible risk, are not likely to underestimate the risk, and that the actual risk may be much lower; even, in some cases, zero. In short, it is important to communicate to the public and to decision makers that when conservative procedures and models are used, the human risk estimates are likely to be overestimated.

During the early years of risk assessment, background levels of the contaminant were often overlooked, even though the impact on decision-making might well have been significant. For example, in a preliminary decision regarding the necessary level of clean-up at a State Superfund site (a rural community), the agency suggested that soil levels of a cyclodiene be reduced to 100 ppb. The goal was to keep the theoretical cancer risk to inhabitants below 1 in 1,000,000. However, the administrator decided not to require any remediation when it was recognized that the background levels of some cyclodienes in many areas in the United States exceeded 500 ppb. The convincing argument was that the adipose tissue level of cyclodienes of persons who lived in the community would be no different after remediation than before since the incremental contribution due to the contaminated soil was negligible when compared to the background uptake of this chemical for all Americans.

In recent years, our experience has shown that the hazard may not always be as it appears. For example, at several sites where lead or PCB contaminated soil was removed and later destroyed, there was no resulting change in the blood levels of these contaminants in either the children or the adults. How could this have occurred? One of the primary routes of uptake is through dust in the home, which is transferred there from the soil. Thus, often cleaning the homes is often more important than removing the contaminated soil from the community; and certainly one must accompany the other. In addition, even when soil was consumed little if any of the chemical was absorbed in the stomach since it was so well bound to the soil, eg, low bioavailability. In many locations, this type of rather simple but practical solution may be the only financially plausible one for dealing with soil contaminated by persistent chemicals. These include simply paving over a contaminated soil (like mine waste that covers hundreds of acres) and then conducting a thorough cleaning of the homes.

Our lack of understanding regarding the uncertainty of model-estimated cancer risks need to be communicated in a thorough and an understandable fashion. For example, the goal of some environmental standards, such as the maximum contaminant levels (MCLs) for drinking water, is to keep the maximum plausible cancer risk between 1 in 100,000 and 1 in 1,000,000. However, it might be useful to note that about 30% of all Americans will eventually develop cancer and about 25% will eventually die from it. Accordingly, a $1 \times 10^{-6}$ risk is equivalent to ensuring that the lifetime cancer risk for persons exposed to this level of contamination will be no greater than 250,001 in 1,000,000 (25.0001%), rather than the background rate of 250,000 in 1,000,000 (25%). If society demands this standard of care, that is its choice; however, both society and its risk managers should be aware of the relative magnitude of various risks before deciding to spend money on one hazard vs. another. Even if the EPA were to regulate all carcinogens in air, soil, and water at levels generally considered insignificant, the decrease in the cancer incidence in the United States would probably be negligible (a reduction of about 0.25–1.3% of the annual cancer mortality).

Risk characterizations are much more useful if they contain cost/benefit analyses (eg, for each dollar spent, how much are the risks likely to be reduced for various portions of the population?). Most risk scholars and risk managers believe that these risk/benefit versus cost analyses are the primary justification for performing health risk assessments. For these applications, the use of Monte Carlo techniques has been invaluable (Evans et al, 1994).

We now recognize that the hallmark of a good risk characterization is a discussion of the uncertainties in the risk estimates. Since 1990, many improvements have been made concerning how to conduct quantitative, rather than qualitative, uncertainty analyses and how to present them. The key element of these analyses is a statistical evaluation of each of the various parameters and the implication with respect to the risk estimate for various segments of the population. Although at first blush this may sound like a scientific nuance, the public and the court's now insist that they understand the level of confidence in our predictions.

A key trait of a high quality risk characterization is the accurate and unbiased discussion of our confidence in the risk estimates. Often, regulatory agencies and the press have erroneously stated or implied that the results of low-dose models actually predict the increased cancer risk for exposed individuals. As noted previously, because statistical models cannot account for the many biological mechanisms (including repair), they cannot be accurate predictors of the actual cancer risk. Risk estimates should not be portrayed as anything more than relative indicators of risk. For example, when the Food and Drug Administration uses the risk level of 1 in 1,000,000, it is confident that the risk to humans is virtually nonexistent, rather than 1 in 1,000,000 exposed persons is likely to develop cancer.

Presentation of complete risk characterization will have many beneficial consequences. It will lead to a better appreciation of the strengths and limitations of the risk assessment process by regulators, legislators, journalists, and the public. It will improve our ability to compare and rank health risks, from chemicals and from other sources. It may improve the scientific credibility of the risk assessment process as scientists see more of their data and judgments used to evaluate environmental hazards. Presentation of the range of risk estimates and their scientific validity will also allow risk managers to do what they are paid to do; make policy decisions. It is time that risk assessors begin a policy of "full disclosure" by conducting complete risk characterization (National Research Council, 1996).

## ALTERNATIVE APPROACHES TO HEALTH RISK ASSESSMENT

Some environmentalists and politicians have questioned the acceptability of risk assessment as a policy tool (Silbergeld, 1993). The reason is that the mere use of risk assessment is considered an admission that a certain amount of risk is acceptable; though, the imposition of any risk is unlawful under certain statutes and unethical in many circumstances. Without question, this is an intimidating position that policy makers have had difficulty refuting. However, it is problematic since it assumes that there may be enough discretionary monies available to virtually eliminate exposure to most risks, included unwanted man-made chemicals.

Perhaps the key point raised by the environmental community is that there are alternatives to risk as-

sessment that are worthy of continued discussion within the international arena. The first alternative is to return to technology-based approaches. This has, in fact, been adopted in the United States in the 1992 Amendments to the EPA Clean Air Act. The second alternative is a return to banning substances or legislating a prohibition on the emission of chemicals from industrial settings. Both of these approaches rely exclusively on the hazard identification process and are very dependent on the skills of the analytical chemist, since any measurable quantity could initiate action. In support of this approach, some have argued that bans are the only successful means to significantly reduce environmental risks. The chemicals DDT, PCB, and lead in gasoline are often identified as major success stories of the banning process.

The third alternative to current approaches that appeals to some environmentalists is to adopt simpler rules for conducting health risk assessments. For example, the European approach involves applying a safety or uncertainty factor to the NOEL from the best animal study and assuming that this will yield a value which, if followed, will prevent the adverse effect. This scheme places an equal weight on both carcinogenic and noncarcinogenic chemicals. The advantage is that it is fast and efficient, but a perceived disadvantage is that it concedes that some level of exposure is probably safe for virtually all persons. In California and a few other US states, risk assessment methods have been standardized so that they can be conducted rapidly and inexpensively.

The fourth alternative that some environmentalists have advocated is one that relies upon public pressure to minimize the hazard. The best documented approaches are California's Proposition 65 and California's Assembly Bill AB-2588, wherein acceptable levels of exposure are established using a single method and anyone that appears to expose persons above this concentration must report this to the agency and the person being exposed (Copeland et al, 1994). This scheme sidesteps the problems of using risk assessments to demonstrate that hazards are most important; instead, control of industrial emissions is brought about through public pressure. Many within the environmental community believe that this approach is quite workable.

## CASE STUDIES

Risk assessment methods have been used for a number of years to help address questions about "how safe is safe" for many different contaminated media. These include pesticide residues on foods as well as chemicals in ambient air, groundwater, surface water, soils, sediment, pharmaceutical drugs, and workplace air. In one form or another, risk assessment has been used to address these issues since the early 1950s. However, the systemic integration of exposure assessment, low-dose extrapolation models, pharmacokinetics, and statistics (eg, modern day risk assessment) only became routine after 1975.

The following two examples illustrate how the risk assessment methodology can be used to evaluate an occupational and an environmental hazard.

## EXAMPLE A
## (Occupational)

2-Methoxyethanol has been used as a solvent for more than 30 years. From 1950 to 1975, this solvent, which is also known as 2-ME and ethylene glycol monomethylether, was used in the chemical industry, and in the late 1970s, the semiconductor industry also began to use it. From 1955 to 1980, limits for workplace air (TLVs and PELs) were based on the solvent's systemic toxicity. The Threshold Limit Value (TLV) was 5 ppm for most years from 1960 to 1980. In the 1980s, it became clear that it could cause embryotoxicity and that it might be a reproductive hazard in animals.

In 1986, the question was raised regarding what airborne concentration of 2-ME was likely to be safe (ie, not likely to pose a developmental hazard or other potentially serious adverse effects in workers). The following approach was used:

### Known:
1. A segment II study of the developmental hazard in rodents showed that 10 ppm (in air) was the no observed effect level (NOEL).
2. Another study examined reproductive end points in rats, rabbits, and mice following inhalation exposures. Pregnant rats and rabbits were exposed to airborne concentrations of 0, 3, 10, and 50 ppm and mice to 0, 10, and 50 ppm during the period of organogenesis. Maternal toxicity and reduced birth weight were noted in rats and mice at 50 ppm. There were no treatment-related effects on litter size, resorption rate, or fetal weight in either species. No treatment-related adverse effects were noted on either the mothers or offspring of either species at 10 ppm or lower.
3. In rabbits, more pronounced decreases in maternal weight gain were noted at 50 ppm, accompanied by a significant increase in the resorption rate and a decrease in fetal body weight. Malformations were observed in 63% of the fetuses from rabbits exposed to 50 ppm with almost all the organ systems being affected. An air concentration of 10 ppm was determined to be the NOEL for this study in rabbits.
4. The available data indicate that rats are usually about as susceptible to developmental toxicants as humans; but occasionally humans are 5- to 10-fold more susceptible.

## Rationale for an Occupational Exposure Limit (OEL)
1. The most sensitive toxic effect (eg, end point with the lowest NOEL) was fetal malformation and reduced birth weight. These effects were seen in mice, rats, or rabbits exposed to airborne concentrations of 50 ppm.
2. All good quality studies of animals identified an adverse effect at doses higher than 10 ppm in air (8 hr/d [eg, 10 ppm seemed a solid NOEL]).
3. The classic approach to setting an occupational exposure limit (OEL) is to apply about a 100-fold safety factor to the animal NOEL. This is based on the assumption that humans are 10-fold more susceptible than the rodent (the rodent-to-human extrapolation factor) and that another 10-fold factor is often applied to account for differences in individual sensitivity among humans. In this case, due to our high level of understanding of the relationship between the blood levels in rats and humans, a factor of 5 seemed appropriate.
4. Another approach (which has gained popularity and support) is to use physiologically based pharmacokinetic equations or models to use animal data to predict the human response. It is known that at the same blood concentrations, humans and animals tend to respond similarly. Mice have a 2-fold lower steady-state blood concentration for a given airborne concentration of 2-ME than humans.
5. Since it appears that in rats the offspring (D) is more susceptible than the adult (A) to the toxic effects, that the lowest observed adverse effect level (LOEL) for toxicity in the adult is 50 ppm, and the LOEL for developmental effects is also 50 ppm for the conceptus, this yields an A over D ratio of 1.0; that is, adverse effects on the offspring were observed only when maternal toxicity was also apparent. This value means that toxicity in adults is a relatively good predictor of developmental effects and that only a small additional uncertainty factor is appropriate (eg, a factor of 3 [Figure 47–8]).

## Calculation of an Occupational Exposure Limit (OEL)
From this information, an OEL can be estimated for humans:

$$OEL = \frac{Animal\ NOEL}{(UF_1)(UF_2)(UF_3)(UF_4)}$$

NOEL = 10 ppm in three different animal species.

$UF_1$ = 5 to account for the possibility that humans are more susceptible than rodents.

$UF_2$ = 1.0 since rodent blood levels are *not* greater than humans at a given airborne concentration (in

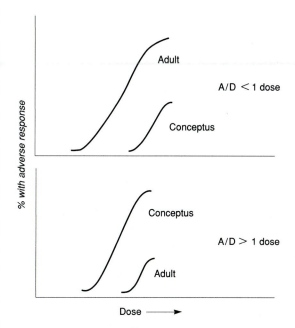

**Figure 47–8.** Relation between adult and developmental affective doses. In the plot in which A/D is less than 1, toxic effects are seen in the pregnant animal at doses lower than those that adversely affect the conceptus. In contrast, when the A/D ratio is greater than 1, the conceptus is much more sensitive to the effects of the chemical than the mother (based on Johnson, 1988).

fact, human blood concentrations are about 10- to 100-fold less than rats for a given dose).

$UF_3 = 3$ to account for the potentially greater susceptibility of the conceptus.

$UF_4 = 10$ to account for the possibility that the most susceptible human is more susceptible than the typical human (this also helps account for the inability to fully appreciate the range of susceptibilities in the rodent population, since only 20 rats per dose are usually studied).

From this, the recommended OEL for humans (for 8 hours of exposure, for a 5-day work week) is as follows:

$$OEL = \frac{10\ ppm}{(5)(1)(3)(10)} = 0.066\ ppm$$
$$OEL = 0.1\ ppm$$

## EXAMPLE B
(Environmental)

Virtually thousands of sites in the United States have contaminated soil due to previous industrial activity or leaking underground storage tanks. Over the past 20 years, many approaches have been used to identify concentrations of these industrial chemicals in soil that should not pose a human or ecological risk. A few years ago, it was recognized that the level of contamination that is safe depends on how people are likely to use the site. For example, contamination of soil in a residential area may result in exposures to children and pets, while similarly contaminated soil at a chemical plant might have limited potential for human exposures (Paustenbach et al, 1992). Soil used for agriculture would need to be safe for grazing animals but would not need to be low enough to protect children who might eat the soil. These distinctions are important, since in residential areas about 85% of the human risk due to contaminated soil (for nonvolatile chemicals) can be related to ingestion of soil and house dust by children.

The following is an example of how risk assessment methods can be used to set clean-up levels for soil. Similar methods are used to set acceptable concentrations of contaminants in airborne dust, groundwater, fish, and other media.

### Known:

1. Residential soil is contaminated with dioxin (2,3,7,8-TCDD).
2. Humans can be exposed via ingestion of soil/dust, airborne dusts, gardening, and dermal contact.
3. Dioxin is a potent, acute toxicant in animals and an extremely potent animal carcinogen.
4. The NOEL in the highest quality animal study that assessed carcinogenicity is 0.001 g/kg/d.
5. The NOEL for any other toxic effect (in animals) is 10 μg/kg/d. If one applies a 100- or 1000-fold safety factor to it, the resulting safe dose for noncancer effects is still higher than the dose that poses a theoretical cancer risk of 1 in 100,000 (eg, $1 \times 10^{-7}$ μg/kg/d), as predicted using a low-dose extrapolation model. Therefore, cancer is the most sensitive adverse effect to protect against. If the cancer risk is low (ie, negligible) then there should be no other health concerns.
6. The rat appears to be as susceptible as any other animal species to the cancer hazard posed by dioxin. For a number of reasons, in general, the rodent is considered a good predictor of the cancer risk in humans. In addition, the human epidemiology data suggest that humans are less susceptible to the cancer hazard than rodents (Aylward et al, 1996).

### Assumptions & Rationale for Setting a Soil Clean-up Level

1. Assume that residents living at the site with dioxin-contaminated soil could be exposed 365 days per year for a duration of 30 years.
2. Soil ingestion pathway parameters are as follows: children are assumed to eat 100 mg per day of house dust and soil from ages 2–6 years (an Agency default assumption). The EPA value for the adult years (7–30) in residence is less,

approximately 50 mg/d. The oral bioavailability of TCDD in soil is assumed to be 40% (0.40).

3. Inhalation pathway exposure parameters are as follows: the typical adult inhalation rate 20 $m^3$ for a 24-hour day (childrens' inhalation rate is 10 $m^3$/d). The airborne particulate concentration from local soils is $7.57 \times 10^{-4}$ mg/$m^3$. Thus, the soil inhalation rates would be $15.14 \times 10^{-3}$ mg/d for an adult and $7.57 \times 10^{-3}$ mg/d for a child.

4. Gardening (vegetable ingestion) pathway parameters are as follows: the typical vegetable ingestion rate is 50 g per day. Although virtually no dioxin is taken up by plants, a soil-to-plant transfer coefficient for dioxin of 0.00145 is used. The percentage of vegetables from home gardens is 38% (0.38).

5. Dermal contact exposure parameters are as follows: the average skin surface area exposed to soil is assumed to be 2,836 $cm^2$ per day for adults and 2,199 $cm^2$ per day for children. The soil adherence factor is assumed to be 1.0 mg per $cm^2$. The dermal bioavailability of TCDD is less than 1% (0.01).

6. The USEPA (1996) oral slope factor for 2,3,7,8-TCDD is $9.7 \times 10^3$ kg per day per mg (Keenan et al, 1991) and the inhalation slope factor is $1.16 \times 10^5$ (USEPA, 1996).

## Calculation of Risk from Individual Pathways for a Child/Adult

The chronic (cancer) risks for the various exposure pathways (soil ingestion, vegetable ingestion, dermal contact, and dust inhalation) due to the dioxin in the soils can be estimated as follows:

### A. Soil Ingestion:

$$RISK = \frac{SF_o \cdot C_{soil} \cdot EF \cdot B_o}{10^6 \, mg/kg \cdot AT}$$
$$\cdot \left( \frac{Ing_{S,a} \cdot ED_a}{BW_o} + \frac{Ing_{S,o} \cdot ED_o}{BW_o} \right)$$

Where:
a = Adult
c = Child
$C_{soil}$ = the acceptable dioxin concentration in soil (mg/kg)
BW = body weight (15 kg for child; 70 kg for adult)
AT = averaging time (70 years = 25,550 days)
$SF_o$ = slope factor for 2,3,7,8-TCDD ($9.7 \times 10^3$ for ingestion)
EF = exposure frequency (365 d/y)
ED = exposure duration (6 years for child + 24 years as adult, or 30 years = total)
$B_o$ = oral bioavailability (0.40)
IngS = soil ingestion rate (soil ingestion: 100 mg/d for a child, 50 mg/d for an adult)

Risk = $10^{-5}$ (1 in 100,000) incremental lifetime cancer risk

So,

$$10^{-5} = \frac{(9.7 \times 10^3)(C_{soil})(365)(0.40)}{(10^6 \, mg/kg)(25,550)}$$
$$\cdot \left( \frac{(50)(24)}{70} + \frac{(100)(6)}{15} \right)$$

As a result,
$C_{soil}$ = 0.0032 mg/kg (protects against soil ingestion hazard)

### B. Vegetable Ingestion:

$$RISK = \frac{SF_o \cdot C_{soil} \cdot EF \cdot B_o \cdot f_V \cdot k_V}{10^6 \, mg/kg \cdot AT}$$
$$\cdot \left( \frac{Ing_{V,a} \cdot ED_a}{BW_o} + \frac{Ing_{V,a} \cdot ED_o}{BW_o} \right)$$

Where:
$Ing_V$ = vegetable ingestion rate (50,000 mg/d)
$f_V$ = fraction of vegetables that are homegrown (0.38)
$k_V$ = soil to vegetable transfer coefficient (0.00145)

So,

$$10^{-5} = \frac{(9.7 \times 10^3)(C_{soil})(365)(0.40)(0.38)(0.00145)}{(10^6 \, mg/kg)(25,550)}$$
$$\cdot \left( \frac{(50,000)(24)}{70} + \frac{(50,000)(6)}{15} \right)$$

$C_{soil}$ = 0.0088 mg/kg (protects against vegetable ingestion hazard)

### C. Dermal Contact:

$$RISK = \frac{SF_D \cdot C_{soil} \cdot EF \cdot B_D \cdot AF}{10^6 \, mg/kg \cdot AT}$$
$$\cdot \left( \frac{SA_a \cdot ED_a}{BW_a} + \frac{SA_c \cdot ED_c}{BW_c} \right)$$

Where:
$SF_D$ = slope factor for 2,3,7,8-TCDD ($9.7 \times 10^3$ for dermal contact)
$B_D$ = dermal bioavailability (0.01)
AF = soil adherence factor (1.0 mg/$cm^2$)
SA = exposed skin surface area (2,199 $cm^2$/d for child; 2,836 $cm^2$/d for adult).

So,

$$10^{-5} = \frac{(9.7 \times 10^3)(C_{soil})(365)(0.01)(1.0)}{(10^6 \, mg/kg)(25,550)}$$
$$\cdot \left( \frac{(2,836)(24)}{70} + \frac{(2,199)(6)}{15} \right)$$

$C_{soil} = 0.0039$ mg/kg (protects against dermal hazard)

### D. Inhalation of Dust From Soil:

$$RISK = \frac{SF_I \cdot C_{soil} \cdot PC \cdot EF \cdot B_I}{10^6 \, mg/kg \cdot AT}$$
$$\cdot \left( \frac{Inh_a \cdot ED_a}{BW_a} + \frac{Inh_c \cdot ED_a}{BW_c} \right)$$

Where:

$SF_I$ = slope factor for 2,3,7,8-TCDD ($1.16 \times 10^5$ for inhalation)

PC = airborne particulate concentration ($7.57 \times 10^{-4}$ mg/m$^3$)

$B_I$ = inhalation bioavailability (1.0)

Inh = air inhalation rate(10m$^3$/d for child; 20 m$^3$/d for adult)

So,

$$10^{-5} = \frac{(1.16 \times 10^5)(C_{soil})(7.57 \times 10^{-4})(365)(1.0)}{(10^6 \, mg/kg)(25,550)}$$
$$\cdot \left( \frac{(20)(24)}{70} + \frac{(10)(6)}{15} \right)$$

$C_{soil} = 0.73$ mg/kg (protects against soil dust inhalation hazard)

## Calculation of Acceptable Soil Concentration at a Given Risk

Since the total risk is cumulative for the four pathways, the acceptable soil concentration at a given target risk for all pathways $(C_{soil})_{ALL}$ can be determined by combining the above equations and solving as follows:

$$(C_{soil})_{ALL} = \left[ \sum_{i=1}^{n} \frac{1}{(C_{soil})_i} \right]^{-1}$$

Where,

i = Pathway (soil ingestion, vegetable ingestion, dermal contact, dust inhalation)

$$\text{or, } (C_{soil})_{ALL} = \left[ \frac{1}{(C_{soil})_{Ing,S}} + \frac{1}{(C_{soil})_{Ing,V}} + \frac{1}{(C_{soil})_{Der}} + \frac{1}{(C_{soil})_{Inh}} \right]^{-1}$$

So,

$$(C_{soil})_{ALL} = \left[ \frac{1}{0.0032 \, mg/kg} + \frac{1}{0.0088 \, mg/kg} + \frac{1}{0.0039 \, mg/kg} + \frac{1}{0.73 \, mg/kg} \right]^{-1}$$

$(C_{soil})_{ALL} = 0.0015$ mg/kg = 1.5 ppb

Thus, a soil concentration of TCDD can be estimated for a given risk.

Acceptable Soil Concentration = 1.5 parts per billion (risk of 1 in 100,000).

## REFERENCES

Albert RE: Carcinogen risk assessment. US Crit Rev Toxicol 1994;24:75.

Aylward LL, Hays S, Karch NJ, Paustenbach DJ: Evaluation of the relative susceptibility of animals and humans to the cancer hazard posed by 2,3,7,8-tetrachlorodibenzo-p-dioxin (TCDD) using internal measures of dose. Environ Science Tech 30:3534–3543.

Baes III, CF, Sharp RD, Sjoreen A, Shor WR: *A Review and Analysis of Parameters for Assessing Transport of Environmental Released Radionuclides Through Agriculture*. ORNL-5786. United States Dept. of Energy. Oak Ridge Nat'l. Lab. Oak Ridge, TN, 1984.

Breyer S: *Breaking the Vicious Circle: Towards Effective Risk Regulation*. Harvard Press, 1994.

Burmaster DE, Anderson PD: Principles of good practice for the use of Monte Carlo Techniques in Human Health and Ecological Risk Assessments. Risk Analysis 1994; 14:477.

Carnegie Commission on Science, Technology, and Government: *Risk and the Environment: Improving Regulatory Decision Making*. The Carnegie Corporation, 1993.

Center for Risk Analysis: *Historical Roots of Health Risk Assessment*. Harvard University Press, 1994.

Commission on Risk Assessment and Risk Management: *Risk Assessment and Risk Management in Regulatory Decision-making*. National Research Council; Washington, D.C., 1996.

Copeland TL et al: Use of probabilistic methods to understand the conservatism in California's approach to assessing health risks posed by air contaminants. J Air Waste Mgt Assn (JAWMA) 1994;44:1399–1413.

Copeland TL et al: Comparing the results of a Monte Carlo analysis with EPA's reasonable maximum exposed individual: A case study of a former wood treatment site. Regul Toxicol Pharmacol 1993;18:275.

Copeland TL et al: Use of Monte-Carlo techniques to understand the conservatism in California's approach to assessing air toxics. J Air Waste Mgt Assn 1994;44:1399.

Crump KS, Hoel DG, Langley CH, Peto R: Fundamental carcinogenic processes and their implications for low dose risk assessment. Cancer Res 1976;36:2973–2979.

Finkel AM, Golding, D: *Worst Things First: The Debate*

*Over Risk Based National Environmental Priorities.* Washington, D.C., Resources for the Future Press, 1994.

Finley BL, Paustenbach DJ: The benefits of probabilistic exposure assessment: three case studies involving contaminated air, water, and soil. Risk Analysis 1994; 14(1):53–73.

Finley BL et al: Recommended distributions for exposure factors frequently used in health risk assessment. Risk Analysis 1994;14(4):533–553.

Gray GM: Complete risk characterization. Risk in Perspective, Harvard Center for Risk Analysis 1994;2(4):1.

Johnson EM: Cross-species extrapolations and the biologic basis for safety factor determinations in developmental toxicology. Regul Toxicol Pharmacol 1988;8:22–36.

Keenan R, Paustenbach D, Wenning R, Parsons A: Pathology reevaluation of the Kociba et al. 1978 bioassay of 2,3,7,8-TCDD: implications for risk assessment. J Toxicol Environ Health 1991;34:279–296.

Leung HW, Paustenbach DJ: Physiolgically based pharmacokinetic and pharmacodynamic modeling in health risk assessment and characterization of hazardous substances. Toxicol Letters 1995;79:55.

McKone TE, Bogen KT: Predicting the uncertainties in risk assessment. Environ Sci Technol 1991;25:16–74.

McKone TE, Daniels JI: Estimating human exposure through multiple pathways from air, water, and soil. Reg Toxicol Pharm 1991;13:36.

Moolgavkar SH, Dewanji A, Venzon DJ: A stochastic two-stage model for cancer risk assessment: The hazard function and the probability of tumor. Risk Anal 1988; 8:383.

National Academy of Science (NAS): *Science and Policy in Risk Assessment.* National Academy of Sciences Press, 1994.

National Research Council: *Understanding Risk: Informing Decisions in a Democratic Society.* National Academy Press, 1996.

National Research Council: *Issues in Risk Assessment.* National Academy of Sciences Press, 1993.

Occupational Safety & Health Administration: Updating Permissible Exposure Limits (PELs) for Air Contaminants. Federal Register, Washington D.C., 1996;61(16): 1948–1950.

Office of Technology Assessment (OTA): Researching Health Risks. US Congress Office of Technology Assessment, OTA-BBS-570, 1993.

Paustenbach DJ: The practice of health risk assessment in the United States (1975–1995): How the US and other countries can benefit from that experience. Human Ecolog Risk Assess 1995;1:29.

Paustenbach DJ: A survey of health risk assessment. Pages 27–124 in: Paustenbach DJ (editor): *The Risk Assessment of Environmental and Human Health Hazards: A Textbook of Case Studies.* John Wiley and Sons, 1989.

Paustenbach DJ et al: A proposed approach to regulating contaminated soil: Identify safe concentrations for seven of the most frequently encountered exposure scenarios. Regul Toxicol Pharm 1992;16:21–56.

Paustenbach DJ: Health risk assessment and the practice of industrial hygiene. Amer Ind Hyg Assoc J 1990;51(7): 339–351.

Paustenbach DJ, Clewell HJ, Gargas M, Andersen ME: A physiological pharmacokinetics model for carbon tetrachloride. Toxicol Appl Pharm 1988;96:191–211.

Reitz RH, Andersen M, Gargas M: A PB-PK model for vinyl chloride. Toxicol Appl Pharm 1996;

Robinson JC, Paxman DG, Rappaport SM: Implications of OSHA's reliance on TLVs in developing the air contaminants standard. Am J Ind Med 1991;19:3–13.

Silbergeld EK: Risk assessment: The perspective and experience of the US environmentalists. Environ Health Perspectives 1993;101:100.

Tengs TO, Adams ME, Pliskin JS, Safran DG, Siegel JE, Weintein MC, and Graham JD: 1995. *Five-Hundred Life Saving Interventions and Their Cost-Effectiveness.* Risk Analysis.

Thompson KM, Burmaster DE, Crouch EAC: Monte Carlo techniques for quantitative uncertainty analysis in public health risk assessments. Risk Analysis 1992;12:53.

United States Environmental Protection Agency: Draft Guidelines for Carcinogenic Risk Assessment. Federal Register 61:17,960, 1996.

USEPA (US Environmental Protection Agency): Guidelines for Exposure Assessment. Federal Register 57: 22888-22938, 1992.

# A       Biostatistics & Epidemiology

*Marc B. Schenker, MD, MPH*

It is apparent to anyone who reads the medical literature today that some knowledge of biostatistics and epidemiology is a necessity. This is particularly true in occupational and environmental health, in which many of the findings are based on epidemiologic studies of subjects exposed to low levels of an agent. Research has become more rigorous in the area of study design and analysis, and reports of clinical and epidemiologic research contain increasing amounts of statistical methodology. The purpose of this Appendix is to provide a brief introduction to some of the basic principles of biostatistics and epidemiology.

# I.  BIOSTATISTICS

## DESCRIPTIVE STATISTICS

### Types of Data

Data collected in medical research can be divided into three types: nominal (categorical), ordinal, and continuous.

**Nominal (categorical) data** are those that can be divided into two or more unordered categories, eg, sex, race, religion. In occupational medicine, for example, many outcome measures such as cancer rates are considered separately for different sex and race categories.

**Ordinal data** are one step up from nominal data, the difference being a predetermined ordering underlying the categories. Examples of ordinal data are clinical severity, socioeconomic status, or ILO (International Labor Office) profusion category for pneumoconiosis on chest x-rays.

Both nominal and ordinal data are examples of discrete data. They take on only integer values.

**Continuous data** are data measured on an arithmetic scale. Examples include height, weight, blood lead, and forced expiratory volume. The accuracy of the number recorded depends on the measuring instrument, and the variable can take on an infinite

number of values within a defined range. For example a person's height might be recorded as 72 inches or 72.001 inches or 72.00098 inches, depending on the accuracy of the measuring instrument.

### Summarizing Data

Once research data have been collected, the first step should be to summarize them. The two most common ways of summarizing data are measures of location, or central tendency, and measures of spread, or variation.

**A.  Measures of Central Tendency:**

**1.  Mean–**The mean (x) is the average value of a set of interval data observations. It is computed using the following equation:

$$\bar{x} = \frac{\sum_{i=1}^{n} x_i}{n}$$

where n = sample size and
    $x_i$ = random variable, such as height, with
    i = 1,...,n.

The mean is strongly affected by extreme values in the data. If a variable has a fairly symmetric distribution, the mean is used as the appropriate measure of central tendency.

**2.  Median–**The median is the "middle" observation, or 50th percentile—ie, half the observations lie above the median and half below. It can be applied to interval or ordinal data. When there are an odd number (n) of observations, the median equals the (n + 1)/2 observation; when there are an even number of observations, the median is halfway between the (n/2) observation and the (n/2) + 1 observation. The median does not have the mathematical niceties of the mean, but it is not as susceptible as the mean to extreme values. If the variable being measured has a distribution that is asymmetric or skewed—ie, if there are a few extreme values at one end of the distribution—the median is a better descriptor than the mean of the "center" of the distribution.

**3.  Mode–**The mode is the most frequently oc-

783

curring observation. It is rarely used except when there are a limited number of possible outcomes.

**4. Frequency distribution**–In discussing measures of location or spread, we often refer to the frequency distribution of the data. A frequency distribution consists of a series of predetermined intervals (along the horizontal axis) together with the number (or percentage) of observations whose values fall in that interval (along the vertical axis). An example of a frequency distribution is presented in Figure A–1.

**B. Measures of Variation:**

**1. Range**–The range is the simplest measurement of variation and is defined as the difference between the highest and lowest values. One disadvantage of the range is its tendency to increase in value as the number of observations increases. Furthermore, the range does not provide information about distribution of values within the set of data.

**2. Variance**–The sample variance ($s^2$) is a measure of the dispersion about the mean arrived at by calculating the sum of the squared deviations from the mean and dividing by the sample size minus one. The equation for deriving sample variance is as follows:

$$s^2 = \frac{\sum_{i=1}^{n}(x_i - \bar{x})^2}{n-1}$$

Variance can be thought of as the average of squared deviations from the mean.

**3. Standard deviation**–The sample standard deviation(s) is equal to the square root of the sample variance.

$$s = \sqrt{\frac{\sum_{i=1}^{n}(x_i - \bar{x})^2}{n-1}}$$

See Table A–1 for examples of the calculation of mean, median, mode, variance, and standard deviation.

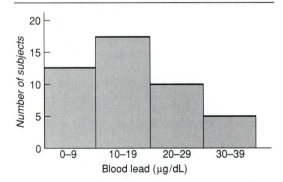

**Figure A–1.** Frequency distribution of subjects by blood lead category.

**Table A–1.** Calculation of mean, median, mode, variance, and standard deviation. (n = 10 workers.)

**$x_i$ = number of years of exposure to asbestos.**

| Worker | $x_i$ | $(x_i - x)$ | $(x_i - x)^2$ |
|---|---|---|---|
| 1. | $x_1$ = 4.0 | –2.2 | 4.84 |
| 2. | $x_2$ = 4.5 | –1.7 | 2.89 |
| 3. | $x_3$ = 5.0 | –1.2 | 1.44 |
| 4. | $x_4$ = 5.0 | –1.2 | 1.44 |
| 5. | $x_5$ = 6.0 | –0.2 | 0.04 |
| 6. | $x_6$ = 6.5 | +0.3 | 0.09 |
| 7. | $x_7$ = 7.0 | +0.8 | 0.64 |
| 8. | $x_8$ = 7.5 | +1.3 | 1.69 |
| 9. | $x_9$ = 8.0 | +1.8 | 3.24 |
| 10. | $x_{10}$ = 8.5 | +2.3 | 5.29 |
| Total: | $\Sigma x_i$ = 62.0 | | $\Sigma(x_i - x)^2$ = 21.6 |

**Mean:** $\bar{x} = \dfrac{62.0}{10} = 6.2$

 **Variance** = $\Sigma(x_i - x)^2/(n - 1) = 21.6/9 = 2.4$
 **Standard deviation** = $\sqrt{2.4} = 1.55$

**Median:**
1. Order the observations from lowest to highest.

2. Median = $1/2 \left( \left[\dfrac{n}{2}\right] \text{observation} + \left( \left[\dfrac{n}{2}\right] + 1 \right) \right.$

 $\left. \text{observation} \right) = 1/2$ (5th observation + 6th observation)

3. Therefore, median = $1/2$ (6.0 + 6.5) = 6.25

**Mode:**
Most commonly occurring observation is 5.0, since it occurs twice and all other observations occur once.

## Sample Versus Population Descriptive Statistics

The descriptive statistics discussed thus far are sample estimates of true population values or parameters. Because we usually do not have the resources to measure variables of interest on entire populations, we instead select a sample from the population of interest and then estimate the population mean from the sample mean or the population variance from the sample variance. The population mean is usually represented by the Greek letter $\mu$ and the population variance by the Greek letter $\sigma^2$. One almost never knows the true population values for these parameters and is almost always conducting sample surveys to estimate them.

## The Normal Distribution

The most important continuous probability distribution is the normal or Gaussian distribution, also known as the bell-shaped curve. Many quantitative variables follow a normal distribution, and it plays a central role in statistical tests of hypotheses. Even when one is sampling from a population whose shape departs from the normal distribution, under certain general conditions it forms the basis for statistical testing of hypotheses.

We often transform data to make them more normal in distribution. For example, in occupational exposure studies, the log dose is used rather than the

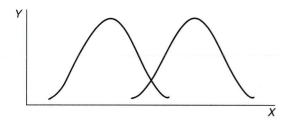

**Figure A–2.** Two normal distributions with different means but identical standard deviations.

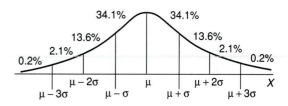

**Figure A–4.** Standard normal distribution.

dose because the log dose more closely approximates a normal distribution. A particular normal distribution is defined by its mean and variance (or standard deviation). Two normal distributions with different means but the same variance will differ in location but not in shape (Figure A–2). Two normal distributions with the same mean but different variances will have the same location but different shapes or "spreads" about the mean value (Figure A–3). Note that the normal distribution is unimodal, bell-shaped, and symmetric about the mean.

The normal distribution has several nice properties that make it amenable to statistical analysis, and variables that follow a normal distribution are for that reason preferred. Thus, data are often transformed to make them more normal, eg, log dose.

The population encompassed by 1 standard deviation (s) on either side of the mean in a normally distributed population will include approximately 67% of the observations in that population (Figure A–4); the population between 2 s on either side of the mean will include approximately 95% of the observations; and that between 3 s on either side of the mean encompasses more than 99% of the observations in the population (Figure A–4). This property of the normal distribution is particularly useful when a researcher or clinician is trying to identify patients with high or low values in response to a certain test. If one knows the mean for that particular test and has some idea of what the standard deviation is, the range within which one would expect (let us say) 95% of patients

to fall can be determined, and a patient with values outside this range might need to be examined further.

To utilize this property of the normal distribution, the sample should be large enough—eg, 20 observations or more—to provide reasonably certain estimates of mean and standard deviation.

> **Example I:** If the mean hematocrit in a clinical population is 42% with a standard deviation of 3%—and assuming hematocrit follows a normal distribution—one would expect 95% of the clinic population to have hematocrits between 42% ± (2 × 3%) or (36, 48)%. A patient falling outside this range could be identified for further testing.

Another principle relevant to normal distribution is the **central limit theorem,** which holds that no matter what may be the underlying distribution of x, the particular variable of interest, the sample mean (x) will have a normal distribution if the sample size (n) is large enough. Thus, if x itself comes from a population with a mean value $\mu$ and population standard deviation s, then x (calculated from a sufficiently large sample of size n) will have a normal distribution with the same population mean $\mu$ and a smaller population standard deviation equal to $(\sigma/\sqrt{n})$. One can then test hypotheses concerning the sample mean x, because it is known to have a normal distribution and its mean and standard deviation are also known. The standard deviation of x is called the standard error of the mean (SEM).

Since one is usually concerned with estimating the true population mean from the sample mean x, it is important to know how good an estimate the sample mean is of the true mean. Every time a sample of size n is selected from the population and x is calculated, a different value for x will be obtained and thus a different estimate of $\mu$. If this were done over and over again and many x's were generated, the x's themselves would have a normal distribution centered on $\mu$ with standard deviation equal to $(\sigma/\sqrt{n})$. In practice, one does not calculate several x's to estimate $\mu$—only one is calculated. The SEM quantifies the certainty with which this one sample mean estimates the population mean. The certainty with which one estimates the population mean increases with sample

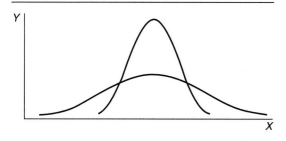

**Figure A–3.** Two normal distributions with identical means but different standard deviations.

size, and it can be seen that the standard error decreases as n increases. Furthermore, the more variability in the underlying population, the more variable will be the estimate of μ. It can also be seen that the standard error increases as σ increases. The "true" SEM is σ/√n, and the sample estimate of the standard error of the mean is s/√n, where s is the sample standard deviation.

Many investigators summarize the variability in their data with the standard error because it is smaller in value than the standard deviation. However, the standard error does not quantify variability in the population; it quantifies the uncertainty in the estimate of μ, the population mean. An investigator describing the population sampled should use the standard deviation to describe that population. The standard error of the mean is used in testing hypotheses about the population mean—as will be discussed later.

> **Example II:** Suppose blood lead is measured on 20 patients. Assume the sample mean (x) equals 20 μg/dL and the sample standard deviation (s) equals 5 μg/dL with sample size (n) of 20. If blood lead has a normal distribution in this sample, one would expect 95% of the population to lie within 2 s of the mean. Thus, if the investigator's sample was a representative one, 95% of the population will have blood leads between 20 ± (2 × 5) (ie, between 10 and 30 μg/dL). These numbers quickly summarize the distribution and give the readers a range against which to compare their own patients. However, investigators often summarize their data with the mean and the standard error of the mean and report that "blood lead in this sample population was 20 ± (2 × (5/√20))." This would lead a reader to believe that 95% of blood leads would be expected to fall between 17.8 and 22.2 μg/dL if one did not know the difference between the standard deviation and the standard error of the mean. In reality, 17.8 and 22.2 μg/dL describe a quantity known as the 95% confidence interval for the true mean blood lead μ: it does not describe a range of expected values. The reader of the report usually wishes to compare a patient's blood lead with an expected range of values for blood lead, ie, the mean ± 2 s.

## INFERENTIAL STATISTICS

In general, there are two steps to be followed in data analysis. The first is to describe the data by using descriptive statistics such as the mean, median, variance, and standard deviation. The second step is to test specific hypotheses that were formulated *before* conducting the research project. This is done by formulating a **null hypothesis** and an **alternative hypothesis,** wherein the null hypothesis is "no difference exists" and the alternative hypothesis is "difference exists."

An example of a null hypothesis might be, "There is no difference in pulmonary function between groups of underground miners and surface miners." The alternative hypothesis would be, "There is a difference between the two groups."

Once the hypotheses are formulated, the appropriate statistical test can be performed. Some of the most commonly used methods will be discussed below.

## The Case of Two Groups: The *t*-Test

In many instances an investigator is interested in comparing two groups to determine whether they differ on average for some continuous variable. For example, an investigator might be interested in determining whether exposure to organic solvents has an effect on psychomotor performance such as reaction time. To do this, one would select a sample of a group of industrial painters who are exposed to such solvents and compare their test performances with those of a group of workers not exposed to such solvents. Obviously, even if there are truly no differences between two employee groups in how they perform on such a test, the sample mean test scores will probably be unequal simply because of random fluctuation.

The main question is, "Are the differences larger than one would expect by chance if there truly is no difference in the reaction times?"—ie, do the samples come from one underlying population, not two? The null hypothesis in this situation is that the true mean reaction time in the painter group equals the true mean reaction time in the nonpainter group.

The alternative hypothesis is that the underlying true means are unequal. This is usually called a two-sided alternative hypothesis, because we are not specifying the direction of the inequality. In the example, average reaction time in the painter group might be faster or slower than average reaction time in the nonpainter group. Differences in either direction are examined in testing the null hypothesis.

The appropriate statistical test in this situation is the two-sample *t*-test. Two independent samples have been drawn—ie, the individuals in one sample are independent of the individuals in the other. The *t*-test has the following form:

$$t = \frac{\overline{x}_1 - \overline{x}_2}{SE\,(\overline{x}_1 - \overline{x}_2)}$$

**where x$_1$ = sample mean group 1 and**
**x$_2$ = sample mean group 2.**

Note that the numerator is the difference of sample means and the denominator is the standard error of this quantity. Dividing by the SE standardizes the difference in sample means by the variability present in the data. If the difference in the means was very large but the data from which it was calculated was highly variable, the *t*-statistic would reflect this and would be adjusted accordingly. The *t*-statistic reduces down as shown below:

$$t = \frac{\overline{x}_1 - \overline{x}_2}{\sqrt{\left(\dfrac{s_1^2}{n_1}\right) + \left(\dfrac{s_2^2}{n_2}\right)}}$$

where $s_1^2$ = variance in group 1 and $s_2^2$ = variance in group 2.

Use of the *t*-statistic assumes that the two samples have the same underlying population variance $\sigma^2$. Thus, a pooled estimate of the variance is calculated and substituted into the *t*-statistic. This pooled estimate $s_p^2$ has the following form:

$$s_p^2 = \frac{(n_1 - 1)\, s_1^2 + (n_2 - 1)s_2^2}{(n_1 + n_2 - 2)}$$

Therefore, the two-sample *t*-statistic is as follows:

$$t = \frac{\overline{x}_1 - \overline{x}_2}{\sqrt{\left(\dfrac{s_p^2}{n_1}\right) + \left(\dfrac{s_p^2}{n_2}\right)}}$$

Note that the pooled estimate of the variance is simply a weighted average of the variances from sample 1 and sample 2. Thus, if one sample is much larger than the other, more weight is given to its estimate of $\sigma^2$ because it is assumed to be more reliable since it is based on a larger sample size. Note further that if the two samples are of equal size, the pooled variance is simply the sum of the two sample variances divided by 2. From the format of the *t*-test, one can see that if the two sample means are similar in value, the numerator of *t* will be close to zero—and, consequently, the value of *t* would be small, leading to the conclusion that the null hypothesis is true and that there is probably only one underlying distribution from which the two samples come. If one obtains a large value for the *t*-statistic, it is likely that the two samples come from two different underlying distributions, and one would therefore want to reject the null hypothesis.

How large does *t* have to be to reject the null hypothesis? Tables of the *t* statistic indicate what value of *t* would cause the null hypothesis to be rejected. Even when the null hypothesis is true and there really is no difference between the groups being compared, there is the possibility that a large value of *t* might occur owing to random chance alone. One would like the probability of this occurrence to be small, ie, less than 5%.

To find the proper value of *t* for a particular study, a quantity known as the **degrees of freedom** is necessary. The degrees of freedom are equal to $(n_1 + n_2 - 2)$.

Once the degrees of freedom are known, the value of *t* may be obtained from the *t* table and compared to the *t* statistic calculated in the study. If the study *t* statistic is larger than the tabled cutoff value, one can conclude that this is unlikely to have happened under the null hypothesis, which is therefore rejected.

Bear in mind that the alternative hypothesis was the two-sided alternative, meaning that the two group means were simply *different* but not specifying the direction of the difference. Consequently, in the *t*-table, two cutoff points are actually obtained, since both very large negative and very large positive values of *t* are of interest. The *t*-distribution is symmetric, so that the two cutoff points are simply $\pm (t)$. If the study *t*-value is larger than $+t$ or smaller than $-t$, the null hypothesis is rejected.

An example problem is worked below to give the flavor of the *t*-test and how it is used.

**Example III:** Two-sample t-tests. The following tabulation presents the mean change in plasma cholinesterase concentration from baseline levels for 15 pesticide applicators and 14 unexposed controls.

| | N | Mean Decline (%) | Standard Deviation |
|---|---|---|---|
| Applicators | 15 | 25 | 11 |
| Controls | 14 | 10 | 8 |

*Do the data present sufficient evidence from which to conclude that the mean decline in cholinesterase is different for the two groups?*

*The null hypothesis is that there is no difference in cholinesterase change between the two groups. The alternative hypothesis is that there is a difference in cholinesterase change between the two groups.*

*First calculate $s_p^2$:*

$$s_p^2 = \frac{(n_1 - 1)\, s_1^2 + (n_2 - 1)s_2^2}{(n_1 + n_2 - 2)}$$

$$= \frac{(15 - 1)\, 11^2 + (14 - 1)\, 8^2}{(15 + 14 - 2)}$$

$$= 90.21$$

*Substitute into the formula for t:*

$$t = \frac{\overline{x}_1 - \overline{x}_2}{\sqrt{\left(\dfrac{s_p^2}{n_1}\right) + \left(\dfrac{s_p^2}{n_2}\right)}}$$

$$= \frac{25 - 10}{\sqrt{\left(\dfrac{90.21}{15}\right) + \left(\dfrac{90.21}{14}\right)}}$$

$$= \frac{15}{\sqrt{12.458}}$$

$$= 4.25$$

*Therefore, t = 4.25 and df = $n_1 + n_2 - 2 = 27$.*

*The study t-value of 4.25 with 27 degrees of freedom is compared with the tabled t value of ± 2.05, which has a 5% chance of occurring when the null hypothesis is true. Since +4.51 is larger than +2.05, the null hypothesis is rejected—ie, there is a statistically significant difference in the mean change in plasma cholinesterase from baseline between the two study groups.*

## Paired *t*-Test

The above discussion concerns the two-sample *t*-test and is appropriate for the situation in which two independent groups are being compared. Another common situation occurs when there are paired samples—ie, the two observations are not independent of one another.

For example, suppose a researcher is measuring change in pulmonary function (eg, $FEV_1$) over a work shift and there are 20 subjects in the study. (See example below.) The researcher would measure $FEV_1$ among the subjects before and after the work shift. Clearly, the before and after measurements are not independent, and one would like to take advantage of the fact that all individual (nonexposure) characteristics have been controlled. To do this, the *difference* in $FEV_1$ (before-after) is calculated for each subject. Since the *difference* is the only observation made per subject, the data set has now gone from 40 observations (2 per subject) to 20 observations (1 per subject). If there is no effect of work shift on $FEV_1$, one would expect the difference in $FEV_1$ for each subject to be small in value or close to zero. If the null hypothesis is not true and work shift exposure does change $FEV_1$, the differences will not be close to zero. The *t*-statistic calculated in this situation is known as the paired *t*-statistic and has the following form:

$$t = \frac{\bar{D}}{(s_D / \sqrt{n})}$$

**where** $\bar{D} = \dfrac{\Sigma D_i}{n}$ = **average difference and**

$s_D$ = **standard deviation of differences.**

$$= \sqrt{\frac{\sum_{i=1}^{n} (D_i - \bar{D})^2}{n-1}}$$

The appropriate null hypothesis is that the true mean of the differences is zero, and the appropriate alternative hypothesis is that the true mean of the differences is not zero. Again, it is a two-sided alternative, and one is looking for large positive or large negative differences. Small absolute values of the *t*-statistic would indicate that the null hypothesis is probably true, and large absolute values of *t* would lead to rejection of the null hypothesis. One goes to

the *t*-table to determine how large a value of *t* is needed to reject the null hypothesis. To enter the table, one needs to know the appropriate degrees of freedom. In the paired *t* situation, there are n–1 degrees of freedom, or the number of pairs minus one.

## Common Errors in Use of the *t*-Test

A common mistake made with the *t*-test is known

---

**EXAMPLE: Paired *t*-test**

A study of painters involved measuring pulmonary function ($FEV_1$; liters) at the beginning (A) and end (B) of a work shift. The results were as follows:

| Case # | $A_1$ | $B_1$ | $D_1 = (A_1 - B_1)$ | $(D_1 - D)$ | $(D_1 - D)^2$ |
|---|---|---|---|---|---|
| 1 | 3.14 | 3.01 | 0.13 | 0.10 | 0.010 |
| 2 | 2.85 | 2.80 | 0.05 | 0.02 | 0.000 |
| 3 | 2.50 | 2.30 | 0.20 | 0.17 | 0.029 |
| 4 | 3.01 | 3.15 | −0.14 | −0.17 | 0.029 |
| 5 | 1.55 | 1.55 | 0.00 | −0.03 | 0.001 |
| 6 | 2.21 | 2.15 | 0.06 | 0.03 | 0.001 |
| 7 | 2.81 | 2.68 | 0.13 | 0.10 | 0.010 |
| 8 | 3.25 | 3.34 | −0.09 | −0.12 | 0.014 |
| 9 | 2.66 | 2.56 | 0.10 | −0.07 | 0.029 |
| 10 | 1.95 | 1.90 | 0.05 | −0.02 | 0.000 |
| 11 | 3.50 | 3.46 | 0.04 | 0.01 | 0.000 |
| 12 | 3.95 | 4.06 | −0.11 | −0.14 | 0.020 |
| 13 | 4.10 | 3.90 | 0.20 | 0.17 | 0.029 |
| 14 | 3.60 | 3.56 | 0.04 | 0.01 | 0.000 |
| 15 | 2.80 | 2.90 | −0.10 | −0.13 | 0.017 |
| 16 | 2.50 | 2.50 | 0.00 | −0.03 | 0.001 |
| 17 | 2.10 | 2.16 | −0.06 | −0.09 | 0.008 |
| 18 | 3.70 | 3.61 | 0.09 | 0.06 | 0.004 |
| 19 | 2.92 | 2.86 | 0.06 | 0.03 | 0.001 |
| 20 | 3.31 | 3.42 | −0.11 | −0.14 | 0.020 |
| | | | 0.54 | | 0.198 |

$$\bar{D} = \frac{\Sigma D_i}{n} = \frac{0.54}{20} = 0.027$$

**Degrees of freedom = n − 1 = 19**

$$s_D = \sqrt{\frac{\sum_{i=1}^{n} (D_i - \bar{D})^2}{n-1}}$$

$$= \sqrt{\frac{0.198}{19}} = 0.102$$

$$t = \frac{\bar{D}}{(s_D / \sqrt{n})} = \frac{0.027}{0.102 / \sqrt{20}} = 1.18$$

Compare the calculated *t* of 1.18 to the tabled *t* of 2.093. Since the calculated *t* is less than the *t* in the table, the null hypothesis (of no change in function over work shift) is not rejected.

---

as the multiple comparison problem. The problem arises when an investigator has several groups to compare and proceeds to compare them two at a time, using the *t*-test each time. In other words, group 1 is compared with group 2 with the *t*-test, then group 2 with group 3, then group 1 with group 3, etc. The problem with proceeding in this fashion is that overall there is more than a 5% chance of mistakenly rejecting the null hypothesis—even though there is only a 5% chance of making this mistake with each individual comparison. This increased probability of making a mistake occurs because multiple tests give the investigator multiple chances to make an error. Thus, the chance of falsely rejecting a null hypothesis is greater than the 5% risk of mistakenly rejecting each comparison taken by itself, even if all the hypotheses are true. There are many ways of adjusting for this situation, known as **multiple comparison procedures.** What is important to remember is that if one does enough of such two-group comparisons, the probability of rejecting the null hypothesis incorrectly at least once increases with the number of such comparisons made and can be quite a bit greater than 5%.

## Analysis of Variance

When the variables under study are of the interval (continuous) type and there are more than two groups under study, the investigator is usually concerned with whether the means in the groups are different from one another. The appropriate statistical method to use in this situation is analysis of variance.

Suppose one were studying three groups of workers occupationally exposed to three different gases. One might want to test whether the particular gases affected mean $FEV_1$ levels differently in the three groups. In this example, individual $FEV_1$ values would be adjusted for nonexposure determinants (age, sex, height, race). The null hypothesis is that the group means for $FEV_1$ are equal, ie, that a particular exposure has no effect on $FEV_1$ values. Obviously, there will be differences between the sample means in each group owing to random fluctuations in $FEV_1$ among individuals.

Are the differences observed in the sample means due merely to random fluctuations or are they due to true differences in $FEV_1$ caused by the gas exposures. To answer this question, one proceeds under the assumption that the gas exposure has no effect and that the three groups are really random samples from the same underlying population. The null hypothesis assumes that any observed differences in the sample means and standard deviations are due simply to random sampling. Analysis of variance tests this null hypothesis by estimating the true population variance in two different ways and comparing these two estimates of the variance. If the three samples do indeed come from the same underlying population, these two estimates of the variance will be very close in value. If the three samples do not all come from the same underlying population, these two estimates will be further apart in value, and this separation is what one hopes to detect.

Certain statistical assumptions are made when an analysis of variance test is performed on a set of data: (1) It is assumed that there has been random assignment to treatment or exposure groups and that the groups are independent; (2) the underlying variance $\sigma^2$ in each group is assumed to be the same (even though the true group means may be different and the sample variances may differ slightly); and (3) the random variable under study—eg, $FEV_1$—has a normal distribution. Conceptually, the method of analysis of variance proceeds as follows:

Once the null hypothesis is formulated, the sample variance is computed within each exposure group. Each of these estimates, computed within an exposure group, is unaffected by differences among the group means. Each "within" group estimate of the variance is estimating $\sigma^2$. These estimates are averaged to obtain one "within" group variance estimate. The values of the individual exposure group means are then used to arrive at a second estimate of $\sigma^2$. In this second case, differences (or variability) among the group means will affect the estimate of $\sigma^2$. If a particular gas exposure has no effect on $FEV_1$, both estimates of $\sigma^2$ should be similar. To test the null hypothesis, a statistic known as the F statistic is calculated. The "F" is simply the ratio of the "between" group variance estimate to the "within" group variance estimate. Since both numbers estimate the same parameter ($\sigma^2$), if the null hypothesis is true, the value of F should be close to 1. If F is significantly larger than 1, one is led to reject the null hypothesis and must conclude that the exposure groups are different in levels of $FEV_1$.

How does one determine how large F must be in order to reject the null hypothesis? Because of random fluctuations in the data, it is possible that a large F-statistic might result even when the null hypothesis is true. However, one would like the chance of this happening to be very small. Tables of the F statistic are available to assist the investigator in selecting a value of F against which the F-statistic calculated from the data can be compared. The tabled value of F is one that would occur less than about 5% of the time if the null hypothesis were true. If the F-statistic calculated from the researcher's data is larger than the one in the table, the results are known to occur less than 5% of the time just by random chance, even when the null hypothesis (no difference in sample groups) is true. Since the observed results are therefore very unlikely to happen under the null hypothesis, the researcher can reject the null hypothesis and say that there is a difference among the groups. A 5% cutoff point is an arbitrary one, and, depending on the individual situation, one could set the cutoff at 1% or 10%. The conventional cutoff point is 5%.

When one is studying *more than two groups* and the data involved are continuous (eg, FEV, blood lead) and the question of interest is whether the groups all come from the same underlying population—ie, have the same mean value—the most appropriate *first test* of the null hypothesis is the analysis of variance. If one fails to reject the null hypothesis with the F-statistic, no further investigation of this null hypothesis is necessary. There are no differences among groups. One does not need to start comparing the mean of group 1 with the mean of group 2, etc. On the other hand, if one performs an analysis of variance on the data and rejects the null hypothesis, then there exist some differences in the outcome ($FEV_1$ or blood lead) among the study groups associated with the particular exposure. One can then use procedures known as multiple comparison tests to identify exactly which group or groups differ significantly from the others.

This is an oversimplified discussion of analysis of variance meant only to develop the concept of this important statistical method. Not enough details have been provided for the reader to be able to perform this test. The purpose is to convey the flavor of the method so that situations in which analysis of variance is the appropriate first analytic procedure will be recognized. The bibliography includes references to texts in which the method is described in greater detail.

## Analyzing Rates & Proportions: The Chi Square Test

In the previous sections, the discussion concerned the analysis of continuous type data. This section begins a discussion of the analysis of categorical data. An example of categorical data is given in the following table of cigarette smoking history among cases of lung cancer and controls with other diseases.

|  | Lung Cancer | Controls |
|---|---|---|
| Cigarette smokers | 450 | 225 |
| Nonsmokers | 20 | 225 |
| Total | 470 | 450 |

It is immediately apparent, without doing any statistical tests, that there is an association of cigarette smoking and lung cancer. The row variable, cigarette smoking, is associated with the column variable, lung cancer. A simple calculation of the proportions of lung cancer and control cases who were cigarette smokers confirms this association. Of the lung cancers cases, 450/457 = 95.7% smoked cigarettes, while 225/450 = 50% of the controls smoked cigarettes.

However, suppose that the table was of mesothelioma and cigarette smoking, and the following results were obtained.

|  | Mesothelioma | Controls |
|---|---|---|
| Cigarette smokers | 80 | 200 |
| Nonsmokers | 40 | 104 |
| Total | 120 | 304 |

In this example, the ratio of cigarette smokers to non-smokers among the mesothelioma cases and the controls is nearly the same, approximately twice as many smokers as non-smokers for both. In this case, one would say that there is no association between the two variables in the table, the column variable (mesothelioma) and the row variable (cigarette smoking). The null hypothesis in this example would be that there is no association between mesothelioma and cigarette smoking, and one would not reject the null hypothesis on the basis of the extremely close proportions of smokers in the mesothelioma and the control groups.

Most situations with categorical data are not as clear-cut as these two examples. In most cases, one cannot simply "eyeball" the data to determine whether the two variables are or are not independent of one another. The statistical test one uses to determine whether or not there is an association in such data is known as the chi square test. An example of a situation in which the chi square test is applied is shown below.

**Example IV:** Three groups of farm workers are studied for the occurrence of new skin rashes during the growing season. The three groups are involved in growing and harvesting (1) grapes, (2) citrus crops, and (3) tomatoes. The workers are followed for the growing season, and the occurrence of new rashes in the three groups is compared to determine if there is an association between exposure (crop) and outcome (rash).

Crop 1, N = 100
Crop 2, N = 200
Crop 3, N = 300

| Response | Exposure (Crop) | | | Total |
|---|---|---|---|---|
|  | 1 | 2 | 3 |  |
| Rash | 30 | 40 | 32 | 102 |
| No rash | 70 | 160 | 168 | 398 |
| Total | 100 | 200 | 200 | 500 |

The null hypothesis in this situation is again the hypothesis of "no difference"—only it is phrased as no association between the row variable (rash) and the column variable (crop).

One can quickly compute from the table that the percentage working on crop 1 with a rash is 30%; on crop 2, it is 20%; and on crop 3, it is 16%. By just eyeballing the data, one would probably think that crop 1 is different from crops 2 and 3. The null hypothesis is there is no association between what crop a worker worked on and whether or not a rash developed. The question is whether the differences in response are due simply to random variation in the data or whether they are larger than one would expect by chance alone if the null hypothesis were true. To test this, the chi square statistic is calculated. As with the $t$-test and F-test, one determines whether this chi square is unlikely to have occurred by chance alone under the null hypothesis. The calculation of the chi square involves first determining an "expected" value for each cell in the table. The expected value is the value one would "expect" to see in the cell if there were no association between row (rash) and column (exposure) variables—ie, that value one would "expect" to see if the null hypothesis were true. The expected value is obtained as follows:

According to the null hypothesis, there are no differences among exposures, so we would expect the same proportion to develop a rash in each group. If this is true, the best estimate of the expected proportion with rashes in each exposure group comes from the overall information given by the row total number with rashes divided by the total number of workers in the study. That would be 102/500 = 0.204. Then, for exposure 1, one expects that 0.204 of the 100 people in exposure group 1 will develop rashes, ie, 20.4 people; for exposure 2, one expects that 0.204 of the 200 people working with crop 2 will develop rashes, ie, 40.8 people; and for crop 3, one expects that 0.204 of the 200 people will develop rashes, ie, 40.8 people. In other words, since under the null hypothesis there is no association between exposure and percentage developing a rash, one expects the same percentage to respond favorably (or unfavorably) in each group. The expected proportion of workers not developing rashes is obtained in the same manner. The best estimate of the proportion not developing a rash in each group is the total number not developing a rash divided by the total number of workers, which equals 398/500 = 0.796. This gives an expected frequency of $100 \times 0.796 = 79.6$ working with crop 1 not developing rashes, 159.2 working with crop 2 not developing rashes, and 159.2 working with crop 3 not developing rashes. Putting the expected values in parentheses alongside the observed values, the table now looks like this:

| Response | Exposure (Crop) | | | |
|---|---|---|---|---|
| | 1 | 2 | 3 | Total |
| Rash | 30 (20.4) | 40 (40.8) | 43 (40.8) | 102 |
| No rash | 70 (79.6) | 160 (159.2) | 168 (159.2) | 398 |
| Total | 100 | 200 | 200 | 500 |

To test the null hypothesis, one looks at the observed and expected numbers in each cell to see how close together the two values are. If the values are close together, one may decide that the null hypothesis is true. If they are very different, one may decide that the null hypothesis is not true. To decide whether the observed and expected values are close together, the chi square statistic is calculated. It has the following form:

$$\chi^2 = \sum_{i=1}^{n}\left[ \frac{(O_i - E_i)^2}{E_i} \right]$$

where $E_i$ = expected value in cell i,
$O_i$ = observed value in cell i,
i = 1,...,n, and
n = number of cells in the table.

Large values of chi square indicate a lack of agreement between observed and expected values; small values of chi square indicate close agreement.

How does one determine what is a large chi square? Just as in the preceding discussions about continuous data, one goes to a table of chi square values. The chi square value that would occur less than 5% of the time if the null hypothesis (no association) were true is identified in the table and compared to the study chi square value. If the study chi square is larger than the table cutoff value, the null hypothesis is rejected, since this is known to occur less than 5% of the time when the null hypothesis is true. If the study chi square value is smaller than the table cutoff value, the null hypothesis is not rejected, since this is known to happen more than 5% of the time when the null hypothesis is true. Alternatively, one could calculate the exact $P$ (probability) value of the study chi square statistic. To use the chi square tables, the degrees of freedom are needed to enter the proper point in the table. The degrees of freedom in the chi square situation are equal to (number of rows–1) times (number of columns–1). When there are two rows and three columns in a table, the degree of freedom is (2–1) times (3–1), which equals two degrees of freedom. One thing to remember is that the chi square statistic works only when the sample is sufficiently large. A rule of thumb is that the chi square is a good approximation when all *expected* values are equal to or greater than 5.

Calculating the chi square statistic for the preceding example, the following results are obtained.

$$\chi^2 = \frac{(70 - 79.6)^2}{79.6} + \frac{(160 - 159.2)^2}{159.2}$$

$$+ \frac{(168 - 159.2)^2}{159.2} + \frac{(30 - 20.4)^2}{20.4}$$

$$+ \frac{(40 - 40.8)^2}{40.8} + \frac{(32 - 40.8)^2}{40.8}$$

$$= 8.08$$

The tabled value of chi square to which the calculated value is compared is 5.99. Since 8.08 is larger than 5.99, the null hypothesis is rejected.

Calculating the chi square statistic is only one method for analyzing categorical data. It is, however, one of the most common statistical tests found in the medical literature.

## The *P*-Value & Statistical Significance

An important quantity in all statistical tests of hypothesis is the *P*-value. The *P*-value is the probability of observing a particular study result (eg, *t*-statistic calculated from study data) by chance alone when the null hypothesis is really true. In the examples thus far, the *P*-value of the test statistic has actually been used without calculating its exact value. The procedure has been to calculate, for example, a *t*-statistic from the study data. One then goes to a table of *t*-values and looks up that value of *t* that will occur less than 5% of the time by chance alone when the null hypothesis is true—ie, one looks up the tabulated *t*-statistic that has a *P*-value of 5%. If the value of the *t*-statistic computed for the sample is smaller than the one in the table, the null hypothesis is not rejected, since that is known to occur more than 5% of the time when the null hypothesis is true—ie, it has a *P*-value greater than 5%. When the computed sample *t*-statistic has a value larger than the one in the table, the null hypothesis is rejected, since that is known to occur less than 5% of the time when the null hypothesis is true. In other words, the sample *t*-statistic has a *P*-value less than 5%, so the null hypothesis is rejected. The exact *P*-value of the sample *t*-statistic can also be obtained from tabulated values, so that one can report *P*-values less than other cutoff values, eg, 1% ($P < 0.01$). When the *P*-value is less than 5%, the result is commonly referred to as being "statistically significant." However, "statistical significance" may not be the same as clinical or public health significance, since the former is affected by the size of the study population but may reflect differences that have no biologic importance.

The researcher in a typical study is interested in comparing an exposed group to a control group and using the observed difference in proportions or mean values to estimate the effect of the exposure. For example, one is interested in determining delta $\delta$, where $\delta$ equals the true mean value of sperm concentration among exposed workers minus the true mean value of sperm concentration in unexposed workers. One then wishes to test whether $\delta = 0$; one may wish to determine whether the (true) proportion with disease from one exposure is equal to the (true) proportion with disease under a second exposure or control. One can then calculate $\delta$ as the difference between these two proportions, again testing to see whether $\delta = 0$.

Even if the treatment and control groups in the study are truly being sampled from one underlying population (ie, if there is no real difference between treatment and control) some differences between the two groups will occur by chance alone. If the observed difference in sample means or proportions has a small probability of occurring by chance alone (assuming no true underlying difference), then the null hypothesis that $\delta = 0$ is rejected. The "rule" for deciding how small that probability has to be before rejecting the null hypothesis is known as the **level of significance** of the statistical test and is designated as alpha $\alpha$.

Thus, the procedure in a typical study is to formulate a null hypothesis ($H_0$), and, usually,

$$H_0: \mu_1 = \mu_2$$
$$\text{also written as } H_0: \delta = \mu_1 - \mu_2 = 0$$

eg, $H_0$: mean sperm concentration with exposure 1 = mean sperm concentration with exposure 2.

or,

$$H_0: p_1 - p_2 = 0$$
$$\text{also written as } H_0: \delta = p_1 - p_2 = 0$$

ie, $H_0$: proportion with disease in exposure 1 = proportion with disease in exposure 2.

The (two-sided) alternative hypothesis is,

$$H_A: \mu_1 \neq \mu_2$$
$$\text{also written as } H_A: \delta = \mu_1 - \mu_2 \neq 0$$

ie, $H_A$: the mean sperm concentrations are not equal under treatments 1 and 2 or

$$H_A: p_1 \neq p_2$$
$$\text{also written as } H_A: \delta = p_1 - p_2 \neq 0$$

ie, $H_A$: the proportions with disease are not equal under treatments 1 and 2.

After the study has been completed, sample estimates of $\mu$ or p are calculated for the two exposure groups. The probability is calculated that a difference as large as the one observed in the study would occur if the null hypothesis were true. This probability is the *P*-value of the test. If the *P*-value is less than $\alpha$ (the significance level), the null hypothesis is rejected. If the *P*-value is not less than $\alpha$, the null hypothesis is not rejected.

## THE TYPES OF MISTAKES ONE CAN MAKE IN DOING A RESEARCH STUDY

There are two types of errors one can make in deriving inferences from a typical research study. They are known as type I and type II errors.

## Type I Error

If one decides to reject the null hypothesis and declare the two groups different when in fact they really are from the same underlying population, this is a type I error. The type I error is equal to the significance level $\alpha$, and the significance level is *established before* the study is done. Thus, $\alpha$ equals the probability that one will reject the null hypothesis when the null hypothesis is true, ie, when the investigator decides what chance of making this kind of mistake is acceptable and sets the $\alpha$ level accordingly. For example, an investigator may decide that it is extremely important not to declare that a disease (eg, cancer) is associated with an exposure unless there is overwhelming evidence of an association from the study. In this case, the $\alpha$ level might be set at 1% instead of 5%, where 5% is the usual value for $\alpha$ used in most studies.

## Type II Error

If a researcher decides not to reject the null hypothesis when, in fact, there is a difference between the two groups, a type II error has been made—ie, a true difference between the two groups has been missed. The type II error is usually designated by $\beta$.

In a research study, the type II error is not a single value. If the null hypothesis is false, this means that exposure does not equal control, ie, $\delta$ is not equal to 0. There are an infinite number of values that this difference could take on. For each different value of the difference $\delta$ between exposed and control, there is a different value for the type II error. If one is interested in determining the probability that one would miss a true difference between exposure and control groups, the exact value of the difference being examined must be specified. Once this is done, the probability that one would fail to reject the null hypothesis given the true nonzero difference between the two groups can be calculated.

## The Power of a Study

One of the most important quantities calculated for a research study is the power of a particular study. The power is the probability that one will correctly reject the null hypothesis when the null hypothesis is truly false. In other words, the power is the probability of correctly recognizing a true difference between the two groups. The power of a study is actually the complement of the type II error $\beta$, ie, power = $1 - \beta$. Thus, the power of a study is different for every different value of $\delta$ that occurs. To calculate the power, one must specify a particular alternative. Power is particularly important when one is evaluating a negative study—a study that finds no difference between the groups.

Suppose the power of a study is 40%. This means that the researcher had a 40% chance of finding a true difference between the exposure groups. If no difference between the exposure groups was found and the power of the study was reported as 40%, the reader might wonder whether that study even had a chance of finding a difference between exposures if the exposures were truly associated with different outcomes.

The power of a statistical test is determined or affected by three quantities: (1) the magnitude of the type I error $\alpha$; (2) the size of the exposure effect $\delta$ the researcher is interested in detecting; and (3) the sample size of the study. Quantities (1) and (2) can be used to estimate the sample size needed in a study for a specified study power.

As the size of the type I error becomes smaller, the power of the study likewise becomes smaller. The type I error is the probability of incorrectly declaring a difference when there really is none. If it becomes harder to make this mistake (ie, $\alpha$ is smaller), it becomes harder to reject the null hypothesis in general, and power involves correctly rejecting the null hypothesis.

When a study is set up to look for a very large exposure effect $\delta$, it is relatively easy to detect this large effect, and the chances are great that the null hypothesis will be correctly rejected. The opposite occurs when one is looking for a very small $\delta$. Thus, power increases as $\delta$ increases.

As sample size increases, the variability of the measure of exposure effect decreases. Consequently, the test statistic increases in value, making it easier to exceed the cutoff point for rejecting the null hypothesis. This increases the chances of correctly rejecting the null hypothesis, and so power increases as sample size increases.

A handy table for remembering the quantities discussed in this section is shown below:

| | $H_0$ true (no difference) | $H_0$ false (difference exists) |
|---|---|---|
| $H_0$ study (declare no difference) | Correct decision | Type II error $\beta$ |
| $H_0$ reject (declare a difference) | Type I error $\alpha$ | Power $1-\beta$ |

## REFERENCES

The three books listed below are excellent introductory texts for clinicians who wish to learn the basic concepts and vocabulary of biostatistics. All three cover the elementary descriptive and analytic statistical methods useful for understanding today's medical literature.

### INTRODUCTORY TEXTS

Campbell MJ, Machin D: *Medical Statistics: A Common Sense Approach,* 2nd ed. New York, NY Wiley, 1993.

Glantz SA: *Primer of Biostatistics.* McGraw-Hill, 1992.

Ingelfinger JA et al: *Biostatistics in Clinical Medicine,* 3rd ed. McGraw-Hill, 1994.

The following four books are also introductory statistical textbooks but are more technically difficult than the preceding group; they cover more statistical procedures in greater depth. The books differ somewhat in the amount of mathematics used, but nothing beyond college algebra is require to cover the material as presented.

### MORE ADVANCED TEXTS

Armitage P, Berry G: *Statistical Methods in Medical Research,* 2nd ed. Blackwell, 1987.

Dawson-Saundres B, Trapp RG: *Basic & Clinical Biostatistics,* 2nd ed. Appleton & Lange, 1994.

Rosner BA: *Fundamentals of Biostatistics,* 4th ed. Duxbury, 1995.

Shedecor, GW, Cochran WG: *Statistical Methods,* 8th ed. Iowa State Univ Press, 1989.

## II. EPIDEMIOLOGY

Epidemiology is the study of the distribution and determinants of health- and disease-related conditions in populations. It is concerned with both epidemic (excess of normal expectancy) and endemic (always present) conditions.

The basic premise of epidemiology is that disease is not randomly distributed across populations. Not only is it important to know what sort of disease a particular person has—it is necessary also to know what sort of person has a particular disease. While the practice of much of occupational medicine is concerned with the pathogenesis of disease and the treatment of individuals with diseases, the focus of occupational epidemiology is on groups of individuals—with or without diseases—in an attempt to infer the causes that precede specific diseases and to determine what occupational or other lifestyle factors can be manipulated to eliminate specific diseases or reduce the prevalence of the disease.

There are three major types of epidemiologic studies: descriptive, analytic, and experimental.

**Descriptive** epidemiologic studies characterize person, place, and time. (1) Person: What are the personal characteristics of people who get a particular disease?—eg, age, race, sex, occupation, socioeconomic status, immune status. (2) Place: Where do they live or work or travel?—eg, international, national, and local comparisons, urban/rural, climate, altitude. (3) Time: When does the illness occur?—eg, temporal variation, seasonal fluctuations. Descriptive studies do not test hypotheses but nevertheless are powerful tools for characterizing disease distributions and associations.

**Analytic** studies attempt to determine the etiologic factors associated with a disease by calculating estimates of risk: (1) What exposures do people with the disease have in common?—eg, smoking, exogenous hormone use, diet, radiation, asbestos. (2) How much is risk increased by such exposures (using relative risk as the measure of excess risk)? (3) How many cases could be avoided if the exposure were eliminated (using attributable risk as the appropriate measure)? Analytic studies involve testing specified hypotheses.

**Experimental** studies involve a search for strategies for altering the natural history of disease. Examples of experimental studies are intervention trials to reduce risk factors, screening studies aimed at identifying the early stages of disease, and clinical trials of different treatment modalities to improve prognosis.

### MORTALITY & MORBIDITY

The two basic measures of disease in a population are mortality rates and morbidity rates. Examples of different types of mortality rates and how each is calculated are given in Table A–2. Morbidity is measured by calculating either prevalence or incidence rates. Prevalence is the number of existing cases of a disease at a given time divided by the population at risk for that disease at that time. This result is commonly multiplied by 100,000 to derive the prevalence rate per 100,000 population.

For purposes of etiology, the incidence rate is a more important measure of morbidity and is equal to the number of *new cases* of a disease occurring over a defined interval divided by the midinterval population at risk for that disease (multiplied by 100,000).

While mortality data are available throughout the world—with different completeness depending on the quality of death registration systems—incidence rates can be calculated only for those diseases for which there are population-based registries of disease or for which special studies have been conducted. The National Cancer Institute has a program of cancer registries around the United States that provides information on cancer incidence covering approximately 10% of the US population. Accurate enumeration of the population at risk—available from census data—is vital for deriving valid estimates of both mortality and morbidity rates. Rates can be specific to any subgroup of interest, defined by age, sex, race, or other characteristics. For example, the incidence rate for endometrial cancer among white women aged 50–54 in the United States in 1976 was 30 per 100,000, compared with 13.6 per 100,000 among black women of the same age. One must remember that in calculating a rate, the events in the numerator

**Table A–2.** Measures of mortality.

$$\text{Crude death rate } = \frac{\text{Number of deaths in year (all causes)}}{\text{Total population}} \times 1000$$

eg, U.S. 1977 = 8.8 ÷ 1000 population or 878.1 ÷ 100,000 population

$$\text{Cause-specific death rate } = \frac{\text{Number of deaths from specific cause in year}}{\text{Total population}} \times 100,000$$

eg, Cancer in U.S. 1977 = 178.7 ÷ 100,000 population

$$\text{Age-specific death rate } = \frac{\text{Number of deaths among persons of specified age group in year}}{\text{Population in specified age group}} \times 100,000$$

eg, Cancer in age group 1–14 = 4.9 ÷ 100,000

$$\text{Infant mortality rate } = \frac{\text{Number of deaths among children less than 1 year of age in year}}{\text{Number of births in year}} \times 1000$$

eg, U.S. 1977 = 14.1 ÷ 1000 live births (12.3 for whites; 21.7 for black and other)

must be drawn from the population specified in the denominator—ie, those in the denominator must be at risk for the disease. Thus, for endometrial cancer, men would not be included in the denominator.

Some problems to keep in mind about current disease data include the following:

(1) The only complete registry for all causes is for deaths, and the cause-of-death assignment on the death certificate is often inaccurate. In addition, for a disease whose case-fatality ratio is low (ie, a disease unlikely to result in death when it occurs), the death rate is a gross underestimate of the incidence of the condition in the community. An example of this would be nonmelanoma skin cancer.

(2) Morbidity reporting, even when it is legally mandated, as is the case for certain infectious diseases (eg, tuberculosis, sexually transmitted diseases), often results in severe under-reporting.

(3) Complete and accurate population-based morbidity registries are limited in geographic coverage.

## ADJUSTMENT OF RATES

In attempting to compare disease rates across population groups or to assess changes in rates over time, the effect of differential age distribution in the two populations whose rates are being compared should be taken into account. Disease risk is almost always a function of age; differences in crude rates (ie, rates not adjusted for age) across populations may reflect age differences rather than differences in occupational or environmental factors of interest.

Age-specific rates are not subject to that shortcoming, provided the range in each age group is relatively narrow. It is cumbersome, however, to compare rates among populations across many age strata. Age adjustment or standardization provides a summary measure of disease risk for an entire population that is not influenced by variations in age distribution.

There are two methods for age adjustment: a direct method, which applies observed age-specific rates to a standard population; and the indirect method, which applies age-specific rates from a standard population to the age distribution of an observed population. In discussing the methods for adjusting rates, cancer will be used as the disease being studied.

The **direct method** of age adjustment is appropriate when each of the populations being compared is large enough to yield stable age-specific rates. For example, the direct method is used for comparison of cancer rates over time in the United States. Crude mortality rates showing a dramatic increase in cancer over the past few decades would seem to provide strong evidence of a cancer epidemic. It needs to be ascertained, however, to what extent the aging of the country's population has contributed to the apparent epidemic or to what extent other factors, such as an increase in cancer-causing agents in the environment, might be responsible.

The first three columns of Table A–3 show the actual age distributions of the US population in 1940 and 1970, the percentage of the population in each group in the two periods, the corresponding number

**Table A–3.** Age adjustment by direct method, using cancer mortality data for the United States, 1940 and 1970.[1]

| Age Group | Actual Population (1) | Actual Population (2) | Number of Cancer Deaths (3) | Age-Specific Death Rates Per 100,000 (4) | Standard Population (5) | Expected Number of Cancer Deaths (6) |
|---|---|---|---|---|---|---|
| **1940** | | | | | | |
| <40 | 87,737,829 | 66.7 | 10,283 | 11.72 | 217,093,330 | 25,443 |
| 40–49 | 17,053,068 | 13. | 18,071 | 105.97 | 41,149,961 | 43,607 |
| 50–59 | 13,100,511 | 10. | 33,279 | 254.03 | 34,177,557 | 86,821 |
| 60–69 | 8,534,997 | 6.5 | 43,686 | 511.85 | 24,143,606 | 123,579 |
| 70–79 | 4,073,514 | 3.1 | 38,160 | 936.78 | 13,352,179 | 125,080 |
| 80+ | 1,139,143 | 0.9 | 14,721 | 1,292.29 | 4,934,355 | 63,766 |
| Totals | 131,639,062 | 100. | 158,200[3] | | 334,850,988 | 468,296[3] |
| **1970** | | | | | | |
| <40 | 129,355,501 | 63.7 | 16,096 | 12.44 | 217,093,330 | 27,006 |
| 40–49 | 24,096,893 | 11.9 | 26,075 | 108.21 | 41,149,961 | 44,528 |
| 50–59 | 21,077,046 | 10.4 | 61,143 | 290.09 | 34,177,557 | 99,146 |
| 60–69 | 15,608,609 | 7.7 | 90,099 | 577.24 | 24,143,606 | 139,367 |
| 70–79 | 9,278,665 | 4.6 | 88,826 | 957.31 | 13,352,179 | 127,821 |
| 80+ | 3,795,212 | 1.9 | 49,333 | 1,299.87 | 4,934,355 | 64,140 |
| Totals | 203,211,926 | 100. | 331,572[2] | | 334,850,988 | 502,008[2] |

[1] Public Health Service, Vital Statistics of the United States, 1940 and 1970 (National Center for Health Statistics, Rockville, MD).
[2] Crude death rate = [sum of column 3 + sum of column 1] $\times 10^5$ = 163.2 per 100,000. Age-adjusted death rate = [sum of column 6 + sum of column 5] $\times 10^5$ = 149.9 per 100,000.
[3] Crude death rate = [sum of column 3 + sum of column 1] $\times 10^5$ = 120.2 per 100,000 population. Age-adjusted death rate = [sum of column 6 + sum of column 5] $\times 10^5$ = 139.8 per 100,000 population.

of actual cancer deaths, and the age-specific death rates. Crude death rates per 100,000 population were 120.2 for 1940 and 163.2 for 1970, an increase of over 30%. Comparison of the age-specific rates, however, shows only minor increases between the two time periods. It should be noted that the percentage of the population in all age groups over 40 was higher in 1970 than in 1940.

To remove the variable effect of age using the direct method of adjustment, a "standard" population is chosen. The number of people in each age group of the standard population is then multiplied by the appropriate age-specific rate in each of the study populations. This generates the number of deaths one would expect in each age group if the populations had similar age distributions. The expected number of deaths is then summed over all age groups; the sum is divided by the total standard population; and the result is multiplied by 100,000. The choice of a standard population is arbitrary; it might be the combined population of the two groups whose rates are being compared, only one of those populations, or any other population.

In our example, the standard was the combined population of the United States in 1940 and 1970, shown in column 5 of Table A–3. The age-specific rates for each period (column 4) were applied for each age group to the standard population, yielding the expected number of deaths shown in column 6. Age-adjusted rates are then calculated by dividing the sum of expected deaths for each period by the total standard population. The resulting adjusted rates are 139.8 per 100,000 for 1940 and 149.9 per

100,000 for 1970. Thus, the magnitude of the increase in the crude rates has been reduced from about 30% to 7%. It can be concluded that age is an important factor in the increased cancer rates in the United States, though age alone does not entirely explain changes over time.

When the group of interest is relatively small and thus likely to have unstable age-specific rates, it is more appropriate to use the indirect than the direct method of age adjustment. This is most commonly the situation with investigation of cause-specific mortality in an occupational cohort. The **indirect method** is frequently employed to compare the cancer incidence or follow-up experience of a study group with that expected based on the experience of a larger population or patient series. With the indirect method, the age-specific rates from a standard population are multiplied by the number of person-years at risk in each group in the study series. The number of observed deaths is then compared with the number expected by means of a ratio.

The **standardized mortality ratio (SMR)** is an example of indirect standardization. In calculating an SMR, the age-specific rates from a standard population (eg, county, state, country) are multiplied by the person-years at risk in the study population (eg, industry employees) to give the expected number of deaths. The observed number of deaths divided by the expected number (times 100) is the SMR (see the example in Table A–4). An SMR may also control for time-specific mortality rates by indirect standardization.

Thus, the equation for an SMR is as follows:

**Table A–4.** Age adjustment by indirect method in computation of standardized mortality ratio (SMR).

| Age | Observed Deaths (1) | Person Years (2) | U.S. Population Rates (per $10^5$) (3) | Expected Deaths = (2) × (3) |
|---|---|---|---|---|
| 20–29 | 1 | 5,000 | 20.6 | 0.1 |
| 30–39 | 0 | 15,000 | 22.7 | 0.3 |
| 40–49 | 4 | 60,000 | 45.3 | 2.7 |
| 50–59 | 2 | 40,000 | 94.3 | 3.8 |
| 60–69 | 12 | 70,000 | 224.4 | 15.7 |
| | Σ Obs = 19 | | | Σ Exp = 22.6 |

SMR = [Σ Obs/Σ Exp] × 100 = [19/22.6]100 = 84

$$SMR = \left[\frac{\Sigma\, a_i}{\Sigma\, E(a_i)}\right] \times 100$$

$$= \left[\frac{Observed}{Expected}\right] \times 100$$

where $a_i$ = the number of people with a specific death in the *i*th stratum of age (and time), and

$E(a_i)$ = the expected number of deaths based on the age-specific (and time-specific) rates in the reference population.

The result is multiplied by 100, so that when observed deaths equal expected deaths, the SMR is 100, and the differences from 100 represent the percentage difference in mortality in the study population compared with that of the reference population.

Indirect standardization may also be used to adjust incidence rates for age or other factors. Thus, incident cases of a disease within a workplace could be expressed as the **standardized incidence ratio (SIR)**, as follows:

$$SIR = \left[\frac{Observed\ number\ of\ new\ cases}{Expected\ number\ of\ new\ cases}\right] \times 100$$

Although it is most common to adjust rates for age and time, the direct and indirect methods of adjustment can be used to adjust for population differences in other factors as well, such as sex, race, socioeconomic status, or stage of disease.

## Design Strategies for Analytic & Experimental Studies

Descriptive epidemiology provides disease rates for different groups. It identifies segments of the population—by age, sex, time, occupation, marital status, geographic area of residence, or other parameters—whose unique experience suggests etiologic hypotheses worthy of pursuit through rigorous analytic studies. Descriptive epidemiology tells *who* gets the disease *where* and *when* and is the basis of analytic epidemiology, which in turn focuses on specific questions, such as the following:

*What* exposure do people with the disease have in common, compared with people without the disease?

*Why* does exposure induce or promote disease?

*How much* is risk increased by such exposure?

*How many* cases might be avoided were the exposure eliminated?

The last question addresses the ultimate objective of epidemiologic research: to identify risk factors so that intervention might either prevent the occurrence of the disease (primary prevention) or lead to early detection (secondary prevention).

The three basic strategies for analytic epidemiology are (1) the cohort study, (2) the case-control study, and (3) the experimental study (clinical trial).

Cohort and case-control studies are observational: the investigator does not control exposure or modify behavior of the study subjects. In the experimental study, the investigator intervenes by introducing treatment or other exposures to study their impact on the disease experience.

# TYPES OF EPIDEMIOLOGIC STUDIES

## THE COHORT STUDY

In the design of a cohort study, a disease-free group of individuals characterized by a common experience or exposure is identified and followed forward over time, or prospectively, to determine whether disease occurs at a rate different from that in a cohort without the exposure. The **relative risk (RR)** of disease associated with the exposure can then be calculated:

$$RR = \frac{Incidence\ rate\ in\ the\ exposed\ group}{Incidence\ rate\ in\ the\ nonexposed\ group}$$

A frequently cited example of the prospective cohort design is the follow-up study of British physicians whose smoking habits were ascertained by means of a mailed questionnaire. The doctors were grouped according to smoking habits, and their deaths were subsequently monitored. Lung cancer rates for those exposed to various levels of smoking were then compared with the rates for nonsmokers by means of the relative risk. Other examples of cohort studies include investigations of long-term cancer incidence among atomic bomb survivors exposed to varying degrees of radiation and deaths among British coal miners.

Theoretically, the prospective cohort study is ideal because the hypothesized cause or exposure precedes the effect—ie, disease—and because disease rates and relative risks can be calculated directly provided that a suitable comparison group is built into the study or otherwise available for calculation of rates in the nonexposed population. In addition, the exposure of interest can be accurately recorded at the time of exposure: it is not based on recall of past events. This approach has been popular in occupational studies in which the disease experience of workers exposed to putatively hazardous substances has been compared with that of other workers without the exposure or with that of the general population.

In practice, however, because of the expense, the time involved, and the number of subjects required, the model prospective cohort study is relatively rare. To avoid some of these constraints, a **historical cohort study** might be done whereby a group of persons who in the past experienced an exposure of interest is identified and their disease record up to the present is investigated. An example is the follow-up of mortality among insulation workers exposed to asbestos. The population of union insulation workers in the 1940s was identified, and their cause-specific mortality rate through the 1970s was determined. Mortality rates for lung cancer and other causes in this population were tabulated and compared with those expected on the basis of mortality rates for all US men. Because the historical cohort study is really a retrospective approach, the terms cohort study and prospective study should not be used synonymously.

## Measures of Association in a Cohort Study

Three measures of association will be discussed using the symbols and numbers provided in Tables A–5 and A–6. Let us assume that one is doing a study of smokers and nonsmokers and following them to see who develops lung cancer over some defined period of time.

**A. Relative Risk (RR):** Relative risk is the risk of disease in people exposed to a factor relative to the risk in people not exposed and is a measure of the strength of association between an exposure and a disease.

**Table A–5.** Presentation of data from a cohort study.

| | | Disease | | |
|---|---|---|---|---|
| | | Present | Absent | |
| Exposure | Yes | a | b | a + b |
| | No | c | d | c + d |

$$RR = \frac{\text{Disease rate in the exposed population}}{\text{Disease rate in the nonexposed population}}$$

$$= \frac{\dfrac{a}{a+b}}{\dfrac{c}{c+d}} = \frac{\dfrac{63}{10^5}}{\dfrac{7}{10^5}} = 9$$

A relative risk greater than 1 implies a positive association of the disease with exposure to the factor; a relative risk less than 1 implies a negative association (protective effect) of exposure to the factor with disease.

The results in the above example suggest that the risk of lung cancer among smokers is 9 times greater than the risk for nonsmokers. Relative risk is important for testing etiologic hypotheses.

**B. Attributable Risk (AR):** Attributable risk is the rate in the exposed population minus the rate in the nonexposed population.

$$AR = \frac{a}{a+b} - \frac{c}{c+d}$$

$$= \frac{63}{10^5} - \frac{7}{10^5} = \frac{56}{10^5}$$

ie, 56 of the 63 lung cancer deaths that occur annually among 100,000 smokers (ie, 89%) are attributable to smoking. Because a disease may have multiple risk factors that interact with each other, the sum of attributable risks may be greater than 100%.

Attributable risk is important for counseling individuals with risk factors.

**C. Population Attributable Risk (PAR) Percentage:** PAR percentage is the proportion of a disease in a population related to (or "attributable to") a given exposure.

$$PAR = \frac{P_c (RR - 1)}{P_c (RR - 1) + 1}$$

**Table A–6.** Example of data collected in a cohort study of lung cancer and smoking.

| | Develop Lung Cancer | Do Not Develop Lung Cancer | |
|---|---|---|---|
| Smokers | 63 | 99,937 | 100,000 |
| Nonsmokers | 7 | 99,993 | 100,000 |

where $P_e$ = the proportion of the population exposed to the risk factor and
RR = relative risk.

Assuming that 40% of the population smokes ($P_e$) and that the relative risk (RR) of lung cancer associated with smoking is 9, then

$$= \frac{0.4\ (9-1)}{0.4\ (9-1)+1} = \frac{3.2}{4.2} = 76.2\%$$

That is to say, 76% of cases of lung cancer in the general population are attributable to smoking. Population attributable risk is important for public health policy and planning, ie, in estimating what percent of cases in a population could be eliminated by removing an exposure.

## CASE-CONTROL STUDY

The case-control study is the most frequently used design in analytic epidemiology. It determines the risk factors associated with a particular disease by comparing a group of subjects (cases) who have the disease with one or more control groups composed of subjects who do not have the disease. Risk factors studied may be permanent, such as gender or ethnicity; they may be current, such as present drug use; or they may be historical, such as previous employment. The difference in the frequency distribution of the risk factors between the case and control groups is examined, and the magnitude of the association of these factors with the disease under study is estimated.

Case-control studies are a commonly used design in occupational epidemiology to evaluate multiple exposures associated with a single outcome. For example, an investigator may be interested in the many occupational and non-occupational causes of lung cancer. Conversely, a study of many health outcomes associated with a single exposure or workplace would be investigated by a cohort design.

The case-control study is always retrospective. The investigator starts by identifying diseased and nondiseased individuals (ie, the effect) and looks backward for the presence or absence of attributes or exposures (ie, the causes) in these individuals.

For example, to study the relationship between asbestos exposure and mesothelioma, a case-control study would compare the history of asbestos exposure in a group of mesothelioma patients with the history of asbestos exposure in a group of subjects who do not have mesothelioma. The cohort study, in contrast, first identifies a group of disease-free individuals classified for absence or presence of the risk factor or exposure of interest and then follows these individuals over time to compare the incidence of disease in the exposed and unexposed groups. A co-

hort study of the relationship between asbestos and mesothelioma would first classify a group of nondiseased persons according to their asbestos exposure and follow them to determine whether the asbestos exposed subjects had a higher incidence of mesothelioma over time than the nonexposed subjects.

Case-control studies generally can be done more rapidly and less expensively than cohort studies. The time required to complete the study is the time needed to assemble the necessary data; the investigator does not need to wait for cases of the disease to appear. This usually results in lower personnel costs. The study is also less costly because fewer subjects are necessary to test a hypothesis.

For example, suppose half of the general population is exposed to a risk factor (eg, cigarette smoking) and half is not. If a disease has an annual incidence rate of 100 per 100,000 in the exposed and 10 per 100,000 in the nonexposed population, a study of 100 cases and 100 controls would probably reveal the increased risk of disease associated with exposure to the factor. Uncovering 100 cases of disease in a cohort study would mean following 10,000 exposed people for 10 years. The more rare the disease, the greater the relative advantage of the case-control study.

### Source & Selection of Cases

In defining a case, the diagnostic criteria should be clear and permit selection of a homogeneous group of cases. For example, in cancer studies, microscopic confirmation of disease and clearly defined criteria for classification by histologic type of cancer greatly enhance the validity and generalizability of the study findings. The case group is usually composed of (1) all persons with the disease seen at a particular medical facility or group of facilities in a specified period, or (2) all persons with the disease found in a community or in the general population in a specified period. Whatever the source of the cases, they should be newly diagnosed (or incident) cases of the disease. Inclusion of prevalent (diagnosed in the past) cases will increase the sample size but will complicate analysis and interpretation of results. Prevalent cases are "survivors" and are therefore not representative of all people who develop a disease. Inclusion of prevalent cases may identify factors that result from the disease rather than factors that are causally related to its development.

### Source & Selection of Controls

The four most common sources of the control group are (1) the general population, (2) hospital patients, (3) relatives of cases, and (4) associates or friends of cases.

The **general population** control group is appropriate if all or most cases occur in a specific geographic area—eg, a county—in which event the controls represent the same target population as the cases. Using general population controls presents certain problems: potentially lower response rates than from other types of control groups and from the case group, differing quality of information if the interview setting differs for the cases and the controls, and higher costs.

The **hospital patient** control group is selected from patients at the same hospital or clinic that the cases attended. This control group may share the selective factors that influenced the cases to come to a particular hospital or clinic, eg, residence, ethnicity, or income. These patients (the controls) are readily available, have time to spare, and are more cooperative. The disadvantage of the hospital control group is that it is composed of people who are ill and who will differ from the general population with regard to factors often associated with disease, such as smoking habits and drug use. In addition, the factors that cause patients to attend a particular hospital may not be the same for all diseases. For example, a hospital with a national reputation for treating Hodgkin's disease may have patients with this disease from all over the country, whereas its population of coronary disease patients may come only from the region surrounding the hospital; thus, the two patient groups may differ greatly. Similarly, healthy people attending a hospital screening clinic may differ markedly in ethnic, socioeconomic, or other factors from the inpatient population of that hospital. One consideration in selecting controls is whether to draw them from the hospital's entire patient population or to exclude patients who have diseases related to factors under study. For example, in a case-control study of the relationship between lung cancer and smoking, it would seem logical to exclude from the control group persons who have emphysema, because emphysema is related to smoking, the factor under study. There is also the problem of not knowing whether factors being studied are related to diseases present in hospital controls. Selecting controls from many diagnostic categories would minimize this problem.

**Spouses and siblings** are the relatives most commonly used as controls because of similarity in ethnicity and environment with the case group. Moreover, sibling controls are genetically similar to the cases. Spouses as controls are appropriate if there is an approximately equal number of male and female cases and the age range of cases is such that a high proportion of spouses are likely to be alive. When siblings are the controls, one sibling should be selected per case. Using all available siblings would result in the control group's having many characteristics related to large family size, and these factors may confound any observed associations. Similarly, cases who have no siblings must be excluded so that the case group is not weighted with the characteristics of one-child families.

A control group of **associates of cases** such as neighbors, coworkers, friends, or schoolmates has the advantage of being composed of generally healthy individuals who are similar to the case group in lifestyle characteristics—eg, neighborhood controls are usually of the same socioeconomic status as the cases. However, such associates might be more similar to cases than members of the general population with respect to risk factors under investigation, thus impairing the ability of the study to detect true differences in exposure between people with and without disease. Other disadvantages of associates as controls are the effort necessary to identify them, a response rate different from that of cases, and probable variations in the quality of information obtained from cases and controls.

## Sampling

Once the source of the control group has been determined, one must decide on the method of selecting the controls. Either all eligible individuals are selected from a specific group—though this is usually not required—or a sample is selected. Whenever sampling is employed, its protocol should be defined and adhered to throughout the sampling. Examples of common sampling strategies are (1) random sampling, (2) systematic sampling, and (3) paired sampling.

In **random sampling,** each member of the source group has an equal chance of being represented in the control group. For example, all individuals might be assigned a number, and the sample would be selected using a table of random numbers.

In **systematic sampling,** the source group for controls is assumed to have an ordered sequence, and every $n$th individual is selected. As long as the sequence of the source group is not related to an important study variable, the resulting characteristics of a systematic sample are similar to those of a random sample.

In addition to random or systematic sampling, a popular method of selecting controls is **paired sampling.** In paired sampling, one or several controls are selected for each case based on a defined relationship to the case. For example, if we use hospital controls, the person who was admitted immediately before or after the case might be chosen for the control group. The investigator may choose to select for each case one or more controls who are individually matched with the case on characteristics such as sex, age, or socioeconomic status—which, if not controlled, might lead to spurious associations in the final results. For example, as a neighborhood control, the resident of the nearest dwelling to the right of the case's house who is of the same sex and age ($\pm$ 5 years) as the case might be selected. Such matching at the outset of the study is one way of taking into account any variables known to be associated with both the disease and the exposure of interest.

## Sources of Bias

Bias is defined as deviation from the truth of results or of inferences or processes leading to such deviation.

While bias is more common in case-control studies, it may occur also in cohort studies—eg, outcome measures may be obtained differently in exposed and unexposed subjects. The principle is the same: Any difference in the way information is obtained from the study groups may bias the results of the study.

**A. Selection Bias:** The appropriate control group should be judiciously chosen to avoid selection bias. Under the null hypothesis, cases and controls have been equally "exposed" to the study factor. Therefore, the cases and controls must be comparable and representative of the same underlying population, so that if we reject the null hypothesis and determine that cases differ from controls on the study factor, it is not because we selected them to be different by using a biased procedure. Since the case group is usually chosen first, selection bias is avoided by a careful choice of the appropriate control group.

As an example of how selection bias can occur, suppose we are studying the relationship between Alzheimer's disease and previous exposure to lead. We choose our case group from the inpatient population of a private hospital and our control group from the outpatient clinic of the same hospital. Once we have selected our cases and controls, we discover that they differ dramatically with respect to socioeconomic status—the inpatient population being predominantly upper middle class and the clinic population predominantly lower class. Thus, if we find that the cases and controls differ in terms of prior lead exposure, we would not know whether this is a true difference or whether the difference is due to other factors related to socioeconomic status.

Selection bias can also occur if the control group is composed of people who volunteer for the study, since volunteers differ in significant ways from nonvolunteers, eg, they may be more educated, more active in community affairs, less likely to be smokers.

**B. Interviewer (Data Collection) Bias:** In interviewing study subjects about past exposures or events, the interviewer who knows the disease status of the individual (case or control) may unconsciously pose questions or probe for answers in a different manner. For example, in a case-control study of factors related to lung cancer, an interviewer might pursue in greater depth questions concerning asbestos exposure when obtaining work or environmental histories from cases than from controls.

To avoid this bias, the procedure used to collect information should be identical for cases and controls. The data collector should ideally be unaware of the hypotheses being tested and whether the subject is a case or control; however, in collecting information of a medical or personal nature, it is often difficult to avoid learning of the person's disease status. Every effort must therefore be made to keep interviews as comparable as possible (eg, place, length, and format of questionnaire, attempts to gain cooperation and accurate information, and other aspects of the interview). Each interviewer should see an equal number of cases and controls.

**C. Recall Bias:** When a study subject is asked to recall past exposures or events, recall might depend on the person's current disease status. For example, a person with lymphoma is more likely to recall remote exposure to pesticides than a control subject without cancer. To minimize recall bias in this instance, one might try to obtain independent verification of previous exposure. It is also advantageous to use information recorded before the time of diagnosis wherever possible. In using data from interviews in which the case has a serious illness and the control has not, the items on which cases and controls can be compared with the greatest confidence are those least subject to recall bias. For example, prior surgery is a more objectively reported event than prior drug use.

## Confounding

The phenomenon of confounding is another explanation for an apparent association between an exposure and a disease and may also cause no association to be observed when a true association actually exists. As with bias, confounding may occur in any type of analytic epidemiologic study. When confounding occurs, an extraneous factor is associated with the exposure and is an independent cause of the disease being studied. In this situation, an observed association between an exposure and a disease is in fact due wholly or in part to the association of the exposure with the confounding factor, which in turn is a cause of the disease. If the confounding factor is not differentially associated with the exposed subjects or is not a cause of the disease, it cannot be a confounding factor.

An example of a confounding factor would be cigarette smoking in a study of an occupational exposure and lung cancer. Cigarette smoking is a known cause of lung cancer. If the cigarette smoking prevalence were greater (or less) in the population exposed to the agent, failure to control for smoking in the study design or analysis would lead to an apparently greater (or lesser) association between the exposure and lung cancer.

## ANALYSIS OF CASE-CONTROL STUDIES

Data from the case-control study are conventionally arrayed so that cases and controls can be compared on exposure to a hypothesized etiologic factor:

|  |  | Disease Status |  |
|---|---|---|---|
|  |  | Cases | Controls |
| Exposure { | Yes | a | b |
|  | No | c | d |
|  |  | a + c | b + d |

The **incidence** of disease among the exposed and nonexposed cannot be calculated using case-control data because the cases and controls in the study rarely reflect the true proportions of diseased and nondiseased persons in the population. (The investigator usually selects roughly equal numbers of cases [a + c] and controls [b + d] in the study, whereas there are many more nondiseased than diseased people in the population.) Therefore, relative risk of disease associated with exposure cannot be calculated directly in a case-control study, as it was for the cohort study. However, an estimate of the relative risk, known as the **odds ratio,** can be calculated if the proportion of diseased people in the general population is small compared with the proportion of nondiseased (almost always true). Recall that the true relative risk using data from a cohort or incidence study is as follows:

$$RR = \frac{\dfrac{a}{a+b}}{\dfrac{c}{c+d}}$$

where a = the number of cases among the exposed group in a cohort study,
b = the number of noncases among the exposed group.
c = the number of cases among the nonexposed group, and
d = the number of noncases among the nonexposed group.

In a cohort study, as in the general population, "a" is *very* small relative to "b." Similarly, "c" is *very* small relative to "d." Thus, in the general population (and the usual cohort study), a/(a + b) ≅ a/b and c/(c + d) ≅ c/d. Consequently, the formula for relative risk reduces to

$$\frac{\dfrac{a}{b}}{\dfrac{c}{d}} = \frac{ad}{bc} = \textit{odds ratio (estimated relative risk)}$$

## Example

*100 men with lung cancer and 100 controls are interviewed regarding smoking history*

|  | Cases | Controls |
|---|---|---|
| Smokers | 80 | 30 |
| Nonsmokers | 20 | 70 |
|  | 100 | 100 |

$$\text{Odds ratio} = \frac{ad}{bc} = \frac{80 \times 70}{30 \times 20} = \frac{5600}{600} = 9.3$$

*Since the odds ratio is an estimate of relative risk, one can conclude that these data show a ninefold-increased risk of lung cancer in smokers compared to nonsmokers.*

**Population attributable risk (PAR)** (ie, the proportion of all instances of the disease in the population that can be attributed to the exposure of interest) can be estimated from case-control studies, using the following equation:

$$PAR = \frac{p\,(OR - 1)}{p\,(OR - 1) + 1}$$

where p = the proportion of the population with exposure of interest (estimated from controls as b ÷ [b + d]), and
OR = the estimated relative risk (odds ratio) associated with the characteristic.

### Matched Case-Control Studies

Controls are frequently selected in a case-control study so as to be individually matched to the cases as to characteristics such as age, sex, race, or socioeconomic status that are known to be related to the disease. Matching helps make the two groups similar with respect to factors other than the exposure of interest in the study and thus serves to reduce the likelihood of spurious associations. The investigator must be careful, however, not to overmatch, ie, to match cases and controls on factors related to the exposure of interest; overmatching can artificially reduce—may even eliminate—true exposure differences between diseased and nondiseased individuals in the study. It should be obvious that cases and controls cannot be compared in the analysis with respect to any characteristics on which they have been matched.

The data in a matched pairs analysis are organized as shown below:

|  |  | Controls | |
|---|---|---|---|
|  |  | Exposed | Not exposed |
| *Cases* | Exposed | r | s |
|  | Not exposed | t | u |

where r = the number of pairs in which both case and control are exposed to the factor (concordant),

s = the number of pairs in which the case but not the control is exposed to the factor (discordant),

t = the number of pairs in which the control but not the case is exposed to the factor (discordant), and

u = the number of pairs in which both case and control are not exposed to the factor (concordant).

To compute the **odds ratio** (estimated relative risk) for a matched pairs study, only the discordant pairs enter into the calculation:

$$\text{Odds ratio} = \frac{s}{t}$$

$$\text{where } t \neq 0$$

## Example

*One hundred and seventy-five children aged 5–15 years admitted to hospital in 1968 with acute asthma were matched on age, sex, race, and date of admission to 175 controls. All children or their parents in the study were interviewed regarding personal habits and home characteristics during the month preceding admission. The results regarding environmental tobacco smoke (ETS) exposure were as follows:*

|        |         | Controls |        |        |
|--------|---------|----------|--------|--------|
|        |         | Yes ETS  | No ETS | Totals |
| *Cases* | Yes ETS | 10       | 57     | 67     |
|        | No ETS  | 25       | 95     | 108    |
|        |         | 35       | 152    | 187    |

$$\text{Odds ratio} = \frac{s}{t} = \frac{57}{25} = 2.3$$

*These data show that children who have asthma have a 2.3 times greater odds of environmental tobacco smoke exposure than do children without an acute asthma admission.*

## THE EXPERIMENTAL STUDY

The experimental study is the type of design most familiar to clinical investigators, but it is rarely encountered in occupational epidemiology. Unlike the cohort and case-control studies, which are observational in nature—ie, the investigator observes exposed individuals for the development of disease or diseased individuals for past exposures—in an experimental study the investigator manipulates exposures and studies the impact upon disease. The intervention can occur at different points in the natural course of

the disease. Subjects are normally randomly assigned to the different interventions in an experimental study. Ideally, study outcomes should also be determined by individuals blind to the exposure status of the subjects.

Experimental clinical trials are often undertaken among individuals with the same disease who are assigned to different treatment groups. An example is the CARET study, in which men with asbestos exposure, who are at increased risk of lung cancer, are randomly assigned to receive beta-carotene or a placebo. The study was undertaken to determine whether beta-carotene decreases the risk of developing lung cancer.

Alternatively, intervention might occur in the form of a screening program offered to one group of people at risk of disease and not to another similar group.

An example of this type of intervention study is the National Cancer Institute's Cooperative Screening for Early Lung Cancer Program. Men aged 45 and older with a history of heavy cigarette smoking were assigned to a dual-screened group receiving chest x-rays and sputum cytologic testing or to a group receiving only chest x-rays. The objective was to determine whether the addition of sputum cytologic testing to regular chest radiography resulted in earlier detection and improved lung cancer survival.

## CAUSAL ASSOCIATION

An epidemiologic study may demonstrate an association that is not valid because of chance, bias, or confounding, as previously discussed. If the association is believed to be valid—ie, the disease occurrence is in fact not equal among the exposed and unexposed subjects—and the association cannot be explained by chance, bias, or confounding, the investigator must consider whether the data support a cause and effect association.

This process involves consideration of the study itself and all existing data on the subject. Factors that should be considered in evaluating whether an association is causal include (1) the strength of the association; (2) whether dose-response relationships are present; (3) consonance with existing knowledge, ie, other studies demonstrating the same finding; (4) biological credibility, ie, whether there is a proposed biological mechanism; and (5) the time sequence, ie, whether cause precedes effect.

While uncertainties will always exist following an epidemiologic study, action on the findings of a study will depend in part on how strongly the data support a causal association and on the need for action versus the consequences of obtaining more data.

# REFERENCES

## EPIDEMIOLOGY

The books listed below are excellent general introductory texts in epidemiology and cover basic descriptive and analytic methods. Examples provided throughout are drawn from classic epidemiologic studies.

Checkoway H, Pearce N, Crawford-Brown DJ: *Research Methods in Occupational Epidemiology.* Oxford Univ Press, 1989.

Fletcher RH, Fletcher SW, Wagner EH: *Clinical Epidemiology,* 2nd ed. Williams & Wilkins, 1988.

Friedman GD: *Primer of Epidemiology,* 4th ed. McGraw-Hill, 1994.

Hennekens CH, Buring JE: *Epidemiology in Medicine.* Little, Brown, 1987.

Last JM (editor): *A Dictionary of Epidemiology,* 3rd ed. Oxford Univ Press, 1995.

Lilienfeld DE, Stolby PD: *Foundations of Epidemiology,* 3rd ed. Oxford Univ Press, 1994.

Monson RR: *Occupational Epidemiology,* 2nd ed. CRC Press, 1990.

Rothman KJ: *Modern Epidemiology.* Little, Brown, 1986.

## CASE-CONTROL STUDIES

The following references describe in detail the methodologic issues and statistical theory underlying the design and analysis of case-control studies as used in epidemiologic research. Many examples drawn from published studies are presented.

Breslow NE, Day NE: *Statistical Methods in Cancer Research.* International Agency for Research on Cancer, 1980.

Fleiss JL: *Statistical Methods for Rates and Proportions.* Wiley, 1981.

Schlesselman JJ: *Case Control Studies: Design, Conduct, Analysis.* Oxford Univ Press, 1982.

# B

# Clinical Practice Guidelines for Musculoskeletal Injuries in Adults[1]

## Purpose and Scope

Low back problems affect virtually everyone at some time during their life. Surveys indicate a yearly prevalence of symptoms in 50 percent of working age adults; 15-20 percent seek medical care. Low back problems rank high among the reasons for physician office visits and are costly in terms of medical treatment, lost productivity, and nonmonetary costs such as diminished ability to perform or enjoy usual activities. In fact, for persons under age 45, low back problems are the most common cause of disability.

Acute low back problems are defined as activity intolerance due to lower back or back-related leg symptoms of less than 3 months' duration. About 90 percent of patients with acute low back problems spontaneously recover activity tolerance within 1 month. The approach to a new episode in a patient with a recurrent low back problem is similar to that of a new acute episode.

The findings and recommendations included in the *Clinical Practice Guideline* define a paradigm shift away from focusing care exclusively on the pain and toward helping patients improve activity tolerance. The intent of this *Quick Reference Guide* is to bring to life this paradigm shift. The guide provides information on the detection of serious conditions that occasionally cause low back symptoms (conditions such as spinal fracture, tumor, infection, cauda equina syndrome, or non-spinal conditions). However, treatment of these conditions is beyond the scope of this guideline. In addition, the guideline does not address the care of patients younger than 18 years or those with chronic back problems (back-related activity limitations of greater than 3 months' duration).

## Initial Assessment

- Seek potentially dangerous underlying conditions.

- In the absence of signs of dangerous conditions, there is no need for special studies since 90 percent of patients will recover spontaneously within 4 weeks.

A focused medical history and physical examination are sufficient to assess the patient with an acute or recurrent limitation due to low back symptoms of less than 4 weeks duration. Patient responses and findings on the history and physical examination, referred to as "red flags" (Table 1), raise suspicion of serious underlying spinal conditions. Their absence rules out the need for special studies during the first 4 weeks of symptoms when spontaneous recovery is expected. The medical history and physical examination can also alert the clinician to non-spinal pathology (abdominal, pelvic, thoracic) that

[1]Source: Pages 1–7 in: Quick Reference Guide for Clinicians. Number 14. Acute Low Back Problems in Adults: Assessment and Treatment. Clinical Practice Guideline. U.S. Department of Health and Human Services. Public Health Service. Agency for Health Care Policy and Research. Rockville, MD. AHCPR Publication No. 95-0643. December 1994.

can present as low back symptoms. Acute low back symptoms can then be classified into one of three working categories:

- ■ **Potentially serious spinal condition**—tumor, infection, spinal fracture, or a major neurologic compromise, such as cauda equina syndrome, suggested by a red flag.

- ■ **Sciatica**—back-related lower limb symptoms suggesting lumbosacral nerve root compromise.

- ■ **Nonspecific back symptoms**—occurring primarily in the back and suggesting neither nerve root compromise nor a serious underlying condition.

## Table 1. Red flags for potentially serious conditions

| Possible fracture | Possible tumor or infection | Possible cauda equina syndrome |
|---|---|---|
| **From medical history** | | |
| Major trauma, such as vehicle accident or fall from height. Minor trauma or even strenuous lifting (in older or potentially osteoporotic patient). | Age over 50 or under 20. History of cancer. Constitutional symptoms, such as recent fever or chills or unexplained weight loss. Risk factors for spinal infection: recent bacterial infection (e.g., urinary tract infection); IV drug abuse; or immune suppression (from steroids, transplant, or HIV). Pain that worsens when supine; severe nighttime pain. | Saddle anesthesia. Recent onset of bladder dysfunction, such as urinary retention, increased frequency, or overflow incontinence. Severe or progressive neurologic deficit in the lower extremity. |
| **From physical examination** | | |
| | | Unexpected laxity of the anal sphincter. Perianal/perineal sensory loss. Major motor weakness: quadriceps (knee extension weakness); ankle plantar flexors, evertors, and dorsiflexors (foot drop). |

## Medical History

In addition to detecting serious conditions and categorizing back symptoms, the medical history establishes rapport between the clinician and patient. The patient's description of present symptoms and limitations, duration of symptoms, and history of previous episodes defines the problem. It also provides insight into concerns, expectations, and nonphysical (psychological and socioeconomic) issues that may alter the patient's response to treatment. Assessment tools such as pain drawings and visual analog pain-rating scales may help further document the patient's perceptions and progress.

A patient's estimate of personal activity intolerance due to low back symptoms contributes to the clinical assessment of the severity of the back problem, guides treatment, and establishes a baseline for recommending daily activities and evaluating progress.

Open-ended questions, such as those listed below, can gauge the need for further discussion or specific inquiries for more detailed information:

■ *What are your symptoms?*

Pain, numbness, weakness, stiffness?

Located primarily in back, leg, or both?

Constant or intermittent?

■ *How do these symptoms limit you?*

How long can you sit, stand, walk?

How much weight can you lift?

■ *When did the current limitations begin?*

How long have your activities been limited? More than 4 weeks?

Have you had similar episodes previously?

Previous testing or treatment?

■ *What do you hope we can accomplish during this visit?*

## Physical Examination

Guided by the medical history, the physical examination includes:

■ General observation of the patient.

■ A regional back exam.

■ Neurologic screening.

■ Testing for sciatic nerve root tension.

The examination is mostly subjective since patient response or interpretation is required for all parts except reflex testing and circumferential measurements for atrophy.

## Addressing Red Flags

Physical examination evidence of severe neurologic compromise that correlates with the medical history may indicate a need for immediate consultation. The examination may further modify suspicions of tumor, infection, or significant trauma. A medical history suggestive of non-spinal pathology mimicking a back problem may warrant examination of pulses, abdomen, pelvis, or other areas.

## Observation and Regional Back Examination

Limping or coordination problems indicate the need for specific neurologic testing. Severe guarding of lumbar motion in all planes may support a suspected diagnosis of spinal infection, tumor, or fracture. However, given marked variations among persons with and without symptoms, range-of-motion measurements of the back are of limited value.

Vertebral point tenderness to palpation, when associated with other signs or symptoms, may be suggestive of but not specific for spinal fracture or infection. Palpable soft-tissue tenderness is, by itself, an even less specific or reliable finding.

## Neurologic Screening

The neurologic examination can focus on a few tests that seek evidence of nerve root impairment, peripheral neuropathy, or spinal cord dysfunction. Over 90 percent of all clinically significant lower extremity radiculopathy due to disc herniation involves the L5 or S1 nerve root at the L4-5 or L5-S1 disc level. The clinical features of nerve root compression are summarized in Figure 1.

■ *Testing for Muscle Strength.* The patient's inability to toe walk (calf muscles, mostly S1 nerve root), heel walk (ankle and toe dorsiflexor muscles, L5 and some L4 nerve roots), or do a single squat and rise (quadriceps muscles, mostly L4 nerve root) may indicate muscle weakness. Specific testing of the dorsiflexor muscles of the ankle or great toe (suggestive of L5 or some L4 nerve root dysfunction), hamstrings and ankle evertors (L5-S1), and toe flexors (S1) is also important.

■ *Circumferential Measurements.* Muscle atrophy can be detected by circumferential measurements of the calf and thigh bilaterally. Differences of less than 2 cm in measurements of the two limbs at the same level may be a normal variation. Symmetrical muscle bulk and strength are expected unless the patient has a neurologic impairment or a history of lower extremity muscle or joint problem.

■ *Reflexes.* The ankle jerk reflex tests mostly the S1 nerve root and the knee jerk reflex tests mostly the L4 nerve root; neither tests the L5 nerve root. The reliability of reflex testing can be diminished in the presence of adjacent joint or muscle problems. Up-going toes in response to stroking the plantar footpad (Babinski or plantar response) may indicate upper motor-neuron abnormalities (such as myelopathy or demyelinating disease) rather than a common low back problem.

■ *Sensory Examination.* Testing light touch or pressure in the medial (L4), dorsal (L5), and lateral (S1) aspects of the foot (Figure 1) is usually sufficient for sensory screening.

## Figure 1. Testing for lumbar nerve root compromise.

| Nerve root | L4 | L5 | S1 |
|---|---|---|---|
| Pain | 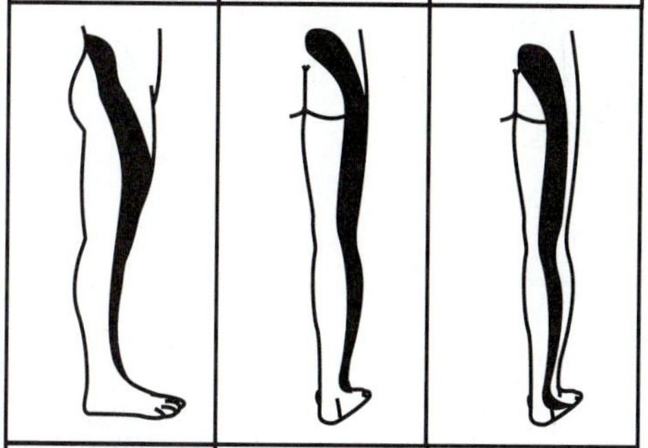 | | |
| Numbness | 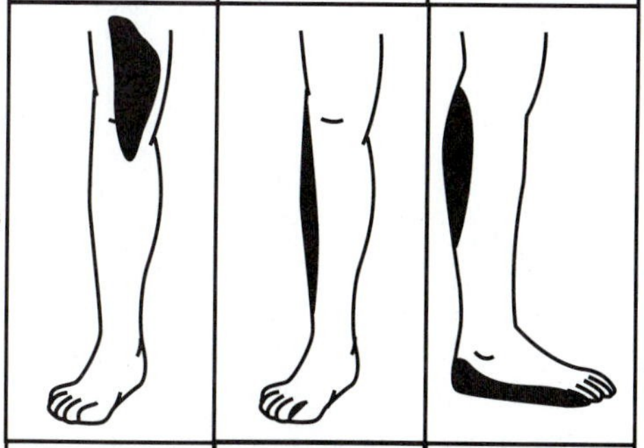 | | |
| Motor weakness | Extension of quadriceps. | Dorsilflexion of great toe and foot. | Plantar flexion of great toe and foot. |
| Screening exam | Squat & rise. | Heel walking. | Walking on toes. |
| Reflexes | Knee jerk diminished. | None reliable. | Ankle jerk diminisned. |

# Clinical tests for sciatic tension

*The straight leg raising (SLR) test* (Figure 2) can detect tension on the L5 and/or S1 nerve root. SLR may reproduce leg pain by stretching nerve roots irritated by a disc herniation.

## Figure 2. Instructions for the Straight Leg Raising (SLR) Test

(1) Ask the patient to lie as straight as possible on a table in the supine position.

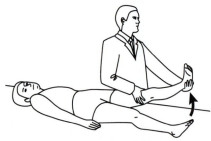

(2) With one hand placed above the knee of the leg being examined, exert enough firm pressure to keep the knee fully extended. Ask the patient to relax.

(3) With the other hand cupped under the heel, slowly raise the straight limb. Tell the patient, "If this bothers you, let me know, and I will stop."

4) Monitor for any movement of the pelvis before complaints are elicited. True sciatic tension should elicit complaints before the hamstrings are stretched enough to move the pelvis.

(5) Estimate the degree of leg elevation that elicits complaint from the patient. Then determine the most distal area of discomfort: back, hip, thigh, knee, or below the knee.

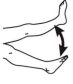

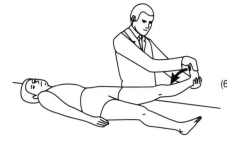

(6) While holding the leg at the limit of straight leg raising, dorsiflex the ankle. Note whether this aggravates the pain. Internal rotation of the limb can also increase the tension on the sciatic nerve roots.

Pain below the knee at less than 70 degrees of straight leg raising, aggravated by dorsiflexion of the ankle and relieved by ankle plantar flexion or external limb rotation, is most suggestive of tension on the L5 or S1 nerve root related to disc herniation. Reproducing back pain alone with SLR testing does not indicate significant nerve root tension.

***Crossover pain*** occurs when straight raising of the patient's well limb elicits pain in the leg with sciatica. Crossover pain is a stronger indication of nerve root compression than pain elicited from raising the straight painful limb.

***Sitting knee extension*** (Figure 3) can also test sciatic tension. The patient with significant nerve root irritation tends to complain or lean backward to reduce tension on the nerve.

## Figure 3.  Instructions for sitting knee extension test.

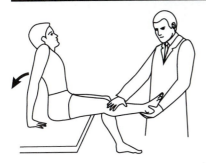

With the patient sitting on a table, both hip and knees flexed at 90 degrees, slowly extend the knee as if evaluating the patella or bottom of the foot. This maneuver stretches nerve roots as much as a moderate degree of supine SLR.

# Index